848-6383

ANATOMY IN SURGERY

Anatomy in Surgery

PHILIP THOREK, M.D., F.A.C.S., F.I.C.S.

Clinical Professor of Surgery (Formerly Assigned to Gross and Topographic Anatomy), University of Illinois College of Medicine; Diplomate of the American Board of Surgery; Professor of Topographic Anatomy and Clinical Surgery, Cook County Graduate School of Medicine; Member of the American Association of Anatomists; Fellow, American College of Chest Physicians; Surgeon-in-Chief of the American Hospital

753 Illustrations, 210 in Color

DRAWN BY CARL T. LINDEN

Formerly Assistant Professor in Medical Illustration, University of Illinois College of Medicine, Chicago

SECOND EDITION

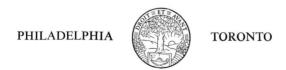

PHILADELPHIA   TORONTO

J. B. LIPPINCOTT COMPANY

TO MY PARENTS

Foreword

In this book on surgical anatomy, the author has deviated considerably from the usual plan and has presented the material with a stronger surgical viewpoint. Obviously, it will appeal primarily to surgeons and particularly to those in training because operative technic is included with the anatomy. The entire body is covered in the anatomic discussion and the principles of technic described for the important operations. This method of presentation of anatomic data has an obvious advantage in that it correlates the anatomy with the technical phase of surgery; without question, the young surgeon will find that this integration will make it much easier for him to remember the important anatomic details. The author is to be complimented in the efficiency of the correlation of anatomy and surgery.

The text is written in a clear and refreshing style; it is obvious that the author is a trained and effective teacher. The accuracy of thought and the continuity of expression are definite proof that the author has spent an enormous amount of time in preparing the text as well as in choosing the illustrations.

Another attractive feature in this volume is the caliber of illustrations, all of which have been furnished by one artist. The drawings are excellent and are to be commended for their clarity and accuracy. It is a relief to note the large size of lettering for the labels; this feature makes it easy to find and identify the various details of a drawing. About half of the illustrations are in color—a feature which adds greatly to their value.

Anatomy is an important phase of surgery and is very necessary in the training of a surgeon. Years ago it was perhaps overemphasized in the prerequisites of a surgeon. During recent years when a knowledge of physiology was found to be so important to the surgeon, anatomy has to a great extent been neglected. The pendulum is threatening to swing too far and give the young surgeon the idea that he need not spend time on anatomy. The time will never come when anatomy will be unimportant to the surgeon; the young surgeon must always appreciate this. It may be safe to prophesy that several decades hence the surgeons' work will be confined largely to the correction of congenital deformities and the treatment of traumatic injuries. If this situation should come to pass, the relative importance of anatomy to the surgeon will again become very prominent and justly so.

For the above reason the young surgeon should find this volume decidedly helpful in his training period; since anatomy is a science which unfortunately is readily forgotten, the older surgeon likewise should find the contents very useful. The author is to be congratulated on having prepared a volume with so many fine qualities.

WARREN H. COLE

Preface to the Second Edition

In this second edition of *Anatomy in Surgery,* I have welcomed the opportunity to improve the book and make it more useful. Since this is a study of anatomy as related to surgery, it becomes necessary to add the anatomic application to the newer cardiovascular surgery and to some of the surgery involving such organs as the liver.

New illustrations have been added to this edition wherever needed. Where it was thought that some of the former illustrations could be improved, Carl Linden's ability to depict such material clearly was a most welcome asset. Great patience was taken to place the illustrations as close as possible to the descriptive text.

Like its predecessor, this edition does not deal with surgical technics. Those procedures which are presented stress mainly the surgical anatomy as it is applied to the given procedure.

At times I have been criticized for oversimplification. Such criticisms must be accepted graciously if one believes that it is better to understand a little than to misunderstand a lot. I have found the use of mnemonics and alliterations to be helpful in attempting to remember and comprehend so complicated a subject as anatomy. It is easy to get lost in the study of anatomic anomalies and variations. Numerous treatises and books deal adequately with the subject of anomalies. In this book, therefore, the most common anatomic arrangements have been included, as well as the more common anomalies, particularly those which have some clinical bearing.

No author is omniscient, and no book is all-inclusive. I suspect that some readers will object to the omission of certain structures or subjects. I would be extremely grateful for any constructive criticism.

Throughout the preparation of this edition, the personnel of the J. B. Lippincott Company has given me the same wholehearted co-operation and encouragement which I have enjoyed in working with them for almost two decades. I wish particularly to thank Stanley A. Gillet, Walter Kahoe and Helen Steiner for the parts they played in indexing, suggestions and proofreading, respectively.

PHILIP THOREK, M.D.

Preface to the First Edition

This book on surgical anatomy is the culmination of seventeen years' experience in teaching gross and topographic anatomy and surgery. I have had the good fortune of constant daily contact with both the undergraduate student at the University of Illinois College of Medicine and the postgraduate student at the Cook County Graduate School of Medicine. It was only through personally appreciating the dilemma of the medical student and his desire to know clinical surgery, as well as the avidity of the postgraduate student for additional anatomic knowledge, that the idea for this book presented itself.

When the text was started twelve years ago, my notes previously prepared for lectures and anatomic demonstrations formed the nucleus for this work. Fifteen years of clinical observations as seen at the operating table provided additional data.

It is intended that *Anatomy in Surgery* might act as a means of narrowing the gap which exists between freshman anatomy and operative surgery. An attempt has been made to clarify this complex subject by a simple method of presentation and correlation. Punctilious attention has been given to the anatomic details, both in the text and in the illustrations. All of the drawings are original; many are presented in third-dimensional views; and all are closely analogous to the text. If any reference sources have not been properly acknowledged it is indeed an unintentional oversight.

I am deeply indebted to the artist, Mr. Carl Linden. His untiring efforts, understanding, wholehearted and sincere co-operation have made working with him a memorable experience. The creative talent which he possesses and his ability to depict true anatomic relationships are responsible for the illustrations of this book.

I am most grateful to Miss Mary Y. Nugent for her invaluable assistance in preparing the manuscript, arranging material and reading the proof.

I wish to thank the officers and the personnel of the J. B. Lippincott Company, particularly Mr. Walter Kahoe, Mr. Stanley A. Gillet and Mr. Edwin H. Bookmyer, whose splendid co-operation and keen interest have made this work possible.

PHILIP THOREK

A List of Basic References

1. Anson, *An Atlas of Human Anatomy,* Saunders

2. Brash and Jamieson, *Cunningham's Manual of Practical Anatomy,* Oxford

3. Brash and Jamieson, *Cunningham's Text-Book of Anatomy,* Oxford

4. Braus, *Anatomie Des Menschen,* Springer

5. Callander, *Surgical Anatomy,* Saunders

6. Corning, *Lehrbuch Der Topographischen Anatomie,* Bergmann

7. Goss, *Gray's Anatomy of the Human Body,* 27th ed., Lea and Febiger

8. Grant, *Atlas of Anatomy,* Williams and Wilkins

9. Grant, *Method of Anatomy,* Williams and Wilkins

10. Jamieson, *A Companion to Manuals of Practical Anatomy,* Oxford

11. Jamieson, *Illustrations of Regional Anatomy,* Williams and Wilkins

12. Jones and Shepard, *Manual of Surgical Anatomy,* Saunders

13. Keibel-Mall, *Human Embryology,* Lippincott

14. McGregor, *Synopsis of Surgical Anatomy,* Williams and Wilkins

15. Patten, *Human Embryology,* Blakiston

16. Schaeffer, *Morris' Human Anatomy,* Blakiston

17. Sobotta, *Atlas of Human Anatomy,* Stechert

18. Spalteholz, *Hand Atlas of Human Anatomy,* Lippincott

19. Toldt, *An Atlas of Human Anatomy,* Macmillan

20. Treves and Rogers, *Surgical Applied Anatomy,* Cassell

Contents

SECTION 1: HEAD

SECTION 3: THORAX

SECTION 4: ABDOMEN

Section 5: PELVIS

SECTION 6: MALE PERINEUM AND EXTERNAL GENITALIA

SECTION 7: FEMALE PERINEUM AND EXTERNAL GENITALIA

SECTION 8: SUPERIOR EXTREMITY

SECTION 9: INFERIOR EXTREMITY

Section 10: VERTEBRAL COLUMN, VERTEBRAL (SPINAL) CANAL, SPINAL CORD

Scalp

SCALP PROPER

The scalp is made up of the soft parts which cover the skull from one temporal line to the other and from the eyebrows in front to the superior nuchal lines behind. It is of particular interest to the surgeon because injuries and infections in this region may involve the skull, the sinuses, the meninges or the brain, and superficial cysts and vascular tumors may be found between its layers. It consists of 5 layers. If one spells the word "SCALP," these layers can be remembered (Fig. 1):

    S—Skin
    C—Connective tissue (dense)
    A—Aponeurosis (occipitofrontalis)
    L—Loose connective tissue
    P—Periosteum (pericranium)

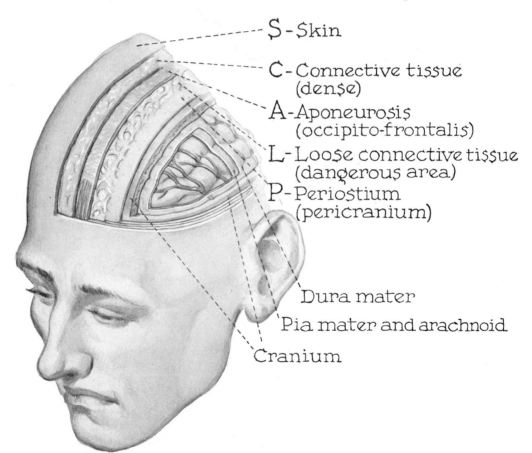

S - Skin

C - Connective tissue (dense)

A - Aponeurosis (occipito-frontalis)

L - Loose connective tissue (dangerous area)

P - Periostium (pericranium)

Dura mater

Pia mater and arachnoid

Cranium

FIG. 1. Diagrammatic representation of the 5 layers of the scalp and the deeper structures. The word "SCALP" is spelled when one recalls the first letter of each layer. The loose connective tissue layer is the "dangerous area" since the emissary veins are located here and it is in this plane that pus or blood may spread.

1

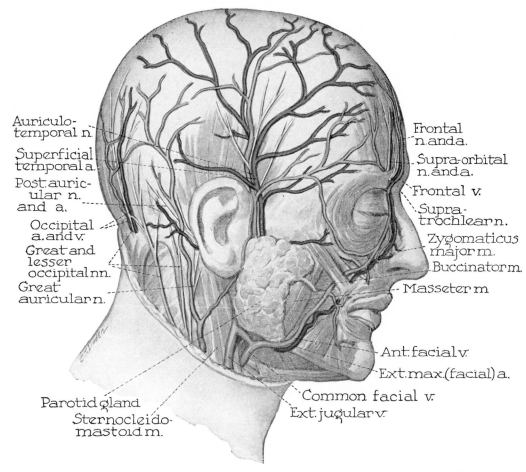

Auriculo-temporal n.

Superficial temporal a.

Post. auric-ular n. and a.

Occipital a. and v.

Great and lesser occipital nn.

Great auricular n.

Frontal n. and a.

Supra-orbital n. and a.

Frontal v.

Supra-trochlear n.

Zygomaticus major m.

Buccinator m.

Masseter m.

Ant. facial v.

Ext. max. (facial) a.

Common facial v.

Ext. jugular v.

Parotid gland

Sternocleido-mastoid m.

FIG. 2. The vessels and the nerves of the scalp and the side of the face. All the nerves of the scalp are sensory, with the exception of the facial nerve, which supplies the epicranius muscle.

SKIN

The skin of the scalp is very thick and contains numerous hairs and sebaceous glands. The hairs pass through it to an unusual depth, so that on reflecting the skin, the hair roots are cut across and can be seen and felt on its deep surface. The sebaceous glands may give rise to sebaceous cysts (wens). The skin is firmly attached to the underlying dense connective tissue layer, and because of this it is removed with difficulty.

CONNECTIVE TISSUE

The dense connective tissue is the superficial fascia and acts as a firm bond of union between the skin above and the aponeurosis below. In this dense, fibrous and unyielding layer run the superficial nerves and blood vessels of the scalp. This tissue holds the vessels firmly in place and prevents them from retracting; thus profuse bleeding results when the scalp is injured. Because of the great vascularity of the scalp it is rarely necessary to cut away any avulsed portions, as the flap usually retains its viability. Due to the compactness of the tissue, subcutaneous hemorrhage cannot spread extensively, and inflammation is associated with little swelling but much pain.

APONEUROSIS

The aponeurotic layer has been called the epicranial aponeurosis (occipitofrontalis muscle or galea aponeurotica). It consists of two frontal and two occipital bellies, connected by the epicranial aponeurosis. The occipitalis arises from bone, but the frontalis has no bony origin. The occipital portion takes its origin from the outer half of the superior nuchal line; the frontalis arises from the skin and the subcutaneous tissues of the eyebrows and the root of the nose, where it blends with the orbicularis oculi. The muscles are continuous over the temporal fascia and have no well-defined lateral margins. The epicranial muscle belongs to the muscles of expression, since the posterior bellies draw the entire scalp backward and the anterior produce the characteristic transverse wrinkles in the skin of the forehead. The frontal bellies are supplied by the temporal branches of the facial nerve, and the occipital by the posterior auricular branches of the same nerve. The aponeurosis is felt as a dense and strong membrane which is connected to the frontalis in front and to the occipitalis behind, and on each side it passes superficial to the temporal fascia to become attached to the zygomatic arch. If a scalp wound gapes, the examining physician may be certain that the galea has been divided transversely, since the skin is attached to this structure so firmly that otherwise no gaping would be possible.

Loose Connective Tissue

The loose connective tissue has been referred to as the subepicranial connective tissue space. It lies between the aponeurotic layer above and the pericranium below and is really not a true space but a potential one. The important emissary veins connecting the venous sinuses in the skull with the veins of the scalp traverse this dangerous area. This loose areolar tissue permits free movements of the scalp and allows large collections of blood or pus to accumulate under the scalp without undue tension. The first three layers of the scalp can be easily separated from the pericranium through this space, and the knowledge of this plane permitted the Indians to become so clever at "scalping." The space is closed posteriorly by the attachments to the superior nuchal line and laterally to the zygomatic arch; since the frontalis has no attachment to bones anteriorly, it is open in this direction. Due to this lack of attach-

ment anteriorly, bleeding may occur into the loose connective tissue layer in head injuries; after a day or two of slow gravitation, the hemorrhage appears first in the upper eyelids and later in the lower.

Periosteum

The pericranium (periosteum) refers to the outer or external periosteum of the skull. It is loosely attached to the surface of the skull bones except at the suture lines and over the temporal fossae. At the suture lines it dips between the bones as a suture membrane which is blended with the periosteum of the interior of the skull, this latter being known as the outer layer of the dura. Collections of fluid beneath the pericranium can easily strip it but cannot pass beyond the suture line, and for this reason any swelling, such as cephalhematoma, will maintain the shape of the bone to which it is related. Surgeons do not hesitate to remove this layer, because the blood supply to the skull can be provided through the attachment of muscles.

VESSELS, NERVES AND LYMPH VESSELS

Arteries. The vessels of the scalp (Fig. 2) are numerous and they anastomose freely. The arteries are derived from both the internal and the external carotids. Anteriorly, the supratrochlear and the supraorbital arteries ascend over the forehead, accompanied by the nerves of the same name. Both are branches of the ophthalmic artery (internal carotid). Their terminal branches anastomose with each other, with their fellows of the opposite side and with the superficial temporal (external carotid) of the same side. Laterally, the superficial temporal artery ascends in front of the ear (tragus), accompanied by the auriculotemporal nerve. It divides into anterior and posterior branches which supply large areas of scalp, and then it anastomoses with the corresponding vessels of the opposite side. Posteriorly, there are two arteries on each side, the posterior auricular and the occipital. The posterior auricular ascends behind the auricle and supplies that structure and adjoining parts of the scalp; the occipital extends over the occipital area accompanied by the greater occipital nerve. Since the arteries of the scalp anastomose so freely with each other and those of the opposite side, they form potential collaterals following ligation of the external or the common carotid artery on one side.

Veins. The supratrochlear and the supraorbital veins unite to form the anterior facial vein (p. 111), which makes an important communication with the superior ophthalmic.

Nerves. The nerves of the scalp (Fig. 2) are arranged in five groups which, considered from before backward, are: (1) The *supratrochlear,* appearing through the supratrochlear notch of the frontal bone and supplying the region of the glabella; (2) the *supraorbital,* which emerges through the supraorbital notch or foramen of the frontal bone, runs upward over the forehead and supplies the scalp as far as the crown of the head; (3) the *auriculotemporal,* which passes in front of the tragus of the ear and supplies the side of the scalp; (4) the *posterior auricular,* supplying a small area behind the ear; (5) the *great occipital,* which supplies the large area of skin over the occipital region and extends forward to the vertex. The lesser occipital nerve may or may not extend into the scalp.

All the nerves of the scalp are sensory with the exception of the facial, which supplies the epicranius muscle. The supratrochlear, the supra-orbital and the auriculotemporal are branches of the trigeminal; the great auricular, the lesser and the great occipital are of spinal origin. Any of these may be affected by referred or neuralgic pains, the occipital and the supra-orbital being involved most commonly. Since the nerves of the scalp approach it from all directions and overlap, it is rarely possible to produce an adequate local anesthesia by a single nerve block. The area to be anesthetized must be ringed by a series of injec-

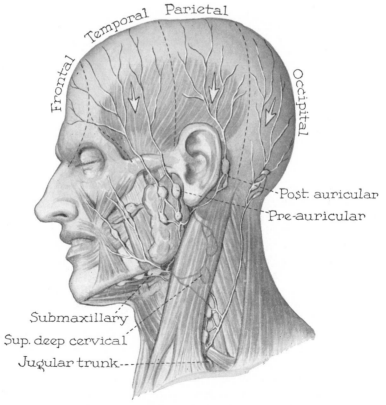

FIG. 3. Regional lymph drainage of the scalp. This represents a general plan which is subject to many variations.

tions. Like the vessels, the nerves travel in the subcutaneous tissue; hence, the solution must be placed in this layer and not in the subaponeurotic layer where it would spread with great ease but would not produce anesthesia.

Lymph Vessels. The lymph vessels of the scalp and the face (Fig. 3) drain downward from the occipital region to the occipital glands, from the parietal and the temporal regions to the preauricular and the post-auricular glands, and from the frontal region to the submaxillary glands. Infected wounds, pediculi and furuncles usually cause the lymphadenitis associated with scalp pathology.

CIRSOID ANEURYSM

Reid and Andrus believe that cirsoid aneurysms are abnormal arteriovenous communi-

cations. Ligation of the surrounding vessels improves the condition but rarely cures it; therefore, excision is the treatment of choice. Hemorrhage is the greatest danger.

Technic (Fig. 4). Short individual incisions are placed over the pulsating vessels leading to the aneurysm. These usually include the superficial temporal artery and vein, the occipital artery and vein, the supraorbital vessels and the frontal vein. These are ligated and divided. A continuous locked suture is placed around the mass to control bleeding. A U-shaped incision is made within the hemostatic suture, and a skin flap is reflected upward, thus exposing the aneurysm. The mass of vessels is carefully excised. The encircling hemostatic suture is removed bit by bit, all bleeding points are controlled, and the skin flap is sutured into place.

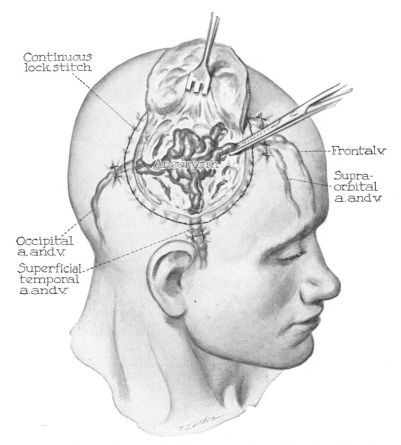

Continuous
lock stitch

Frontal v.

Supra-
orbital
a. and v.

Aneurysm

Occipital
a. and v.

Superficial
temporal
a. and v.

FIG. 4. Operation for cirsoid aneurysm. Short individual incisions are placed over the main pulsating vessels which lead to the aneurysm; these are ligated and divided. A continuous lock stitch is placed around the mass, and the aneurysm is removed.

Skull

EMBRYOLOGY

The brain of the fetus is surrounded by a membranous capsule which is continuous with a similar capsule surrounding the spinal cord. Chondrification begins in the base, but ossification begins in the calvarium (supra-orbital portion) before the chondrifying process has progressed very far. Bones which are formed in membrane are the frontal, parietal, squamous temporals, the greater wings of the sphenoid (except their roots) and the occipital above the nuchal lines. Centers appear for these bones about the 7th week. In general, the older basal portion of the skull is preformed in cartilage, but the facial and the roofing bones are formed intramembranously.

At birth the skull reveals a lack of firmness between the bone sutures so that considerable movement can be produced, thus facilitating the "molding" which takes place during childbirth. The most striking feature of the neonatal skull is the marked disproportion between the cranium and the facial skeleton. At birth the facial region covers only one eighth of the skull as compared with one half in the adult.

FONTANELLES

The fontanelles (Fig. 5) are unossified spaces which appear at the angles of the parietal bones. The *anterior fontanelle* is 4-sided and is bounded by the margins of the 2 frontal and the 2 parietal bones. Intracranial pulsations may be transmitted through this tissue and are usually visible in infants. Extension of the bony margins closes this fontanelle before the age of 2 years. The *posterior fontanelle* is 3-sided and is bounded by the occipital and the 2 parietal bones; its sides pass laterally into the *lambdoid sutures* and its apex to the *sagittal suture*. It is usually closed during the first year of life. These membranous areas exist in the midline of the cranium and are of great value in determining the position of the fetal head during labor. Fontanelles are also present at the pterion and the asterion.

The suture between the 2 frontal bones of the newborn child disappears around the 3rd year of life but may persist indefinitely, giving rise to a *metopic suture*.

SKULL PROPER

The word "skull" refers to the entire skeleton of the head and the face, including the mandible. "Cranium" refers to the skull minus the mandible. "Calvarium" refers to the skull after the bones of the face have been removed (that portion which is above the supra-orbital ridges).

The skull as a whole is slightly flattened from side to side. When viewed from above it appears to be smooth, but from below it is very uneven. It is oval in shape, wider behind than in front, and is composed of flattened or irregular bones that are joined together immovably, with the exception of the mandible. The skull is made up of 24 bones, including the mandible and the bones of the head and the face. The bones consist of 2 tables or plates of compact substance which enclose a layer of spongy bone between them known as the diploë. The diploë contains marrow and is supplied by numerous small diploic branches that arise from the arteries of the scalp and the dura mater. The veins of the diploë anastomose with each other to form the main diploic veins. In some of the bones the diploë is absorbed, leaving cavities which are referred to as air sinuses and are situated between the tables of compact bone. The sinuses communicate with the cavity of the nose and have a mucous lining that is also continuous with the nasal cavity.

The exterior of the skull should be viewed

from 5 different positions, each of which is referred to as "norma": norma verticalis (from above); norma basalis (from below); norma frontalis (from in front); norma occipitalis (from behind); norma lateralis (from the side).

NORMA VERTICALIS

(Fig. 6.) The top of the skull shows portions of 4 bones: the frontal, the occipital, the right and the left parietals. They are united by serrated bony seams called sutures, which have interlocking jagged sawlike edges. The suture that unites the frontal to the 2 parietal bones runs across the skull from side to side in a crownlike arrangement and is known as the *coronal suture*. That suture which unites the occipital to the 2 parietal bones resembles the Greek capital letter lambda which looks like an inverted "V" and is known as the *lambdoid suture*. "Sagitta" means arrow, and the lambdoid suture and the *sagittal suture*, with the anterior fontanelle, have a definite resemblance to an arrow. The meeting point between the coronal and the sagittal sutures is called the *bregma*. At birth the parts of the frontal and the parietal bones around the bregma are not

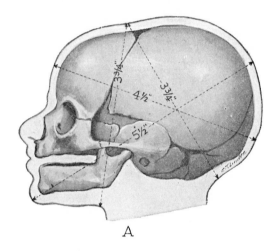

A

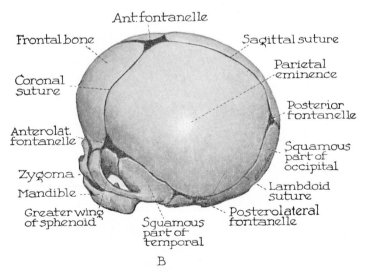

Ant. fontanelle

Frontal bone

Sagittal suture

Coronal suture

Parietal eminence

Anterolat. fontanelle

Posterior fontanelle

Zygoma

Squamous part of occipital

Mandible

Lambdoid suture

Greater wing of sphenoid

Squamous part of temporal

Posterolateral fontanelle

B

FIG. 5. The fetal skull: (A) Lateral view, showing average measurements. (B) Oblique view, showing the sutures and the fontanelles.

fully ossified; because of this a lozenge-shaped membranous area results which is called the anterior fontanelle. This yields to the touch, and the pulse rate can be counted here. That point at which the sagittal and the lambdoid sutures meet is called the *lambda* and marks the site of the posterior fontanelle. The *vertex,* the highest point of the skull, is on the sagittal suture near its middle. The *parietal foramen* is a small opening present on either side of the sagittal suture; it is usually big enough to admit a pin, and a small artery and vein pass through it. This vein connects the veins of the scalp with the superior sagittal sinus; hence, an infection from the scalp may travel along this vein and involve the sinus. It is interesting to note that the sagittal suture is less serrated between the two parietal foramina.

Norma Basalis

(Fig. 7.) This view is obtained when the skull is turned upside down, thus exposing the external surface of its base. The anterior part of this aspect is occupied by the *bony palate,* which is formed by the palatine

processes of the maxillae and the horizontal plates of the palatine bones.

In the median plane anteriorly, the *incisive fossa* receives the openings of the lateral incisive canals, which transmit the terminal parts of the greater palatine vessels to the nose and the descending terminal branches of the long sphenopalatine nerves. Anterior and posterior median incisive canals are sometimes present. The *greater palatine fossa,* which transmits the greater palatine vessels and nerves, is found in the postero-lateral corner near the last molar. The *lesser palatine fossae* lie immediately behind the greater. Behind and above the hard palate are the *choanae* (the posterior bony apertures of the nose). These are separated from each other by the vomer and are bounded laterally by the medial pterygoid plate.

The *pterygoid plates* are a pair of large lateral and medial processes projecting downward from the roots of the greater wings of the sphenoid bones. Between these processes is an interval known as the *pterygoid fossa,* which opens posteriorly and is about half an inch in width. The free border of the medial plate ends below in a hook called the

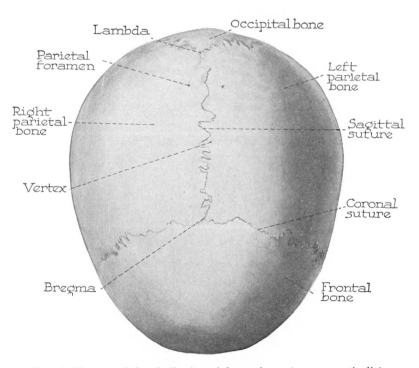

Fɪɢ. 6. The top of the skull, viewed from above (norma verticalis).

hamulus. This gives attachment at its tip to the pterygomandibular ligament, and by its posterior border to the upper fibers of the superior constrictor muscle of the pharynx. The tensor palati tendon twists around its lateral and anterior aspects. The lateral plate gives origin to the lateral pterygoid muscle on its lateral surface and to the medial pterygoid on its medial surface. Lateral to the structures just described is the roof of the infratemporal fossa.

Posterolateral to the plates, the *foramen ovale* is found, which is quite large and transmits the mandibular nerve, the accessory meningeal artery and some small veins that connect the cavernous venous sinus with the pterygoid venous plexus. Some lymph vessels from the meninges also pass through this foramen, as does the lesser superficial petrosal nerve at times. Posterolateral to the foramen ovale is the *foramen spinosum,* which transmits the middle meningeal vessels. The *zygomatic arch* is a prominent feature of this aspect. At its caudal end is found the articular fossa, which receives the articular process of the mandible. The *foramen lacerum* is a large and jagged aperture located at the base of the medial pterygoid plate. The *carotid canal,* which is posterolateral to the foramen lacerum, is a tunnel in the petrous portion of the temporal bone through which the internal carotid artery travels on its way to the cranial cavity. From its opening the canal leads upward for a short distance, bends to become horizontal and runs in a medial direction and forward to open into the foramen lacerum. The canal is in immediate relationship to the middle and the internal ears. The thumping sounds that one hears in the head during moments

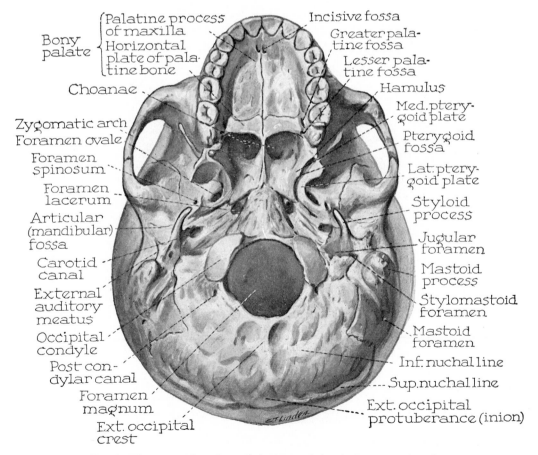

FIG. 7. The external surface of the base of the skull (norma basalis).

of excitement or after violent exertion are due to the beating of the internal carotid artery against the bone that separates it from the internal ear (Fig. 74 A).

The *jugular foramen* is a large opening with uneven margins situated directly behind the carotid canal. The largest structure in this foramen is the internal jugular vein. Other structures associated with it will be reviewed when the interior of the base of the skull is discussed. The jugular foramen is opposite the external auditory meatus, and that part of the bone which bounds the foramen forms the floor of the middle ear. It is important to keep this relationship in mind since, in diseases of the middle ear, infec-

tion may pass through the bone and attack the internal jugular vein.

Directly lateral to the foramen is the *styloid process*. Two ligaments (the stylohyoid and the stylomandibular) and 3 muscles (the styloglossus, the stylohyoid and the stylopharyngeus) are attached to this process. The stylohyoid ligament runs from its tip to the hyoid bone, and the stylomandibular ligament extends from the front of it to the posterior border of the mandible. The stylomandibular ligament is a thickened part of the fascia that covers the anteromedial aspect of the parotid gland. The *stylomastoid foramen* is found immediately at the base of the styloid process and is the foramen that trans-

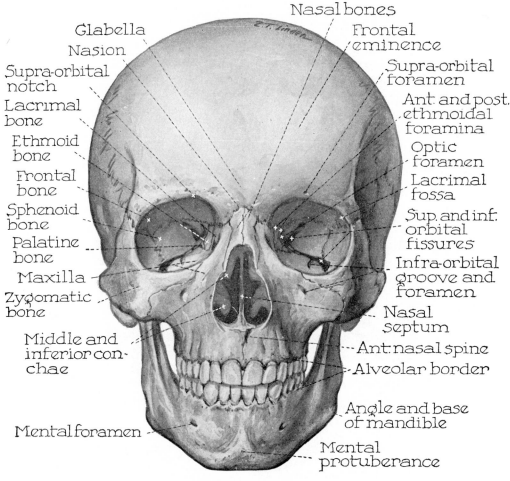

Glabella
Nasion
Supra-orbital notch
Lacrimal bone
Ethmoid bone
Frontal bone
Sphenoid bone
Palatine bone
Maxilla
Zygomatic bone
Middle and inferior conchae
Mental foramen

Nasal bones
Frontal eminence
Supra-orbital foramen
Ant. and post. ethmoidal foramina
Optic foramen
Lacrimal fossa
Sup. and inf. orbital fissures
Infra-orbital groove and foramen
Nasal septum
Ant. nasal spine
Alveolar border
Angle and base of mandible
Mental protuberance

FIG. 8. Front view of the skull (norma frontalis). It is made up of 6 regions: frontal, orbital, nasal, zygomatic, maxillary and mandibular.

mits the facial nerve from the brain to the exterior of the skull. The stylomastoid branches of the posterior auricular vessels are also transmitted by this foramen.

The *mastoid process* can be palpated under cover of the lobule of the auricle but is not recognizable as a bony structure until the end of the 2nd year. The *mastoid foramen,* which is variable in size and position, is found posterior to the mastoid process. It transmits a vein to the transverse sinus and a small branch of the occipital artery to the dura mater.

The *foramen magnum,* the largest bony foramen in the skull, is the opening through which the medulla oblongata, or lowest subdivision of the brain, becomes continuous with the spinal cord. Its level is approximately the same as that of the mastoid process on the side of the head, and it is opposite a point on the back of the neck midway between the external occipital protuberance and the spine of the second cervical vertebra.

The *occipital condyles* are the large, smooth and rather oblong protuberances that lie at the margins of the foramen magnum. They articulate with the atlas, and nodding movements of the head take place at the

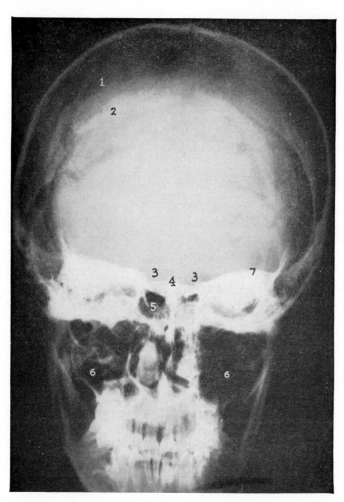

FIG. 9. X-ray study of the front of the skull (posteroanterior projection): (1) parietal bone, (2) coronal suture, (3) frontal sinuses, (4) crista galli, (5) sphenoid bone and sinus, (6) zygoma, (7) lesser wing of sphenoid bone.

joints between the atlas and the condyles.

The *anterior condylar canal* is above the lateral margin of the anterior part of the condyle. It is usually hidden by the condyle, and the skull must be tilted before the opening can be seen. The anterior condylar canal is smaller than the jugular foramen and is the opening that transmits the hypoglossal nerve. The *posterior condylar canal,* when present, passes above the posterior part of the condyle and opens into the posterior fossa. It transmits an emissary vein that connects the sigmoid venous sinus with the suboccipital venous plexus.

Behind the foramen magnum a bony crest is noted, known as the *external occipital crest,* which ends in an elevation called the *external occipital protuberance* (inion). From the region of the midpoint on this crest the *inferior nuchal line* curves laterally on each side, but the line is often poorly defined and difficult to see. The *superior nuchal line* curves laterally on each side from the external occipital protuberance and separates the scalp area above from the area for the neck muscles (nuchal area) below.

NORMA FRONTALIS

(Figs. 8 and 9.) The front of the skull, uneven in contour, is made up of 6 regions: (1) frontal (forehead); (2) orbital; (3) nasal; (4) zygomatic; (5) maxillary (upper jaw); (6) mandibular (lower jaw).

Frontal Region. The forehead, or frontal region, is formed by the frontal bone. Superiorly, it merges into the top of the skull; inferiorly, it is limited by the orbits and the root of the nose. The depression at the nasal root is called the *nasion;* it is found at the point in the median plane where the 2 nasal bones articulate with the frontal bone, and is opposite the anterior extremity of the brain.

Directly above the orbital margins are 2 elevations, the *superciliary arches.* These give prominence to the eyebrows and are more elevated in the male. The elevation that exists between the superciliary arches (between the eyebrows) is called the *glabella,* so designated because the overlying skin is bald or glabrous.

Behind the superciliary arch and in the anterior part of the frontal bone a large air space is usually found; it is known as the *frontal sinus.* The *frontal eminence* is the most convex part of each frontal bone and is situated about 2 fingerbreadths above the lateral end of the superciliary arch.

The *supra-orbital foramen* or notch is located immediately above the upper border of the orbital opening at the junction of its medial with its lateral two thirds. It transmits the nerve and the vessels of the same name. The supra-orbital margin ends laterally in a prominent projection called the zygomatic process of the frontal bone; it articulates with the zygomatic bone. The zygomatic process is easily felt at the lateral end of the eyebrows and may be a serviceable landmark, since it marks a line that curves upward and backward from it and is known as the anterior part of the temporal line. In thin people this line can be both felt and seen.

Orbital Region. Each orbit is a deep cavity which resembles an irregular cone and may be likened to a pyramid having 4 walls, an apex and a base. The bones that form the orbital pyramid are the maxillary, zygomatic, sphenoid, frontal, palatine, ethmoid and lacrimal. The medial walls are parallel and separated by the nasal cavity; the lateral are at right angles to each other. The apex of the pyramid is marked by the *optic foramen.* Probes passed through these foramina meet at right angles near the dorsum sellae. The base of the pyramid is the opening on the face and the boundaries are the margins of the orbit.

The *roof,* or superior wall, of the orbit is concave and is formed mainly by the orbital plate of the frontal bone and posteriorly by the lesser wing of the sphenoid. It separates the orbit from the sinus anteromedially and from the anterior cranial fossa elsewhere. The lacrimal gland occupies a fossa in the anterolateral part of the roof. At the medial angle the trochlea is attached. This is a small fibrocartilaginous ring through which the tendon of the superior oblique muscle passes. The point of attachment is usually marked by a small pit or spicule of bone called the trochlear fossa or spine.

The *floor,* or inferior wall, is formed by the orbital plate of the maxilla. This plate also forms the roof of the subjacent maxillary sinus. A great part of the floor is separated from the lateral wall posteriorly by the *inferior orbital fissure.* The anterior end of this fissure is closed, but the posterior meets the medial end of the superior orbital fissure at the apex of the orbit. The inferior fissure transmits the maxillary nerve (which becomes the infra-orbital nerve), the infra-orbital vessels, the zygomatic nerve, nervous twigs from the sphenopalatine ganglion to the lacrimal gland, the periosteum of the orbit, and a vein connecting the ophthalmic veins with the pterygoid venous plexus in the infratemporal fossa. The *infra-orbital groove* leads forward on the floor for a short distance from the fissure and then tunnels through the floor to reach the *infra-orbital foramen,* which transmits the nerve and the vessels of the same name.

The *lateral wall* is formed by the orbital process of the zygomatic bone and the orbital surface of the great wing of the sphenoid. Between the lateral wall and the roof, near the apex of the orbit, the *superior orbital fissure* is found. Through this fissure the oculomotor, the trochlear, the ophthalmic division of the trigeminal and the abducens nerves enter the orbital cavity, accompanied by orbital branches of the middle meningeal artery. Passing backward through this fissure are the ophthalmic veins and the recurrent branch of the lacrimal artery which reach the dura mater. The superior orbital fissure separates the lateral orbital wall from the roof, and the inferior fissure separates this wall from the floor. Of the 4 walls, the lateral is the thickest and the only one that is not in close contact with the paranasal sinuses; resection of this wall gives safe access to the contents of the orbital cavity.

The *medial wall* is very frail and is formed, from before backward, by the frontal process of the maxilla, the lacrimal bone, the lamina papyracea of the ethmoid and a small part of the body of the sphenoid in front of the optic foramen. This wall contains the *lacrimal fossa,* which lodges the lacrimal sac, the *anterior ethmoidal foramen,* which transmits the nasociliary nerve and the anterior ethmoidal vessels, and the *posterior ethmoidal foramen,* which accommodates the posterior ethmoidal nerve and vessels. The medial wall is in close contact with the sphenoid sinus posteriorly and the ethmoid sinuses anteriorly, these sinuses separating the orbit from the cavity of the nose. The *apex,* which is situated at the back of the orbit, corresponds to the *optic foramen.* This short cylindrical canal transmits the optic nerve and the ophthalmic artery. The ophthalmic vein passes through the superior orbital fissure; hence, it does not travel with its artery.

Injury or infection in the orbital cavity may travel in the following ways: superiorly, to the frontal sinus or the anterior cranial fossa, which contains the frontal lobe of the brain; inferiorly, to the maxillary sinus; medially, near the apex, to the sphenoid sinus; farther forward to the ethmoid sinuses, which separate the orbit from the cavity of the nose, and within the orbital margins to the floor of the fossa for the lacrimal sac; laterally, through the posterior part of the orbit to the middle cranial fossa, which lodges the temporal lobe of the brain, and more anteriorly to the anterior part of the temporal fossa.

Nasal Region. The bony part of the external nose is best seen from the norma frontalis. The nasal cavity itself is discussed elsewhere (p. 83). The osseous part of the nose is formed by the 2 nasal bones in the bridge of the nose and on each side by the frontal process of the maxilla, which lies behind the nasal bone. This part of the maxilla also forms the medial margin of the orbital opening. The nasal cavity is divided by a thin median partition or *septum* into right and left halves. The principal part of the septum seen through the anterior bony aperture is the perpendicular plate of the ethmoid that forms the upper part; it is usually bent to one side or the other. The side walls of the nasal cavity are uneven because of 3 rough, curled, bony plates called *conchae,* which project downward from each side wall. That portion of the cavity that lies below and lateral to each concha is called a meatus of the nose (superior, middle and inferior). The superior concha is too far back to be seen through the anterior aperture, but the middle and the inferior conchae and meatuses are visible (Fig. 63).

Zygomatic and Maxillary Regions. These form the cheek bones and the upper jaw regions, respectively. The upper jaw region is situated between the orbits and the teeth. The *anterior nasal spine* is a sharp spur of bone which projects forward from the 2 maxillae at the lower margin of the anterior aperture of the nose. The maxilla ends inferiorly in the *alveolar border,* which has slight ridges marking the roots of the anterior teeth, the most prominent of which are the canines. The canine tooth is the third, counting from the middle in front (Fig. 8).

Near the lower margin of the orbit and almost immediately above the canine fossa is the *infra-orbital foramen,* which transmits the infra-orbital vessels and nerve and is located about one fingerbreadth lateral to the side of the nose. The *zygomaticofacial foramen* appears as a small opening on the zygomatic bone immediately below the lateral part of the lower margin of the orbit. It transmits the zygomaticofacial branch of the zygomatic nerve and a small branch of the lacrimal artery. The large single air space found inside the maxilla is called the maxillary sinus (antrum of Highmore); it communicates with the nasal cavity. This sinus is of considerable practical importance and will be discussed elsewhere (p. 91).

Mandibular Region. The mandible is the largest and strongest bone of the face and it contains the lower teeth. The bone develops in 2 symmetrical halves, which fuse early and ossify during the first year. It consists of a horseshoe-shaped body and a pair of flat, broad rami that stand up from the posterior part of the body. Two processes project upward from the upper border of each ramus: an anterior called the *coronoid process,* and a posterior designated as the *condyloid process,* which is divided into a head and a neck (Figs. 8 and 10).

The external surface of the body of the bone is marked in the median line by a faint ridge, the *symphysis menti,* or line of junction of the 2 embryologic pieces of bone. The ridge divides below and encloses a triangular eminence known as the *mental protuberance,* the base of which is depressed in the center but raised on either side to form the mental tubercles. In the region of the protuberance the bone is bent forward to form the *chin.* The alveolar is the upper border, so called because it is occupied by a row of pits or alveoli, 16 in number, which form the sockets for teeth. The lower border is the *base* of the mandible. It is smooth and rounded. The mental foramen, which transmits the mental vessels and nerves, is found about 1 inch from the symphysis and midway between the upper and the lower borders.

The internal surface of the body of the mandible is concave from side to side and contains the mylohyoid line, which gives origin to the mylohyoid muscle. The *angle* of the mandible is that point at which the posterior border of the ramus joins the lower border of the body. It is subcutaneous and is easily felt 2 or 3 fingerbreadths below the lobule of the ear. The thin, sharp coronoid process gives attachment along its edges and on its deep surface to the temporalis muscle; the more posteriorly situated condyloid process articulates with the articular fossa on the infratemporal surface of the squamous temporal. Articular cartilage covers its superior and anterior aspects but not the posterior. The lateral aspect of the condyloid process is covered by the parotid gland, which is situated immediately in front of the tragus. When a finger is placed in front of the tragus, and when the mouth is alternately opened and closed, the movements of the condyloid process can be felt. The notch, situated between the coronoid and the condyloid processes, is known as the mandibular notch; it transmits the nerve and the vessels to the masseter muscle.

About the center of the *medial* surface of the ramus of the mandible the mandibular foramen is found. It leads into a canal which passes downward and forward in the substance of the bone and carries the inferior alveolar vessels and nerve to the teeth. A spur of bone, known as the *lingula,* usually

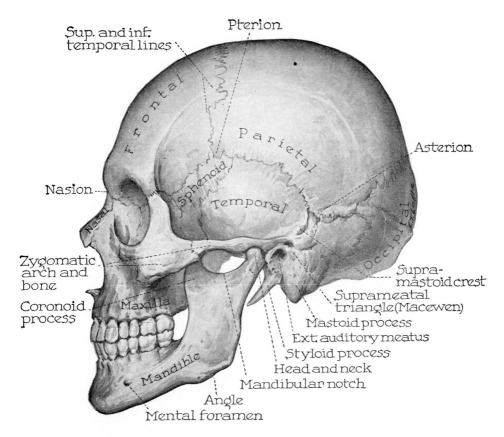

FIG. 10. Side view of the skull (norma lateralis). This part of the skull is formed by 5 bones: frontal, parietal, occipital, temporal and the great wing of the sphenoid. The face is situated below and in front.

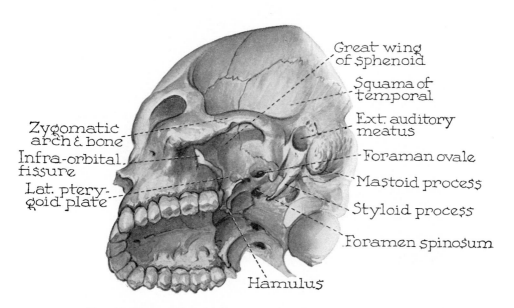

FIG. 11. Temporal and infratemporal region viewed from below.

overlaps this foramen. The mylohyoid groove, lodging the mylohyoid nerve and artery, commences behind the lingula and runs for about 1 inch obliquely downward and forward on the ramus.

Norma Lateralis

(Figs. 10, 11, 12.) Some anatomy textbooks prefer to discuss a superior and an inferior temporal line, but these markings are so indistinct that the term *"temporal line"* is sufficient for surgical considerations. This line starts at the zygomatic process of the frontal bone, curves upward and backward and is easily felt on the living subject in its anterior and upper parts. Posteriorly, it curves downward and forward into the *supramastoid crest*. It gives attachment to the epicranial aponeurosis, the temporal fascia and the uppermost fibers of the tem-

poralis muscle. The *pterion* is that region where the frontal, the great wing of the sphenoid, the parietal and the temporal bones meet. A point on the pterion about 4 cm. above the zygoma and 2.5 cm. behind the frontal process of the zygomatic bone overlies the anterior division of the middle meningeal artery.

The *infratemporal crest* on the great wing of the sphenoid is a horizontal anteroposterior ridge which separates the temporal fossa above from the infratemporal fossa below. The temporal fossa is a wide space outlined by the temporal line and the zygomatic arch; it contains the temporalis muscle, its vessels and nerves and the zygomaticotemporal nerve. This is the thinnest and weakest region of the skull. Since the middle meningeal artery passes through here, many cases of fractures associated with injury to the vessel

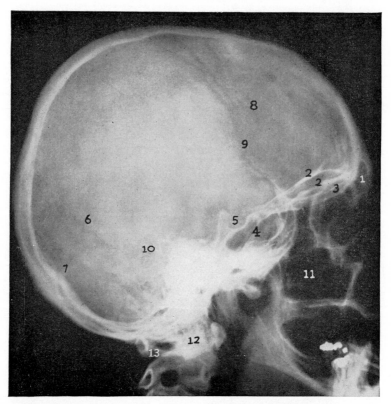

Fig. 12. X-ray study of the skull (lateral projection): (1) frontal sinus, (2) superior orbital plate, (3) orbit, (4) sphenoid sinus, (5) sella turcica, (6) lambdoid suture, (7) internal occipital tuberosity, (8) coronal suture, (9) middle meningeal channel (artery), (10) mastoid, (11) maxillary sinus, (12) odontoid process of axis, (13) atlas.

are common. The importance of and the approach to this region are discussed in a subsequent section (p. 24).

The *infratemporal fossa* is a wide space behind the maxilla, below the infratemporal crest and lateral to the pterygoid plates. It communicates with the temporal fossa through the gap which exists between the zygoma and the rest of the skull. The gap is traversed by the temporalis muscle as it descends to its insertion. The fossa contains the pterygoid muscles, the internal maxillary artery and its middle meningeal branch, the mandibular nerve and its branches, the chorda tympani nerve and the pterygoid venous plexus.

Two fissures are present in the depth of the fossa: the *infra-orbital fissure,* which lies horizontally and connects the infratemporal fossa with the orbit; and the *pterygomaxillary fissure,* which is placed vertically and transmits the terminal part of the maxillary artery. The pterygomaxillary fissure leads medially into the pterygopalatine fossa.

The *zygomatic arch* is quite evident and can be felt running from the prominence of the cheek to the tragus. It is formed by the zygomatic process of the temporal and the temporal process of the zygomatic bone. The tendon of the temporalis passes medial to the arch to gain insertion into the coronoid process of the mandible. The upper border of the arch gives attachment to the temporal fascia, and the lower border and medial surface give origin to the masseter muscle. The posterior root of the process is continued backward above the external auditory meatus as the *supramastoid crest.* Below the posterior root of the arch is an elliptical orifice known as the *external auditory meatus,* which is bounded in front, below and behind by the tympanic part of the temporal bone.

Lateral to this and not seen in the dried skull, the cartilaginous segment of the external auditory meatus is attached. The bony meatus is barely wide enough to admit an ordinary pencil. It passes in a medial direction and slightly forward and opens into the middle ear in an oblique manner so that the tympanic membrane, which closes the opening, looks downward and forward as well as in a lateral direction. The outer orifice is also oblique, the upper margin overhanging the lower. The medial end of the meatus is closed during life by a tense vibrating membrane, called the *tympanic membrane,* which separates the meatus from the tympanic cavity (middle ear).

Between the posterosuperior part of the meatus and the posterior root of the zygomatic arch the *suprameatal triangle* (Macewen) is found. It lies immediately behind the upper part of the external meatus and, although small and often inconspicuous, it is important because the tympanic antrum lies about ½ inch medial to it. The antrum is a cavity in the temporal bone which is surgically important in diseases of the *mastoid process.* This process can be palpated under cover of the lobule of the auricle. It is absent at birth and does not begin to appear until the 2nd year of life. A line drawn from one mastoid to the other passes immediately below the foramen magnum.

NORMA OCCIPITALIS

(Fig. 7.) The back of the skull is horseshoe-shaped and extends from the tip of one mastoid process, over the vault, to the tip of the other. The bones that take part in its formation are parts of the 2 parietals, the occipital and the mastoid portion of the temporal, with its mastoid process. Some parts have already been seen from the norma verticalis, namely, the parietal eminences, the posterior part of the sagittal suture, the parietal foramina, the lambda and the lambdoid suture.

The *occipitomastoid suture* descends between the occipital bone and the mastoid temporal. The *mastoid foramen* is seen on or near this suture and transmits an emissary vein which connects the veins on the outside of the skull with the sigmoid venous sinus.

The *external occipital protuberance* (inion) is usually well marked in the median plane at the lower part of the back of the skull. It can be felt in the living person immediately above the nape of the neck and acts as a useful guide.

The *superior nuchal line* is the curved ridge that arches laterally to either side of the protuberance. This protuberance, together with the right and the left superior

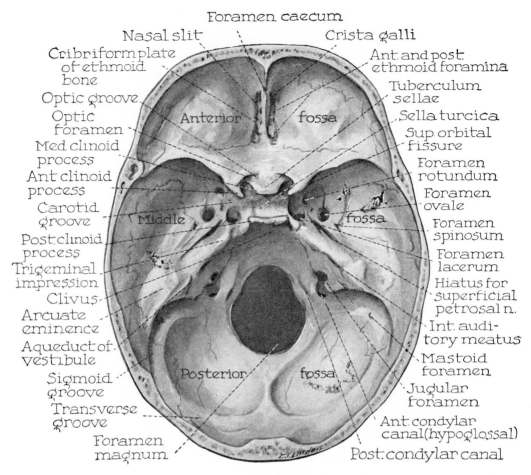

Foramen caecum

Nasal slit
Cribriform plate of ethmoid bone
Optic groove
Optic foramen
Med.clinoid process
Ant.clinoid process
Carotid groove
Post.clinoid process
Trigeminal impression
Clivus
Arcuate eminence
Aqueduct of vestibule
Sigmoid groove
Transverse groove
Foramen magnum

Crista galli
Ant. and post. ethmoid foramina
Tuberculum sellae
Sella turcica
Sup. orbital fissure
Foramen rotundum
Foramen ovale
Foramen spinosum
Foramen lacerum
Hiatus for superficial petrosal n.
Int. auditory meatus
Mastoid foramen
Jugular foramen
Ant. condylar canal (hypoglossal)
Post. condylar canal

Anterior   fossa

Middle

fossa

Posterior   fossa

Fig. 13. The upper surface of the base of the skull. The anterior fossa is on a higher plane than the middle fossa, and the middle is higher than the posterior; in this way three terraces are formed.

nuchal lines, marks the division between the back of the head and the back of the neck.

The *lambda* is the point of junction between the sagittal and the lambdoid sutures; it marks the position of the posterior fontanelle in the fetal skull.

INTERIOR OF THE SKULL

SKULL CAP

The inner aspect of the skull has a top part or skull cap and a floor or base (Fig. 13). The *skull cap* is concave and presents depressions for the convolutions of the cerebrum and many furrows for the branches of the meningeal vessels. Along the midline is a longitudinal groove, narrow in front at the frontal crest, where it begins, but broader behind. This lodges the superior sagittal sinus, and its margins afford attachments for the falx cerebri. Bordering the sagittal groove, granular pits are seen which increase with age and occasionally are of sufficient depth to pass through the diploë to the outer table. They lodge and are eroded by the arachnoid granulations. In addition there are numbers of minute nutrient foramina.

BASE OF THE SKULL AND THE CRANIAL FOSSAE

The *base* of the skull on its inner surface shows a natural subdivision into *3 cranial fossae:* anterior, middle and posterior. Since the anterior fossa is on a higher plane than the middle, and the middle is higher than the posterior, there is a natural tendency toward the formation of 3 terraces.

The *anterior cranial fossa* is limited posteriorly by the posterior edges of the lesser wings of the sphenoid and in the median part by the anterior edge of the optic groove of the sphenoid. It lodges the frontal lobes of the brain and the olfactory bulbs and tracts. The floor of the fossa is depressed in its median part, where it constitutes the roof of the nasal cavity. The median part is formed by the cribriform plate of the ethmoid bone, through which the *crista galli,* or cock's comb, rises. It is an upward continuation of the nasal septum and gives attachment to the anterior end of the falx cerebri.

The *foramen caecum* is a small pit found directly in front of the crista. In early life the superior longitudinal sinus communicates with the veins of the nose through this foramen, but in the adult it is usually closed, hence its name—caecum (blind). The cribriform plate is perforated like a sieve by numerous olfactory nerves, which are clothed in an arachnoid sheath and arise from the olfactory cells in the nasal mucosa.

At the side of the cribriform plate the *anterior* and the *posterior ethmoidal foramina* are found. They mark the medial ends of two short canals that lead from the orbital cavity and open at the side of the cribriform plate; they transmit the anterior and the posterior ethmoidal arteries and the anterior ethmoidal nerve. The anterior ethmoidal artery and nerve, after passing through the foramina, run on the cribriform plate and then descend into the nose through the *nasal slit* which is found at the side of the front of the crista galli. Anterolateral to the median area, the roof of the frontal sinus and the roof of the orbit are found.

Fractures of the anterior fossa may involve the cribriform plate and be accompanied by lacerations of the meninges and the mucous membrane of the roof of the nose. Such an injury gives rise to epistaxis, accompanied or followed by a discharge of cerebrospinal fluid. There may result some loss of smell due to laceration of the olfactory nerves as they pass upward from the nose and, if dural injury is present, it affords a route whereby infection can travel to the intracranial region from the nose. Meningitis or abscess in the frontal lobe may be a sequela of this type of fracture. If the cribriform plate does not heal after fracture and if a dural laceration remains unrepaired, there may be a continuous discharge of cerebrospinal fluid from the nose, known as cerebrospinal rhinorrhea. When the fracture involves the orbital plate of the frontal bone, subconjunctival hemorrhage is a characteristic feature, and the hemorrhage may seep within the orbit, producing an exophthalmos. The frontal sinus may also be involved.

The *middle cranial fossa* is shaped like a butterfly, having a small median and two lateral expanded concave parts. The median part is formed by the upper surface of the body of the sphenoid. The *sella turcica* is the saddle-shaped area that accommodates the pituitary gland. Anteriorly is the ridge known as the *tuberculum sellae,* on either side of which is an *anterior clinoid process.* Immediately anterior to this process the *optic foramen* is situated at the end of the *optic groove.* The posterior part of the sella turcica is formed by the crest of the dorsum sellae, ending laterally in the *posterior clinoid process* (Fig. 13).

The lateral part of the floor of the middle cranial fossa is formed by the greater wing of the sphenoid, the upper aspect of the petrous part of the temporal and a portion of the squamous part of the temporal bone. These lateral parts lodge the temporal lobes of the brain. The *superior orbital fissure* transmits to the orbital cavity the oculomotor, the trochlear, the ophthalmic division of the trigeminal and the abducens nerves, some filaments from the cavernous plexus of the sympathetic system and the orbital branch of the middle meningeal artery. From the orbital cavity this fissure also transmits the ophthalmic veins and a recurrent branch of the lacrimal artery to the dura mater.

On either side of the sella is the *carotid groove* for the internal carotid artery. Three foramina run almost parallel with this groove. These are, from anterior to posterior and from medial to lateral: the *foramen rotundum* for the passage of the maxillary nerve, the *foramen ovale* for the mandibular nerve, the accessory meningeal artery and the lesser petrosal nerve, and the *foramen spinosum* for the passage of the middle meningeal vessels and a recurrent branch of the mandibular nerve.

Medial to the foramen ovale is the *foramen lacerum,* a short, wide canal rather than a foramen, its lower part being filled by a layer of fibrocartilage. Its upper and inner parts transmit the internal carotid artery, which is surrounded by a plexus of sympathetic nerves. The petrous portion of the temporal bone forms a large and important part of the floor of the fossa. The highest part of this bone is known as the *arcuate eminence* and marks the position of the superior semicircular canal. Lateral to the eminence and immediately adjoining the squamous portion of the bone, the *tegmen tympani* is found. This is a very thin plate of bone which roofs the tympanic antrum, the tympanic cavity and the auditory tube. The important relationship of the thin tegmen tympani intervening between the inferior surface of the temporal lobe of the brain and the tympanic cavity cannot be overemphasized. This bone is the only barrier which exists between a diseased middle ear and the membranes of the brain or the brain itself.

The *hiatus* for the *greater superficial petrosal nerve* is a small slit seen lower down on the anterior surface and about midway between the apex of the petrous temporal and the side of the skull. It communicates with the facial canal in the interior of the bone and transmits a slender nerve from which it takes its name. This nerve has its origin from the facial in the substance of the temporal bone and runs in a medial direction forward to the foramen lacerum. The *trigeminal impression* is found at the upper aspect of the apex of the petrous temporal and is represented by a slightly hollowed-out area. In it is lodged the trigeminal ganglion, which extends forward over the upper and the lateral parts of the foramen lacerum.

The middle fossa is the commonest site of fracture of the skull because of its position and because it is weakened by numerous foramina and canals. Frequently, the tegmen tympani is fractured, and the tympanic membrane torn. Then blood and cerebrospinal fluid are discharged from the external auditory meatus and appear at the ear. The facial and the auditory nerves may be involved. At times the walls of the cavernous sinus are lacerated, and cranial nerves 3, 4 and 6, which lie in relation to its lateral wall, may also be injured. Fractures involving the middle cranial fossa may also pass through the sphenoid bone or the base of the occipital bone and cause bleeding into the mouth.

The *posterior cranial fossa* is the largest and deepest of the cranial fossae and lodges the hind brain (cerebellum, pons and medulla oblongata). Its floor is formed by the basilar, the condylar and the squamous parts of the occipital bone; its lateral wall, by the posterior surface of the petrous and the medial surface of the mastoid part of the temporal bone.

The *foramen magnum* is the most prominent feature of the fossa. At the anterolateral boundary of the foramen the *anterior condylar canal* is found which transmits the hypoglossal nerve. This nerve arises by several roots of origin, and the canal is frequently divided into two parts by a small bar of bone. The foramen magnum transmits a number of structures, the most important being the medulla oblongata, the meninges, the vertebral arteries and the ascending parts of the accessory nerves. This foramen marks the lowest part of the posterior cranial fossa.

FIG. 14. The two methods used to expose the brain, its coverings and vessels.

Trephine operation: (A) skin flap formed, turned down and trephine in place; (B) removal of trephined "button" of bone; (C) incision into dura mater; (D) dural flap formed and reflected; (E) closure of dura.

Osteoplastic craniotomy: (1) soft tissues incised, bone exposed and trephine openings made; craniotome divides the bone; (2) bone is fractured at the base of the flap; (3) dura is divided and underlying structures exposed; (4) dural closure.

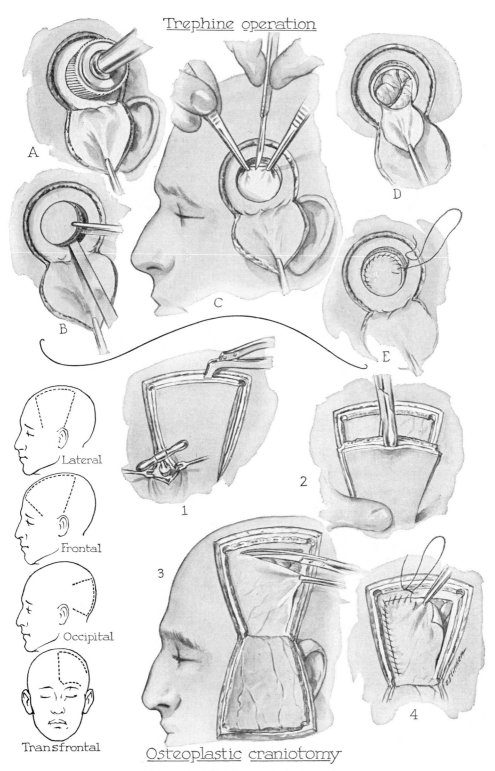

Trephine operation

A

B

C

D

E

Lateral

Frontal

Occipital

Transfrontal

1

2

3

4

Osteoplastic craniotomy

FIG. 14. (*Caption on facing page*)

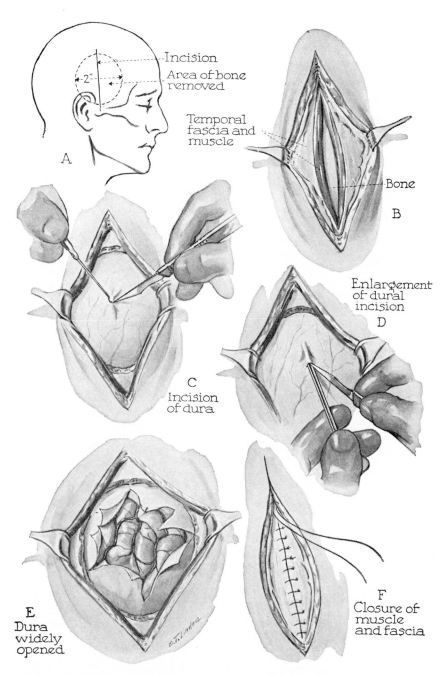

FIG. 15. Subtemporal decompression: (A) Line of incision and amount of
bone to be removed; the incision is placed about three fifths of an inch in front
of the tragus and extends upward and slightly backward for about 4 inches;
(B) temporal muscle and fascia are incised, exposing temporal bone; (C) part
of the temporal bone has been removed, and the dural hook has been placed;
(D) dural opening enlarged on a grooved director; (E) and (F) are self-
explanatory.

The *clivus* is the broad, sloping surface that exists between the anterior margin of the foramen magnum and the root of the dorsum sellae; it is related to the pons and the medulla oblongata. The *internal auditory meatus* is found at the posterior aspect of the petrous temporal and runs laterally into the bone. Through it pass the motor and the sensory roots of the facial nerve, the auditory nerve, the internal auditory branch of the basilar artery and the auditory vein which joins the inferior petrosal sinus.

The *jugular foramen* is situated between the lateral part of the occipital and the petrous part of the temporal bone. It is a large aperture with irregular margins and transmits three sets of structures. At times small spicules of bone project from its margin and may divide it partly or completely into corresponding compartments. The anteromedial compartment transmits the inferior petrosal sinus and a meningeal branch of the ascending pharyngeal artery. The middle compartment transmits the glossopharyngeal, the vagus and accessory nerves. The posterolateral compartment is larger than the other two and transmits the sigmoid sinus as it becomes the internal jugular vein, and a meningeal branch of the occipital artery. The inferior petrosal sinus, which passes through the anterior part of the foramen, becomes the internal jugular vein immediately outside of the skull. The *transverse groove* begins at the side of the internal occipital protuberance and sweeps around the cranial vault to the lateral end of the upper margin of the petrous temporal. It then joins the *sigmoid groove,* which curves downward and descends along the side wall of the skull and extends in a medial direction to end at the jugular foramen. The right transverse groove is wider than the left because it usually receives the sagittal sinus.

The *mastoid foramen* is an aperture of variable size which leads from the exterior of the skull into the sigmoid groove on the side wall of the posterior cranial fossa. Through it a mastoid vein and the mastoid emissary vein and the mastoid branch of the occipital artery pass. The *aqueduct of the vestibule* (aqueductus vestibuli) is found about ½ inch lateral to the internal auditory meatus.

Fractures of the posterior fossa are probably more important than such injuries in the other fossae, since it is here that a small fissure fracture may prove to be fatal. The bone is thin in places and, since there is no outlet for the escape of blood or cerebrospinal fluid as in the anterior and the middle fossae, these fractures may be overlooked. Some days after the injury, blood may be noted over the mastoid process. Fractures of the base of the skull involving the hypoglossal canal may be manifested by paralysis of one side of the tongue.

SURGICAL CONSIDERATIONS

TREPHINING OPERATIONS

Two methods are usually employed to expose the brain: trephining and osteoplastic resection (Fig. 14).

In trephining operations a circular disk of a cranial bone is removed by use of a trephine. The main indications for such operations are hemorrhage, abscess, fracture, evacuation of cerebrospinal fluid, or as a preliminary step to further brain surgery. A U-shaped or linear incision is made. If the former is used, its convexity is placed toward the crown of the head and the pedicle toward the base. The size of the flap is much larger than the bone which is to be removed. The incision passes through the skin, the superficial fascia, the muscle and the periosteum to the bone, and hemostasis is accomplished as the operation proceeds. With the trephine site cleared, a piece of bone is removed and, if a larger opening is needed, it may be obtained by removing pieces of bone from the circumference with a rongeur forceps. The dura is exposed and can be opened, but any large dural vessels should be ligated first. The necessary operative procedure is carried out, and the dural flap is sutured back into its normal position. The bone may or may not be replaced, and the wound is closed in layers.

OSTEOPLASTIC CRANIOTOMY

Osteoplastic craniotomy implies the raising of a portion of skull which may be replaced when the operation is completed. Lateral, frontal, transfrontal, occipital and suboccipital osteoplastic flaps have been described, depending upon the area to be operated (Fig. 14). The incision passes through all the soft tissues down to the bone. Vessels are clamped and ligated, and the periosteum is detached for a short distance along the line of the contemplated bone incision. Openings are made along the bone margins by means of a drill, a burr or a small trephine, and the bone that intervenes is divided by a saw or rongeur forceps. The base of the pedicle is steadied, usually with the left hand. The upper portion of the flap is grasped with a cranial claw forceps, and with a quick jerk the bone is fractured. The flap thus created is turned back, and the dura is opened by means of a similar but smaller flap. The necessary operative procedure is carried out, the dura is closed by fine interrupted sutures, and the bone flap with its attached soft parts is replaced and sutured into position.

SUBTEMPORAL DECOMPRESSION

(Fig. 15.) A *subtemporal decompression* is really a craniectomy, which implies the removal of a portion of the skull, leaving a permanent gap. Such a procedure is necessary in about 10 per cent of all cases of severe head injuries where it is desired to give the brain room for expansion. The permanent bone defect should be covered over, if possible, by muscle so that a herniation of the brain does not result. Since the temporal muscle is conveniently situated, the decompression is usually made subjacent to it, hence the name "subtemporal decompression."

In this operation the skin incision, beginning at the zygoma, is placed three fifths of an inch in front of the tragus and extends upward and slightly backward for about 4 inches. The temporal fascia and muscle are incised to the bone in line with the scalp incision, the muscles and the fascia are retracted, and a piece of temporal bone a little over 2 inches in diameter is removed. The middle meningeal artery may cause troublesome bleeding (p. 38). The dura is palpated to determine the degree of tension; if it is high, the dura should be opened. However, some surgeons prefer to reduce the tension first by ventricular puncture. Sutures are placed in the muscle before the dura is opened but are not tied and may be brought

together quickly to prevent rupture of the cerebral cortex. A fine hook is placed in an avascular dural area, which is incised. The dural opening may be enlarged by incising on a grooved director. If the tension is high, the brain protrudes with great force, and care must be taken to prevent a cortical rupture. As soon as the dura has been incised adequately, the muscles are brought together, followed by closure of the fascia and the skin.

INTRACRANIAL HEMORRHAGE

(Fig. 16.) A line known as the eye-ear line, or *Reid's base line,* is utilized in cranial topography. It extends from the lower margin of the orbit to the upper border of the external auditory meatus. Some anatomists prefer to refer to a horizontal plane known as the Frankfurt plane for such orientation.

Extradural Hemorrhage. Extradural hemorrhage is usually caused by an injury to the middle meningeal artery or one of its branches. This vessel arises from the internal maxillary artery and enters the cranium via the foramen spinosum. It passes upward and forward for a short distance over the great wing of the sphenoid and soon divides into anterior and posterior branches, which ramify upon the dura and supply the greater part of its lateral and superior surfaces. The anterior branch, which is the larger, continues obliquely forward over the great wing to the antero-inferior angle of the parietal bone, in which it forms a deep groove. It ascends in this groove behind the anterior margin of that bone almost as far as the sagittal suture. The posterior branch passes upward and backward over the squamous portion of the temporal bone. The artery is accompanied by its two venae comites. The *anterior branch* is found readily through an opening which is made 1½ inches behind the external angular process of the frontal bone and a similar distance above the upper border of the zygoma (Fig. 16-A). This is the branch that is damaged most frequently and, since it is closely related to the motor area of the cortex, injury to it might produce a loss of power in the muscles of the opposite side of the body. The *posterior branch* can be reached through a trephine hole 1 inch above the external auditory meatus (the midmeatal point). In

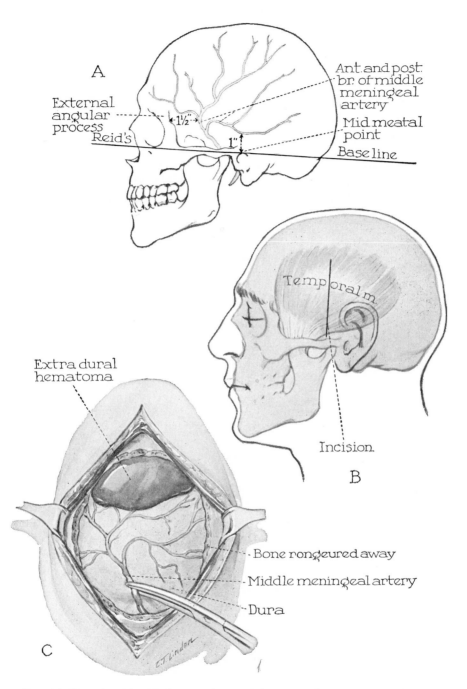

FIG. 16. Extradural hemorrhage: (A) cranial topography, location of the anterior and posterior branches of the middle meningeal artery; (B) incision for ligation of the middle meningeal artery; (C) extradural hematoma located and vessel clamped.

ligating the *middle meningeal artery,* either a vertical or a horseshoe-shaped incision (Fig. 16) can be used. The skin incision should be continued vertically downward toward the zygoma, and the temporal muscle is divided. Only when the bone opening is sufficiently large should the clot be removed; this usually requires an opening of about 2 inches in diameter. The bleeding vessel is located and ligated by passing a needle about it, clamping with a Cushing clip or coagulating with an electrosurgical needle. The muscle, the fascia and the skin are closed with fine sutures. Drainage is not indicated in these cases.

Subdural Hemorrhage. When subdural hemorrhage is present, it might become necessary to explore through a trephine opening to locate the point of hemorrhage. After the skull has been opened, the dura is tense and plum colored, signifying extravasated blood beneath it. The exploratory trephine hole is enlarged, the dura is opened, and necessary hemostatic measures are carried out.

Brain

EMBRYOLOGY

In the early embryo a primitive neural groove extending along the dorsal surface is converted into a tube by the elevation and the fusion of the neural folds. The cranial end of the neural tube forms the brain; it expands and constricts to form a series of three communicating sacs which are the primary brain vesicles known as the forebrain (prosencephalon), the midbrain (mesencephalon) and the hindbrain (rhombencephalon), the last being continuous with the

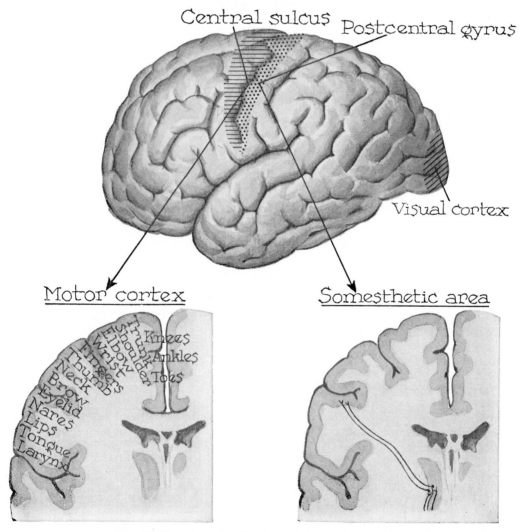

Central sulcus   Postcentral gyrus

Visual cortex

Motor cortex   Somesthetic area

Trunk Shoulder Elbow Wrist Fingers Thumb Neck Brow Eyelid Nares Lips Tongue Larynx Knees Ankles Toes

Fig. 17. Functional localizations of the cerebral cortex.

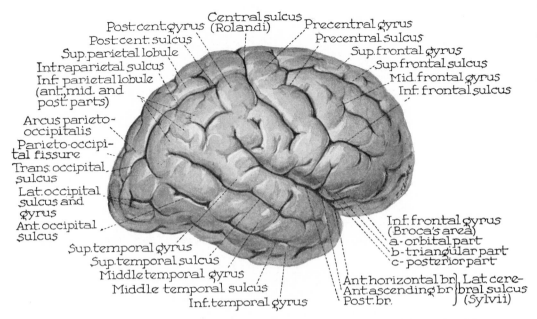

Central sulcus
Post. cent. gyrus (Rolandi)
Post. cent. sulcus
Sup. parietal lobule
Intraparietal sulcus
Inf. parietal lobule
(ant., mid. and
post. parts)
Arcus parieto-
occipitalis
Parieto-occipi-
tal fissure
Trans. occipital
sulcus
Lat. occipital
sulcus and
gyrus
Ant. occipital
sulcus
Precentral gyrus
Precentral sulcus
Sup. frontal gyrus
Sup. frontal sulcus
Mid. frontal gyrus
Inf. frontal sulcus
Inf. frontal gyrus
(Broca's area)
a - orbital part
b - triangular part
c - posterior part
Ant. horizontal br] Lat. cere-
Ant. ascending br } bral sulcus
Post. br.] (Sylvii)
Sup. temporal gyrus
Sup. temporal sulcus
Middle temporal gyrus
Middle temporal sulcus
Inf. temporal gyrus

FIG. 18. Lateral surface of the right cerebral hemisphere, viewed from the side.

spinal medulla. The cavity of the tube thus formed subsequently becomes the ventricular system and the central canal of the spinal cord, and the walls of the tube become the nerve elements of the brain and the spinal cord. The forebrain becomes the cerebral hemispheres and the optic vesicles; the midbrain develops into the brain stem connecting the cerebrum with the pons and the cerebellum, and the hindbrain forms the cerebellum, the pons and the medulla oblongata.

BRAIN PROPER

The average weight of the human brain in the adult male is approximately 1,380 grams; of the female, approximately 1,250 grams. Increasing rapidly during the first 4 years of life, the brain reaches its maximum weight about the 20th year and decreases slowly as age progresses.

When inspected from above, the only parts visible are the *cerebral hemispheres*. The *longitudinal fissure* separates the two hemispheres, except in its central part where the *corpus callosum* forms its floor. The fissure contains the *falx cerebri,* which projects into it from the cranial vault. The surfaces of the cerebral hemispheres are interrupted by many sulci (fissures) that separate the vari-

ous convolutions (gyri) from one another. The sulci are produced by infolding of the cerebral cortex, in this way increasing the amount of cortical substance without increase in the surface of the hemispheres. Various convolutions are associated with various functions, and the different functional areas show structural differences in their cortex (Fig. 17).

CEREBRAL HEMISPHERES AND LOBES

(Fig. 18.) These hemispheres occupy the anterior and the middle cranial fossae, and each is composed of 5 lobes: frontal, parietal, temporal, occipital and central (island of Reil, insula). The falx cerebri, which separates the cerebral hemispheres, is a fold of dura mater that projects downward from the vault of the skull. The hemispheres are separated from the cerebellum by another fold of dura mater called the *tentorium cerebelli* (Fig. 23).

1. The *frontal lobe* on the lateral surface is bounded posteriorly by the *central sulcus* (fissure of Rolando). This sulcus is important because the convolution in front of it contains the higher centers for control of movements of the opposite side of the body.

It is easily identified because it is the only sulcus of any length that lies between two parallel and almost vertical convolutions. Its upper end cuts the superomedial border of the hemisphere, and its lower end is separated from the posterior ramus of the lateral sulcus by a bridge of cortex.

Inferiorly the *lateral cerebral sulcus* (fissure of Sylvius) separates the frontal from the temporal lobe. It passes upward and backward, and its posterior end bends upward into the parietal lobe.

On the superolateral surface of the frontal lobe the *precentral gyrus* is bounded by the central sulcus, around the lower end of which it joins the *postcentral gyrus*; in front it is bounded by the *precentral sulcus*, containing the higher centers that control the movements of the opposite side of the body. It should be noted that in the cortex the body is represented in the inverted position, hence, the centers for the lower limbs occupy the uppermost part of the convolution. Below the lower limb come the trunk, the upper limb, the neck and finally the head. Corresponding muscles of opposite sides of the body are connected with the cortex of both cerebral hemispheres; an example of this is the movements of both eyes. Therefore, it is understood that such movements are not affected by unilateral lesions of the internal capsule. Movements and not individual muscles are represented in the cortex. The *superior* and *inferior frontal sulci* run forward from the precentral sulcus and divide this area into *superior, middle* and *inferior gyri*. The inferior frontal gyrus reveals the *anterior horizontal* and the ascending rami of the *lateral sulcus*. The cortical area associated with these two limbs is known as Broca's area and is associated with the function of speech. This area consists of an orbital part below the horizontal ramus, a triangular part between the two rami, and a posterior part behind the ascending ramus that is directly continuous with the cortex at the lower end of the precentral gyrus. In right-handed people the left side of this region is better developed.

2. The *parietal lobe* is limited in front by the central sulcus, behind by the artificial boundary of the occipital lobe and the lateral parieto-occipital sulcus, above by the superomedial border and below by the posterior horizontal limb of the lateral cerebral fissure and its backward prolongation. These boundaries are somewhat artificial and not entirely definite.

The *postcentral sulcus* lies parallel with and a little behind the central sulcus; the *postcentral gyrus,* containing the *sensory* projection centers, is placed between them. A tumor involving this area produces diminution in various sensations, and the patient loses his ability to localize a painful stimulus or to be certain of its intensity; he may have difficulty determining the weight, the size and the texture of various objects and materials.

From the postcentral sulcus the *intraparietal sulcus* passes directly backward and in this way demarcates a *superior parietal lobule* from an *inferior*. Lesions of the inferior parietal lobule produce the interesting sign of asterognosis (inability to correlate and interpret various sensory impressions). This lobule is divided from below by 3 upturned ends: the posterior ramus of the lateral sulcus, and the superior and middle temporal sulci. As a result of this the ends of these sulci are capped by arched gyri which are called the anterior, the middle and the posterior parts of the inferior parietal lobule (supramarginal, angular and postparietal gyri). The postparietal gyrus is not always as evident as the other two. Wordblindness, the inability to understand written words, is a characteristic finding associated with a lesion of the angular gyrus of the left side in right-handed individuals. Lesions of the upper parietal lobe are associated with inability to recognize the form or nature of objects. Some authorities prefer not to include the postcentral gyrus in the parietal lobe. With lesions of this gyrus the patient loses his ability to localize a painful stimulus or to measure its intensity. If this area is irritated, there may be numbness, needle-and-pin sensation or "shocks of electricity" in his extremities. At times such sensory attacks are initiating symptoms of the jacksonian type of motor convulsions. Optic radiations pass through a portion of the parietal lobe on their way to the visual center; hence, a deeply placed tumor may produce a

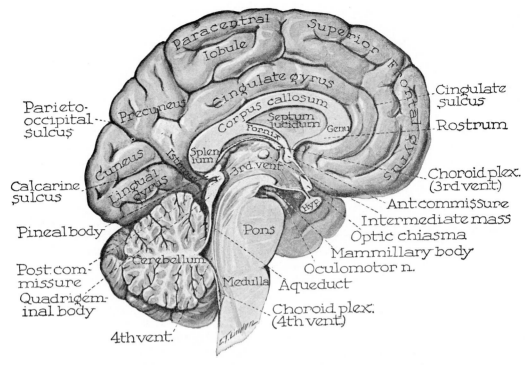

Fig. 19. Medial aspect of the brain, sectioned in the sagittal plane.

contralateral homonymous visual field defect (half-blindness of the corresponding sides of both retinae).

3. The *temporal lobe* is bounded above by the posterior horizontal limb of the lateral cerebral sulcus. Where this fissure turns up, the line of the posterior limb must be continued backward until it cuts the arbitrary line marking off the front of the occipital lobe. Posteriorly, this line separates the temporal from the occipital lobe. The temporal lobe has *three gyri* (superior, middle and inferior), which are separated from each other by *two sulci* (superior and inferior temporal sulci). The *superior temporal sulcus* runs parallel with the posterior ramus of the lateral sulcus, and its posterior end turns upward and into the parietal lobe, where it is surrounded by the angular gyrus (inferior parietal lobule). The *superior temporal gyrus* lying immediately above the same-named sulcus contains the higher auditory centers. Since the temporal lobes occupy the middle fossa of the skull, they are susceptible to injury in basal fractures. Lesions involving the superior temporal gyrus may also be asso-

ciated with an inability to understand the spoken word (word-deafness). The *middle temporal gyrus* lies below the superior temporal sulcus and is bounded inferiorly by the *middle temporal sulcus,* which is usually interrupted.

4. The *occipital lobe* is arbitrarily marked off by drawing a line downward and a little forward from the parieto-occipital fissure to the inferolateral border of the hemisphere. The surface of the lobe is quite variable. The *transverse* and *lateral occipital sulci* divide this lobe into the *superior,* the *middle* and the *inferior gyri.* The superior occipital gyrus is connected anteriorly to the superior parietal lobule by the parieto-occipital arc. The middle occipital gyrus is continuous above with the inferior parietal lobule and in front with the middle temporal gyrus. The inferior occipital gyrus is connected in front with the inferior temporal gyrus.

Investigators believe that the chief function of the occipital lobe is concerned with vision. A destructive lesion in this region produces a contralateral homonymous hemianopsia. Certain visual hallucinations may result from irritation of the occipital lobe and are usually described by patients as colors of the rainbow, bright lines, flashes of light or brilliant lightning patterns.

5. The *central lobe* can be seen only when the edges of the lateral cerebral fissures are pulled apart. Even this maneuver does not completely expose the lobe, since certain parts that will be described later (p. 38) must also be removed. The lobe is surrounded by the *circular sulcus* and is overlapped by parts of cortex which are called *opercula,* of which there are four: temporal, orbital, frontal (pars triangularis) and frontoparietal.

Medial Surface of the Cerebral Hemisphere (Fig. 19). If the two cerebral hemispheres are divided by a main vertical incision, the great (white) commissure known as the *corpus callosum* stands out as a striking landmark. This is about 4 inches long and extends to within 1½ inches of the anterior and 2½ inches of the posterior extremities of the hemisphere. The anterior part of the corpus callosum, known as the *genu,* bends upon itself and ends below in a point called the *rostrum.* The hind part of the corpus is called the *splenium,* and the intermediate part forms the *body* (truncus). The fibers that run through it are principally transverse ones and are mainly association fiber tracts that connect the two cerebral hemispheres. Tumors involving the corpus callosum usually produce the same symptoms as those in the frontal lobe because of their close anatomic position.

The rostrum is connected to the upper part of the optic chiasma by a narrow sheet of gray matter called the *lamina terminalis.* The genu contains fibers running forward and medially into the frontal lobe, thus forming the *forceps minor.*

The body of the corpus lies at the bottom of the longitudinal fissure in the median plane and at each side of this forms the roof of the lateral ventricles. The splenium covers the dorsal aspect of the midbrain, and the great cerebral vein separates the splenium above from the pineal body below. The fibers of the splenium arch backward and medially into the occipital lobe on either side, forming the *forceps major.* The intermediate fibers that exist between the forceps major and minor are known as the *tapetum.* Below the

middle third of the corpus callosum the body of the *fornix* is found. As this structure passes forward, its anterior pillar arches downward until it is lost in the lower part of the brain, terminating in the mammillary body of its own side. The fornix forms the efferent tract from the hypocampus of one hemisphere to that of the other and to the brain. A thin membrane, *septum lucidum* (septum pellucidum), stretches from the anterior convexity of the fornix to the concavity of the corpus callosum. It consists of two layers with a slitlike cavity between, is not lined by ependyma, and forms a partition between the anterior horns of the lateral ventricles.

Behind the fornix and at the most anterior part of its arch, the *interventricular foramen* (foramen of Monro) is found. This appears as an open aperture bounded by the fornix in front and the optic thalamus behind and provides a communication between the lateral and the third ventricles. This is brought about by a V-shaped arrangement in which the two limbs anteriorly communicate with the lateral ventricles on either side, and the junction of the two open into the third ventricle via the foramen of Monro (Fig. 24).

The *anterior commissure,* located a little below the foramen and in front of the fornix, appears as a small rounded bundle of fibers, the posterior aspect of which can be seen in the anterior wall of the third ventricle. The concavity of the fornix arches around the front of the *optic thalamus* and forms the lateral wall of the third ventricle. The thalamus is joined to its counterpart by the interthalamic connexus (middle commissure) which is really not a commissure since it is formed by gray matter.

The *posterior commissure* is a layer of white fibers that connects the two thalami posteriorly. It forms the posterior boundary of the third ventricle and is placed just above the upper opening of the aqueduct of the midbrain (Sylvius). The *pineal body* is situated directly above and posterior to the posterior commissure.

The *sulcus cinguli* begins below the rostrum and follows the curvature of the corpus callosum and is separated from it by the *gyrus cinguli.* The sulcus turns upward in the region of the splenium and cuts the superomedial border of the hemisphere just behind the upper end of the central sulcus. The *medial gyrus* lies immediately in front of this upper end of the central sulcus, forming the medial surface of the frontal lobe and containing the higher motor centers that control the movements of the lower limb of the opposite side of the body. This latter portion of the gyrus is referred to as the *paracentral lobule,* behind which is found the *precuneus.* The lobule is bounded posteriorly by the parieto-occipital sulcus; it forms the medial surface of the parietal lobe and is separated from the occipital lobe by the parieto-occipital sulcus. The gyrus is separated from the parietal lobe by the interrupted suprasplenial (subparietal) sulcus.

The *calcarine sulcus* passes forward from the occipital lobe and just above the infero-medial border of the hemisphere. It joins the parieto-occipital sulcus so that these 2 sulci enclose a triangular area of cortex known as the *cuneus,* which forms the medial surface of the occipital lobe. From the point of union of the 2 sulci the calcarine sulcus runs forward into the gyrus cinguli, the narrow part of which is termed the *isthmus.* The *lingual gyrus* lies below the calcarine sulcus as far back as the occipital lobe.

INFERIOR SURFACE OF BRAIN, CEREBELLUM AND MEDULLA OBLONGATA

(Fig. 20.) The inferior surface of the brain consists of two parts: the anterior (orbital) and the posterior (tentorial). The *anterior surface* of the frontal lobe rests upon the floor of the anterior cranial fossa, thereby

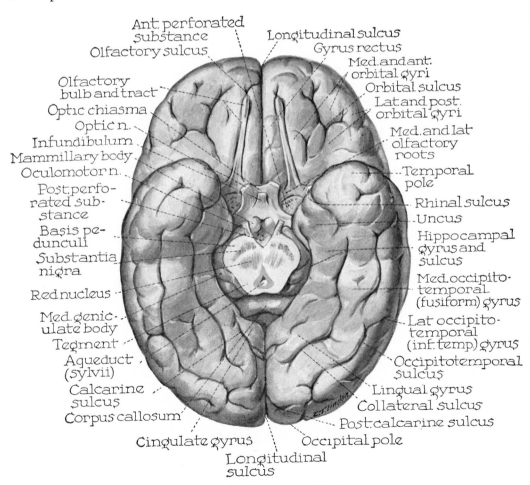

FIG. 20. Inferior surface of the brain.

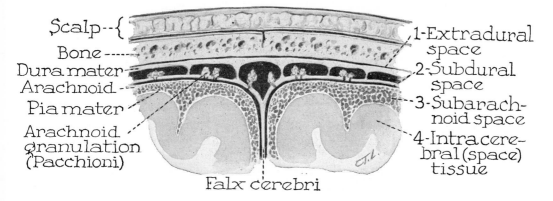

Scalp--{
Bone-----
Dura mater-
Arachnoid--
Pia mater-
Arachnoid granulation (Pacchioni)

1-Extradural space
2-Subdural space
3-Subarachnoid space
4-Intracerebral (space) tissue

Falx cerebri

FIG. 21. Diagrammatic frontal section through the scalp, the skull, the meninges and the brain. The arachnoid villi invade the dura, and the subarachnoid space is trabeculated. The 4 intracranial spaces should be noted.

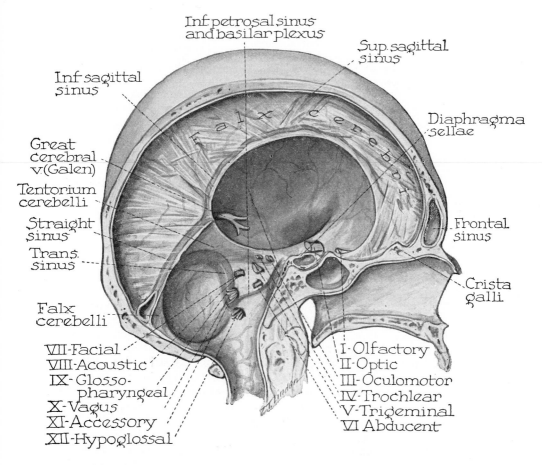

Inf. petrosal sinus and basilar plexus
Sup. sagittal sinus
Inf. sagittal sinus
Diaphragma sellae
Great cerebral v (Galen)
Tentorium cerebelli
Straight sinus
Trans. sinus
Falx cerebelli
Frontal sinus
Crista galli

VII-Facial
VIII-Acoustic
IX-Glosso-pharyngeal
X-Vagus
XI-Accessory
XII-Hypoglossal

I-Olfactory
II-Optic
III-Oculomotor
IV-Trochlear
V-Trigeminal
VI Abducent

FIG. 22. The 4 membranes formed by the infolding of the dura mater (falx cerebri, falx cerebelli, tentorium cerebelli and diaphragma sellae). The venous sinuses and the cranial nerves are also shown.

coming into relationship with the orbit, the frontal sinus and the nasal cavity. It is bounded behind by the stem of the lateral sulcus. The *orbital gyri* and *sulci* occupy this area. Very little is known about the functions of this portion of the brain.

The *posterior surface* lies on the floor of the middle cranial fossa and in the tentorium cerebelli, thus coming into relationship with the tympanic antrum. Its medial part is formed by the *hippocampal gyrus,* which is continuous posteriorly with the gyrus cinguli at the isthmus. The anterior extremity of this gyrus forms a projection called the *uncus,* which receives incoming olfactory fibers and is associated with olfactory impressions. The *rhinal sulcus* separates the uncus from the temporal lobe.

The hippocampal gyrus is bounded laterally by the *collateral sulcus.* The *lingual gyrus* begins near the occipital pole, lying posterior to the hippocampal gyrus and medial to the collateral sulcus.

The *medial occipitotemporal (fusiform) gyrus,* lateral to the lingual and hippocampal gyri, is bounded laterally by the occipitotemporal sulcus. Lateral to this sulcus the *lateral occipitotemporal (inferior temporal) gyrus* is found.

The *olfactory bulb* continues backward as the *olfactory tract,* which passes along the medial border of each orbital area, parallel with the great longitudinal sulcus. Inferiorly, the olfactory bulb rests upon the cribriform plate of the ethmoid, through which the olfactory nerves from the nasal mucous membrane pass. The olfactory tract divides into *medial* and *lateral olfactory roots.* Directly posterior to these roots is found the *anterior perforated substance,* which transmits numerous arteries and veins to and from the interior of the brain.

The *optic chiasma* results from the crossing of the optic nerves and lies posteromedial to the anterior perforated space. The *optic tracts* continue backward from the chiasma and disappear under cover of the uncus. If the optic commissure is gently retracted backward, a very delicate layer, *lamina terminalis,* is seen. This may be torn easily and, if injured, the cavity of the third ventricle is exposed. Immediately behind the optic chiasma the *tuber cinereum* is located. While poorly developed in the human, it is particularly well developed in certain types of fish whose sense of taste dominates the sense of smell. The *infundibulum* (stalk of the hypophysis) is at its summit. Behind the tuber cinereum the two small white *mammillary bodies* are seen whose nuclei form important olfactory centers.

The *posterior perforated substance* is situated immediately behind the mammillary bodies and is perforated by branches of the posterior cerebral arteries which supply the thalami. The *cerebral peduncles,* two large bundles of white substance lying close together at the superior margin of the pons, gradually diverge as they travel upward to form the *interpeduncular fossa,* disappearing beneath the optic tracts. These two great bundles associate the cerebral hemispheres with all the structures below them.

The structures about to be described can be seen best if the temporal lobe is retracted, and as this is done the optic tract can be followed backward around the lateral side of the peduncle, where it broadens and divides into lateral and medial roots. The lateral root ends in the *lateral geniculate body* and the *superior corpus quadrigeminum,* which it reaches through the superior brachium. These nuclei constitute the lower visual centers (Fig. 38). The medial root ends in the *medial geniculate body* and has no connection with vision. Behind and above the geniculate bodies is the overhanging hind end of the optic thalamus known as the *pulvinar.* This is associated with the lower visual centers.

The *corpora quadrigemina* are 4 round bodies that are found on the dorsal aspect of the midbrain immediately below and medial to the pulvinar. The superior corpora quadrigemina (colliculus superior) are larger than the inferior and have the pineal body situated just above them in such a way that the colliculus superior of one side is separated from that of the other. Each of the 4 corpora has a brachium or ridge running lateral from it.

The lateral geniculate body, the superior corpora quadrigemina and the pulvinar are known collectively as the *lower visual centers.* The lateral geniculate body is the most important component of this group, since it is a relay station on the visual pathway from the retina to the visual cortex. The inferior quadrigeminal bodies are associated with auditory pathways. A medial groove separates the ventral part of the peduncle, forming the *basis* or *crusta pedunculi*. The dorsal part of the peduncle is known as the *tegmentum* and contains important afferent pathways and the *red nucleus*. The tegmentum and the base of the peduncle are separated on each side by a band of deeply pigmented gray matter that is known as the *substantia nigra*. The *aqueduct of Sylvius* appears in the mid-line nearer the dorsal side, and the *splenium* (hind end of the corpus callosum) is situated more posteriorly.

The interpeduncular fossa occupies a central position and is bounded in front by the optic chiasma, anterolaterally by the optic tract and posterolaterally by the cerebral peduncles. The contents of this fossa from before backward are the tuber cinereum with its infundibulum, the corpora mammillaria and the posterior perforated space. All these structures take part in the formation of the floor of the third ventricle.

The *cerebral* peduncles attach the cerebrum to the pons; the *cerebellar* peduncles attach the cerebellum to the pons and the medulla (Fig. 19). The *pons varolii* is placed above the medulla, below the cerebral peduncles and between the lateral halves of the cerebellum. It is about 1½ inches long and 2 inches wide; its ventral surface reveals a midline groove (basilar sulcus) for the basilar artery. The pons also presents transverse markings and openings for the entrance of vessels and forms part of the floor of the 4th ventricle. Its dorsal surface is smaller than its anterior and is continuous with the posterior surface of the medulla.

The *cerebellum* (Fig. 19) occupies the posterior cranial fossa. It is separated from the cerebral hemispheres above by the tentorium cerebelli and in front is related to the pons and the medulla oblongata, from which it is separated by the fourth ventricle. It is closely related to the sigmoid sinus and the tympanic antrum on each side. The cerebellum consists of a median strip, called the vermis, and two hemispheres. It resembles the cerebrum in structure in that gray matter forms a layer of cortex placed on the surface

and not centrally, as in the spinal cord and the brain stem.

The *medulla oblongata* extends from the foramen magnum to the lower border of the pons. It connects the spinal cord below to the pons above. Anteriorly, it rests upon the basilar part of the occipital bone and posteriorly lies in a depression between the hemispheres of the cerebellum, which is called the *vallecula cerebelli*. The posterior aspect of the medulla is conveniently divided into upper and lower halves, the upper forming the lower part of the floor of the 4th ventricle, while the lower is directly continuous with the posterior part of the spinal cord. The medulla, approximately 1¼ inches long, is pyramidal in shape, having its apex at the spinal cord and its base at the pons. It presents anterior and posterior median fissures that are continuous with those of the cord.

MENINGES

(Figs. 21, 23.) The brain and the spinal cord are surrounded by three enveloping membranes, which are known from inside out as the pia mater, the arachnoid mater and the dura mater. Their names suggest their qualities: the dura is tough and firm, the arachnoid resembles a spider's web, and the pia represents a very thin, clinging, skin-like structure that hugs the surface of the brain and follows its irregularities. The dura and the arachnoid do not dip into the fissures but fit the brain as a child's mitten fits its hand; on the other hand, the pia mater dips into each fissure and fits the brain very much as a glove fits the hand, since each finger has its own indentation (see venous sinuses of the dura mater, p. 47).

The *dura mater* (Figs. 22, 23) is the most external membrane of the brain; it consists of two layers that are firmly blended with each other except in certain locations. The more superficial of these layers is the endocranium, which is a periosteum (endoperiosteum). Through the openings in the skull it is continuous with the external periosteum (pericranium). The endoperiosteum is the layer that is intimately related to the bones of the skull and in no way takes part in the formation of the falx cerebri or the tentorium cerebelli. Bulging arachnoid granulations (enlarged villi of the arachnoid projecting through the layers of the dura mater) project from each side of the median sagittal plane and produce the pits found on the parietal bone. The middle meningeal vessel ascends in the dura and produces a groove in the parietal bone. The deeper or inner layer of dura is smooth and lined by endothelial cells. It resembles a serous membrane and is separated from the superficial layers by a small amount of fibrous tissue. The venous sinuses and the meningeal vessels separate the 2 layers of dura. By a process of infolding and reduplicating itself, the inner layer of dura forms 4 membranes that subdivide the cranial cavities. These membranes are the falx cerebri, the falx cerebelli, the tentorium cerebelli and the diaphragma sellae.

The sickle-shaped *falx cerebri* is placed vertically between the 2 hemispheres of the cerebrum and is a reduplication of the inner layer of the dura. It consists of 2 layers of serous dura. Its upper border is convex and attached to the crista galli in front; it extends back to the internal occipital protuberance and between these two points is attached to the internal surface of the skull. Its lower border is attached to the tentorium cerebelli behind but otherwise remains free to project between the cerebral hemispheres in front of the tentorium. The falx is narrow in front and becomes wider as it is traced backward. The superior sagittal sinus appears in its upper border; its lower border contains the inferior sagittal sinus and aids the tentorium in the support of the straight sinus.

The *falx cerebelli* passes vertically from the tentorium to the foramen magnum and separates the 2 cerebellar hemispheres. It attaches posteriorly to the internal occipital crest, where it encloses the occipital sinus. Construction of the falx cerebelli is exactly the same as that of the falx cerebri.

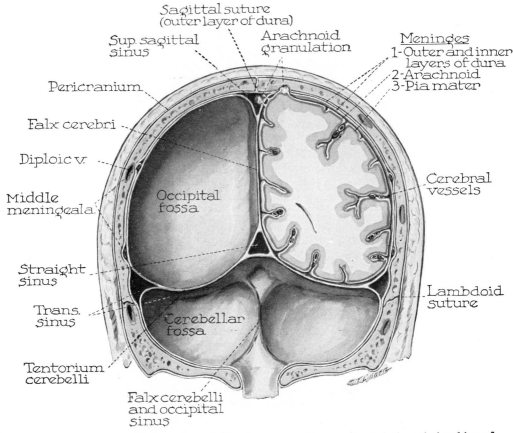

Fig. 23. Coronal section through the foramen magnum, showing the relationships of the meninges, the venous sinuses and the blood vessels.

The *tentorium cerebelli* is a tentlike fold of a double layer of serous dura mater, forming a partition between the cerebellum and the posterior part of the cerebral hemispheres. It forms a roof for the cerebellum and a floor for the occipital lobe and the posterior part of the temporal lobe of the cerebrum. Anteriorly, a wide gap known as the tentorial notch permits the passage of the midbrain. Because of this arrangement the tentorium possesses a free inner and an attached outer border. This outer border has 3 attachments: to the margins of the groove of the transverse sinus of the occipital bone; to the margins of the groove for the superior petrosal sinus on the petrous portion of the temporal bone; to the posterior clinoid process of the sphenoid bone. The free border runs forward to the anterior clinoid process, and the upper layer of the tentorium becomes continuous with the falx cerebri in the median plane.

The *diaphragma sellae* is also a fold of inner layer of dura mater with a foramen in its center. Its lateral border is attached to the clinoid processes; its medial border forms the boundary of the foramen of the diaphragma sellae and also surrounds the infundibulum. The superior surface of the diaphragm is in relation to the base of the brain; its inferior aspect is related to the hypophysis, which is bound by it to the hypophyseal fossa.

The *arachnoid mater,* a delicate membrane enveloping the brain and medulla spinalis, lies between the pia mater internally and the dura mater externally. It does not dip into the various sulci on the surface of the brain, but is carried into the longitudinal fissure by the falx cerebri. Over the convolutions the arachnoid and the pia are in close contact but are separated at the sulci by the subarachnoid space, which contains the cerebrospinal fluid and is crossed by a gauzy retinaculum of cobweblike fibers connecting the two membranes (Fig. 21). At the base of the brain this network is much reduced and the two membranes are widely separated to form the so-called *subarachnoid cisternae*. The three main cisternae are:

1. The *cisterna cerebromedullaris* (cisterna magna) is a cavity resulting from the arachnoid's bridging the inferior surface of the cerebellum and the dorsal surface of the medulla oblongata. It is continuous below with the spinal subarachnoid space. Cerebrospinal fluid passes directly into this cistern from the fourth ventricle by means of the foramen of Magendie (median aperture).

2. The *cisterna pontis,* a space lying in front of the pons and the medulla oblongata, is continuous with the subarachnoid space about the medulla and has been referred to as "Hilton's water bed," since it forms a water cushion to protect the brain. The roots of the lower 8th cranial nerves traverse this cavity.

3. The *cisterna interpeduncularis,* a wide cavity formed by the arachnoid as it extends across and between the two temporal lobes, encloses the cerebral peduncles and contains the arterial circle of Willis. Some consider it part of the cisterna basalis, which connects it to a smaller cisterna in front of the optic chiasma. The arachnoid granulations are seen best in old age, where they produce pitting of the parietal bone. When hypertrophied, they are called *pacchionian bodies*. Although they appear to originate in the dura, they are really villous processes of the arachnoid that push the dura mater ahead of them. They serve as channels for the passage of cerebrospinal fluid into the venous system and at times may become large enough to produce pressure signs.

The *pia mater* is the innermost of the three meninges and is in reality the membrane of nutrition. It is closely attached to the surface of the brain and dips into the depths of all the sulci, carrying branches of the cerebral arteries with it. The larger blood vessels of the brain lie in the subarachnoid space, but the smaller ones ramify the pia and proceed into the substance of the brain proper. At certain locations the pia mater sends strong vascular duplications into the brain; these spread over the cavities of the third and the fourth ventricles and are known as the choroid telae. The choroid tela of the 3rd ventricle extends into each lateral ventricle. The blood vessels on the border projecting into the lateral ventricle are enlarged into a plexus known as the choroid plexus of the lateral ventricle, from which the greater amount of cerebrospinal fluid is formed.

INTRACRANIAL SPACES

(Fig. 21.) The 4 intracranial spaces are: the extradural (exterior to the dura); subdural (beneath the dura); subarachnoidal (beneath the arachnoid); the intracerebral (within the brain tissue proper).

1. The *extradural space* is only a potential one because the dura touches the internal surface of the skull. The meningeal vessels (p. 24) are in this space, and if they are injured, bleeding takes place between the dura and the skull. If this bleeding is permitted to continue, the dura is slowly stripped away from the bone. Bleeding into this space is usually *arterial* and therefore rapid and often fatal. If the arachnoid is intact and the subarachnoid space has not been entered, there is no blood in the cerebrospinal fluid.

2. The *subdural space* is situated between the dura and the arachnoid. Hemorrhage into this space may result from injury to large arteries such as the middle cerebral or internal carotid, but this is rare, rapidly fatal and of no practical importance. It is much more important to consider subdural hemorrhage as *venous,* since the large sinuses, such as the superior longitudinal and lateral, may be torn when the dura is injured. If the arachnoid is also torn, as it may be over the great cisterns at the base of the brain, blood escapes into the subarachnoid space and will appear in the cerebrospinal fluid.

3. The trabeculated *subarachnoid space* is situated between the arachnoid and the pia mater; cerebrospinal fluid circulates here. The space is not wide over the convexity of the brain, but is quite extensive at the base of the skull where the cisternae are formed. These form a "water bed" of subarachnoid fluid upon which the brain floats. Only the anterior third of the brain rests directly upon bone (the orbital plates of the frontal bone).

4. Involvement of the *intracerebral "space"* is really involvement of brain substance proper. Theoretically, the subpial space is that potential interval that exists between the pia and the brain and is of no practical importance. Attempts to strip the pia mater

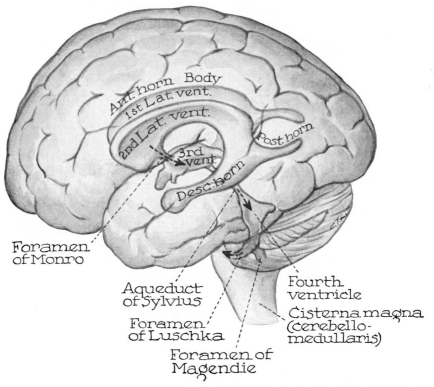

FIG. 24. The ventricular system. The horns and the body of the first and the second lateral ventricles are pictured in relation to the brain.

from the brain are often unsuccessful, since brain tissue comes away with the intimately attached pia. Bleeding into the brain proper may be traumatic in origin or may be the result of spontaneous rupture of an artery in its interior. Since the pia is frequently torn with these hemorrhages, frank blood appears in the cerebrospinal fluid.

VENTRICULAR SYSTEM AND CEREBROSPINAL FLUID

The circulation of the cerebrospinal fluid is associated with (1) the ventricular system and (2) the subarachnoid space. The spinal fluid is formed in the ventricular system and absorbed in the subarachnoid space.

The *ventricular system* (Fig. 24) is com-

posed of four ventricles, two of which are lateral. Normally, these spaces communicate freely with each other through well-defined openings. Each lateral ventricle is situated within a cerebral hemisphere and is sub-divided into an anterior horn (in the frontal lobe), a body (in the parietal lobe), a posterior horn (in the occipital lobe), and a descending horn (in the temporal lobe). Each communicates with the third ventricle by a single opening known as the foramen of Monro. This foramen has a V-shaped arrangement of two limbs, each draining its respective lateral ventricle. It is situated in the anterior horn and is the only means of exit for the lateral ventricles. The 3rd ventricle empties into the 4th by means of the

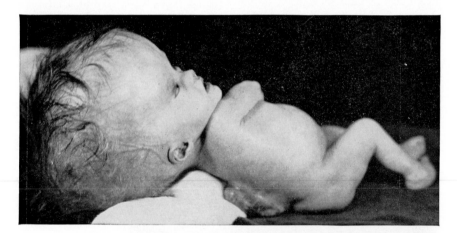

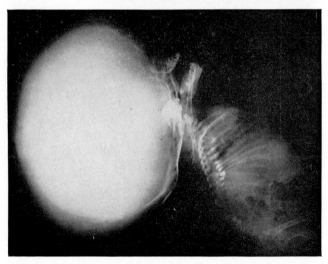

FIG. 25. Photograph and roentgenogram of a hydrocephalic infant. A spina bifida is also present.

aqueduct of Sylvius, which is about ½ inch long and quite narrow, being only slightly larger than the lead of a pencil. This aqueduct, passing through the midbrain, enters the anterior part of the 4th ventricle; it is the only source of exit for the 3rd and both lateral ventricles. Because of its location and its small size, it is the weakest and most important point of the entire ventricular system. The 4th ventricle is situated in the posterior cranial fossa, the cerebellum forming its roof and the pons and the medulla its floor. It connects with the subarachnoid space by three openings: the two lateral foramina of Luschka and a median foramen of Magendie. The two lateral foramina of Luschka open into the cisterna lateralis, and the foramen of Magendie into the cisterna magna (cisterna cerebellomedullaris). In this way the ventricular system becomes connected with the subarachnoid space. The fluid, having gained entrance into this space and the cisternae, circulates freely around the cerebrum and the cerebellum, finally passing down the spinal subarachnoid space. Cerebrospinal fluid is formed by the choroid plexus, mainly in the lateral ventricles; from this point it passes through the foramen of Monro into the 3rd ventricle and finally into the subarachnoid space, where it comes in contact with the arachnoid villi, which absorb it and return it to the venous stream in the dural sinuses.

The total amount of cerebrospinal fluid has been estimated to be between 90 and 150 cc. in adults. If there is a block along the route of the ventricular system, the condition of hydrocephalus results (Fig. 25). If such a block is located at a lateral ventricle entrance into the 3rd ventricle, distention of one ventricle would result; if the block is at the aqueduct of Sylvius, a distention of both

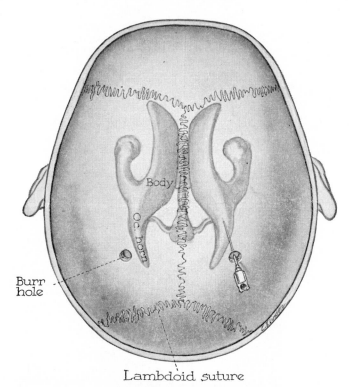

Body

Oc. horn

Burr hole

Lambdoid suture

FIG. 26. Ventriculography. Two small incisions are made 1 inch to each side of the midline and 2 inches above the lambdoid suture. Two burr holes are placed at these points, and the dura is nicked. Then a ventricular needle is introduced into the lateral ventricle at the junction of the body and the occipital horn. Cerebrospinal fluid is replaced with air.

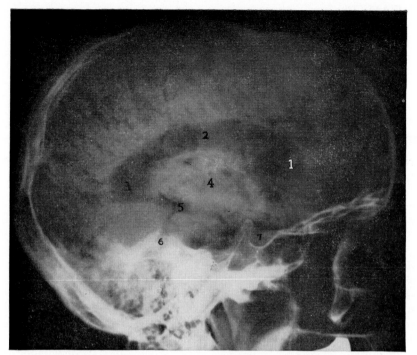

FIG. 27 A. Encephalogram in lateral projection: (1) anterior horn, (2) body of the lateral ventricle, (3) posterior horn, (4) third ventricle, (5) descending horn, (6) fourth ventricle, (7) sella turcica.

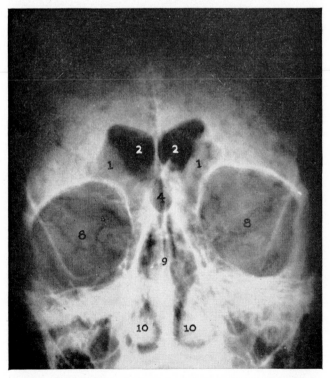

FIG. 27 B. Encephalogram in anteroposterior projection: (1) anterior horn, (2) body of the lateral ventricle, (4) third ventricle, (8) orbit, (9) nasal septum, (10) inferior turbinates.

lateral and the 3rd ventricles would result; if the obstruction is at the openings in the 4th ventricle (Magendie and Luschka), distention of all ventricles will ensue. The type of block may be determined by ventriculography.

SURGICAL CONSIDERATIONS

Two procedures, ventriculography and encephalography, are valuable diagnostic aids, especially in the localization of brain tumors and obstruction of the ventricular system (Figs. 26 and 27).

ENCEPHALOGRAPHY

Encephalography consists of withdrawing cerebrospinal fluid by means of a lumbar puncture needle and introducing air. The air slowly ascends and produces an outline of the ventricular system which can be seen on a roentgenogram. It is important to utilize a manometer during the procedure so that the cerebrospinal pressure is measured. As a rule, from 20 to 25 cc. of air is introduced; the outlines of the ventricles are seen, and any abnormality is noted. Encephalography should not be used when there is an increase in intracranial pressure.

VENTRICULOGRAPHY

Ventriculography (Fig. 26) is a more formidable procedure but is the method of choice. It involves two incisions and two perforations of the skull. The technic consists of making two small incisions in the scalp about 1 inch on either side of the mid-line and about 2 inches above the lambdoid suture. The lips of each incision are retracted, and a small burr hole is made. The dura is exposed, carefully nicked with a small crucial incision, and a ventricular needle is introduced. This is passed downward, forward and inward in such a way that the lateral ventricle is entered in the region of the junction of its body with the occipital horn. Thus, a study of the cerebrospinal fluid

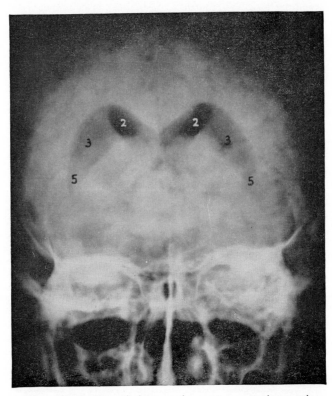

FIG. 27 C. Encephalogram in postero-anterior projection: (2) body of the lateral ventricle, (3) posterior horn, (5) descending horn.

is permitted, as well as temporary relief from intracranial pressure. Fluid is removed and replaced by a somewhat smaller volume of air, the average amount of air injected being from 50 to 120 cc. After this, lateral and anteroposterior roentgenograms are taken (Fig. 27 A and B). The lateral view may show deformity of the anterior or the posterior horns by tumors situated in the frontal or occipital regions. The anteroposterior view may reveal a deflection of the ventricles from the midline or a filling defect of the third ventricle. During this procedure it is best to have the patient in the sitting or semisitting position.

CISTERNAL PUNCTURE

In *cisternal puncture* (Fig. 28) the patient may be in a sitting position or lying on one side with the head placed somewhat forward. The first palpable cervical spinous process is located in the midline, and a point is taken immediately above it. The needle is then inserted in a forward and upward direc-

tion. The upward path parallels an imaginary line that joins the external auditory meatus with the nasion; as the needle advances it strikes the posterior *occipito-atloid* ligament. In the adult this is at a depth of between 4 and 5 cm. Piercing of the ligament by the needle is usually felt, and then the cistern is entered. The medulla is about 1 inch anterior to the posterior occipito-atloid ligament.

ARTERIAL SUPPLY

(Fig. 29.) The arterial supply of blood is furnished to the brain by 4 vessels: 2 vertebral and 2 internal carotid arteries. The *vertebral artery,* a branch of the subclavian, after ascending and perforating the dura, unites with the same vessel of the opposite side to form the *basilar.* This vessel lies in the basilar groove of the pons and at its superior margin divides into 2 terminal branches known as the *posterior cerebral arteries.* The *internal carotid,* after penetrating the dura, reaches the base of the brain

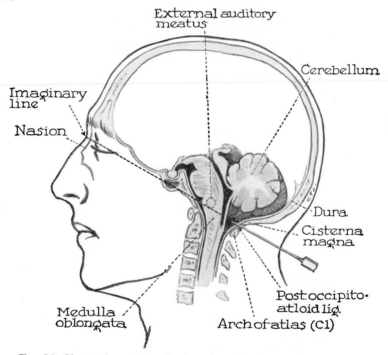

FIG. 28. Cisternal puncture. An imaginary line is constructed between the external auditory meatus and the nasion. The needle enters above the spinous process of the 1st cervical vertebra, parallels this line and enters the cisterna magna. The medulla is about 1 inch anterior to the posterior occipito-atloid ligament.

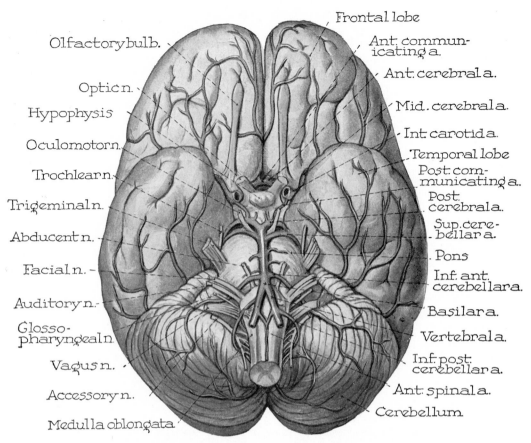

Olfactory bulb.

Optic n.

Hypophysis

Oculomotor n.

Trochlear n.

Trigeminal n.

Abducent n.

Facial n.

Auditory n.

Glosso-
pharyngeal n.

Vagus n.

Accessory n.

Medulla oblongata

Frontal lobe

Ant. commun-
icating a.

Ant. cerebral a.

Mid. cerebral a.

Int. carotid a.

Temporal lobe

Post. com-
municating a.

Post.
cerebral a.

Sup. cere-
bellar a.

Pons

Inf. ant.
cerebellar a.

Basilar a.

Vertebral a.

Inf. post.
cerebellar a.

Ant. spinal a.

Cerebellum

FIG. 29. The arterial supply as seen from the base of the brain, and the formation of the circle of Willis. The cranial nerves are shown in relation to the vessels.

at the angle between the optic nerve and the optic tract, then divides into 2 branches: *anterior* and *middle cerebral arteries*. These are connected by communicating vessels to form the *arterial circle of Willis,* which lies within the interpeduncular subarachnoid cistern. The arterial circle is formed in the following way: anteriorly, the anterior communicating artery joins the 2 anterior cerebral arteries, and the posterior communicating artery connects the internal carotid with the posterior cerebral artery; posteriorly, the basilar artery bifurcates into the two posterior cerebral arteries to complete the circle. The so-called circle is really heptagonal in shape. Two separate sets of branches arise from the cerebral arteries: (1) the *central branches,* which are very numerous and slender, pierce the surface of the brain to supply the internal parts of the

cerebrum, including the basal nuclei, and do not anastomose with one another; (2) the *cortical branches* ramify over the surface of the cerebrum and supply the cortex, anastomose in the pia, and are not sharply cut off from one another. The anterior cerebral artery supplies the superior and the middle frontal convolutions and the entire medial surface of the hemisphere as far back as the parieto-occipital fissure. It also supplies the leg center of the paracentral lobule and the highest point of the precentral convolution. The middle cerebral artery is a direct continuation of the internal carotid; it runs upward and outward to the Sylvian fissure and supplies most of the exposed surface of the hemisphere, the insula and the internal capsule. It also supplies the bulk of the motor area of the brain, the cortical center for hearing, part of the center for vision and the

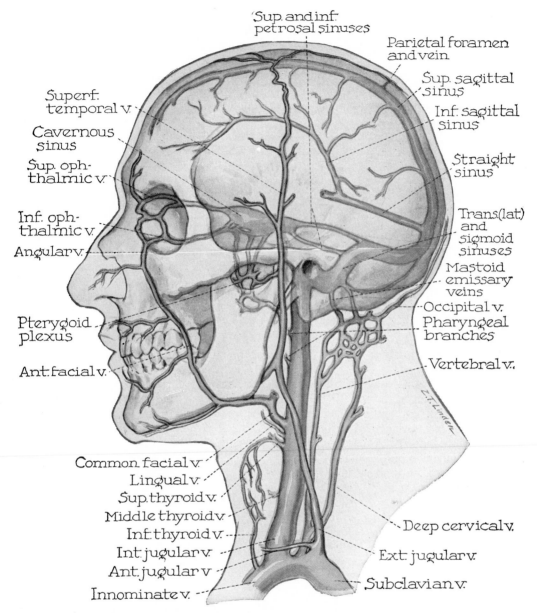

Sup. and inf. petrosal sinuses

Parietal foramen and vein

Sup. sagittal sinus

Inf. sagittal sinus

Straight sinus

Trans.(lat.) and sigmoid sinuses

Mastoid emissary veins

Occipital v.

Pharyngeal branches

Vertebral v.

Superf. temporal v.

Cavernous sinus

Sup. oph-thalmic v.

Inf. oph-thalmic v.

Angular v.

Pterygoid plexus

Ant. facial v.

Common facial v.

Lingual v.

Sup. thyroid v.

Middle thyroid v.

Inf. thyroid v.

Int. jugular v.

Ant. jugular v.

Innominate v.

Deep cervical v.

Ext. jugular v.

Subclavian v.

Fig. 30. Veins of the head and the brain. Three of the emissary veins (parietal, mastoid and ophthalmic) are shown with their intracranial communications. Since the blood flow can travel in either direction, infection may also pass both ways. The angular vein, which drains the upper lip or "dangerous area of the face," is of particular importance because of its communication with the cavernous sinus.

motor speech area of the left hemisphere. It gives off the lenticulostriate artery, which is the vessel most frequently ruptured in cases of cerebral hemorrhage. This vessel has been referred to as the "artery of apoplexy" (Charcot). The posterior cerebral artery supplies the middle and the inferior temporal gyri, the medial part of the occipital lobe and the lower surface of the temporosphenoidal lobe.

VEINS OF THE HEAD AND THE BRAIN

(Fig. 30.) The veins of the head and the brain may be divided as follows: (1) the emissary veins, which connect the veins of the inside of the skull with those of the head, the face and the neck; (2) the diploic veins, which form venous plexuses situated between the inner and the outer tables of the skull; (3) the cerebral and the cerebellar veins, which drain the venous blood of the cerebrum and the cerebellum; (4) the venous dural sinuses, which are placed between the layers of the dura mater.

EMISSARY VEINS

The *emissary veins* connect the intracranial and the extracranial veins. Since blood may flow in either direction, infection may also travel both ways. This double direction of blood flow equalizes the venous pressure in the sinuses and the superficial veins. The more important emissary veins include:

1. The parietal vein, which passes through the parietal foramen at the top of the skull and joins the occipital vein via the superior sagittal sinus. It is of marked surgical importance as the path by which a relatively simple scalp infection may result in a thrombophlebitis or sinus thrombosis involving the superior sagittal sinus.

2. The emissary veins of the foramen caecum connect the beginning of the superior sagittal sinus with the veins of the frontal sinus and the root of the nose. By means of this route infection may travel from either of the latter two structures to the superior sagittal sinus. These veins are seen more constantly in children than in adults.

3. The mastoid is the most constant of the emissary veins; it connects the occipital or posterior auricular vein with the transverse (lateral) sinus. It is of surgical importance because of the frequency with which mastoid disease takes place and may result in infection of the transverse (lateral) sinus.

4. The ophthalmic veins are considered as emissary veins which drain into the cavernous sinus. Blood can flow in the reverse direction in these vessels and pass to the face and infratemporal fossa.

It is in connection with these emissary veins that the *anterior facial vein* becomes of utmost importance, the latter communicating with the cavernous sinus through the ophthalmic veins. The anterior and the posterior facial veins join in the neck to form the common facial vein, which pierces the deep fascia and ends in the internal jugular; at times it may cross the sternocleidomastoid muscle and end in the external jugular vein. That part of the anterior facial vein which passes along the side or angle of the nose has been called the *angular vein*. It is important because it drains the so-called "dangerous area of the face." Boils and carbuncles commonly occur in this region and should such lesions be opened, death may result from involvement of the cavernous sinus; the internal jugular vein may also become infected in such cases. Since these veins have no valves, infected thrombi become detached as a result of the constant motion brought about by talking and masticating, causing a spread of the infection into the interior of the skull.

There are other emissary veins that are of less practical importance, namely, the veins of the hypoglossal canal, the condyloid canal, the foramen ovale, the foramen lacerum, the foramen of Vesalius and the emissary veins accompanying the middle meningeal artery.

DIPLOIC VEINS

The *diploic veins* (Fig. 31) form venous plexuses between the inner and the outer tables of the skull. In the skull of the child the bone consists of a single layer in which numerous veins grow and communicate with each other. Marrow is found around these branching and communicating vessels, and this ingrowth results in the formation of an outer table of skull, an inner table and the diploë situated between them. The veins form a plexus that is drained by four diploic venous trunks on each side: the *frontal* diploic vein drains into the supra-orbital vein; the *anterior parietal* (*temporal*) drains into the sphenoparietal sinus; the *posterior parietal* (*temporal*) drains into the lateral sinus; the *occipital* also drains into the lateral sinus. Diploic markings may be confused with fractures on a roentgenogram of the skull (Fig. 32). In the parietal region the so-called "parietal spider" is seen, a spiderlike arrangement of these veins. There are no diploic arteries, since the arterial blood supply comes by way of the meningeal and the pericranial arteries.

Cerebral and Cerebellar Veins

The *cerebral* and the *cerebellar veins* (Fig. 33) are veins of the brain proper. They do not accompany the arteries; they have no valves, no muscle tissue around them, and their walls are extremely thin. They are lodged for the greater part in the grooves on the surface of the brain and are covered by arachnoid. The superior veins run upward toward the superior sagittal sinus, turn forward and run parallel with the sinus for a short distance before entering it. The cerebral veins are divided into external and internal groups, depending upon whether they drain the outer surface or the inner part of the hemisphere. The external veins are named the middle, the superior and the inferior cerebral veins. The internal veins draining the deeper parts of the hemisphere are the terminal ones and the great cerebral *vein of Galen* (Fig. 22).

Venous Dural Sinuses

Venous sinuses of the dura mater (Figs. 22, 23, 30, 34) are spaces between the 2 layers of dura mater which collect blood and return it to the internal jugular vein. Into these spaces spinal fluid is also drained from the subarachnoid space through the arachnoid villi and granulations. Sinuses differ from other venous structures in the body in that their walls consist of a single layer of endothelium, as a result of which there is no tendency for them to collapse. Seven of these sinuses are paired, and 5 are unpaired. The unpaired sinuses are the superior sagittal,

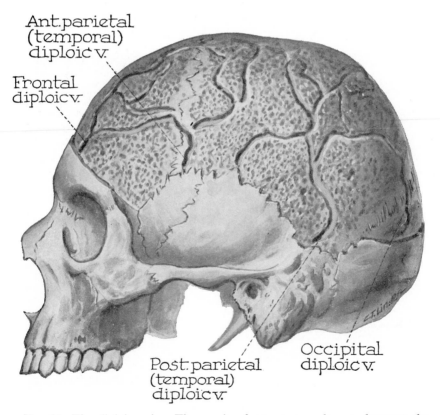

Ant. parietal (temporal) diploic v.

Frontal diploic v.

Post. parietal (temporal) diploic v.

Occipital diploic v.

Fig. 31. The diploic veins. These veins form venous plexuses between the outer and the inner tables of the skull. Four diploic venous trunks drain these plexuses. The outer table of compact bone has been removed to demonstrate the veins.

inferior sagittal, straight, intercavernous and basilar. The paired sinuses are the spheno-parietal, cavernous, superior petrosal, inferior petrosal, occipital, transverse and sigmoid. Only those that are of practical and surgical importance will be considered.

The *superior sagittal (longitudinal) sinus* is in a somewhat exposed position along the insertion of the falx cerebri. It begins in front of the crista galli at the foramen caecum, where it occasionally communicates with the veins of the nasal mucous membrane. It then passes upward and backward in the upper border of the falx cerebri until it reaches the internal occipital protuberance, where it lies a little to one side of the median plane, usually on the right. Here it forms a dilatation known as the *confluence of sinuses* (torcular Herophili), at which point the superior sagittal, the transverse, the occipital and the straight sinuses all meet. Here the superior sagittal bends acutely to the right, occasionally to the left, and becomes

continuous with the transverse sinus. Lateral expansions of the sinus (*lacunae lateralis*) are found on each side. These lacunae receive meningeal and diploic veins, and the superior sagittal sinus receives emissary veins, diploic veins and those veins which drain the cerebral hemispheres. As the superior sagittal sinus runs posteriorly, it grooves the internal aspect of the skull, and its surface marking may be indicated by a line drawn over the median line of the vertex from the root of the nose to the external occipital protuberance.

The *inferior sagittal sinus* passes backward in the lower border of the falx cerebri. It unites with the great cerebral vein at the free margin of the tentorium cerebelli to form the straight sinus.

The *straight sinus* travels backward along the attachment of the falx cerebri to the tentorium. At the internal occipital protuberance it bends acutely to the left, occasionally to the right, to form the tranverse sinus. It

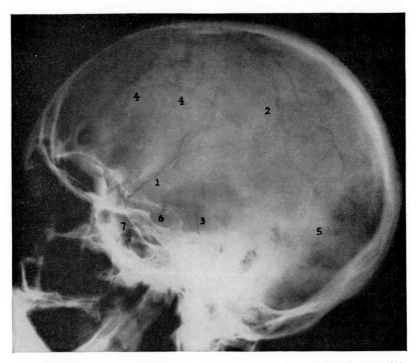

FIG. 32. Lateral roentgenogram of the skull, demonstrating the arterial channels, the diploic veins and a fracture line: (1) middle meningeal groove, (2) plexus of diploic veins, (3) fracture line over the squamous portion of the temporal bone, (4) coronary suture, (5) lambdoid suture, (6) sella turcica, (7) sphenoid sinus.

receives tributaries from the posterior part of the cerebrum, the cerebellum and the falx cerebri.

The *transverse (lateral) sinus*, which is a paired structure, begins at the internal occipital protuberance. The right is usually continuous with the superior sagittal sinus and the left with the straight sinus. It receives the superior petrosal sinus and a few inferior cerebral and cerebellar veins. It is bounded by the 2 layers of tentorium and the outer layer of dura mater and runs hori-zontally at first in a lateral direction and then forward. It lies in the transverse groove of the skull and in the attached margin of the tentorium.

The *sigmoid sinus* is a continuation of the transverse sinus and receives its name from the S-shaped curves which it makes. Some authors believe the term "transverse" should be restricted to that part of the sinus that passes between the internal occipital protuberance and the posterior inferior angle of the parietal bone. The remaining part of the

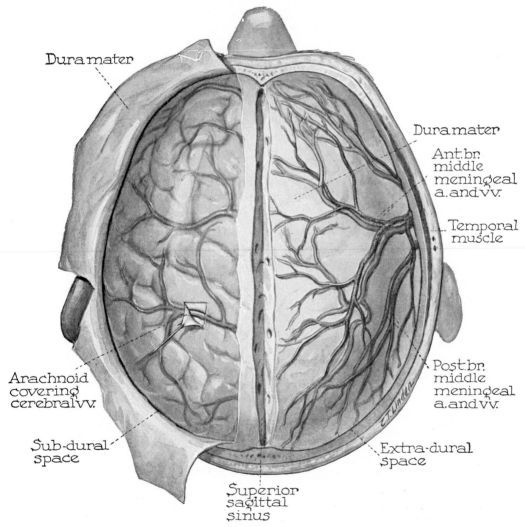

FIG. 33. The cerebral veins, viewed from above. The superior sagittal sinus has been opened, and the dura mater has been reflected on the left side, exposing the subdural space. The intact dura on the right side reveals the relationship of the extradural space and the middle meningeal vessels. A small flap of arachnoid has been reflected to show the position of the cerebral veins.

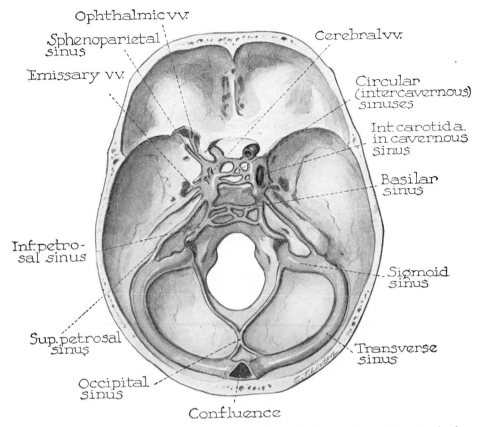

Ophthalmic vv.

Sphenoparietal sinus

Emissary vv.

Cerebral vv.

Circular (intercavernous) sinuses

Int. carotid a. in cavernous sinus

Basilar sinus

Inf. petro-sal sinus

Sigmoid sinus

Sup. petrosal sinus

Transverse sinus

Occipital sinus

Confluence

FIG. 34. Venous sinuses at the base of the skull. The right internal carotid artery is shown surrounded by the cavernous sinus.

sinus (to the jungular foramen) is known as the sigmoid sinus, which curves downward, leaves the tentorium, passes between the two layers of dura and ends at the jugular foramen, where it becomes the internal jugular vein. The continuation of the sinus as the internal jugular explains the propagation of a transverse sinus thrombosis. This justifies the ligation of the internal jugular to prevent the spread of septic emboli to the heart. The superior petrosal sinus joins it at its first bend, and the inferior petrosal at its termination. It forms an important posterior relation of the tympanic antrum. In suppurative conditions of the tympanic antrum or cavity this sinus may become the site of a septic process that travels through the cerebellar tributaries and forms a cerebellar abscess. It is separated from the mastoid cells by only a very thin plate of bone; hence, diseases from the middle ear into the mastoid

cells can form a suppurative process that involves the sinus (sinus thrombosis). Its communications are numerous and important; it is connected by the mastoid emissary vein with the occipital vein, by the occipital sinus with the transverse sinus and by the posterior condylar emissary vein with the suboccipital plexus.

The *cavernous sinus* is situated to either side of the body of the sphenoid bone and is continuous with the ophthalmic veins in front. Posteriorly, it divides into the superior and the inferior petrosal sinuses. It surrounds the internal carotid artery. Injury in this area may result in the formation of an arteriovenous aneurysm which produces stasis in the superior ophthalmic vein. This may bring about a pulsating exophthalmos due to pulsations of the cartoid artery transmitted to the engorged venous spaces. Cavernous sinus thrombosis may follow inflammatory lesions of the face and the upper lip, the extension taking place through the facial, the nasal and the ophthalmic veins. This sinus is intimately related to the gasserian ganglion and may be injured during operations on the latter. Infections involving the cavernous sinus are frequently accompanied by basilar meningitis.

The *circular sinus* consists of the two transverse venous connections between the cavernous sinuses. The *sphenoparietal sinus* runs along the lesser wing of the sphenoid to the superior sagittal sinus. The *occipital sinus* is extremely variable in size and lies in the attached border of the falx cerebelli. The *basilar sinus* is a wide trabeculated space behind the dorsum sellae which unites the cavernous and the inferior petrosal sinuses of opposite sides. It also communicates below with the spinal veins.

HYPOPHYSIS

EMBRYOLOGY

(Fig. 35.) The hypophysis or, in older terminology, the pituitary body developmentally consists of two different parts: a buccal or glandular portion which is derived from the roof of the mouth and lies anteriorly; and a nervous portion derived from the brain. The anterior part is an upgrowth (Rathke's pouch) from the roof of the primitive pharynx (stomodeum). Normally, the stalk that connects the anterior lobe to the roof of the mouth disappears completely because of the rapid growth of the body of the sphenoid bone, but occasionally this stalk may persist as the craniopharyngeal canal. At the site of Rathke's pouch or along the persisting craniopharyngeal canal, cysts may develop that are lined with squamous epithelium (craniopharyngeomas). After the anterior lobe has become isolated, a rapid proliferation of its cells takes place which displaces the gland. The posterior lobe is of nervous origin and is derived from the brain. It grows in a downward direction from the floor of the third ventricle and forms the infundibulum.

ADULT HYPOPHYSIS

The adult gland measures 13x8 mm. and can be likened to an apple: the stem is the infundibulum that connects it to the brain, and the skin is the dura mater that ensheaths it. The *anterior lobe* consists of a pars anterior and a pars intermedia, which are separated from each other by a narrow groove, a remnant of the diverticulum from which this lobe developed. The anterior lobe is the larger of the two and grows backward around each side of the posterior; it is hollowed out posteriorly to accommodate that lobe and, therefore, assumes a kidney shape. It is very vascular, blood vessels reaching it along the infundibulum from the arterial circle.

The *pars intermedia*, the middle part, contains a few blood vessels, small masses of colloid material, and some finely granulated cells.

The *posterior lobe*, arising as a downgrowth from the brain, contains no nerve cells but has numerous neuroglial cells and fibers and small collections of colloid material. Pituitrin is secreted in this lobe, but the secretion of the anterior lobe is concerned with growth and the production of prolans, which are intimately related to the other endocrine glands.

The hypophysis lies in the sella turcica within duplications of the dura, which forms an osteofibrous compartment. The deep layer of dura dips into the sella; laterally, it meets the superficial leaf, which passes over the gland to form the diaphragm. The lateral walls of the fossa form the medial walls of the cavernous sinuses. The superficial layer of dura, forming the diaphragma sellae, produces a roof for the gland; the roof contains a central aperture; and through it the infundibulum connects the posterior lobe to the tuber cinereum. The 2 anterior and the 2 posterior clinoid processes surround the gland as a 4-poster bedstead in which the pituitary body rests.

Four venous sinuses form a square that encloses the gland: the cavernous on each side and the anterior and the posterior intercavernous sinuses in front and behind. In the outer wall of the cavernous sinus lie the 3rd, the 4th, the ophthalmic branch of the 5th, and the 6th cranial nerves. The internal carotid artery is situated beneath and within the meshes of the sinus. Anteroinferiorly, the gland is related to the sphenoid sinus. When

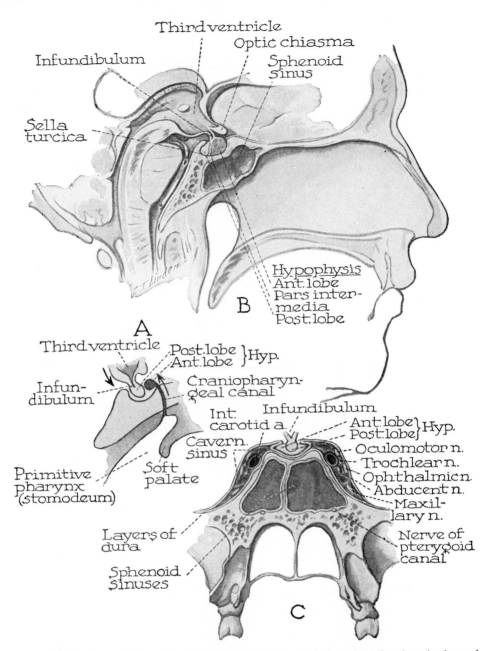

FIG. 35. The hypophysis: (A) embryogenesis; (B) sagittal section showing the hypophysis in the sella turcica and its relations to the optic chiasma; (C) frontal section through the hypophysis and the cavernous sinus, showing the normal relations between these and 4 of the cranial nerves.

FIG. 36. Two approaches to the hypophysis. (A) The intracranial approach: an osteoplastic flap is formed through a frontoparietal approach. The dura is incised, the cortex protected, and the frontal lobe gently elevated. The tumor and the optic nerves are exposed. (B) The transphenoidal operation: an incision is made between the upper lip and the gum. The mucoperiosteum is separated from each side of the septum, and the latter is removed. The anterior wall of the sphenoid sinus is nibbled away until the floor of the sella turcica is encountered. The latter is removed, the dura is exposed, and the hypophysis, with its pathology, is identified.

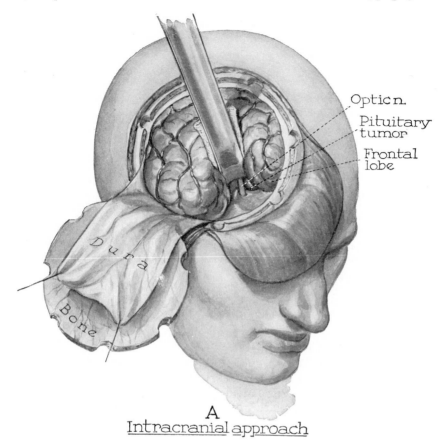

Optic n.

Pituitary
tumor

Frontal
lobe

Dura

Bone

A
Intracranial approach

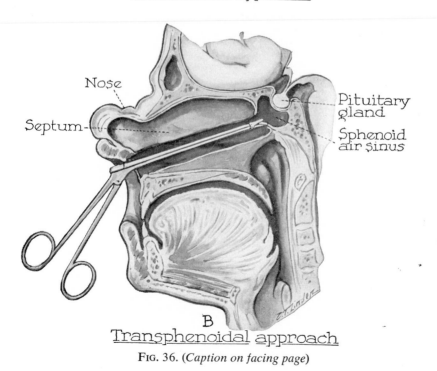

Nose

Septum

Pituitary
gland

Sphenoid
air sinus

B
Transphenoidal approach

FIG. 36. (*Caption on facing page*)

the sinus is large, only a thin plate of bone separates it from the gland; hence, the larger the sinus the more extensive is its relation to the hypophysis.

The optic chiasma lies superior to the hypophysis and, therefore, is related to the infundibulum rather than the gland proper. As the infundibulum passes upward posterior to the chiasma, it is in contact with its posterior edge and undersurface. The chiasma is nowhere in direct contact with the bone.

SURGICAL CONSIDERATIONS

Two main routes are utilized to expose the hypophysis: an intracranial and a nasal (Fig. 36). Most authorities believe that the nasal route is impractical since the exposure of the gland is poor and the danger of infection is increased.

Intracranial and Transphenoidal Operations. The *intracranial approach* takes the transfrontal route or one of its modifications. A more lateral approach in which an osteoplastic flap is utilized (Fig. 36 A) is described by Heuer. This begins 3 cm. behind the external angle of the orbit, is carried just within the hair line to about 1 inch from the longitudinal sinus, where it turns backward and then curves downward posteriorly to the parietal eminence to a point 4 cm. behind the helix. In reality this is a frontoparietal approach that combines both frontal and lateral routes. The dura is incised, the cortex protected, and the frontal lobe gently elevated, exposing the optic nerve or the optic commissure and the hypophysis. Some authors describe an extradural approach, but this is not as useful, since certain tumors may be missed because of the lack of exposure and because the region posterior to the optic nerve and the internal carotid artery cannot be seen properly.

In a *transphenoidal operation* (Fig. 36 B) an incision is made in the mucous membrane between the upper lip and the gum. The anterior edge of the nasal septum is exposed, the mucoperiosteum is separated from each side of the septum, and the latter is removed. The anterior wall of the sphenoid sinus is encountered and nibbled away until the bulging floor of the sella turcica is exposed. When this has been removed, the dura is incised, and the pituitary gland with its pathology is revealed and treated.

Cranial Nerves

The cranial nerves are 12 pairs of symmetrically arranged nerve trunks that are attached to the base of the brain. They leave the skull via various foramina at its base and are distributed for the greater part to the head. Some of these nerves may be described as traveling in a direction away from the brain; some of them convey impulses in a reverse direction. On leaving the brain each cranial nerve is invested by a sheath of pia mater, traverses the subarachnoid space, pierces the arachnoid and receives an additional sheath from the latter-mentioned membrane. It next enters a canal in the dura mater; this leads to the foramen in the skull through which the nerve leaves the cranium. It is invested by a sheath of dura which is continuous with the epineurium covering the nerve trunk proper. The dural aperture and the foramen do not necessarily correspond to each other in location since some of the nerves (the 4th and the 6th) run an intra-

dural course of some length before they leave their foramina. These nerves are not only numerically designated from before backward but are also distinguished by their specific names, which are based on their distributions or functions.

1. **Olfactory Nerves** (Fig. 37). These nerves, about 15 to 20 in number, arise from the upper third of the nasal mucous membrane, pass through the cribriform plate of the ethmoid bone and enter the substance of the olfactory bulb, which lies in contact with the orbital surface of the frontal lobe of the brain. The olfactory tract runs backward from the bulb and ends in the corpus callosum. The lateral branch of the tract terminates in the uncus, and the medial branch ends in the subcallosal gyrus. Some medial olfactory striae course through the olfactory portion of the anterior commissure to the opposite olfactory bulb. Lesions that affect the uncinate area of the

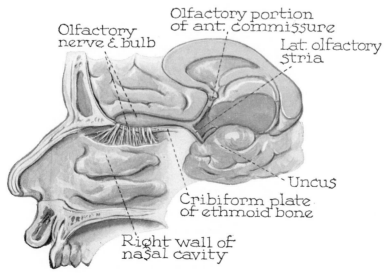

FIG. 37. The olfactory nerve.

temporal lobe may start with unpleasant olfactory prodromes, which are followed by a dreamy state; such attacks have been called uncinate gyrus fits.

2. **Optic Nerve** (Fig. 38). This nerve extends from the posterior aspect of the eyeball to the optic chiasma. In its course it passes through the optic foramen, accompanied by the ophthalmic artery, which lies to its outer and lower side. After gaining entrance to the cranium it converges toward the nerve of the opposite side, which it joins to form the *optic chiasma*. In the optic chiasma those fibers that arise from the nasal side of the retina decussate with the corresponding fibers of the opposite side, but the fibers arising from the temporal side of the retina do not.

The *optic tracts* arise on each posterolateral angle of the chiasma and are continuations of the optic nerves. Each tract consists of fibers arising in the temporal half of the retina of the same side and the nasal half of the retina of the opposite side. These tracts divide into lateral and medial roots; the lateral end in the gray matter of the lateral geniculate body and the superior corpus quadrigeminum. The medial root ends in the medial geniculate body and has no connections with vision. From the lateral geniculate body new fibers arise and enter the internal capsule; here they assume the name of optic radiations and pass backward and terminate in the *higher visual centers* in the visual cortex (postcalcarine and calcarine sulci). As the optic nerve passes from the brain, it receives its perineural sheath from the pia mater, an outer covering from the dura and an inner covering from the arachnoid. These sheaths remain separated, and the two enclosed spaces may be involved separately. Increased pressure from the subarachnoid space in the cranial cavity is transmitted to the subarachnoid space around the optic nerve; the central vein and artery become compressed, resulting in an engorgement of the retinal veins and a diminution of the artery. This condition is known as papilledema.

3. **Oculomotor Nerve** (Figs. 39, 41). This nerve travels from the cavernous sinus to the orbit. After reaching the orbit through the lower part of the superior orbital fissure, it immediately divides into superior and inferior divisions. The superior division supplies the superior rectus and the levator palpebrae superioris muscles; the inferior supplies the inferior oblique and the medial and inferior recti. From the inferior division a short nerve passes to the ciliary ganglion,

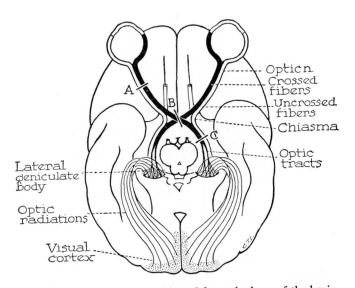

FIG. 38. The optic nerves, viewed from the base of the brain. A lesion at A would involve the nerve and result in blindness; at B the chiasma would be involved, resulting in bitemporal hemianopsia; at C, injury to the optic tract would produce a homonymous hemianopsia.

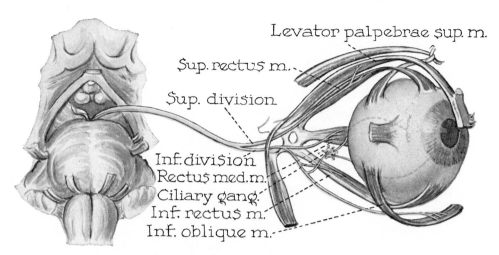

FIG. 39. The oculomotor nerve (diagrammatic).

the ciliary muscle and the sphincter pupillae. The oculomotor nerve supplies all the extrinsic muscles of the eye with the exception of the external rectus and the superior oblique. A lesion of the 3rd nerve results in ptosis of the upper lid (paralysis of the levator palpebrae superioris); dilated pupil (the sympathetic fibers are unopposed); loss of accommodation (paralysis of the ciliary muscle) and external strabismus (unopposed action of the external rectus and the superior oblique muscles).

4. **Trochlear Nerve** (Fig. 40). This is the smallest of the cranial nerves. It lies a little below and lateral to the oculomotor nerve and supplies the superior oblique muscle. Its course is almost the same as that of the 3rd nerve. At the superior orbital fissure it lies above the muscles. The trochlear nerve is rarely involved alone; but when this does occur, the patient experiences difficulty in moving the eye in an outward and downward direction. It has been stated that this nerve supplies the "down and out" muscle, since the action of the superior oblique is to rotate the eye outward and downward. This is an excellent test for the 4th nerve since the patient, in attempting to look downward and outward, will see double.

5. **Trigeminal Nerve** (Figs. 41, 42). This is the thickest of the cranial nerves and has a wide distribution. It has a large sensory root upon which the semilunar (gasserian) ganglion is situated, the ganglion resting in a fossa on the superior surface of the petrous

bone near its apex. The three main divisions of the nerve—ophthalmic, maxillary and mandibular—arise from this ganglion. The motor root lies inferolateral to the sensory root and does not enter the ganglion. Both roots arise from the lateral part of the inferior surface of the pons. The 5th nerve resembles a spinal nerve in that it has two roots—a sensory and a motor—with a gan-

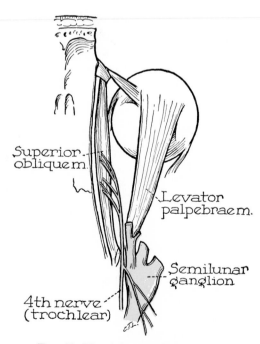

FIG. 40. The right trochlear nerve, seen from above. Its fibers enter the superior oblique muscle.

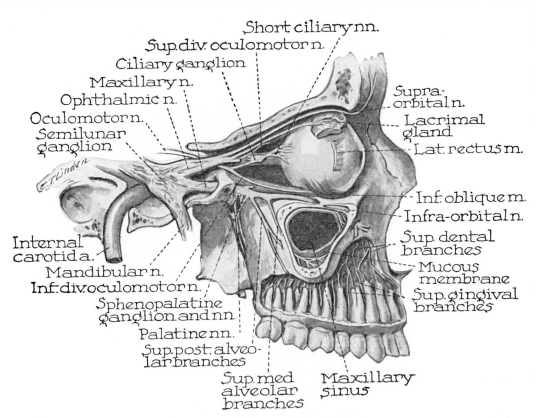

Short ciliary nn.
Sup. div. oculomotor n.
Ciliary ganglion
Maxillary n.
Ophthalmic n.
Oculomotor n.
Semilunar ganglion
Internal carotid a.
Mandibular n.
Inf. div. oculomotor n.
Sphenopalatine ganglion and nn.
Palatine nn.
Sup. post. alveolar branches
Sup. med. alveolar branches
Supra-orbital n.
Lacrimal gland
Lat. rectus m.
Inf. oblique m.
Infra-orbital n.
Sup. dental branches
Mucous membrane
Sup. gingival branches
Maxillary sinus

FIG. 41. The trigeminal nerve and the semilunar (gasserian) ganglion. The lateral wall of the orbit has been removed, and the maxillary sinus has been opened.

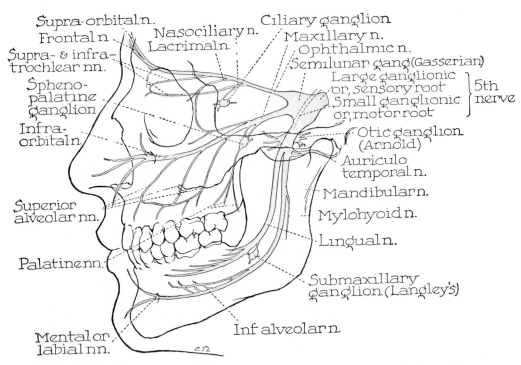

Supra-orbital n.
Frontal n.
Supra- & infra-trochlear nn.
Spheno-palatine ganglion
Infra-orbital n.
Nasociliary n.
Lacrimal n.
Ciliary ganglion
Maxillary n.
Ophthalmic n.
Semilunar gang. (Gasserian)
Large ganglionic or, sensory root
Small ganglionic or, motor root
} 5th nerve
Otic ganglion (Arnold)
Auriculo temporal n.
Mandibular n.
Mylohyoid n.
Lingual n.
Superior alveolar nn.
Palatine nn.
Submaxillary ganglion (Langley's)
Mental or labial nn.
Inf. alveolar n.

FIG. 42. Diagram of the trigeminal nerve and the semilunar (gasserian) ganglion.

glion on the sensory. The nerve provides the sensory supply to the face and the anterior half of the scalp and sends motor branches to the four muscles of mastication (except the buccinator) and to four other muscles: tensor palati, tensor tympani, mylohyoid and anterior belly of the digastric. There are five ganglia on the 5th nerve: the semilunar on the nerve trunk, the ciliary on the ophthalmic division, the sphenopalatine on the maxillary division, the otic on the mandibular division, and the submaxillary (Langley's) also on the mandibular division. All these ganglia, with the exception of the semilunar, receive motor, sensory and sympathetic fibers.

The *semilunar (gasserian) ganglion*, the sensory ganglion of the 5th nerve, occupies a space between the outer and the inner layers of dura known as the *cave of Meckel* (cavum trigeminale), which is in reality a diverticulum of the inner layer of dura. There are two layers of dura above and two layers below the ganglion, the two layers being fused. The foramen which transmits the middle meningeal artery is on the outer side of the ganglion and must be encountered before the ganglion is reached by the temporal route. The cavernous sinus and the internal carotid artery are found medially. The motor root makes no connections with the ganglion but passes through the foramen ovale and on the outside of the skull joins the mandibular division. Posterior to the cave the superior petrosal sinus is located as it widens to join the cavernous sinus. The sphenoparietal sinus is found anteriorly as it joins the cavernous sinus. Because of these relationships, the ganglion should be approached through the middle region of the outer aspect of the cave.

The ophthalmic is the smallest division of the 5th nerve. After giving off a small twig to the dura mater, it passes forward in the lateral wall of the cavernous sinus and enters the orbit through the superior orbital fissure. In the fissure it splits into three branches: frontal, nasociliary and lacrimal. The lacrimal and the frontal branches enter the orbit above the muscles; the nasociliary passes between the two heads of the lateral rectus.

The *lacrimal nerve* travels along the lateral part of the orbit and supplies the lacrimal gland, the conjunctiva and the skin of the upper eyelid.

The *frontal nerve* divides into supra-orbital and supratrochlear nerves that lie beneath the roof of the orbit. The supra-orbital nerve reaches the scalp after passing through the supra-orbital notch (foramen) and then divides into medial and lateral branches that supply the scalp. The supratrochlear nerve runs above the pulley of the superior oblique muscle. The frontal nerve supplies the mucous membrane of the frontal sinus, the skin of the upper eyelid, the scalp and the forehead.

The *nasociliary nerve* leaves the orbit by the anterior ethmoidal foramen and then changes its name to the anterior ethmoidal nerve. It passes over the cribriform plate of the ethmoid bone and enters the nose through the nasal slit. In the nose it gives off a medial branch to the nasal septum and a lateral branch which reaches the face after passing between the nasal bone and the upper cartilage. This nerve supplies the skin on the lower part of the nose. The branches of the nasal nerve in the orbit are the twigs to the ciliary ganglion, the ciliary nerves to the eyeball and the infratrochlear nerve.

The *ciliary ganglion* is a small reddish body, situated between the lateral rectus and the optic nerve; it receives a sensory root from the nasociliary branch of the ophthalmic, a motor root from the lower division of the oculomotor, and a sympathetic nerve from the plexus around the internal carotid artery. It gives off from 12 to 14 short ciliary nerves which supply the muscles and the iris.

The *maxillary division* of the trigeminal nerve resembles the ophthalmic in that it is purely sensory. It leaves the middle cranial fossa through the foramen rotundum and reaches the pterygopalatine fossa. After crossing the fossa the nerve leaves by way of the inferior orbital fissure to occupy the inferior orbital groove and canal. It appears on the face at the infra-orbital foramen as the infra-orbital nerve; here it divides into the following terminal branches: a small meningeal branch to the dura mater; two ganglionic branches to the sphenopalatine ganglion; zygomatic branches to the orbit through the inferior orbital fissure, which divides into the zygomaticotemporal and zygomaticofacial; posterior superior alveolar to the molar teeth; infra-orbital, which supply the three molars, the canine and the incisors; and facial, which supply the lower eyelids (palpebral), the side of the nose (nasal) and the upper lip (labial).

The *sphenopalatine ganglion* (Meckel) is associated with the maxillary division of the 5th nerve. The sensory roots of the ganglion arise from the maxillary division of the trigeminal nerve, and the motor and the sympathetic fibers from the nerve of the pterygoid canal (Vidian). The branches of the ganglion are orbital (secretomotor fibers to the lacrimal gland), pharyngeal, nasal and palatine.

The *mandibular nerve* is the largest division of the trigeminal. It consists of a sensory portion derived from the trigeminal ganglion, and a motor root. These two portions pass separately through the foramen ovale but rejoin immediately to form a common trunk. After giving off a meningeal branch, the nervous spinosus, which enters the cranium through the foramen spinosum, the trunk furnishes a twig to the medial pterygoid and divides into anterior and posterior divisions. The anterior division consists mainly of motor fibers and divides into deep temporal nerves, the nerves to the masseter, the lateral pterygoid nerves and the buccal nerve. The posterior division gives off the two roots of the auriculotemporal and divides into the lingual and the inferior alveolar nerves. The only motor fibers in this division are those that form the mylohyoid branch of the inferior alveolar. The anterior division has been referred to as the lingual division, and the posterior has often been called the inferior dental. As both of these divisions run downward they are concealed by the external pterygoid muscle and the ramus of the mandible and are distributed to the tongue, the gums, the lower teeth and the muscles of mastication.

The *lingual nerve* travels forward to the anterior two thirds of the tongue, to which it is distributed.

The *inferior alveolar nerve*, larger than the lingual, enters the mandibular canal through the mandibular foramen, passes through the ramus and the body of the mandible and distributes its branches to the lower teeth. Two ganglia—the otic and the submaxillary—are associated with the mandibular division of the 5th nerve. The otic is very small and difficult to find; it lies immediately below the foramen ovale in front of the middle meningeal artery and sends muscular branches to the tensor tympani and the tensor palati. The submaxillary (Langley's) ganglion is also associated with the mandibular division, lying on the outer surface of the hyoglossus muscle and joining the lingual nerve. Although the 5th nerve is mainly sensory, it may be tested by utilizing its motor branches to the masseter muscle. When the nerve is involved the masseter will not protrude on the affected side if the patient clenches his teeth.

6. **Abducens Nerve** (Fig. 43). The 6th cranial nerve supplies only one muscle, the lateral rectus, and resembles the 4th nerve in that it is very slender. It originates at the base of the pons and emerges from its lower border. Soon after its origin it crosses either superficial or deep to the antero-inferior cerebellar artery. This is an important relation,

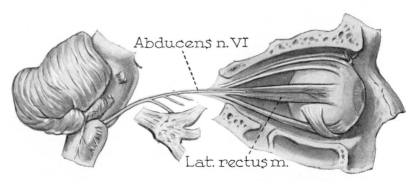

Fig. 43. The right abducent nerve (diagrammatic).

because a hardened and arteriosclerotic artery in this region may press upon the nerve, causing its paralysis. The nerve passes almost vertically up the back of the petrous portion of the temporal bone, where it may be involved in fractures of the base of the skull; it then takes a sharp bend, enters the cavernous sinus and, after leaving the sinus, passes through the superior orbital fissure into the orbit with the 3rd and the 4th nerves. Involvement of the 6th nerve paralyzes the lateral rectus muscle of the same side. This means that the now unopposed medial rectus can displace the eyeball inward, resulting in an internal strabismus. This nerve may also be involved in cases of increased intracranial pressure.

7. **Facial Nerve** (Fig. 44). This nerve is seen when the cerebellum is removed. It is the motor nerve to the face and contains no cutaneous branches. Leaving the brain at the lower border of the pons and accompanying the auditory 8th nerve into the internal auditory meatus, it passes through the temporal bone and leaves the skull through the stylomastoid foramen.

In the temporal bone it gives off the *great superficial petrosal nerve*, which sends sensory fibers to the mucous membrane of the soft palate and secretory fibers to the mucous glands; the *nerve to the stapedius muscle;* and the *chorda tympani*, which passes through the tympanic cavity, joins the lingual nerve and thus supplies taste and sensation fibers to the anterior two thirds of the tongue and secretory fibers to the submaxillary and sublingual glands.

At the exit from the stylomastoid foramen the facial nerve gives off the posterior auricular nerve and a branch which divides into two twigs supplying the stylohyoid muscle and the posterior belly of the digastric.

The *posterior auricular nerve* ascends behind the ear and supplies the posterior and the superior auricular muscles and the occipital belly of the occipitofrontalis. Having given off its branches in the temporal bone and at the exit from the stylomastoid foramen, the facial nerve supplies its terminal branches to the face. Here it divides into two main divisions: a temporofacial and a cervicofacial. A controversy exists at present as to whether the facial nerve runs through the parotid gland or whether it passes around the isthmus of the gland, thus being "sandwiched" between the so-called superficial and deep lobes of the gland. In my experience at both the dissecting and the operating tables,

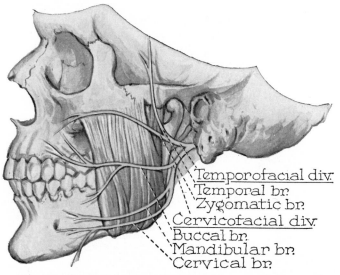

FIG. 44. The facial nerve. It divides into two divisions: the temporofacial and the cervicofacial. These give rise to the 5 terminal branches which form the pes anserinus (goose's foot). Its relations to the parotid gland are seen in Figures 87 and 88.

I usually have found that the nerve passes through the gland. This is considered more fully on page 120 where the parotid gland is discussed.

The two divisions break up into a nerve plexus which has been called the *pes anserinus* (goose's foot). These terminal nerves forming the plexus emerge at the anterior border of the parotid gland and radiate over the side of the face in a fanlike manner (Figs. 87 and 88). The temporofacial division gives rise to 2 terminal branches: *temporal* and *zygomatic*. A temporal branch appears at the upper border of the gland and supplies the frontalis muscle and the facial muscles which are situated above the zygoma. The zygomatic branches are divided into a smaller upper branch, which passes forward from the upper anterior border of the parotid to the zygomatic bone and supplies the adjoining facial muscle, and a lower zygomatic branch, which appears at the anterior border of the gland and runs with the transverse facial vessels to the muscles of the upper lip and the nose.

The cervicofacial division gives rise to the *buccal,* the *mandibular* and the *cervical branches*. The buccal branch appears at the anterior border of the gland and supplies the buccinator and the orbicularis oris muscles. The mandibular branch supplies the lower lip and the chin. The cervical branch appears at the lower border of the gland and supplies the platysma and the depressors of the lower lip. Intracranial lesions of the facial nerve are characterized by involvement of only the lower half of the face; cra-

nial lesions may result from middle-ear diseases or fractures of the face or the skull. Extracranial lesions result in facial paralysis, as seen in Bell's palsy, in which condition the involved side of the face is flat and expressionless; the patient is unable to whistle, blow out his cheeks, wrinkle his forehead or show his teeth. In its course the facial nerve makes connections with the auriculotemporal and the great auricular nerves.

8. **Auditory (Acoustic) Nerve** (Fig. 45). The 8th nerve consists of two parts: the cochlear, which carries auditory impulses, and the vestibular, which has to do with equilibrium. At the lower border of the pons the roots are combined into a single trunk which leaves the posterior cranial fossa by way of the internal auditory meatus, where it divides into an upper part with only vestibular fibers. The cochlear nerve is distributed to the cochlear duct and the spiral organ; the vestibular fibers are distributed to the semicircular ducts, the utricle and the saccule. Lesions of the 8th nerve may produce complete deafness on the same side and a loss of equilibrium.

9. **Glossopharyngeal Nerve** (Fig. 46). The 9th nerve emerges from the brain in such a way that its uppermost rootlets of origin are situated just below the 8th nerve, and the lowermost are practically continuous with the 10th. It passes upward and outward to the jugular foramen, through which it leaves the skull. In this foramen it is enclosed in a special dural compartment, and the 10th and the 11th nerves and the jugular vein are posterior to it. The glosso-

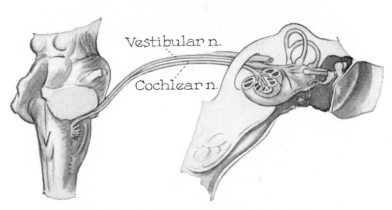

Vestibular n.

Cochlear n.

FIG. 45. The auditory nerve (diagrammatic).

pharyngeal then passes downward and forward between the internal and the external carotid arteries, winds around the stylopharyngeus muscle and reaches the undersurface of the base of the tongue, going beneath the hyoglossus muscle. It supplies taste and sensations to the posterior third of the tongue and supplies the epiglottis, the soft palate, the tonsils and the pillars of the fauces. Lesions of this nerve produce anesthesia of the posterior third of the tongue as well as of the pharynx.

10. **Vagus (Pneumogastric) Nerve** (Fig. 47). In this nerve the rootlets of origin are continuous above with those of the 9th. The nerve leaves the cranium through the middle compartment of the jugular foramen and occupies the same sheath of dura as does the accessory nerve. The vagus descends between the internal carotid artery and the internal jugular vein; it enters the carotid sheath and travels downward, lying behind and between the common carotid artery and the internal jugular vein.

The *right* vagus passes over the first part of the subclavian artery and reaches the thorax behind the right innominate vein. In the superior mediastinum it is found to the right of the innominate artery and the trachea, and posterior to the superior vena cava. It continues along the lateral aspect of the trachea to the posterior mediastinum, where it splits into several branches at the back of the root of the lung; these form the posterior pulmonary plexus. From this plexus the vagus continues as two cords, which pass on to the esophagus to unite with the vagus of the opposite side, forming the esophageal plexus. The nerve leaves this plexus as a single trunk, descending behind the esophagus and passing through the corresponding opening in the diaphragm to become distributed to the posterior surface of the stomach. Communicating fibers are fur-

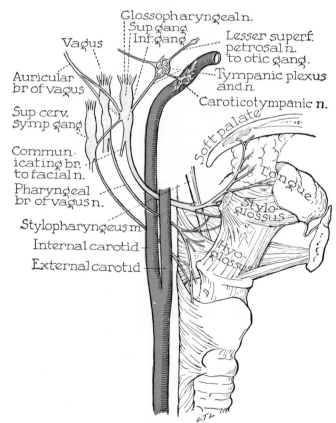

FIG. 46. The glossopharyngeal nerve. Its communications with surrounding nerves are shown.

nished to the celiac, the splanchnic and the renal plexuses.

The *left* vagus enters the thorax between the left common carotid and the subclavian arteries, posterior to the left innominate vein and the left phrenic nerve. After crossing to the left of the aortic arch it breaks up at the back of the root of the lung into the posterior

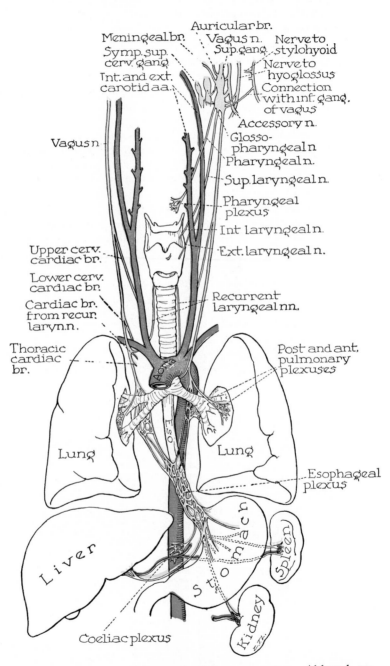

Fig. 47. The right and the left vagus nerves. Although an esophageal plexus is demonstrated in the illustration, nevertheless, it is believed by some anatomists that the vagi do not form a true plexus in this region, but rather reveal individual nerve filaments.

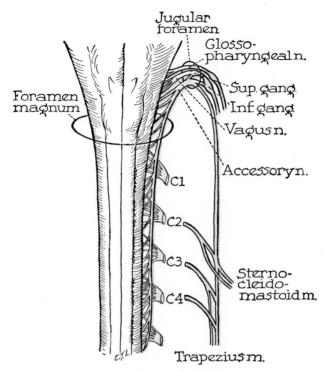

FIG. 48. The spinal accessory nerve.

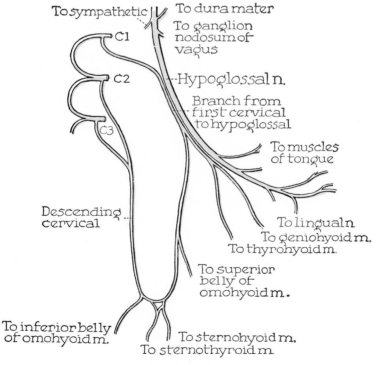

FIG. 49. Plan of the hypoglossal nerve.

pulmonary plexus. From this plexus the two efferent nerves pass over the descending thoracic aorta and reach the esophagus as the esophageal plexus. The continuing nerve passes through the esophageal orifice and travels over the anterior surface of the stomach, sending branches into the gastro-hepatic ligament to form the hepatic plexus. The laryngeal nerves that arise from the vagus will be discussed in the section on the larynx (p. 192). The most typical sign of a lesion of the vagus is paralysis of its recurrent laryngeal branch. Such a lesion produces an immobile vocal cord fixed in the cadaveric position on the affected side.

11. **Spinal Accessory Nerve** (Fig. 48). The 11th cranial nerve originates partly from the brain and partly from the spinal cord, hence its name, spinal accessory nerve. The cerebral part arises from the medulla oblongata and leaves in company with and below the vagus; the spinal part arises from the anterior column of gray matter of the spinal medulla and leaves the cord as low as the 6th cervical nerve. The spinal portion ascends in the spinal canal to enter the cranium through the foramen magnum, joins the accessory part and then leaves the skull through the middle compartment of the jugular foramen lying posterior to the vagus and the glossopharyngeal nerves. It passes over the internal jugular vein, beneath the posterior belly of the digastric muscle, then pierces the sternocleidomastoid muscle and runs over the posterior triangle of the neck to enter the trapezius. In the sternocleidomastoid it communicates with the 2nd cervical, and in the trapezius with the 3rd and the 4th cervical nerves. Lesions of this nerve paralyze the sternocleidomastoid, but paralysis of the trapezius varies according to how much of it is supplied by the 3rd and the 4th cervicals; also the scapula is displaced downward, and its vertebral border is imperfectly approximated to the midline when the shoulders are braced back. The nerve may be injured in operations on the neck, especially in removal of tuberculous glands that surround it.

12. **Hypoglossal Nerve** (Fig. 49). This nerve leaves the skull through the anterior condylar canal and enters the neck behind the internal jugular vein and the internal carotid artery; it passes beneath the posterior belly of the digastric muscle, crosses the external carotid artery on the first part of the lingual artery and then enters the submandibular triangle. At this point it disappears beneath the mylohyoid muscle and runs upon the hyoglossus muscle just beneath the submandibular duct. Lying medial to the lingual artery, it reaches the tongue.

The *descending branch* of the 12th nerve passes down in the anterior wall of the carotid sheath, where it joins with the descending cervical nerves (2nd and 3rd) to form the ansa hypoglossi. The 12th nerve is the motor nerve to the tongue and also supplies the sternohyoid, the sternothyroid and the omohyoid muscles. When it is involved, the corresponding half of the tongue becomes atrophied, and if the patient is asked to protrude his tongue, the healthy side causes it to deviate toward the side that has been paralyzed.

Special Senses

THE EYE AND ITS APPENDAGES

Eyelids, Layers and Practical Considerations

The *eyelids* (palpebrae) are two thin, movable folds, the upper being the larger, more movable and furnished with a muscle known as the *levator palpebrae superioris*, which elevates the lid. Both eyelids are covered by skin superficially and by mucous membrane (conjunctiva) over the deep aspect. When the eye is opened an elliptical space, the *palpebral fissure*, remains between the lid margins. The lids are united laterally and medially by corresponding palpebral commissures (canthi). The *lateral palpebral commissure* (external canthus) is more acute than the medial and is placed directly against the globe (Fig. 50). The *medial commissure*, or internal canthus, is prolonged for a short distance toward the nose, and here the 2 eyelids are separated by a triangular space known as the *tear lake (lacus lacrimalis)*. This lacus is bounded above and below by the lacrimal parts of the eyelid and laterally by a crescentic fold of conjunctiva known as the *plica semilunaris*, which is considered as a remnant of the third eyelid. In the lacus there is a reddish elevation, the *caruncle*, composed of modified skin and containing a few fine hairs, sebaceous and sweat glands.

Near the medial angle of the eye, where the eyelids meet, the eyelashes stop abruptly; at this point are found rounded elevations known as *lacrimal papillae*. When the eyelid is everted the small opening (*punctum lacrimale*) is seen on the summit of each papilla. The puncta are in close apposition with the conjunctivae, and each leads into the *lacrimal canaliculus (duct)*, which passes medially to the lacrimal sac. The eyelashes arise from the mucocutaneous junction of the lids, and directly behind them the opening of the *tarsal gland* can be seen.

The eyelids have 6 layers (Fig. 51):

1. **Skin.** The skin of the eyelids is extremely thin; there probably is no thinner skin at any other place in the body. The eyelashes project from the lid margin at the mucocutaneous border. Associated with these hairs are sebaceous glands, called the *glands of Zeis*, which open into each hair follicle. The *glands of Moll* are sweat glands and likewise open into or beside the hair follicles.

2. **Loose Subcutaneous Tissue Layer.** This subcutaneous tissue layer is extremely loose and easily distended with blood or exudate so that any effusion into it becomes apparent immediately. Involvement of the sebaceous glands of hair follicles in the skin and the subcutaneous tissues results in the common condition known as a sty (hordeolum). There is little or no subcutaneous fat in the eyelids.

3. **Layer of Striped Muscle.** The layer of striped muscle is made up of the palpebral fibers of the *orbicularis oculi muscle*. It acts as the sphincter of the palpebral fissure. (The levator palpebrae situated in the upper lid is attached along the upper margin of the tarsal plate.)

4. **Areolar Layer (Submuscular).** The sensory nerves lie in this layer; therefore, in producing anesthesia of the lid it is necessary to inject deeply to the orbicularis muscle. This areolar space is continuous above with the dangerous area of the scalp.

5. **Tarsal Plate.** The tarsae are 2 thin plates of dense connective tissue about 1 inch long; they are present in each eyelid. They contribute to the form and the support of the lids and are connected with the lateral wall of the orbit by the lateral (external)

tarsal ligament and with the medial wall by the medial (internal) tarsal ligament. The tarsae are further connected with the upper and the lower orbital margins by an aponeurotic layer of connective tissue called the *palpebral fascia* (orbital septum). The superior tarsal plate receives the main insertion of the *levator palpebrae superioris*. The meibomian sebaceous glands (tarsal glands) are located in the plate proper and are identified as yellow streaks when the lid is examined from the conjunctival side. These glands open on the lid margin, and their secretion guarantees an airtight closure of the lid, thus preventing maceration of the skin by tear moisture. An obstructed hair follicle (sty) will protrude on the front of the lid but an obstructed tarsal (meibomian) gland or chalazion will protrude onto the globe of the eye as a tarsal cyst.

6. **Conjunctiva.** This layer of mucous membrane attaches the eyeball to the lid. The lines along which the reflection of the conjunctiva takes place from lid to eyeball are termed the *superior* and the *inferior fornices*. The area where the conjunctiva lines the posterior surface of the lid is known as the *palpebral conjunctiva*, and where it covers the globe of the eye it is called the *bulbar conjunctiva*. The conjunctiva is firmly adherent to the tarsal plate but is loosely attached to the sclera over the globe of the eye.

The *arterial supply* of the lids is derived from the superior and the inferior palpebral branches of the ophthalmic artery, which form a rich vascular anastomosis. The *veins* of the lids drain into the ophthalmic veins by way of subconjunctival or retrotarsal veins. The *lymphatics* drain laterally to the preauricular glands and medially to the facial and the submaxillary groups. The chief *motor nerve* of the lids is the facial to the orbicularis oculi muscle; if this nerve is injured, it impairs the important sphincter action of the muscle in closing the lids. The oculomotor nerve supplies the levator palpebrae muscle, and in the event of its paralysis, a ptosis or inability to lift the lid results.

LACRIMAL APPARATUS

The lacrimal apparatus consists of the lacrimal glands, 2 lacrimal ducts, the lacrimal sac and the nasolacrimal duct (Figs. 50, 52).

Lacrimal Gland. This gland is situated in a depression in the superolateral angle of the

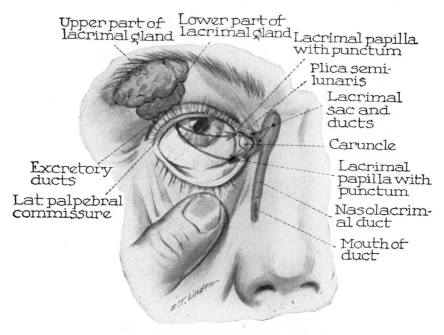

FIG. 50. The right eye and the lacrimal apparatus.

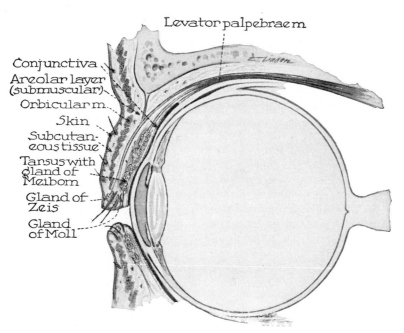

Levator palpebrae m.

Conjunctiva

Areolar layer
(submuscular)

Orbicular m.

Skin

Subcutan-
eous tissue

Tarsus with
gland of
Meibom

Gland of
Zeis

Gland
of Moll

FIG. 51. Diagram of the 6 layers that form the eyelids.

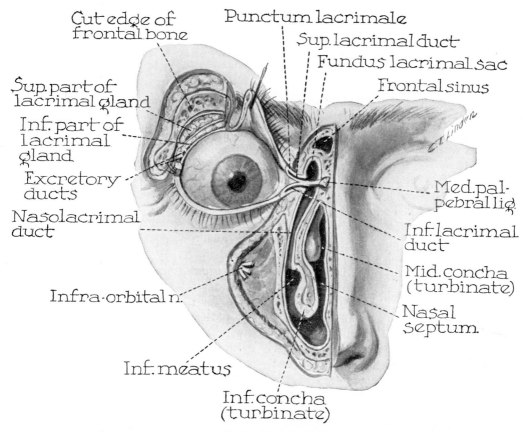

Cut edge of
frontal bone

Punctum lacrimale

Sup. lacrimal duct

Fundus lacrimal sac

Frontal sinus

Sup. part of
lacrimal gland

Inf. part of
lacrimal
gland

Excretory
ducts

Nasolacrimal
duct

Med. pal-
pebral lig.

Inf. lacrimal
duct

Mid. concha
(turbinate)

Nasal
septum.

Infra-orbital n.

Inf. meatus

Inf. concha
(turbinate)

FIG. 52. The lacrimal apparatus. The right half of the upper eyelid and part of the
right frontal bone and the nose have been removed.

orbit; it is oval in shape, about the size and the shape of an almond, and is divided by the aponeurosis of the levator palpebrae superioris into two portions: a superior and an inferior. The *superior* or orbital portion is longer and is fixed to a depression in the orbital plate of the frontal bone. In front it lies against the orbital septum, through which access is gained for removal of this portion of the gland. Behind, it rests on the tendon of the levator palpebrae muscle. The *inferior* or palpebral portion is smaller and joins the orbital portion behind. It lies on the palpebral conjunctiva, to which it is adherent and through which its ducts open. These two portions of the glands pour tears into the upper fornix by means of 8 to 12 tiny ducts. The tears travel over and lubricate the eyeball, pass into the lacrimal ducts to the lacrimal sac, then down the nasolacrimal duct and into the nose.

Lacrimal Ducts (Canaliculi). These ducts are situated one in each eyelid, starting at tiny orifices called the *puncta lacrimalia*. The ducts are about 1 cm. long, passing first vertically and then almost horizontally inward to join the lacrimal sac. The course of the duct is important to know when one is attempting to pass a probe.

Lacrimal Sac. This is situated in the lacrimal fossa formed by the frontal process of the superior maxilla and the lacrimal bone. The dome of the sac, known as the fundus, projects above the internal tarsal ligament. This ligament may be rendered prominent by drawing on the skin laterally; immediately behind it the sac will be found.

Nasolacrimal Duct. This duct is the downward continuation of the lacrimal sac. It is about ¾ inch long and descends in a bony groove that is formed by the superior maxilla, the lacrimal and the inferior turbinate bones. In the region of the maxilla the duct is in close contact with the maxillary sinus; its direction is backward, outward and downward and may be identified by a line from the inner angle of the eye to the first upper molar tooth of the same side. The continuity of the duct with the mucous membrane of the nose explains the extension of diseases from the nose into the lacrimal passages. Its opening in the nose is under cover of the anterior part of the inferior nasal concha.

Surgery of the Gland, the Sac and the Ducts. Although infections and tumors of the lacrimal gland are somewhat unusual, involvement of the tear-conducting passages is common. This is known as *dacryocystitis*. As a rule, some obstructing agent in the nasolacrimal duct is the cause of the inflammatory process. Obstruction of the duct may be produced by infections of the nasal fossa or the paranasal sinuses. A prominent symptom in all diseases of the tear-conducting apparatus is epiphora or tearing.

Normally, the *lacrimal duct* admits a probe about 3.5 mm. in diameter, which can be passed medially through the lower punctum. Probing has been used to relieve obstructions, but it should not be attempted in inexperienced hands. If this procedure fails, then more radical ones may be advised, such as establishing a communication between the sac and the middle nasal passage (Toti's operation) or extirpation of the lacrimal sac.

Removal of the lacrimal sac is performed as a last resort in persistent cases of dacryocystitis. The incision begins at a point about 3 mm. above and internal to the inner canthus and is carried downward and outward about 1 inch. After division of the skin, the margins are dissected, and an attempt is made to locate the anterior lacrimal crest. The fascia is incised, and when the sac is exposed, it is separated from the periosteum of the lacrimal fossa. The ducts are divided, the extremities of the sac freed and excised as low as possible in the nasolacrimal duct.

Excision of the lacrimal gland is reserved for those cases where the lacrimal sac has been removed, leaving no channel for drainage of tears and resulting in troublesome watering of the eye. Excision of the superior portion of the gland may be made through a curved incision parallel with the outer half of the orbital margin. The incision passes through the skin, the connective tissue and the orbital fascia down to the periosteum. The wound edges are retracted, bringing into view the lacrimal gland, which is grasped by forceps and brought as far into the wound as possible. Then the gland is freed, and the lacrimal artery is clamped and ligated. To remove the inferior or accessory lacrimal gland, a small horizontal incision is made over the contour of that gland. Retraction of the wound edges brings the gland into view; then it is dissected from its bed and removed.

ORBIT

The orbital cavity has been likened to a quadrilateral pyramid, the base being in front, and the summit behind. The orbits are bony cavities, situated between the anterior portion of the cranium and the face, and are separated by the nasal fossa. Each orbit contains the globe of one eye and its appendages. The orbital cavity is closed in front by the eyelids, which are separated from the globe of the eye by folds of conjunctiva. The eyeball occupies the anterior part of the orbit, and the posterior portion is filled with fat, fascia, muscles, vessels and nerves, which are appendages of the eye. The anterior and the posterior portions are divided from each other by the so-called capsule of Tenon (p. 77), which is the membranous sac enveloping the posterior portion of the eyeball and forming a socket in which it moves. The walls of the orbit are very thin and are lined with periosteum, called *periorbita*, which is continuous through the optic foramen with the dura mater. Pathologic effusion may detach the periosteum from the bone, since it is attached loosely. At the lacrimal groove it splits to enclose the lacrimal sac. The 4 walls are in contact with 4 fossae: the anterior cerebral above, the maxillary sinus below, the nasal medially and the temporal laterally. Therefore, involvement of the orbital cavity may encroach upon any of these 4 regions, and vice versa. Since, with the exception of its frontal aspect, the orbit is surrounded by bone, tumors developing here will take the path of least resistance and push the eyeball forward, producing the condition of *exophthalmos.*

Lateral, Temporal and Intracranial Approaches. *Kronlein's operation* affords a *lateral temporal orbital approach* to the retroocular space and is a procedure by which an orbital tumor may be removed, leaving the eye in place. An appropriate incision which extends to the bone is made, the central part of the incision exposing the orbital margin. The periosteum is separated from the outer wall of the orbit, and the contents of the latter are retracted gently. The sphenomaxillary fissure is located and marked. An incision through the bone is then made by means of a chisel or an electric saw from a point a little above the external angular process of the frontal bone extending to the anterior end of the fissure; a second incision extends from the base of the orbital process of the malar bone backward to the same point. The resulting wedge-shaped piece of bone can be swung outward, exposing the periosteum lining the lateral wall of the orbit, thus permitting exploration of the orbital contents. If greater access is required, the external rectus muscle can be divided and later united. After removal of the tumor, the bone is rotated into place, the periosteum is sutured, and the skin incision is sewed in the usual manner.

For *orbital decompression,* Naffziger and Jones have described an *intracranial approach* to the orbit. The operation gives adequate space for such conditions as progressive exophthalmos. In this procedure bilateral frontal flaps are resected, the dura is elevated over the frontal lobe, and the roof of the orbit is removed, together with the superior portion of the optic foramen. The projection of the frontal and the ethmoidal sinuses into the orbital plate should be determined preoperatively by means of roentgenograms. Any orbital contents under pressure bulge through the newly made opening in the bone. Also, the orbital fascia is opened. This approach has been utilized in operative procedures involving the retroocular space.

EYEBALL

The eyeball is situated in the anterior part of the orbit, nearer the roof than the floor, and somewhat closer to the outer than the inner wall. It is approximately 1 inch in all diameters. Behind, it rests upon the capsule of Tenon, which forms a socket in which it may move freely; in front, it comes in contact with the posterior surface of the eyelid. It has least protection on its outer side.

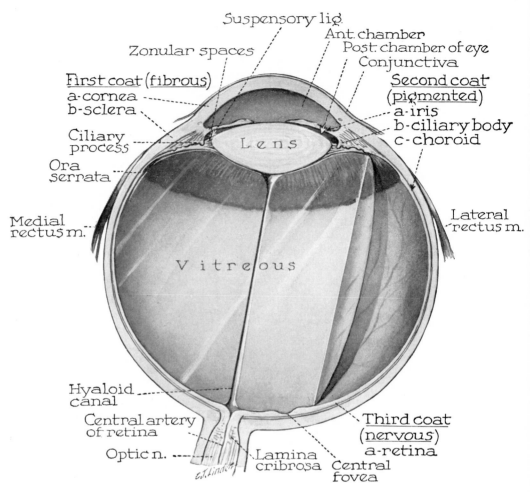

FIG. 53. Horizontal section of the right eye. The eyeball has 3 coats (fibrous, pigmented and nervous) and 3 refractive media (aqueous humor, vitreous humor and lens).

Coats and Media

The eyeball consists of 3 coats which enclose 3 refractive media (Fig. 53). The first coat is fibrous and contains the sclera and the cornea; the second is pigmented and contains the choroid, the ciliary body and the iris; the third coat is nervous and contains the retina. The refractive media are the aqueous humor, the vitreous humor and the lens.

Sclera. The sclera forms a tough fibrous external capsule which encloses the posterior five sixths of the eyeball and is continuous in front with the cornea. Although it is a thick, nondistensible membrane, it thins out where the optic nerve enters and becomes a sieve-like membrane called the *lamina cribrosa.* Around the entrance of the optic nerve, several small openings are seen; these permit passage of the ciliary nerves and arteries. These arteries arise from the posterior ciliary branches of the ophthalmic artery. The *long ciliary branches* pass between the choroid and the sclera to supply the iris and the ciliary regions; the *short ciliary arteries* terminate in the choroid. The smaller veins come together to form 4 or 5 main trunks, the *venae vorticosae,* which perforate the sclera and leave it midway between cornea and the optic nerve where they drain into the ophthalmic veins. Beyond the margin of the cornea, the sclera can be seen through the conjunctiva as the "white" of the eye.

The anterior ciliary arteries pierce the sclera near the corneoscleral junction (Fig. 59).

Cornea. This anterior transparent part of the outer coat of the eyeball occupies about one sixth of the circumference of the globe and is continuous with the opaque sclera. It has been likened to a little watch glass whose curvature is greater than that of the sclera. It has no blood vessels but derives its nutrition from the lymph which circulates in its numerous lymphatic spaces. At the corneoscleral junction is an important line known as the *limbus*. In operations on the iris and the lens, incisions are made close to it. The superficial surface of the cornea is covered by a layer of stratified epithelium that is continuous with the conjunctiva; posteriorly, it is limited by a *posterior elastic membrane* (Descemet's membrane) which is covered by a layer of mesothelium, this being in contact with the aqueous humor (Fig. 54). At the peripheral margin the fibers of this membrane divide into 3 groups: the innermost

fibers turn medially into the iris and form the *ligamentum pectinatum iridis*, which have been referred to as the pillars of the iris; the middle fibers form the site of origin of the ciliary muscle; the outermost fibers become continuous with the sclera. At the corneoscleral junction a circular venous space is seen; this occupies the region of the anterior chamber in the deeper part of the coat. It is known as the *sinus venosus sclerae* (canal of Schlemm); it communicates with the scleral veins and with the aqueous humor, the latter communication taking place through the spaces of Fontana. The cornea is supplied by the ophthalmic division of the 5th nerve via surrounding conjunctival and ciliary branches. These nerves give the warning of an injury or a foreign body in the eye. If this nerve should be injured or divided, as in removal of a gasserian ganglion, the cornea becomes insensitive, may ulcerate, and eventually the eye may be lost.

The second coat of the eyeball is the

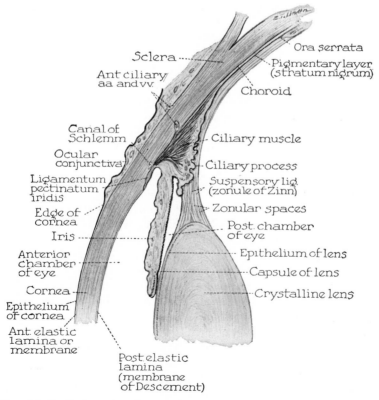

FIG. 54. Sagittal section through the upper half and the front of the eyeball.

vascular tunic, which consists, from behind forward, of the choroid, the ciliary body and the iris, all of which are continuous with each other and, therefore, are often affected simultaneously. This layer has also been referred to as the *iridociliary-choroidal tunic* or the *uveal tract*.

Choroid. The choroid extends from the optic nerve to the *ora serrata*, the latter being the jagged edge where the true retina ends. Externally, the choroid is in contact with the sclera; internally, it is attached to the retina. It is the nourishing coat of the eyeball and is composed mainly of blood vessels; its internal layer contains pigment cells which may give rise to melanosarcoma. The vessels in the choroid may be visible in ophthalmoscopic examinations; in the fundus of the eye they produce the red background against which the retinal vessels stand out. The veins of the choroid are external to the arteries and form 4 or 5 principal trunks, the *venae vorticosae*.

Ciliary body. This consists of the ciliary muscle and the ciliary processes. The body is triangular on sagittal section and is a continuation of the choroid, which it connects to the margin of the iris. The body has been referred to as the "dangerous area" of the eye, since wounds here can involve the iris, the choroid, the retina or the cornea. Inflammation of the body in one eye may be followed by sympathetic ophthalmia involving the ciliary body of the opposite eye. The *ciliary muscle* makes up the outer side of the triangle of the ciliary body and consists of flat bundles of unstriped muscle, the outermost running anteroposteriorly and the inner circularly. The nerve to this muscle originates from the oculomotor. The fibers of the muscle run backward from the corneoscleral junction to the choroid; when they contract they pull the choroid forward, thus relaxing the suspensory ligament, which in turn allows the lens to become more convex. Therefore, the ciliary muscle is the muscle of accommodation.

Ciliary processes. These processes, about 70 in number, are of the same structure as the rest of the choroid and consist essentially of blood vessels that are forward continuations of those of the choroid. They also have a considerable amount of pigment and some glandlike structures which, according to one theory, are supposed to form the aqueous humor.

Iris. The iris corresponds to the diaphragm of a camera and has a central opening, the *pupil*, which regulates the amount of light to reach the retina. The iris separates the anterior chamber of the eye from the posterior and has been called a "curtain" which divides the space between the cornea and the lens into anterior and posterior chambers. It is visible through the cornea, and the pigment in it determines the color of the individual's eye. It is attached at its periphery to approximately the middle of the anterior surface of the ciliary body and does not arise from the corneoscleral junction but farther back. This fact is utilized in a number of operations in this region.

The iris is composed of a delicate stroma of connective tissue which contains blood vessels, nerves, pigment cells and two groups of involuntary muscle fibers. The first set of muscle fibers is the circular sphincter group (sphincter pupillae), contraction of which narrows the pupil. The nerve supply is by the oculomotor via the short ciliary nerves. This first set of muscle fibers is approximately 1 mm. broad and is situated around the pupillary margin. The second group is a less clearly defined dilator set of muscles (dilator pupillae) which lies near its posterior surface. Its fixed point is at the root of the iris, and it is supplied by the sympathetic nerves. In inflammatory lesions that affect the iris (iritis), adhesions may form either in front of the cornea (anterior synechia) or posteriorly to the capsule of the lens (posterior synechia). The vessels to the iris arise from the long and the short anterior ciliary arteries. The nerve supply is derived from the long and the short ciliary nerves.

Retina. The expanded termination of the optic nerve forms the innermost coat of the eye. It should be considered as a part of the brain, since it arises from a hollow outgrowth of the forebrain. Therefore, the optic nerve is a nerve tract that connects one part of the brain with another. It extends forward almost as far as the ciliary processes, at which point it ends in an irregular edge known as the *ora serrata*. From this point forward it continues as a thin layer as far as the ciliary processes. This prolongation contains no nerve fibers and is known as the ciliary part of the retina. The retina is attached to the choroid at only two points: the entrance of the optic nerve and the ora serrata. This accounts for its easy separation from the choroid. Under normal conditions the retina is transparent and not visible, making the subjacent choroid visible as the red background of the eye as seen through the ophthalmoscope (Fig. 55). The point of entrance of the optic nerve is known as the *optic disk (papilla)*; this is located a

little below and to the medial side of the posterior pole of the eyeball. The normal disk presents a slight central depression, the physiologic cup or excavation, which marks the point of divergence of entering optic nerve fibers and the entry of retinal vessels. At the edge of the disk a variable amount of pigment is normally present. The disk is considered as the physiologic "blind spot" of the retina. The *macula lutea (yellow spot)* is found above and to the lateral side of the disk and forms a yellowish, circular area that is devoid of blood vessels. In contradistinction to the disk, it is the area of "most distinct vision." The macula is from 1 to 2 mm. in diameter and has in its center

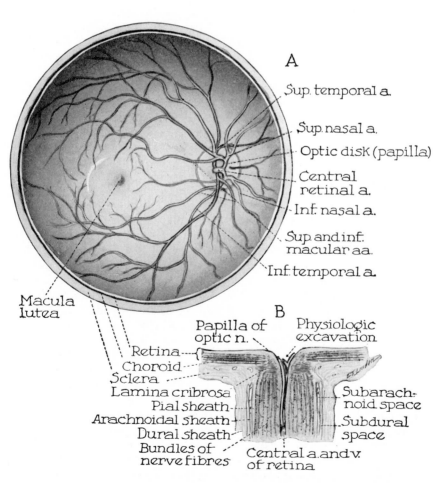

FIG. 55. (A) The right eyeground. (B) Horizontal section of the terminal part of the optic nerve and its entrance into the eyeball.

a tiny depression called the *fovea centralis*. The *central artery of the retina* is a branch of the ophthalmic, entering the optic nerve about 2 cm. from the eyeball and running within it as far as the retina, which it enters about the middle of the disk. In the fetus this vessel extends as far as the lens and passes through the vitreous, but previous to birth that position which is beyond the retina disappears and remains as the hyaloid canal (Fig. 53). After emerging through the disk, the central artery divides into superior and inferior branches, each of which subdivides into temporal and nasal branches. The branches and the central artery are end vessels; if an embolus plugs them, sudden blindness results. Because of the transparency of the retina, these vessels are clearly visible through the ophthalmoscope and afford an ideal opportunity for study. The veins follow the same distribution as the arteries, are somewhat broader and empty into the ophthalmic veins that form the cavernous sinus in the retro-orbital region. Pulsation is normal in these veins but is not normal in the arteries. The retina proper consists essentially of nuclei and processes of 3 layers of nervous tissue which have been placed one on top of the other and form synapses. They have been referred to as the visual cells (rods and cones), the bipolar cells and the ganglion cells.

Detachment of the retina results in blindness in the corresponding field of vision. Operations have been devised to re-attach it. One such procedure is the use of small electropunctures that are placed in the sclera. This results in adhesions which should bind the previously separated retina to the choroid.

Aqueous Humor (Fig. 53). This clear fluid occupies the space between the cornea in front and the lens behind. The iris divides this space into 2 chambers: anterior and posterior. The *anterior chamber* is bounded in front by the cornea, behind by the iris and opposite the pupil by the anterior part of the lens. The *posterior chamber* is situated between the posterior aspect of the iris and the lens. The aqueous humor that fills these 2 chambers should be regarded as the lymph of the eye, although its composition is not that of true body lymph, since it contains less albumin and does not clot unless pathologically altered. The 2 chambers communicate freely with each other through the pupil. It is believed that the aqueous humor is secreted into the posterior chamber by the ciliary body and then passes through the pupil into the anterior chamber, from which it is drained away by the sinus venosus sclerae (canal of Schlemm) to the anterior ciliary veins.

Vitreous body. This soft, gelatinous substance fills the whole of the eyeball behind the lens. This jellylike material supports the retina behind and is hollowed in front for the reception of the lens. It is enclosed in a delicate and transparent structure called the *hyaloid membrane*, which is in contact with the retina but from which it may be separated readily except at the optic disk. As this membrane passes anteriorly, it becomes thickened and irregular where it receives the ciliary processes that fit into its corresponding furrows. At the margin of the lens the membrane divides into a posterior layer, which lines the hollowed anterior aspect of the vitreous body, and an anterior layer, which is attached to the anterior aspect of the lens. The *hyaloid canal* extends from the optic disk through the vitreous as far as the capsule of the lens and is the remnant of a passage for the central artery of the retina that was present in the fetus.

Lens. This biconvex, transparent, colorless body is situated between the aqueous humor in front and the vitreous humor behind. It is in contact with the iris anteriorly and is about one third of an inch in diameter and one fifth of an inch thick. A capsule surrounding it is attached to the ciliary processes in the neighborhood of its circumference by the *suspensory ligament (zonula ciliaris)*. The latter is derived from the hyaloid membrane. Contraction of the ciliary muscle draws the hyaloid membrane forward; this relaxes the suspensory ligament, resulting in a greater convexity of the anterior surface of the lens. The ability of the lens, by virtue of its elastic structure, to change its refractive power is known as the *power of accommodation*. Loss of such elasticity is known as *presbyopia*. The lens may be displaced anteriorly into the aqueous chamber, from which location it can be removed through a corneal incision; it may be displaced posteriorly into the vitreous chamber, usually resulting in glaucoma. If the sclera is ruptured, the lens can be seen immediately below the conjunctiva. Opacity of the lens results in cataract formation.

ORBITAL FASCIA (TENON'S CAPSULE)

Orbital fascia (Fig. 56). This thickened, aponeuroticlike connective tissue suspends the structures of the orbit. It extends from the optic foramen forward to the circumference of the orbit, blends with the periosteum and gives rise to prolongations that ensheath almost every structure contained in the bony orbit. The principal parts of the aponeurosis are the fascia of the bulb (Tenon's capsule), sheaths of the muscles and check ligaments.

Fascia of the Bulb. This reduplication of the orbital fascia surrounds the posterior two thirds of the eyeball. It surrounds the optic nerve behind, merges into its sheath and furnishes tubular sheaths to the orbital muscles where they attach to the globe. Anteriorly, it is in contact with the outer surface of the sclera; posteriorly, it is in relation to the orbital fat. The fascia is important because (1) it forms a partition that divides the orbital cavity into anterior and posterior compartments; (2) it provides a practical joint in which the eyeball moves like the head of a bone; (3) it permits an enucleation of the eye without opening the posterior compartment and therefore lessens the danger of meningeal infection; (4) it acts as a barrier to the spread of infection or hemorrhage between the eyeball and the retroocular space; (5) it is an efficient socket for a prosthesis (artificial eye) after enucleation of the eyeball.

At that point where the lateral and the medial recti perforate the fascia, strong capsular expansions spread to the corresponding walls of the orbit. This arrangement checks lateral and medial rotation of the eye, hence the name "check ligaments." These ligaments are of surgical importance because they limit the degree of retraction of the muscles after an enucleation of the eyeball or a tenotomy. They are connected to each other by a thickened hammock of fascia that is situated below the eye. This thickened part is known as the *suspensory ligament of Lock-*

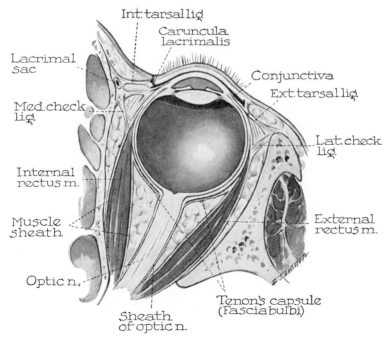

FIG. 56. The orbital fascia and its principal parts (Tenon's capsule, check ligaments and muscle sheaths).

wood. This band, with the orbital periosteum, aids in the support of the eyeball after excision of the maxilla; therefore, it should be identified and preserved. The posterior compartment of the orbit or that part that is behind Tenon's capsule contains the muscles of the eye, the ophthalmic artery and vein, the nerves of the orbit and fat.

MUSCLES

(Fig. 57.) The muscles of the orbit include the 4 recti (superior, inferior, medial and lateral), the 2 obliqui (superior and in-ferior) and the levator palpebrae superioris. Six of the 7 orbital muscles arise from the margins of the optic foramen, each by a single head, except the lateral rectus, which has 2 heads. A common tendinous ring is found around the circumference of the optic foramen for the origin of these muscles. The lower inner portion of this ring is known as the *ligament of Zinn*.

Rectus Muscles. The 4 rectus muscles insert into the sclera as at the 4 points of the compass, the tendon of each piercing the fascia bulbi (Tenon) as it inserts. They

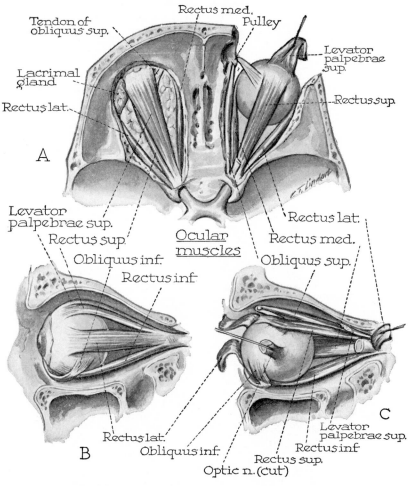

FIG. 57. The muscles of the orbit. (A) Viewed from above, with the orbital roofs removed; on the right side, the orbital fat has been dissected away. (B) Left side, lateral view with the muscles intact. (C) Left side, lateral view; the levator palpebrae superioris and the lateral rectus muscles have been severed. The optic nerve has also been cut, revealing the medial rectus muscle.

pass forward from their common origin at the tendinous ring to form a conelike muscular capsule for the optic nerve and the posterior half of the eyeball. The lateral rectus pulls the eye laterally (outward), and the medial does the reverse. However, the actions of the superior and the inferior recti are not so simple. Because of the relationship to the vertical axis and the line of pull, the superior rectus does not produce pure upward movement but a combination of upward and medial rotation. In a similar manner the inferior rectus produces a combination of downward and medial rotation.

Superior Oblique Muscle. This muscle arises a little above the upper margin of the optic foramen. It passes to the inner angle of the orbit, where it becomes a rounded tendon, and continues through the fibrocartilaginous ring (pulley) that is situated in the trochlear fossa. It then makes a sharp hairpin turn, passes beneath the superior rectus and inserts into the outer and posterior part of the globe of the eye, either between the superior and the lateral recti muscles or under the superior rectus. Contraction of this muscle rotates the eyeball so as to make the pupil look downward, but in addition to this it produces a certain degree of lateral rotation. Pure downward rotation of the eyeball can be produced only when the superior oblique and the inferior rectus work together.

Inferior Oblique Muscle. This muscle arises from the orbital floor just lateral to the opening of the nasolacrimal canal and inserts either under the lateral rectus or between the lateral and the superior recti. Its action makes the pupil look upward and lateral. If it is desired to look straight upward, the inferior oblique and the superior rectus must work together.

Levator Palpebrae Superioris Muscle. This muscle is situated immediately under the orbital roof. It arises from this roof anterior to the optic foramen and inserts into the upper lid. Its fibers fuse with the orbital septum and the upper border of the superior tarsal plate and skin. Its action is to raise the lid, thus working in opposition to the orbicularis oculi muscle. The orbicularis has been considered as the sphincter, and the levator as the dilator of the eye.

VESSELS AND NERVES

Ophthalmic Artery (Figs. 58, 59). This vessel arises from the internal carotid immediately after the latter leaves the cavernous sinus. It passes forward through the optic foramen below and lateral to the optic nerve. In the orbit the artery turns around the lateral side of the nerve, crosses directly above it and then travels forward, parallel with the nasociliary nerve. It ends at the medial angle of the eye by dividing into the supra-orbital and the supratrochlear branches. The branches of the ophthalmic artery are:

The *central artery of the retina (arteria centralis retinae)* (Fig. 59), arising from the ophthalmic while it still lies below the optic nerve, runs in the substance of the nerve to the optic disk, where it divides into branches that supply the retina. These are end arteries and can be identified in the living eye with the ophthalmoscope.

The *ciliary arteries* form a posterior and an anterior group. The posterior group ramifies in the choroid coat; two of them, the long posterior ciliary arteries, run forward to the ciliary zone, where they form an anastomotic circle with the anterior ciliaries. The anterior group pierces the sclera near the corneoscleral junction, thus forming an arterial ring that supplies branches to the ciliary body and iris.

The *supratrochlear and supra-orbital arteries* leave the orbit with the supratrochlear and the supra-orbital nerves, respectively. They supply the superficial tissues of the forehead where they anastomose with branches of the superficial temporal (external carotid) artery.

The ophthalmic artery also gives off muscular and palpebral branches and a branch to the lacrimal gland.

Ophthalmic veins (Fig. 30). These are two in number: the superior and the inferior. The *superior ophthalmic vein* accompanies the artery. Beginning at the union of the supratrochlear and the supra-orbital veins and anastomosing with the anterior facial vein, it passes through the superior orbital fissure and ends in the cavernous sinus. The *inferior ophthalmic vein* lies below the optic nerve, and one of its branches communicates with the pterygoid plexus via the inferior orbital fissure. The other branches of the ophthalmic vein leave the orbit through the lower part of the superior orbital fissure and terminate by joining the cavernous sinus.

Orbital Nerves (Fig. 58). These include the optic (the 3rd, the 4th and the 6th, constituting the motor nerves to the eye muscles), and the ophthalmic division of the 5th, which is the sensory supply to the orbit.

The *optic nerve* is about 2 inches long and extends from the optic chiasma to the eyeball. In its course it may conveniently be divided into 3 parts: the intracranial (in the cranial cavity), the intra-osseous (in the optic foramen) and the intra-orbital (in the orbit). In the cranial cavity the nerve lies on the front part of the diaphragma sellae and then on the anterior portion of the cavernous sinus. The anterior perforated substance, the

olfactory nerve and the anterior cerebral nerve all cross and lie above this nerve. The internal carotid artery is at first below and then becomes lateral to it. The ophthalmic artery arises from the internal carotid, inferomedial to the nerve, but soon crosses to its lateral side. In the optic foramen the nerve is surrounded by a continuation of the dura, the arachnoid and the pia, which accompany it to the posterior aspect of the eyeball. Since the nerve is separated from the sphenoid air sinus by only a thin plate of bone, a retrobulbar neuritis may develop in diseases affecting the sinus. In the orbit the nerve is surrounded by the orbital fat, and at the optic foramen it is surrounded by the origin of the ocular muscles. The nasociliary nerve, the ophthalmic artery and the superior ophthalmic vein cross the nerve superiorly from without inward; the nerve to the inferior oblique muscle lies below it. The ciliary ganglion can be located on the outer side of the nerve, between it and the

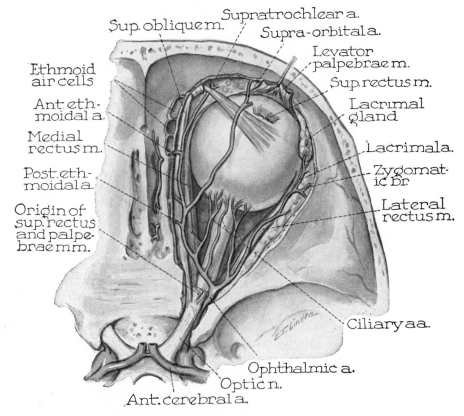

FIG. 58. The right ophthalmic artery and the optic nerve, as seen from above.

lateral rectus muscle. Where the nerve enters the eyeball, it is surrounded by the long and the short ciliary nerves (Fig. 59). The central artery of the retina arises from the ophthalmic artery near the optic foramen and passes forward in the dural sheath of the nerve. With its accompanying vein, it then crosses the subarachnoid space to enter the nerve on its under and inner aspect and runs directly in its substance. The subarachnoid space of the cranial cavity is directly continuous with the subarachnoid space around the optic nerve; because of this continuity, an increase of pressure in the intracranial subarachnoid space may be transmitted to the intra-orbital space. As a result of this, the central vein and artery may become compressed, resulting in an engorge-

ment of all the retinal vessels, diminution of the size of the arteries, and later exudation that produces the condition known as *choked disk* or *papilledema*. The nerve pierces the sclera at a point medial to the posterior pole of the eyeball and, having spread through the sclerotic and the choroid coats, spreads out to form the inner layer of the retina. The muscles of the orbit are supplied by 3 cranial nerves: the 3rd (oculomotor), the 4th (trochlear) and the 6th (abducent).

The *oculomotor nerve* (Fig. 39) supplies all the muscles of the orbit with the exception of the superior oblique and the lateral rectus. Through the ciliary ganglion it also supplies the sphincter muscle of the iris and the ciliary muscle (the muscle of visual ac-

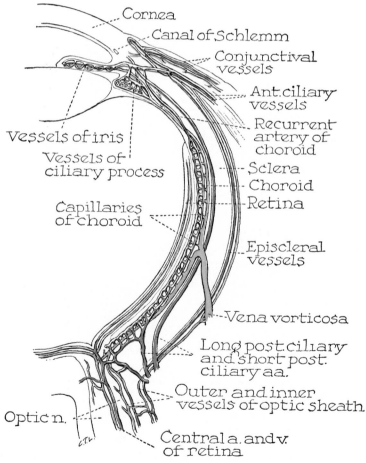

Cornea
Canal of Schlemm
Conjunctival vessels
Ant. ciliary vessels
Recurrent artery of choroid
Sclera
Choroid
Retina
Episcleral vessels
Vena vorticosa
Long post. ciliary and short post. ciliary aa.
Outer and inner vessels of optic sheath
Central a. and v. of retina

Vessels of iris
Vessels of ciliary process
Capillaries of choroid
Optic n.

Fig. 59. Vessels of the ocular globe (diagrammatic, after Leber).

commodation). If this nerve is involved, the following conditions will result: ptosis or drooping of the upper eyelid because of a paralysis of the levator palpebrae superioris; an external strabismus due to unopposed action of the external rectus and inability to turn the eyeball up or down; dilation of the pupil because of paralysis of the sphincter of the pupil; loss of accommodation due to paralysis of the ciliary muscle, and at times a slight prominence of the eyeball because of unopposed action of the superior oblique plus paralysis of all but one rectus muscle. The oculomotor nerve passes forward in the upper part of the lateral wall of the cavernous sinus to the superior orbital fissure and enters the orbit between the two heads of the lateral rectus muscle.

The *trochlear nerve* (Fig. 40) takes a course similar to the oculomotor but lies slightly below and to the lateral side of the 3rd nerve. It enters the orbit at the superior orbital fissure above the muscles and supplies only the superior oblique muscle.

The *abducens nerve* (Fig. 43) lies below the artery as it approaches the superior orbital fissure. Here it enters the orbit between the two heads of the lateral rectus, which it supplies.

The *ciliary ganglion* has a sensory supply (nasociliary branch of the ophthalmic nerve), a motor supply (inferior division of the oculomotor nerve) and sympathetic fibers (cavernous plexus on the internal carotid artery). If a local anesthetic is injected into the region of the ciliary ganglion, the resulting anesthesia will permit surgery upon the eyeball.

Surgery (Enucleation of the Eyeball) (Fig. 60). The object of enucleation is to

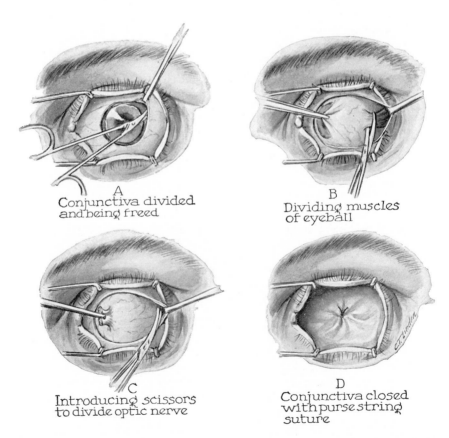

A
Conjunctiva divided and being freed

B
Dividing muscles of eyeball

C
Introducing scissors to divide optic nerve

D
Conjunctiva closed with purse string suture

FIG. 60. Enucleation of the eyeball: (A) division and separation of the conjunctiva, (B) division of the ocular muscles, (C) severing the optic nerve, (D) closure of conjunctiva.

remove the eyeball and leave the muscles to coalesce and form a stump upon which the artificial eye may rest and move. As much conjunctiva as possible should be preserved. The lids are retracted by means of a retention speculum, and the conjunctiva is grasped in such a way as to form a fold radiating toward the limbus. This fold is divided, as is the remaining conjunctiva in its entire extent adjacent to the limbus. The conjunctiva is separated from the globe beyond the insertion of the ocular muscles. Tenon's capsule is divided over the insertion of one of the muscles, and the tendon of that muscle is picked up, drawn away from the eyeball and divided. The other muscles are handled in similar fashion. The eyeball is retracted toward the nose, and a pair of curved blunt scissors is passed backward until the optic nerve is encountered. The nerve is divided, the eyeball is delivered from its socket, and the oblique muscles are severed near the sclera. After control of hemorrhage the conjunctiva is closed, and the operation is completed.

NOSE

EXTERNAL NOSE

(Fig. 61.) The external nose forms a tri-angular pyramid; its upper angle, which connects directly with the forehead, is referred to as the *root*, and its free angle as the *apex* or *tip*. The mobile lateral walls of the pyramid expand to form the *wings (alae)*, which are supplied with sebaceous and sweat glands. The *base* of the nose presents two elliptical orifices *(nares)* which are separated from each other by an anteroposterior *septum* called the *columna*. Small stiff hairs *(vibrissae)* found along the margins of the nares arrest the passage of foreign substances that may be carried in during inspiration. The *dorsum* of the nose is formed by the union of the two lateral surfaces in the midline. The *bridge* is the upper part of the dorsum that is supported by the nasal bones.

Skin. The skin is thin and lax over the root and the greater part of the dorsum, but over the alae it becomes thick and very adherent to the deeper parts; it has a rich

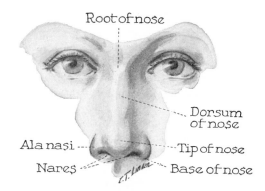

FIG. 61. The external nose.

blood supply; so it is well suited for plastic surgery. Wounds in this region heal well.

Nerves. The skin over the root of the nose is supplied by the nasal branch of the first division of the 5th nerve, which also supplies the skin over the alae and the region of the nostrils. The greater part of the side of the nose is supplied by the second division of the 5th nerve and is the seat of painful neuralgia when that trunk is involved. The anatomic fact that the nasal nerve is a branch of the ophthalmic trunk and has intimate connections with the eye explains the lacrimation that follows painful infections about the nostrils.

Arteries. The arteries of the nose are derived from the facial, which supplies the side of the nose, the alar and the septal branches to the septum and the alae, and the ophthalmic artery which sends branches to the root and the dorsum.

Veins. The veins follow the course of the arteries. Those at the root empty into the ophthalmic veins and then into the cavernous sinus. Inflammation in this region, such as furunculosis and erysipelas, may travel by means of this communication into the intracranial circulation and send septic emboli into the brain.

INTERNAL NOSE

Nasal Cavities. Two chambers are situated one on each side of the median plane. They are especially adapted for detecting odors and warming and filtering the air that passes to the lungs. The cavities communicate in front with the exterior by means of the *anterior nares* and behind with the nasal part of the pharynx by means of the *choanae* (posterior nares) (Fig. 158). Inside the aperture of the nostrils is a slight dilation known as the *vestibule*. The nasal cavities are placed below the middle part of the anterior cranial fossa and above the mouth, being separated from the latter by the palate; laterally, they are in relation to the orbit and the maxillary antrum. The nasal cavities present a roof, a floor, a medial wall (septum), a lateral wall and anterior and posterior openings.

Roof. The roof (Fig. 62) of each nasal cavity or fossa is about one eighth of an inch in width, is horizontal in the middle and slopes in front and behind. The sloping anterior part is formed by the frontal and the nasal bones and the nasal cartilages; the central portion is horizontal and is formed by the cribriform plate of the ethmoid; the sloping posterior part is formed by the anterior and lower surface of the body of the sphenoid. The anterior part corresponds to the slope of the bridge of the nose. The intermediate part is thin and delicate, is perforated by olfactory nerves and ethmoidal vessels and is located immediately beneath the anterior cranial fossa. Fracture of this part may result in meningitis. The posterior sloping part of the sphenoid sinus is located over the posterior aspect of the roof in the body of the sphenoid. Traction on a polyp attached to the roof of the nasal cavity may cause a breaking of this thin wall, resulting in a communication with the cranial cavity. Meningoceles that may project through the roof into the nasal cavity have been mistaken for nasal polyps.

Floor. The floor of the nasal cavity represents its larger part and is much wider than the roof. It is concave from side to side and its anterior three fourths is formed by the palatine process of the maxilla and the posterior fourth by the horizontal plate of the palatine bone (Fig. 62). The incisive canal is located anteriorly and is pierced by the so-called *foramina of Stensen and Scarpa,* which transmit the nasopalatine nerve. The floor is horizontal and measures about 3 inches in length from the tip of the nose to

the posterior border of the septum; it is about ½ inch wide.

Medial Wall or **Septum.** This forms a median vertical partition between the two nasal cavities. It is usually deflected from the median plane, thus reducing the size of one nasal cavity and increasing the other. It is formed posteriorly by the vomer, antero-superiorly by the perpendicular plate of the ethmoid, and antero-inferiorly by the septal cartilage. As this cartilage extends backward, it fits into the angle between the ethmoid and the vomer. Tiny projections or crests of the palatine, the maxillary, the frontal, the nasal and the sphenoid bones form peripheral parts of the bony septum. The mucous membrane of the septum is not particularly adherent. The olfactory nerve supplies the upper part of the septum, and trigeminal branches are distributed over the entire septal area. These branches include an interior nasal branch (ophthalmic nerve) and the long sphenopalatine (nasopalatine) nerve that arises from the maxillary (spheno-palatine ganglion) (Fig. 65). This nerve travels downward and forward on the septum, its branches passing through the incisive foramina to supply the mucous membrane of the anterior part of the hard palate.

Lateral Wall. This (Fig. 63) reveals 3 elevations caused by the superior, the middle and the inferior conchae (turbinate bones). Below and lateral to each concha, the corresponding nasal passage or meatus is found. Above the superior concha is the *spheno-ethmoidal* recess, a narrow space into which the sphenoid sinus opens. The scroll-shaped conchae project in a more or less horizontal direction from the lateral wall so that their free margins point downward and inward. The superior and the middle conchae arise from the ethmoid bone, but the inferior is an independent bone. The lateral nasal wall is formed by the frontal process of the maxilla, the lacrimal bone, the ethmoid, the nasal surface of the maxilla, the inferior nasal concha, the perpendicular plate of the palatine bone, and the medial pterygoid plate of the sphenoid. The *superior concha,* the smallest, is situated on the upper and back part of the lateral wall, its anterior extremity lying beneath the middle of the cribriform plate of the ethmoid bone. It does not overhang sufficiently to obscure the superior meatus, of which it forms the upper boundary. The *middle concha* extends farther than the superior and has free anterior and inferior borders. It reaches as far forward as the anterior extremity of the cribriform plate and overhangs and completely conceals the middle meatus. The *inferior concha* is an independent bone that articulates with the maxilla and the perpendicular plate of the palatine, in this way forming part of the medial wall of the maxillary sinus. Its overhanging free border covers the inferior meatus and almost reaches the floor of the nasal cavity. Its posterior end lies about 1 cm. in front of the pharyngeal orifice of the auditory (eustachian) tube. This bone may interfere with the introduction of an instrument into the eustachian tube. Its anterior end is about ¾ inch behind the orifice of the nostril. Swelling of the inferior concha usually signifies a sinus disease, most commonly the antrum, since pus from the antrum runs over it and results in inflammatory changes. The posterior end of

the concha at times reveals a polypoid growth that fills the surrounding space.

Superior Meatus. This is a short, narrow fissure in the front of which the posterior ethmoidal cells open. The *middle meatus* is situated below and lateral to the middle concha and cannot be seen unless that concha has been detached or displaced upward. The meatus continues anteriorly to a shallow depression, the *atrium,* located above the vestibule. On the lateral wall of this meatus appears the *ethmoid bulla,* a rounded elevation that is caused by the bulging of the middle ethmoid cells that open immediately above the meatus; the size of the bulla varies with that of the contained cells. Below and in front of the bulla is a groove called the *hiatus semilunaris* whose anterior end leads into the *infundibulum.* The latter is a short passage by means of which the frontal sinus enters the middle meatus. The anterior ethmoid sinuses may open into the infundibulum or directly into the hiatus; the maxillary sinus opens into the posterior aspect of the hiatus, but its orifice is usually hidden by the lower border of the groove. There may be an accessory opening of this

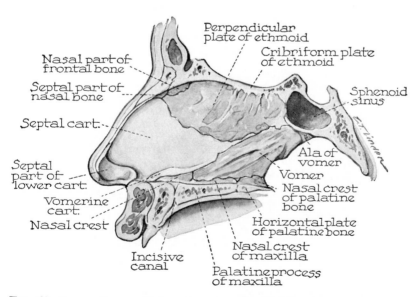

FIG. 62. Paramedian sagittal section through the left nasal fossa, showing the roof, the floor and the nasal septum of the nasal cavity.

sinus into the middle meatus behind the hiatus; the middle ethmoid air cells usually open directly onto the bulla. In summary, then, it may be stated that the anterior and the middle ethmoid cells, the frontal and the maxillary sinuses and the infundibulum all open into the middle meatus.

Inferior Meatus. This lies between the inferior concha and the floor of the nose. The *nasolacrimal duct* opens into it under cover of the anterior part of the inferior concha, this opening being about ¾ inch above the nasal floor. The spheno-ethmoid recess has been referred to as the "highest meatus" and lies between the superior concha and the roof of the nose; into this space the sphenoid sinus opens.

Cartilages. The cartilages of the nose

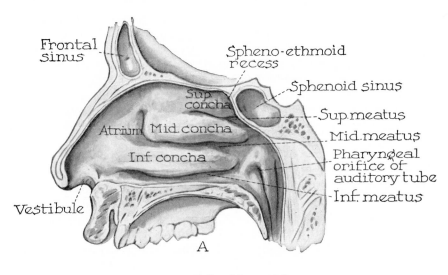

A

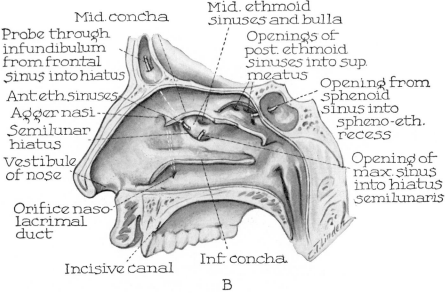

B

FIG. 63. The lateral wall of the right nasal cavity. (A) The middle and the inferior meatuses have been labeled but cannot be seen because the middle and the inferior conchae conceal them. (B) Portions of the conchae have been removed, and the communications with the paranasal sinuses are represented diagrammatically.

(Fig. 64) are 5 in number: 1 septal, 2 upper and 2 lower. Additional small flakes of cartilage are found in the upper part of the ala, but the lower has none.

The *septal cartilage* (Fig. 62) is broad and quadrangular, with the following attachments: the posterosuperior border is attached to the perpendicular lamina of the ethmoid; the postero-inferior to the vomer and the maxillae; the anterosuperior to the nasal bones above and the fibrous tissue below; the antero-inferior to the septal process of the lower nasal cartilage.

The *upper nasal cartilage* is triangular and has these attachments: superior border to the nasal bone and frontal process of the maxilla; inferior to the lower cartilage; the anterior border is continuous with the septal cartilage above but separated from it by a fissure below.

The *lower nasal cartilage* is large and oval and is located above the anterior part of the nostril; it has a septal process that turns backward in the lower part of the septum.

Anterior Aperture. This aperture of the nose is pear-shaped and is formed by the nasal bones and the anterior border of the maxilla that ends in the anterior nasal spine.

The *posterior nares* (*choanae*) (Fig. 158) are each bounded laterally by the internal pterygoid lamina, medially by the vomer, above by the body of the sphenoid and the ala of the vomer, and below by the horizontal plate of the palate.

The *vestibule* of the nose is the dilation inside the nostril that is lined by a squamous epithelium and from the lower border of which the vibrissae grow; it is bounded above by a ridge that separates it from the atrium, a depressed area in front of the middle meatus, which is in turn bounded by another ridge called the *agger nasi* (Fig. 63). The latter is formed by the superior turbinated crest on the frontal process of the superior maxilla.

Mucous Membrane. This is continuous with all the cavities communicating with it. The superior or olfactory portion is thin and less resistant; it covers the cribriform plate of the ethmoid and contains the endings of the olfactory nerves. The respiratory portion is thicker, more vascular, and at times forms a little padlike mass of mucous membrane that is often mistaken for a polyp. The thickness of this membrane, especially over the middle and the inferior conchae, makes nasal cavities and apertures of the nose smaller in the living than they appear in the skeleton. The mucous membrane is lined by columnar epithelium that is ciliated in the respiratory portion but nonciliated in the olfactory part. The respiratory part of the nasal mucous membrane enables the air to obtain warmth and moisture in its passages through the nose, and it also accounts for the manner in which the nasal cavity becomes occluded in the early stages of a common cold. The membrane is supplied by many glands that are most conspicuous over the lower and back parts of the outer wall and over the posterior and inferior parts of the septum. These glands may hypertrophy and become very active, and they are capable of providing a copious, watery secretion. When filled with blood, the mucous membrane of the nose swells and obliterates the interval between the bone and the septum. If the membrane becomes the seat of chronic inflammation, the upper part may become edematous and protrude from the ethmoidal region or from the middle turbinate in the form of polypi. The mucous membrane has been looked upon as mucoperiosteum and perichondrium because it is closely adherent to the underlying bone and cartilage by a fibrous layer.

VESSELS AND NERVES

Blood Supply. The blood supply of the nasal mucous membrane (Fig. 65A) is derived chiefly from the terminal part of the *internal maxillary artery* by its largest branch, the *sphenopalatine artery*. This vessel enters the nasal cavity through the sphenopalatine foramen and, after supplying branches to the lateral wall, travels downward and forward on the septum, accompanied by its corresponding nerve. An additional blood supply is provided by the *ophthalmic artery* through its anterior and posterior ethmoidal branches. The veins accompany the arteries and form a rich network beneath the mucous membrane, especially in the region of the middle and the inferior conchae. The *ethmoidal veins* drain into the superior sagittal sinus. The *nasal veins* drain into the *ophthalmic veins* and then into the cavernous sinuses. In this way an intracranial and intranasal communication is made, explaining the danger of an infected process in the nose that may extend to the meninges and the brain.

Lymph Drainage. This is accomplished by way of the deep cervical glands, following the path of the internal jugular vein.

Nerves. The nerves (Fig. 65B) associated with the nasal cavities are derived from two sources: (1) the *olfactory nerves,* which pass through the openings in the cribriform plate of the ethmoid and supply the mucous membrane of the upper third (olfactory portion) of the nasal cavities; these are non-medullated fibers and pass to the olfactory bulb; (2) the *sensory nerves* for the nasal cavity, which arise from the ophthalmic branch of the trigeminal. The ophthalmic nerve, by means of its *anterior ethmoidal branch,* gives off a branch to the septum which runs downward on the inner surface of the nasal bone over the atrium and the middle meatus; it supplies the mucous mem-

brane in this region and the cutaneous lining of the vestibular part, and appears between the nasal bones and the upper nasal cartilages to supply the skin. The *maxillary nerve* also aids in the sensation of this part of the respiratory tract via the sphenopalatine ganglion.

PRACTICAL CONSIDERATIONS

FRACTURES, RHINOSCOPY, EPISTAXIS, POLYPI AND SEPTAL DEFORMITIES

Nasal Fractures. Frequently the nasal bones are broken by direct violence. The fracture most commonly found is through the lower third of the bones where they are thinnest and have the least support. Since there is no muscle pull, the deformity that occurs is due entirely to the direction of the force; if the mucous membrane of the nose is torn, there might be an associated emphysema. Union takes place with great rapidity.

Anterior rhinoscopy is achieved by means of a light from a forehead mirror or lamp shining through a speculum introduced into the anterior cartilaginous part of the nose. The structures that may be seen and exam-

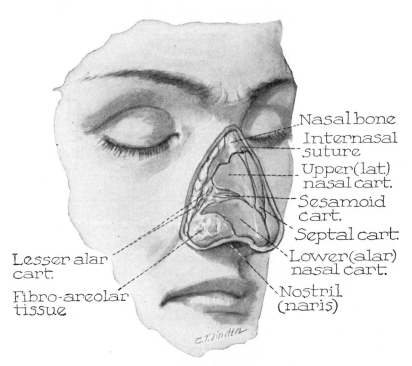

Nasal bone
Internasal suture
Upper (lat) nasal cart.
Sesamoid cart.
Septal cart.
Lower (alar) nasal cart.
Nostril (naris)

Lesser alar cart.
Fibro-areolar tissue

C.T. Linden

FIG. 64. Cartilages of the nose.

ined through this view are the inferior meatus, the anterior end of the inferior and the middle turbinates and the septum. The superior turbinate does not protrude far enough to be visualized.

Posterior rhinoscopy is accomplished by passing a small mirror over the tongue and behind the soft palate into the pharynx. Reflected light is used and the following structures are seen: the posterior nares, the septum, the middle turbinate, part of the superior and the inferior turbinates, part of the inferior meatus, the middle meatus, the eustachian tube, the mucous membrane of the roof and the upper part of the nasopharynx.

Epistaxis (Nose Bleeds). The vascularity of the nose is great, and trauma is frequent, which explains the frequency of nose bleeds, although many other causes exist. If the

bleeding originates from the anterior portion of the septum, as it most frequently does, it may be stopped by pressure through the anterior nares. Packing of the posterior nares is accomplished by passing a soft rubber catheter into the nostril until it appears in the pharynx, where it is grasped and drawn out through the mouth. Then a strong ligature is attached to the tip of the catheter and a pledget of gauze to the other end of the ligature about one foot from the tip of the catheter. Next, both catheter and ligature are withdrawn from the nostrils. The silk ligature is drawn out of the nostril, and traction is put on it so that the gauze pack is applied forcibly to the bleeding area in the posterior region. This traction can be maintained by tying the ligature over a pledget of gauze at the nostril. A second ligature can be attached to the posterior pledget, and this

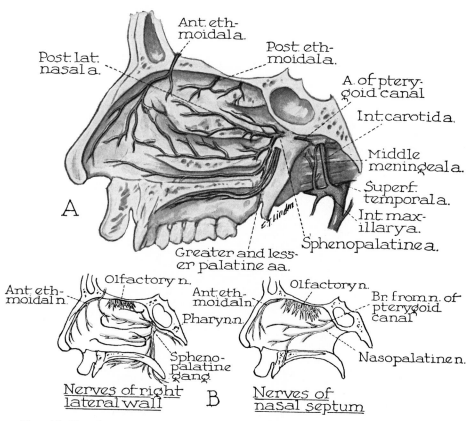

Fig. 65. Vessels and nerves of the nose: (A) blood supply to the lateral wall of the right nasal cavity, (B) nerve supply to the right lateral wall and the septum of the nose.

is left hanging out of the mouth so that removal of the pack can be accomplished by traction on the second ligature. These ligature ends may be placed over the ear for convenience.

Polypi have a predilection for the nasal fossae and may block the nostrils, thus interfering with respiration. They may press outward, widen the nose and project through the anterior or posterior nares. If the nasal duct is pressed upon by a growth in the nose, epiphora or tearing may be an early symptom. Polypi have been known to press on the palate and encroach on the mouth. Their removal can be accomplished by grasping the polyp in a forceps, applying a snare wire

about its base and dividing it. Very often polypi are the result of disease of the bone and then require procedures that include removal of the bone or drainage of the sinus.

Deformities of the Septum (Fig. 66). To some degree these are the rule rather than the exception among civilized people. Only in a small proportion are symptoms present that require correction. Submucous resection is now the accepted procedure. The incision is usually convex forward and should be so placed that a sufficient piece of cartilage is left in front to support the tip of the nose. Then a suitable elevator is inserted between the mucoperichondrium and the cartilage, and the former is lifted carefully over the

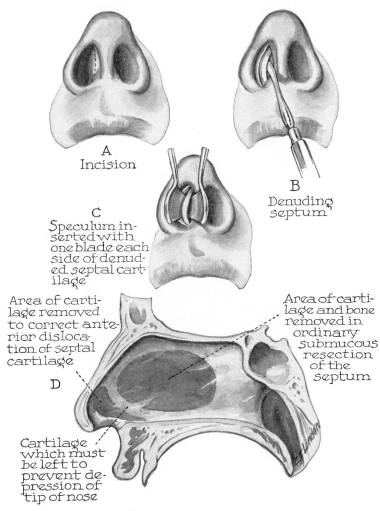

A
Incision

B
Denuding septum

C
Speculum inserted with one blade each side of denuded septal cartilage

Area of cartilage removed to correct anterior dislocation of septal cartilage

D

Area of cartilage and bone removed in ordinary submucous resection of the septum

Cartilage which must be left to prevent depression of tip of nose

FIG. 66. Submucous resection for the correction of a deviated septum.

whole extent of the cartilaginous deviation. The necessary part and amount of cartilage is then removed. The flaps are allowed to fall together, and packing is inserted into each nasal cavity. This ensures apposition of the raw surfaces.

PARANASAL SINUSES

(Figs. 67, 68, 69.) The paranasal sinuses are irregular air spaces or diverticula originating from buds of mucous membrane that sprout from the nasal cavities and grow into the diploic layer of certain bones. Each sinus takes its name from the bone in which it is situated: maxillary (antrum of Highmore), frontal, ethmoid and sphenoid. These sinuses are enclosed in compact bone. They communicate with the nasal cavities with which their mucous membranes are continuous and are filled with air. They communicate with the nasal cavities by means of narrow orifices that may become occluded because of congested mucous membrane. Like the mucous lining of the nose, the membrane lining the sinuses is covered with ciliated epithelium. The anatomy of the paranasal sinuses is somewhat inconstant, since there is no definite constancy in their size, shape and type. Under normal conditions during respiration there is an interchange of air between them.

MAXILLARY SINUS (ANTRUM OF HIGHMORE)

This maxillary sinus is the largest of the paranasal sinuses and is the first to appear. Although it begins to develop about the 4th month of intra-uterine life, it continues to grow in the adult, acquiring its maximum development in the 2nd or the 3rd decade. The sinus varies considerably in size in different individuals, but the following have been given as the average dimensions: anteroposterior, 1¼ inches; transverse, 1 inch; vertical, 1½ inches.

Situated in the interior of the superior maxilla, the base of this pyramidal cavity is

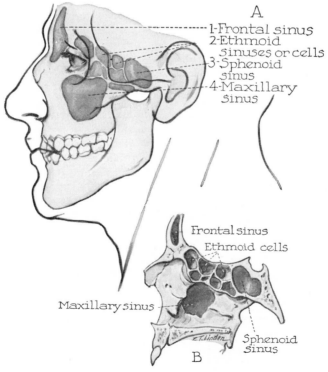

FIG. 67. Paranasal sinuses: (A) surface projection of the sinuses, (B) sagittal section (semidiagrammatic), showing the 4 paranasal sinuses.

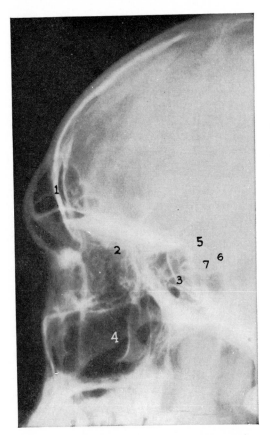

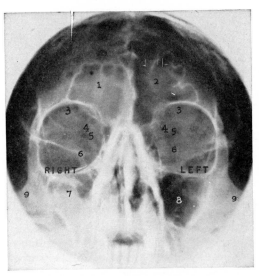

FIG. 69. X-ray projection for the upper half of the orbit, showing an effusion in the right maxillary and the frontal sinuses. These should be compared with the normal sinuses on the left side: (1) right frontal sinus, obliterated by effusion; (2) left frontal sinus, normal appearance; (3) roof of the orbit; (4) lesser wing of the sphenoid; (5) sphenoidal fissure; (6) greater wing of the sphenoid; (7) right maxillary sinus, obliterated by effusion; (8) left maxillary sinus, normal appearance; (9) zygoma.

FIG. 68. Normal x-ray appearance of the paranasal sinuses in a lateral projection: (1) frontal sinuses, (2) ethmoid cells, (3) sphenoid sinus, (4) maxillary sinuses, (5) anterior clinoid processes of the sella turcica, (6) posterior clinoid processes of the sella turcica, (7) sella turcica.

formed by the lateral wall of the nasal cavity, and the apex extends to the zygomatic process; its roof is formed by the orbital wall, which is frequently ridged by the infra-orbital canal, and its floor by the alveolar process. In front the pyramid is bounded by the facial surface of the superior maxilla and behind by the zygomatic surface of the same bone. This sinus lies lateral to the lower half of the nasal cavity in front of the pterygopalatine and the infratemporal fossae, below the orbit and above the molar teeth.

The infra-orbital nerves and vessels lie in the roof of the sinus, and their branches to the incisor, the canine and the premolar teeth descend in the anterolateral wall. This nerve produces infra-orbital facial pain when the maxillary sinus is diseased.

The floor formed by the alveolar margin is about ½ inch below the nose, and in it are seen elevations produced by the roots of some of the upper teeth, the most usual being the 1st and the 2nd molars. It is possible that all true maxillary teeth (canine to the "wisdom") may be in relation to it. At times the roots actually project into the sinus, but as a rule they produce a bulge into the floor and are separated from the cavity by a thin layer of spongy bone. This relationship between teeth and sinus explains the production of maxillary disease by infected teeth and also the establishment of drainage for an empyema of the sinus by removal of one of these teeth. The floor of the sinus is not smooth, since it presents incomplete septa that form pockets in which inflammatory products may stagnate. Such pockets may be inaccessible to treatment and must be handled individually. The nerves and the vessels to the molar teeth descend in the lower part of the posterior wall of the antrum. The sinus drains into the infundibulum of the middle meatus of the nose by means of a maxillary ostium; this opening varies from a tiny slit to a complete replacement of the floor of the infundibulum. The maxillary sinus is more frequently the site of disease than are any of the other accessory sinuses (Fig. 69). Infection may take place through the upper molar alveoli and by way of the nose. Tumors of the antrum are not too uncommon; hence, knowledge of the surrounding anatomy is important. A malignant tumor may grow rapidly and by pressure upward can encroach upon the eyeball; growth downward may involve the palate and loosen the teeth; inward extension would obstruct the nostril, and backward involvement would invade the pharynx. Such growths should be treated by excision of the superior maxilla.

Surgery (Fig. 70). Acute nasal infections that are severe or have a tendency to persist may extend to the maxillary sinus as well as to any of the other sinuses. Carious teeth projecting into the sinus cavity may also be the cause of such infections, or extension from adjacent sinuses (frontal, sphenoid and ethmoid) can be the inciting agent. If pus is present in the maxillary sinus, it may be visible at the middle meatus.

Of all the nasal sinuses, the maxillary is the easiest to irrigate. This can be done by one of four methods: by entering the natural opening (ostium) or by perforating the naso-antral wall directly beneath the inferior turbinate. Since the natural opening is placed at too high a level for pus to escape, it may remain stagnant. Therefore, it becomes necessary to explore or drain the antrum via another route. A needle is introduced through the nostril and is passed outward and backward. It pierces the bone under cover of the inferior turbinate (inferior nasal concha) and enters the sinus at a much lower level than the natural orifice of the cavity.

The sinus may also be entered through the region of a tooth which is at fault after that tooth has been extracted and a hole drilled upward through its socket and into the sinus. This dental approach was used for many years in empyema of the antrum, but unfortunately infections recurred from the mouth. This, plus insufficient drainage, has resulted in its being discarded by some authorities.

Another approach to the maxillary sinus —by many believed to be the best—is that which passes through the outer oral wall. The head is turned to the sound side, and the lip is retracted upward and backward. An incision is made over the roots of the teeth from the canine to the 2nd molar, and the periosteum is divided in the same line and separated from the bone. The facial wall of the antrum is opened by means of a small chisel, and the interior is curetted. Drainage into the nares may be instituted by removing the anterior part of the inferior turbinate.

FRONTAL SINUSES

The frontal sinuses, bilaterally placed cavities of variable extent situated anteriorly between the two plates of the frontal bone, have been considered as extensions of the anterior ethmoid cells. The anterior wall of each sinus is responsible for the prominence of the forehead, which is situated above the eyebrow.

Although not present at birth and not usually recognizable until the 7th year of life, this sinus may appear as early as the age of 2 years.

It is separated from its fellow by a complete bony septum which is often deviated to one side so that one sinus is larger.

The septum thins as the sinuses grow and at times may even disappear by absorption. This sinus is about 1 inch in both height and width but may be much wider and considerably higher and has been known to extend backward between the two tables of the roof of the orbit.

In its peripheral parts there are small partitions that form loculae and produce an irregular outline. The sinus presents a posterosuperior wall, an anterior wall and a floor. The posterosuperior wall is thin, contains no diploë and separates the sinus from the meninges and the frontal convolutions of the brain. The anterior wall looks onto the forehead and contains diploë. Because of the presence of these diploë, infectious processes involving the bone (osteomyelitis) spread more readily in this wall than in the posterior.

The floor in the frontal sinus separates it from the orbit, the nose and the anterior ethmoid sinuses. The sinus opens into the nose via the infundibulum, a narrow canal that passes between the anterior ethmoid air cells. The sinus then opens into the hiatus semilunaris (Fig. 63). Due to the close relationship of sinuses and their openings, an infection in one sinus can, and usually does, spread to another. Therefore, it is not uncommon for an opening of the maxillary sinus

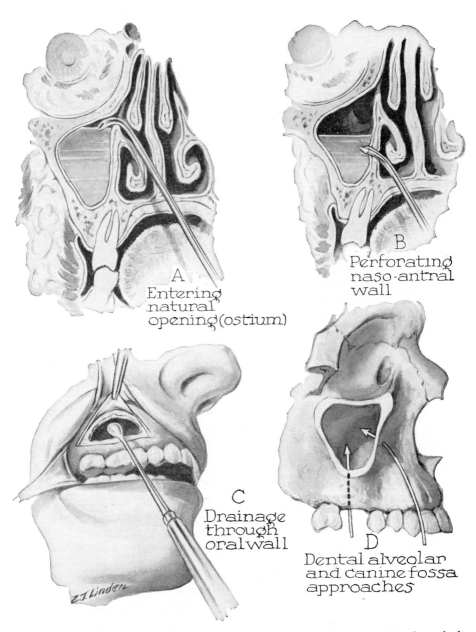

FIG. 70. Surgery of the maxillary sinus: (A) via the natural opening, (B) through the naso-antral wall, (C) the outer oral wall approach, (D) dental approaches.

to receive pus from the frontal and the anterior ethmoid cells as it travels along the hiatus semilunaris. The maxillary sinus thus becomes involved and produces its usual symptoms, which may divert attention from the true source of the infection (frontal or anterior ethmoid sinus disease).

A fracture over the frontal sinus can be depressed without injuring the cranial contents, but such fracture may be associated with emphysema of the surrounding tissues due to communication with the nose.

Inflammation of the mucous lining of the frontal sinus may be secondary to an infection in the nose; conversely, when pus forms within this sinus, it may drain into the nasal fossa. If the communication with the nose is blocked because of swelling of the lining membrane, it may give rise to serious complications by destroying the internal table and infecting the cranial contents; it may even perforate the wall of the orbit and produce serious eye complications. An early diagnosis of the presence of pus in the frontal sinus calls for opening into the sinus by trephining over the supra-orbital margin.

Extranasal and Intranasal Approaches. Interference with the normal ventilation or drainage of the frontal sinus is usually associated with marked edema in the region of the middle meatus, and the middle turbinate becomes tightly compressed against the lat-

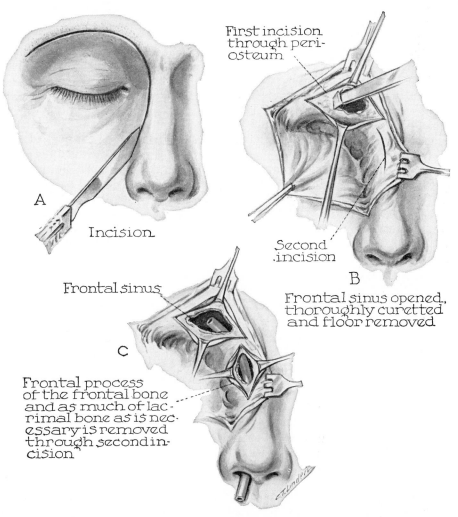

A   Incision

First incision through periosteum

Second incision

B   Frontal sinus opened, thoroughly curetted and floor removed

Frontal sinus

C

Frontal process of the frontal bone and as much of lacrimal bone as is necessary is removed through second incision

Fig. 71. Extranasal approach to a diseased frontal sinus.

eral wall. A deviation of the nasal septum also aggravates the condition, and if the inflammatory process becomes purulent, empyema of the sinus results. When the frontal duct is open, pus passing along the semilunar hiatus may involve the opening of the maxillary sinus and produce a sinusitis here. Since the anterior ethmoidal cells open with the frontal duct into the infundibulum of the semilunar hiatus, these cells too may become involved in frontal sinus disease. Osteomyelitis or abscess of the frontal bone may result and can terminate in meningitis.

An *intranasal* operation for sinus disease is utilized by some and is described under surgery of the ethmoid cells (p. 97).

The *extranasal* or external approach is usually performed in the following way (Fig. 71): the eyebrow is shaved, and an incision is made, beginning at the temporal end, extending to the middle of the root of the nose and then curving downward to the base of the nasal bone. The soft parts are freed from the bone, and then two incisions are made in the periosteum. The first is placed just above and parallel with the supra-orbital margin; the second passes over the frontal process of the maxillary bone. These two incisions do not meet. The frontal sinus is opened, thoroughly curetted, and its floor removed. The frontal process of the frontal bone and as much of the lacrimal bone as is necessary are removed through the second incision. This gives access to the ethmoid cells, and the ethmoid sinus is curetted. The operation also permits access to the anterior wall of the sphenoid sinus. Drainage is instituted by means of a tube that is placed in the upper wound, carried under the bridge of the bone through the nose and out at the nostril.

SPHENOID SINUS

The sphenoid sinus, a large cavity situated in the body of the sphenoid bone, is divided into right and left halves by a complete bony septum usually bent to one side (Fig. 67). Each half has been referred to as a sphenoid sinus, and each has its own opening. The sinus may be limited to the anterior part of the bone, but usually occupies the whole of its body, extending into the wings of the sphenoid, the pterygoid process and even into the basilar process of the occipital bone.

Formation of the sinus begins in the 5th month of intrauterine life as a recess of the nasal cavity but does not extend into the body of the sphenoid until the 7th year.

Both sinuses have important relationships above, below, in front and laterally. Above the sphenoid sinus, the pituitary body and the optic nerve are found, the nerve at times forming a ridge inside the sinus. This close relationship causes the optic nerve to be involved in sphenoid sinusitis, giving rise to sudden loss of vision (retrobulbar neuritis). The sinus is bounded below by the nose. In front, the wall of the sinus separates it from the ethmoid air cells, and laterally the cavernous sinuses containing the internal carotid artery and the 6th nerve are located. The abducens, the oculomotor and the trochlear nerves, and the ophthalmic and the maxillary divisions of the trigeminal nerve may be involved in disease of the sphenoid sinus, which is considered a "danger spot" in the skull because of these important surrounding structures. Each half of the sinus has an orifice of its own that opens into the highest meatus, the spheno-ethmoid recess.

Surgery. The sphenoid sinuses may be drained by an external route as described in operations involving the frontal sinuses, or through a nasal route (Fig. 72B). In the *nasal route* the posterior half of the middle turbinate is removed, and a small hook or curette is introduced upon the anterior superior wall of the nasal cavity. The point of this curette is carried downward and then turned forward and outward toward the eye of the involved side. It is firmly pressed into the posterior ethmoid labyrinth and then drawn forward and downward. The posterior wall of the labyrinth is entirely broken down. The sphenoid sinus is located, entered, and its anterior wall removed.

ETHMOID SINUSES (CELLS)

There are from 8 to 10 very thin-walled intercommunicating cavities occupying the greater part of the ethmoid labyrinth and known as the ethmoid sinuses. The boundaries of these sinuses are completed by the frontal, the palatine, the sphenoid bones and the superior maxilla.

They have been divided arbitrarily into three sets: anterior, middle and posterior. The anterior ethmoid sinuses open into the middle meatus on the floor of the hiatus semilunaris; the middle ethmoid sinuses open into the middle meatus on the surface of the bulla ethmoidalis; the posterior, into the superior meatus.

Above the ethmoid sinuses are the meninges and the frontal convolutions in the anterior cranial fossa; in the front is the frontal sinus; behind is the sphenoid; below, the nose; and laterally, the orbit. The ethmoid cells in each labyrinth may vary from 4 large cells to 17 small ones, the average number being 9.

These spaces are separated from their surrounding structures by extremely thin plates of bone (lamina papyracea); because of this, infection may spread to the surrounding parts quite readily. This explains why ethmoiditis is the most common cause of

orbital cellulitis. The relations of the ethmoid air sinuses to the cranial cavity are more extensive than those of the frontal and the sphenoid; hence, meningitis, subdural abscess, cerebral abscess and sinus thrombosis may complicate ethmoiditis. It should be recalled that the frontal sinus has been considered as one of the anterior ethmoid cells.

Nasal Approach. Acute inflammation of the ethmoid cells at times is associated with acute rhinitis (common cold) and diseases of the frontal and the maxillary sinuses. The diseased ethmoid sinus can be opened and drained externally by procedures that have been described for frontal sinus drainage, but more frequently the nasal route is used (Fig. 72A). A curette is introduced into the nasal cavity through the vestibule and carried to the anterior attachment of the middle turbinate. This is pressed firmly downward from the orbit and removes the anterior aspect of the turbinate. The curette is carried through the turbinate, the hiatus semilunaris removed, and entrance gained to the anterior

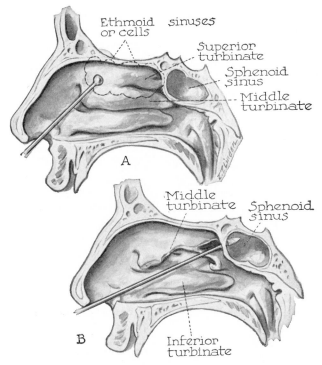

FIG. 72. Surgery of the sphenoid and the ethmoid sinuses: (A) nasal approach to the ethmoid sinuses (cells); (B) nasal approach to the sphenoid sinus.

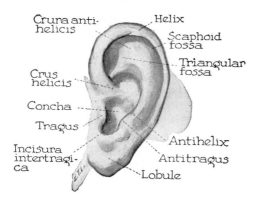

Cruna anti-
helicis
Crus
helicis
Concha
Tragus
Incisura
intertragi-
ca
Helix
Scaphoid
fossa
Triangular
fossa
Antihelix
Antitragus
Lobule

FIG. 73. The external ear.

ethmoid labyrinth. These cells are removed from before backward by the curette; usually, the entire middle turbinate is removed.

AUDITORY APPARATUS

For the purpose of description the ear is divided into 3 parts: external, middle, and internal.

EXTERNAL EAR

The external ear (Fig. 73) is made up of the auricle (pinna) and the external auditory meatus. Its purpose is to collect and convey sound waves to the tympanic membrane (ear drum).

Auricle. This contains a cartilaginous framework that permits it to retain its characteristic form, but at its most dependent point, the lobule, the cartilage is replaced by fibrofatty tissue.

The *helix* is the outer margin or rim of the auricle that forms the rolled superior and posterior margins and continues into the lobule. On the posterosuperior aspect of the helix a small tubercle known as *Darwin's tubercle* is found.

The *antihelix* forms a curved ridge that runs somewhat parallel with the helix, ends below in a small tubercle called the *antitragus* and bifurcates above into two limbs that form the boundary of a shallow depression known as the *fossa triangularis*.

The *concha* is the centrally placed deep cavity of the auricle; this is divided into an upper and a lower part by a ridge known as the *crus helicis*, the upper part lying over *Macewen's triangle*. If a fingertip is placed

into this upper part of the concha, it will come into contact with a depressed area of bone that forms the floor of Macewen's triangle, which is bounded above by the suprameatal crest. The lower part of the concha leads into the external auditory meatus and is bounded by the *tragus*, which forms a backward projection somewhat semilunar in shape, and partially obscures the opening of the meatus.

The *incisura intertragica*, a notch, bounds the tragus inferiorly and separates it from the antitragus. The antihelix forms the posterior boundary of the concha.

The *skin* of the lateral surface of the auricle is supplied by the great auricular nerve over its lower third and the auriculotemporal nerve over its upper two thirds; the medial surface is supplied over its lower third by the great auricular and over its upper two thirds by the lesser occipital nerves.

There are intrinsic and extrinsic *ligaments* in the auricle, the former maintaining the cartilage in position, and the latter attaching the auricle to the temporal bone.

There are also intrinsic and extrinsic *muscles* that are rudimentary and of no practical importance. The small intrinsic muscles are 6 in number, and all are supplied by the facial nerve.

The auricle receives its *arterial supply* from the external carotid by way of the *posterior auricular artery* behind and the superficial temporal artery in front. Its *venous drainage* is by means of the superficial temporal veins in front and the external jugular below.

The *lymph vessels* of the ear rarely drain into the retro-auricular glands but drain into the mastoid glands, which are situated at the tip of the mastoid process where the efferent lymphatics pierce the sternocleidomastoid and enter the deep cervical chain. The external aspect of the auricle drains into the preauricular gland, then into the deep cervical chain.

External Auditory Meatus (Fig. 74). This canal extends from the concha to the tympanic membrane; it is about 1¼ inches long, the first half being cartilaginous and the remainder osseous. On looking into this tube its entire length cannot be visualized, because its floor rises for a short distance and then recedes; in its midportion there is a slight backward and inward curve. The lower wall of the canal is longer than its upper, and it is narrowest about its middle.

If examination of the external auditory meatus is desired, it is necessary to straighten out its tortuous course by pulling upward and backward on the auricle.

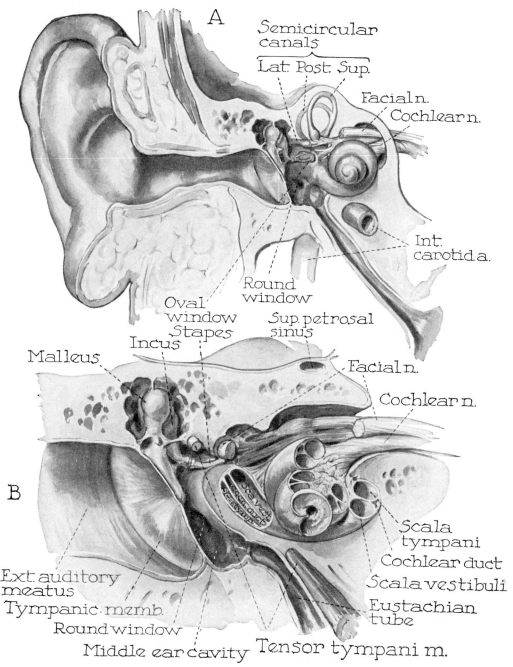

FIG. 74. Diagram of a frontal section through the right external, the middle and the inner ear: (A) external, middle and internal ear, coronal section; (B) enlarged diagram of the middle and the internal ear, with the cochlea cut.

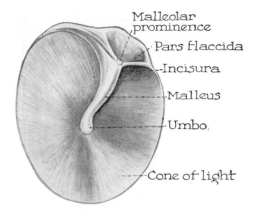

Malleolar prominence

Pars flaccida

Incisura

Malleus

Umbo

Cone of light

Fig. 75A. The right tympanic membrane (ear drum).

The *skin* of the cartilaginous portion is supplied with hair follicles and sebaceous and ceruminous glands. Since it is firmly bound down to the perichondrium and the periosteum, infections of the canal give rise to severe pain but little swelling.

The *cutaneous nerve supply* to this region is derived from the auriculotemporal nerve and the auricular branch of the vagus nerve.

The meatus has superior, anterior and posterior relationships. The *superior wall* is separated from the middle cranial fossa by a thin plate of bone; hence, suppuration in the meatus may penetrate this bone and cause meningitis. The *anterior wall* is in relation to the parotid gland, and abscesses of this gland can extend into the meatus. The lower jaw also lies in front of the canal so that injuries, such as falls on the chin, may fracture this wall and produce hemorrhage from the meatus, which may be confused with bleeding from the ear as seen in basal skull fracture. The *posterior wall* is bony and separates the meatus from the mastoid cells; pus from these cells may discharge into it.

Tympanic Membrane

The tympanic membrane (ear drum) separates the external and the middle ears and consists of outer (cutaneous), inner (mucous) and intermediate (fibrous) layers. The cutaneous layer is continuous with the skin of the external auditory canal, and the inner mucous membrane is continuous with the lining of the tympanic cavity.

The tympanic membrane forms the lateral protecting wall of the tympanic cavity and transmits the vibrations of sound waves along the auditory ossicles to the labyrinth. It is placed obliquely so that its outer or lateral surface faces downward, forward and laterally, forming an angle of about 45° with the floor of the meatus (Fig. 74). As a result of this obliquity, the floor and the anterior wall of the meatus are longer than the roof and the posterior wall. The membrane bulges into the middle ear; hence, its lateral surface is concave. The deepest part of this concavity is called the *umbo* and corresponds to the tip of the handle of the malleus.

Otoscopic Examination. On otoscopic examination, a healthy tympanic membrane is of a pearly gray color (Fig. 75A). Its circumference, except in the upper part, is somewhat thickened and fits into a groove in the temporal bone. The unattached upper part of the circumference measures about 5 mm. and forms a "gap" known as the *tympanic notch* or *incisura*. Over this area the membrane has no strong fibrous partition but is merely represented by the continuation of the covering of the auditory canal which overlies the mucosa lining the tympanic cavity. Therefore, the upper part of the membrane is thin and loose and is called the *pars flaccida* or *Shrapnell's membrane*. From the umbo, the handle of the malleus can be seen through the membrane, running upward and forward to the periphery.

When the tympanic membrane is examined by reflected light the "cone of light" is seen which has its apex at the umbo and extends downward and forward to the periphery. This luminous triangle undergoes changes in diseases of the ear. A rather constant landmark is a small bulge that lies in the anterosuperior region and is known as the *malleolar prominence*; from this, anterior and posterior malleolar folds emerge, forming the boundaries for the flaccid portion of the membrane.

The handle of the malleus runs from the malleolar prominence downward and backward as far as the umbo. The long crus of the incus, although lying on a deeper plane, can be seen lying behind and parallel with the handle of the malleus. The chorda tympani passes across the upper portion of the membrane. The ear drum is divided into four quadrants by two imaginary oblique lines: one is drawn downward and backward along the line of the handle of the malleus, the other at right angles to the first, downward and forward through the umbo. In this way two superior and two inferior quadrants are developed.

The membrane is normally held taut by the tensor tympani muscle. If the membrane ruptures from violent pressure, it usually gives way at the antero-inferior quadrant or in the region of the malleus. Perforations of the inferior quadrants are usually caused by otitis media. Since the largest blood vessels are found in the region of the handle of the malleus, redness is seen here most frequently. The ear drum is supplied by two nerves: the auriculotemporal, which supplies its anterior half; and the auricular branch of the vagus, which supplies the posterior half.

Myringotomy. The *incision of the drum membrane (myringotomy)* (Fig. 75B) should be made under direct vision; it starts at the bottom and follows the periphery of the drum backward and upward. Starting at 6 o'clock, it passes through 7, 8, 9, 10 and stops at 11 o'clock, thus avoiding important structures and providing adequate drainage. At its starting point such an incision avoids an abnormal jugular bulb, and at its upper end it avoids the incudostapedial articulation and the chorda tympani.

MIDDLE EAR

The middle ear (tympanic cavity) (Fig. 76), an air space in the petrous portion of the temporal bone, is lined by mucous membrane and contains the auditory ossicles (malleus, incus and stapes) which transmit sound vibrations from the tympanic membrane to the internal ear. The tympanic cavity is about ½ inch in length and height and about one tenth to one sixth of an inch wide.

Its uppermost part, the *epitympanic recess* or attic, lies above the level of the tympanic membrane and contains the head of the malleus and the body of the incus. In the walls of this recess are found several small compartments that may harbor infections which become chronic because of inadequate drainage. The roof of the epitympanic recess is a thin plate of bone called the *tegmen tympani*, which separates the recess from the middle cranial fossa.

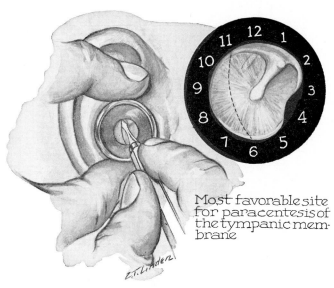

Most favorable site for paracentesis of the tympanic membrane

FIG. 75B. Paracentesis of the right tympanic membrane (myringotomy). The incision extends between 6 and 11 o'clock.

The middle ear has a roof, a floor and 4 walls: lateral, medial, anterior and posterior.

The **roof** is formed by the tegmen tympani, a thin plate of bone separating it from the middle cranial fossa and the temporal lobe of the brain.

The **floor** is narrow and consists of thin bone separating the tympanic cavity from the jugular fossa.

The **lateral wall** is formed mainly by the tympanic membrane, which does not reach the roof of the cavity, the upper part of this wall being formed by the squamous portion of the temporal bone.

The **medial wall** (Fig. 74) separates the tympanic cavity from the internal ear and presents the following: The *foramen ovale* (fenestra vestibuli) leads into the vestibule and is occupied by the base of the stapes. The *promontory*, a rounded projection formed by the first turn of the cochlea, is placed below the foramen ovale. The *foramen rotundum* (fenestra cochlea) lies at the bottom of a funnel-shaped depression that is situated behind the promontory and is closed by a membrane known as the *secondary tympanic membrane* which covers an

aperture in the bone leading to the scala tympani of the cochlea. Finally, the *prominence of the facial canal* is produced by the facial nerve running backward along the upper part of the medial wall, then turning downward in the medial wall of the aditus.

The **anterior wall** opens directly into the *auditory (eustachian) tube*. This tube runs downward, forward and medially into the nasopharynx, except in children where the direction of the tube is practically horizontal. The middle ear is most commonly infected by micro-organisms which pass along the eustachian tube from an infected nasopharynx. Above, the tube lodges the tensor tympani muscle, and the bone to its medial side makes up the lateral wall of the carotid canal.

The **posterior wall** presents a large aperture above known as the *aditus*; this leads to the tympanic antrum. Below this the *pyramid* is found just behind the foramen ovale and contains the stapedius muscle, the tendon of which projects through the apex.

Since the middle ear is frequently diseased, its relation to important structures and various paths through which infection

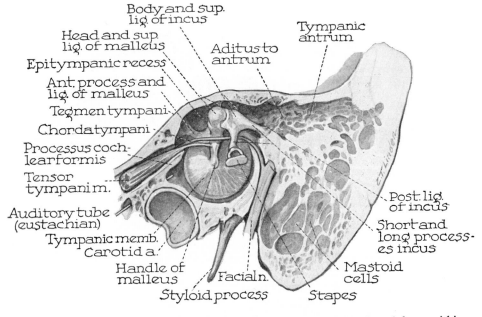

Fig. 76. Sagittal section of right tympanic cavity (middle ear), viewed from within.

may travel becomes important. Infection may result in: (1) erosion through the roof, causing meningitis or intracranial abscess; (2) involvement through the tympanic floor encroaching upon the internal jugular vein and causing fatal hemorrhage or septic thrombophlebitis; (3) erosion of the anterior wall, followed by ulceration into the carotid artery with fatal hemorrhage; (4) extension to the prominence of the facial canal on the medial wall, resulting in permanent facial paralysis; (5) involvement of the internal ear with resultant permanent deafness; (6) infection of the mastoid antrum and cells (mastoiditis).

The **muscles** of importance in this region are the tensor tympani and the stapedius. The *tensor tympani muscle* lies in a small canal above the eustachian tube, taking its origin from the cartilage of this tube. Its tendon bends at right angles around a bony pulley, runs laterally across the cavity of the middle ear and is inserted into the medial side of the manubrium of the malleus. It is innervated by the mandibular nerve (otic ganglion), and its action is indicated by its name. The *stapedius muscle* is lodged in the pyramid, from the apex of which its tendon issues, and is inserted into the posterior part of the neck of the stapes. This muscle draws the neck of the stapes backward and is innervated by the facial nerve.

Auditory Ossicles (Fig. 76). There are three auditory ossicles: malleus, incus and stapes; they form a bony chain across the middle ear, passing from the tympanic membrane to the foramen ovale.

The *malleus* (hammer) has 5 parts: (1) a head, which is the thickened upper part and contains a facet on its posterior surface for articulation with the body of the incus; (2) a neck, which is a constriction below the head; (3) the handle (manubrium), which is a long, tapering process passing downward and backward, closely attached in its whole extent to the tympanic membrane and continuing backward to the umbo; (4) the lateral process, which arises from the root of the handle and projects laterally; it attaches to the tympanic membrane by the anterior and the posterior malleolar folds that bound the flaccid part of the ear drum;

(5) the anterior process, a slender spicule that passes from the neck downward and forward to the squamotympanic fissure.

The *incus* (anvil) is a bone that has been likened to a 2-fanged tooth that has 3 parts: (1) a body that articulates in front by a funnel-shaped facet with the head of the malleus; (2) the short process attached to the margin of the aditus; (3) the long process, which passes downward, behind and parallel with the handle of the malleus. The tip projects medially and terminates in the lentiform nodule that articulates with the head of the stapes. The shadow of the long process at times may be seen in the posterior part of the membrane on otoscopic examination.

The *stapes* (stirrup) consists of a head that faces laterally and articulates with the lentiform nodule of the incus; the neck, where the tendon of the stapedius is inserted; the limbs that arise from the constricted neck and pass medially to the extremities of the base, the anterior limb being shorter and straighter than the posterior; the base that dips into the foramen ovale is kidney-shaped, the more convex border of the kidney appearing uppermost, and is held firmly in place in the foramen by an annular ligament. The bones are connected by joints lined by synovia and are bound together and secured to the walls of the cavity by the following ligaments: the anterior ligament of the malleus, passing between the lateral process and the posterior malleolar fold; the superior ligament of the malleus, passing between the head of the malleus and the roof of the tympanic cavity; the posterior ligament of the incus, passing between the short process of the incus and the posterior wall of the tympanic cavity; the annular ligament of the stapes, connecting the base of the stapes with the apex of the foramen ovale.

The tympanic cavity contains folds of mucous membrane that extend from the inner walls to the ossicles. The continuation of this mucous membrane with that lining the auditory tube, the mastoid antrum and the mastoid air cells explains the ever-present danger of pharyngeal infections spreading to the tympanic cavity, ear bones and air spaces.

Tympanic (Mastoid) Antrum. The *tympanic* antrum is a large recess situated in the posterior part of the petrous portion of the temporal bone. It is about the size of a small pea and is really a large mastoid air cell (Fig. 76).

The *aditus* (aditus ad antrum), an oval slit with its long axis nearly vertical and measuring about a ¼ inch, connects the epitympanic recess with the antrum. Any obstruction of this narrow aperture favors stasis and retention of inflammatory exudates that may find their way to the mastoid cells. Both the aditus and the antrum lie just below the tegmen tympani. Since the aditus opens close to the roof of the antrum, it is not in an efficient place to drain that cavity.

The tympanic antrum is relatively larger and more superficial in the child than in the adult. *Superiorly*, it has a roof that is the backward continuation of the tegmen tympani and is, therefore, in close relationship to the middle cranial fossa and the temporal lobe of the brain. Involvement of this wall may cause a subtemporal abscess. Its *anterior* wall has in its upper part an opening which communicates with the epitympanic recess; this opening has been referred to above as the aditus. Its *posterior* wall opens into mastoid air cells and separates the antrum from the sigmoid (transverse) sinus and the cerebellar hemisphere. The *lateral* wall is formed by the squamous part of the temporal bone, is about ½ inch thick in the adult, is the wall of surgical approach and projects laterally in that part of the temporal bone that is covered by the auricle.

Above the promontory and even above the fenestra vestibuli is found the *canal for the facial nerve (aqueduct of Fallopius)*. This canal contains the facial nerve as it travels in its intrapetrous portion. It also forms a ridge, the wall of which is so extremely thin that the nerve may be seen through it. Above the fenestra ovalis the facial canal, together with the external semicircular canal, form the inner boundary of the aditus. This is an important relationship and should be kept in mind in any operative procedure in this region. At the medial wall of the aditus the facial canal curves downward and opens on the inferior surface of the temporal bone at the stylomastoid foramen.

The *chorda tympani nerve* passes forward between the handle of the malleus and the long process of the incus, reaching a small opening in front of the upper part of the tympanic ring.

The *mastoid process* does not exist at birth but begins its development at the end of the first year. As it grows, its diploë is gradually replaced by air cells.

The *mastoid cells* usually occupy the whole of the mastoid process, which has a very thin coating of compact bone. In the upper part the cells communicate with the antrum; at the middle of the mastoid process they increase in size. Since the mastoid cells are developed as outgrowths from the mucous membrane of the middle ear and the antrum, they are lined by the membrane and are filled with air from these cavities. The cells near the apex of the mastoid are smaller and do not communicate with those above; the lowermost cells contain marrow and not air and represent the unaltered diploë of the cranial bones. Infection from the tympanic cavity may invade these cells, spread down the mastoid process and invade the deepest-lying cells. If the formation of air cells (pneumatisation) is complete, the entire mastoid process is composed of these large air spaces; this is known as the pneumatic type of mastoid. However, if pneumatisation is interfered with so that the cells do not develop, the diploic type of mastoid process results, in which the structure resembles the other cranial bones (outer and inner tables with diploë between). When this occurs, the antrum is the only cell present. The sclerotic type of mastoid process is one in which the process is composed of very dense compact bone and is usually the result of a chronic infection that has interfered with the absorption of the diploë and the pneumatisation process. It results in an acellular mastoid that is extremely hard.

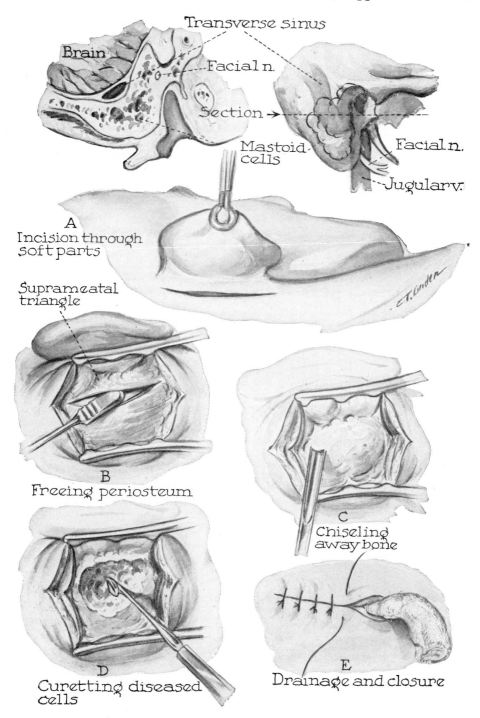

FIG. 77. Simple mastoid operation (antrotomy). The two uppermost figures reveal the surgical anatomy in the region to be explored. Note the level at which the section is taken in the figure on the right and then shown in cross section in the figure on the left. Figures A to E depict the steps in the operation.

CLINICAL AND SURGICAL CONSIDERATIONS

Mastoiditis, Simple and Radical Mastoid Surgery

In **mastoiditis**, suppurating mastoid cells can involve the lateral sinus. This involvement may be the result of contamination of the small veins that reach the sinus through the bone or by direct infection from a perisinus abscess. From the lateral sinus, extension can take place to the internal jugular vein or even to the other side of the skull by way of the confluence of sinuses. Mastoid disease may extend upward through the roof of the antrum, involve the brain and the meninges and result in meningitis, extradural or brain abscesses.

Mastoiditis usually follows an acute disease of the tympanic cavity because of the mucous membrane continuity. Once the mastoid cells have become involved, the infection may spread in one of many ways, traveling either to the transverse sinus or to the meninges and the brain; the facial nerve may become involved, or the cortex of the mastoid process itself might be perforated.

In performing a **simple mastoid operation (mastoidectomy or antrotomy)**, it is possible to injure vital structures (Fig. 77). If the opening in the antrum extends too far upward, the middle cranial fossa may be opened; if too far backward, the transverse sinus is entered, and if the opening is placed too deep, the facial nerve may be injured. In doing this operation, an incision is made about ½ inch posterior to and parallel with the insertion of the auricle; separation of the soft parts from the bone subperiosteally is carried anteriorly to the posterior margin of the auditory canal, superiorly and anteriorly to the suprameatal spine and posteriorly far enough to expose the mastoid process. Chiseling is begun in an angle formed by the temporal line above and the posterior bony wall of the canal in front. The chisel should always chip in a direction parallel with the auditory meatus. After the antrum is opened, it is explored, and the opening is enlarged as desired. The diseased cells and carious bone are removed; the wound is irrigated, dried and packed. Closure with drainage follows.

The **radical mastoid operation** converts the mastoid antrum, the cells and the middle ear into a single cavity, and all the ossicles except the stapes are removed.

Auditory (Pharyngotympanic, Eustachian) Tube. The pharyngotympanic tube is an osseocartilaginous tube about 1½ inches long which connects the tympanic cavity with the nasopharynx (Fig. 74). The posterior third is bony, and the anterior two thirds partly cartilaginous and partly fibrous. The mucous membrane lining the tube is continuous with that of the middle ear and the pharynx.

Through this tube the air pressure on both sides of the ear drum is equalized; should the tube become obstructed by edema, etc., air cannot enter, and a negative pressure results in the tympanic cavity. With the atmospheric pressure on the outer side of the drum, the membrane retracts into the cavity and a sensation of fullness in the ear results. The course of the tube is downward, medially and forward from the tympanic cavity, its narrowest part, the isthmus, lying at the junction of the cartilaginous and bony parts.

The cartilaginous portion opens from the lateral wall of the nasal fossa close to the pharyngeal opening and presents medial and lateral walls which lie so close together that only a slitlike cavity results.

The bony part of the tube is in relation superiorly to the canal of the tensor tympani muscle, anterolaterally to the petrotympanic fissure, and posteromedially to the carotid canal and its contents (Fig. 76). Normally, the pharyngeal orifice is closed. During swallowing and yawning it opens by means of the action of the tensor veli palatini muscle. The tympanic orifice is located in the anterior wall of the tympanic cavity below the canal for the tensor tympani muscle.

Inflation of the middle ear may be accomplished by *Valsalva's method*. The patient closes the mouth and the nose and forcibly blows out the cheeks. This drives air through the auditory tube, a sense of fullness is felt in the ears and hearing is diminished because of the resulting distention of the tympanic membrane. The same may be accomplished by the *Politzer method*, where the nozzle of a Politzer bag is inserted into the nostril, and the nose is closed. The patient then swallows, and the bag is compressed, forcing air into the tympanum.

INTERNAL EAR

The internal ear (labyrinth) is situated in the petrous portion of the temporal bone and is concerned with sound perception, orientation and balancing (Figs. 78, 79). It consists of two labyrinths, a bony labyrinth which contains a membranous one. For the greater part, the membranous labyrinth is not in contact with its bony labyrinth but is surrounded by a fluid known as perilymph.

The **bony labyrinth** is about 3 mm. thick. It is as hard as ivory and consists of the cochlea, the vestibule and the semicircular canals (Fig. 79).

The **cochlea** resembles a small shell that makes 2½ turns. It may also be likened to a spiral staircase that makes its turns around a central pillar called the *modiolus*. The promontory on the medial wall of the tympanic cavity is formed by the first coil of the cochlea. The base of the cochlea passes backward and medially to form part of the floor of the meatus. The apex of the cochlea is directed forward and lateralward. A spiral ledge of bone projects from the modiolus and divides the cochlea into a *scala vestibuli* in front and a *scala tympani* behind (Fig. 74). The aqueduct of the cochlea passes from the scala tympani through the petrous bone to the notch at the margin of the jugular foramen. This duct brings the perilymph of the bony labyrinth and the cerebrospinal fluid of the subarachnoid space into communication. The cochlea opens posteriorly into the bony vestibule, which contains the membranous saccule and the utricle.

Vestibule. The central part of the bony labyrinth is situated behind the cochlea, in front of the semicircular canals and medial to the tympanic cavity. On its lateral (tympanic) wall is the *fenestra vestibuli*, which is closed by the stapes. Medially, it communicates with the posterior cranial fossa through the aqueduct of the vestibule. The 5 openings of the semicircular canals are found in the posterior part of the vestibule. On the lateral wall the secondary tympanic membrane closes the fenestra of the cochlea, thus separating the perilymphatic space from the tympanic cavity.

Semicircular Canals. The 3 bony semi-

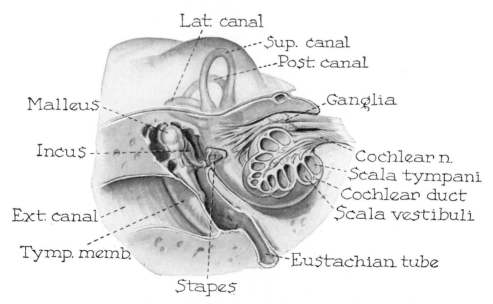

FIG. 78. The middle and the internal ear, seen from above.

circular canals are horseshoe-shaped, contain the membranous semicircular ducts and open into the posterior part of the vestibule. They are from 12 to 22 mm. in length, and each is less than 1 mm. in diameter, except at one end where they form a bulge known as the ampulla. They are named superior, posterior and lateral. The superior is nearly coronal, the posterior nearly sagittal, the lateral nearly horizontal. The anterior part of the lateral canal lies in the medial wall of the aditus immediately above the canal for the facial nerve. These 3 canals open into the vestibule by only 5 apertures because the medial end of the superior joins the upper end of the posterior, forming a single canal known as the common crus.

Membranous Labyrinth. This lies within the bony labyrinth and consists of sacs that contain a fluid known as *endolymph* (Fig. 79C). It has the same general form as has the bony labyrinth but is somewhat smaller and is separated from the bony walls by a fluid known as *perilymph*. It differs in form slightly from the bony labyrinth in the region of the osseous vestibule where the mem-

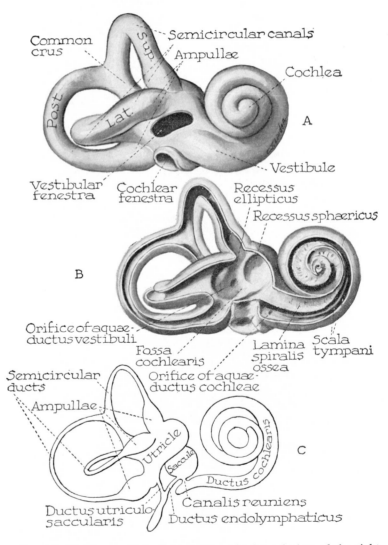

Fig. 79. The internal ear (labyrinth): (A) lateral view of the right bony labyrinth, (B) interior of the right bony labyrinth, (C) the membranous labyrinth.

branous labyrinth consists of 2 membranous sacs: the utricle and the saccule. This labyrinth consists of the cochlear duct, the saccule, the utricle, and 3 semicircular ducts.

Cochlear Duct. This contains the spiral organ of Corti, which is the essential part of the organ of hearing. The membranous cochlea is a membranous tube which consists of 3 parts: scala tympani, scala vestibuli and duct of the chochlea. The last contains the spiral organ to which the cochlear nerve is distributed. The cochlear duct lies lateral to the scala vestibuli and is separated from it by the *vestibular membrane*, which passes from the spiral lamina upward and laterally to the roof of the scala. A triangular section results; this is bounded medially by the vestibular membrane, laterally and above by the lateral wall of the cochlea and below by the basilar lamina. The elongated *spiral ganglion* is situated in a canal that runs around the modiolus at the base of the spiral lamina. The peripheral branches from the ganglion pass to the organ of Corti; the central branches leave the bone through the foramina at the base of the internal auditory meatus and constitute the cochlear part of the auditory nerve. The organ of Corti presents the important functional element in the hair-bearing cells which receive the ending of the cochlear nerve. Posteriorly, the duct of the cochlea is connected with the saccule by the *canalis reuniens*, and it terminates in a blind cone-shaped extremity.

Utricle and **Saccule.** These two membranous sacs are situated in the bony vestibule and are indirectly connected to each other. The utricle, the larger of the two sacs, is situated in the posterior and upper parts of the vestibule and receives the apertures of the membranous semicircular canals posteriorly; a narrow duct called the *ductus utriculosaccularis* leaves it. The saccule is smaller and rounder, and the narrow *ductus endolymphaticus* leaves its posterior end to join the ductus utriculosaccularis. The junction of these two ducts ends in a small blind sac called the *saccus endolymphaticus* which is situated in the aqueduct of the vestibule close to the dura mater on the posterior surface of the petrous portion of the temporal bone.

Semicircular Ducts. These ducts are about one third the size of the semicircular canals, but in number, shape and form they are similar, and each presents an ampulla at one end. They open by 5 orifices into the utricle, one opening being common to the medial end of the superior duct and the upper end of the posterior duct. With the utricle, the semicircular ducts receive the terminal branches of the vestibular nerve. The ducts, the utricle and the saccule are all held in position by numerous fibrous bands which stretch across the space between them and the osseous walls.

The various parts of the membranous labyrinth communicate with each other and contain a fluid called endolymph. It represents a closed system and does not communicate with the subarachnoid space.

The **acoustic nerve** (Fig. 78) divides in the internal auditory meatus into two main branches: the vestibular and the cochlear. The posterior or vestibular branch supplies the utricle, the saccule and the ampullae of the semicircular canals. The inferior or cochlear branch is distributed to the cochlea.

The **cochlear nerve** divides into numerous filaments which pass through foramina which lead to small canals; these canals pass through the modiolus and then radiate laterally between the bony layer of the spiral lamina to the spiral organ of Corti.

For practical purposes, all pyogenic involvement of the labyrinth results from middle-ear infections. Functional changes in the labyrinth indicate invasion and possible meningeal involvement. Since the labyrinth is so small and the nerve endings so close, diffuse suppuration would destroy them and abolish their activity.

HEAD

Face

EMBRYOLOGY

At the anterior end of the embryo an opening called the stomodeum appears during the latter part of the first month of intra-uterine life. The face is formed from five processes surrounding this opening: one frontonasal, two maxillary and two mandibular processes (Fig. 80). The mandibular processes grow medially, fuse and unite in the midline, forming the lower jaw or mandible. When a failure of fusion of these processes occurs, a fissure of the lower lip results. The fusion of the upper processes converts the single stomodeal orifice into the cheeks, the whole upper lip except the philtrum (the vertical groove in the middle of the upper lip), most of the upper jaw and the palate. The appearance of an olfactory pit divides the frontonasal process into a medial and two lateral nasal processes. The medial process forms the septum of the nose, the philtrum and premaxilla; the lateral processes form the side of the nose but take no part in the formation of the upper lip. By imperfect fusion various defects result, such as harelip, macrostoma, microstoma, cleft palate, etc.

SKIN, BLOOD AND NERVE SUPPLY

Skin. The skin of the face is thin, vascular, movable and abundantly supplied with sebaceous and sweat glands. The absence of deep fascia in the anterior aspect of the face permits muscles arising from the bone to be inserted directly into the skin. The glands situated in the skin lie in immediate relationship to the subjacent loose areolar tissue, and it is the presence of this loose tissue, unsupported by deep fascia, that permits the rapid spread of edema. Over the lower part of the nose, however, the skin is firmly bound to the underlying cartilage, and inflammations here are extremely painful. The skin over the chin resembles the integument of the scalp in that it is very dense and adherent to the parts beneath.

Because of its mobility and vascularity, the skin of the face is especially adaptable to plastic operations and sound healing. The "dangerous area" of the face is triangular and bounded by lines that join the root of the nose with the angles of the mouth. The venous drainage from this area enters the angular vein, which communicates with the cavernous sinus via the superior

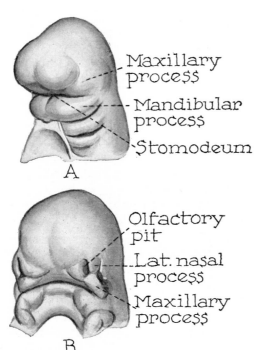

FIG. 80. Embryogenesis of the face: (A) before the appearance of the olfactory pit; (B) after the appearance of the olfactory pit.

ophthalmic vein. Therefore, boils or carbuncles in this region may produce a cavernous sinus thrombosis (Fig. 30).

Blood Supply. The blood supply of the face is free, and anastomoses are numerous (Fig. 2). The arterioles have a rich supply of sympathetic vasomotor nerves from the superior cervical ganglion, and because of this, blushing and blanching occur readily in emotional states. The main artery of the face is the *facial* (*external maxillary*), which is a branch of the external carotid. It appears at the base of the jaw immediately in front of the masseter muscle, passes upward in a tortuous manner toward the angle of the mouth and the side of the nose, and terminates near the inner canthus of the eye, where it anastomoses with the nasal branch of the ophthalmic artery. It crosses the lower jaw, the buccinator muscle, the upper jaw and the levator angulis oris; it is covered superficially by the platysma, the risorius, the zygomaticus major and minor and the levator labii superioris. In its lower part the artery rests directly on the mandible and is covered only by skin and the risorius muscle. Leaving the mandible, it travels on the surface of the buccinator and a little higher is crossed by the zygomaticus major muscle. In the interval between these two muscles it is covered only by skin and superficial fascia. Its accompanying veins lie behind it on the masseter. The cervical branch of the facial nerve enters the face superficial to the artery. A rich anastomosis occurs between the vessels of the two sides, and an additional anastomosis exists between the facial artery and the arteries which accompany the cutaneous branches of the 5th nerve on the face (ophthalmic and internal maxillary arteries).

The facial artery supplies *superior* and *inferior labial arteries* which pass medially in the upper and the lower lips; they are situated in the submucous tissue about ¼ inch from the mucocutaneous junction, where their pulsations can be felt easily. Each anastomoses with its fellow of the opposite side and forms an arterial ring around the lips. During operations these vessels may be controlled by grasping the lip between the fingers and the thumb. The superior labial artery supplies a small branch to the nasal septum.

Because of the marked vascularity, extensive areas of facial skin, torn in lacerating wounds, often retain their viability and may be sutured back into place.

The *anterior facial vein* is the companion vein of the facial artery. It is formed near the inner angle of the eye by the union of the supra-orbital and supratrochlear veins and passes behind the artery, taking a less tortuous but more superficial course. It makes three important connections: with the diploic veins through the frontal diploic veins; with the pterygoid plexus through the deep facial veins; and with the cavernous sinus through the superior ophthalmic vein. The vein itself terminates in the internal jugular vein. The important relationship between this vessel and the "dangerous area" of the face has been stressed.

Nerves. The nerves of the face are branches of the *facial,* which supplies the muscles of expression, and the *trigeminal,* which supplies the integument and the muscles of mastication (Figs. 41 and 44).

The entire skin of the face, with the exception of the area over the lower half of the ramus of the mandible, which is supplied by the great auricular nerve, is innervated by the 3 divisions of the trigeminal nerve. Since the face is developed from 3 rudiments, the frontonasal, the maxillary and the mandibular processes, each possesses its own sensory nerve. These nerves make up the 3 divisions of the trigeminal: the ophthalmic, the maxillary and the mandibular (Fig. 41).

The *ophthalmic,* or first division of the trigeminal nerve, has 5 cutaneous branches: (1) The *supra-orbital nerve* leaves the orbit through the supra-orbital notch or foramen about 2 fingerbreadths from the median line. It divides into lateral and medial branches which supply the central portion of the upper eyelid, and then ascends to innervate the skin of the forehead and the scalp as far back as the vertex. It is accompanied by the supra-orbital branch of the ophthalmic artery. (2) The *supratrochlear nerve* emerges about one fingerbreadth from the median plane and supplies the medial part of the upper eyelid and a small area of the forehead above the root of the nose. (3) The *infratrochlear nerve* emerges from the orbit above the medial palpebral ligament and supplies a small area of skin around the upper eyelid and the adjacent part of the nose. (4) The *external nasal nerve* emerges on the face at the lower border of the nasal bone and supplies the skin of the nose as far down as its tip. (5) The *lacrimal nerve* supplies the lateral part of the upper eyelid and the corresponding part of the conjunctiva.

At times a nasociliary division of the ophthalmic nerve is described; it has been referred to in this text as the infratrochlear or the external nasal nerve.

The *maxillary,* or second division of the trigeminal nerve, has the following branches: (1) The *infra-orbital nerve,* a direct continuation of the maxillary, emerges from the infra-orbital foramen, passes under cover of the levator labii superioris and is accompanied by a small artery. It divides into terminal branches: the palpebral for the lower lid, nasal for the posterior part of the nose, labial for the upper lip, and buccal for the cheek. (2) The *zygomaticofacial nerve* appears through the foramen of the same name as a twig and supplies the skin over the bony prominence of the cheek. (3) The *zygomaticotemporal nerve* passes through the foramen of the same name, pierces the temporal fascia near the zygomatic bone and supplies the skin of the anterior part of the temple.

The *mandibular,* or third division of the trigeminal nerve, has 3 branches which reach the skin: (1) The *mental nerve* emerges through the mental foramen and is situated deep to the depressor anguli oris; it sends its terminal branches to the lower lip, the chin and the skin over the body of the mandible. (2) The buccal nerve appears at the anterior border of the ramus of the jaw below the level of the parotid duct and travels almost to the angle of the mouth. It supplies the skin over the cheek, and the branches that pierce the buccinator supply the mucous membrane of the cheek. (3) The *auriculotemporal nerve* is accompanied by the superficial temporal artery and passes under cover of the parotid gland. As its name implies, it supplies cutaneous branches to the auricle and the temporal region, but it also supplies the modified skin which lines the external auditory meatus and cover the outer surface of the tympanic membrane. The terminal branches on the scalp may reach as high as the vertex.

The mandibular nerve supplies the skin over the lower jaw but extends onto the external ear and upward to the side of the head.

The branches of the 5th nerve which appear on the face communicate with branches of the 7th. For this reason a lesion in the territory of the 5th may cause a reflex spasm involving the facial muscles and producing a so-called facial tic. These conditions are treated best by removing the irritating cause, but they may require temporary interruption of the reflex arc by crushing the 7th nerve where it leaves the stylomastoid foramen. Trigeminal neuralgia is manifested by acute pain in the parts supplied by branches of the 5th nerve and may be due to carious teeth, sinus disease or irritative lesions within the cranium. In some cases of intractable neuralgia where all sources of possible peripheral irritation have been removed, it may be necessary either to resect nerves where they leave their bony canals or inject them with alcohol. If a lesion completely involves the 5th nerve, an extensive anesthesia of the same side of the face results which extends exactly to the midline. The muscles of mastication of the same side are also paralyzed, but the buccinator, which is supplied by the 7th nerve, remains intact. If only the 1st and the 2nd divisions of the 5th nerve are severed, the loss is entirely sensory, but if the 3rd division is cut, there is a sensory loss as well as a paralysis of mastication.

The *facial nerve,* supplying motor branches to the muscles of expression (Fig. 85), also sends fibers to the stapedius, the stylohyoid, the posterior belly of the digastric, the scalp muscles, the auricle and the face, including the buccinator and the platysma; it provides secretory fibers to the salivary glands and sensory (taste) fibers to the tongue and the palate. Developmentally, the 7th is the nerve of the hyoid arch; therefore, it supplies all the muscles derived from it. It leaves the skull at the stylomastoid foramen, turns forward, laterally and slightly downward, then enters the parotid isthmus and passes between the superior and the deep lobes of the gland. It lies superficial to the external carotid artery and the posterior facial vein and may be injured in operations in this region or on the parotid gland. The terminal branches of the nerve appear at the margins of the parotid and spread like the rays of an open fan or a goose's foot (pes anserinus). The 5 terminal branches are: (1) The *temporal branch* appears at the upper border of the gland and runs upward and forward to supply the facial muscles above the zygoma and the frontalis muscle. (2) The *zygomatic branch* emerges from the anterior border of the parotid above the parotid duct and supplies the muscles below the eye. (3) The *buccal branch* passes below the duct and supplies the buccinator and the orbicularis oris; it communicates with the buccal branch from the mandibular division of the trigeminal nerve. (4) The *mandibular branch* emerges still lower and supplies the muscles of the chin and the lower lip. (5) The *cervical branch* appears at the lower end of the parotid, passes within a fingerbreadth of the angle of the jaw between the platysma and the deep fascia, supplies the platysma and then sends twigs up to the muscles of the lower lip.

Coleman believes that there is a complicated and intricate intermingling of the various branches of the facial nerve so that the fibers meant for one group find their way to another.

CLINICAL AND SURGICAL CONSIDERATIONS

Trigeminal Neuralgia. Trigeminal neuralgia (tic douloureux, facial neuralgia) is a neuralgia of the 5th cranial nerve which is associated with severe pain along one or more of its divisions. Some surgical measures have been adopted to alleviate or cure the condition, among them alcohol injection into the nerve or into the gasserian ganglion and, if this fails, division of its sensory route. Most authorities have abandoned operations on the ganglion, since good results are obtained by section of the sensory root. The first division of this nerve is rarely at fault, but involvements of the 2nd and the 3rd divisions are frequent.

Injection of the Maxillary Nerve. Injection of the maxillary nerve should be done where the nerve emerges from the foramen rotundum into the pterygopalatine fossa. Two points should be marked (Fig. 81 A): the first is marked in the angle between the anterior border of the coronoid process and the lower border of the zygomatic arch; the second is marked in the angle between the upper border of the zygoma and its frontal process. Then these two lines are joined by a straight line, and a needle is inserted at the first point and passed upward and inward at an angle of 45° with the horizontal. The needle is kept in the direction of the line constructed and passes behind the mandible to enter the pterygopalatine fossa. It will strike the bone which forms the margin of the foramen rotundum about 2 or 3 inches from the surface. The injection, first of procaine and then of alcohol, is made at this point.

Injection of the Mandibular Nerve (Fig. 81 A, B). This is done at the foramen ovale. The needle is inserted at the center of and under the zygomatic arch and then directed slightly forward. It will strike the outer lamella of the pterygoid process. Then the needle is withdrawn slightly and directed backward, where it will enter the foramen ovale.

Injection of the Gasserian (Semilunar) Ganglion (Fig. 82). This is made through the foramen ovale and is done in the following way: a mark is made on the skin of the face about 3 cm. to the side of, and a similar distance above, the angle of the mouth. An imaginary line is drawn from this proposed point of entrance to the pupil, and a second line is drawn from this point to the auricular tubercle of the same side. The needle is introduced and advanced toward the center of the zygomatic arch in the plane joining the point of entry of the needle to the pupil when the patient is viewed from the front. The needle strikes the infratemporal bony plane and then is withdrawn gently and pushed up in a more posterior direction; this is continued until, when viewed from the front, the needle is in the plane of the first line and, when viewed from the side, in the plane of the second line. It then enters the foramen ovale and there will encounter the ganglion.

Division of the sensory root of the 5th nerve (Fig. 83) was perfected by Frazier. A vertical incision is made which divides the skin, the temporal fascia and the underlying muscle. The periosteum is incised and detached from the temporal bone by means of a periosteal elevator; a burr hole is made through the temporal bone and enlarged with bone forceps. The dura is separated from the base of the skull, and a retractor elevates the brain from the base of the middle fossa. The middle meningeal artery is exposed, cut and ligated as it emerges into the middle fossa through the foramen spinosum. The dura is

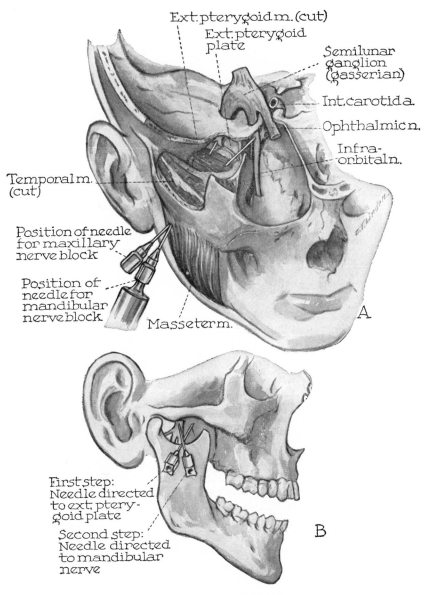

Fig. 81. Injection of the maxillary and the mandibular nerves: (A) direction of needle for the injection of the maxillary and the mandibular nerves, (B) injection of the mandibular nerve.

stripped until the 3rd division of the 5th nerve and the edge of the foramen ovale are exposed; the sheath of the nerve is incised and gently pushed upward and backward until the gasserian ganglion is seen. A small flap of arachnoid is turned downward, exposing the fan-shaped fibers of the sensory root. The sensory fibers are drawn outward, exposing the motor root. The sensory root is divided behind the ganglion.

MUSCLES

The facial muscles are placed around the orifices of the eye, the ear, the nose and the mouth and act as sphincters or dilators

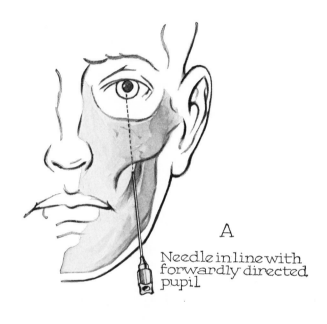

A

Needle in line with forwardly directed pupil

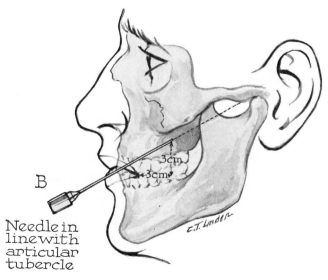

B

Needle in line with articular tubercle

Fig. 82. Injection of the gasserian ganglion.

(Fig. 84). All are innervated by the 7th (facial) nerve. It is extremely difficult to memorize this confusing group; hence, it is best to locate *two* landmarks around which the muscles are arranged. The *two* landmarks are the *two* orbicularis muscles, namely, the orbicularis oculi and the orbicularis oris. *Two* muscles are associated with the nose, *two* muscles with the zygoma, *two* are levators of the lip, *two* are at the angle of the mouth, *two* are placed at the lower lip, and the *two* remaining muscles are associated with the chin and the cheek.

Orbicularis Oculi. This muscle has 3 parts, namely, the orbital, the palpebral and the lacrimal. The *orbital portion* passes in circular form from the medial palpebral ligament and the adjacent part of the frontal bone across the forehead, the temple, the cheek and back to the medial ligament where it started. Since these fibers have no lateral attachments, they draw the lids medially. They are responsible for the "crow's feet" usually seen at the lateral angles of the eye.

The *palpebral portion,* arising from the medial palpebral ligament, which is a short fibrous cord stretched horizontally from the medial commissure of the eyelids to the adjoining part of the maxilla, curves laterally in both eyelids. The fibers of this part are inserted into the lateral palpebral raphe and are located within the lid proper and in front

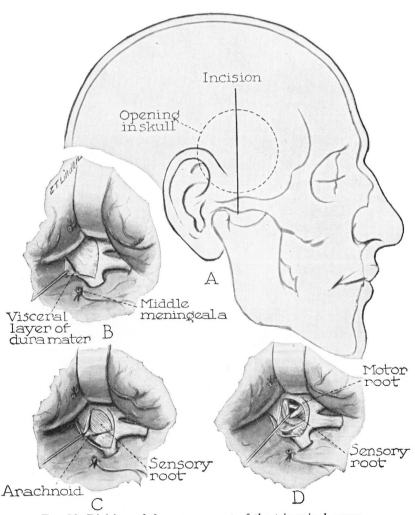

FIG. 83. Division of the sensory root of the trigeminal nerve.

of the palpebral fascia. They usually act involuntarily and close the lids in sleeping and in blinking.

The *lacrimal part* (Horner's muscle, tensor tarsi) is made up of fibers which pass medially behind the tear sac and attach to the posterior lacrimal crest, keeping the lids closely applied to the eyeballs. This part of the orbicularis oculi can also contract independently of the other two portions, and by this independent action wrinkles the skin around the eye, giving partial protection from light or wind. Those fibers which insert into the skin of the eyebrow draw it down as in frowning and also draw the eyebrows closer together, producing one or more vertical furrows in the middle of the forehead.

Orbicularis Oris. This sphincter muscle of the mouth forms the greater part of the substance of the lips. Its fibers encircle the oral aperture and extend upward to the nose and downward to the groove which is situated between the lower lip and the chin. Many of its fibers are derived directly from the buccinator; others from the depressors and the elevators of the angles of the mouth. This complex arrangement makes possible the varied movements of the lips, such as, pressing, closing, pursing, protruding, inverting and twisting.

Muscles Associated With the Nose. These two muscles are the procerus and the compressor nares.

The *procerus* muscles unite. They arise from the fascia covering the lower parts of the nasal bones, broaden and insert into the skin between and above the eyebrow. Their fibers interlace with the frontal bellies of the

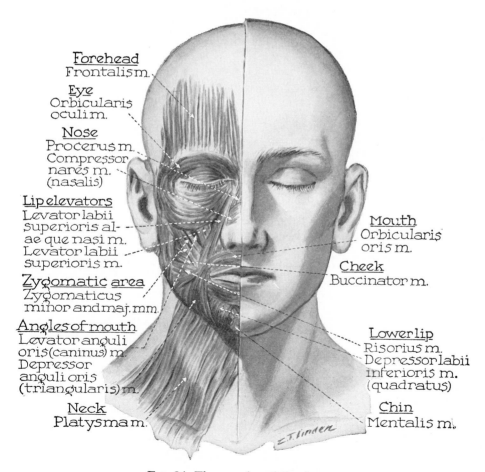

FIG. 84. The muscles of the face.

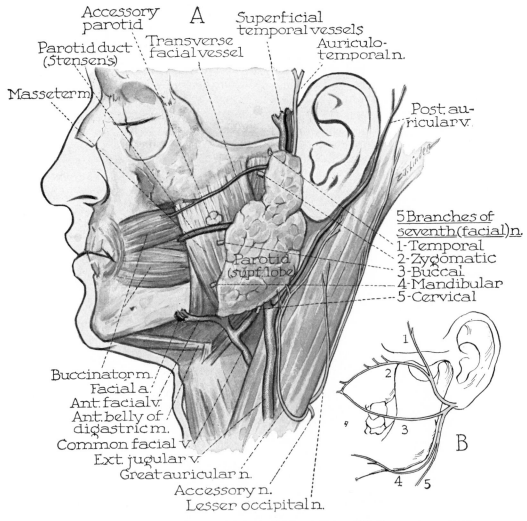

FIG. 85. The parotid gland: (A) superficial relations, (B) the most common pattern formed by the fine branches of the facial nerve.

occipitofrontalis. By their contraction they draw down on the skin of the root of the nose and produce transverse wrinkling.

The *compressor nares* muscle originates from the side of the bony aperture of the nose and spreads out as a fan-shaped muscle just above it. It joins its fellow of the other side, thus forming a sling across the bridge of the nose. It compresses the nostril, and its action is especially well demonstrated in the crying of infants. (Two other muscles, the dilator naris and the depressor septi nasi, are also found in this area but are small and clinically unimportant.)

Muscles Associated With the Zygomatic Area. These two muscles are the zygomaticus minor and the zygomaticus major.

The *zygomaticus minor* arises from the zygomatic bone and is closely related to the lateral margin of the levator labii superioris. This is a mere muscular slip and is often absent.

The *zygomaticus major* is both longer and thicker than the minor and runs obliquely from the zygomatic bone to the angle of the mouth. The major has been referred to as the "smiling muscle."

Lip Elevators. These two muscles are the levator labii superioris alaeque nasi and the levator labii superioris.

The *levator labii superioris alaeque nasi* is a small muscle lying along the attachment of the nose; it divides and inserts into the ala and the upper lip. It aids in dilation of the nostril and elevates the upper lip.

The *levator labii superioris* muscle is thin, fairly wide and descends from the infra-orbital margin into the upper lip. It is over-lapped by the orbicularis oculi.

Muscles Associated With the Angle of the

Mouth. These two muscles are the levator anguli oris (caninus) and the depressor anguli oris (triangularis).

The *levator anguli oris* lies deep to the levator superioris; it arises from the upper jaw below the infra-orbital foramen, inserts partly into the skin of the angle of the mouth and blends with the orbicularis oris. It also lies deep to the zygomatic major.

The *depressor anguli oris* muscle is placed

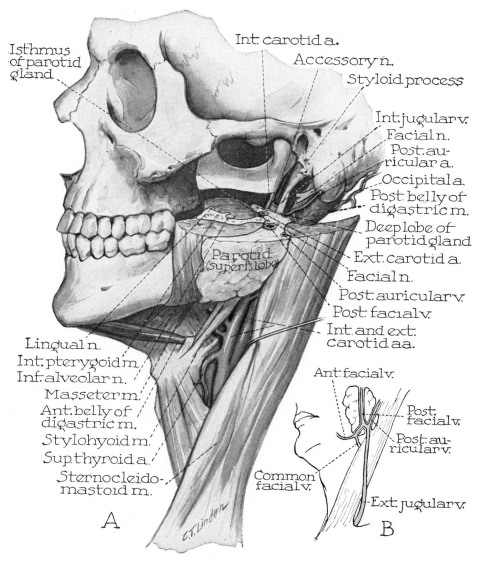

FIG. 86. Deep relations of the parotid gland: (A) the ramus of the mandible has been cut across transversely, showing the superficial and deep lobes of the gland connected by the isthmus; (B) venous pattern commonly found in the gland substance.

superficially. It is triangular in shape, its base corresponding to its insertion in the neighborhood of the angle of the mouth.

Muscles Associated With the Lower Lip. These two muscles are the risorius and the depressor labii inferioris.

The *risorius* lies horizontally opposite the angle of the mouth but may be continuous with the posterior fibers of the platysma or may arise independently from the fascia covering the masseter muscle. Its fibers converge at the angle of the mouth, where they are inserted into the skin. By drawing the angle of the mouth in a lateral direction, the muscle plays a large part in the production of a smile and has been referred to as the "grinning muscle."

The *depressor labii inferioris muscle* is short and wide, lies in front of the depressor anguli and is overlapped by it. Its medial groove meets and decussates with that of its fellow above the transverse groove on the lip, leaving a triangular space which is filled by the mentalis.

Muscles Associated With the Chin and the Cheek. The *mentalis* muscle passes from the lower incisor downward to the skin over the chin. When it contracts, it raises the skin over this area, thereby accentuating the transverse fold.

The *buccinator* muscle is situated more deeply and forms the fleshy stratum of the cheek. Its fibers pass horizontally forward to the angle of the mouth. The mucous membrane of the cheek and the lips lines its inner surface. The muscle arises from the alveolar margins of both upper and lower jaws external to the molar teeth and more posteriorly from the pterygomandibular raphe. The uppermost and lowermost fibers pass directly into the upper and the lower lips, respectively; but the middle fibers decussate, the upper half running into the lower lip and the lower half into the upper lip. At the angle of the mouth the muscle blends with the orbicularis oris. It retracts the mouth angle and therefore is considered as the antagonist of the orbicularis oris. Since the buccinator is supplied by the facial nerve, it is not classified as a muscle of mastication; however, it is used during mastication to press the cheek against the teeth and to prevent the food from escaping into the vestibule of the mouth. It also aids in the action of blowing and sucking. The buccopharyngeal fascia is a thin sheet that clothes the surface of the buccinator muscle and extends backward to cover the constrictor muscles of the pharynx. The parotid duct on its way to the vestibule of the mouth pierces this fascia, the buccinator and the mucous membrane of the mouth.

The *buccal fat pad,* also referred to as the suctorial pad, is situated on the buccinator muscle. It is a mass of fat, encapsulated in fascia, which lies on the muscle partly tucked in between the buccinator and the masseter. The buccal nerves, small vessels and the parotid duct pierce it. It thickens the cheek and helps to reduce atmospheric pressure during sucking. It is much larger in infants than in adults, and the rounded fullness of a baby's cheek is largely due to it.

PAROTID REGION

Although the parotid gland may be considered as a constituent of the neck, its relations to the face are more numerous and of greater practical importance.

Parotid Gland

(Figs. 85, 86.) The parotid gland is the largest of the salivary glands; it fills the parotid space and sends a process forward over the masseter muscle. Its fibrous capsule sends septa into the interior of the gland, dividing it into lobules and making removal difficult at times. In this respect it differs from the submaxillary gland, which is loosely enveloped and easily shelled out. In front of the styloid process and from the medial surface of the gland is a pharyngeal prolongation which is closely related to the wall of the pharynx and to the great vessels in the parapharyngeal space. The fascial septum separating this aspect of the gland from the carotid sheath may be broken through by pathologic erosions or malignant tumors as well as sharp instruments.

The parotid gland has the following relationships: superficially, it is covered by skin, superficial fascia lymph glands, fibrous capsule and branches of the great auricular nerve. The *upper border* is in contact with the external auditory meatus and the temporomandibular joint; abscesses of the gland may perforate into either of these structures. The *anterior border* is grooved by the masseter, the ramus of the mandible and the internal pterygoid muscle. The *posterior border* is in contact with the mastoid process and the sternocleidomastoid muscle. The *lower border* overlaps the internal and the external carotid arteries and the internal jugular vein. The *deep surface* is in contact with the digastric and the styloid muscles, the internal and the external carotid arteries, and the 9th, the 10th, the 11th and the 12th cranial nerves. Confusion still exists concerning the relationship between the facial nerve and the parotid gland (Fig. 87). In 1912 Gregoire described a superficial and a deep lobe of the parotid gland joined by an isthmus that was situated above the facial nerve. In 1917 McWhorter also described two lobes, but, in his opinion, the isthmus lay between the main divisions of the nerve. In 1945 McCormack, Cauldwell and Anson confirmed this work. In 1948 McKenzie stated that there were several isthmuses connecting the superficial and the deep lobes of the parotid gland. The branches of the facial nerve passed between these isthmuses so that the superficial and the deep lobes of the

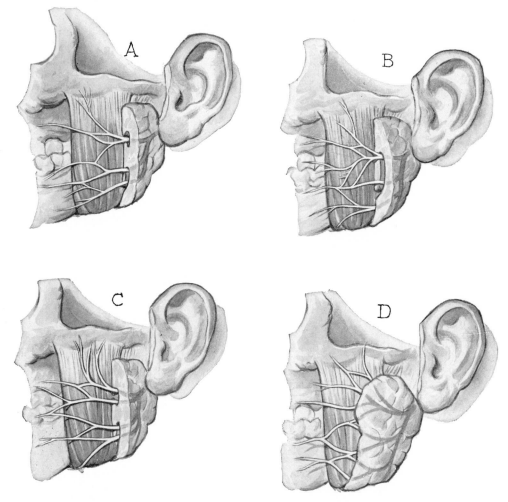

Fig. 87. Some of the variations between the parotid gland and the facial nerve.
 A. The two parotid lobes are united by an isthmus.
 B. The lobes are united above.
 C. A combination of a and b
 D. No division into superficial and deep lobes. The nerve courses through the "one-lobed" parotid gland.

gland could be joined at various locations. It is difficult to determine which of these views is correct, and the surgeon working in this area will have to keep the various patterns in mind as he performs surgery on the parotid gland. The *socia parotidis* is an accessory part of the parotid gland which lies immediately above its duct and on the masseter muscle.

The *fibrous capsule* of the parotid is derived from the investing layer of deep cervical fascia which splits at the lower pole of the gland to ensheath it. The deeper of these two layers passes under the gland and attaches to the base of the skull; the superficial layer passes anterior to the masseter muscle and attaches to the lower border of the zygomatic arch. This layer has been referred to as the parotideomasseteric fascia and accounts for the intense pain caused by inflammatory swellings of the gland. That part of the fascia which connects the styloid process to the angle of the mandible has been called the stylomandibular ligament and separates the parotid and the submaxillary glands.

Nerve and Blood Supply. The *auriculotemporal nerve* is a sensory branch of the mandibular division of the 5th, which supplies the skin in front of the ear. Its course is as follows: ascending upward through the temporal region to the vertex of the skull, the nerve emerges from the upper border of the parotid, crosses the root of the zygoma between the external ear and the condyle of the jaw and divides into its temporal branches. It may be compressed by tumors or swellings in the parotid gland and produce exquisite pain radiating over the temple as high as the vertex.

The 7th or *facial nerve,* emerging from the stylomastoid foramen, divides into its two main branches, which embrace the isthmus of the parotid gland. From here these branches redivide and radiate from the border of the gland in the form of a goose's foot (pes anserinus) (Fig. 85 B). This has been discussed elsewhere (p. 62).

Although *veins* are variable (Fig. 86 B), they follow a fairly constant course in the substance of the parotid gland. The *posterior facial vein* aids in the formation of two other veins—the external jugular and the common facial. At its lower end and while in the parotid, the posterior facial divides into an anterior and a posterior branch. The anterior branch joins the anterior facial vein to form the common facial, and the posterior joins the posterior auricular to form the external jugular vein.

The *external carotid artery* ascends from under cover of the digastric and the stylohyoid muscles and comes into relationship with the posteromedial surface of the parotid. Here it gives rise to a posterior auricular artery and then enters the gland, passing from the posteromedial to its anteromedial surface. At the back of the neck of the mandible it divides into internal maxillary and superficial temporal branches. The *superficial temporal artery* arises under cover of the parotid gland, emerges at its upper border, accompanied by a corresponding vein and the auriculotemporal nerve (Fig. 2). It ascends across the root of the zygoma, where its pulsations may be felt readily; it continues upward on the temporal fascia and divides into anterior and posterior branches, which supply the scalp. In addition to many small branches which supply the parotid gland, the auricle and the facial muscles, the superficial temporal supplies a *transverse facial artery* which runs forward on the masseter muscle, emerges at the anterior border of the gland and continues parallel with and above the parotid duct.

The *lymph glands* of the parotid region may be divided into two groups: a superficial, which is superficial to the parotid sheath and constitutes the preauricular group draining the temporal and the frontal regions of the scalp, the outer portion of the eyelid and the outer aspect of the ear. A deeper group makes up the parotid group, which is scattered through the gland substance and drains the upper and posterior parts of the nasopharynx, the soft palate and the middle ear. These relationships are important because swellings of the parotid gland may be confused with enlarged and infected lymph glands in this region.

Parotid (Stensen's) Duct (Fig. 85). The *duct* of the parotid gland begins at the anterior part, passes forward on the masseter muscle about one fingerbreadth below the zygoma and is accompanied by the transverse facial artery above and the buccal branch of the facial nerve below. It bends abruptly around the anterior border of the masseter, pierces the substance of the buccinator muscle, runs obliquely forward between the buccinator and the mucous membrane of the mouth and opens on a papilla opposite the upper 2nd molar tooth. It may be felt best when the jaws are clenched, because it then can be rolled against the tense masseter muscle. The duct is about 2½ inches long and ⅛ inch in diameter, its orifice being its narrowest part. The bend the duct makes

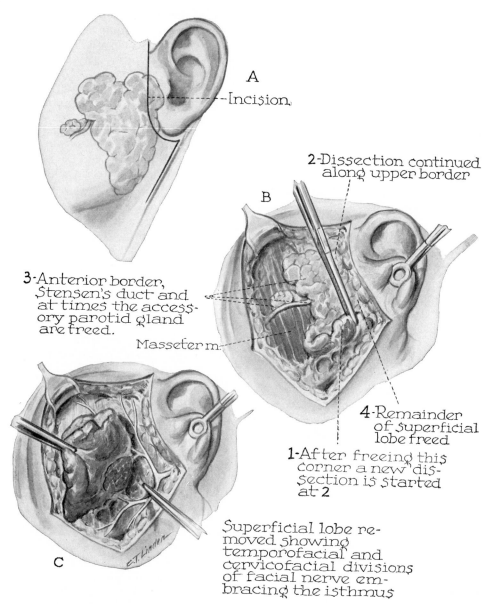

A
--Incision.

2-Dissection continued along upper border

B

3-Anterior border, Stensen's duct and at times the accessory parotid gland are freed.

Masseter m.

4-Remainder of superficial lobe freed

1-After freeing this corner a new dissection is started at 2

Superficial lobe removed showing temporofacial and cervicofacial divisions of facial nerve embracing the isthmus

C

Fig. 88. Parotidectomy: (A) Incision which also may be utilized for preliminary ligation of the external carotid artery. (B) Mobilization of the superficial lobe. The numbers indicate the order in which this dissection takes place. (C) Division of the isthmus. The operation may end at this stage if only the superficial lobe is involved, or it may be continued by putting traction on the isthmus and removing the deep lobe. The branches of the facial nerve are visualized and protected.

around the anterior border of the masseter may be so sharp that the buccal segment remains at right angles to the masseteric part. This should be kept in mind if a probe is passed along the duct from the mouth. Its course can be marked by the middle third of a line which joins the lobule of the ear to the midpoint between the red margin of the upper lip and the ala of the nose.

SURGICAL CONSIDERATIONS

PAROTIDECTOMY

Most authorities believe that mixed tumors of the parotid gland are potentially malignant and, therefore, should be subjected to complete extirpation.

In **total parotidectomy,** a long incision is made in front of the ear and as close as possible to the cartilage (Fig. 88). The inferior end of this incision turns around the lobule, extends to the mastoid process and then downward along the anterior border of the sternocleidomastoid muscle. Bailey is of the opinion that one of the first steps should be the ligation of the external carotid artery, which makes the operation easier and safer.

The anterior skin flap is reflected forward to the mandible. The submaxillary salivary gland within its capsule is utilized as a landmark, and the posterior belly of the digastric is identified.

Mobilization of the superficial parotid lobe is the next step and is accomplished best by commencing at the anterior extremity of its lower border. Sistrunk has advised isolating the inframandibular branch of the facial nerve first as it passes along the angle of the jaw, but many surgeons have found difficulty in locating the nerve before the gland has been properly freed.

The anterior extremity of the lower border is considered a safe area and is an excellent place to commence dissection (Fig. 88 B). After freeing this corner, a new dissection is started at the extreme posterior end of the upper border of the gland. The ear is retracted backward, and a cleavage plane is found which allows the gland to be dissected upward and forward. In this location the temporal artery is found, but if the external carotid has been ligated, the temporal can be

dissected up with the parotid gland or left in situ, whichever is easier.

The dissection continues along the upper border, and the gland is lifted from the zygomatic arch. At this stage a sharp lookout is kept for the uppermost part of the pes anserinus. It is important to preserve the upper branches that go to the orbital region. These lie on the masseter muscle, and once the correct cleavage plane is found, there is no great difficulty, since the nerves have a tendency to adhere to the muscle rather than the gland. As the dissection continues along the anterior border, Stensen's duct and at times the socia parotidis are freed from the masseter. In the middle region the mid-portions of the pes are seen and freed as far as possible. The antero-inferior border of the gland which was mobilized as the first step is now grasped and retracted upward. Dissection then proceeds toward the mastoid process, using the digastric muscle as a guide. At this step the main trunk of the facial nerve usually can be identified. With this under vision and the gland mobilized on all sides, the isthmus and its limitations can be made out by vision or palpation. Then the free superficial lobe is retracted forward, and the isthmus is divided from behind forward. This having been done, the facial nerve and its divisions will usually become apparent. Stensen's duct is divided, if this has not been done already. The facial nerve can be held aside by fine retractors or ligatures passed beneath it, and the deep lobe is removed by separating it from the great vessels of the neck and the pharyngeal wall. Sometimes bleeding occurs from the large tributaries of the jugular vein during this stage and it may become necessary to ligate the jugular. The surgeon must remember that this is only one of many technics described. The various anatomic descriptions of this region (p. 122) resulted in different surgical approaches. Eddey has presented an operation in which he described three isthmuses of the parotid gland, stating that the facial nerve is completely surrounded by glandular tissue. Riessner uses the so-called "upper branch" of the facial nerve as a safe guide for parotid gland removal. Many other technics can be studied by anyone interested in the surgery of this area.

Parotid Abscess

A parotid abscess may be drained through an incision (Blair) which commences about 1 inch anterior to the ear and is carried downward behind and below the angle of the jaw. This is deepened through the capsule of the gland, and then the parenchyma can be opened by blunt dissection. The deep part of the gland may be drained by lifting the lower pole forward. It may become necessary to drain the space between the masseter and the superficial lobe of the gland, and

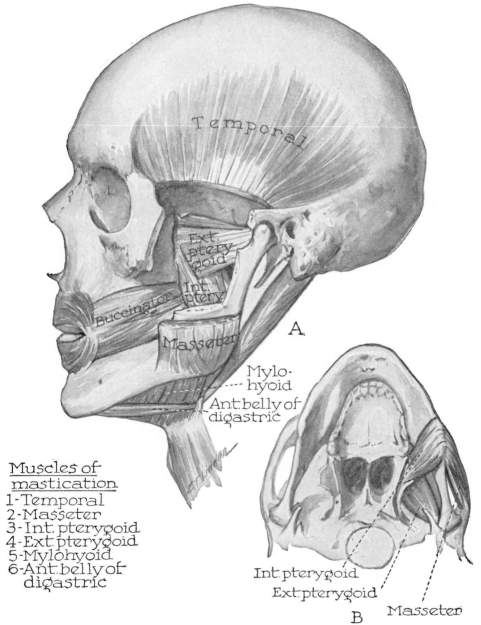

Fig. 89. The 6 muscles of mastication. (A) Viewed from left side; the zygomatic arch and part of the mandible have been removed. The temporal muscle has been cut for the purpose of exposing the pterygoid muscles. (B) Viewed from below to show the course and the attachments of the external and internal pterygoid muscles.

this too can be accomplished through the same incision. Some surgeons have advised the use of a horizontal incision for the drainage of such an abscess.

TEMPORAL AND INFRATEMPORAL REGIONS

MUSCLES OF MASTICATION

The muscles of mastication (Fig. 89) include the temporal, the masseter, the external and the internal pterygoids, the mylohyoid and the anterior belly of the digastric. All of these are supplied by the trigeminal nerve (mandibular branch). Since they do not appear over the same region of the face, only those concerned with the temporal and the infratemporal regions will be discussed here.

Temporal Fascia. This strong aponeurotic layer covers the upper aspect of the temporal muscle, attaches above to the superior temporal line and splits below into two layers attached to the lateral and the medial margins of the upper border of the zygoma. The space thus formed is occupied by fatty tissue and some small blood vessels.

Temporal Muscle. This muscle arises from the whole of the temporal fossa (frontal, parietal, squamous portion of the temporal and greater wing of the sphenoid bones), and its fibers converge on a gap that exists between the zygoma and the side of the skull. The fibers pass downward deep to the zygomatic arch, then beneath the masseter, and become inserted into the margins of the deep surface of the coronoid process. Some anterior fibers descend beyond the coronoid to reach the anterior border of the ramus of the mandible. A true view of the muscle can be obtained only if the temporal fascia is removed and if the zygoma is divided and turned downward together with the masseter muscle. The muscle is a powerful elevator of the mandible, and its posterior fibers act as a retractor of the same bone. Nowhere else in the body is a group of muscles opposed by so weak a group of opponents as in this region. The temporal, the masseter and the internal pterygoid muscles produce the great biting and grinding power, but their opponents which depress the mandible (external

pterygoid, digastric, mylohyoid and geniohyoid) are able to afford only weak resistance. Therefore, when a state of spasm is produced, the stronger group prevails. Should this spasm be clonic, a chattering of the teeth occurs, but if the spasm is tonic, the mouth is rigidly closed, and the condition known as trismus or lockjaw results. This locking of the jaw is a frequent symptom of tetanus but is also found in any condition that might produce an irritation of the mandibular branch of the trigeminal nerve, as is sometimes seen in caries of the lower teeth or during the cutting of a lower wisdom tooth.

Masseter Muscle. This muscle is held firmly by the masseter fascia, which binds it to the margins of the ramus and the body of the mandible; the muscle covers nearly the entire lateral surface of the ramus of the mandible. An expansion of the fascia overlies the fat pad of the cheek and holds it against the buccinator muscle. The parotid duct lies within the fascia and is protected by it. The muscle arises by two closely associated heads: a superficial and a deep, which arise from the surface of the zygomatic arch. It is inserted into the lateral surface of the ramus and the coronoid process of the mandible. The muscle raises and protrudes the mandible, and its fibers may be felt well if the jaws are clenched firmly. The transverse facial vessels, the parotid duct and branches of the facial nerve all lie on its lateral surface, and the parotid gland overlaps it posteriorly. The muscle does not cover the head and the neck of the mandible (Fig. 2).

Pterygoid Muscles. These muscles (Fig. 89 B) lie on a deeper plane and are almost completely hidden by the ramus of the mandible. Only a small part of the external pterygoid can be seen through the mandibular notch.

Many authors prefer to consider the *internal (medial) pterygoid muscle* as being associated with the masseter, and these two muscles have been likened to the two bellies of the digastric. The fibers of the internal pterygoid originate from the medial surface of the lateral pterygoid lamina and by a small slip from the tuberosity of the maxilla. They pass downward and backward and insert into the medial surface of the ramus of

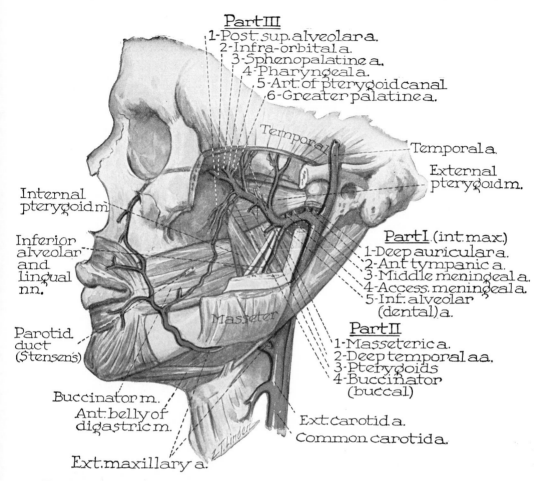

Part III
1-Post. sup. alveolar a.
2-Infra-orbital a.
3-Sphenopalatine a.
4-Pharyngeal a.
5-Art. of pterygoid canal
6-Greater palatine a.

Temporal a.

External
pterygoid m.

Internal
pterygoid m.

Inferior
alveolar
and
lingual
nn.

Part I (int. max.)
1-Deep auricular a.
2-Ant. tympanic a.
3-Middle meningeal a.
4-Access. meningeal a.
5-Inf. alveolar
(dental) a.

Part II
1-Masseteric a.
2-Deep temporal aa.
3-Pterygoids
4-Buccinator
(buccal)

Parotid
duct
(Stensen's)

Buccinator m.
Ant. belly of
digastric m.

Ext. carotid a.
Common carotid a.

Ext. maxillary a.

Fig. 90. The internal maxillary artery. The vessel is divided into 3 parts by the external pterygoid muscle. Part I is known as the mandibular portion; Part II, the pterygoid; and Part III, the pterygopalatine portion. The branches of each part are numbered and represented.

the mandible from the mandibular foramen to the angle. The muscle elevates the mandible, protrudes it and pulls it to the opposite side. Superficial to this muscle is the ramus of the mandible, the external pterygoid, the lingual and the inferior dental nerves, the maxillary and the inferior dental vessels and the sphenomandibular ligament. Deep to it are the tensor palati and the levator palati, the superior constrictor of the pharynx and the eustachian (auditory) tube.

The *external (lateral) pterygoid muscle* originates by two heads: the lower from the lateral surface of the lateral pterygoid lamina, and the upper from the undersurface of the great wing of the sphenoid. The fibers are directed backward and become inserted in the digital fossa on the front of the neck of the mandible and to the capsule and the disk of the mandibular joint. In this way its contraction opens the mouth by sliding the condyle forward and protruding the jaw. One muscle acting alone pulls the chin over the opposite side. The internal maxillary artery crosses the lower head of the muscle obliquely and, as a rule, runs superficial to it.

Buccinator. This forms the muscle layer of the cheek and is discussed here for the sake of completion. It arises from the outer alveolar margins of both the upper and the lower jaws in the region of the molar teeth and passes to the angle of the mouth, where it blends with the orbicularis oris. The middle fibers decussate at the angle of the mouth, so that the uppermost fibers pass to the lower lip and vice versa. It is supplied by the buccal branches of the facial nerve. By its action of retracting the angle of the mouth and flattening the cheek, it compresses the cheek so that during mastication food is pushed beneath the molar teeth. Compression of the cheek against the gums prevents masticated food from becoming lodged there. In paralysis of the facial nerve it becomes necessary for the patient constantly to dislodge the food with his finger. This muscle also aids in the act of blowing and whistling. Its superficial surface is covered with buccal pharyngeal fascia, and its deep surface is lined with the mucous membrane of the cheek. Posteriorly, it is covered by the buccal fat pad, which separates it from the masseter and the temporal muscles, anteriorly, by the superficial fascia, which contains the facial artery, the anterior facial vein, the buccal nerve and artery and the buccal branches of the facial nerve. The muscle is pierced by the parotid duct and twigs from the buccal nerve.

VESSELS AND NERVES

Internal Maxillary Artery. This artery (Fig. 90) arises from the external carotid opposite the neck of the mandible and under cover of the parotid gland. It passes forward deep to the neck of the bone and superficial to the sphenomandibular ligament. Between the mandible and the sphenomandibular ligament it is accompanied by its vein and lies superficial to the inferior alveolar (dental) nerve. It goes upward and forward superficial to the external pterygoid between it and the temporal muscle, or deep to the external pterygoid, between it and branches of the mandibular division of the 5th nerve. It then passes medially between the two heads of the pterygoid and through the pterygomaxillary fissure into the pterygopalatine fossa, to end in its numerous terminal branches.

The external pterygoid muscle divides the maxillary artery into three parts. The first is known as the mandibular portion; it lies between the neck of the mandible and the sphenomandibular ligament, taking a horizontal course forward nearly parallel with and a little below the auriculotemporal nerve. In this location it is imbedded in the parotid gland and usually crosses in front of the inferior alveolar nerve. The second part is called the pterygoid portion, and here the artery may lie lateral or medial to the external pterygoid muscle. This part of the artery usually runs obliquely forward and upward under cover of the ramus of the mandible and passes on the superficial surface of the muscle. The vessel then passes between the two heads of origin of this muscle and enters the pterygopalatine fossa. Part three of the vessel, the pterygopalatine portion, lies in the pterygopalatine fossa in relation to the sphenopalatine ganglion. The branches which arise from the first part of the artery are associated with foramina; those which come from the second part are associated with muscles, and the branches of the third part are again associated with foramina.

The branches of the first part of the internal maxillary artery are:

1. The *deep auricular artery,* which passes to the external auditory meatus.

2. The *anterior tympanic,* which enters the pterotympanic fissure to the middle ear.

3. The *middle meningeal,* which arises from the upper border of the maxillary bone and runs upward and deep to the external pterygoid muscle. As it ascends it is embraced by the two heads of the auriculotemporal nerve; it enters the middle cranial fossa through the foramen spinosum and upward and forward on the squamous temporal and great wing of the sphenoid bone toward the antero-inferior angle of the parietal bone, where it divides into anterior and posterior branches. The anterior branch travels upward across the great wing of the sphenoid toward the pterion and then on the parietal bone behind the coronal suture near the motor cortex. The posterior branch passes upward and backward on the squamous temporal to the middle of the lower border of the parietal bone and then breaks up into its terminal branches.

4. The *accessory meningeal,* also referred to as the *small meningeal artery,* has a similar course and may be a branch of the above-

mentioned vessel; it enters the middle cranial fossa through the foramen ovale and supplies the dura mater and the trigeminal ganglion.

5. The *inferior alveolar (dental) artery* passes downward behind the inferior alveolar nerve and between the sphenomandibular ligament and the mandible. It supplies a mylohyoid branch and then enters the mandibular foramen to supply the teeth and the lower jaw. Its terminal branch appears on the face accompanied by the mental nerve.

There are 4 branches of the second portion of the internal maxillary artery:

1. The *masseteric artery* passes laterally through the mandibular notch to the masseter muscle and also supplies the mandibular joint.

2. The *deep temporal* has 2 branches, anterior and posterior, which ascend between the temporalis muscle and the pericranium; they supply the muscle and anastomose with the middle temporal artery.

3. The *pterygoid arteries* are irregular in number and origin and supply the pterygoid muscles.

4. The *buccinator (buccal) artery* travels forward with the buccal nerve between the internal pterygoid and the jaw to supply the buccinator muscle, the skin and the mucous membrane of the cheek.

The 6 branches of the third portion of the internal maxillary artery are:

1. The *posterosuperior alveolar,* which descends over the posterior surface of the maxilla, sends branches to the gums, the buccinator muscle, through the bone to the molars, the premolars and the maxillary sinus.

2. The *infra-orbital artery,* really a continuation of the parent trunk, is accompanied by the maxillary nerve through the infra-orbital canal, appearing on the face beneath the levator labii superioris. In the canal it sends branches to the orbit and an anterior dental branch which accompanies the nerve and supplies the front teeth. On the face it supplies the lacrimal sac and the medial angle of the orbit.

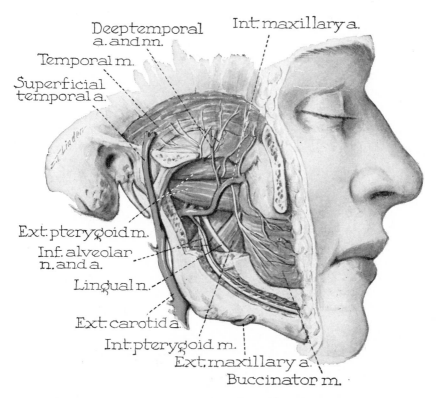

FIG. 91. The lingual and the inferior alveolar (dental) nerves.

3. The *greater palatine artery* passes through the greater palatine canal with the nerve of the same name, then along the hard palate in a groove about ½ inch from the teeth, and finally through the lateral incisive foramen to the nose.

4. The *pharyngeal artery* is very small and passes backward through the pharyngeal canal accompanied by the pharyngeal nerve. It is distributed to the upper part of the pharynx and the auditory tube.

5. The *artery of the pterygoid canal (Vidian)* passes backward along the pterygoid canal with its corresponding nerve. It is distributed to the upper part of the pharynx and to the auditory tube, sending a small branch into the tympanic cavity which anastomoses with the other tympanic artery.

6. The *sphenopalatine artery* enters the nasal cavity through the sphenopalatine foramen and supplies the mucous membrane of the nasal cavity, the adjacent sinuses and the pharynx. At the back part of the superior meatus it supplies posterior lateral nasal branches which spread forward over the conchae and the meatus, anastomosing with the ethmoidal arteries and nasal branches of the descending palatine artery. It ends on the nasal septum as posterior septal branches which anastomose with the ethmoidal arteries and the septal branches of the superior labial. One branch descends in a groove on the vomer to the incisive canal and anastomoses with the descending palatine artery.

Pterygoid Venous Plexus. This rich network of veins is located around the lateral pterygoid muscle; veins corresponding to the maxillary artery empty into it. From its posterior end a maxillary vein passes backward to unite with the superficial temporal, forming the posterior facial vein. The plexus makes the following communications: with the cavernous sinus through the foramen ovale; with the anterior facial through the deep facial vein; with the inferior ophthalmic veins through the inferior orbital fissure (Fig. 30).

Mandibular Division of the Trigeminal Nerve. In the parotid region this plays an important role. It leaves the skull through the foramen ovale in the greater wing of the sphenoid bone and differs from the other two divisions in that it is a mixed nerve (Fig. 41). The sensory part arises from the gasserian ganglion, and the motor part is the motor root of the 5th nerve. The two roots pass through the foramen ovale and almost immediately unite into one trunk which is covered by the external pterygoid muscle. It lies on the surface of the tensor palati (veli palatina) muscle, which separates the nerve from the auditory (eustachian) tube and the nasopharynx. The middle meningeal artery lies lateral to and a little behind it. The trunk divides into anterior and posterior divisions.

The undivided trunk gives off a recurrent nerve and the nerve to the internal pterygoid muscle. The recurrent nerve (nervus spinosus) passes back into the foramen spinosum and supplies the dura and the mastoid air cells. The nerve to the internal pterygoid muscle is self-explanatory. From the anterior division, mainly muscular, are derived the deep temporal, the masseteric, the external pterygoid and the long buccal branches. From the posterior division, mainly sensory, are derived the auriculotemporal, the inferior dental (alveolar) and the lingual nerves. Although the anterior division of this nerve gives off muscular branches to the temporal, the masseter and the external pterygoid muscles, the long buccal nerve is essentially sensory; it passes down between the two heads of the external pterygoid muscle, pierces the anterior part of the temporal muscle, traverses the suctorial fat pad, and then branches outward to the skin of the face and inward to the mucous membrane of the cheek.

Auriculotemporal Nerve. This nerve has been discussed elsewhere (p. 60). It is a sensory branch of the mandibular nerve which forms an anastomosis with the facial nerve and otic ganglion. It emerges from the upper border of the parotid and crosses the root of the zygoma between the external ear and the condyle of the jaw, where it divides into its temporal branches. This nerve is sometimes resected in persistent neuralgias and is easily found where it crosses the zygoma, lying between the ear and the temporal artery. By means of its communication with the otic ganglion, secretory fibers result; these supply the parotid gland; hence, the rationale for division of it in an attempt to close a parotid fistula. Auricular branches of this nerve pass to the upper ear and the external auditory meatus. Referred pain from these branches may be so severe that the ear drum may be opened unnecessarily when one of the molar teeth is at fault.

Lingual Nerve. This nerve (Fig. 91) passes downward deep to the external and on the surface of the internal pterygoid muscle. In this part of its course it is in front of the inferior alveolar nerve and is joined by the chorda tympani (7th nerve), which contains taste fibers that are carried by the lingual to the anterior two thirds of the tongue. As the nerve continues downward and forward it lies between the mandible and the internal pterygoid, and farther forward is under cover of the mucous membrane of the mouth on the superior constrictor and the styloglossus

muscles. It passes forward between the mylohyoid and the hyoglossus and arrives between the sublingual gland and the genioglossus muscle, where it crosses the submandibular duct and supplies the gums and the anterior two thirds of the tongue (Fig. 106 A). One should not be confused between taste and sensation if one recalls that the lingual nerve supplies the anterior two thirds of the tongue with its sensory fibers, but this nerve carries fibers from the facial nerve by way of the chorda tympani, which supply taste fibers to the same region of the tongue (Fig. 98). Resection of the lingual nerve is at times necessary for the relief of intense pain which is associated with carcinoma of the tongue.

Inferior Alveolar (Dental) Nerve. This nerve passes downward deep to the external pterygoid muscle but superficial to the sphe-

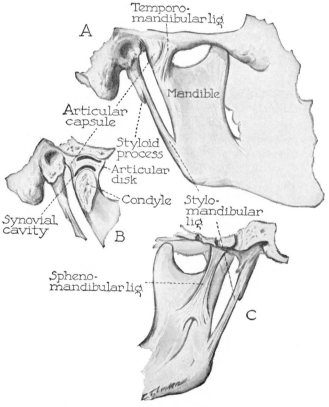

FIG. 92. The temporomandibular joint: (A) lateral view, right side; (B) exposure of the joint and the articular disk, following removal of the temporomandibular ligament and part of the condyle of the mandible; (C) medial view, showing the stylomandibular and the sphenomandibular ligaments.

nomandibular ligament and is accompanied by the dental vessels. Immediately before entering the mandibular foramen it gives off the nerve to the mylohyoid muscle; this descends in a groove on the deep surface of the mandible in company with the mylohyoid vessels. This nerve reaches the posterior edge of the mylohyoid, passes superficial to that muscle and ends by supplying the mylohyoid and the anterior belly of the digastric. In the inferior dental canal it sends branches to the roots of the lower teeth and gums. The nerve finally emerges through the mental foramen as the mental nerve (Fig. 91).

TEMPOROMANDIBULAR JOINT

The temporomandibular (temporomaxillary, mandibular) is a synovial joint that is formed by the head of the mandible with the articular fossa and the eminence of the temporal bone. The articulating surfaces are completely separated by an *articular disk* which divides the joint cavity into an upper and a lower chamber (Fig. 92 B). The joint is surrounded by a lax capsule which envelops the bony articular surface and furnishes attachment to the interposed cartilage. The laxity of this capsule enables free joint movements. Over its lateral aspect the capsule is markedly thickened and strengthened by the *temporomandibular ligament* (external lateral ligament) (Fig. 92 A), which stretches from the zygoma and the tubercle at its root to the lateral and the posterior surfaces of the neck of the mandible. The ligament is covered by the upper part of the parotid gland and is in relation to the superficial temporal vessels. The articular disk is attached around its circumference to the capsular ligament. However, there is an exception to this attachment, since the disk receives part of the insertion of the external pterygoid muscle in front. The lower disk surface is concave to fit into the head of the mandible, but its upper surface undulates to fit the fossa and the eminence. The disk can become loose or detached and, as it slips back and forth, may produce an audible click (clicking jaw). At times it may become detached at one end and is then apt to double on itself, in which event it becomes impacted between the joint surfaces and causes locking; the symptoms may become so discomforting and embarrassing that removal of the disk is necessary.

Two accessory ligaments described as bands and giving additional ligamentous support to the joint are the sphenomandibular and the stylomandibular.

The *sphenomandibular ligament* (*internal lateral ligament*) lies on a deeper plane than the joint, distinct from the medial part of the articulation, and is a thin and fairly long band stretching from the spine of the sphenoid bone to the edge and the margins of the mandibular foramen (Fig. 92 C). Medially, its upper part is separated by fat from the wall of the nasopharynx, and its lower part lies on the internal pterygoid muscle. Laterally, it is related to the mandibular joint, and the mandible is separated from the ligaments, from above downward, by the auriculotemporal nerve, the external pterygoid muscle, the maxillary vessels and the inferior dental vessels and nerves. Although these structures separate the ligament from the joint, the chorda tympani nerve lies deep to the ligament.

The *stylomandibular ligament* is a thickened part of the cervical fascia that covers the deep surface of the parotid gland. It extends from the styloid process to the posterior border and angle of the mandible and separates the parotid from the submandibular gland.

The *synovial membrane* is in two separate parts, since it has two separate cavities to line. The upper synovial cavity is the more extensive because of the greater size of the articular fossa of the temporal bone. The membrane, although reflected onto the articular disk, disappears from this part in the adult.

The construction of the temporomandibular joint permits a wide range of movements. Elevation is produced by the masseter, the internal pterygoid and the temporalis muscles; depression by the digastric, the mylohyoid, the geniohyoid and the platysma, protrusion by the pterygoids, the anterior part of the temporalis and fibers of the masseter; retraction by the posterior fibers of the temporalis and the deeper fibers of the masseter. Grinding movements are produced by the

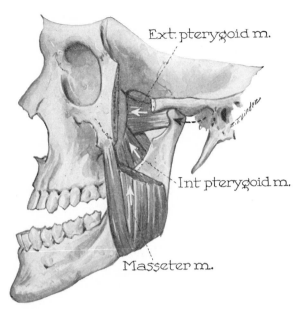

FIG. 93. Anterior dislocation of the mandible. The condyle has been drawn over the articular eminence into the zygomatic fossa by the contraction of the external pterygoid. Then the mandible is drawn upward and fixed in place by masseter, internal pterygoid and temporalis muscles.

pterygoids of opposite sides acting alternately. The construction of the joint permits a forward dislocation, either unilateral or bilateral, which can occur when the mouth is widely opened. Such dislocations have occurred during a blow struck on the lower front teeth, or during laughing, yawning, vomiting and also in the dentist's chair. When the mouth is opened widely, the con-dyles and the interarticular fibrocartilage glide forward. Normally, the condyles should not reach as far as the summit of the articular eminence, but when the mouth is opened widely all parts of the capsule except the anterior are made tense, and if at this time the external pterygoid muscle contracts vigorously, the condyle is drawn over the articular eminence onto the zygomatic fossa

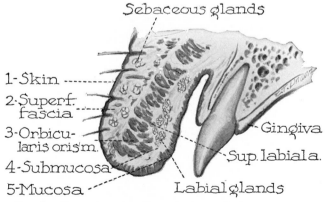

FIG. 94. Sagittal section through the upper lip. The 5 layers which constitute each lip are shown.

and the interarticular cartilage remains behind. As soon as it reaches its new position, it is drawn up immediately by the internal pterygoid, the temporal and the masseter muscles and is thereby spastically fixed in place (Fig. 93).

MOUTH AND REGIONS THAT SURROUND IT

LIP REGION

The *lips* are two fleshy folds that circumscribe the mouth and close the buccal cavity in front. At the sides they unite to form the commissures. The lips consist of 5 layers (Fig. 94):

1. **Skin.** The layer of skin is fairly thick and adherent to the subjacent connective tissue and muscular layers. It contains hair follicles and sebaceous glands and is frequently the site of furuncles. The lower lip is a favorite site for epitheliomas.

2. **Superficial Fascia.** This fascia is a connective tissue layer which contains some fat. Since it is arranged loosely, considerable edema may take place when the lips are bruised or inflamed.

3. **Orbicularis Oris Muscle.** This essential muscle of the lips is arranged in an elliptical manner around the buccal orifice, the extremities of the upper and the lower portions meeting at the lip commissures. It acts as a sphincter of the mouth. Because the general direction of these muscle fibers is circular, a vertical incision in this area causes separation of the wound edges. Since it is supplied by the facial nerve, paralysis interferes with articulation, prevents tight closure of the mouth and as a result allows saliva to drip from the paralyzed corner.

4. **Submucous Tissue.** The submucosa is the layer that contains vessels and mucous labial glands. An arterial circle is formed in this tissue; this arises from the upper and the lower *labial branches* of the facial artery (external maxillary). The pulsations of these vessels can be felt by grasping the lip between the finger and the thumb. This circle provides a rich blood supply for the lips and is nearer the free than the attached border. Since these arteries anastomose freely, it is well to tie both ends when they are severed. Due to their vascularity, the lips are often the site of nevi and other vascular tumors.

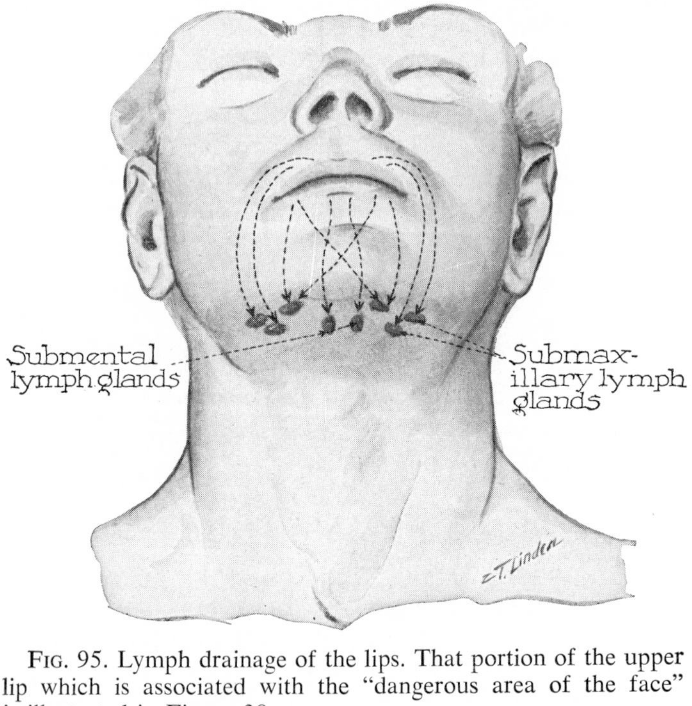

FIG. 95. Lymph drainage of the lips. That portion of the upper lip which is associated with the "dangerous area of the face" is illustrated in Figure 30.

The *mucous glands* situated in this layer are large, numerous, and can be felt with the tip of the tongue and seen when the lip is everted. The ducts of the glands open into the mucous membrane, and should they become occluded, an opalescent bluish "mucous cyst" develops as a result of distention of the gland.

The *veins* accompany the arteries and flow into the facial vein. By means of this flow a communication, the importance of which has been stressed before, exists between the lips and the intracranial circulation.

The *lymphatics* (Fig. 95) of the upper lip drain into the submaxillary nodes; those of the median portion of the lower lip drain into the submental glands; and those of the lateral portion pass directly into the submaxillary. Metastatic involvement of the submental and the submaxillary nodes continues to the superior and the inferior chains of deep cervical glands.

The *motor nerves* of the lips are derived from the facial, and the sensory branches supply the skin and the mucous membrane through the trigeminal by way of the infraorbital, the buccal and the mental branches.

5. **Mucous Membrane.** This constitutes the innermost layer of the lip and is covered with stratified epithelium.

Operation for single harelip

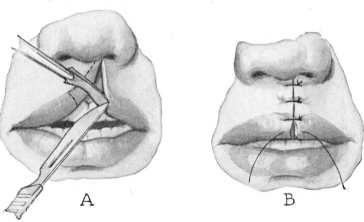

A   B

Operation for double harelip

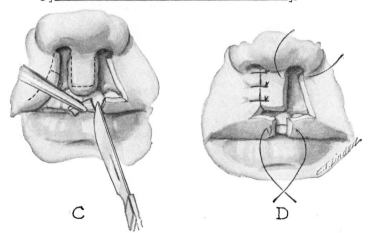

C   D

FIG. 96. Operations for single and double harelip.

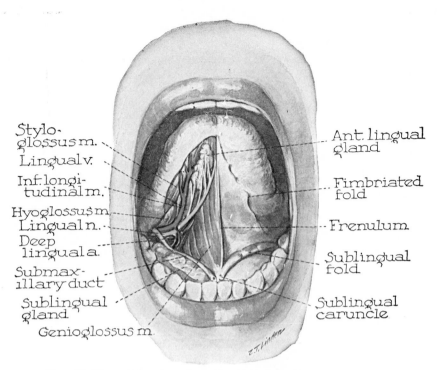

Stylo-
glossus m.

Lingual v.

Inf. longi-
tudinal m.

Hyoglossus m.

Lingual n.

Deep
lingual a.

Submax-
illary duct

Sublingual
gland

Genioglossus m.

Ant. lingual
gland

Fimbriated
fold

Frenulum

Sublingual
fold

Sublingual
caruncle

FIG. 97. The sublingual region. The mucosa has been removed on
the right side to expose the deeper structures.

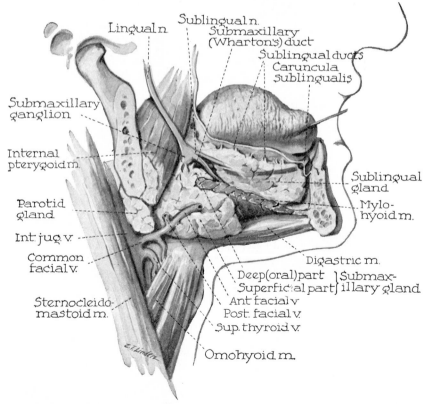

Lingual n.

Sublingual n.

Submaxillary
(Wharton's) duct

Sublingual ducts

Caruncula
sublingualis

Submaxillary
ganglion

Internal
pterygoid m.

Parotid
gland

Int. jug. v.

Common
facial v.

Sternocleido-
mastoid m.

Sublingual
gland

Mylo-
hyoid m.

Digastric m.

Deep (oral) part ⎫ Submax-
Superficial part ⎬ illary gland

Ant. facial v.

Post. facial v.

Sup. thyroid v.

Omohyoid m.

FIG. 98. The sublingual and the submaxillary salivary glands: sagittal section, showing the relations between glands, ducts, vessels and nerves.

SURGICAL CONSIDERATIONS

HARELIP

Operations for unilateral harelip (Fig. 96 A, B) depends upon the size of the defect. If small, and if the parts are freely movable, all that is necessary is to pare the margins and approximate the wound. The incision should include skin, mucous membrane and all the intervening tissue. If the parts are immobile and the defect more nearly complete, then more complicated and involved procedures must be done.

Operation for double harelip (Fig. 96 C, D) is a rather extensive one, and the surgeon should be specially trained and ready to meet any difficulties that arise. The central defect is prepared by incising its edges throughout its entire length and thickness; then the lateral margins are incised so that their approximation with the central part of the defect and with each other becomes possible.

Harelip is frequently associated with clefts in the hard and the soft palates. Surgical correction for this condition is described elsewhere (p. 145).

CARCINOMA OF THE LIP

Carcinoma of the lip is usually of the squamous-cell type. It arises from the mucocutaneous junction and is almost always found on the lower lip. The treatment may be surgical or by irradiation. If surgery is chosen, a V-shaped excision is employed, extending well into healthy tissue. However, this method is advisable only for small and early growths. For larger lesions, not only must the primary growth be removed, but also the associated glands: the submaxillary, the submental and, at times, the deep cervical chain. Enlarged nodes of the neck may involve one or both sides and are usually removed at a second stage by a radical operation en bloc. This involves an extensive suprahyoid dissection.

MOUTH PROPER

The mouth cavity is conveniently divided by the arch formed by the teeth and the gums into the vestibule, which lies between the gums and the cheeks, and the mouth proper, which lies behind and within the arch of the teeth.

The mouth proper lies within the arch of the teeth and communicates with the vestibule by means of an interval situated behind the last molar tooth. It is bounded in front and at the sides by the gums and the teeth, above by the hard and the soft palates, below by the tongue and the sublingual region and opens posteriorly into the pharynx via the isthmus.

Sublingual Region (Fig. 97). The two sublingual regions make up the floor of the mouth. Each is represented as a deep groove lying between the mandible and the root of the tongue and placed on the mylohyoid and the hyoglossus muscles. The anterior two thirds of the tongue rises from the floor, and the *frenulum linguae* appears as a median fold which connects the tongue to the floor. On each side of the frenulum the lingual vein appears as a prominent blue line. If the frenulum is made prominent by pressing the tip of the tongue against the hard palate, two small papillae will be noted at either side and at its summit, each representing the openings of the ducts of the submaxillary glands. The sublingual fold, a ridge of mucous membrane, passes laterally and backward from the papilla and overlies the sublingual gland. Each sublingual compartment contains the sublingual gland, an anterior prolongation of the submaxillary gland, the submaxillary duct, the lingual and the hypoglossal nerves and the sublingual vessels.

The *sublingual gland* is indicated by the sublingual fold (plica) which is found between the alveolus and the anterior part of the tongue. It takes an oblique forward and inward course to the *sublingual caruncle* near the frenulum. It not only indicates the position of the sublingual gland but also marks the line of the submaxillary (Wharton's) duct and the lingual nerve. The sublingual is the smallest of the salivary glands and rests on the mylohyoid muscle in the sublingual fossa close to the symphysis (Fig. 98). Its posterior end is in contact with the anterior prolongation of the submaxillary gland. The submaxillary duct, the lingual and the hypoglossal nerves and the sublingual vessels are situated between the sublingual gland and the root of the tongue. When the submaxillary gland is pressed on from the outside, its anterior prolongation can be felt through the mucous membrane slightly in front of the angle of the jaw. This prolongation forms a continuous glandular mass with the sublingual gland.

The many *sublingual ducts* open separately into the floor of the mouth. One of the larger ones on the posterior part opens into or by the side of the submandibular gland.

Ranula is a term that has been applied loosely to all cysts appearing in the floor of the mouth, but many observers believe that it should be restricted to cysts that originate in connection with the ducts of the salivary glands. It is a retention cyst which appears as a bluish mass filled with a mucouslike substance and is associated with a blockage of the submaxillary (Wharton's) or sublingual duct.

The *submaxillary duct* arises from the medial surface of its gland and accompanies it under the mylohyoid muscle; it passes diagonally across the medial aspect of the sublingual gland and adheres to it. In its course the hyoglossus and the genioglossus muscles lie medial to it, the hypoglossal nerve below, and the lingual nerve at first above, crossing it superficially at the anterior border of the hyoglossus, and then turning upward and deep. The lingual artery is under cover of the mylohyoid muscle but is crossed superficially by branches of the hypoglossal nerve and at its termination by the lingual nerve and the submaxillary duct.

Vestibule and Buccal Cavity. The *vestibule* lying between the gums and the cheeks, communicates with the mouth behind the last molars.

Stensen's duct opens into the vestibule opposite the second upper molar on a small papilla which can be felt with the tip of the tongue. About the circumference of the vestibule, the superior and the inferior cul-de-sacs

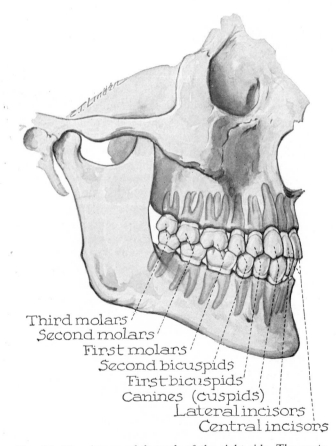

Third molars
Second molars
First molars
Second bicuspids
First bicuspids
Canines (cuspids)
Lateral incisors
Central incisors

Fig. 99. The sixteen adult teeth of the right side. The roots have been represented in phantom.

are formed by the reflection of the mucous membrane of the lips and the cheeks on the upper and the lower alveolar arches.

The *buccal cavity* is an area between the inferior margin of the orbit and the lower jaw, extending from the masseter muscle to the fold of the nose and the commissure of the lip. The cheeks (buccae) resemble the lips in their structure, having the same 5 layers: (1) the *skin;* (2) *superficial fascia* containing the zygomaticus major, the risorius and the platysma muscles; the parotid duct is surrounded by mucous glands, vessels and branches of the facial and the trigeminal nerves; (3) the *muscular layer* (buccinator) is covered with the buccopharyngeal fascia and is pierced by the parotid duct; (4) the *submucous layer* contains the mucous buccal glands; and (5) the *mucous membrane* is made up of stratified epithelium.

In the region of the cheek the subcutaneous fat increases to form the so-called *suctorial fat pad* located on the buccinator muscle and partly under and in front of the masseter; it is larger in the child, where it gives rotundity to the baby's cheeks and is useful in the act of sucking. This fat is continuous with the temporal and the lateral regions of the face.

The *lymphatics* from the anterior part of the cheek end in glands below the mandible; those from the posterior part end in glands on the surface of and inside the parotid gland.

The *nerves* of the cheek are branches of the facial supplying the muscles; the labial branches of the infra-orbital, the buccal and the mental nerves supply the skin and the mucous membrane with sensory fibers.

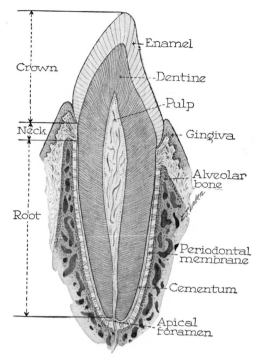

FIG. 100. Vertical section of a tooth, showing its structure.

The *external maxillary (facial) artery* is the only important vessel to the cheek; it crosses forward on the buccinator muscle and becomes the angular artery at the corner of the mouth.

Gums. The gums (gingivae) consist of dense vascular fibrous tissue which is covered by mucous membrane and is attached to the alveolar margins of the jaw. They are continuous with the mucosa of the oral vestibule

FIRST DENTITION

	MOLAR	MOLAR	CANINE	INCISOR	INCISOR	INCISOR	INCISOR	CANINE	MOLAR	MOLAR
Upper:	2nd	1st	1	2nd	1st	1st	2nd	1	1st	2nd
Lower:	2nd	1st	1	2nd	1st	1st	2nd	1	1st	2nd
Month of appearance:	24	12	18	9	7	7	9	18	12	24

SECOND DENTITION

	MOLARS	PREMOLARS	CANINE	INCISORS	INCISORS	CANINE	PREMOLARS	MOLARS
Upper:	3rd, 2nd, 1st	2nd, 1st	1	2nd, 1st	1st, 2nd	1	1st, 2nd	1st, 2nd, 3rd
Lower:	3rd, 2nd, 1st	2nd, 1st	1	2nd, 1st	1st, 2nd	1	1st, 2nd	1st, 2nd, 3rd
Year of appearance:	18, 12 6	10, 9	11	8, 7	7, 8	11	9, 10	6, 12, 18

externally and the palate or floor of the mouth internally. The submucous base is continuous with the alveolar periosteum which dips into each tooth socket, thus forming the root membrane (pericementum). Although quite vascular, the gums are not very sensitive. A portion of gingivae projects into each interdental space and surrounds the necks of the teeth. When caries attacks a tooth, the infection may spread and give rise to a subperiosteal abscess known as a *gum boil*. Because of the dense membrane under which the pus forms, intense pain results.

The term *epulis* is applied to a class of tumors connected with the gums and the alveolar processes. This may be a simple hypertrophy of the fibrous tissue of the gums and is then known as a fibrous epulis, or may spring from the periosteum, then becoming a malignant tumor.

Teeth. The *teeth* begin to appear at the 6th month of life, but the rudiments of both temporary and permanent teeth are present at birth. They are developed from the skin, the dentine being derived from the dermis and the covering enamel from the epidermis. There are two periods of dentition.

The result of the *first dentition* is 20 temporary or so-called deciduous (milk) teeth which appear between the 6th and the 24th months, the lower ones preceding the uppers. There are 4 incisors, 2 canines and 4 molars in each jaw but no premolars. The table on page 139 is a dental formula for the temporary teeth, with the dates of eruption expressed in months.

An interval of 4 years follows the first dentition, and at the age of 6 the *permanent teeth* (*second dentition*) begin to erupt and continue to appear until the 25th year. These statements can be simplified by saying that the first temporary teeth appear in the 6th or 7th months, and the first permanent teeth in the 6th or 7th year. In the second denti-

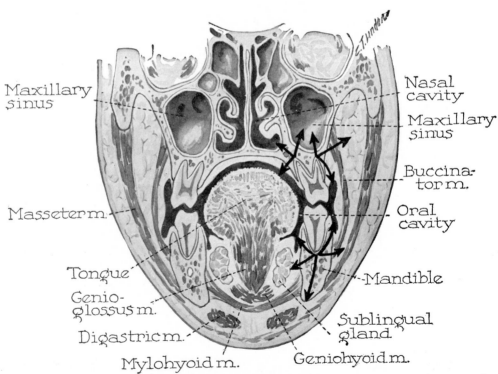

Maxillary sinus — Nasal cavity — Maxillary sinus — Buccinator m. — Masseter m. — Oral cavity — Tongue — Genioglossus m. — Mandible — Digastric m. — Sublingual gland — Mylohyoid m. — Geniohyoid m.

Fig. 101. Alveolar abscesses and their possible paths of invasion. In the upper jaw, the infection may spread to the external bony plate, into the mouth, the nasal cavity or the maxillary sinus. In the lower jaw, abscesses may burrow between periosteum and soft tissue, or between periosteum and bone, and then discharge on the neck, between the jaw and the chin; pus may also find its way to the floor of the mouth, resulting in Ludwig's angina (see Fig. 107).

tion, the first or 6-year molars erupt first, the 12-year molars second, and the 18-year molars or wisdom teeth third. Wisdom teeth may erupt late in life or not at all, failure of eruption often being the cause of cysts of the jaw.

The table at bottom of page 139 is a dental formula for the permanent teeth, with the date of eruption expressed in years.

There are 32 permanent teeth, 16 in each jaw, consisting of 4 varieties (Fig. 99): (1) The *incisors* or cutting teeth. The crown of these is chisel-shaped; the labial surface, convex; and the lingual, concave. The upper and particularly the central upper incisors are large, but the lower ones are the smallest of all the teeth. The roots of the incisors are single. The upper incisors overlap the lower, and from this point onward, with the exception of the last molar, every tooth in the upper jaw bites against two lower teeth. (2) The *canine* teeth are distinguished by their somewhat pointed crowns. The labial surface is convex, and the lingual slightly concave. The root is single and long, that of the upper canine being longer than that of

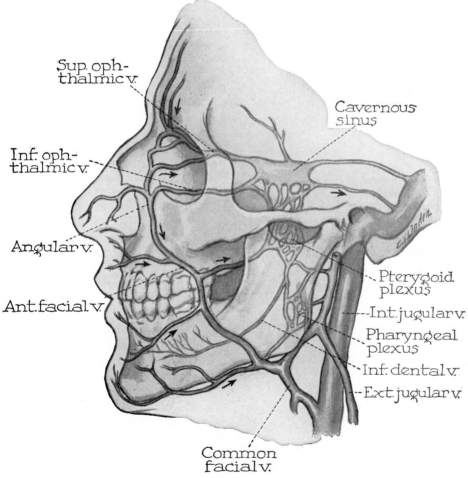

Fig. 102. The venous drainage of the teeth and possible paths of extension of a thrombophlebitis. The veins of the upper jaw drain in two directions: the anterior drains into the anterior facial vein, and the posterior into the pterygoid plexus. Following a tooth extraction, these infections may travel to the pterygoid or the pharyngeal plexus. Pterygoid plexus infections can extend to the inferior ophthalmic veins or through the foramina lacerum and ovale. In cavernous sinus thrombosis following anterior teeth infections, the thrombophlebitis usually spreads from the anterior facial vein through the orbit via the ophthalmic veins, usually the superior.

any other tooth, thereby producing the canine eminence on the anterior surface of the maxilla. The upper canines are larger than the lowers and are known as the "eye" teeth. (3) The *bicuspids,* or premolars, acquired their name because of the two cusps which they present, one being lingual and the other labial. Each has a single root which shows a tendency to divide, especially in the first upper bicuspid. (4) The *molars* are distinguished as the 1st, the 2nd and the 3rd; these are the grinding teeth. The upper molars have 4 cusps and the lower have 5. All are characterized by their large crowns and are the largest of all the teeth but diminish in size from the 1st to the 3rd. Each has 2 or 3 roots, which occasionally are united in the last molar. As a rule, a difference may be noticed between the molars of the maxilla and those of the mandible. Normally, the upper molars possess 3 roots and the lower have 2. The upper molars have either 3 or 4 projecting tubercles, and the lower usually have 5.

Each tooth (Fig. 100) has a *crown* covered with enamel, a *neck* encircled by gum, and a *root* imbedded in the jaw. At the apex of each root is found the *apical foramen,* which is a pinpoint opening leading through a widening canal to the *pulp cavity.* This is filled with tooth pulp, a vascular connective tissue with numerous little nerves and vessels which reach it via the apical foramen. Each tooth consists of: (1) *enamel,* which is the insensitive covering of the crown; (2) *dentine,* the exquisitely sensitive yellowish basis of the tooth; (3) *cement* (crusta petrosa), a bony covering for the root and the neck of the tooth; (4) *pulp,* which is a fibrous material containing the nerves and the vessels; (5) *periodontal membrane,* which is continuous with the lamina propria of the gum and is attached to both the cement and the alveolar wall.

The teeth are rooted in the alveolar cavities or sockets and are firmly maintained there. These sockets, and particularly the lower ones, are much nearer the outer than the inner table, as evidenced by their palpable bulging into the vestibule. The thinness of this outer plate explains the perforation of root abscesses onto the vestibular surfaces and also the fractures of the outer plate during tooth extractions.

The maxillary teeth are supplied by branches of the *maxillary* and the *infraorbital* nerves. The *lymph vessels* of these teeth end in glands on the surface of the parotid and below the mandible. The mandibular nerve supplies the mandibular teeth; and their lymph vessels end in glands below the mandible and in the carotid triangle.

An *alveolar abscess* (Fig. 101) is a collection of pus located at the apex of the tooth. The infection in the pulp cavity invades the space between the root and the socket. The pus escapes through the surface offering the least resistance, usually the external alveolar plate lateral to the apex of the tooth. However, it may burrow and form a sinus some distance from the point of origin. Abscesses are less likely to occur in the upper jaw, where the blood supply is good; if such an abscess forms, it may extend into the maxillary sinus or the nasal cavity. In the lower jaw pus may make a path between the periosteum and the soft tissue or between the periosteum and the bone. Pus burrowing in such directions may discharge on the neck beneath the jaw and the chin, or into the floor of the mouth, producing a Ludwig's angina (p. 150). An abscess of the wisdom tooth may penetrate the lateral tissues at the angle of the jaw or occasionally pass downward into the neck, forming a large abscess in the submaxillary region.

Veins of the lower jaw (Fig. 102) drain into the inferior dental vein, which in turn drains into the pterygoid plexus. Those from the upper jaw drain in two directions: the anterior veins drain into the anterior facial, and the posterior into the pterygoid plexus. Following tooth extraction, ascending infections may involve the pterygoid or pharyngeal plexuses; from here they may travel to the cavernous sinus via the vein of Vesalius (Fig. 30). On the other hand, a thrombophlebitis of the pterygoid plexus may travel through the veins which communicate with the inferior ophthalmic vein. In cavernous sinus thrombosis following infections of the anterior teeth there is a tendency for the infection to spread via the anterior route: the anterior facial and angular veins through the orbit via the ophthalmic veins, and especially by the way of the superior.

In the condition known as *pyorrhea alveolaris,* a purulent inflammation of the dental periosteum is present. The process involves the gingivae and the walls of the alveoli. Recession of the gums takes place until the teeth and their gingival and alveolar connections become loosened and finally fall out. As soon as the tooth is removed, the inflammatory symptoms usually subside.

Hard and Soft Palates (Fig. 103). The *palate* forms the superior wall or roof of the buccal cavity. It consists of two portions: in front, a hard palate which has an osseous base, and, posteriorly, a soft palate composed of fibrous tissue.

The *hard palate* is covered by mucous membrane and forms a partition between the buccal and the nasal cavities. It is formed by the palatine processes of the maxilla and the horizontal plate of the palatine bone. The mucous membrane is peculiar in that it is practically one with the periosteum which covers the bone (mucoperiosteum). Therefore, in dissecting it, the bone is laid bare, since the mucous membrane and the periosteum cannot be separated. The membrane is thin in the midline but thicker at the sides, the increased thickness being due to the presence of numerous glands that lie beneath the surface laterally but are absent toward the midline. Because of its toughness, the membrane is easy to manipulate when flaps are being formed in the operation for cleft palate.

The main *blood supply* of the hard palate is derived from the descending palatine branches of the internal maxillary artery, which emerges from the posterior palatine canal near the inner side of the last molar; it then passes forward and inward, ending in the anterior palatine canal. The artery is so situated that it is easily injured when incisions are made for operations in cleft palate. Should this occur, delayed healing or even sloughing of the flaps may result. Therefore, in dissecting such flaps, the vessel may be spared if the incision is placed as close as possible to the gingival border and, as it is extended posteriorly, it should wind about the last molar. The artery runs closer to the bone than to the mucous surface. Some surgeons advocate that the vessel be ligated deliberately as a preliminary step in the treatment of cleft palate and that actual repair be postponed for some weeks until a collateral circulation has become established.

The mucous membrane of the hard palate is noted for its numerous rugosities. The median *raphe* is very distinct and terminates in front in the incisive papilla which overlies the anterior palatine foramen. On each side of the raphe are the transverse ridges which form the *palatine rugae.* These vary in number and in prominence and become less distinct as age advances.

The *soft palate,* or vellum, is attached to the posterior edge of the hard palate and consists of connective tissue, muscles, blood vessels, nerves and glands. It is a fleshy curtain that hangs down in the isthmus of the fauces and shuts the mouth from the pharynx during nasal breathing. In deglutition or mouth breathing it is raised to a horizontal position to close the buccal portion of the pharynx from the nasopharynx and in this way prevents food from entering the nasopharynx. If the palate is paralyzed and cannot be raised, the nasopharynx is unprotected, and fluids are liable to be regurgitated through the nose. Although the anterior border of the palate is attached, its posterior is free and presents in the midline a downward projection called the *uvula.* The soft palate is attached to the lateral wall of the pharynx on each side and is uniformly about ¼ inch thick. Its framework is formed by the *palatal aponeurosis,* which is attached to the posterior edge of the bony palate, is joined by the tendons of the palati muscles and finally becomes lost between the muscles.

There are 5 *muscles* of the soft palate: 2 descend from it to the tongue and the pharynx (glossopalatine and pharyngopalatine), 2 descend to the palate from the base of the skull (levator palati and tensor palati), and one lies in its substance (musculus uvulae) (Fig. 103).

1. The *levator palati muscle* originates from the lower surface of the apex of the petrous bone and the medial surface of the eustachian tube. It inserts into the upper aspect of the palatal aponeurosis.

2. The *tensor palati muscle* originates from the scaphoid fossa of the sphenoid bone

and the lateral aspect of the eustachian tube. Its tendon winds around the hamulus and pierces the buccinator to form a broad attachment to the palatal aponeurosis and to the posterior border of the hard palate.

3. The *palatoglossus* or *glossopalatinus muscle* arises from the undersurface of the palatine aponeurosis, descends in front of the tonsils in the glossopalatine arch and is inserted into the posterior aspect and side of the tongue.

4. The *palatopharyngeus* or *pharyngopalatinus muscle* arises from the posterior border of the bony palate and from the palatine aponeurosis, then descends behind the tonsil in the pharyngopalatine arch. It is inserted partly into the posterior border of the thyroid lamina and partly into the posterior wall of the pharynx. As it descends, it is in intimate contact with the inner surface of the constrictor muscles and lies posteromedial to the stylopharyngeus.

5. Each *musculus uvulae* arises from the posterior nasal spine and the palatine aponeurosis and inserts into the uvula. Two small muscular slips lie on either side of the midline in the substance of the uvula.

The actions of the tensor and the levator muscles are indicated by their names. The palatoglossi muscles aid in the elevations of the dorsum of the tongue and in the closure of the oropharyngeal isthmus during the first stage of deglutition. The palatopharyngeal muscles aid in the elevation of the larynx and thus shorten the pharynx in the second stage of deglutition. The uvular muscle shortens and raises the uvula.

The muscles of the soft palate are supplied by several *nerves*. The levator palati, the muscle uvulae and the palatopharyngeus are supplied, with the muscles of the pharynx, by the spinal accessory nerve; the palatoglossus, by the hypoglossal nerve,

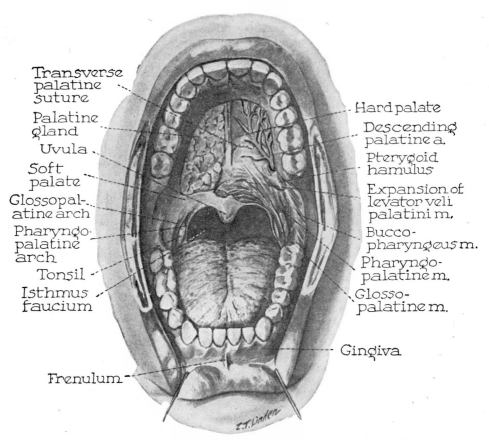

FIG. 103. The palate. The palatine glands have been removed on the left side to show the vascular supply.

which also supplies the muscles of the tongue; the tensor palati is supplied, together with the tensor tympani, by the third division of the 5th nerve through the otic ganglion.

The nerve supply to the mucous membrane of the soft palate is derived from branches descending from the sphenopalatine ganglion (maxillary nerve). These have been referred to as the lesser and the middle palatine nerves.

The *blood supply* of the soft palate is derived from branches of the ascending pharyngeal, maxillary and facial arteries.

SURGICAL CONSIDERATIONS

STAPHYLORRHAPHY AND URANOPLASTY

(Fig. 104) Different types of cleft palate require different management. The name "staphylorrhaphy" is given to the operation

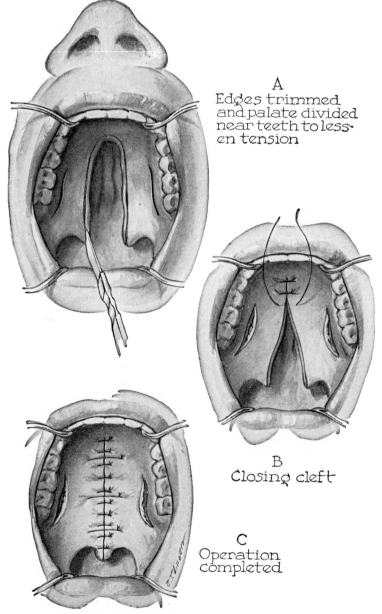

A
Edges trimmed
and palate divided
near teeth to lessen tension

B
Closing cleft

C
Operation
completed

FIG. 104. The surgical correction of cleft palate.

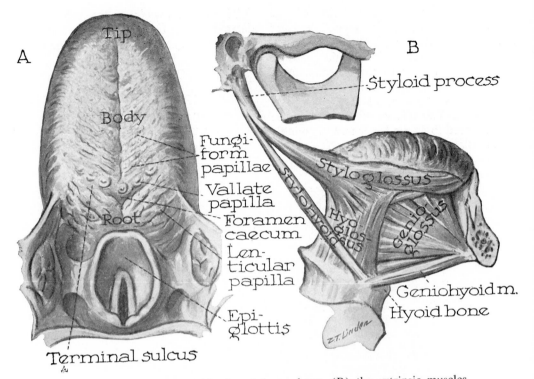

Fig. 105. The tongue: (A) viewed from above, (B) the extrinsic muscles.
The glossopalatine muscle is shown in Figure 103.

that approximates a cleft in the soft tissue, and "uranoplasty" to that which corrects a defect in the bone. The soft parts are divided on the hard palate to the bone and then separated from it. The soft and the hard tissue edges are freshened, the edges of the soft tissues are separated from the underlying bone and smoothly trimmed with a sharp scalpel. The soft parts are brought together by sutures, the periosteum being included. At times retention sutures are necessary to maintain proper tension. The important features of the operation are proper mobilization and freshening of the margins of the cleft associated with approximation of the soft parts to close the defect.

Tongue (Vessels and Nerves). The tongue is a solid mass of muscle covered by mucous membrane and attached to the floor of the mouth, the hyoid bone and the mandible. Situated below the palate, above the floor of the mouth proper and in front of the pharynx, it is divided into two parts which differ developmentally, structurally and function-

ally, in nerve supply and in appearance. The anterior two thirds, called the oral part or *body*, has also been referred to as the buccal portion; the posterior third is the pharyngeal part or *root*. The boundary between the oral and the pharyngeal parts is marked on the dorsum of the tongue by an inverted V-shaped groove called the terminal sulcus, the apex of which corresponds to a depression known as the *foramen caecum* (the upper end of the thyroglossal tract).

The *dorsal surface* (Fig. 105 A) of the buccal part of the tongue presents a rough mucous membrane with numerous papillae, but the dorsal surface of the pharyngeal portion is relatively pale and presents masses of lymphoid nodules called "lingual tonsils." These form the lowest part of the ring of lymphatic tissue that encircles the pharynx (Waldeyer's ring).

The three types of *papillae* characteristic of the mucous membrane of the anterior two thirds of the tongue are:

1. The *vallate papillae,* 10 to 12 in number, which lie immediately in front of the

sulcus terminalis. Since they run anteriorly and parallel with the sulcus, they too are arranged as an inverted V. Each is a short cylinder surrounded by a circular trench, the outer wall of which is raised to resemble a collar. Serous glands open into the trench, and taste buds lie in their walls.

2. The *fungiform papillae* are smaller than the vallate and appear as bright-red spots, more numerous at the tip and the margin. They are furnished with taste buds and consist of a rounded head attached by a narrow base.

3. The *filiform papillae* are the smallest and most numerous of the lingual papillae. They cover the anterior two thirds of the tongue and give it its characteristic velvety appearance. Posteriorly, they are arranged in rows parallel with the sulcus terminalis, but they are transverse in the middle of the tongue and become irregular anteriorly. They contain the touch corpuscles.

The *inferior surface* of the tongue (Fig. 97) has no papillae and is smooth. It is connected with the floor of the mouth by the frenulum, on each side of which is the lingual (ranine) vein; the vessel is visible through the mucous membrane. Laterally, there is a fringed fold called the *fimbriated fold*. These folds converge toward the tip and indicate the position of the deep lingual (ranine) artery, which is placed deeper than the vein.

The *muscle substance* of the tongue (Fig. 105 B) is divided into right and left halves by a median fibrous septum, each half being made up of both intrinsic and extrinsic muscles. The extrinsic muscles move the tongue and alter its shape, but the intrinsic only alter its shape. The 4 *extrinsic muscles* are the *genioglossus* which protrudes the tongue, the *styloglossus* which retracts it, the *hyoglossus* which depresses it, and the *glossopalatine* which elevates the root of the tongue. The 4 intrinsic muscles are the *longitudinalis superior*, the *longitudinalis inferior*, the *transversus* and the *verticalis*.

The motor nerve of the tongue (Fig. 106 A) is the *hypoglossal*, which supplies the entire musculature except the glossopalatine which is supplied by the pharyngeal plexus. The *glossopharyngeal nerve* supplies both taste and sensory fibers to the posterior third of the tongue. The *lingual nerve* (trigeminal) supplies sensory fibers to the anterior two thirds, but the *chorda tympani* (facial) is incorporated in the lingual and supplies part of the tongue with taste fibers. Because of this arrangement, the semilunar ganglion may be removed and taste remain unaffected. If the hypoglossal nerves are injured, as may occur in excision of the tongue for carcinoma or in fracture of the jaw, the genioglossi become paralyzed, and the tongue falls backward and may produce suffocation. If only one genioglossus is paralyzed, the protruded tongue is thrust to the paralyzed side, thus indicating the side of the lesion.

The *lingual artery* supplies the tongue (Fig. 106 A); it is a branch of the external carotid and arises between the superior thyroid and the facial arteries. It makes a characteristic short upward hook and disappears under cover of the posterior border of the hyoglossus muscle. Before reaching this muscle it is applied to the middle constrictor of the pharynx and then passes between the hyoglossus and the genioglossus. The hyoglossus separates it from the 12th nerve. The artery turns upward and, after supplying branches to the sublingual gland, terminates as the *profunda artery,* running forward in the lower part of the tongue as far as its tip. Its only anastomosis is at the tip, and because of this the tongue can be bisected almost bloodlessly.

Four *veins* pass backward to form the lingual vein. They are: (1) the *ranine,* the chief vein of the tongue, which crosses the anterior surface of the hyoglossus muscle obliquely; (2) an accompanying vein which runs with the hypoglossal nerve on the outer surface of the hyoglossus muscle; (3) and (4) two *venae comites* of the lingual artery which accompany the artery on the deep surface of the hyoglossus muscle. After these 4 veins converge to form the lingual, they cross the loop of the lingual artery and both carotids and end in the internal jugular; at times they may terminate in the common facial vein.

The *lymph drainage* (Fig. 106 B) of the tongue may be divided into 4 groups: namely, apical, marginal, central and posterior or basal.

1. *Apical Group.* These lymph vessels

start at the tip of the tongue and pass in two directions: directly to the submental glands, and to the jugulo-omohyoid (supra-omohyoid) gland.

2. *Marginal Group.* Many of these vessels pass down on the outer surface of the hyoglossus muscle. The group drains the side of the tongue and passes to the submandib-

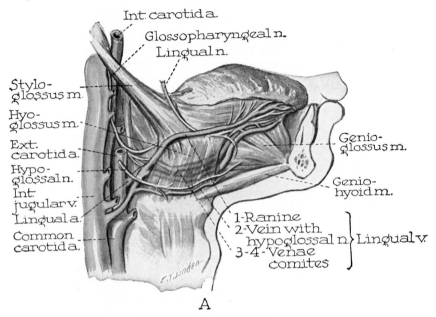

Int. carotid a.
Glossopharyngeal n.
Lingual n.
Stylo-glossus m.
Hyo-glossus m.
Ext. carotid a.
Hypo-glossal n.
Int. jugular v.
Lingual a.
Common carotid a.
Genio-glossus m.
Genio-hyoid m.
1-Ranine
2-Vein with hypoglossal n. } Lingual v.
3-4-Venae comites
C.T.Linden

A

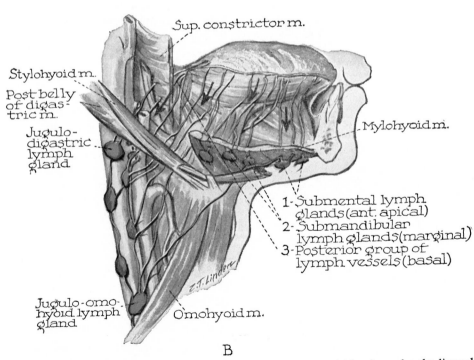

Sup. constrictor m.
Stylohyoid m.
Post belly of digastric m.
Jugulo-digastric lymph gland
Mylohyoid m.
1-Submental lymph glands (ant. apical)
2-Submandibular lymph glands (marginal)
3-Posterior group of lymph vessels (basal)
Jugulo-omo-hyoid lymph gland
Omohyoid m.
C.T.Linden

B

FIG. 106. Nerves and vessels of the tongue: (A) nerves and blood supply; the lingual vein is formed by 4 veins; (B) lymph drainage of the tongue; the central group of lymph vessels is not shown.

ular gland and to the glands of the deep cervical chain. There may be lymph nodes lying on the hyoglossus in relation to these vessels; these may be palpated if a finger is placed in the floor of the mouth and the fingers of the other hand placed beneath the jaw bone.

3. *Central Group.* These are the vessels that drain the area of the tongue immediately to either side of the median raphe. They pass directly downward in the midline between the genioglossi muscles and then to either

the right or the left deep cervical glands.

4. *Posterior (Basal) Group.* The vessels of this group drain the posterior part of the tongue, many of them passing freely from one side to the other. They enter the deep cervical chain.

In carcinoma of the tongue, cancer cells may pass freely to the lymph vessels, then to the lymph glands, and may involve both sides of the neck. Therefore, it is necessary that all glands receiving lymph from the tongue be eradicated.

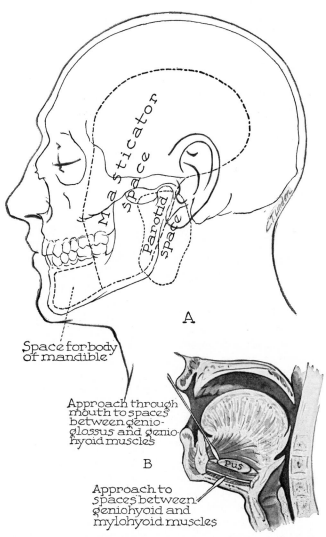

FIG. 107. Infections about the face and the mouth: (A) the 3 muscular fascial spaces, (B) approach to abscesses above and below the geniohyoid muscle.

PRACTICAL CONSIDERATIONS

THREE MUSCULAR FASCIAL SPACES AND ONE VASCULAR VISCERAL SPACE

Coller and Yglesias have emphasized the fact that the fasciae in this region are attached to periosteum, enclose facial muscles and form closed spaces. In this way the spaces are separated from cervical fascial spaces, and infections do not spread into the neck but remain limited. However, the fasciae which surround the viscera and the vessels are continuous between the face and neck so that infections may travel from one to the other. These authors have described three muscular fascial spaces and one vascular visceral space (Fig. 107 A).

Space of the Body of the Mandible. This fascial space exists between the superficial and the deep divisions of the middle muscular fascia. It has an important bearing on infections of this bone and, because of the fascial attachment, osteomyelitis of the body of the mandible is prevented from spreading either superficially or deep. An infection in this location may do one of three things: discharge into the mouth, spread to the masticator space, or remain localized. The space is drained through the mouth by means of an incision that goes through the gingival mucous membrane of the vestibule or by an incision through the skin along the inferior border of the body of the bone.

Masticator Space. The second space is occupied by the ramus of the mandible. It is bounded externally by the masseter, internally by the pterygoids and superiorly by the temporal muscle. Infections in this space may travel upward either to the so-called superficial or to deep temporal spaces. The temporal spaces may be drained by incisions that are carried through the skin, the subcutaneous tissue and the temporal fascia. If the malar bone or the zygoma are involved, resection of either may be necessary.

Parotid Space. This is the third fascial space of the face. It is occupied by the parotid gland. Drainage of this space can be accomplished by an incision that is made in front of the ear and passes downward behind and below the jaw. The external surface of the parotid is thus exposed without injury to the facial nerve if the dissection is kept external to the glandular substance. If it is desirable to drain the space between the masseter muscle and the superficial part of the parotid gland, a horizontal incision is made at the level of and parallel with the superior border of the mandible.

Visceral Vascular Fascial Space. This is the lateral pharyngeal space. It is bounded anteriorly by the medial wall of the masticator space, laterally by the parotid space, posteriorly by the carotid sheath and medially by the submaxillary gland. Since this is not one of the enclosed facial fascial spaces, infection may travel and involve the internal carotid artery, producing severe hemorrhage, or it can produce septic thrombosis of the internal jugular vein. Drainage may be external through the parotid space or internal through the lateral pharyngeal wall. Infection in this space can spread readily to the viscerovascular spaces of the neck and the mediastinum.

UPPER AND LOWER LIP INFECTIONS

Infections in the upper lip should not be incised or squeezed. Many surgeons advocate ligation of the angular vein, but this is still a moot question. If pus is present, some advise drainage. Meningitis and the occurrence of cavernous sinus thrombosis should always be kept in mind (Fig. 30).

Infections in the lower lip are less dangerous than those of the upper. Cavernous sinus thrombosis rarely occurs from infections in this region because the veins lie at a deeper level and are more efficiently splinted by muscle and bone. Two anatomic spaces are formed in the floor of the mouth (Fig. 107 B). The superficial space lies between the genioglossus and the geniohyoid muscles and is divided into two compartments by a median fascial septum. The second space lies at a deeper level and is situated between the geniohyoid and the mylohyoid muscles. It, too, is divided in the middle by a fascial septum. *Ludwig's angina* constitutes involvement of these spaces, with elevation of the tongue and inflammation of the mucous membrane over the involved area. If the infection is unilateral, the tongue is pushed to the opposite side, but if bilateral, it is pushed upward toward the roof of the mouth. The treatment of Ludwig's angina consists of early drainage instituted in the involved space; hence, it is important to determine whether the abscess is below or above the geniohyoid. If the abscess is below this muscle, the region under the chin is prominent, and an incision should be made through the skin, the subcutaneous tissue and the mylohyoid muscle into the abscess cavity. If the swelling is diffuse, the incision should follow the lower border of the mandible in order that both sides of the fascial septum or both sides of this space can be dealt with properly. If the infection is situated above the geniohyoid muscle, it usually points under

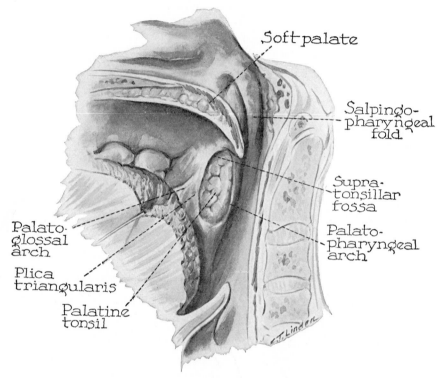

Fig. 108. The palatine tonsil and its relations, shown in sagittal section.

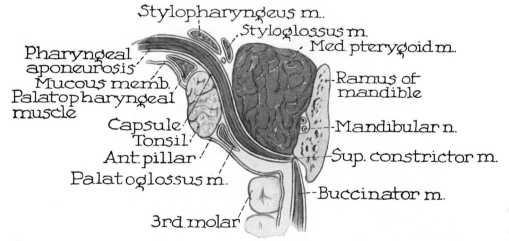

Fig. 109. The relations of the palatine tonsil to its capsule and the surrounding structures.

the tongue and then can be drained through the floor of the mouth, the incision passing through the mucous membrane and the genioglossus muscle. Both sides of the fascial septum should be explored.

PHARYNX

Tonsils

(Figs. 108, 109.) The term "tonsil" usually applies to the faucial or palatine tonsils. The tonsillar region, although anatomically located in the anterolateral pharynx and properly belonging to it, is considered as an intermediate area between the buccal cavity and the oral division of the pharynx. The tonsils are two masses of lymphoid tissue placed in the *fossa tonsillaris* and located on the surface at a point a little above the angle of the mandible. They lie between the palatoglossal and the palatopharyngeal arches, above the back part of the tongue and below the soft palate. Each tonsil has *two* surfaces (medial and lateral), *two* borders (anterior and posterior), and *two* poles (superior and inferior).

The **medial surface** is free and can be seen through the mouth when the tongue is depressed. It faces inward and presents from 12 to 30 rounded or slitlike openings called the *tonsillar crypts*. Tiny plugs of food, debris or pus often fill and identify these openings. This surface is covered with mucous membrane in the form of squamous epithelium which invades the substance and lines the crypts.

The **lateral** is the attached surface. It is covered by a fascia derived from the pharyngeal aponeurosis, which is referred to as the capsule of the tonsil. This is attached laterally by loose areolar tissue to the inner surface of the superior constrictor of the pharynx. Lateral to the superior constrictor are the ascending palatine, the pharyngeal and the tonsillar arteries; the medial pterygoid muscle is situated lateral to these. One or more veins descend over the lateral surface of the capsule. The superior constrictor

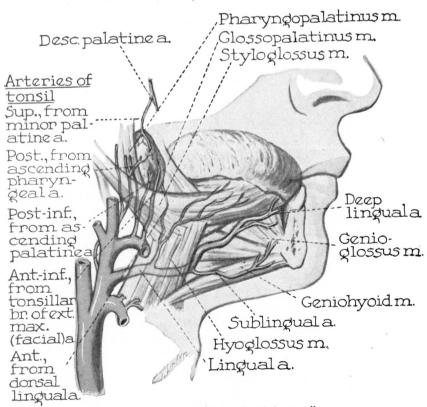

Fig. 110. The blood supply of the tonsil.

separates the tonsil from the facial artery at that point where the artery begins to arch downward.

Poles. The *upper pole* of the tonsil invades the lateral surface of the soft palate, and the *lower* is continuous with the lingual tonsil.

Borders. The *anterior border* is in contact with the palatoglossus muscle, and the *posterior* with the palatopharyngeus muscle.

The **blood supply** (Fig. 110) of the tonsil is very profuse, the main vessel being the *tonsillar artery,* a branch of the facial (external maxillary). This vessel enters the tonsil from its lateral aspect and near its lower pole. Other small vessels aid in the blood supply, anastomosing freely with one another. They are the ascending palatine (facial), dorsalis linguae (lingual), greater palatine (maxil-

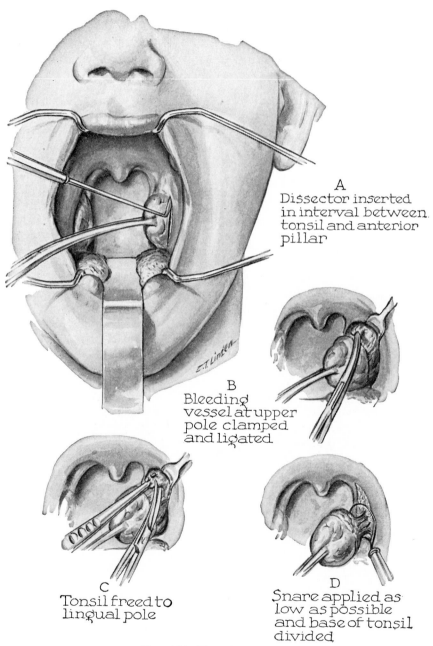

A
Dissector inserted in interval between tonsil and anterior pillar

B
Bleeding vessel at upper pole clamped and ligated

C
Tonsil freed to lingual pole

D
Snare applied as low as possible and base of tonsil divided

FIG. 111. Tonsillectomy.

lary) and the ascending pharyngeal arteries.

The **veins** form a plexus which surrounds the capsule, pierce the superior constrictor and end in the pharyngeal plexus, which is a tributary of the internal jugular vein.

The **lymphatics** leave the gland, pierce the superior constrictor and end in the superior deep cervical chain. One gland is situated below the posterior belly of the digastric and the angle of the jaw. It lies on the carotid artery in the angle formed by the junction of the common facial with the internal jugular vein and has been referred to as the jugulo-digastric gland (tonsillar gland of Wood). This may be enlarged not only in nonspecific infections, but by the tubercle bacillus when it gains entrance by way of the tonsil.

The **nerve supply** to the tonsil is derived from the glossopharyngeal nerve and the pharyngeal plexus.

SURGICAL CONSIDERATIONS

Tonsillectomy and Peritonsillar Abscess. When a tonsil is removed, its capsule should remain attached to it. This exposes the constrictor muscle and not the aponeurosis of the pharynx. Therefore, the capsule is removed with the tonsil because it is firmly blended with that organ.

In tonsillectomy, traction on the gland pulls it forward without dragging the pharyngeal wall and the internal carotid artery. This is explained by the laxity of the tissue which exists between the gland and the superior constrictor. However, in patients who have suffered repeated attacks of quinsy, this lax tissue may be replaced by dense adhesions. Tonsillar hemorrhage following surgery is the result of bleeding from the tonsillar vessels proper, since the possibility of injuring the internal carotid is most remote and the external carotid lies still farther externally.

In *tonsillectomy* (Fig. 111), after proper exposure with a mouth gag and tongue depressor, a tenaculum is applied to the palatal pole, and traction made downward and medially. This maneuver makes visible the interval between the tonsil and its anterior pillar. A sharp dissector enters this space along the anterior pillar and incises just beneath the mucous membrane which covers the tonsil. Retraction of the anterior pillar with blunt dissection will expose the blue-white capsule. If sharp dissection is preferred, the point of the scissors is applied toward the tonsil side, and an attempt is made to remain in the avascular cleavage plane. The tonsil is freed down to its lingual pole. A snare is then applied as low as possible on its base, tightened, and the base divided. A retractor is applied to the anterior pillar for the purpose of inspection, and pledgets of gauze or cotton are introduced for hemostasis by pressure. If active arterial bleeding is present, the severed artery is grasped and tied with a fine suture.

In the treatment of *peritonsillar abscess,* an imaginary line should be drawn from the base of the uvula to the last molar of the same side. An incision is made at the junction of the anterior one third with the posterior two thirds along the arcus palatinus. This incision is spread with forceps, and the pus is allowed to flow out. Some surgeons advocate entering the tonsillar fossa (Fig. 108) with a curved sharp-pointed forceps. The approach between the tonsil and the anterior pillar seems to be an easier method of draining the supratonsillar fossa.

Neck in General

The numerous vessels, nerves and visceral structures found in the neck make this region both interesting and important to the surgeon. The upper limits of the neck are the lower border of the jaw, a line extending from the angle of the jaw to the mastoid process, and the superior curved line of the occipital bone. The lower limits are the sternal notch, the clavicles and a transverse line from the acromioclavicular joint to the spinous process of the 7th cervical vertebra. The contour of the neck varies with age and sex, being well rounded in women and children but more angular in men; hence, the landmarks are more conspicuous in the male. In extension, the anterior part of the neck is lengthened, and in flexion it is shortened, so that the distance between its movable parts from the sternum to the lower jaw varies as does the relationship of these parts to the vertebrae. Therefore, it is necessary in giving relative positions of landmarks to suppose that the neck is midway between flexion and extension, this being the natural upright position unless otherwise stated. The anterior portion of the neck contains the respiratory tube (larynx and trachea) and the alimentary tube (pharynx and esophagus); the great vessels and nerves are located on the sides, and the posterior portion contains the cervical segment of the spine and surrounding musculature. The infrahyoid region extends from the hyoid bone above to the suprasternal notch below and is limited laterally by the anterior border of the sternocleidomastoid muscles.

EMBRYOLOGY

Visceral Arches

The branchial (visceral) arches are best developed in the human embryo about the last half of the 3rd week of intra-uterine life, at which time they appear as parallel bars (Fig. 112). Six such arches are present, and they occupy a region which later becomes the neck. They represent the gill apparatus mechanism of water breathing vertebrates in which the respiratory function is performed by means of a rich vascular tissue that lines the clefts. Water passes through these fringes, permitting the exchange of the oxygen of the water and the carbon dioxide of the blood. In higher vertebrates with the acquisition of aerial respiration, a loss of function in these gill arches takes place, and the number is reduced from 7 as seen in fish to 6 in man. The 5th and the 6th arches are blended with the surrounding structures so that they are not visible externally as distinct bars. Each arch has an outer covering of ectoderm (squamous epithelium), an inner covering of entoderm (columnar epithelium) and an intermediate mass of mesoderm. Between the bars, internal and external depressions are found. The internal depressions are called *visceral pouches,* and the external are known as *visceral clefts*; the cleft membrane is formed between the two depressions. Each arch is supplied with a plate of cartilage, a muscle mass, a nerve and an artery.

First, or Mandibular, Arch. This is supplied by the mandibular branch of the 5th nerve and the external maxillary artery. Its muscle mass develops into the muscles of mastication, which are supplied chiefly by the mandibular nerve. This arch becomes differentiated into a shorter upper maxillary process and a longer lower mandibular one, both of which play a large part in the formation of the face. The cartilage of the first arch, referred to as Meckel's cartilage, is almost entirely replaced by the mandible, but its end persists and forms two of the ear bones, the malleus and the incus.

Second, or Hyoid, Arch. This is supplied

by the facial nerve, and its artery is the external carotid. Its muscle mass becomes the muscles of facial expression and the platysma. The cartilage of the 2nd arch is known as the cartilage of Reichert. From it are developed the Stapes, the Styloid process, the Stylohyoid ligament and the Smaller cornu of the hyoid bone; hence, it can be called the "S" arch.

Third, or Thyrohyoid, Arch. This is supplied by the glossopharyngeal nerve and the internal carotid artery. The muscle mass of this arch becomes the stylopharyngeus muscle, and the cartilage develops into the body and the greater cornu of the hyoid bone.

Fourth, Fifth and Sixth Arches. These arches are unnamed and somewhat indefinite. However, the 4th arch gives rise to the cricothyroid muscle which is supplied by the external branch of the superior laryngeal nerve. The muscle mass of the 5th arch forms some of the intrinsic muscles of the larynx which are supplied by the recurrent laryngeal nerve. The cartilages of the 4th and the 5th arches become the framework of the larynx. The thyroid cartilage originates from arches 4 and 5; the cricoid, the arytenoids, the rings of

the trachea and the bronchi are formed from the 6th arch.

The arches enclose the primitive pharynx within which develop the important "T" structures: Tongue, Tonsils, Tube (eustachian), Thyroid, Thymus and paraThyroids.

CERVICAL SINUS

The 2nd visceral arch, growing faster than the arches below it, soon overhangs them and forms a deep groove known as the cervical sinus (Fig. 113). The downgrowing 2nd arch eventually meets and fuses with the 5th, resulting in a space lined by squamous epithelium which normally disappears. However, if this space persists, a *branchial cyst* results. If the 2nd arch fails to meet the 5th, an opening called a *branchial fistula* is found along the anterior border of the sternocleidomastoid muscle which is most commonly placed above the sternoclavicular joint. The cleft membrane always forms a septum between such a cyst or fistula and the pharynx. Since a branchial fistula is situated below the 2nd arch and above the 3rd, its course can be readily understood, passing between the internal and the external carotid

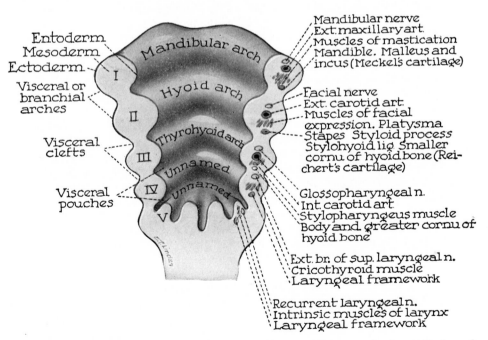

FIG. 112. Arrangement and structure of the visceral arches in the fetus. Each arch has a nerve, an artery, a plate of cartilage and a muscle mass. The structures to which each of these gives rise have been named in the drawing.

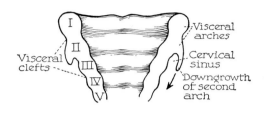

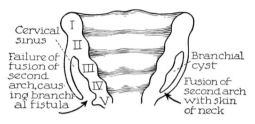

FIG. 113. Formation of a branchial cyst and a branchial fistula in the embryo.

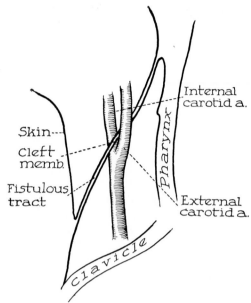

FIG. 114. The course of a branchial fistula (diagrammatic).

arteries (Fig. 114). The facial and the hypoglossal nerves lie superficial to the fistulous tract, and the glossopharyngeal nerve lies deep to it. If the fistula extends upward to the pharyngeal recess it will pass between the stylohyoid and the stylopharyngeus muscles.

SURGICAL CONSIDERATIONS

Branchial cysts should be completely excised and, since there is little adherence to the surrounding structures, these procedures are usually quite simple. A transverse incision is made in a skin crease of the neck so that there is minimal scarring, the proper cleavage plane is found, and the cyst is removed.

Branchial Fistulae. Excision of branchial fistulae (lateral cervical fistulae) tends to be more difficult, since there is adherence to surrounding tissues (Fig. 115). It is wise to inject such a fistula with methylene blue and determine whether or not the dye appears inside the pharynx; this also marks the fistulous tract. These operations may be long and difficult. Since complete exposure is necessary, a longitudinal incision along the anterior border of the sternocleidomastoid muscle is advised which extends from the external fistulous opening below to the angle of the jaw. The fistulous tract is dissected from below upward, and the great vessels and the surrounding nerves are protected.

An assistant's finger may be inserted through the mouth to press the region of the internal opening of the fistula toward the surgeon. The incision is deepened through the skin, the superficial fascia and the platysma. Then the superficial layer of deep cervical fascia is incised along the anterior border of the sternocleidomastoid which is freed and retracted posteriorly. The fistulous tract is dissected from below upward to the lower border of the posterior belly of the digastric which is retracted upward. The fistula may pass lateral to both carotids or may dip between them. The pharyngeal part of the dissection requires exact anatomic exposure. Some surgeons have suggested a stepladder type of operation, making multiple transverse incisions.

BONY CARTILAGINOUS FRAMEWORK

The bony cartilaginous framework of the neck consists of the hyoid bone, the thyrohyoid membrane, the thyroid cartilage, the cricothyroid membrane, the cricoid cartilage and the trachea (Fig. 116).

Hyoid Bone. This has no immediate relation with the skeleton; it lies in the soft part of the neck at the root of the tongue and possesses great mobility. Mosher has noted the importance of the greater cornu and has stated that 16 major structures of the neck (the glossopharyngeal, the recurrent laryngeal and the phrenic nerves excepted) are in close relation to it. The hyoid bone is on

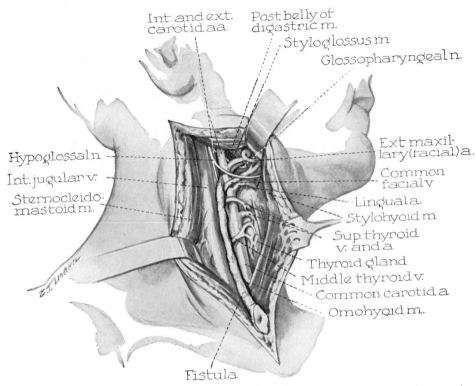

FIG. 115. Excision of a branchial fistula. The incision extends along the anterior border of the sternocleidomastoid muscle from the fistulous opening below, to the angle of the jaw above. The posterior belly of the digastric muscle and the anterior border of the sternocleidomastoid muscle are retracted in opposite directions, giving adequate exposure. In this case the fistula passes between the external and the internal carotid arteries. The tract is dissected from below upward.

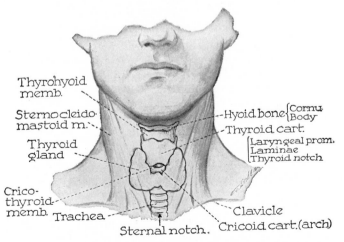

FIG. 116. The bony and cartilaginous framework of the neck.

a level with the 3rd cervical vertebra, and its body is approximately on a level with the angles of the jaw. The upper borders of the cornu are excellent guides to the lingual arteries. Therefore, the hyoid bone is of great surgical importance as a landmark. The external laryngeal muscles and several muscles of the tongue and the floor of the mouth attach to it.

Thyrohyoid Membrane. This membrane is situated between the hyoid bone and the thyroid cartilage. It acts as a ligament which suspends the larynx from the hyoid and attaches to the posterior border of the bone and its greater cornu. The interval between the bone and the cartilage varies from 1 to 1½ inches.

Thyroid Cartilage. This consists of 2 laminae which are separated behind but united in front to form a projection called the *laryngeal prominence* or *Adam's apple*. The anterior borders of the laminae are joined at their lower halves, but the upper halves are separated and form the V-shaped *thyroid notch* which can be felt through the skin. This is an important landmark, since the common carotid arteries usually bifurcate at this level. An oblique line is usually visible on the posterior part of the lateral aspect of the lamina, and it is to this line that the sternothyroid muscle inserts and the thyrohyoid muscle takes its origin.

Cricothyroid Membrane. This membrane closes the space separating the cricoid and the thyroid cartilages. It is lozenge shaped, is widest in the midline and tapers toward the side. Through this space the simplest and most rapid tracheotomy may be performed for the immediate relief of suffocation.

Cricoid Cartilage. This cartilage forms a complete ring encircling the larynx, below the thyroid cartilage. Its narrow anterior part, or arch, is easily felt through the skin and lies on a level with the 6th cervical vertebra. The posterior part, or lamina, is much deeper, projects upward and occupies the lower part of the gap between the two laminae of the thyroid. At this level is the junction of the pharynx and the esophagus, the larynx and the trachea, and here also the common carotid is crossed by the omohyoid muscle. It is also a useful guide in controlling serious hemorrhage from either carotid ar-

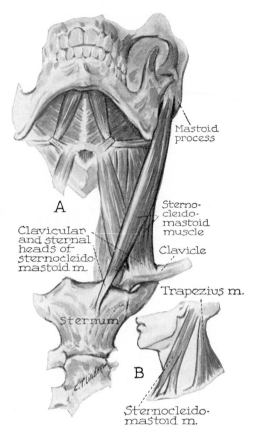

Fig. 117. The sternocleidomastoid muscle. This structure is the most important surgical landmark in the neck.

tery, since at this level pressure may be maintained against the tubercle of the 6th cervical vertebra.

STERNOCLEIDOMASTOID MUSCLE

The sternocleidomastoid muscle is the most important surgical landmark in the neck (Fig. 117). It arises by two heads: the sternal head originates in front of the manubrium sterni by means of a rounded tendon, and the clavicular head takes origin from the upper border and front of the medial third of the clavicle by muscle fibers. The muscle inserts on the outer surface of the mastoid process and the lateral third of the superior nuchal line. Its nerve supply is derived from the spinal part of the spinal accessory and the 2nd and the 3rd cervical nerves. When both muscles contract, the head becomes flexed on the vertebral col-

umn, but contraction of one muscle rotates
the head to the opposite side and draws it
down toward the chest. The sternocleidomastoid separates the anterior from the posterior triangle of the neck, and many structures which are considered as contents of
these triangles actually lie under the muscle.
These structures are the common and the
internal carotid arteries, the internal jugular
vein, the vagus nerve, the scalenus anterior
muscle and the cervical plexus. The triangular interval existing between the sternal and
the clavicular heads is very evident in thin
individuals and appears as a slight depression. Beneath the lower end of this depression
and just above the sternoclavicular joint lies
the common carotid on the left side and the
bifurcation of the innominate artery on the
right. The carotid sheath is under cover of
its lower part and along its anterior border
above. Along its posterior border, the nerves
of the cervical and the brachial plexuses are
found. The spinal part of the spinal accessory nerve extends backward and downward
through its deep fibers.

DEEP CERVICAL FASCIA (FASCIA COLLI)

The important *deep cervical fascia* consists
of 3 layers: superficial (general investing or
enveloping fascia), middle (pretracheal fascia) and deep (prevertebral fascia) (Figs.
118, 119).

SUPERFICIAL LAYER (GENERAL INVESTING OR ENVELOPING FASCIA)

**The superficial layer of deep cervical
fascia** is characterized by its tendency to
divide, hence its synonyms: investing or
enveloping layer. This fascia splits to envelop
two muscles (trapezius and sternocleidomastoid), *two* salivary glands (submaxillary
and parotid) and *two* spaces (space of Burns
and a space above the clavicle in the posterior triangle). It extends from the ligamentum nuchae posteriorly to the midline
anteriorly where it becomes continuous with
its fellow of the opposite side. As it leaves
the ligamentum nuchae, it splits to envelop
the trapezius muscle, reuniting at the muscle's
anterior border to form the roof of the pos-

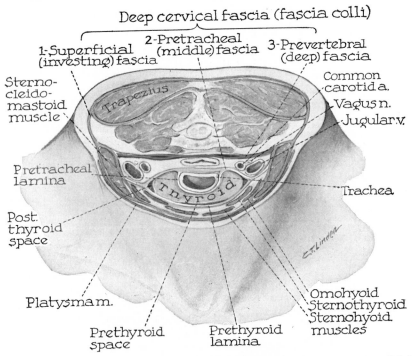

FIG. 118. The deep cervical fascia in cross section. The first or superficial
investing layer has been colored red; the second or pretracheal layer is
yellow; the third or prevertebral layer is blue.

terior triangle. It divides again at the posterior border of the sternocleidomastoid muscle, the two layers joining at its anterior border to form the roof of the anterior triangle.

This layer of fascia is attached above to the external occipital protuberance, the superior nuchal line, the mastoid process (base), the zygomatic arch and the lower border of the mandible. Below it is attached to the acromion process and spine of the scapula, the clavicle and the manubrium sterni. Its enveloping of the submaxillary gland is accomplished by a splitting of the fascia at the lower border of the gland, the superficial layer attaching to the lower bor-

der of the mandible and the deep layer to the mylohyoid line (Figs. 120 and 118). The submaxillary *lymph glands* are inside of this sheath and in immediate contact with the submaxillary *salivary gland*; therefore, in the removal of the lymph glands for tuberculosis or carcinoma, the salivary gland also should be sacrificed.

The parotid investment is brought about by a splitting which takes place at the lower border of the parotid gland, the deeper layer passing deep to the gland and attaching to the base of the skull. The superficial layer passes superficial to the gland and attaches to the zygomatic arch; this layer is

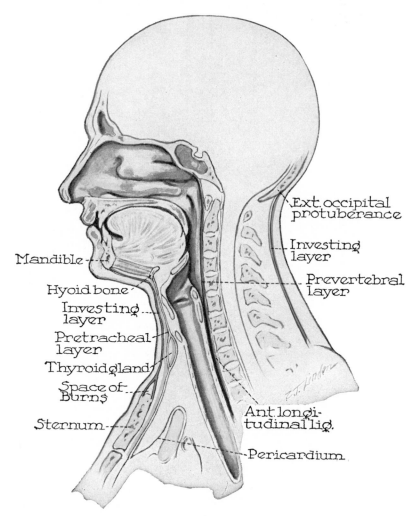

Fig. 119. The deep cervical fascia in longitudinal section. The same color identification of the 3 layers as was used in Figure 118 is utilized here.

very dense, and any swelling of the under-lying parotid gland causes tension and pain (mumps).

The superficial fascia splits below to form 2 spaces: the first is over the lower part of the *posterior triangle* where it is attached to the clavicle; between its layers are found the descending supraclavicular veins and part of the external jugular vein. The second space is over the lower part of the *anterior triangle* where it splits and attaches to the front and the back of the manubrium sterni, forming the *suprasternal space of Burns* (Figs. 119, 120). This contains the sternal head of the sternocleidomastoid muscle, the communica-tion of the anterior jugular veins (jugular arch), lymph glands and fat.

MIDDLE LAYER (PRETRACHEAL FASCIA)

This layer is part of the general investing fascia and arises from the deep surface of the sternocleidomastoid muscle. It passes in front of the carotid system (internal jugular vein, common carotid artery and vagus nerve) and divides into the prethyroid and the pre-tracheal layers or laminae (Figs. 121 and 118).

Prethyroid Layer. This is a thin lamina which passes in front of the thyroid gland and attaches to it along an irregular line at the junction of the middle and the posterior thirds of the superficial surfaces of each lat-eral lobe. Therefore, it passes in front of the superior thyroid vessels above and the in-ferior thyroid veins below. Laterally, it is

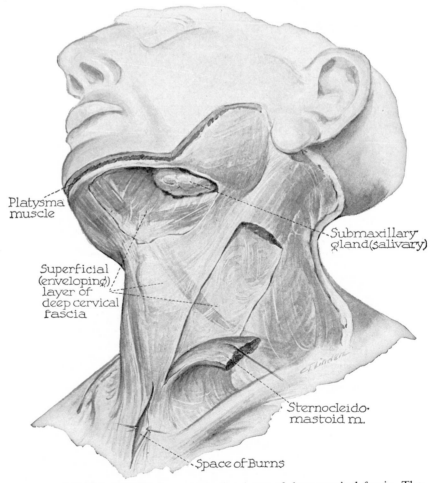

Platysma muscle

Superficial (enveloping) layer of deep cervical fascia

Submaxillary gland (salivary)

Sternocleido-mastoid m.

Space of Burns

FIG. 120. The superficial or enveloping layer of deep cervical fascia. The illustration demonstrates the "fascial envelopes" formed for the submaxil-lary salivary gland and sternocleidomastoid muscle.

separated from the surface of the gland and from the pretracheal fascia proper by an interval filled with loose areolar tissue which has been aptly referred to by Sloan as the *posterior thyroid space* (Fig. 118). This triangular space is limited anteriorly by the prethyroid lamina, posteriorly by the pretracheal layer proper and medially by the thyroid gland. It is necessary to enter this space before attempting to mobilize the lobe and dislodge it medially.

Pretracheal Layer Proper. This layer passes in front of the trachea and extends behind the posterolateral border of the thyroid, thus forming the posterior boundary of the posterior thyroid space. Its fibers converge on the thyrotracheo-esophageal area where they become dense and thick and fix the thyroid gland to this area. There is no cleavage plane at this point. This has been called the pedicle of the thyroid, and from here the fascia continues medially over the trachea and the larynx to join the pretracheal layer of the opposite side.

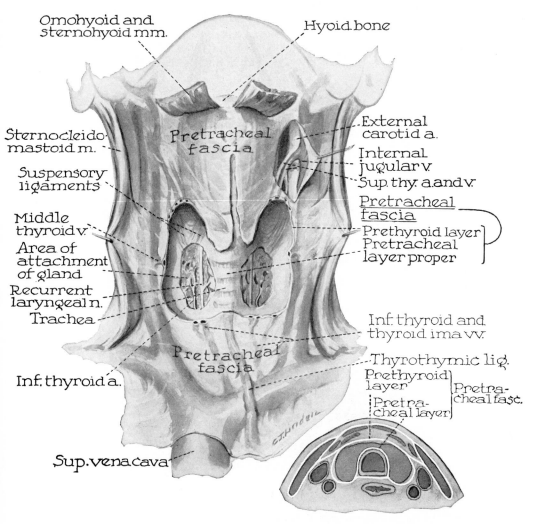

FIG. 121. The pretracheal fascia. This fascia is a part of the general investing fascia; it arises from the deep surface of the sternocleidomastoid muscle. After passing in front of the carotid system, it attaches to the thyroid gland and then splits into 2 layers: an anterior prethyroid layer and a posterior pretracheal layer. The thyroid has been removed to show the distribution of the fascia. The inset shows the division of the fascia into 2 layers.

The vertical extent of the pretracheal fascia is from the hyoid bone above to the superior mediastinum below where it blends with the fibrous pericardium (Fig. 119).

The suspensory ligaments of the thyroid gland are thickened portions of the pretracheal fascia that run from the upper and inner parts of the gland to the cricoid cartilage. The ligaments form a sling that anchors the gland to the larynx which must be severed before the thyroid can be mobilized properly.

DEEP LAYER (PREVERTEBRAL FASCIA)

The prevertebral fascia (Figs. 118, 119) also arises from the general investing fascia and is much thicker than the pretracheal. It passes behind the carotid system and covers the muscles that are applied to the cervical

vertebrae (longus colli, longus capitis, scalenus anterior, medial and posterior, etc.). It is attached to the base of the skull above and continues into the thorax where it blends with the anterior longitudinal ligament of the spine. The great vessels of the neck lie on this fascia, and the phrenic nerve and the anterior rami of the cervical nerves are behind it. As the roots of the brachial plexus and the subclavian artery pass under the scalenus anterior muscle they carry the prevertebral fascia with them into the axilla as the axillary sheath.

BUCCOPHARYNGEAL FASCIA

The buccopharyngeal fascia (Fig. 122) is a layer of connective tissue that passes around the sides and the back of the pharynx

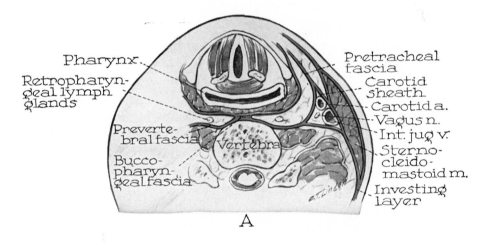

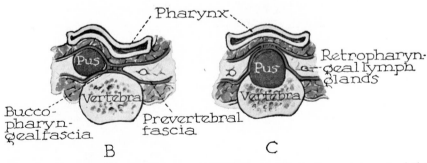

FIG. 122. The buccopharyngeal fascia. (A) This fascia binds the upper part of the pharynx to the prevertebral fascia directly in the midline. (B) Acute retropharyngeal abscess involves the lymph glands in front of the prevertebral fascia and because of the attachment of the buccopharyngeal fascia presents to either side of the midline. (C) The chronic abscess, usually from tuberculosis of a cervical vertebra, is behind the prevertebral fascia and appears in the midline.

and binds the middle of the back of the pharynx to the prevertebral fascia. This anatomic fact aids in the diagnosis and the treatment of retropharyngeal abscesses.

In the *unilateral* variety or acute retropharyngeal abscess, a group of inflamed lymph glands break down which lie in the interval between the prevertebral and the buccopharyngeal fasciae. They drain the nasopharynx and bulge on one side of the midline because of the midline attachment of the two fascia. The *midline* variety or chronic retropharyngeal abscess usually results from tuberculosis of a cervical vertebra and starts behind the prevertebral fascia. Should it bulge into the pharynx it would be centrally located; it may then travel laterally behind the prevertebral fascia and point at the posterior border of the sternocleidomastoid.

SUBMENTAL TRIANGLE

The submental triangle (Fig. 123) has as its base the body of the hyoid bone and as its apex the symphysis of the mandible. It is bounded laterally by the anterior bellies of the digastric muscles. The roof of the triangle is made up of the investing layer of deep cervical fascia, and its floor is formed by the mylohyoid muscles with their median raphe. The triangle contains the *submental lymph* glands, which drain the superficial tissue below the chin, the central part of the lower lip, the adjoining gums, the anterior part of the floor of the mouth, and the tip of the tongue. The efferent vessels from these glands pass to join the submandibular (submaxillary) lymph glands. When they enlarge or become abscessed they are usually prevented from rising into the mouth by the mylohyoid muscles.

Wide incisions may be made into this area because there are no important structures that can be injured. After incising the investing layer of deep cervical fascia, location of the digastric and the mylohyoid muscles will immediately orient the surgeon.

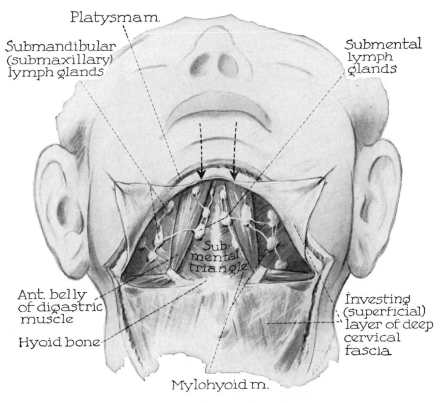

FIG. 123. The submental triangle. The superficial layer of deep cervical fascia has been incised to show the lymph drainage of the triangle.

Anterolateral Region of the Neck

ANTERIOR TRIANGLE

The anterior triangle (Fig. 124) of the neck is bounded in front by the midline of the neck, which extends from the symphysis of the mandible above to the sternal notch below; behind, by the anterior border of the sternocleidomastoid; above, by the lower border of the mandible and a line drawn backward from its angle to the posterior boundary. This triangle is subdivided into 3 subsidiary triangles by the anterior and the posterior bellies of the digastric and the superior belly of the omohyoid.

The digastric triangle is bounded by the anterior belly of the digastric in front, the posterior belly of the same muscle behind, and the border of the mandible above.

The carotid triangle is bounded by the superior belly of the omohyoid below, the sternocleidomastoid behind and the posterior belly of the digastric above.

The muscular triangle is bounded by the superior belly of the omohyoid above, the sternocleidomastoid below, and the midline of the neck in front.

Submental Triangle. That region of the neck which is bounded by the body of the hyoid bone below and the anterior bellies of the digastric on each side forms the submental triangle.

SUPERFICIAL STRUCTURES (SKIN, SUPERFICIAL FASCIA, PLATYSMA AND LYMPH NODES)

Skin. The skin of the neck is loosely attached, especially anteriorly. Since it is well supplied with blood vessels, it favors plastic surgery. The skin that covers the posterior region is very thick, adherent and contains numerous sebaceous glands, which explains the frequency of furuncles and carbuncles in this area.

Superficial Fascia. This fascia of the neck consists of fat and connective tissue. It is not clearly defined and is difficult to demonstrate.

Platysma Myoides. This rhomboidal muscle lies *in* the superficial fascia of the neck (Fig. 125). It originates from the fascia of the pectoralis major and the deltoid and inserts into the lower border of the mandible; its fibers converge as they pass upward and medially. Some of the fibers reach the face and mingle with the risorius and other depressor muscles. Its posterior border is free, covers the lower anterior part of the posterior triangle and continues across the base of the jaw to the angle of the mouth. Its anterior border decussates behind the chin. Since it is a muscle of expression, it is supplied by the cervical branch of the facial nerve which reaches its deep surface. Branches of the anterior cutaneous nerve of the neck pierce it. In some individuals it is well developed and in others it is difficult to find. It is lacking in the midline of the neck; therefore, it cannot be sutured in this location. Between the muscle and the underlying superficial layer of deep cervical fascia lie the anterior and the external jugular veins and the cutaneous nerves of the neck. Incisions in the neck bleed freely before the deep fascia is cut, because the retraction of the divided platysma holds the cut veins open and prevents them from retracting. However, when the deep fascia is divided, the veins are able to retract, and most of the oozing stops.

Lymph Nodes. The external jugular lymph nodes are usually found as a cluster lying upon and near the external jugular vein as it approaches the region of the parotid gland. They are superficial to the superficial layer of the deep cervical fascia and, when not diseased, are small or even absent. They receive lymph from the external ear in the parotid region and drain into the deep nodes which lie upon the carotid sheath beneath

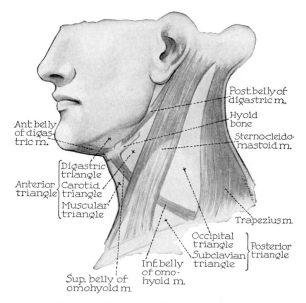

Post. belly of
digastric m.

Hyoid
bone

Sternocleido-
mastoid m.

Ant. belly
of digas-
tric m.

Digastric
triangle

Anterior | Carotid
triangle | triangle

Muscular
triangle

Trapezius m.

Occipital
triangle

Subclavian
triangle

Posterior
triangle

Inf. belly
of omo-
hyoid m.

Sup. belly of
omohyoid m.

FIG. 124. The triangles of the neck.

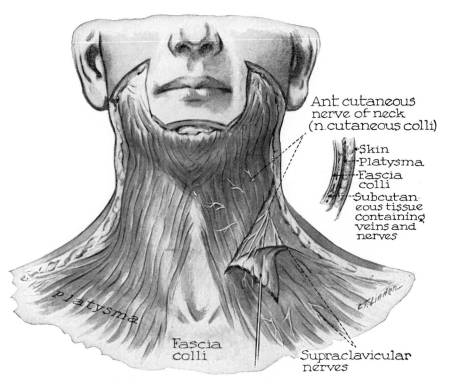

Ant. cutaneous
nerve of neck
(n. cutaneous colli)

Skin
Platysma
Fascia
colli
Subcutan-
eous tissue
containing
veins and
nerves

platysma

Fascia
colli

Supraclavicular
nerves

FIG. 125. The platysma muscle. A wedge of muscle has been cut out on the left
to show the underlying nerves. The inset shows the true position of the platysma,
in the superficial fascia.

the sternocleidomastoid muscle. Since they are on and not under the deep fascia, it is a safe and simple procedure to eradicate or incise them, but the position of the external jugular vein should be kept in mind.

NERVES

Four superficial nerves associated with the posterior border of the sternocleidomastoid muscle; they supply the skin of this region (Fig. 126). They are derived from the anterior primary rami of the 2nd, the 3rd and the 4th cervical nerves through the branches of the cervical plexus, which lies under cover of the muscle.

Lesser Occipital. The lesser occipital nerve (2nd cervical) appears at the junction of the middle and the upper thirds of the posterior border of the sternocleidomastoid where it hooks around the accessory nerve; it passes upward and backward along the posterior border of that muscle to supply the skin over the lateral part of the occipital region.

Great Auricular. The great auricular nerve (2nd and 3rd cervicals) appears at a slightly lower level, runs parallel with the external jugular vein and enters the nuchal region posterior to the ear; it supplies the skin over the angle of the jaw, the parotid gland, the postero-inferior half of the lateral and the medial aspects of the auricle, and the skin over the mastoid region.

Anterior Cutaneous. The anterior cutaneous nerve (cutaneous colli, 2nd and 3rd cervicals) appears close to the great auricular nerve but runs transversely forward across the sternocleidomastoid and beneath the external jugular vein; it supplies the region about the hyoid bone and the thyroid cartilage.

Supraclavicular. The supraclavicular nerve (3rd and 4th cervicals) appears at a slightly lower level than the preceding ones. The anterior (medial) supraclavicular travels downward and medially across the lower part of the sternocleidomastoid; the middle (intermediate) runs across the clavicle, and the posterior (lateral) extends downward and laterally across the trapezius and the acromial end of the clavicle.

The last four cranial nerves, in their extracranial courses, are located in the region of the digastric muscle (Fig. 127).

Vagus. The vagus (10th cranial) nerve leaves the skull through the jugular foramen and at its exit is closely related to the 9th, the 11th and the 12th nerves; the internal jugular vein lies posterior to it, and the internal carotid artery is anterior. In the neck the vagus supplies the alimentary and the respiratory tubes by means of its branches— the pharyngeal, the superior and the recurrent laryngeal.

Glossopharyngeal. The glossopharyngeal nerve (9th cranial) leaves the skull through the jugular foramen with the vagus and the accessory, but in its own sheath of dura mater. It descends between the internal jugular and the internal carotid vessels to the lower border of the stylopharyngeus around which it winds and then passes forward between the internal and the external carotid arteries. Its one motor branch supplies the stylopharyngeus muscle.

Spinal Accessory. The spinal accessory nerve (11th cranial) has a double origin: spinal and cranial. The spinal part arises from the upper 5 or 6 segments of the spinal cord, and the cranial is accessory through the vagus. It makes an abbreviated appearance in the carotid triangle between the digastric and the sternocleidomastoid muscles. As it enters the deep surface of the sternocleidomastoid about 2 inches below the tip of the mastoid process, it is surrounded by lymph glands and is accompanied by the sternocleidomastoid branch of the occipital artery. It appears about the middle of the posterior border of the sternocleidomastoid muscle and here again is surrounded by lymph glands. The accessory nerve supplies the sternocleidomastoid and the trapezius; its cervical branches are entirely sensory.

Hypoglossal. The hypoglossal nerve (12th cranial) is the motor nerve of the tongue. It emerges from the skull through the anterior condylar (hypoglossal) canal in the occipital bone and is in close contact with the 9th, the 10th and the 11th cranial nerves. It lies between the internal jugular vein and the internal carotid artery and, as it descends, is closely related to the vagus until it appears at the lower border of the posterior belly of the digastric. Here it turns forward and medially and crosses, in turn, the internal

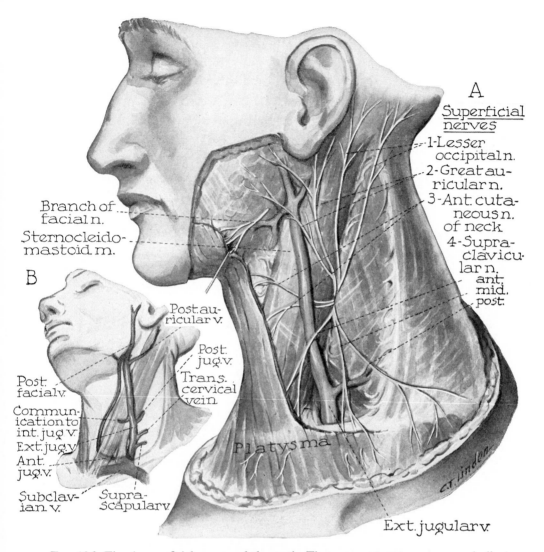

A
Superficial
nerves
1-Lesser
occipital n.
2-Great au-
ricular n.
3-Ant. cuta-
neous n.
of neck
4-Supra-
clavicu-
lar n.
ant.
mid.
post.

Branch of
facial n.
Sternocleido-
mastoid m.

B

Post. au-
ricular v.

Post.
jug. v.
Trans.
cervical
vein

Post.
facial v.
Commun-
ication to
int. jug. v.
Ext. jug. v.
Ant.
jug. v.

Subclav-
ian v.
Supra-
scapular v.

Platysma

Ext. jugular v.

FIG. 126. The 4 superficial nerves of the neck. These are cutaneous nerves and all ot them are related to the posterior border of the sternocleidomastoid muscle. The inset shows the plan of the veins in this region.

carotid, the occipital and the external carotid arteries and the loop of the lingual artery. As it crosses the lingual artery, the hypoglossal nerve is crossed superficially by the common facial vein, passes deep to the posterior belly of the digastric and the submaxillary gland and enters the submandibular region where it is distributed to the muscles of the tongue. As the nerve continues forward, it comes to lie superficial to the hyoglossus muscle which separates it from the lingual artery, then continues in an intermuscular cleft between the hyoglossus and the

mylohyoid to the muscles of the tongue (Fig. 106-A).

The *ascending branch of the hypoglossal nerve* leave its parent trunk where it bends forward to cross the carotid vessels.

The *descending branch* continues downward on the surface of the internal and the common carotid arteries and is imbedded in the anterior wall of the carotid sheath.

From its lateral side it is joined by the descending cervical nerve (2nd and 3rd cervicals) which arises from the cervical plexus, and the nerve loop so formed constitutes the *ansa hypoglossi.* Branches from this ansa are distributed to the sternohyoid, the sternothyroid and both bellies of the omohyoid. The thyrohyoid receives its own nerve from the first cervical via the hypoglossal.

Cervical Plexus. This plexus should not be confused with the cervical sympathetic groups (Fig. 128). The plexus lies on the scalenus medius and the levator anguli scapulae under cover of the sternocleido-

mastoid muscle. It is formed by the upper 4 cervical nerves, all but the first of which divides into 2 parts. A branch from each nerve joins the superior cervical ganglion. These nerves are combined in irregular series of loops under cover of the sternocleidomastoid. The roots of the plexus lie deep to the prevertebral fascia and are frequently injured in radical neck surgery. The terminal branches pierce the fascia and continue to

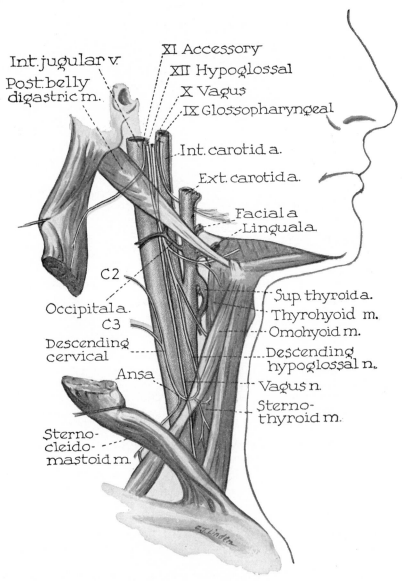

FIG. 127. The last 4 cranial nerves in their extracranial courses. These nerves are closely related to the posterior belly of the digastric muscle. The formation of the ansa hypoglossi is also shown.

the muscles which they supply and the nerves with which they connect. The superficial cutaneous branches radiate from the plexus and appear in the supraclavicular region as they wind around the posterior margin of the sternocleidomastoid muscle.

Phrenic Nerve. Of the muscular or deep branches, the phrenic is the most important. It is derived from the 4th cervical, but receives additional fibers from the 3rd and the 5th. It passes downward in the neck and lies deep to the prevertebral fascia, traveling on

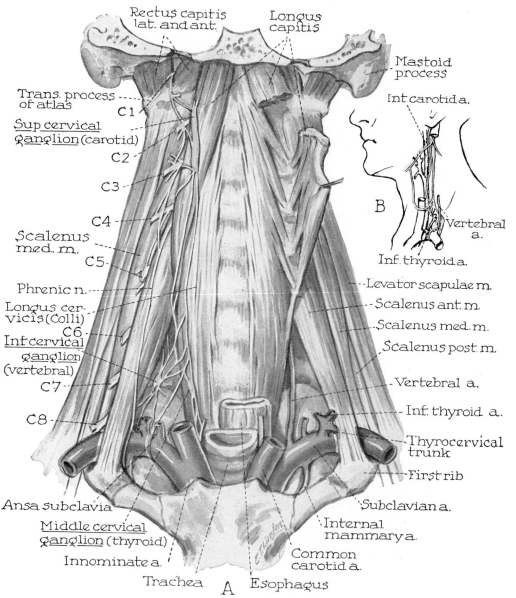

Rectus capitis lat. and ant.

Longus capitis

Mastoid process

Trans. process of atlas

C 1

Int. carotid a.

Sup. cervical ganglion (carotid)

C2

C3

C4

Scalenus med. m.

C5

B

Vertebral a.

Inf. thyroid a.

Phrenic n.

Levator scapulae m.

Scalenus ant. m.

Longus cervicis (Colli)

C6

Scalenus med. m.

Inf. cervical ganglion (vertebral)

Scalenus post. m.

C7

Vertebral a.

Inf. thyroid a.

C8

Thyrocervical trunk

First rib

Ansa subclavia

Subclavian a.

Middle cervical ganglion (thyroid)

Internal mammary a.

Innominate a.

Common carotid a.

Trachea   A   Esophagus

Fig. 128. The cervical sympathetics. This group consists of 3 ganglia with their connecting branches. The ganglia are known as superior, middle and inferior and have been called carotid, thyroid and vertebral, respectively, from their almost constant association with these arteries. The inset shows these relationships. The cervical plexus should not be confused with the cervical sympathetic group. The plexus is formed by the upper 4 cervical nerves and lies on the scalenus medius muscle.

the anterior scalene muscle; it enters the thorax at the root of the neck on its way to the diaphragm.

Superficial Branches of the Cervical Plexus. These branches, all cutaneous, are the cutaneous colli, the lesser occipital, the great auricular and the descending supra-clavicular nerves (Fig. 126). The *deep* branches are muscular and divide into anterior and posterior branches. The *anterior* branch supplies the thyrohyoid, the genio-hyoid, the rectus capitus lateralis, the rectus capitis anterior, the longus capitis, the longus colli, the scalenus anterior and the intertrans-

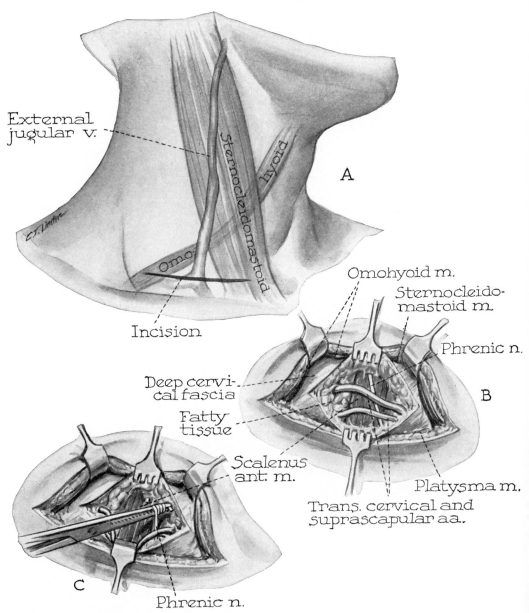

FIG. 129. Phrenic avulsion. (A) the incision starts at the posterior border of the sterno-mastoid muscle, one fingerbreadth above the clavicle. (B) The deep cervical fascia is incised, and the subfascial fat, which is an important guide, is identified. The transverse cervical and suprascapular arteries clamp the phrenic nerve onto the scalenus anterior muscle. (C) The phrenic nerve is avulsed.

versalis. The *posterior* branch supplies the sternocleidomastoid, the levator scapulae, the trapezius and the scalenus medius muscles. Communicating branches also are found which travel to the sympathetics and the hyoglossal muscle.

Cervical Sympathetic. This group (Fig. 128) consists of 3 ganglia with connecting branches which form a chain lying behind the carotid sheath and upon the prevertebral fascia. It extends from beneath the mastoid process to the 1st rib. The ganglia are known as the superior, the middle and the inferior and have been called, respectively, carotid, thyroid and vertebral from their almost constant association with these arteries.

The *superior* or *carotid* is the largest ganglion in the neck. It lies in front of the transverse processes of the 2nd and the 3rd cervical vertebrae on the longus capitis and behind the carotid sheath. It is fusiform in shape and sends a branch downward to connect with the middle ganglion.

The *middle* or *thyroid* ganglion is the smallest of the 3, and some authors state that it is inconstant or absent. This error may be due to the fact that the ganglion sometimes occupies a lower position, nearer the inferior ganglion of which it has been considered a part. It lies on a level with the 6th cervical vertebra in front of or behind the inferior thyroid artery.

The *inferior* or *vertebral* ganglion is next in size to the superior. It is found behind the vertebral artery, between the neck of the 1st rib and the transverse process of the 7th cervical vertebra. At times it unites with the first thoracic sympathetic ganglion to form the stellate ganglion. Since it is beneath the vertebral artery, just as the latter is given off from the subclavian, it makes surgical approach to the ganglion difficult. Some of the fibers that connect the middle with the inferior cervical ganglion descend in front of the subclavian artery and then upward behind it to form the so-called *ansa subclavia*.

SURGICAL CONSIDERATIONS

Phrenic Avulsion. The phrenic nerve is usually described as originating from the 4th cervical; however, it has been found originating from the 1st, the 2nd, the 3rd, the 5th and the 6th cervicals and the 1st dorsal nerves. Accessory phrenics are present at times, and for this reason the operation of avulsion is to be preferred. Fibers of the 5th cervical traveling with the nerve to the subclavius muscle are the most common varieties of accessory phrenics found. During avulsion the phrenicopericardial vessels may be torn, producing an internal hemorrhage.

An incision about 2 inches long is made, starting at the posterior border of the sternocleidomastoid muscle and is placed about a fingerbreadth above the clavicle (Fig. 129 A). If greater exposure is desired, a longitudinal incision about 3 to 4 inches long is placed along the posterior border of the sternocleidomastoid muscle. The incision is deepened through the platysma where the superficial cervical nerve and the external jugular vein come into view; these may be divided or retracted.

The posterior border of the sternocleidomastoid is identified and cleansed, as is the belly of the omohyoid. The deep cervical fascia which forms a cover for the scalenus anterior is identified and incised, and the underlying adipose tissue is noted. This fat is an important guide, since the muscle is not immediately visualized when the cervical fascia has been severed.

The subfascial fat is dissected free, and the scalenus anticus is exposed. As the muscle is cleared, the phrenic nerve appears toward its medial aspect as a thin, white cord running downward and slightly toward the midline.

The transverse cervical and suprascapular arteries clamp the phrenic nerve down onto the scalenus anterior in this fatty tissue (Fig. 129 B). These vessels should be looked for and retracted, since they might cause annoying hemorrhage and make exposure difficult (p. 172). Pinching the phrenic produces pain in the neck, the shoulder or the arm and dilation of the corresponding pupil. After proper identification, the nerve can be divided, resected, injected or avulsed by slowly winding the distal end on a hemostat (Fig. 129 C). The thoracic duct should be protected while operating on the left phrenic nerve.

Stellate Ganglionectomy. This is particularly useful in dealing with amputation stump neuralgia, painful traumatic arthritis and causalgia when these are associated with vasospasm which responds to diagnostic procaine injections. It has also been utilized in

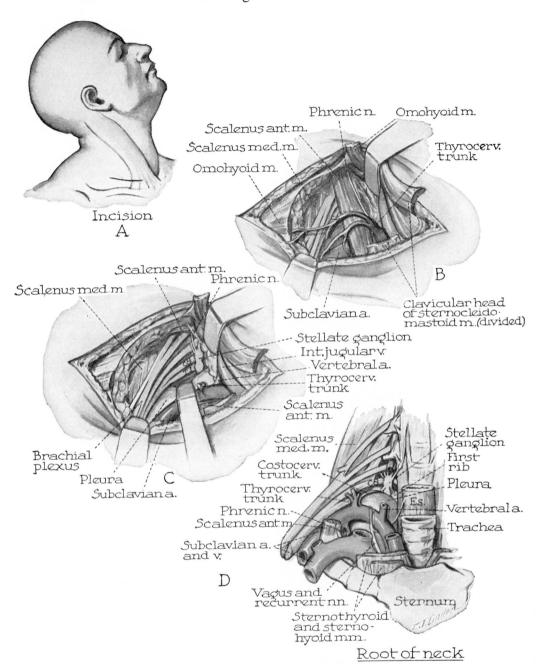

Phrenic n.   Omohyoid m.

Scalenus ant. m.

Scalenus med. m.

Omohyoid m.

Thyrocerv. trunk

Incision

A

B

Clavicular head of sternocleido- mastoid m. (divided)

Scalenus ant. m.

Phrenic n.

Scalenus med. m.

Subclavian a.

Stellate ganglion

Int. jugular v.

Vertebral a.

Thyrocerv. trunk

Scalenus ant. m.

Scalenus med. m.

Stellate ganglion

First rib

Pleura

Costocerv. trunk

Thyrocerv. trunk

Brachial plexus

Pleura

Subclavian a.

C

Phrenic n.

Scalenus ant. m

Subclavian a. and v.

Es.

Vertebral a.

Trachea

D

Vagus and recurrent nn.

Sternum

Sternothyroid and sterno- hyoid mm.

Root of neck

FIG. 130. Stellate ganglionectomy. (A) Transverse incision placed a fingerbreadth above the clavicle and continued laterally 2 inches from the sternal head of the sternocleidomastoid muscle. (B) The clavicular head of the sternocleidomastoid, the omohyoid and the deep cervical fascia have been divided, exposing the scalenus anticus muscle and the phrenic nerve. The subfascial fat is the important landmark in this part of the dissection. (C) The scalenus anticus muscle has been divided, and the thyrocervical trunk ligated and severed. With downward retraction of the subclavian artery and the apex of the lung, the stellate ganglion becomes visible. (D) Anatomic relations in the root of the neck.

angina pectoris, bronchial asthma and hyperhidrosis. Many technics have been used in cervical sympathectomies and ganglionectomies, but the following is one of the most common methods employed.

A transverse incision is made about a fingerbreadth above the clavicle and is carried laterally 2 inches from the sternal head of the sternocleidomastoid muscle (Fig. 130 A). The clavicular head of the muscle is divided, thus centering the incision over the vertebral artery. The omohyoid, which travels obliquely across the field, is divided and the deep cervical fascia exposed and incised. The carotid sheath is retracted anteriorly, and

the phrenic nerve is located on the scalene anterior muscle; this, too, is retracted toward the midline (Fig. 130 B). The anterior scalene muscle is cut just above its insertion into the 1st rib, which exposes the upper 3 thoracic ganglia and the proximal portion of the subclavian artery with its thyrocervical trunk and vertebral branches. The thyroid axis is ligated and cut, and the subclavian artery is retracted downward. The stellate ganglion can now be visualized; it is adherent to the lateral surface of the 7th cervical and the 1st thoracic vertebrae.

The thoracic duct should be protected when the operation is performed on the left

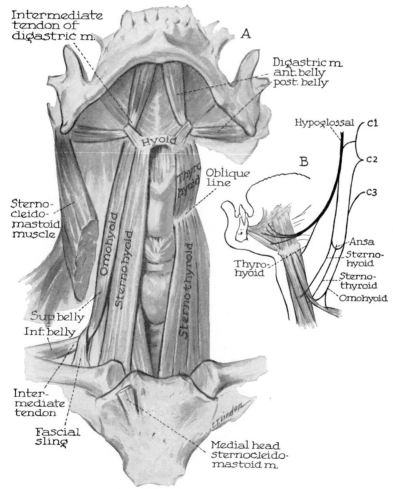

FIG. 131. The 4 infrahyoid muscles: (A) the 2 superficial muscles are seen on the right side and the 2 deeper ones on the left; (B) the nerve supply.

side. Sibson's fascia, which attaches the apex of the pleura to the posterior part of the 1st rib, is cut. The entire apical pole can then be freed by blunt dissection to about the level of the 3rd rib. This should permit visualization of the inferior cervical and the first thoracic ganglia (Fig. 130 C).

It should be remembered that this may appear as a double ganglion, which is shaped like a dumb-bell with an isthmus, or may appear as a single mass. Its lower part lies in front of and against the head of the 1st rib; its upper pole is connected with the lower trunk of the brachial plexus by fine rami which give it a star-shaped appearance, hence the name "stellate." It is dissected free, and the nerve chain is followed down as far as the 3rd thoracic ganglion. The incision is closed in layers.

MUSCLES

Infrahyoid. The infrahyoid muscles have been referred to as the depressors of the larynx and also as the "strap" or "ribbon" muscles. The 4 muscles making up this group are the sternohyoid, the omohyoid, the sternothyroid and the thyrohyoid. The first two lie side by side and cover the other two (Fig. 131 A). All are supplied by branches of the anterior rami of the 1st, the 2nd and the 3rd cervical nerves by means of the hypoglossal nerve and the ansa hypoglossi which approach the muscles from the lateral side. The nerves pass between the superficial and the deep muscles and enter their opposed surfaces (Fig. 131 B).

Sternohyoid. This muscle arises from the posterior surface of the manubrium sterni and the adjoining part of the clavicle, continues upward and medially and inserts into the medial part of the lower border of the body of the hyoid bone. At its origin it is separated from its fellow of the opposite side by an interval of 4 to 6 cm., but as they ascend they gradually converge so that at the point of insertion both muscles lie in contact with each other. The interval between the two muscles is filled by the pretracheal fascia. Contraction of this muscle depresses the hyoid bone.

Omohyoid. The omohyoid muscle consists of an inferior belly, an intermediate tendon and a superior belly. It lies in the same plane as the sternohyoid. The inferior belly arises from the upper border of the scapula and the suprascapular ligament, crosses the posterior triangle of the neck and passes deep to the sternocleidomastoid and ends as the *intermediate tendon.* It lies on the surface of the carotid sheath and is bound to the clavicle by the deep cervical fascia which forms a fascial sling. Its tendon gives origin to the superior belly which passes upward and medially superficial to the common carotid artery and along the lateral border of the sternohyoid. It becomes inserted into the lower border of the body of the hyoid bone. The omohyoid abruptly bends away from the sternohyoid below the level of the cricoid cartilage. Unlike the digastric, the two bellies of the omohyoid are supplied by the same nerve, since the inferior belly is a backward extension of the superior. Its action depresses the hyoid bone and draws it backward and laterally.

The two deeper muscles, thyrohyoid and sternothyroid, are divided into a muscle above and one below the oblique line of the thyroid cartilage where both attach (Fig. 131).

The sternothyroid is of considerable surgical importance. It is perhaps the most important surgical landmark in thyroid surgery and, if identified properly, can aid in finding the correct cleavage plane. It must be emphasized that a distinct cleavage plane exists between the sternohyoid and the sternothyroid muscles, and very often the surgeon believes that he has cut both muscles when in reality only the more superficial sternohyoid has been severed. If the thyroid gland is enlarged, the sternothyroid becomes so thin that it is not clearly visualized. If this should occur, then the true capsular structures and the cleavage planes are lost, and the operation proceeds with great difficulty and much hemorrhage. The muscle arises from the posterior aspect of the manubrium sterni, extends upward deep to the sternohyoid and covers the lobe of the thyroid gland. It is inserted into the oblique line on the lamina of the thyroid cartilage. The lower border converges on its fellow as it descends until their medial borders just meet at the center of the manubrium. Its contraction depresses the larynx.

The thyrohyoid muscle is a short, quadrilateral structure which appears to be a continuation of the sternothyroid. It arises from the oblique line on the thyroid cartilage, passes upward and is inserted into the lower margin of the hyoid bone. The muscle is fairly thick, covers the thyrohyoid membrane and projects laterally to the omohyoid. It depresses the hyoid bone, but when the bone is fixed by the suprahyoid muscles, it acts as an elevator of the larynx.

The digastric muscle constitutes another important surgical landmark and guide in the upper part of the neck. Its name suggests that it has 2 bellies that are connected by a common tendon.

The *anterior belly* runs forward, medially and upward from the common tendon to attach to the lower border of the mandible near the midline. It is placed on the surface of the mylohyoid muscle and is partly overlapped by the submaxillary gland.

The *posterior belly* arises from the mastoid part of the temporal bone and is covered by the mastoid process and the sternocleido-mastoid muscle, but as it passes downward, forward and medially it becomes visible. It crosses superficially to the internal jugular

vein, the accessory, the vagus and the hypo-glossal nerves, the occipital, the internal and the external carotids and the facial (external maxillary) arteries.

The common or so-called *intermediate tendon* is attached to the body of the hyoid by a pulleylike band of fascia. This tendon perforates the stylohyoid muscle, lies on the hyoglossus muscle and is overlapped by the submaxillary gland. The latter is a good guide to the intermediate tendon, and the inter-mediate tendon in turn is a good guide to the hyoglossus muscle. The nerve supply of the muscle is derived from two sources. The posterior belly is supplied by the facial nerve as it leaves the stylomastoid foramen, and the anterior belly by the nerve to the mylo-hyoid from the trigeminal nerve. Therefore, the posterior belly receives its nerve supply from the 7th cranial; and the anterior belly, from the 5th cranial nerve.

VESSELS AND CAROTID SHEATH

The general investing layer of the deep cervical fascia gives rise to 2 sheaths which originate from the deep surface of the sterno-

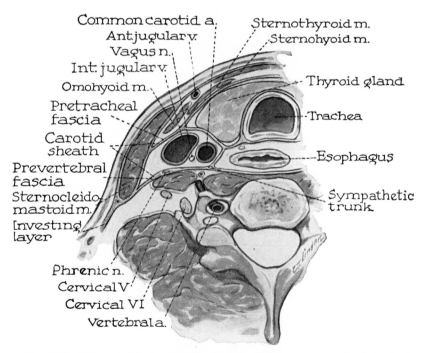

FIG. 132. The carotid sheath. This is formed by the pretracheal fascia in front and the prevertebral fascia behind; both fasciae originate from the general investing layer of deep cervical fascia.

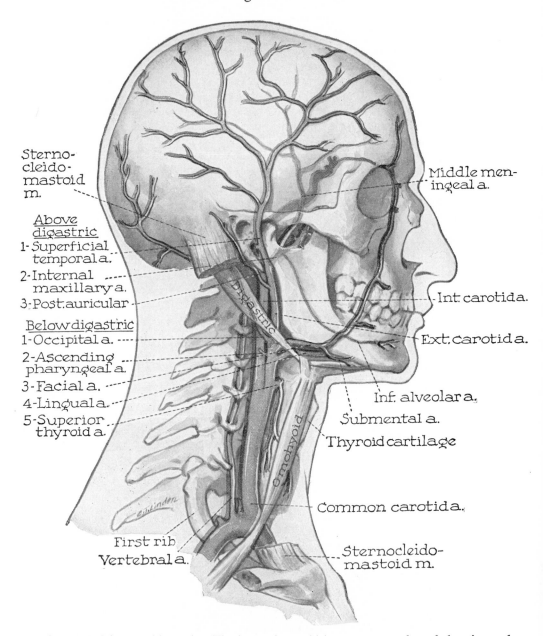

Sterno-
cleido-
mastoid
m.

Above
digastric
1- Superficial
temporal a.
2- Internal
maxillary a.
3- Post. auricular

Below digastric
1- Occipital a.
2- Ascending
pharyngeal a.
3- Facial a.
4- Lingual a.
5- Superior
thyroid a.

First rib
Vertebral a.

Middle men-
ingeal a.

Int. carotid a.

Ext. carotid a.

Inf. alveolar a.
Submental a.
Thyroid cartilage

Common carotid a.

Sternocleido-
mastoid m.

Fig. 133. The carotid arteries. The internal carotid is more posterolateral than internal, and as it ascends it lies medial to the external carotid. The external carotid has 8 branches, 5 of which are below and 3 above the digastric muscle.

cleidomastoid (Fig. 132). These 2 offshoots are the pretracheal and the prevertebral layers. Between them and near their origin are found the common carotid artery, the internal jugular vein and the vagus nerve. The fascia immediately surrounding these structures, the pretracheal in front and the prevertebral behind, forms the carotid sheath, which extends from the base of the skull to the root of the neck. The sympathetic trunk is imbedded in its posterior wall, the descendens hypoglossi in the anterior wall, and the descendens cervicalis, the cervical branches of the vagus and the internal jugular vein pierce it. Although the structures are surrounded by this tubelike fascia, they also are imbedded in fibrous tissue that is derived from it so that each structure has its own coat. The vein is external to the artery and almost entirely covers it. The sheath is applied to the side of the cervical viscera, namely, the esophagus, the pharynx and the thyroid gland.

Carotid Arteries. (Fig. 133) The *common carotid artery* arises differently on the two sides: the right arises as a terminal branch of the innominate behind the sternoclavicular joint; the left originates in the thorax from the arch of the aorta, passes upward and to the left and enters the neck behind the left sternoclavicular joint. This is the largest artery in the neck; and as it passes from behind the sternoclavicular joint, it runs upward and backward under cover of the anterior border of the sternocleidomastoid muscle in the direction of the mandible. When it reaches the level of the upper border of the thyroid cartilage it forms a dilation known as the *carotid bulb* and then divides into its 2 terminal branches: the internal and the external carotid arteries.

The carotid body and the carotid sinus are 2 sensory structures which are frequently confused; they are associated with the region of the carotid bifurcation (Fig. 134). The *carotid body* is a small flattened structure measuring about 2.5 by 6 mm. It is usually found on the posteromedial side of the common carotid artery where it is held firmly in place by connective tissue. It contains numerous nerves and nerve endings and at one time was regarded as part of the chromaffin system. It does not secrete epinephrine, and its cells do not have a chromaffin reaction. Its nerve supply is not via the sympathetic system. The carotid body represents a specialized sensory organ (vascular chemoreceptor) which responds to chemical changes in the blood and thereby affects cardiovascular output and respiration. Hypoxia and anoxia stimulate this body, resulting in an increase in blood pressure, cardiac rate and respiratory movements. On occasion, tumors arise in the carotid body, which have been referred to as "glomus" tumors. This is a misnomer, since it is not a tumor of arteriovenous origin. The removal of carotid body tumors may be extremely difficult and associated with morbidity and/or mortality.

The *carotid sinus* is usually located at the

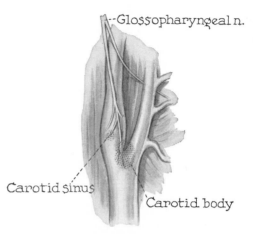

Fig. 134. The carotid sinus, the carotid body, and their relationships to the glossopharyngeal nerve.

base of the internal carotid artery and is composed of numerous and complicated sensory nerve endings. In contrast with the carotid body (chemoreceptor), the carotid sinus is a pressoreceptor. Its nerve endings are stimulated by pressure as by the pressure of blood itself. Stimulation of this sinus causes a reduction of blood pressure and a slowing of the heart rate. At times this sinus becomes unduly sensitive to pressure so that a mere turning of the head may drop the blood pressure, slow the heart and produce loss of consciousness. Denervation of the sinus may abolish this so-called carotid sinus syndrome.

The nerve to both the carotid body and the carotid sinus is the *intercarotid nerve* (Hering); it arises from the glossopharyngeal nerve. Some authorities are of the opinion that this nerve supply may be connected with the vagus, the hypoglossal or the superior cervical ganglion.

Throughout the course of the common carotid artery it is imbedded with the internal jugular vein and the vagus nerve, in the connective tissue that constitutes the carotid sheath. The vein lies on the lateral side of the artery and when full of blood overlaps it anteriorly. The vagus nerve lies posteriorly between the artery and the vein.

Usually the only branches of the common carotid are its terminal ones, but occasionally, when its bifurcation is at a higher level, the ascending pharyngeal or the superior thyroid may arise from it.

Anteriorly, in addition to the superficial structures, this artery is covered by the anterior border of the sternocleidomastoid muscle. Between the muscle and the artery in the lower part of the neck the following structures intervene: the superior belly of the omohyoid, the sternohyoid and the sternothyroid muscles. In the upper part of its course the descending ramus of the hypoglossus and the ansa hypoglossi are imbedded in the anterior wall of the sheath, and the common facial vein usually crosses the artery at its termination.

Posteriorly, the artery is related to the anterior tubercles of the transverse processes of the lower 4 cervical vertebrae and the muscles that attach here, namely, the scalenus anterior and the longus capitis. It is separated from these structures by the prevertebral fascia and the sympathetic trunk. In the lower part of the neck it lies in front of the vertebral artery as it ascends to the foramen and the transverse process of the 6th cervical vertebra and in front of the inferior thyroid artery, which arches medially to the thyroid gland. On the left side the thoracic duct crosses behind the vessel and below the inferior thyroid artery.

Medially, it is related to the inferior constrictor muscle of the pharynx and the thyroid gland. The lobe of the thyroid either lies medial to the artery separating it from the esophagus, the pharynx, the trachea and the larynx or forms a direct anterior relation.

Laterally, it is related to the internal jugular vein and the vagus nerve.

The internal carotid artery is the larger of the 2 terminal branches of the common carotid. It is distributed to the brain and to the eye and its appendages. From its origin at the upper border of the thyroid cartilage it passes to the carotid canal of the temporal bone. It turns forward in the cavernous sinus, perforates the dura mater on the inner side of the anterior clinoid process and divides into the anterior and the middle cerebral arteries. Below the posterior belly of the digastric the artery is overlapped by the anterior border of the sternocleidomastoid and the more superficial structures; the hypoglossal nerve, the occipital artery and the common facial vein are interposed between it and the muscle. Above, the artery ascends under cover of the posterior border of the

digastric and the stylohyoid and is crossed by the posterior auricular artery. It passes beneath the styloid process and the stylopharyngeus muscle. These 2 structures are placed between the artery and the parotid gland in which the external carotid artery and the posterior facial vein are imbedded. The internal carotid has no branches in the neck. It may be difficult to distinguish between the internal and the external carotid arteries. Even in a well-planned operation for ligation, one has been mistaken for the other; hence, the following points should be noted: the internal carotid furnishes no branches in the neck, but the external has 3 anterior branches; the vessel is not really internal but at its origin is posterolateral to the external vessel; as it ascends it passes to the medial side of the external carotid toward the lateral wall of the pharynx.

The external carotid artery is the smaller of the 2 terminal branches of the common carotid and extends from the upper part of the thyroid cartilage to the neck of the mandible where it divides into its 2 terminal branches—the superficial temporal and the maxillary (internal) arteries. This carotid has been called "external," not because of its location, which is really internal and superficial to the internal carotid, but because of the fact that it is distributed to parts outside of the skull. Near the angle of the jaw it is crossed by the posterior belly of the digastric and the stylohyoid muscles. Above this it is at first deep to and then enclosed by the substance of the parotid gland where it terminates opposite the neck of the mandible by dividing into its 2 terminal branches. In its short course before entering the substance of the parotid, it is applied to the inferior and the middle constrictor muscles. The vessel has 8 branches: 5 below the digastric muscle and 3 above it (Fig. 133).

The 5 branches *below* the digastric muscle are:

1. The *superior thyroid artery,* which arises from the anterior aspect of the external carotid near its origin. It passes downward and forward under cover of the omohyoid, the sternohyoid and the sternothyroid muscles, parallel with but superficial to the external laryngeal nerve. It reaches the upper pole of the thyroid gland to which it is distributed. Its branches are the infrahyoid, the

superior laryngeal, the sternocleidomastoid, the cricothyroid, the isthmic, the glandular and the muscular.

2. The *lingual artery* arises opposite the greater cornu of the hyoid bone, makes an upward loop, disappears under cover of the hyoglossus muscle and enters the submandibular (submaxillary) region (p. 147). The loop of this artery is crossed superficially by the hypoglossal nerve.

3. The *facial (external maxillary) artery* arises near the angle of the mandible, is directed upward and forward on the superior constrictor muscle, beneath the digastric; it continues in a groove on the deep surface of the submandibular gland to the body of the mandible and ascends to the face, anterior to the masseter muscle (p. 111).

4. The *ascending pharyngeal artery* arises from the deep aspect of the external carotid close to its origin and continues upward, medial to the internal carotid on the side wall of the pharynx. It is usually small and supplies the pharynx, the soft palate and the meninges.

5. The *occipital artery* arises from the posterior aspect of the external carotid opposite the facial and continues upward and backward deep to the posterior belly of the digastric. It is crossed by the transverse part of the hypoglossal nerve at its origin, follows the posterior belly of the digastric and is in contact with the skull medial to the mastoid notch, lying deep to the process in the muscles that attach to it. It anastomoses with the deep cervical branch from the costocervical trunk and thus forms a link between the subclavian and the carotid systems.

The branches of the external carotid artery *above* the digastric muscle are 3 in number. The *posterior auricular artery* generally arises at or above the upper border of the muscle and in the parotid region. It becomes superficial as it crosses the base of the mastoid process and ascends behind the auricle. It supplies the area of the auricle on the back of the scalp. The 2 terminal branches of the carotid, the *superficial temporal* and the *"internal" maxillary,* have been discussed elsewhere (p. 128).

The *superficial relations* of the external carotid artery are: in the carotid triangle the vessel is covered by skin, superficial fascia, platysma, branches of the anterior cutaneous nerve of the neck, the cervical branch of the facial nerve and the deep fascia. Beneath the deep fascia, the artery is crossed by the common facial and lingual veins and the hypoglossal nerve. At the upper part of the triangle the anterior branch of the posterior facial vein crosses the artery. After leaving the carotid triangle, the vessel is partially covered by the angle of the mandible and is crossed by the posterior belly of the diagastric and the stylohyoid muscles. Within the substance of the parotid gland the posterior facial vein is superficial to the artery, and both of these vessels are crossed in turn by branches of the facial nerve. In its entire course the vessel is accompanied by numerous sympathetic ganglia which constitute the *external carotid plexus.*

Collateral anastomoses between the internal and the external carotids are usually adequate to maintain circulation after ligation of either of the vessels. Many anastomotic connections exist between the arteries of the ophthalmic region of the internal carotid and the facial region of the external. Communications exist between the external carotid artery and the thyrocervical trunk through the superior thyroid branch of the former and the inferior thyroid branch of the latter. A communication between the vertebral and the internal carotid arteries via the posterior communicating artery of the circle of Willis is also present. Other communications between the lingual, the facial, the occipital, the posterior auricular and the ascending pharyngeal arteries connect the external carotids of the 2 sides. The internal carotid arteries communicate across the base of the brain by the anterior communication artery and with the basilar trunk. When the common carotid is ligated, circulation is not interfered with anatomically or clinically unless the anastomotic paths are disturbed by vascular degenerative changes due to age or other pathologic processes.

External and Internal Jugular Veins. (Figs. 135, 136) The *external jugular vein* varies in size. It is formed below the lobule of the ear by the union of the posterior auricular vein with a branch of the posterior facial. It begins at the lower part of the parotid gland, runs almost vertically downward, crosses the sternocleidomastoid muscle obliquely, and in the angle between the

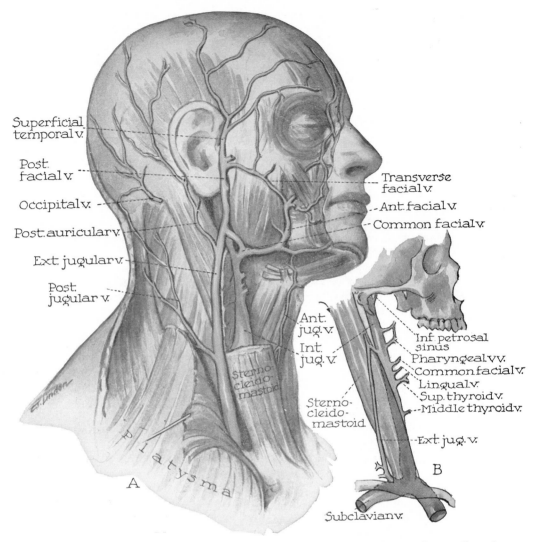

Superficial temporal v.

Post. facial v.

Occipital v.

Post. auricular v.

Ext. jugular v.

Post. jugular v.

Sterno cleido mastoid

Platysma

A

Transverse facial v.

Ant. facial v.

Common facial v.

Ant. jug. v.

Int. jug. v.

Sterno-cleido-mastoid

Inf. petrosal sinus

Pharyngeal vv.

Common facial v.

Lingual v.

Sup. thyroid v.

Middle thyroid v.

Ext. jug. v.

B

Subclavian v.

FIG. 135. Lateral view of the veins of the neck: (A) the platysma has been reflected to show the external jugular vein, and the sternocleidomastoid has been cut to show the internal jugular; (B) tributaries of the internal jugular vein.

clavicle and the posterior border of that muscle pierces the deep cervical fascia to which it is firmly bound; it then joins the subclavian vein. It lies upon the superficial layer of deep cervical fascia, beneath the platysma muscle, and at times may be absent or very small. It is so closely associated with the platysma that when the latter is reflected, the vein remains attached to it. If one external jugular is large the other is small; and if both are large, then the internal jugulars are correspondingly small. The external communicates with the internal jugular via a branch which turns around the anterior

border of the sternocleidomastoid. At times, it receives a posterior jugular vein from the back of the neck. At its termination the external jugular is joined by the transverse cervical, the suprascapular and the anterior jugular veins.

The *internal jugular vein* begins at the jugular foramen about ½ inch below the base of the skull, as a continuation of the sigmoid (transverse) sinus. It passes downward and forward through the neck and ends behind the upper border of the sternal end of the clavicle where it meets the subclavian and forms the innominate vein. It is dilated markedly at its origin, forming the superior bulb that lies in the jugular foramen and the fossa. This bulb is larger on the right side because the superior sagittal sinus usually turns to the right. The inferior bulb is a dilation of the vein below a bicuspid valve which is situated about ½ inch above the clavicle. The junction of the internal jugular and the subclavian veins is separated from the lower part of the sternoclavicular joint by the 2 infrahyoid muscles.

The tributaries (Fig. 135 B) *of the veins* in this region are: (1) *The inferior petrosal sinus*, which helps to drain the cavernous sinus and leaves the skull through the anterior part of the jugular foramen to join the upper end of the internal jugular.

2. *The pharyngeal veins* from the plexus on the side of the pharynx pass either superficially or deeply to the internal carotid artery and join the internal jugular vein in the upper part of the neck.

3. *The common facial vein* is the largest and most important tributary of the internal jugular. It is formed by the union of the anterior and the posterior facial veins and continues downward and backward just above the level of the upper border of the thyroid

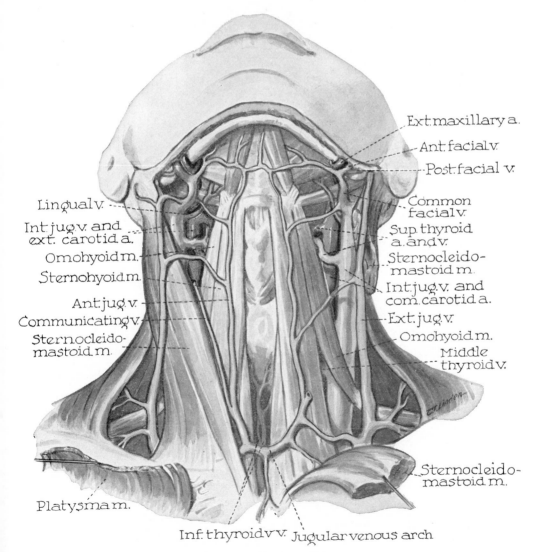

Ext. maxillary a.

Ant. facial v.

Post. facial v.

Lingual v.

Int. jug. v. and ext. carotid a.

Omohyoid m.

Sternohyoid m.

Ant. jug. v.

Communicating v.

Sternocleido-mastoid m.

Common facial v.

Sup. thyroid a. and v.

Sternocleido-mastoid m.

Int. jug. v. and com. carotid a.

Ext. jug. v.

Omohyoid m.

Middle thyroid v.

Sternocleido-mastoid m.

Platysma m.

Inf. thyroid v. v.   Jugular venous arch

FIG. 136. The anterior, the external and the internal jugular veins. The sternocleidomastoid muscle has been cut and reflected on the left side.

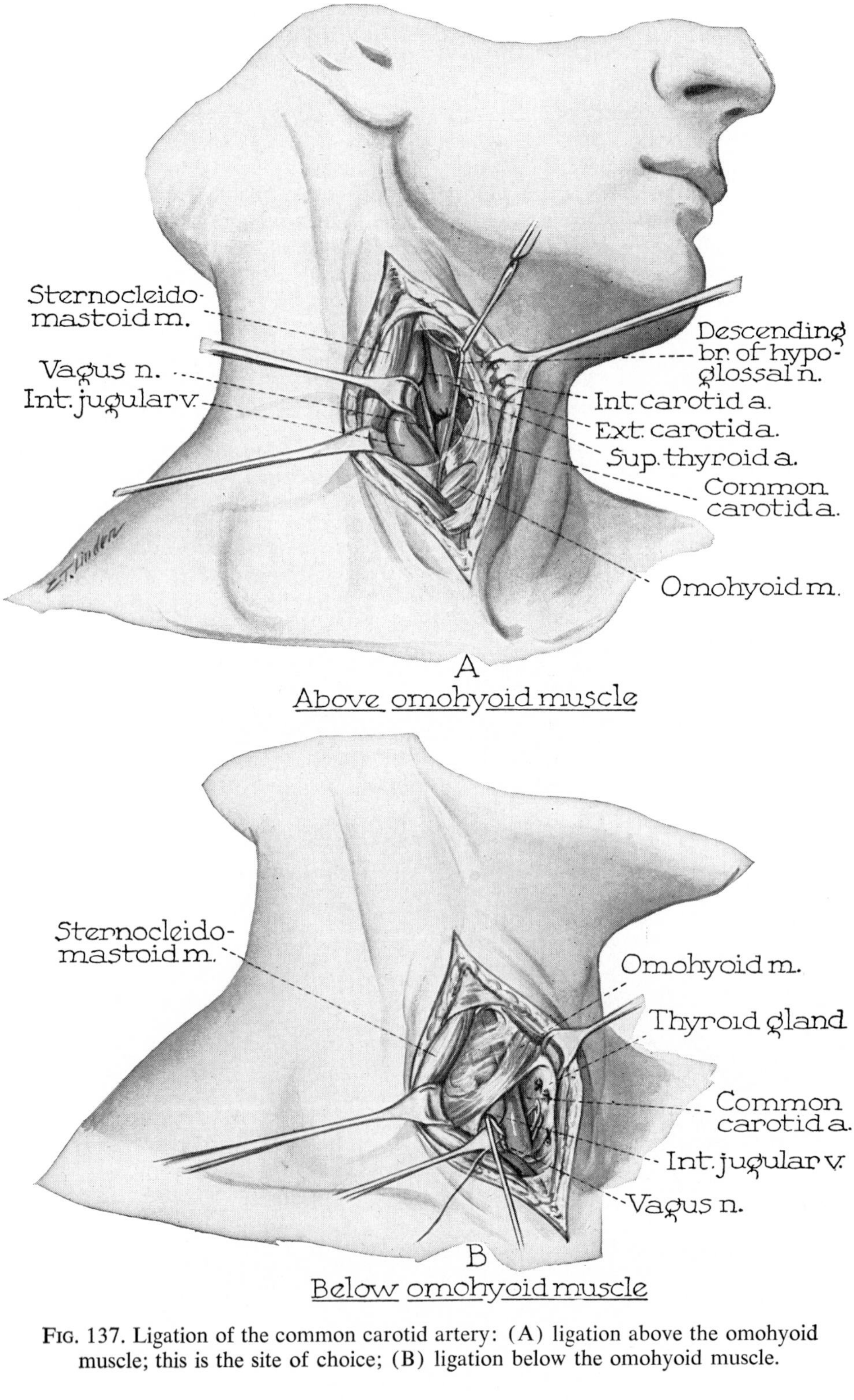

Sternocleido-
mastoid m.

Vagus n.

Int. jugular v.

Descending
br. of hypo-
glossal n.

Int. carotid a.

Ext. carotid a.

Sup. thyroid a.

Common
carotid a.

Omohyoid m.

A
Above omohyoid muscle

Sternocleido-
mastoid m.

Omohyoid m.

Thyroid gland

Common
carotid a.

Int. jugular v.

Vagus n.

B
Below omohyoid muscle

Fig. 137. Ligation of the common carotid artery: (A) ligation above the omohyoid
muscle; this is the site of choice; (B) ligation below the omohyoid muscle.

cartilage. It passes superficially to the hypoglossal nerve as that structure crosses the loop of the lingual artery. At times it receives the thyroid and the lingual veins and then is referred to as the "thyrolingual facial trunk."

4. *The lingual vein,* when it does not form a tributary of the common facial, enters the internal jugular opposite the greater cornu of the hyoid bone.

5. *The superior thyroid vein* ascends from the upper pole of the thyroid gland in company with the corresponding artery. At the pole there are numerous small tributaries of this vein which form a trunk at a higher level. It crosses superficially to the common carotid artery and joins either the common facial or the internal jugular vein.

6. *The middle thyroid vein* passes laterally and deeply to the infrahyoid muscles. It crosses superficially to the common carotid artery and ends in the internal jugular at the level of the cricoid cartilage.

The internal jugular vein is enclosed in the carotid sheath. Its uppermost part lies behind the internal carotid artery and posterolateral to the last 4 cranial nerves. As the vein descends, it lies laterally to the common carotid and overlaps it; hence, in exposing the artery its sheath should be opened toward the inner side to avoid injuring the vein.

Superficial Relations of the Internal Jugular Vein. These relations are the most complicated and the most important surgically. Throughout the greater part of its course the internal jugular lies under the sternocleidomastoid muscle, but in its extreme upper portion it is deep to the parotid gland.

Inferiorly, the infrahyoid muscles are situated between the vessel and the sternocleidomastoid. In its upper part it is separated from the parotid gland by the styloid process, the stylopharyngeus and the stylohyoid muscles and the posterior belly of the digastric. In this region it is crossed superficially by 2 arteries and a nerve (posterior auricular and occipital arteries and accessory nerve). At a lower level it is crossed by the sternocleidomastoid branch of the occipital artery. After leaving the parotid and the digastric at the upper angle of the carotid triangle, it disappears under the sternocleidomastoid but is separated from the muscle by many structures, namely, numerous lymph glands along its entire course, the descendens cervicalis nerve at the level of the thyroid cartilage, the sternocleidomastoid branch of the superior thyroid artery, the intermediate tendon of the omohyoid at about the level of the cricoid cartilage and, lastly, the sternohyoid and the sternothyroid muscles.

Medially, the vein is related to the vagus nerve and the common carotid artery below, and to the 9th, the 10th, the 11th and the 12th cranial nerves and the internal carotid artery above.

Posteriorly, as the vein descends, it crosses the transverse process of the atlas and lies lateral to the tips of the lower transverse processes. In succession, it rests on the levator scapulae, the scalenus medius and the scalenus anterior muscles and is separated from them by the carotid sheath and the prevertebral fascia. The latter-named fascia is situated between the vein and the loops of the cervical plexus above and the phrenic nerve below.

SURGICAL CONSIDERATIONS

Ligations of Carotid Arteries and Internal Jugular Vein. (Fig. 137) The indications for ligation of the *common carotid artery* are wounds of the carotid artery or its branches, aneurysms, angiomas, inoperable tumors of the face, the neck and the skull, hemorrhage from distal branches and at times hydrocephalus and epilepsy. Ligation of the common carotid artery can be dangerous, especially in elderly people, since it may be followed by diplopia, blindness, convulsions, coma, hemiplegia or death. The point of election is above the omohyoid muscle; however, ligation below may be necessary in injuries of the artery. Collateral circulation takes place by means of the communications between the carotids of the 2 sides, both inside and outside the skull, and by the enlargement of branches of the subclavian artery. The chief communications outside the skull are the superior thyroid above with the inferior thyroid below, and the descending branch of the occipital above with the

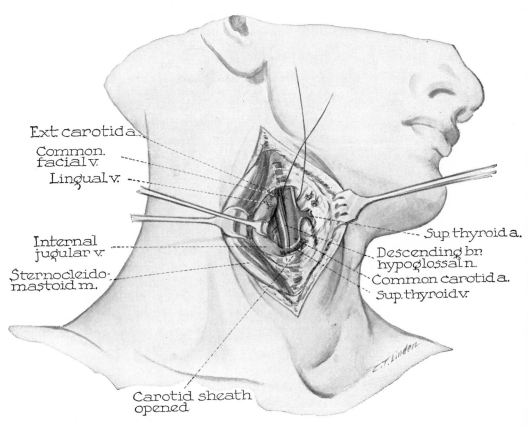

Ext. carotid a.
Common.
facial v.
Lingual v.

Internal
jugular v.
Sternocleido-
mastoid m.

Sup. thyroid a.
Descending br.
hypoglossal n.
Common carotid a.
Sup. thyroid v.

Carotid sheath
opened

E.T. Linden

FIG. 138. Ligation of the external carotid artery; the usual site is between the superior thyroid and the lingual arteries.

deep cervical and the ascending branch of the transverse cervical below. Within the skull the vertebral artery compensates for the carotid.

In *ligation above the omohyoid,* the head is rotated toward the opposite side, and at the anterior border of the sternocleidomastoid muscle a 3-inch incision is made, the center of which is placed at the level of the cricoid cartilage. Superficial vessels are ligated; if necessary, the anterior and the external jugular veins are tied and divided. The deep fascia is severed; the sternocleidomastoid is retracted in an outward direction. The omohyoid muscle is exposed, and the carotid tubercle is felt where it lies in the angle between the sternocleidomastoid and the omohyoid. Pulsations of the artery can be felt in this angle. The jugular vein lies to the lateral side of the artery and overlaps it; the superior thyroid, the lingual and the

facial veins may cross the artery at its upper end, and it may be necessary to ligate them. Some authorities believe that the internal jugular vein should also be ligated. The descending branch of the hypoglossal nerve may be identified on the anterior aspect of the carotid sheath and it is exposed and displaced medially. If the omohyoid muscle interferes with exposure or ligation, it may be severed or retracted in a downward direction. The sheath is opened to the inner side, and the artery is exposed. A ligature should be passed from without inward, keeping close to the artery, especially in back, so that the vagus nerve is not included in the ligature.

Ligation below the omohyoid is much more difficult and is done only in case of necessity. The skin incision is longer and is usually extended to the jugular notch. If the sternocleidomastoid protrudes, it may be detached in the region of its sternal or clavicular head after severing the superficial layer of deep cervical fascia. The ribbon muscles that cover the thyroid gland are exposed, and the lateral margin of the sternothyroid is retracted medially with the thyroid and the trachea which lie behind it. The middle layer of deep cervical fascia, forming a sheath for the omohyoid muscle, is incised along the inferior margin of the muscle; this space reveals a few thyroid veins which usually require ligation. The inferior thyroid artery, passing beneath the carotid sheath, can usually be spared. The internal jugular vein is retracted laterally, the artery is freed, and a ligature is passed around it. If one hugs the artery, the recurrent laryngeal nerve can be avoided.

Ligation of the external carotid artery (Fig. 138) is indicated for wounds, aneurysms, as a palliative measure for malignant growths, and as a preliminary step to operations in the field supplied by its branches. After ligation below the digastric muscle, the collateral circulation is brought about by the inferior with the superior thyroid arteries, the deep cervical from the costocervical with the occipital, the transverse cervical with the occipital, branches of the 2 vertebrals, and branches of the 2 internal carotids through the circle of Willis.

The usual site of ligation is between the superior thyroid and the lingual trunks, but it may be performed proximally to the superior thyroid. Since the latter vessel may arise from the common carotid, it is wise to expose the origin of both carotids. A skin incision is made, extending for about 3 inches from the angle of the jaw to the upper border of the thyroid cartilage, in front of the anterior border of the sternocleidomastoid muscle. Skin, platysma and superficial fascia are divided, exposing the anterior border of the sternocleidomastoid. Since the common facial and lingual veins often cross the operative field, they are sought, ligated and divided. The superficial layer of deep cervical fascia is incised to mobilize the sternocleidomastoid muscle which is drawn backward. The carotid sheath is exposed and opened. In the connective tissue of the sheath the descending branch of the hypoglossal nerve is seen

and is displaced medially, and the internal jugular vein is retracted laterally. Between them the bifurcation of the common carotid artery can usually be seen. Since the first part of the external carotid lies medial to the internal, the 2 vessels may be mistaken unless it is remembered that the external carotid is the only vessel that gives off branches. After the latter is exposed, it is ligated on a level with the greater cornu of the hyoid bone. It is best to pass the ligatures from the internal carotid side and to guard against including the descending hypoglossal nerve as well as the superior laryngeal nerve. The wound is closed in layers.

Ligation of the internal carotid artery has been done for wounds, aneurysms or pulsating exophthalmus due to an arteriovenous aneurysm between the artery and the cavernous sinus. Collateral circulation takes place through the circle of Willis. The internal carotid, running to the base of the occiput without giving off any lateral branches, can be exposed in its lower part in the same manner described for the external carotid artery (p. 184). However, if it must be ligated near the base of the skull, the operation is a most extensive one, since exposure must take place above the posterior belly of the digastric, and here the vessel lies very deep. The internal carotid artery is identified near the bifurcation of the common carotid and then traced upward. The digastric muscle is retracted upward, and the external carotid inward. The ligature is passed from without inward, avoiding the internal jugular vein, the vagus nerve and the sympathetic trunk. Some authorities advise primary placement of a ligature around the common carotid to be used only in case of absolute necessity.

Ligation of the internal jugular vein has been resorted to in such conditions as transverse sinus thrombosis to prevent extension of infection into the general circulation. In its lower portion the vein is found quite easily, but identification becomes more difficult as it travels cephalad, since its tributaries become more numerous. The ligation of one or both jugular veins has been carried out without any appreciable difficulty. The vein may be found readily by incising along the anterior border of the sternocleidomastoid muscle; it is the most superficial structure in the carotid sheath.

Obstructing lesions in vessels supplying the brain may be associated with episodes of syncope and/or transient neurologic symptoms. Corrective or palliative procedures are now available to correct such difficulties associated with major or with "little" strokes. When obstruction of the internal carotid artery has been demonstrated, a bypass graft may be indicated (Fig 139 A). Another method of correcting these problems is removal of the obstructing agent (thromboendarterectomy) and widening of the vessel lumen by inserting an elliptical patch (Fig. 139 B).

THYROID GLAND

Embryology. (Fig. 140) At the junction of the posterior third with the anterior two thirds of the tongue, the *foramen caecum* is noted as a small depression. From this site at an early stage of fetal life, a solid column of cells grows downward, becomes canalized

and forms the *thyroglossal duct,* from which the thyroid gland is formed. The duct passes down exactly in the midline between the genioglossi muscles as far as the upper border of the thyroid cartilage, where it turns to one or the other side of the midline. From this point on its course is represented by the pyramidal lobe. The question whether the thyroglossal duct passes in front of, through, or behind the body of the hyoid bone seems to have been answered by Frazer who has shown that it is placed in front of the bone and then takes a recurrent course up behind the hyoid before continuing downward. For this reason many advocate removal of the midportion of the hyoid to make certain that the entire tract is eliminated. If the duct remains open after birth, thyroglossal cysts develop either above the thyroid cartilage where they are usually centrally placed, or below the cartilage where they are usually found to the left of the midline. Since the thyroglossal duct never opens onto the surface of the neck at any stage of its develop-

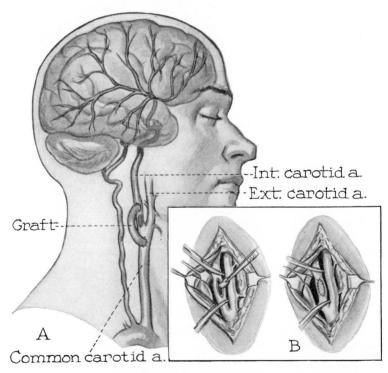

FIG. 139. Obstruction of the internal carotid artery. (A) A bypass graft has been placed. (B) Removal of the offending clot and widening of the vessel by an elliptical patch.

ment, congenital thyroglossal fistula is impossible. However, fistulae do occur as a result of bursting or opening of a thyroglossal cyst onto the surface. Accessory thyroid glands may occur anywhere along the line of the duct and are sometimes found at the back of the tongue (lingual thyroids).

Thyroid Gland Proper (Fig. 141). The adult thyroid is a ductless gland. It is a highly vascular, solid organ related to the pretracheal fascia, that binds it to the larynx and causes it to rise and fall during the act of swallowing. It possesses its own true fibrous capsule, which is continuous with the stroma of the gland. The thyroid consists of a pair of lateral lobes which are joined across the median line by the isthmus. Each lateral lobe extends from the middle of the thyroid

cartilage to the 6th tracheal ring, is pyramidal in shape with its apex upward and measures 2 inches in length, 1¼ in width and ¾ inch in thickness. These measurements are greatly altered by pathologic conditions. The lobe is related medially to the thyroid and the cricoid cartilages, the cricothyroid and the inferior constrictor muscles, the trachea, the esophagus and the external and the recurrent laryngeal nerves. Some describe the medial surface as being related to 2 tubes (esophagus and trachea), 2 nerves (recurrent and external laryngeal) and 2 muscles (inferior constrictor and cricothyroid) (Fig. 141 C). The lobe is related posteriorly to the common carotid and the inferior thyroid arteries and the longus cervicis muscle. Superficially, it is covered by the sternohyoid, the omo-

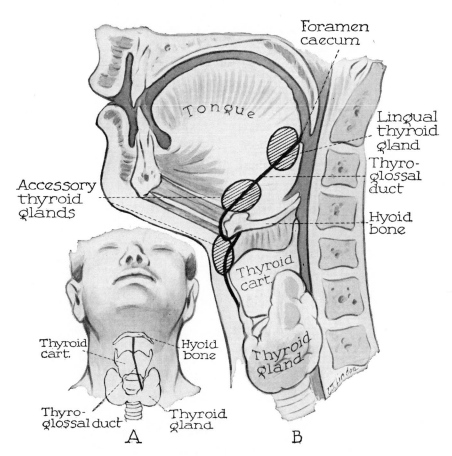

FIG. 140. Embryology of the thyroid gland: (A) course of the thyroglossal duct, (B) lateral view of the thyroglossal duct and possible locations of accessory thyroid glands.

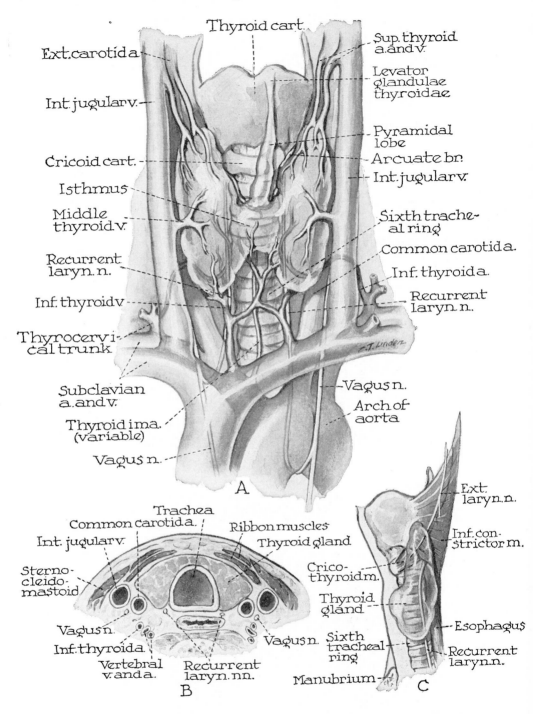

Fig. 141. The thyroid gland. (A) The gland has been presented as a transparent structure to show the relations of the vessels and nerves. The path of the inferior thyroid artery can be followed. (B) Cross section through the isthmus of the thyroid gland. (C) The thyroid gland viewed from the left side. The gland is in relation to 2 nerves (recurrent and external laryngeal), 2 tubes (esophagus and trachea) and 2 muscles (inferior constrictor and cricothyroid).

hyoid and the sternothyroid and is overlapped by the sternocleidomastoid muscle.

The *isthmus,* which occasionally is absent, is a bar of thyroid tissue, varying in width and lying under cover of the skin and the fascia in the median line of the neck. It is situated on the 2nd, the 3rd and the 4th tracheal rings and is nearer the lower than the upper pole. A triangular projection, or *pyramidal (middle) lobe,* extends upward usually from the left side of the upper border of the isthmus and is connected to the hyoid

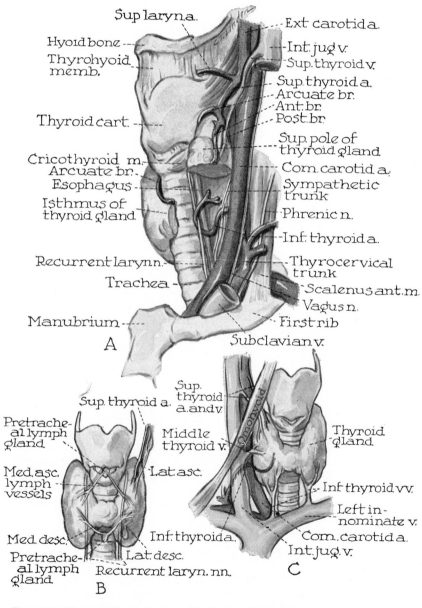

FIG. 142. The vessels of the thyroid gland: (A) the isthmus has been cut and the lower part of the left lobe removed to show the relationships of the superior and the inferior thyroid arteries and the recurrent laryngeal nerve; (B) the lymph drainage of the thyroid gland; (C) the veins of the thyroid.

bone by a fibromuscular slip called the *levator glandulae thyroidae*.

Arteries. The arteries of the thyroid gland are 2 pairs, the superior and the inferior thyroids, and sometimes a single artery, the thyroidea ima (Figs. 141, 142).

The superior thyroid artery is the first branch of the external carotid; it supplies infrahyoid, laryngeal and sternocleidomastoid branches in the carotid triangle. It passes down under cover of the "strap" muscles and at the superior pole of the thyroid gland trifurcates into an anterior branch that supplies the front of the gland, a posterior that goes behind and an isthmic (arcuate) branch that joins its fellow of the opposite side along the upper border of the isthmus. The superior laryngeal nerve is situated only a little higher than the superior thyroid artery and, if the vessel is grasped too high, the nerve may be included in the ligature.

The inferior thyroid artery is a branch of the thyrocervical trunk which arises from the first part of the subclavian. Although the superior vessel enters the superior pole, the inferior thyroid does *not* enter at the inferior pole of the gland. It travels upward along the medial border of the scalenus anterior muscle as far as the level of the 6th cervical vertebra and turns medially behind the vagus nerve and the common carotid artery. It passes in front of the vertebral vessels and, continuing downward, reaches the posterior border of the gland to which it is finally distributed. To do this it makes a hairpin turn, the summit of which varies considerably as to its level. It also supplies the larynx, the pharynx, the trachea, the esophagus and the surrounding muscles. As the artery reaches the thyroid it is crossed either in front or behind by the recurrent laryngeal nerve. A large branch of the vessel ascends along the posterior border of the gland to anastomose with a descending branch from the superior thyroid artery.

The thyroidea ima is a branch from the innominate or the aortic arch. It varies in size from a tiny arteriole to a vessel as large as the inferior thyroid, which it may replace. It passes upward over the anterior surface of the trachea, under cover of the thymus, and reaches the inferior border of the isthmus. Its presence should be kept in mind when performing a low tracheostomy and during thyroid surgery.

The accessory thyroid arteries are small vessels supplying the esophagus, the trachea and the thyroid gland. The 4 major thyroid arteries may be ligated, but the blood supply to the gland remains surprisingly good because of these accessory vessels.

Veins. The veins of the thyroid form a rich plexus situated in front of the gland. As they leave the gland, they form 3 main trunks in the form of superior, middle and inferior thyroid veins.

The superior thyroid vein is the only venous trunk that accompanies the artery of the same name. It leaves the upper part of the gland, taking as its guide the outer border of the omohyoid muscle, crosses the common carotid artery and ends in the internal jugular vein.

The middle thyroid vein has no accompanying artery. It leaves the gland about its midportion, follows the inner border of the omohyoid, crosses the common carotid artery and ends in the internal jugular vein.

The inferior thyroid veins commence at the lower pole of the gland and at the lower border of the isthmus; they pass downward in front of the trachea and may be connected by several transverse branches and end in the left innominate vein.

Nerves. Two nerves are related to the thyroid gland: the superior and the recurrent (inferior) laryngeal. Both are branches of the vagus nerve (Fig. 143).

The superior laryngeal nerve arises from the inferior ganglion (nodosum), passes downward and medially and crosses behind the internal carotid artery. It divides into the internal and the external laryngeal nerves.

The internal laryngeal nerve, the larger of the two branches, is accompanied by the superior laryngeal branch of the superior thyroid artery and with it pierces the thyrohyoid membrane at the posterior border of the thyrohyoid muscle. It is purely sensory and supplies fibers to the floor of the piriform fossa and the mucous membrane of the larynx above the vocal cord.

The external laryngeal nerve accompanies

the superior thyroid artery but is placed on a deeper plane. It passes deeply to the upper pole of the thyroid gland and is distributed to the cricothyroid and the inferior constrictor muscles. During ligation of the superior thyroid vessels, the external laryngeal nerve (nerve to the cricothyroid) is in danger. It may be included in the ligature, and such inclusion would cause a weakness or huskiness of the voice. However, this condition is temporary and becomes normal within a few months.

The recurrent (inferior) laryngeal nerve is a structure of vital importance in thyroid surgery. Considerable variations in its position may take place so that the nerve may penetrate and traverse the gland proper, may be behind the gland, or may remain in the tracheo-esophageal groove (Fig. 144). During thyroid surgery, when the gland is dislocated forward and medially, the nerve usually hugs the side of the trachea. Then it is located not in the tracheo-esophageal groove but on the posterolateral aspect of the trachea. It always passes posterior to the joint that exists between the inferior cornu

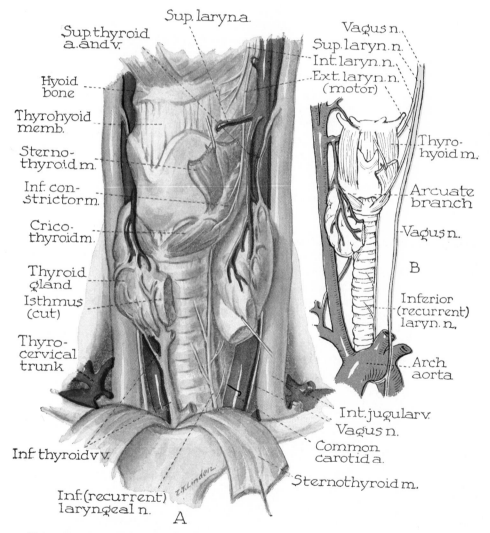

FIG. 143. The nerve supply of the thyroid gland: (A) the thyroid isthmus has been cut to show the course of the recurrent laryngeal nerve; (B) the nerves are shown on the left, and the arteries on the right.

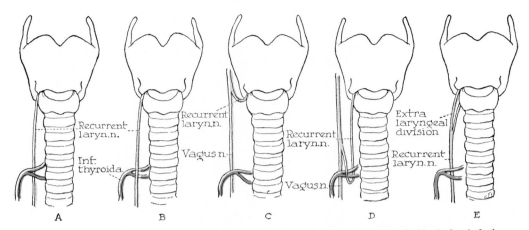

FIG. 144. Possible locations of the recurrent laryngeal nerve: (A) behind the inferior thyroid artery; (B) in front of the inferior thyroid artery; (C) high origin, this accounts for the inability to find the nerve during thyroidectomy; (D) origin around the inferior thyroid artery; (E) extralaryngeal division. In some instances the nerve may pass between the branches of the artery.

of the thyroid and the cricoid. This cartilaginous prominence formed by the joint is a valuable guide to the nerve. On the right side the recurrent leaves the vagus nerve as it crosses the first part of the subclavian artery, turns upward and medially behind that artery and the common carotid and travels in the groove between the trachea and the esophagus. It ascends in this groove to the lobe of the thyroid gland and crosses or is crossed by the inferior thyroid artery. Upon reaching the lower border of the inferior constrictor muscle it passes deeply to it so as to gain access to the muscles of the larynx. It supplies the muscles that act on the vocal folds but also supplies sensory branches to the mucous membrane of the larynx below these folds. Therefore, it is both sensory and motor. On the left side, the nerve arises within the thorax after turning around the arch of the aorta and then ascends in the neck in the tracheo-esophageal groove.

To aid in the exposure of the recurrent laryngeal nerve, M. M. Simon has constructed an anatomic triangle which can be identified readily (Fig. 145). It is bounded by the recurrent laryngeal nerve anteriorly, the common carotid artery posteriorly, and the inferior thyroid artery forms its base. The triangle is dependent on the variations and the anomalies that may take place. The recurrent laryngeal nerve supplies all the in-

trinsic muscles of the larynx with the exception of the cricothyroid.

There is a voluminous and confusing literature concerning the innervation of the larynx. Some of this confusion resulted from the difficulty of interpreting the various positions of a paralyzed vocal cord. To add to the confusion, a completely paralyzed or cadaveric cord may resume normal function, and a presumably incompletely paralyzed vocal cord would remain unchanged—in a position of adduction with good tension—for decades. The variety of responses and positions has been clarified and explained by the works of King and Gregg, who directed attention to the anatomic reasons for these various positions. They state that some recurrent laryngeal nerves divide into two trunks extralaryngeally, thus supplying fibers to the abductor and the adductor muscles, respectively. On the basis of these findings one can assume that if a paralyzed vocal cord is observed in the midline with good tension, the recurrent nerve is divided extralaryngeally, and the posterior division, which supplied the abductor muscle, has been injured. The abductor group of muscles, thus being unopposed, have pulled the vocal cord to the midline. In such a patient there would be no dyspnea, and the speaking voice would be normal. If a vocal cord is completely paralyzed (cadaveric) and is in an inter-

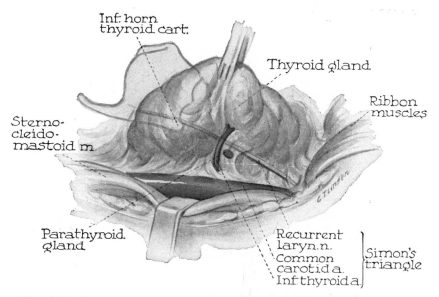

Inf. horn
thyroid cart.

Thyroid gland

Ribbon
muscles

Sterno-
cleido-
mastoid m.

Parathyroid
gland

Recurrent
laryn. n.
Common
carotid a.
Inf. thyroid a.

Simon's
triangle

FIG. 145. Simon's triangle. This aids in the identification of the recurrent laryngeal nerve. It is bounded anteriorly by the recurrent nerve, posteriorly by the common carotid artery, and the inferior thyroid artery forms its base. The inferior horn of the thyroid cartilage also makes an excellent guide to the nerve.

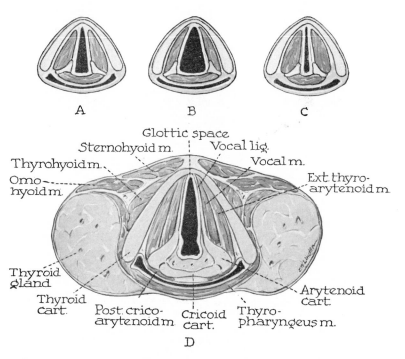

A   B   C

Glottic space

Sternohyoid m.   Vocal lig.

Thyrohyoid m.   Vocal m.

Omo-
hyoid m.   Ext. thyroarytenoid m.

Thyroid
gland

Arytenoid
cart.

Thyroid
cart.

Post. crico-
arytenoid m.

Cricoid
cart.

Thyro-
pharyngeus m.

D

FIG. 146. Transverse sections through the larynx (vocal cord level): (A) normal glottic space; (B) early bilateral abductor paralysis, the patient can breathe but the voice is impaired; (C) late bilateral abductor paralysis, voice improves but dyspnea and inspiratory laryngeal stridor appear; (D) anatomic relations.

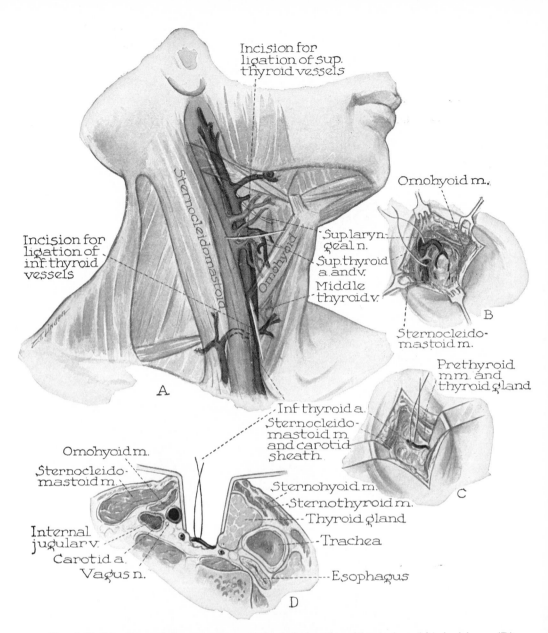

Incision for
ligation of sup.
thyroid vessels

Omohyoid m.

Sternocleidomastoid

Incision for
ligation of
inf. thyroid
vessels

Omohyoid

Sup. laryn-
geal n.

Sup. thyroid
a. and v.

Middle
thyroid v.

B

Sternocleido-
mastoid m.

A

Prethyroid
mm. and
thyroid gland

Inf. thyroid a.

Sternocleido-
mastoid m.
and carotid
sheath

Omohyoid m.

Sternocleido-
mastoid m.

Sternohyoid m.

Sternothyroid m.

Thyroid gland

C

Internal
jugular v.

Carotid a.

Vagus n.

Trachea

Esophagus

D

FIG. 147. Ligations of the superior and the inferior thyroid arteries: (A) incisions, (B) ligation of the superior thyroid artery, (C) ligation of the inferior thyroid artery, (D) transverse section, showing the ligation of the inferior thyroid artery.

FIG. 148 (*Facing page*). Subtotal thyroidectomy. (A) The incision is placed in a transverse skin crease. (B) The investing layer of deep cervical fascia is opened along the anterior border of the sternocleidomastoid muscle. (C) Division of the sternohyoid and the omohyoid muscles on the right. The same is done on the left side. These muscles should be severed high so that their nerve supply (ansa hypoglossi) is not injured. (D) The sternohyoid and the omohyoid muscles have been dissected upward and downward. The sternothyroid on the right side has been severed. (E) Isolation and division of the middle thyroid vein; this permits entrance into the posterior thyroid space. (F) Ligation of the superior thyroid vessels.

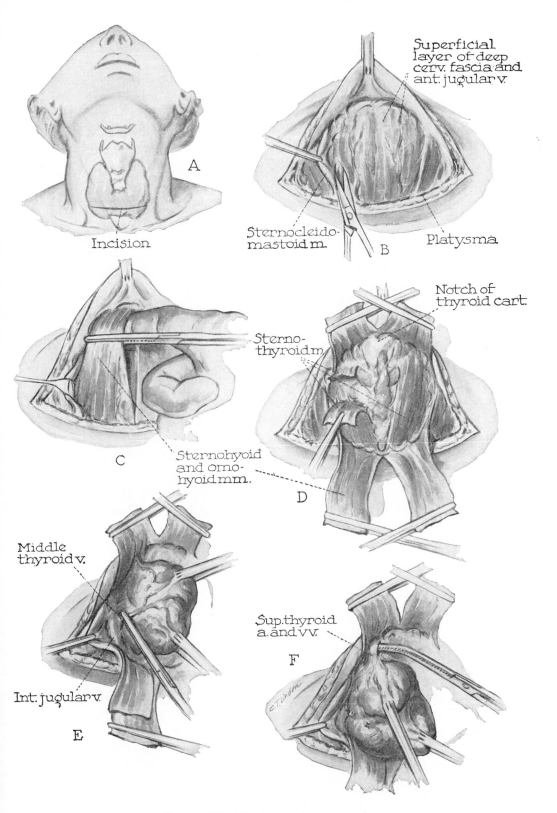

A — Incision

B — Superficial layer of deep cerv. fascia and ant. jugular v.
Sternocleido-mastoid m.
Platysma

C — Sterno-thyroid m.
Sternohyoid and omo-hyoid mm.

D — Notch of thyroid cart.

E — Middle thyroid v.
Int. jugular v.

F — Sup. thyroid a. and vv.

C.T.Linden

FIGURE 148. (*Caption on facing page.*)

197

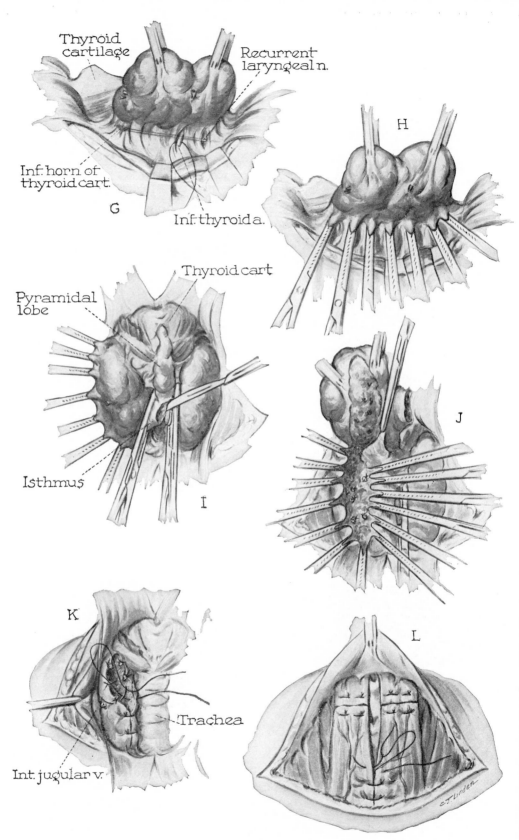

Thyroid
cartilage

Recurrent
laryngeal n.

Inf. horn of
thyroid cart.

Inf. thyroid a.

G

H

Thyroid cart.

Pyramidal
lobe

Isthmus

I

J

K

Trachea

Int. jugular v.

L

Figure 149. (*Caption on facing page.*)

mediate position between abduction and adduction, then it must be assumed that the entire laryngeal nerve has been injured. In such a patient there would be marked hoarseness and an absence of dyspnea. The effects of such an injury could be compensated if the opposite normal cord is capable of crossing the midline. Therefore, it is important to notice on examination of the larynx whether or not a vocal cord fails to move and also to determine its position and tension.

If both recurrent nerves are cut (bilateral abductor paralysis) the vocal cords become lax and cannot be tensed (Fig. 146 B). This results in immediate impairment of voice but rarely causes difficulty in breathing. It is interesting to note that within 3 to 5 months the voice begins to return. This is due to a fibrosis and shrinking of the vocal cords which were previously lax (Fig. 146 C). A few weeks later, the fibrotic process results in fixation of the vocal cords as they approach each other. The fibrotic contraction causes the cords to approach the midline, narrowing the glottic space to a thin slit. As a result of this, dyspnea begins to make its appearance, especially on exertion, resulting in a marked limitation of physical effort.

The sympathetic nerve supply to the thyroid gland is derived from the sympathetic ganglia. The fibers from the middle and the inferior cervical ganglia reach the gland as nervous networks along the superior and the inferior thyroid arteries.

Lymph Drainage. The thyroid gland is drained by 2 sets of *lymph vessels,* the ascending and the descending, each consisting of medial and lateral groups. The *medial group of the ascending vessels* leaves the upper border of the isthmus and passes to the lymph glands situated on the cricothyroid membrane; they are known as the prelaryngeal glands. The *lateral ascending vessels*

leave the upper part of the gland and accompany the superior thyroid artery to the deep cervical chain that is situated at the bifurcation of the common carotid. The *medial descending vessels* pass to the glands on the trachea, the pretracheal glands. The *lateral descending vessels* pass from the deep surface of the thyroid to small glands placed about the recurrent laryngeal nerve.

SURGICAL CONSIDERATIONS

LIGATIONS OF THYROID VESSELS

Ligation of the Superior Thyroid Artery. This can be accomplished either at the trunk or at the poles. Polar ligation is the method of choice, since it gets most of the arterial and venous branches and because the superior laryngeal nerve is in less danger of inclusion. For polar ligation a transverse incision is made in the skin, preferably in a skin crease in the region of the thyroid or cricoid cartilage (Fig. 147 A). Beginning at the medial border of the sternocleidomastoid muscle and extending mesialward for about 2 inches, the incision is carried through the superficial layer of deep cervical fascia; the omohyoid muscle is identified, retracted medially, and the sternocleidomastoid laterally. Deeper dissection will bring the upper pole of the thyroid into view (Fig. 147 B). The superior thyroid artery trifurcates, and there are usually 2 veins for each artery; hence, there may be as many as 9 small vessels at each superior pole. The pole is used as a guide, and this is followed cephalad until the vessels are visualized clearly. The superior laryngeal nerve is usually situated above the point of ligation.

Ligation of the Inferior Thyroid Artery. The most common approach is along the medial border of the sternocleidomastoid, but it has been approached along the lateral border. For the mesial approach, an incision is made along the anterior border of the

---

FIG. 149 (*Facing page*). Subtotal thyroidectomy (*Continued*). (G) Identification of the recurrent laryngeal nerve and ligation of the inferior thyroid artery. (H) Ring of forceps placed into the right lobe. Each hemostat bites into thyroid tissue proper and in this way protects the recurrent laryngeal nerve and the parathyroid glands. (I) Removal of the right lobe, the isthmus and the pyramidal lobe. (J) Protective ring of forceps in place; each hemostat is replaced by a ligature. (K) Approximation of the thyroid remnant. (L) Closure.

sternocleidomastoid muscle (Fig. 147 A). Transverse incisions produce less scarring. The incision is made through the superficial layer of deep cervical fascia, and the sternocleidomastoid muscle is retracted laterally. Dissection is continued in the interval between the carotid sheath and the thyroid gland (Fig. 147 C-D). The middle thyroid vein is severed before the proper cleavage plane is found, and the recurrent laryngeal nerve must be avoided. Isolation and ligation of this vessel as it is done in routine thyroidectomies is described in detail elsewhere (p. 196).

THYROIDECTOMY

Subtotal Thyroidectomy. This operation (Figs. 148-149) is performed frequently, and since technical errors might result in disaster, any anatomic points that make for a safer operation should be stressed. The incision should be so placed that the average string of beads will cover the scar. No fixed point can be mentioned, since necks vary in their length, but generally these incisions should be 1 or 2 fingerbreadths above the sternal notch and extending from one sternocleidomastoid to the other (Fig. 148 A). This is deepened until the subplatysmal cleavage plane is reached.

Having found this avascular plan, the upper flap, consisting of skin, subcutaneous fat and platysma, is grasped and dissected upward, well above the level of the notch of the thyroid cartilage. This exposes the superficial layer of deep cervical fascia and the anterior jugular veins. The anterior borders of the sternocleidomastoid muscles are now identified; the investing layer of deep cervical fascia is incised here (Fig. 148 B). In this way the prethyroid muscles are separated from the sternocleidomastoid which is mobilized. The latter is retracted outward, and adequate exposure of the prethyroid muscles is obtained.

A vertical incision is made in the midline between the two prethyroid muscle bundles and is extended from the thyroid notch to the level of the sternal notch. The sternohyoid and the omohyoid are clamped and divided high, thus protecting their nerve supply (Fig. 148 C). It is an error to state that the prethyroid muscles have been sev-

ered, since the underlying sternothyroid usually remains intact after this step.

A distinct cleavage plane exists between the sternohyoid and the sternothyroid. The sternohyoid and the omohyoid, having been incised, are dissected both upward and downward. The sternothyroid muscle is severed transversely, exposing the thyroid gland (Fig. 148 D).

The last maneuver opens the so-called "surgical capsule" (p. 197). The gland is grasped by forceps, rotated medially, and the internal jugular vein in the carotid sheath is retracted laterally. This maneuver places the thin pretracheal fascia, on the stretch, where it attaches to the thyroid gland, and in this tissue the middle thyroid vein is sought. It is severed and ligated, and the posterior thyroid space is entered (Fig. 148 E). This permits medial dislocation of the gland.

With medial traction on the thyroid, and lateral traction on the carotid sheath, dissection takes place in the proper cleavage plane. The upper pole is identified, as is the entrance of the superior thyroid vessels. These are doubly ligated, off the pole, and severed (Fig. 148 F). Careful separation of the pretracheal layer of pretracheal fascia will reveal the recurrent laryngeal nerve and the inferior thyroid artery (Fig. 149 G). If deemed necessary, the artery is ligated. A ring of forceps is placed around the right thyroid lobe which includes the isthmus; each forceps grasps thyroid tissue proper. The lobe, the isthmus, and the pyramidal lobe are removed above this protective ring (Fig. 149 H,I,J). The clamped thyroid tissue is ligated, and the thyroid that remains is approximated to itself or sutured to the pretracheal fascia (Fig. 149 K). The left lobe is removed in similar fashion. The severed muscles are resutured; and the skin, the superficial fascia and the platysma are approximated as one layer (Fig. 149 L).

Total thyroidectomy is usually done for carcinoma of the thyroid. On the involved side the sternocleidomastoid muscle, the internal jugular vein, the thyroid vessels and all demonstrable lymphatics are included in the dissection and are removed en bloc. Included in this dissection are the prethyroid muscles.

Thyroglossal Duct. This duct originates at

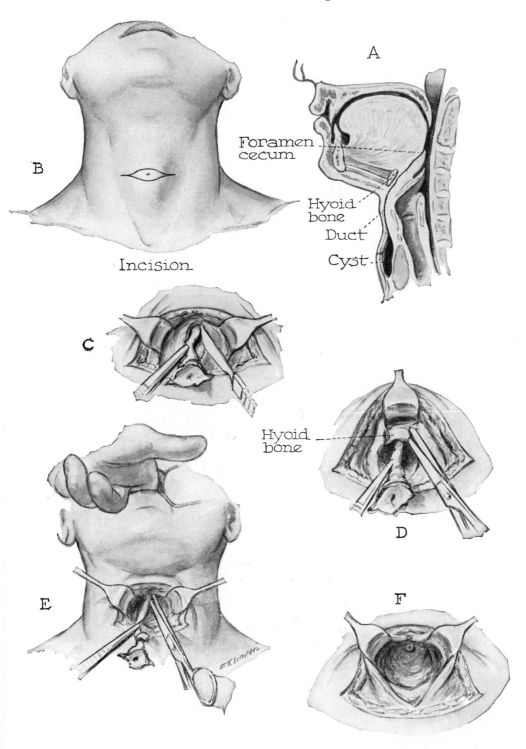

FIG. 150. Removal of a thyroglossal duct: (A) course of a patent thyroglossal duct and cyst; (B) incision; (C) dissection to the hyoid bone; (D) cutting the hyoid bone; (E) an assistant's finger placed in the mouth and pressing on the tongue makes the deeper part of the duct more accessible; (F) dissection completed.

an early stage in fetal life as a depression in the midline of the posterior third of the tongue which is known as the *foramen caecum*. From it a solid cord of cells grows downward which becomes canalized to form the duct that passes downward in the midline of the neck between the genioglossi muscles (Fig. 140). It extends as far as the upper border of the thyroid cartilage and then turns to either side of the midline. This part of its course is represented after birth by the pyramidal lobe of the thyroid gland and a musculofibrous band connecting that lobe to the hyoid bone. Frazer seems to have settled the question as to whether the duct runs in front of, behind or through the hyoid bone.

His works demonstrate that the duct passes in front of the body of the hyoid and then curves up behind the bone before again continuing downward. Therefore, it is important to remove this section of the hyoid bone when removing a patent duct. After passing the thyroid cartilage, the thyroglossal duct expands to form the thyroid gland.

If the duct remains patent, a *thyroglossal cyst* develops. Such a cyst is found usually above the thyroid cartilage and in the midline. Hamilton Bailey has stated that if these cysts develop below the thyroid cartilage, they naturally follow the course of the duct and appear to one or the other side of the midline, usually to the left. Normally, the

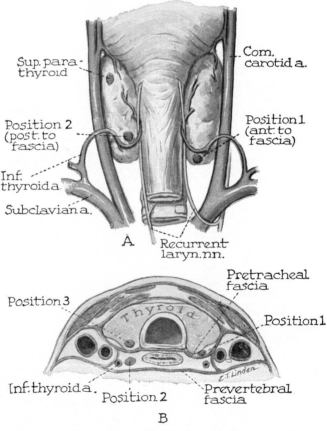

FIG. 151. The parathyroid glands. (A) Posterior view; in position one, the inferior parathyroid is below the inferior thyroid artery, but in position two, it is above the artery. The superior parathyroid in this instance is intraglandular. (B) Cross section. In position one, the gland is anterior to the pretracheal fascia; in position two, it is posterior to this fascia; and in position three, it is intraglandular.

thyroglossal duct does not open onto the surface of the skin of the neck. Therefore, a congenital thyroglossal fistula is not possible, and if a fistula does develop it must be secondary and brought about by a bursting of or an opening into a thyroglossal cyst.

Since the thyroid gland develops from the thyroglossal duct, an accessory or misplaced thyroid may develop anywhere along the line of the duct. The *lingual thyroids* are sometimes found at the back of the tongue in the region of the foramen caecum. The term "ectopic thyroid" means thyroid tissue found in an incorrect position, thus differing from the accessory thyroid (Fig. 140 B).

If a thyroglossal duct swelling appears above the hyoid bone, it is necessary only to split the mylohyoid muscle along its raphe, separate the geniohyoid muscle and remove the tumors. However, if these cysts or tumors appear subhyoid, the dissection must be more radical and include removal of a portion of the hyoid bone.

Thyroglossal cysts, fistulae and sinuses must be removed radically to accomplish a cure (Fig. 150). The cyst is exposed by a transverse incision that is carried down to the sternohyoid muscles. These are divided vertically in the midline, and the cyst is dissected free to the level of the hyoid bone. To expose the sinus completely, a small portion of hyoid bone must be removed in the midline. An assistant's finger placed in the patient's mouth and passed over the back of the tongue enables him to push the foramen caecum and any remaining portion of the sinus tract within reach of the operator. Since the duct is small and cannot be seen clearly, it is best to dissect some of the surrounding tissue with it. Therefore, in the removal it is necessary to include some small portion of the mylohyoid, the geniohyoid and the genioglossus muscles. Deep structures are sutured; divided edges of the hyoid bone are approximated; the wound is closed with or without drainage.

PARATHYROID GLANDS

The parathyroid glands (Fig. 151) are yellowish-brown bodies, the number and the position of which are variable. A superior and an inferior parathyroid are usually present on each side, occupying any position from the back of the pharynx to the superior mediastinum. They are about the size of a small pea and usually lie between the posterior aspect of the lateral lobe of the thyroid and the pretracheal lamina of pretracheal fascia. The parathyroids lie entirely or partially within the substance of the thyroid gland, this being particularly true of the superior, which are then easily removed in thyroidectomy.

The anatomy of the inferior parathyroids is more complex than that of the superior, and the inferior lie in intimate relationship to the inferior thyroid arteries and veins. Their position is variable. Walton has described three rather typical positions of the parathyroids in relation to their surrounding fascial plane: (1) the gland lies below the inferior thyroid artery and is then anterior to the pretracheal fascia; (2) the gland lies above the artery and is then frequently situated deep to the pretracheal fascia and visible only upon incising the fascia; (3) the parathyroids may be in the substance of the thyroid gland proper.

If a tumor develops in a parathyroid in the first-described position, it may pass between the two capsules of the thyroid, along the inferior thyroid veins, in front of the common carotid artery and finally come to lie behind the sternum. If such a tumor is situated behind the pretracheal fascia, it cannot be seen until the fascia is incised and an inspection made even around the circumference of the esophagus. It may even pass into the thorax behind the esophagus. The superior and the inferior parathyroid glands receive their blood supply from the corresponding thyroid vessels.

THYMUS GLAND

Embryologically, the thymus (Fig. 152) appears as 2 entodermal diverticula which arise one on either side of the 3rd branchial pouch. A ventral diverticulum of the 4th pouch may take part in the formation of the gland or entirely disappear. As the 2 diverticula grow they meet and become joined by connective tissue, but there is never any real fusion of thymus tissue proper. Actually, therefore, there are 2 asymmetric thymus glands—a right and a left—which are easily separated by blunt dissection.

The adult thymus gland is a temporary organ that is "sandwiched" between the sternum and the great vessels in the region of the superior mediastinum. It is essentially an organ of the growing period of life which undergoes gradual atrophy after puberty. From birth to puberty it grows relatively slowly; there are tremendous individual variations at any given age. At birth it ranges in weight from 2 to 17 Gm., the average being 13 Gm.; at puberty its average weight is about 37 Gm., but cases have been reported in which it has scarcely been recognizable at this age. In the young adult the average weight is usually reduced to about 25 Gm. The thymus gland is located partly in the neck and partly in the mediastinum, and it is roughly pyramidal in shape with its apex directed upward; in the infant this apex may be in actual contact with the thy-

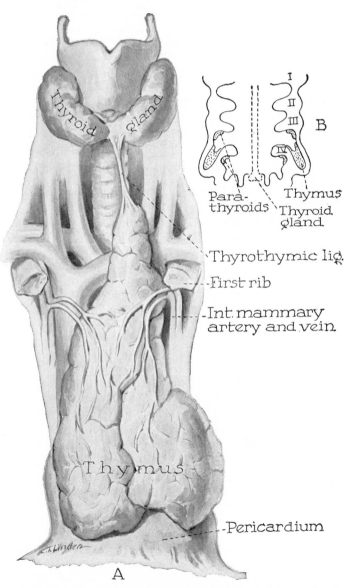

FIG. 152. The thymus gland: (A) enlarged thymus gland extending in front of the pericardium; (B) development of the thymus.

roid gland. It is soft in consistency, and its shape varies with its size and the age of the individual. In infants with short thoraces it is broad and squat, but in adults with long thoraces it is drawn out into 2 irregular flattened bands. It is of pinkish-gray color and has a lobulated surface.

Anteriorly, the thymus gland is related to the sternum and the lower end of the sterno-thyroid muscles. In the young child, its lateral margins may be insinuated between the pleura and the upper costal cartilages.

Posteriorly, it is related from below upward to the pericardium, the ascending aorta,

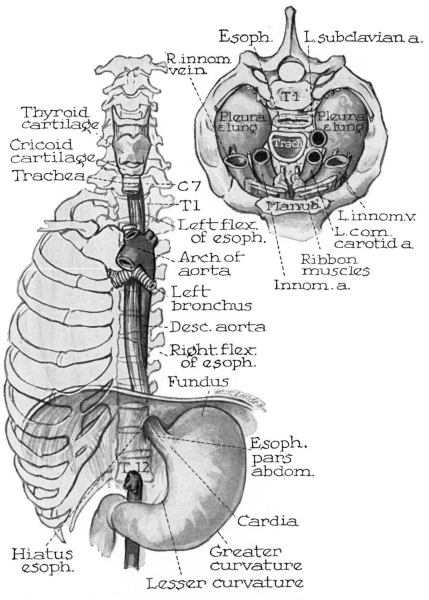

FIG. 153. The cervical part of the esophagus begins opposite the inferior margin of the cricoid cartilage at the level of the body of the 6th cervical vertebra. (*Inset*) Cross section at the level of the first thoracic vertebra. The trachea does not cover the esophagus completely but leaves a part of its left anterior margin exposed; this makes surgical access easier from this side.

the left innominate vein, the trachea and the inferior thyroid veins. It is surrounded by a fibrous capsule that separates it from these structures. It is connected to the thyroid by a strand of tissue called the *thyrothymic ligament*.

The arterial supply of the thymus is received through inconstant branches derived chiefly from the internal mammary artery or its branches.

Veins. These vessels are irregular and drain mainly into the internal mammary or the left innominate.

Lymphatics. The gland has a profuse lymphatic drainage, and certain of the lymphatics open directly into veins without first traversing lymph glands.

Occasionally, the thymus retains its infantile size in the adult and for some unknown reason does not atrophy. In such cases there is a large quantity of lymphoid tissue throughout the body, and the condition is then known as *status lymphaticus*.

Cervical Portion of the Esophagus

(Fig. 153.) The entire esophagus is about 10 inches long and extends from the end of the pharynx through the lower part of the neck and through the superior and the posterior mediastinum. It pierces the diaphragm and enters the stomach opposite the 9th thoracic spine about 1 inch to the left of the midline.

The cervical esophagus is a direct continuation of the pharynx. It commences opposite the inferior margin of the cricoid cartilage at the level of the body of the 6th cervical vertebra. An excellent landmark which locates this point is the carotid tubercle (Fig. 740). The trachea does not cover the esophagus completely but leaves a portion of its left anterior margin exposed, making surgical access easier on this side. As the esophagus descends from the level of the 6th cervical vertebra, it lies in front of the vertebral column and overlaps both longus cervicis (colli) muscles. At the inlet of the thorax the left common carotid is anterior to its left border; the thoracic duct, the left subclavian artery and the pleura are situated on its left side. Higher up the common carotid is also on its left side, and both

are overlapped by the thyroid gland. At times the posterior part of the lateral thyroid lobe may enlarge and insinuate itself upon the anterior surface of the esophagus causing difficulty in swallowing.

The esophagus and the pharynx are loosely attached to the prevertebral fascia and in this way form the retropharyngeal and the retro-esophageal spaces. Abscesses in these spaces are hindered from extending laterally and thus take the path of least resistance, which is downward the mediastinum. Because of its loose connection with the prevertebral fascia and because of its elasticity, this portion of the esophagus can be displaced upward and laterally for a considerable distance.

When the esophagus is empty, it is flattened anteroposteriorly, and its lumen appears only as a slit, but when distended it becomes irregularly cylindrical and presents its typical constriction points, the first and narrowest of which is at its commencement.

SURGICAL CONSIDERATIONS

Esophageal Diverticulum

Shallow and Lahey have done extensive work in this field, and the former has reported a series of cases in which 1-stage diverticulectomy has been accomplished with excellent results (Fig. 154). A longitudinal incision is made along the anterior border of the sternocleidomastoid muscle and is carried through the skin, the superficial fascia and the superficial layer of deep cervical fascia. The sternocleidomastoid is retracted backward until the omohyoid muscle is demonstrated; this is severed at the point where it disappears beneath the sternocleidomastoid. With the omohyoid retracted, the thyroid gland is separated from the internal jugular vein and the common carotid artery. Then the thyroid gland is pulled toward the midline, and the inferior thyroid artery is exposed. This often crosses over the diverticulum or gets in the way of its dissection; hence, it is best to ligate and sever it.

Since a diverticulum is a herniation of mucous membrane through muscle fibers, it should be remembered that there are two weak points in the musculature of the posterior aspect of the pharynx and the esoph-

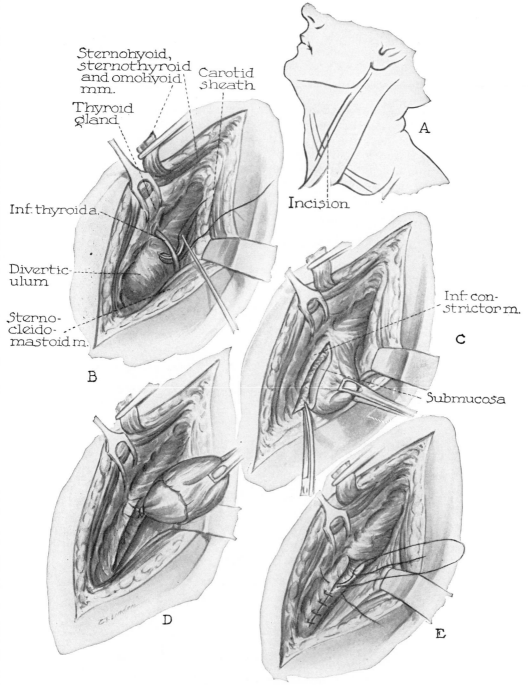

FIG. 154. Esophageal diverticulectomy (one stage). (A) A longitudinal incision is made along the anterior border of the sternocleidomastoid muscle. (B) The omohyoid muscle is severed, and the thyroid gland is retracted medially: the sternocleidomastoid muscle and the carotid sheath are retracted laterally. The inferior thyroid artery is exposed, ligated and severed as it crosses the diverticulum. (C) Fibers of the inferior constrictor muscle are severed, and the sac is mobilized. (D) The sac is ligated close to the pharynx. (E) Closure is effected in layers.

agus; these two points are at the level of the lower fibers of the inferior constrictor, and where the cricopharyngeal muscle diverges from the lowest fibers of the inferior constrictor. These are the two locations where diverticula are most commonly found; however, the approach is usually through the left side of the neck because the esophagus passes to the left of the vertebral bodies.

Shallow has made successful use of the esophagoscope to isolate and aid in the dissection of the diverticulum which is closely bound to the longitudinally running esoph-

agus by the enveloping fibers of the cricopharyngeal muscles. These are separated at the lowest angle of the sac, the fundus is grasped with blunt forceps, and traction is made.

The remaining fibers of the cricopharyngei enveloping the diverticulum are cut. When the neck of the sac is reached, the fibers of the inferior constrictor are seen along the lower border of the neck; these must be severed to mobilize it completely. The neck of the sac is transfixed and ligated, and the sac is removed. This ligation should take

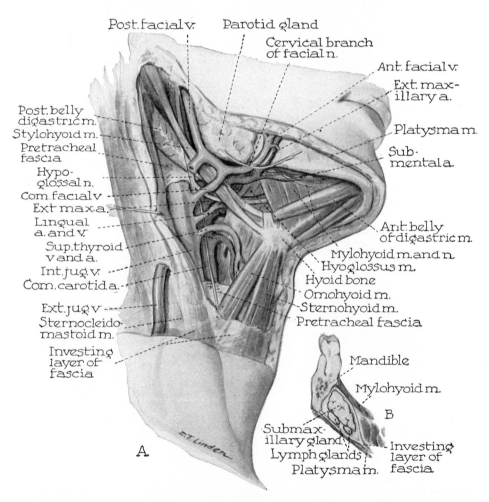

FIG. 155. The submaxillary (digastric) triangle. (A) The superficial layer of deep cervical fascia has been removed, exposing the floor and the contents of the triangle. The submaxillary gland, which overflows the triangle, also has been removed. (B) Coronal section, showing the superficial layer of deep cervical fascia investing the submaxillary gland.

place close to the pharynx. The cricopharyngeus and the inferior constrictor should be closed over the ligated and invaginated sac to prevent a recurrence of the hernia.

SUBMAXILLARY (DIGASTRIC) TRIANGLE

(Figs. 155-156) The submaxillary, or digastric, triangle is bounded by the anterior and the posterior bellies of the digastric and the inferior border of the mandible. The roof is fascial, being formed by the investing (superficial) layer of deep cervical fascia as it passes between the mandible and the hyoid bone. Three muscles make up the floor: the mylohyoid, the hyoglossus and the middle constrictor muscle of the pharynx. These

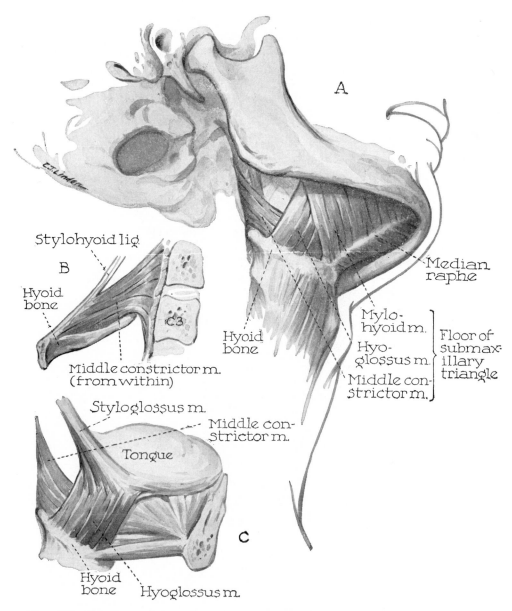

FIG. 156. The floor of the submaxillary triangle: (A) the floor is trimuscular and is formed by the mylohyoid, the hyoglossus and the middle constrictor muscles; (B) the middle constrictor muscle, seen from within; (C) the hyoglossus muscle.

muscles constitute important surgical land-marks and can be identified by the direction of their fibers and the fact that they lie on successively deeper planes.

The fibers of the *mylohyoid muscle* arise from the mylohyoid line of the mandible, run downward and medially and insert into a median raphe which extends from the chin to the hyoid bone. With its fellow of the opposite side it forms a diaphragm oris.

The free oblique posterior fibers reach the hyoid bone and overlap the *hyoglossus muscle,* whose fibers arise from the hyoid, pass directly upward to the lateral surface of the tongue where they attach and inter-digitate with the styloglossus (Fig. 156 C).

The posterior fibers form a free margin which overlaps the *middle constrictor muscle* of the pharynx. The fibers of the latter origi-nate from the cornu of the hyoid bone and are directed horizontally and backward to the median raphe (Fig. 160).

During dissection of this triangle, the fol-lowing structures are encountered: the *skin,* the *superficial fascia,* the *platysma* and the *cervical branch of the facial nerve,* which passes down behind the angle of the man-dible and lies between the platysma and the deep cervical fascia. Incisions made behind the angle of the jaw may injure this nerve and, since it supplies the quadratus labii inferioris, a drop in the angle of the mouth may result. This usually disappears within 3 months.

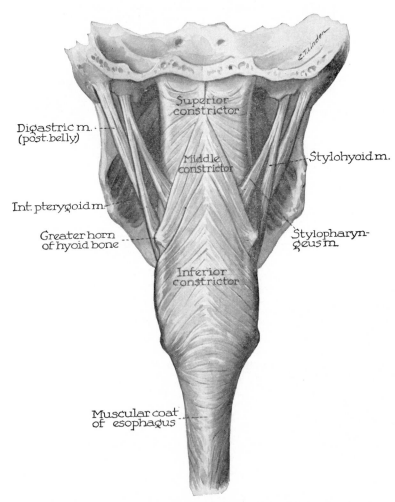

Fig. 157. The pharynx, viewed from behind; with 3 constrictor muscles intact.

The *anterior facial vein* crosses the triangle superficially and at the lower margin of the mandible accompanies the *external maxillary artery*. The deep cervical fascia (investing layer) envelops or invests the *submaxillary salivary gland* which overflows the triangle and conceals the trimuscular floor and the digastric muscle (Fig. 155 B). The gland is separated posteriorly from the parotid by the stylomandibular ligament, which is the thickened part of the parotid fascia between the styloid and the angle of the mandible. The submaxillary gland is indented by the posterior free edge of the mylohyoid muscle and in this way is divided into a superficial and a deep (oral) part (Fig. 98). Its duct (Wharton's) leaves its

deep surface, passes forward deeply to the sublingual gland and opens into the floor of the mouth on the sublingual papilla at the side of the frenulum linguae.

When the submaxillary gland is freed and retracted upward the *mylohyoid nerve* is visible; it is accompanied by the *submental branch of the facial artery*. If the free posterior border of the mylohyoid muscle is identified, the *lingual* and the *hypoglossal nerves* are seen passing behind this border. These nerves are separated by the oral part of the submaxillary gland and its forward-running Wharton's duct. The lingual nerve, Wharton's duct and the hypoglossal nerve run behind the mylohyoid muscle and on the hyoglossus muscle. The hypoglossal nerve is

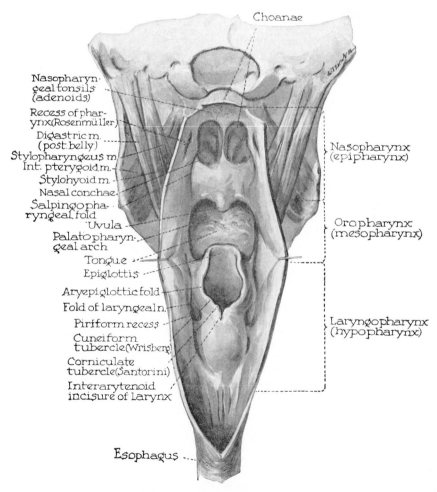

Choanae

Nasopharyngeal tonsils (adenoids)

Recess of pharynx (Rosenmüller)

Digastric m. (post. belly)
Stylopharyngeus m.
Int. pterygoid m.
Stylohyoid m.
Nasal conchae
Salpingopharyngeal fold
Uvula
Palatopharyngeal arch
Tongue
Epiglottis

Aryepiglottic fold
Fold of laryngeal n.
Piriform recess
Cuneiform tubercle (Wrisberg)
Corniculate tubercle (Santorini)
Interarytenoid incisure of larynx

Nasopharynx (epipharynx)

Oropharynx (mesopharynx)

Laryngopharynx (hypopharynx)

Esophagus

FIG. 158. The pharynx viewed from behind, with the 3 constrictor muscles removed.

usually accompanied by 1 or 2 veins. These relationships may be seen when the superficial part of the submaxillary gland is cut away and the mylohyoid muscle is detached at the hyoid bone and median raphe. If the hyoglossus muscle is cut parallel with and above the hyoid bone the *lingual artery* is exposed, lying deep to the hyoglossus muscle while the vein accompanying the hypoglossal nerve lies on this muscle. The vein should not be confused with the artery. An additional vein usually accompanies the lingual artery.

PHARYNX

(Figs. 157, 158, 159) The pharynx is a large vestibule that is common to the respiratory and the digestive tracts. It is a vertically placed musculomembranous tube that extends from the base of the skull to the cricoid cartilage where it becomes continuous with the esophagus. The 6th cervical vertebra marks its lower border posteriorly. It is about 5 inches long and has a transverse diameter greater than the anteroposterior. The widest part (1¾ inches) is opposite the hyoid bone, and the narrowest (¾ inch) is at the esophageal orifice. Since it communicates with the nose, the mouth and the larynx, it has been divided into 3 parts: nasopharynx, oropharynx and laryngopharynx.

Nasopharynx (Epipharynx). This is somewhat cube-shaped and is placed behind the cavity of the nose, above and behind the soft palate. It is part of the respiratory and not of the digestive tract. Its walls, with the exception of the soft palate, are incapable of movement; therefore, the cavity remains patent, and its form never changes.

Its *anterior wall* is formed by the posterior apertures of the nose (choanae) through which it opens into the nasal cavities. These apertures are a pair of oblong openings that slope from the base of the skull downward and forward to the posterior border of the hard palate and are separated by the vomer. By looking through them with a postnasal mirror a view is obtained of the posterior end of the inferior and the middle conchae and the 2 lower meatuses. Each opening is about 1 inch long and ½ inch wide.

The *roof* and the *posterior wall* are considered together as an obliquely sloped surface formed by the body of the sphenoid, the basilar process of the occipital bone and a thick layer of ligamentous fibrous tissue which fills in the angle between the latter and the vertebrae. The roof and the posterior wall are supported by the inferior surface of the body of the sphenoid, the basilar part of the occipital bone and the anterior arch of the atlas below. The posterior wall, especially in childhood, presents a mass of lymphoid tissue known as pharyngeal tonsils (adenoids) which may fill the nasopharynx and hinder or completely block nasal breathing.

The *floor* is made up of the soft palate and the uvula and is the only movable boundary of the nasopharynx. It prevents food from being regurgitated into the nose. Behind the soft palate the nasopharynx is continuous with the oral pharynx through the *isthmus*.

The *lateral wall* presents the opening of the pharyngotympanic tube (eustachian) which is on a level with and about ½ inch behind the inferior nasal concha. The entire side wall measures a little over 1 inch in diameter. The posterior boundary of the eustachian opening presents a prominent elevation (eustachian cushion) which is derived from the cartilaginous portion of the tube, behind which lies the pharyngeal recess (Rosenmüller's fossa). A fold of mucous membrane, the salpingopharyngeal fold, descends from the posterior lip of the orifice and contains the salpingopharyngeus muscle, which gradually disappears as it passes downward.

When adenoids occlude the orifice of the tube, the air in the tympanic cavity gradually becomes absorbed, and deafness may result. The tympanum can be inflated through the pharyngeal orifice of the tube by means of a eustachian catheter. The instrument is passed backward along the floor of the inferior meatus until it reaches the posterior wall of the nasopharynx. If the catheter is rotated laterally through a right angle, its point rises in the pharyngeal recess. Then it may be withdrawn from the nose until the point catches the tubal projection. When a mirror is introduced through the mouth so that the nasopharynx is illuminated by reflected light,

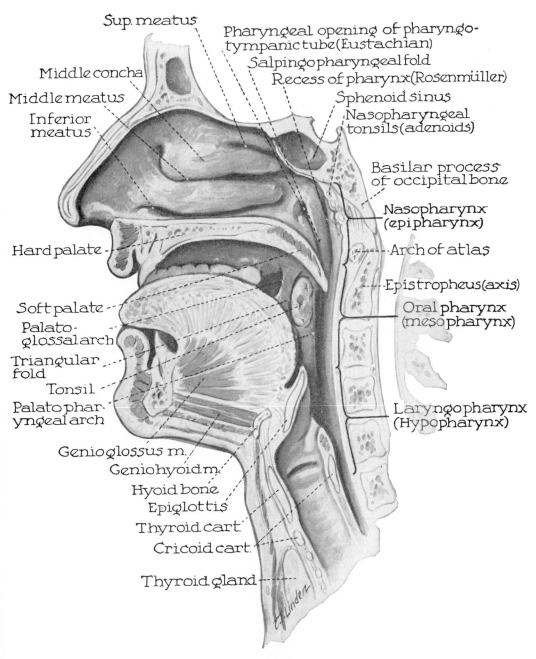

Sup. meatus

Pharyngeal opening of pharyngotympanic tube (Eustachian)

Salpingopharyngeal fold

Recess of pharynx (Rosenmüller)

Middle concha

Middle meatus

Inferior
meatus

Sphenoid sinus

Nasopharyngeal
tonsils (adenoids)

Basilar process
of occipital bone

Nasopharynx
(epipharynx)

Hard palate

Arch of atlas

Epistropheus (axis)

Soft palate

Palato-
glossal arch

Triangular
fold

Tonsil

Palatophar-
yngeal arch

Oral pharynx
(mesopharynx)

Laryngopharynx
(Hypopharynx)

Genioglossus m.

Geniohyoid m.

Hyoid bone

Epiglottis

Thyroid cart.

Cricoid cart.

Thyroid gland

FIG. 159. Sagittal view of the pharynx. The 3 parts of the
pharynx have been subdivided.

a view is obtained of the 4 orifices that open
into the nasal part of the pharynx; the middle
and the superior meatuses of the nose, and
the middle and the superior conchae can be
brought into view and their pathology determined. The side walls and the orifices of the

pharyngotympanic tubes also can be fully
inspected.

Oropharynx (Mesopharynx). This is partly
respiratory and partly alimentary. It is the
posterior continuation of the mouth cavity
that lies behind the mouth and the tongue.

The *anterior wall* presents the opening into the mouth, the lower portion being the pharyngeal part of the dorsum of the tongue that faces directly backward. The epiglottis, which belongs to the laryngeal part of the pharynx and is situated immediately behind the tongue, appears as a leaflike plate of cartilage enveloped in mucous membrane with its upper part standing prominently up and behind the tongue.

The *posterior wall* is smooth and is supported by the body of the axis, which is separated from the pharynx by the prevertebral fascia.

The *lateral wall* is formed by the interval between the palatoglossal and the palatopharyngeal arches that is occupied by the tonsils. A retropharyngeal abscess produces a swelling of the posterior pharyngeal wall that may bulge forward and obstruct the air passages during respiration.

Laryngopharynx (Hypopharynx). This is the longest of the 3 subdivisions; it lies behind the larynx and diminishes in width

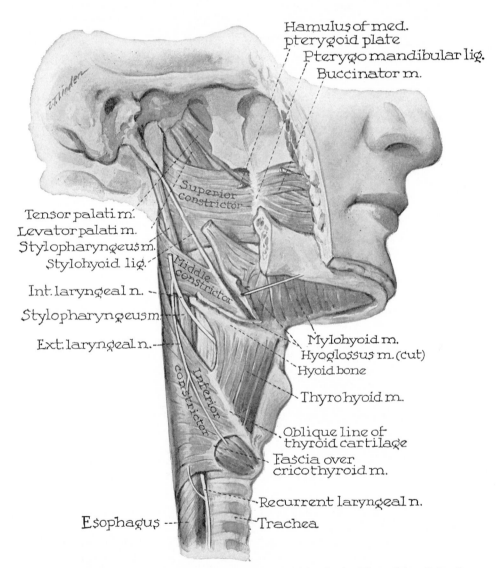

FIG. 160. The muscular coat of the pharynx (side view). The origin of the 3 constrictor muscles is along a continuous line from above downward.

from above downward. Its upper part is common to the digestive and the respiratory tracts, but its lower part, opposite the cricoid, is entirely digestive. Its anterior and posterior walls are in contact except when food is swallowed.

The *anterior wall* is formed by the inlet of the larynx and the posterior aspect of the arytenoid and the cricoid cartilages.

The *posterior wall* is in contact with the anterior and is supported by the bodies of the 3rd, the 4th, the 5th and the 6th cervical vertebrae.

The *lateral walls* are supported by the posterior part of the lamina of the thyroid cartilage and present a small fossa, the *piriform recess,* which is bounded on its medial side by the aryepiglottic fold. The mucous membrane of this area is supplied by the internal laryngeal nerve; hence, if a crumb or a small particle of food lodges in the fossa, uncontrollable coughing results.

Pharyngeal Wall. This wall presents 4 rather distinct layers: buccopharyngeal fascia, muscular, fibrous and mucous coats.

1. *The buccopharyngeal fascia* is a layer of fibrous tissue covering both the buccinator and the pharyngeal muscles. It also invests the constrictor muscles of the pharynx, and between it and the prevertebral fascia a loose areolar tissue is found which forms an easily distensible space in which pus may spread (Fig. 122). This layer contains the venous plexus, which drains the pharynx and communicates with the pterygoid plexus. It enters the jugular vein near the angle of the jaw.

2. *The muscle coat* of the pharyngeal wall is made up of 5 paired voluntary muscles: the 3 constrictors (superior, middle and inferior) which constitute an outer circular layer, and the stylopharyngeus and the palatopharyngeus which constitute an inner longitudinal layer (Fig. 160).

The 3 constrictor muscles are incomplete

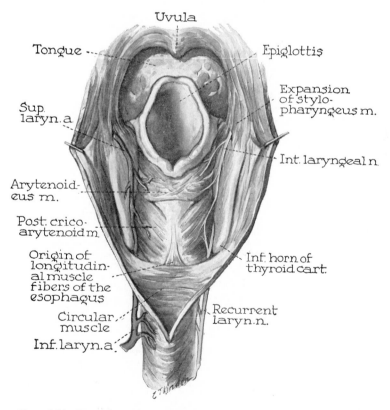

Uvula

Tongue ---

Epiglottis

Sup. laryn. a

Expansion of stylopharyngeus m.

Int. laryngeal n.

Arytenoid-eus m.

Post. crico-arytenoid m.

Origin of longitudinal muscle fibers of the esophagus

Inf. horn of thyroid cart.

Circular muscle

Recurrent laryn. n.

Inf. laryn. a

FIG. 161. Posterior view of the pharynx. The posterior wall has been cut open to show the internal and the recurrent laryngeal nerves and the superior laryngeal artery.

in front, but each widens posteriorly and joins its fellow in the median plane at the median raphe. Each muscle is somewhat fan-shaped and is attached by its front end or handle to the side wall of the nasal, the oral or the laryngeal cavity. Each partly overlaps externally the muscle above it, so that the inferior overlaps the middle, and the middle overlaps the superior. The origin of these muscles is continuous from above down. The *superior constrictor* originates from the lower third of the posterior border of the medial pterygoid plate, the pterygomandibular ligament, the side of the tongue, the mucous

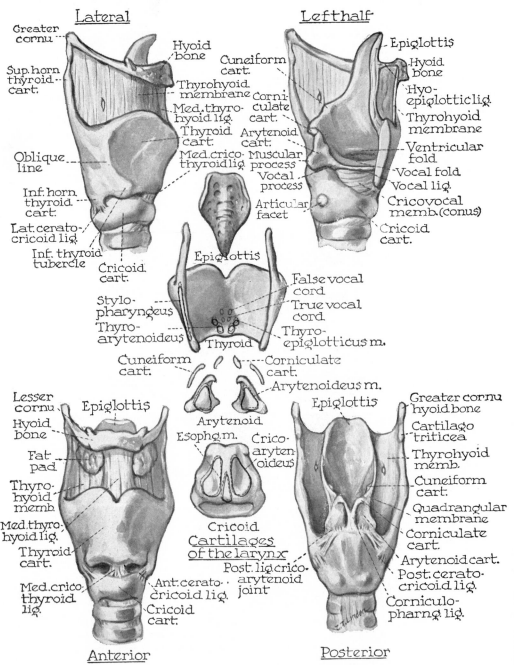

Lateral

Greater cornu
Sup. horn thyroid cart.
Oblique line
Inf. horn thyroid cart.
Lat. cerato-cricoid lig.
Inf. thyroid tubercle
Cricoid cart.

Hyoid bone
Thyrohyoid membrane
Med. thyro-hyoid lig.
Thyroid cart.
Med. crico-thyroid lig.

Cuneiform cart.
Corni-culate cart.
Arytenoid cart.
Muscular process
Vocal process
Articular facet

Left half

Epiglottis
Hyoid bone
Hyo-epiglottic lig.
Thyrohyoid membrane
Ventricular fold
Vocal fold
Vocal lig.
Cricovocal memb. (conus)
Cricoid cart.

Epiglottis

Stylo-pharyngeus
Thyro-arytenoideus
Cuneiform cart.

Thyroid

False vocal cord
True vocal cord
Thyro-epiglotticus m.
Corniculate cart.
Arytenoideus m.

Lesser cornu
Hyoid bone
Fat pad
Thyro-hyoid memb.
Med. thyro-hyoid lig.
Thyroid cart.
Med. crico-thyroid lig.

Epiglottis

Arytenoid
Esophg. m.
Crico-aryten-oideus

Cricoid
Cartilages of the larynx
Ant. cerato-cricoid lig.
Cricoid cart.
Post. lig. crico-arytenoid joint

Epiglottis

Greater cornu hyoid bone
Cartilago triticea
Thyrohyoid memb.
Cuneiform cart.
Quadrangular membrane
Corniculate cart.
Arytenoid cart.
Post. cerato-cricoid lig.
Corniculo-pharng lig.

Anterior   Posterior

FIG. 162. The larynx; 4 views and a disarticulated larynx are shown.

membrane of the mouth and the mylohyoid line. The *middle constrictor* originates from the stylohyoid ligament and the hyoid bone. The *inferior constrictor* arises from the oblique line of the thyroid cartilage and the fascia covering the cricothyroid muscle. They are inserted into a median raphe situated posteriorly, and all are supplied by the pharyngeal plexus through the accessory part of the spinal accessory nerve. The inferior constrictor receives 2 additional nerves: the external and the recurrent laryngeal branches of the vagus.

The *stylopharyngeus muscle* enters the wall of the pharynx between the superior and the middle constrictors (Fig. 157). It meets the *palatopharyngeus muscle* and is inserted with it into the posterior border of the thyroid cartilage. This is visible only after cutting the inferior constrictor muscle. The stylopharyngeus is supplied by the glossopharyngeal nerve, and the palatopharyngeus by the accessory nerve.

3. *The fibrous coat* has been called the pharyngobasilar fascia, the pharyngeal aponeurosis and also the submucous coat. It is strong in its upper part and takes the place of muscle tissue where the superior constrictor is absent. As it passes downward it gradually becomes weaker until it is finally lost as a distinct layer. It forms the principal attachment between the pharynx and the base of the skull.

4. *The mucous coat* consists of a columnar, ciliated epithelium in the nasopharynx and stratified squamous in the lower part.

The various structures pass in a definite arrangement between the constrictor muscles. Between the base of the skull and the superior constrictor are the tensor palati, the pharyngotympanic tube and the levator palati. Between the superior and the middle constrictors are the stylopharyngeus muscle and the glossopharyngeal nerve. Between the middle and the inferior constrictors are the internal laryngeal nerve and the superior laryngeal artery. Between the inferior constrictor and the esophagus are the recurrent laryngeal nerve and the inferior laryngeal artery (Fig. 161).

LARYNX

This upper and specialized portion of the windpipe (Fig. 162) extends from the epi-

glottis to the cricoid; it forms the organ of the voice. At birth it lies opposite the 3rd and the 4th cervical vertebrae but gradually descends until in the adult, it lies opposite the 3rd, the 4th, the 5th and the 6th cervical vertebrae. It is situated in the front and upper part of the neck, below the tongue and the hyoid bone, and between the great vessels of the neck. Above, it opens into the pharynx and below into the trachea. In the midline, it is covered by skin and cervical fascia but laterally is overlaid by the sternohyoid, the sternothyroid, the thyrohyoid and the origin of the inferior constrictor muscles. It consists of cartilages, ligaments and muscles and is lined by mucous membrane. Laterally, it is embraced by the lateral lobes of the thyroid gland, above which it is related to the carotid sheaths. Behind, it rests upon the pharynx which separates it from the body of the 3rd to the 6th cervical vertebrae. After puberty, the larynx is smaller in the female than in the male, the vocal cords in the former being about two thirds the length of the latter.

Cartilages of the Larynx. These are 9 in number (Fig. 162): the epiglottis, the thyroid, the cricoid, 2 arytenoids, 2 corniculates and 2 cuneiforms.

The *epiglottis* is a leaf-shaped lamina of yellow fibrocartilage covering the superior aperture of the larynx. It guards the entrance to the larynx and is situated behind the median thyrohyoid ligament, the hyoid bone and the back of the tongue. Its pointed lower end is attached firmly by the *thyroepiglottic ligament* to the posterior surface of the fused alae of the thyroid cartilage just below the thyroid notch. Its expanded upper end projects upward beyond the hyoid bone and presents a free border covered by mucous membrane both anteriorly and posteriorly. The anterior surface is connected to the dorsum of the tongue by a *median glossoepiglottic* and by *right and left pharyngoepiglottic folds*. The corresponding depression on each side of the median plane forms the *vallecula*. The floor of the vallecula lies immediately above and behind the hyoid bone. The posterior surface of the epiglottis lies in the anterior wall of the vestibule of the larynx.

The *thyroid cartilage* is the largest of the laryngeal cartilages, and its name is derived from the Greek which means "like a shield." It is formed by a pair of broad quadrilateral laminæ that are fused together in front but are widely separated behind. The fusion of these 2 laminae anteriorly in the midline of the neck has a more marked angulation in males and is known as the "pomum Adami" (laryngeal prominence or Adam's apple). The anterior borders of these laminae are united only in their lower halves, the upper halves being separated by a V-shaped *thyroid notch.* The laryngeal prominence and the thyroid notch can be felt easily subcutaneously and thus serve as valuable landmarks. The free and rounded posterior border projects upward as a superior horn and downward as an inferior horn. The superior horn is attached to the tip of the greater cornu of the hyoid bone by a lateral thickened border of the thyrohyoid membrane called the *lateral thyrohyoid ligament.* The inferior horn articulates at its extremity with the side of the cricoid cartilage. An important *oblique line* begins on the lateral surface of the cartilage in front of the root of the superior horn, extends downward and forward and ends behind the middle of the inferior border. This line gives insertion to the sternothyroid muscle and origin to the thyrohyoid muscle. The area in front of it is covered by the thyrohyoid, and the narrower posterior area gives origin to a part of the inferior constrictor muscle of the pharynx. The inferior border of this cartilage is in relation to the circumference of the cricoid cartilage to which it is attached by the cricothyroid membrane. As life progresses this cartilage begins to ossify and may become fractured.

The cricoid cartilage is shaped like a signet ring with the wide part posterior. It is a palpable landmark that indicates the beginning of the trachea and the level of the superior border of the esophagus. Its narrow anterior part, which is palpable through the skin, is called the *arch* and lies on a level with the 6th cervical vertebra. The posterior part, the *lamina,* is much deeper, projects upward and occupies the lower part of the gap between the 2 laminae of the thyroid cartilage. The arch is attached to the thyroid cartilage by the *cricothyroid membrane* and below is fixed to the first tracheal ring by an elastic membrane known as the *cricotracheal ligament.*

The two arytenoid cartilages appear as triangular pyramids, whose apices are directed upward and whose bases articulate with the upper aspect of the posterior portion of the cricoid. They help fill the gap between the 2 laminae of the thyroid cartilage. The posterolateral angle of the base is called the *muscular process* because it provides attachment to the cricoarytenoid muscles. The anterior angle of the base is prolonged forward as a spinelike process called the *vocal process* because the true vocal cords attach here. The 2 *corniculate cartilages* have been referred to as the cartilages of *Santorini.* They are small and conical and are attached to the apex of each arytenoid cartilage. They give attachment to the aryepiglottic folds. The 2 *cuneiform cartilages* have been referred to as the cartilages of *Wrisberg.* They are a pair of little rod-shaped cartilages that are placed in the aryepiglottic folds in front of the corniculate cartilages.

Membranes of the Larynx. The membranes that make up the chief connecting bands of the larynx are the thyrohyoid and the cricothyroid.

The *thyrohyoid membrane* connects the upper border of the thyroid cartilage to the upper part of the posterior surface of the hyoid bone, in this way suspending the larynx from the hyoid. The median portion of this membrane is thickened and is called the *median thyrohyoid ligament;* its cordlike right and left margins are referred to as the *lateral thyrohyoid ligaments.* The median thyrohyoid membrane is pierced by the internal laryngeal nerve and the superior laryngeal vessels on each side. The lateral thyrohyoid ligament passes from the superior horn of the thyroid to the tip of the greater cornu of the hyoid bone, where a small cartilaginous nodule, the cartilago triticea, is found.

The cricothyroid membrane occupies the interval between the cricoid and the thyroid cartilages and consists of a central and 2 lateral portions. The central portion connects the cricoid and the thyroid cartilages and presents a hole in the midline through which the cricothyroid artery sends a branch. This vessel is used as a landmark in laryngeal surgery. The lateral part of the membrane (conus elasticus) is attached below to the upper border of the cricoid cartilage but is free above except at its extremities. It is fixed in front in the angle between the thyroid laminae and behind to the vocal processes of the arytenoids. The free border of the cricothyroid membrane which results is covered by mucous membrane and forms the *true vocal cord*. The ventricular band that is covered by mucous membrane and forms the *false vocal cord* extends from the angle between the thyroid laminae to the anterolateral surface of the arytenoids. These lie above the true vocal cords.

Muscles. The muscles of the larynx are extrinsic and intrinsic.

The extrinsic muscles have been described elsewhere (p. 176); they act upon the voice box as a whole. They are the omohyoid, the sternohyoid, the sternothyroid, the thyro-

hyoid and certain suprahyoid muscles (stylopharyngeus, palatopharyngeus, inferior and middle constrictors of the pharynx).

The intrinsic muscles, on the other hand, confine themselves entirely to the larynx and act on its parts to modify the size of the laryngeal aperture (rima glottidis) and also control the degree of tension of the vocal ligaments. The principal intrinsic laryngeal muscles are the cricothyroid, the arytenoids (transverse and oblique), the posterior cricoarytenoids, the lateral cricoarytenoid and the thyroarytenoid. All of these, with the exception of the transverse arytenoid, are in pairs (Fig. 163).

The cricothyroid muscle is the only intrinsic muscle that lies on the exterior of the larynx. It arises from the lateral surface of

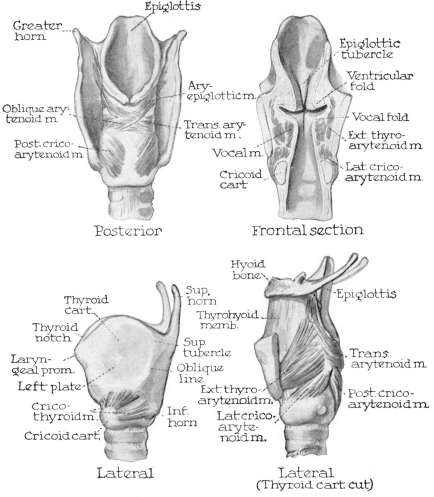

FIG. 163. The intrinsic muscles of the larynx; 4 views are shown.

the cricoid, runs upward and backward and is inserted into the inferior horn of the thyroid cartilage. It bridges the lateral portion of the cricothyroid interval. The cricothyroid muscles are the chief tensors of the vocal ligaments; this action is accomplished by pulling the arch of the cricoid upward around its articulation with the inferior horn of the thyroid cartilage, thus forcing the arytenoids backward and stretching the vocal cords (Fig. 164 B).

The posterior cricoarytenoid is probably the most important of the laryngeal muscles, since its action separates (abducts) the vocal cords, thus widening the rima glottidis. All the other muscles close the larynx by a more or less sphincteric (adduction) action. The cricoarytenoid arises from the back of the cricoid, runs upward and outward to the muscular process of the arytenoid where it inserts. By pulling backward on this process the vocal cords are separated (Fig. 164 A). Bilateral abductor paralysis of these muscles results in suffocation. When both recurrent laryngeal nerves are injured, bilateral abductor paralysis results, and the vocal cords become lax and cannot be abducted. At first this rarely results in dyspnea, but the loss of

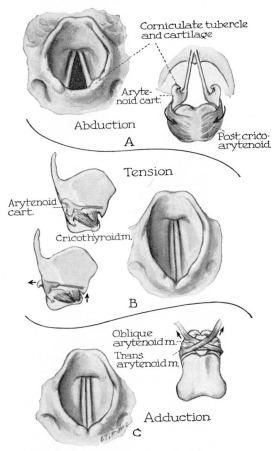

Fig. 164. The action of the intrinsic muscles of the larynx. (A) The action of the posterior cricoarytenoid muscles, separating the vocal cords. (B) By the contraction of the cricothyroid muscle, the vocal ligaments are tensed. (C) Adduction of the vocal cords is brought about by the contraction of the oblique and transverse arytenoid muscles.

voice is immediate. Within 3 to 5 months the voice begins to improve but, unfortunately, dyspnea also makes its appearance. This is the result of atrophy and fibrosis. Within a few weeks the voice becomes more improved, but as the vocal cords continue to fibrose and gradually approach each other the dyspnea becomes severe, especially on exertion. The laryngoscope will reveal the presence of a mere slit.

The transverse arytenoid is the only unpaired muscle of the larynx. It is a thin, flat, muscular band passing from the back of one arytenoid cartilage to the other. When it contracts, it draws the posterior parts of the arytenoids together, helping to close the laryngeal inlet during swallowing (Fig. 164 C).

The oblique arytenoid muscles are a pair of weak muscular slips that lie on the back of the transverse muscle and cross each other, forming a letter X. This muscle continues on as the aryepiglotticus in the aryepiglottic fold in which it reaches the epiglottis. Its action draws the arytenoids together and shortens the aryepiglottic fold. This approximates the arytenoids and the epiglottis. The muscle acts as a sphincter for the laryngeal inlet during swallowing (Fig. 164 C).

The lateral cricoarytenoid muscle arises from the upper aspect of the lateral part of the cricoid, runs upward and backward and is inserted into the muscular process of the arytenoid. These muscles are adductors of the vocal cords and reduce the width of the rima glottidis.

The thyroarytenoid is an upward continuation of the lateral cricoarytenoid. It arises from the deep surface of the thyroid lamina, passes backward and inserts into the anterolateral surface of the arytenoid cartilage. It pulls the arytenoid cartilage forward and slackens the vocal folds. The uppermost fibers of this muscle curve upward into the aryepiglottic fold, are called the thyroepiglottic muscles and join with the aryepiglottic muscles to insert in the edge of the epiglottis. Some of the deepest fibers of the thyroarytenoid form a muscle bundle, the *vocal muscle*; this cannot be separated from the rest of the muscle and actually is the inner

constant part that lies in the vocal lip lateral to the vocal ligament. It draws the vocal process forward, relaxing the vocal ligaments.

The action of the laryngeal muscles is threefold: (1) they open the glottis and permit breathing; (2) they close the glottis and the vestibule during swallowing; (3) they regulate the tension of the vocal cords. The first two actions are automatic and are controlled by the medulla, but the third is voluntary and is controlled by the cerebral cortex. The posterior cricoarytenoids are the only abductors. The lateral cricoarytenoids adduct the cords. The muscles that close the vestibule are the thyroarytenoid, the aryepiglottic and the thyroepiglottic. The muscles that effect the tension of the cords are the cricothyroid, the vocalis and the thyroarytenoid.

Nerves of the Larynx. The nerve supply is derived from the vagus nerve by way of its 2 branches, the superior and the inferior (recurrent) laryngeal, both of which are mixed nerves (Fig. 143).

After a short course, the *superior laryngeal nerve* divides into a thin external and a stouter internal branch.

The external laryngeal nerve is applied to the inferior constrictor muscle and passes deeply to the insertion of the sternothyroid. In its course it passes to and is accompanied by the superior thyroid artery; it sends a few twigs to the inferior constrictor, pierces it and ends by supplying the cricothyroid muscle. The *internal laryngeal nerve* is sensory and pierces the thyrohyoid membrane as several diverging branches. It crosses the anterior wall of the piriform recess and supplies sensory fibers to the larynx above the vocal cords. Nordland and other investigators believe that this nerve innervates the interarytenoid muscle in most cases. Division of the superior laryngeal nerves results in a loss of sensation to the laryngeal mucous membrane, making it difficult or impossible for the patient to perceive a foreign body in the larynx. There is also a weakening or paralysis of the cricothyroid, which produces a huskiness of the voice.

The inferior (recurrent) laryngeal nerve arises at different levels on the 2 sides. On the right it arises in the root of the neck and winds around the subclavian artery, but on the left it arises in the superior mediastinum and winds around the arch of the aorta. It ascends anterior to the tracheo-esophageal groove and can be felt on the lateral aspect of the trachea. It continues upward and becomes intralaryngeal by passing deep to the lower border of the inferior constrictor muscle. The point at which this nerve becomes intralaryngeal is on a level with the inferior horn of the thyroid cartilage.

Vascular Supply of the Larynx. This is derived from the superior laryngeal branch of the superior thyroid artery and the inferior laryngeal branch of the inferior thyroid artery.

Lymphatics. The lymphatics from the upper part end in glands in the carotid triangle, and from the lower part in the glands in front of and besides the larynx and the trachea.

Cavity of the Larynx. This may be divided into 3 compartments: vestibule (supraglottic), middle compartment (glottic area) and an infraglottic area. Some authors have likened the superior aperture of the larynx to a triangle, the base of which is at the

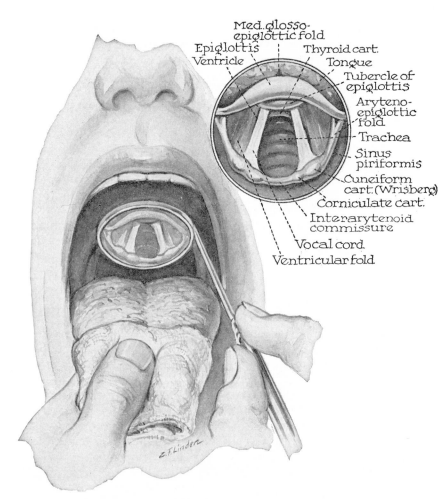

FIG. 165. The inlet of the larynx as seen through a laryngeal mirror. The inset shows the structures magnified and identified.

epiglottis, the sides formed by the aryteno-epiglottic folds, and the apex located at the arytenoid commissure posteriorly.

Inlet of the Larynx. The inlet, or upper aperture, faces almost directly backward so that it is set at right angles to the long axis of the laryngeal tube. It is bounded above by the free margin of the epiglottis, on either side by the aryepiglottic folds of mucous membrane which stretch from the epiglottis to the arytenoid cartilage, and below by the short interarytenoid fold of mucous membrane

(Fig. 165). Two small elevations are noted at the posterior extremity of the aryepiglottic fold. The most anterior protrudes to a higher plane and is the cuneiform cartilage (Wrisberg). The posterior, which is set on a slightly lower plane, is produced by the corniculate cartilage (Santorini), which is situated on the apex of the arytenoid cartilage. These 2 small elevations are easily visible on laryngoscopic examination. The anterior wall of the vestibule is longer than the posterior and is formed throughout by mucous membrane

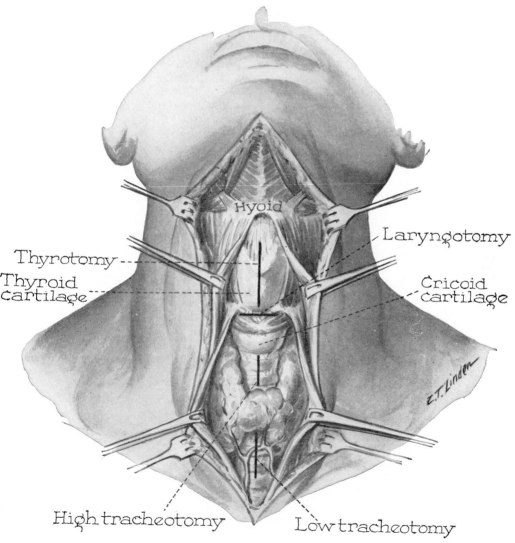

FIG. 166. Thyrotomy, laryngotomy and tracheotomy incisions.

which covers the posterior aspect of the epiglottis. Its central point is marked by a rounded elevation, the *tubercle* of the epiglottis, which is important because it is the most noticeable feature on laryngoscopic examination and is frequently the only structure that is visible in the hands of a novice. The aryepiglottic folds contain the aryepiglottic muscles between its two layers of mucous membrane. Posteriorly, the vestibule is bounded by the arytenoid cartilages and the interarytenoid fold containing the transverse arytenoid muscle. The aryepiglottic and transverse arytenoid muscles are of great importance because they close the inlet of the larynx during the act of swallowing. The *vestibular fold* of mucous membrane passes backward and laterally from the thyroid angle. It contains a small fibrous band, the vestibular ligament (false vocal cord), which stretches from the thyroid angle to the arytenoid cartilage. This fold narrows the lower end of the vestibule.

Glottis. The glottis, or middle compartment, is the narrowest part of the interior of the larynx; it measures nearly 1 inch anteroposteriorly in the adult male and about ¾ inch in the female. It consists of a small sinus, the ventricle or recess, and is situated between the vestibular and the vocal folds. The arytenoid cartilages are posterior and are separated by the interarytenoid notch. Approximately two thirds of the anterior part of the glottis consists of the true vocal cords, the posterior third consisting of the interval between the arytenoid cartilages. The mucosa uniting the 2 arytenoid cartilages forms the posterior or arytenoid commissure and is the usual site of tuberculosis of the larynx.

Vocal Cords. The true vocal cords diverge as they pass posteriorly and extend from the vocal process of the arytenoid to the thyroid angle. They appear as short straight folds that are characterized by the pallor of the covering mucous membrane. This pallor is produced by the absence of loose submucous tissue as well as the absence of blood vessels.

The rima glottidis (*glottic slit*) is that fissure which separates the true vocal cords and the arytenoid cartilages; it is triangular when at rest, linear during phonation and lozenge-shaped in respiration. The glottis is closed after inspiration, thus aiding fixation of the diaphragm during efforts of expulsion (parturition, defecation, urination and vomiting).

The infraglottic, or lowest compartment of the larynx, extends from the true vocal cords to the first tracheal ring. Its walls are made up of the thyroid and the cricoid cartilages and the cricothyroid membrane. In emergency laryngotomy this membrane is incised to gain entrance into the larynx.

SURGICAL CONSIDERATIONS

Thyrotomy (Laryngofissure) (Fig. 166). The incision extends from the hyoid bone above to the cricoid cartilage below; it is placed exactly in the midline and deepened until the isthmus of the thyroid gland is exposed. If necessary, this is divided. When the thyroid cartilage is visualized, a vertical incision is made in the midline through it and the thyrohyoid membrane. Through this incision tumors of the larynx can be removed and treated when removal of the entire larynx is unnecessary. At times this operation also has been used for the removal of foreign bodies that could not be dislodged by other means. The two segments of thyroid cartilage and membranes are sutured together. Some authorities permit the divided cartilage to fall together without suturing.

Laryngotomy has been used as an emergency procedure when the presence of a foreign body or edema necessitates the rapid admission of air into the larynx. It has also been used as a preliminary step in extensive operative procedures. A cyanosed and almost asphyxiated patient can be relieved immediately by this operation, in which a transverse incision is made across the midline of the neck at the level of the upper border of the cricoid cartilage. If the incision is kept close to the upper border, the cricothyroid artery will be avoided. Then it is deepened to and through the cricothyroid membrane, and a laryngotomy tube is inserted. It should be remembered that the cricothyroid space, in children, is so small that it is usually unsuitable for this operation. In extreme emergencies where death from asphyxia appears imminent, the blade of a pocket knife has been successfully plunged directly through the cricothyroid membrane and the opening kept patent by rotating the handle of the knife.

Tracheotomy (tracheostomy) may be an elective or emergency procedure. If elective, it is usually a preliminary step to laryngectomy for malignant disease. However, if it is done as an emergency operation it is utilized where there has been sudden obstruction of the airway as a result of aspiration of a foreign body, edema of the larynx, infections and edema about the throat, or postoperative vocal cord paralysis following injury to both recurrent nerves. Distinction has been made between low and high tracheotomy, the low being below the isthmus of the thyroid and the high above it. Most authorities are of the opinion that the low operation is preferable (Fig. 167). Here an

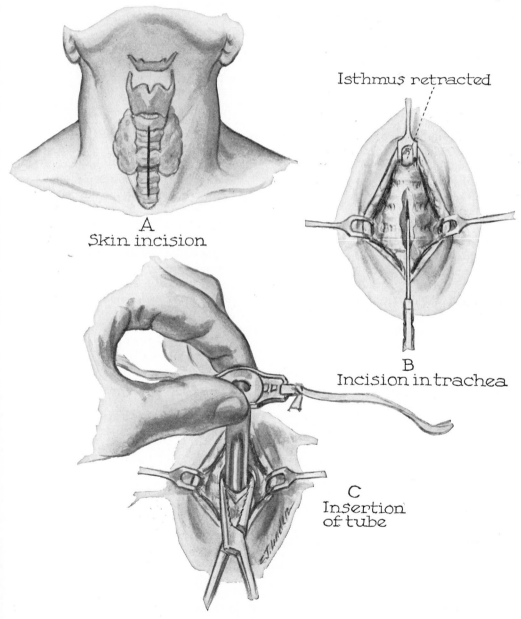

A
Skin incision

Isthmus retracted

B
Incision in trachea

C
Insertion of tube

FIG. 167. Tracheostomy.

incision is made extending from the lower border of the thyroid cartilage downward for about 3 inches in the midline of the neck. The skin and the subcutaneous tissues are divided, and the anterior jugular vein is either ligated or retracted. The sternohyoid muscles are separated in the midline and retracted laterally, exposing the isthmus of the thyroid gland. This in turn is either cut between hemostats or retracted upward, since a low tracheotomy is desirable. At this stage a sharp hook is usually placed beneath the cricoid cartilage in the midline to steady the trachea and pull it forward. Usually the 3rd, the 4th and the 5th tracheal rings are divided from above downward, the opening held open and a tracheotomy tube inserted.

POSTERIOR TRIANGLE

The posterior triangle of the neck is formed as a result of a longitudinal cleavage of what, in embryonic life, was a single muscle plate. This single muscle later becomes the sternocleidomastoid and the trapezius which have a continuous attachment above, extending from the inion to the tip of the mastoid. The attachment is aponeurotic and produces the roughened superior nuchal line. Below, and because of the cleavage, the attachments become disconnected so that the trapezius attaches to the lateral third of the clavicle and the sternocleidomastoid to the medial third.

The posterior triangle is bounded by the posterior border of the sternocleidomastoid muscle, below by the middle third of the clavicle and behind by the anterior border of the trapezius (Fig. 168); the apex of the triangle is the meeting point of the trapezius and the sternocleidomastoid, and when anterior and posterior borders fail to meet on this line, the area is occupied by part of the splenius capitis muscle. The inferior belly of the omohyoid muscle crosses the lower part of the posterior triangle, separating it into an upper, larger occipital triangle and a lower, smaller supraclavicular one. The roof of the posterior triangle is made up of the investing layer of the deep cervical fascia. The floor is muscular and is formed by the following three muscles from above downward: the splenius capitis, the levator scapulae and the scalenus medius. This muscular floor is carpeted by the prevertebral fascia (Fig. 168).

Relations. The triangle is related to the following structures from superficial to deep: skin, superficial fascia, platysma, external jugular vein, posterior border of the sternocleidomastoid muscle, four cutaneous nerves that pierce the investing fascia, the spinal accessory nerve, the posterior belly of the omohyoid muscle, the transverse cervical artery and vein, the transverse scapular artery and vein, the prevertebral fascia, the muscular floor and the nerves that lie upon it.

Skin. The skin of the posterior triangle of the neck is thicker over the upper and posterior part of the triangle than over the lower and anterior part. The *superficial fascia* is usually thin; fat in this region tends to accumulate under the deep fascia rather than superficially.

Platysma Muscle. This muscle lies in the superficial fascia of the side of the neck (Fig. 125). It arises from the deep fascia covering the pectoralis major and the deltoid muscles as low as the 2nd rib. Its fibers pass upward and medially and become inserted into the lower border of the mandible. Some of the upper fibers reach the face, decussate and mingle with the muscles of the lower lip. It can be seen from its course that the platysma leaves the middle line of the neck and the lower part of the anterior triangle uncovered. The nerve supply of the platysma is by way of the cervical branch of the facial nerve. If a skin incision is made along the sternocleidomastoid muscle and the skin and the superficial fascia are reflected carefully either backward or forward, the platysma appears as a very delicate sheet. There is a definite cleavage plane below it, which is filled by loose areolar tissue and in which the external jugular vein is found.

The external jugular vein travels subplatysmally. It varies greatly in size and is formed by the union of the posterior auricular with a branch of the posterior facial vein. It begins in or at the lower part of the parotid gland, passes vertically downward and across the sternocleidomastoid muscle. In the angle between the clavicle and the posterior border of the sternocleidomastoid it pierces the deep fascia and joins the subclavian vein. It receives the following branches: posterior jugular, anterior jugular, oblique jugular, transverse scapular and transverse cervical.

The posterior border of the sternocleidomastoid muscle should be noted because of the nerves in relation to it.

Four superficial nerves pierce the investing layer of deep cervical fascia which is not a strong layer and at times is difficult to display. They can be remembered easily if the landmarks are named from above downward: occiput, ear, neck and clavicle. Thus, there are the lesser occipital, the greater auricular, the anterior cutaneous and the supraclavicular nerves. They all appear from approximately the same point, namely, the posterior border of the middle of the sternocleidomastoid muscle.

The lesser occipital nerve passes upward and along the posterior border of the sternocleidomastoid muscle to reach and supply the skin of the lateral part of the occipital region.

The greater auricular nerve runs parallel with the external jugular vein and supplies the skin that covers the angle of the jaw, the parotid gland, the ear and the skin over the mastoid region.

The anterior cutaneous nerve of the neck appears close to the great auricular nerve and runs transversely forward across the sternocleidomastoid muscle; it divides into ascending and descending branches and supplies most of the skin of the side and the front of the neck. In its course across the sternocleidomastoid it lies either superficially or deeply to the external jugular vein.

The supraclavicular nerves arise a little below the preceding nerve as a single trunk that divides into 3 branches: lateral, intermediate and medial supraclavicular nerves which diverge from one another. The medial branch descends over the medial third of the clavicle and supplies the skin of the front of the chest down to the level of the sternal angle. The intermediate crosses the clavicle and descends on the thoracic wall as far as the 2nd rib. The lateral branch passes over the trapezius muscle and the acromion and innervates the skin on the upper and back parts of the shoulder region.

The spinal accessory nerve is the highest and most important structure in the triangle. It is placed very superficially, lying immediately beneath the investing layer of fascia. It appears at about the middle of the posterior border of the sternocleidomastoid muscle, running under this muscle. Here some small lymph glands surround it, and the lesser occipital nerve takes a recurrent course below it. Branches from the 3rd and the 4th cervical nerves run parallel with the accessory and may be mistaken for it. These cervical nerves also sink into the trapezius muscle and aid in its innervation. The fact that the accessory nerve is the highest structure in the triangle should avoid confusion.

The inferior (posterior) belly of the omohyoid muscle springs from the upper border of the scapula and the suprascapular ligament under cover of the trapezius muscle. It is located about 1 inch above the clavicle, passes upward and enters the posterior triangle at its lower and posterior angle. As it continues forward and slightly upward, it crosses the brachial plexus, continues to the sternocleidomastoid muscle, crosses the scalenus anticus and joins the tendon that connects it to the superior belly of the muscle. The tendon lies under cover of the sternocleidomastoid and on the internal jugular vein. The inferior belly, as it crosses the posterior triangle, lies superficial to the suprascapular nerve, the transverse cervical artery and the brachial plexus. The muscle can be felt through the skin and the fascia a little above the clavicle. Its movements may be seen in a thin person while he is talking. It lies between the investing and the prevertebral layers of the deep cervical fascia and is covered by a specially thickened part of the pretracheal layer. This thickened fascia binds the muscle to the posterior surface of the clavicle and to the 1st rib. In order to dislocate the inferior belly, its fascia should be incised along its upper border and the muscle pulled downward. The nerve supply to the omohyoid is through the ansa hypoglossi.

The transverse cervical artery lies under the omohyoid muscle (Fig. 171). It is a branch of the thyrocervical trunk, and as it passes backward it crosses the scalenus anticus and the phrenic nerve. In its course it

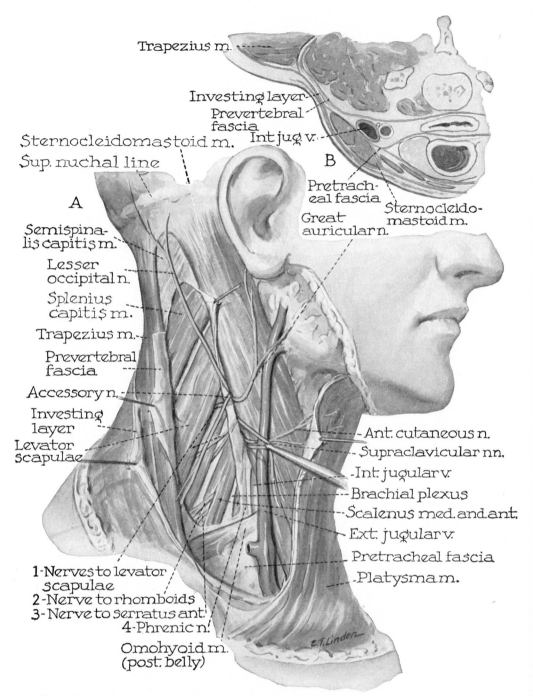

Trapezius m.

Investing layer
Prevertebral
fascia
Int. jug. v.

B

Sternocleidomastoid m.

Sup. nuchal line

A

Pretrach-
eal fascia
Great
auricular n.

Sternocleido-
mastoid m.

Semispina-
lis capitis m.

Lesser
occipital n.

Splenius
capitis m.

Trapezius m.

Prevertebral
fascia

Accessory n.

Investing
layer

Levator
scapulae

Ant. cutaneous n.

Supraclavicular nn.

Int. jugular v.

Brachial plexus

Scalenus med. and ant.

Ext. jugular v.

Pretracheal fascia

Platysma m.

1-Nerves to levator
scapulae
2-Nerve to rhomboids
3-Nerve to serratus ant.
4-Phrenic n.

Omohyoid m.
(post. belly)

E.T. Linden

Fig. 168. The posterior triangle. (A) The floor is trimuscular, being made up of the splenius capitis, the levator scapulae and the scalenus medius. The prevertebral fascia forms a carpet for this floor; the fascia has been incised and retracted in this figure. Four nerves pierce the investing fascia, and 4 nerves lie deep to it. (B) Cross section; the fascia is represented in blue.

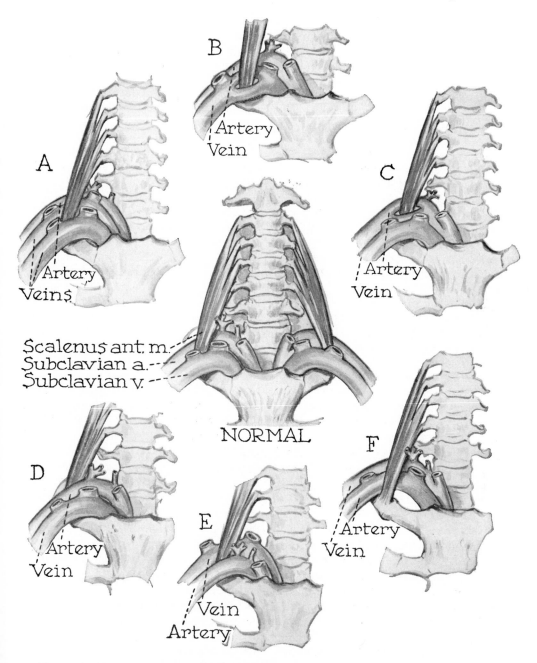

FIG. 169. Variations of the subclavian vessels in the region of the scalenus anterior muscle. E. B. Kaplan has described some of these variations herein depicted. The so-called normal arrangement is noted in the center of the illustration: (A) double subclavian vein arrangement; (B) the formation of a venous ring; (C) the formation of an arterial ring; (D) both the artery and vein pass in front of the muscle; (E) a reversed arrangement in which the vein is behind the muscle and the artery in front of it; (F) both the artery and the vein pass behind the muscle.

also crosses the brachial plexus and the suprascapular nerve. In the occipital triangle it divides into a superficial and a deep branch, the superficial supplying the deep surface of the trapezius muscle, and the deep branch accompanying the levator scapulae muscle to the scapula and taking part in the scapular anastomosis. Occasionally, the transverse cervical artery is small and spends itself in the trapezius; it then is referred to as the superficial cervical artery.

The transverse scapular or suprascapular artery is also found in the lowermost portion of the supraclavicular triangle, and it too is a branch of the thyrocervical trunk. It runs laterally and downward under cover of the sternocleidomastoid, across the scalenus anticus muscle and the phrenic nerve. It passes laterally behind the middle third of the clavicle and in front of the subclavian artery toward the posterior angle of the triangle. From this point on it accompanies the suprascapular nerve to the scapular. Behind the clavicle it is closely accompanied by one or two veins. The suprascapular and the transverse cervical veins run quite superficial to their arteries. Therefore, the arteries are accompanied not by their own veins but by slender venules as they cross the scalenus anticus muscle. The veins end in the external jugular. The suprascapular and the transverse cervical arteries clamp the phrenic nerve onto the scalenus anticus muscle.

The prevertebral fascia forms a carpet that covers the cervical part of the brachial plexus and the subclavian vessels and provides a fascial sheath for them as they enter the axilla. The carpet also covers 4 motor nerves: those to the levator scapulae, the rhomboids, the serratus anterior and the diaphragm. Since the spinal accessory is the highest nerve in the posterior triangle, one may dissect cephalad to it without much risk, since the only other structure in the region of the apex of the posterior triangle is the artery.

The floor of the triangle is muscular. The *levator scapulae muscle* occupies the most central position of the 3 muscles named. It arises from the posterior tubercles of the transverse processes of the upper 4 cervical

vertebrae and is inserted into the vertebral border of the scapula between the root of the spine and the superior angle.

Cephalad to the levator and parallel with it is the *splenius capitis muscle* which arises from the lower half of the ligamentum nuchae and the succeeding vertebral spines. It passes upward and laterally, forming the upper part of the floor, and is inserted into the mastoid process and the adjoining part of the occipital bone, under cover of the sternocleidomastoid muscle.

Caudad to the levator scapulae and parallel with it are the 3 scalenus muscles. The *scalenus medius* arises from the posterior tubercles of all the cervical transverse processes (2nd, 3rd, 4th, 5th and 6th) and is inserted into the upper part of the 1st rib between the groove for the subclavian artery and the neck of the rib. It is best not to consider the *scalenus posterior* as a separate muscle but as that portion of the scalenus medius that passes on to the 2nd rib and inserts there (Fig. 128). The *scalenus anterior* is separated from the medius and the posterior by the brachial plexus and the subclavian artery. It arises from the anterior tubercles of all the transverse processes (3rd, 4th, 5th and 6th). Its posterior border is parallel with and, therefore, hidden by the posterior border of the sternocleidomastoid muscle. It is not considered actually as part of the floor of the posterior triangle, since it is hidden from view. The scalenus anterior inserts into the scalene tubercle (Lisfranc), which is situated on the upper surface of the 1st rib.

Of the structures that lie between the accessory nerve and the omohyoid, the largest and most outstanding is the *brachial plexus*. Its upper part lies in the occipital triangle, but most of the plexus, as it passes through the neck, lies behind the inferior belly of the omohyoid and in the supraclavicular triangle. The formation of this plexus has been discussed on page 635. When the posterior border of the sternocleidomastoid is drawn forward, the nerves forming the plexus are seen emerging from between the scalenus anterior and the medius. This relationship is a useful landmark as it enables these 2 muscles to be identified. The supraclavicular nerve is quite thick and runs downward and backward immediately above the plexus. The nerve to the rhomboids is found a little higher; it pierces the substance of the scalenus medius muscle, runs downward and disappears under cover of the levator scapulae muscle to which it usually gives a branch. Its terminal branches supply the rhomboid muscle. If the upper part of the brachial plexus is pulled forward, the nerve to the serratus anterior commonly called the *long thoracic nerve* is seen. It arises from the back of the brachial plexus and disappears under cover of it. The nerve to the subclavius can be identified here.

PRACTICAL AND SURGICAL ASPECTS

Cervical Rib and Scalenus Syndrome. Adson and Coffey believe that tenotomy of the scalenus anticus muscle is preferable to the more radical resection of the cervical rib. The typical syndrome may occur when no cervical rib is present, and in the absence of such a rib, the condition is referred to as the *scalenus anticus syndrome* (Naffziger). Ochsner, Gage and DeBakey believe that the scalenus anticus syndrome is produced by spasms and contractions of the muscle. They have been able to relieve the symptoms temporarily by injecting the muscle with procaine. The symptoms of compression of the brachial plexus and the subclavian artery are usually pain, numbness, atrophy and circulatory changes (cyanosis, ulcers, gangrene).

A cervical rib attached to the transverse process and the body of the 7th cervical vertebra may vary from a simple bony bulge to a full and well-developed rib (Fig. 170 C). If such a projection is small, its outer extremity may be free and unattached, but if it is longer, it may be joined to the 1st thoracic rib by fibrous attachments.

The operative procedure that has given most success for both cervical rib and scalenus anticus syndrome is executed through an anterior approach that has been described by Adson (Fig. 170). An oblique incision is made about 5 cm. in length, extending upward and backward from the sternoclavicular articulation into the posterior triangle of the neck. The incision is deepened through the fat and the platysma; the tendon of the sternocleidomastoid muscle is exposed at its clavicular attachment and is divided between forceps, the muscular portion being reflected mesially. The tendon of the omohyoid is found and may be either retracted or severed. The scalenus anticus muscle is identified, as is the phrenic nerve which runs obliquely across it from lateral to medial; the nerve is retracted. The borders of the scalenus muscle are dissected free, and its tendinous and muscular fibers are divided close to its insertion. The subclavian artery should be lateral to the scalenus anticus and the pleura medial. As soon as the muscle has been divided, the subclavian artery can be dissected free and will drop forward. A cervical rib, if present, is examined, and if it is causing no pressure, further operative procedure is unnecessary. However, if the rib or its tendinous attachment to the first rib is producing posterior pressure on the brachial plexus, a portion of the rib and the tendon must be removed.

Brachial Plexus Lesions. Brachial plexus lesions are divided into those lesions that involve the entire plexus or only the upper, middle or lower portions of the plexus (p. 638). When the entire plexus is involved either from injury or pressure, the following features are noted: complete anesthesia of the lower part of the arm, the forearm and the hand; flaccid paralysis of the superior extremities with eventual wasting of the muscles.

Erb-Duchenne (upper arm) paralysis is the commonest type of nerve injury, occurring at birth and involving the *5th* and the *6th cervical nerves.* Upper-arm palsy usually results during the course of a complicated delivery with marked downward traction, resulting in a widening of the angle between the head and the shoulder. The injury usually occurs where the 5th and the 6th cervical nerves join to form the upper trunk of the plexus; this is known at Erb's point, which is the spot where 6 nerves meet: 5th cervical, 6th cervical root, anterior division of upper trunks, posterior division of upper trunks, suprascapular nerve and the nerve to the subclavius. The hand hangs at the side in internal rotation with the forearm pronated and the fingers and the wrist flexed. This is referred to by some as the "head-waiter's tip hand." External rotation and abduction are lost at the shoulder, as are flexion and supination of the forearm. Some authorities are of the opinion that when this lesion occurs later in life, there is some associated dulling of sensation over the lower part of the deltoid, the arm and the forearm. The clinical appearance is produced by a paralysis of the abductors and the lateral rota-

tors of the shoulder (deltoid, supraspinatus and infraspinatus) plus a paralysis of the flexors of the elbow (biceps, brachialis and brachioradialis); a weakness of the adductors and the medial rotators of the shoulders (pectoralis major, teres major, latissimus dorsi, subscapularis) also results. The pronator teres, the supinator, the flexors of the wrist and the thenar muscles may be slightly involved.

The *middle-arm type lesion* involves the 7th cervical nerve and produces a paralysis

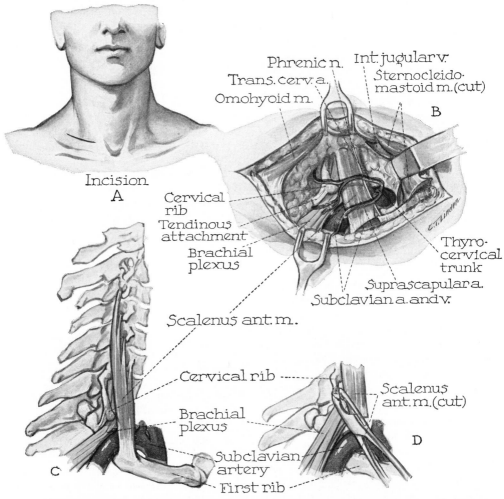

FIG. 170. Sectioning of the scalenus anticus muscle and the removal of a cervical rib: (A) incision; (B) exposure of the scalenus anticus muscle after cutting the clavicular attachment of the sternocleidomastoid muscle; (C) a cervical rib causing pressure on the brachial plexus; (D) removal of a cervical rib.

of the entire radial nerve except its branch to the brachioradialis; there is also a paralysis of the coracobrachialis.

Klumpke (lower-arm) paralysis is usually the result of upward traction on the shoulder. It may also be found in injuries or during breech presentations when the arms are placed over the head. The lesion involves the 8th cervical and the 1st thoracic nerve. It results in a paralysis of the intrinsic muscles of the hand and a paralysis of the flexors of the digits; a "claw" hand results. In addition there is diminished sensation over the medial side of the arm, the forearm and the hand.

Root of the Neck

The region referred to as the root of the neck is really the thoracocervical region that forms a boundary between the neck and the thorax and is occupied by structures that enter or leave the thoracic cavity.

(Fig. 171) The *right common carotid* and the *subclavian arteries* arise from the innominate immediately behind the right sternoclavicular joint which is made up of the sternal end of the first costal cartilage, the medial end of the clavicle and the clavicular notch of the manubrium sterni (p. 179). The joint and the scalenus anterior muscle are landmarks in this region. The *left common carotid* and the *subclavian arteries* arise directly from the aortic arch and after a course of about 1 inch pass into the neck behind the left sternoclavicular joint. On the right side the two infrahyoid muscles intervene between the arteries and the joint, but on the left side the left innominate vein intervenes. On both sides the common carotid is placed in front of the subclavian artery at the entrance to the neck and ends in the carotid triangle by dividing into the internal and the external carotids. It has no collateral branches.

Subclavian Artery. This artery courses through the neck and describes a gentle curve with the convex portion in an upward direction. The scalenus anterior muscle crosses the artery, dividing the vessels into 3 parts: the prescalenus (a part before), retroscalenus (a part behind) and postscalenus (a part after). Therefore, the artery not only occupies the root of the neck but the superior mediastinum as well and becomes the axillary artery at the lateral border of the first rib.

The *prescalenus portion* of the artery passes upward and laterally to the medial border of the scalenus anterior. Anteriorly, the following structures are encountered in a lateral direction: the common carotid artery, the ansa subclavia, the vagus nerve and the internal jugular vein, the latter being separated in part from the artery by the vertebral vein and on the left side by the phrenic nerve. Posteriorly, the artery is intimately related to the cervical dome of the pleura and the apex of the lung. The branches from this part of the vessel are the vertebral, the thyrocervical trunk and the internal mammary. Grant has described a "triangle of the vertebral artery" which has as its base the first part of the subclavian artery, its lateral side is the scalenus anterior, and its medial side the longus cervicis, the apex being made up of the anterior tubercle of the 6th cervical transverse process (Fig. 172). Anatomically, the triangle is seen best when the common carotid artery and the internal jugular vein are divided low. The posterior wall of the triangle, from above downward, is made up of the transverse process of the 7th cervical vertebra, the anterior ramus of the 8th cervical nerve, the neck of the 1st rib, and the cervical pleura which rises to the neck of the 1st rib. The triangle contains the vertebral artery, the vertebral vein which descends in front of the artery and crosses the subclavian artery, the inferior thyroid artery and the ganglionated sympathetic trunk.

The *retroscalenus portion* of the subclavian artery lies behind the scalenus anterior and its superimposed structures. Posteriorly, it is in contact with the cervical dome of the pleura and the apex of the lung. It is located in that triangular space that exists between the anterior and the middle scalene muscles, the base or floor of which corresponds to the 1st rib (Fig. 171 B). Above and lateral to it are the trunks of the brachial plexus; to see these relationships and this part of the artery it is necessary to cut the anterior scalene muscle transversely. Because of the presence

234

of the phrenic nerve, dissection of this muscle cannot be complete if the nerve is not protected properly.

The *costocervical trunk* arises from the posterior aspect of this part of the subclavian artery, passes backward above the pleura to the neck of the 1st rib where it divides into the superior intercostal and the deep cervical arteries (Fig. 171 A).

The *postscalene portion* of the subclavian artery extends from the lateral border of the scalenus anterior to the outer border of the 1st rib. Aneurysm of the subclavian, as a rule, involves this portion and appears as a swelling in the posterior triangle of the neck just above the clavicle. Because of the close proximity of the subclavian vein, an edema of the upper extremity may result. Ligation of

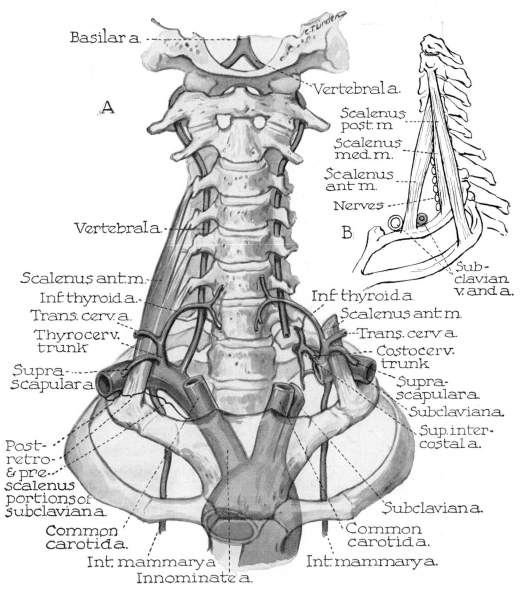

FIG. 171. The arteries in the root of the neck: (A) the subclavian artery is divided into 3 parts by the scalenus anticus muscle; (B) the subclavian artery and vein are separated by the scalenus anticus muscle (side view).

this artery should be carried out in its third part.

Subclavian Vein. This vein has only two parts that correspond to the second and the third parts of the artery; the beginning of the innominate vein substitutes for the first part. This is understandable if it is remembered that the internal jugular vein crosses the first part of the subclavian artery in order to make that union known as the innominate vein. The termination of the internal jugular then crosses and conceals the prescalenus portion of the subclavian artery; hence, no similar part of the subclavian vein exists; the subclavian is a continuation of the axillary vein. At the junction of the sternum with the clavicle the subclavian vein unites with the internal jugular to form the innominate. It begins at the outer border of the 1st rib, runs medially and almost transversely behind the clavicle, lying in front of the subclavian artery which it accompanies throughout its course with the exception of that point where the artery and the vein are separated by the anterior scalene muscle. The vertebral and the internal mammary veins pass directly into it, there being no thyrocervical or costocervical venous trunks. The inferior thyroid veins drain into the innominate vein; the transverse cervical and suprascapular veins open into the external jugular vein. The deep cervical, the ascending cervical and the vein from the

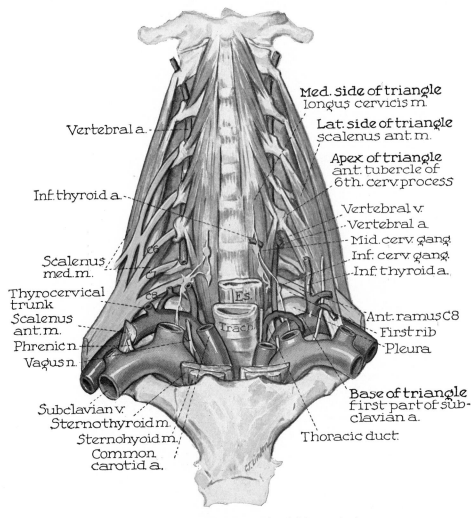

Fig. 172. The vertebral triangle and its contents.

first intercostal space drain into the vertebral before it crosses the subclavian artery to end in the innominate vein. The variations of the subclavian vessels have been described on page 229.

The right innominate vein lies deeply to the inner end of the right clavicle from which it is separated by the sternohyoid and the sternothyroid muscles. It is related to the medial surface of the right pleura and partly overlies the innominate artery. It passes vertically downward into the superior vena cava.

The left innominate vein passes downward behind the upper part of the manubrium to the lower margin of the first right costal cartilage where it ends in the superior vena cava. It is covered in front by the left sternoclavicular joint and on the right is overlapped by the right pleura. Remnants of the thymus intervene between it and the sternum. The vein is on the level of or at times slightly above the upper margin of the manubrium and is endangered in removal of tumors at the root of the neck or in low tracheotomy.

Scalenovertebral Angle. This angle takes the form of an inverted V, is bounded laterally by the scalenus anterior muscle and medially by the longus cervicis (colli) muscle. These two muscles meet at the carotid tubercle (Chassaignac's), which is the well developed anterior tubercle of the transverse process of the 6th cervical vertebra and forms the apex of the triangle (Fig. 172). The roof is formed by the sternocleidomastoid muscle.

The lower part of this angle is crossed by

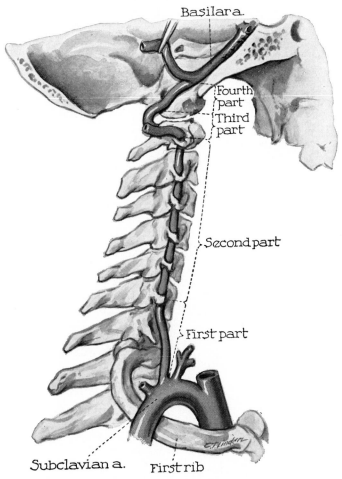

Basilar a.

Fourth part

Third part

Second part

First part

Subclavian a.   First rib

FIG. 173. The vertebral artery; the artery is divided into 4 parts.

the *subclavian artery,* which disappears behind the scalenus anterior muscle but, before disappearing, it gives rise to two large branches from its upper border: the vertebral artery and the thyrocervical trunk. As these two vessels ascend they fill the gap in the scalenovertebral angle.

Vertebral Artery. This is the first and largest branch of the subclavian (Fig. 173). It is divided into 4 parts: the first part passes upward and backward between the scalenus anterior and the longus cervicis muscles and through the foramen in the transverse process of the 6th cervical vertebra; it is surrounded by a plexus of sympathetic nerve fibers and is covered by the vertebral and the internal jugular veins. The second part ascends through the foramina in the transverse processes of the upper 6 cervical vertebrae. The third part emerges from the foramen transversarium of the atlas and passes almost horizontally backward and medially behind the lateral mass of the atlas. The fourth part pierces the spinal dura mater and travels upward into the cranial cavity through the foramen magnum, joining the internal carotid artery to form the circle of Willis.

The vertebral vein descends in front of the artery and may hide it. As it descends, it deviates to the lateral side of the artery and crosses in front of the first part of the subclavian artery; it ends in the posterior aspect of the innominate vein near its origin.

The thyrocervical trunk also arises from the upper part of the subclavian artery at the medial border of the scalenus anterior muscle and at once breaks up into 3 branches: the suprascapular, the transverse cervical and the inferior thyroid arteries. Only the inferior thyroid occupies the scalenovertebral angle. It reaches the level of the 6th cervical transverse process, turns medially and downward and terminates at the posterior border of the lobe of the thyroid gland. The course of this vessel resembles an inverted U. As the artery curves medially it passes over the vertebral vessels and below the carotid system.

The thoracic duct occupies the left side of the scalenovertebral angle. Its course is similar to that of the inferior thyroid artery, but it loops in the reverse direction and at a lower level than does the vessel. In the neck the duct forms an arch that reaches as high as the 7th cervical vertebra, arching behind the carotid system (internal jugular vein, vagus nerve and common carotid artery), and in front of the vertebral system (vertebral vessels). As it passes to the left it also crosses the scalenus anterior muscle and the phrenic nerve. Continuing its course, it crosses the transverse cervical and transverse scapular arteries and usually ends as a single vessel entering the junction of the subclavian and the left internal jugular veins. The duct sometimes divides, one vessel entering the vein on the right and the other entering on the left side.

Bony Thorax

The thorax is shaped like a truncated cone, which is flattened from before backward and contains important organs of respiration, circulation and digestion. Its anterior wall is the shortest and is formed by the sternum and the anterior portions of the first 10 pairs of ribs, with their corresponding costal cartilages. The lateral walls are formed by the ribs, which slope obliquely downward and forward; the posterior wall is made up of the 12 thoracic vertebrae and the ribs as far as their angles (Figs. 174, 175).

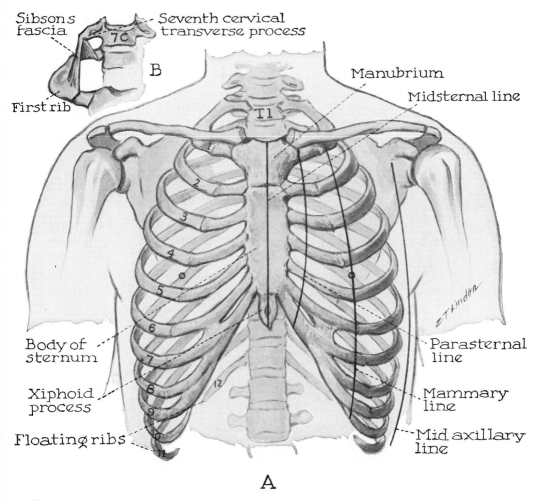

FIG. 174. The bony thorax. (A) Anterior view, with the conventional longitudinal lines shown. (B) Sibson's fascia, which forms the diaphragm for the superior aperture.

239

At birth and about 2 years thereafter the thorax is circular and does not resemble the oval-shaped adult thorax (Fig. 176). Because of this difference, the adult thorax may be increased in thoracic breathing, but this is impossible in the child, since the circumference remains constant in the latter. For this reason, breathing in the first 2 years of life is almost entirely abdominal (diaphragmatic), but as the individual grows older, breathing becomes intercostal (thoracic). Because children's breathing is not thoracic, they are supposed to be more susceptible to postoperative pneumonia. The child restricts his abdominal movements because of pain, thereby interfering with excursions of the diaphragm; this results in poorly aerated lungs, which become filled with accumulated secretions. The child's thorax may be referred to as the "normal" barrel chest of early life. The thorax has a small kidney-shaped superior aperture and a large irregular inferior one.

Superior Aperture. This is the inlet and measures approximately 2 by 4 inches (Fig. 176). It slopes from behind downward and forward. Its boundaries are formed by the body of the first thoracic vertebra, the first ribs, the first cartilages and the upper border of the manubrium sterni. It is kidney-shaped, the first thoracic vertebra representing the hilum. Because of the downward slope of this aperture, the anterior part of the apex of the lung rises above the anterior boundary of the inlet, but its posterior part rises only to the level of the neck of the 1st rib. The diaphragm of the aperture is fascial and is called *Sibson's fascia* (Fig. 174 B). It is pyramidal-shaped and extends from the transverse process of the 7th cervical vertebra to the inner border of the 1st rib and in this way protects the cervical dome of the pleura, which is closely associated with its undersurface. The scalene muscles replace intercostal muscles in this area and are lined internally by Sibson's fascia.

Inferior Aperture. This is the outlet of the thorax. It is large and irregular and bounded by the 12th thoracic vertebra, the lowest ribs, the 7th to the 12th costal cartilages and the xiphisternal joint. It is much wider than the inlet and is occupied by the diaphragm.

Certain **conventional longitudinal** lines are used for the purpose of description and orientation. They run parallel with the long axis of the body and are (Fig. 174):

1. *Midsternal line*—bisects the sternum

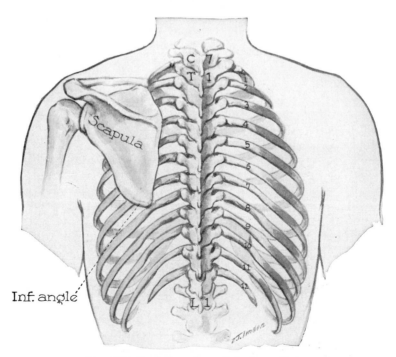

FIG. 175. Posterior view of the bony thorax.

and corresponds to the midline of the back.

2. *Mammary line*—this is dropped from the inner aspect of the clavicle and usually passes through the nipple.

3. *Parasternal line*—lies midway between the midsternal and the mammary lines.

4. *Anterior axillary line*—this runs through the anterior axillary fold.

5. *Posterior axillary line*—passes through the posterior axillary fold.

6. *Midaxillary line*—this is dropped from the middle of the axillary space.

7. *Scapular line*—this runs through the apex of the inferior angle of the scapula.

8. *Paravertebral line*—opposite the tips of the transverse processes of the vertebrae (used in radiology).

RIBS (COSTAE)

The 12 pairs of ribs form a series of obliquely placed bony arches which constitute the greater part of the wall of the thoracic cage. They overhang the upper part of the abdomen, articulate with vertebrae posteriorly and end in costal cartilages anteriorly. They increase in length from the 1st to the 7th and then become progressively shorter.

True Ribs. The first 7 pairs are called true ribs because their cartilages articulate with the sternum.

False Ribs. The cartilages of the last 5 pairs are known as false ribs.

Floating Ribs. The 8th, the 9th and the 10th pairs end by turning upward to join the costal cartilage above, but the 11th and the 12th are free at their extremities and are known as floating ribs.

All the ribs can be felt through the overlying soft structures, with the exception of the 1st, which is hidden by the clavicle, and occasionally the 12th. The 1st rib may be absent or very short. The 2nd rib always can be identified where its cartilage reaches the sternum at the sternal angle. Therefore, when it is necessary to locate a given rib, the 2nd should be found, and the succeeding ribs should be counted from above downward, following a line about 1 inch from the sternum which passes downward and slightly laterally. The ribs vary in length, the longest (7th or 8th) being two or three times as long as the shortest (1st or 12th). The typical ribs are the 3rd to the 9th inclusive, but the 1st, the 2nd, the 10th, the 11th and the 12th have special characteristics.

The so-called typical rib (Fig. 177) articulates with 2 vertebrae, namely, the vertebra to which it corresponds numerically, and the vertebra above this. It has a head, a neck, a tubercle and a shaft; the last-named structure has an angle posteriorly and a costal groove inferiorly. The *head* presents a kidney-shaped articular surface which is divided into two facets by a transverse crest. These facets articulate with the contiguous facets on the lateral aspect of the bodies of the 2 adjacent vertebrae. From the intervening crest or ridge, an interarticular ligament passes to the intervertebral disk. The *neck* is constricted and is about 1 inch long; its upper border is raised into a *crest*. The *tubercle* is located on the back of the junction of the neck and the shaft; below, it reveals a smooth round facet for articulation

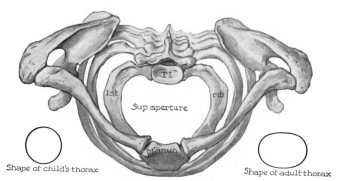

FIG. 176. The bony thorax as viewed from above. The small insets show the transverse section of a child's thorax as compared with that of an adult.

with the corresponding transverse process, and above and behind this is a rough area for the lateral costotransverse ligament. The *shaft* is compressed laterally, giving it internal and external surfaces, which are separated by superior and inferior borders. It not only has a curved but also a twisted appearance. The curvature is greatest posteriorly, and its maximum point is known as the *angle,* which is marked by a ridge on its external surface, the latter being smooth and covered with muscles. The internal surface is also smooth but is covered with pleura; the superior border is rounded, and the inferior border is grooved. The costal groove contains the intercostal vessels and nerves, which are protected by its sharp overhanging outer margin. The *anterior (sternal) extremity* of the shaft is oval in shape and concave for the reception of the costal cartilage.

Special Ribs. This group includes the 1st, the 2nd, the 10th, the 11th and the 12th; they are so-called because they possess special features by which they may be identified.

The *1st rib* has been called the "superlative" rib because it is the highest, broadest, strongest, flattest, most curved and, with the occasional exception of the 12th, the shortest of all the ribs (Fig. 178). Its angle coincides with its tubercle. It is placed almost horizontally so that its surfaces face upward and downward, and it articulates with only one vertebra. The head is small and has only one facet, which articulates with the body of the 1st thoracic vertebra; the neck is relatively long. The tubercle is fairly large and artic-

ulates with the 1st thoracic transverse process. The lower surface of this rib is smooth and devoid of any important landmarks, but the upper surface presents several important features. A roughened area is present for the insertion of the scalenus medius and the origin of the first digitation of the serratus anterior. The front of this rib is crossed by a wide shallow groove, which lodges the subclavian artery. Along the inner border and anteriorly, this arterial groove is limited by the scalene tubercle (*Lisfranc*) where the scalenus anterior muscle inserts. The size of the tubercle varies, in some cases forming a prominent point while in others it is barely recognizable. Anterior to this, a shallow groove is noted, which lodges the subclavian vein. The rib does not contain a costal groove; its lower smooth surface is covered with pleura, and its sternal end is enlarged to receive the lateral extremity of the first costal cartilage.

The *2nd rib* is intermediate in size and shape; it lies between the 1st and the lower ribs; although sharply curved, it is not twisted (Fig. 178). Its angle is just lateral to its tubercle, and its surfaces are oblique. This rib has a poorly marked costal groove and a rough elevation near the middle of its outer surface where the lower part of the first digitation and the whole of the second digitation of the serratus anterior attach. The scalenus posterior is attached behind this point.

The *10th rib* resembles a typical rib but is shorter, and its head usually presents only one facet for the body of the 10th thoracic

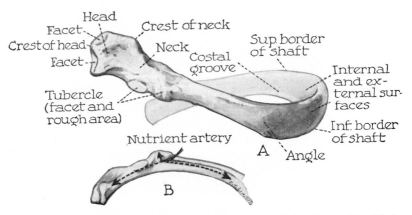

Fig. 177. A typical rib: (A) the individual parts of the rib are identified; (B) the nutrient artery enters just beyond the tubercle.

vertebra. It is the "uncertain" rib, since it may articulate with the 9th cartilage, which may be connected to it by a ligament or may remain free as a floating rib.

The *11th rib* is short and has only a single facet on its head for the 11th thoracic vertebra; it does not have a neck or tubercle, and its costal groove is difficult to see.

The *12th rib* is very short and has only one facet on its head; it lacks a tubercle, an angle and a costal groove. It should be noted that the inner surfaces of both the 11th and the 4th ribs look upward as well as inward.

The blood supply reaches each rib through its own nutrient vessel which enters just beyond the tubercle and runs forward as far as the inner extremity of the bone (Fig. 177 B). An additional supply is obtained from the periosteal vessels. The periosteum of the ribs strips easily from the bone, but that of the sternum does not. H. A. Harris has pointed out that no anastomosis occurs between the vessels of the diaphysis and the epiphysis of the ribs and that the vessels of the former are virtually "end arteries."

Ossification resembles the long bones of the limbs and the bodies of the vertebrae, since it begins to take place in the 2nd fetal month. The process begins near the angle and continues in both directions but fails to reach the sternal end, resulting in costal cartilages.

The ribs, the vertebrae, the sternum and the diploë of the skull are filled with the red blood-forming marrow. It is in these bones and not in the limbs that the blood elements are formed after puberty.

The costal cartilages continue the costal arches in front of the anterior extremities of the ribs. The first 7 cartilages are continued forward and articulate with the sternum. The 8th, the 9th and the 10th anterior extremities end by joining with the costal cartilage above. These form a continuous cartilaginous ridge, known as the *subcostal margin,* which forms a part of the inferior aperture of the thorax. The cartilages increase in length from the 1st to the 7th, and below this point they diminish. When traced downward, the intervals between the cartilages diminish.

STERNUM (BREAST BONE)

The sternum (Fig. 179) is an elongated flat bone which is situated in the midventral line of the thorax and forms the anterior boundary of the thoracic cavity. It is shaped much like an old Roman sword, having a short handle called the *manubrium,* a longer blade called the *body* and a small piece of cartilage at its lower end known as the *xiphoid (ensiform) process.* In early fetal life the sternum is represented by right and left cartilaginous plates with which the rib cartilages articulate (Fig. 179 D). Later, these two plates fuse, but this may be incomplete, resulting in a foramen. Although the

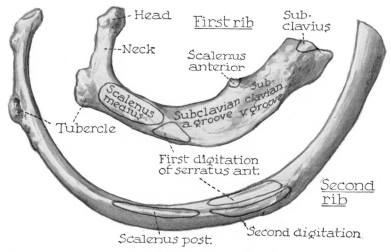

FIG. 178. The 1st and the 2nd ribs as seen from above; the muscular attachments have been identified.

bone becomes ossified in late fetal life, the constituent parts of the body do not begin to fuse until puberty. During its early development it consists of 6 segments (sternebrae), but in the adult the 4 middle sternebrae become fused, resulting in the 3 mature sternal parts named above.

The manubrium is irregularly quadrilateral in shape and is the broadest and most massive part of the bone. Its anterior surface

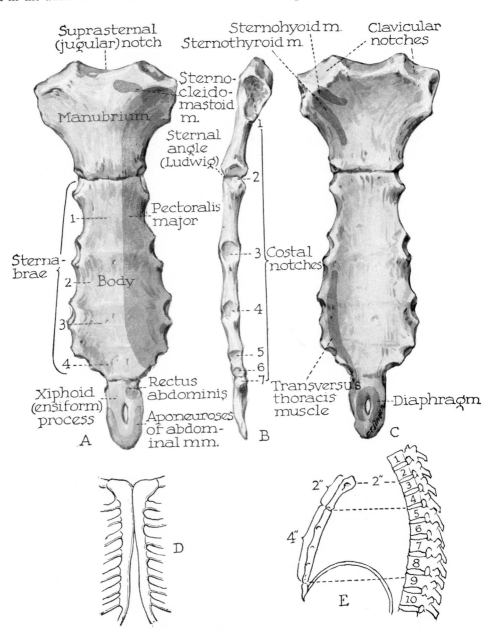

FIG. 179. The sternum. Muscular origins have been colored red, and insertions blue. (A) Front view; the 4 sternebrae and the articulating facets are shown. (B) Side view. The formation of the sternal angle is seen best from this view. (C) Posterior view. This surface is smooth and is related to the pericardium and the pleurae. (D) The 2 embryonic cartilaginous plates from which the sternum is formed. (E) Side view to show the thoracic levels of the jugular notch, the manubriosternal joint and the xiphoid process.

is rough, but the posterior is smooth. The upper border presents 3 notches, 2 of which are called *clavicular notches* which articulate with the clavicles, and a centrally placed *suprasternal (jugular) notch*. The latter can be felt easily through the skin and lies on the same horizontal plane as the disk between the 2nd and the 3rd thoracic vertebrae. At times, the left innominate vein and the "right" innominate artery barely reach above this notch. The manubrium, which is about 2 inches long, lies about 2 inches in front of the second thoracic vertebra (Fig. 179 E).

The body of the sternum is about 4 inches long and is made up of 4 sternebrae. In the adult, lines can be noted which mark the sites of fusion of the sternebrae as they cross the anterior surface of the body, between angular depressions on the sides. The lateral borders show a series of facets for the anterior extremities of the costal cartilages. They are arranged in the following manner: a small facet above, with which a similar facet of the manubrium forms a cavity for the anterior extremity of the 2nd costal cartilage; a facet opposite the extremity of the first transverse ridge for the 3rd costal cartilage, which is formed partly by the first and partly by the second piece; a facet opposite the second ridge, partly on the second segment and partly on the 3rd, for the 4th costal cartilage; a facet for the 5th costal cartilage, partly on the third and partly on the 4th segment, opposite the 3rd transverse ridge and a facet at the side of the 4th segment for the 6th costal cartilage. At the lowest part of the lateral border, a small facet is noted which is completed by a similar one on the xiphoid for the 7th costal cartilage.

The sternal angle (angle of Louis or Ludwig) is that slight angle which is formed where the body and the manubrium meet (Fig. 179 B). It is easily palpated beneath the skin and forms a most important landmark, since it lies over a number of important structures inside the thorax; its surface marks the place of attachment of the 2nd costal cartilage. It forms a convenient starting point to determine the number of a given rib and is on the same horizontal plane as the disk between the 4th and the 5th thoracic vertebrae. The sternomanubrial joint is important in the mechanism of respiration,

since it allows the body of the sternum to move forward and backward like a door, while the manubrium remains stationary.

The medial attachments of the pectorales majores converge from the sternoclavicular joints in front of the manubrium to meet in the midline at the sternal angle; they then pass downward together along the middle of the body and diverge at the level of the 6th costal cartilage. The posterior surface is smooth and related to the pericardium and the pleurae.

Xiphoid (Ensiform) Process. This is the smallest of the 3 sternal divisions and is variable in its appearance; it may be depressed or bent; and sometimes it has a bifid extremity or even may exhibit a perforation. It articulates with the body of the sternum above, but below it ends in a pointed extremity to which the linea alba attaches. Its upper border is at the level of the body of the 9th thoracic vertebra. At birth, the xiphoid (ensiform) process is made up of cartilage but usually becomes incompletely ossified in the adult. Its posterior surface gives attachment to the short anterior fibers of the diaphragm.

MUSCLES WHICH ATTACH TO THE STERNUM

1. *Pectoralis major*—to the marginal area of the anterior surface of the manubrium and the body.

2. *Sternocleidomastoid*—to the anterior surface of the manubrium.

3. *Sternohyoid*—to the posterior surface of the manubrium.

4. *Sternothyroid*—to the posterior surface of the manubrium on a slightly lower level than the forementioned muscle.

5. *Transversus thoracis*—to the posterior surface of the last segment of the body of the xiphoid.

6. *Diaphragm*—to the posterior surface of the xiphoid.

7. *Aponeuroses of the external oblique, the internal oblique and the transversus muscles*—to the lateral border of the xiphoid.

8. *Rectus abdominis*—to the anterior surface of the xiphoid.

Fractures of the sternum are rare, but when present they occur most frequently at the junction of the manubrium with the body; at this point the bone is thinnest. The ligamentous attachments usually protect underlying structures, but at times the upper fragment may pass behind the lower and compress the trachea or injure the aorta.

STERNOCLAVICULAR JOINT

The line of the sternoclavicular joint (Fig. 180) passes from above downward and laterally. The articular surface of the clavicle is larger than the sternal facet; therefore, it comes in contact below with the 1st costal cartilage. In this way the sternal end of the 1st cartilage takes part in the articulation, in addition to the medial end of the clavicle and the clavicular notch of the manubrium sterni.

The joint is surrounded by a rather loose *capsular ligament,* which is lined with synovial membrane and is attached to the margins of the articular surfaces. This ligament is strengthened behind and in front by the *anterior* and the *posterior sternoclavicular ligaments,* whose fibers pass downward and medially from the clavicle to the manubrium and the 1st cartilage.

The *interclavicular ligament* stretches from clavicle to clavicle, across the upper surface of the capsule, and dips in the center to become attached to the floor of the suprasternal (jugular) notch. It is a thickened ligamentous band which is believed to be homologous with the wishbone of the bird.

The *costoclavicular ligament* extends upward, backward and laterally from the 1st costal cartilage to an impression on the lower surface of the sternal end of the clavicle. It forms an important accessory ligament of the joint and helps to limit clavicular movements.

The joint is divided into a medial (inferior) and a lateral (superior) compartment by an articular disk, which is attached to the clavicle in front and behind. This fibrocartilaginous disk, in addition to acting as a buffer which diminishes the shock of blows on the point of the shoulder, also assists in the limitation of movement of the joint and prevents a medial displacement of the clavicle. Synovial membrane lines the two compartments of the joint, and if the articular disk is perforated, the two become continuous.

ARTICULAR RELATIONS

The joint may feel subcutaneous, but in reality it is crossed by the tendon of the sternal head of the sternocleidomastoid muscle. The sternohyoid and the sternothyroid muscles separate it from the great vessels and the vagus nerve. Many large vessels occupy the position behind the joint, because of its great obliquity and the extent of its articulating surfaces. Therefore, on both sides, the internal jugular and the subclavian veins unite to form the innominate vein, directly behind the joint. On the right side the innominate artery divides into the right common carotid and the subclavian, and on the left side the left common carotid and the

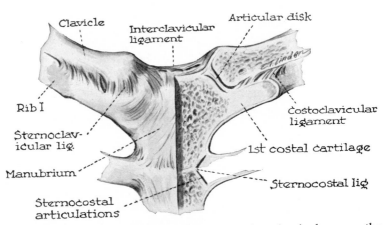

Fig. 180. The sternoclavicular joint. A coronal section is shown on the left half of the illustration. A sternocostal joint is also shown.

left subclavian arteries ascend. On both sides the vagus nerve descends between the veins and the arteries (Fig. 171).

MOVEMENTS

The movements of the sternal ends of the clavicle are always accompanied by movements of the acromial end of that bone, but in the opposite direction. Therefore, when the shoulders are pulled backward, the sternal ends of the clavicle are pushed forward; when the point of the shoulder is depressed, the sternal ends of the clavicle are tilted upward. The movements are associated with those at the acromioclavicular joint. When the shoulder is elevated or depressed the clavicle moves on the articular disk. Elevation of the shoulder is limited by tension of the costoclavicular ligament, and depression by the articular disk and the interclavicular ligament.

In a dislocation involving the joint, the force is usually directed along the long axis of the clavicle so that the sternal end passes forward, tearing the anterior sternoclavicular ligament. The clavicle passes upward and comes to lie in the suprasternal notch, between the sternocleidomastoid in front and the sternohyoid and the sternothyroid behind. If such a dislocation is complete, the costoclavicular ligament is ruptured; then it is difficult to obtain reduction, because of the obliquity of the articular surfaces. Backward dislocation is rare, but if this does occur, the posterior sternoclavicular ligament is torn, and the clavicle compresses the innominate vein, the trachea and, on the left side, the esophagus as well.

STERNOCOSTAL JOINTS

These joints are 7 in number and connect the superior 7 pairs of costal cartilages to the lateral margins of the sternum. Each is enclosed and reinforced by broad anterior and posterior sternocostal ligaments (Fig. 180). The medial supraclavicular nerves (C3, C4) supply the joint, and branches from the internal mammary and the clavicular branch of the thoraco-acromial artery anastomose around it.

INTERCOSTAL SPACES

MUSCLES

The muscles which are associated with the intercostal spaces are the external intercostal, the internal intercostal and the transversus thoracis. Corresponding intercostal nerves and vessels supply them (Figs. 181, 182).

The external intercostal muscle fibers are the thoracic representative of the external abdominal oblique. They pass downward and forward between adjacent borders of 2 ribs and become membranous in the intercartilaginous portion of the space where they assume the name of the *anterior intercostal membrane.* The fleshy interosseous parts extend as far as the tubercles of the rib posteriorly.

The internal intercostal muscle is the thoracic representative of the internal abdominal oblique. These fibers run in the opposite direction to those of the external. The fleshy fibers extend from the sternal ends of the spaces as far as the angles of the ribs posteriorly; here they become membranous and continue as the *posterior intercostal membrane,* which merges with the anterior costotransverse ligaments.

The transversus thoracis muscle is the thoracic representative of the transversus abdominis and should be considered as having 3 parts: the sternocostalis, the innermost intercostal and the subcostal. The *sternocostalis* part has also been referred to as the transversus thoracis and the triangularis sterni; it is the most constant part of the muscle and is located on the back of the anterior wall of the thorax. It arises from the back of the xiphoid and the body of the sternum as high as the 3rd costal cartilage and inserts into the costochondral junction from the 2nd to the 6th rib. Its lowest fibers are horizontal and continuous with the uppermost part of the transversus abdominis muscle. The muscle has three important features: it fails to cross the first two intercostal spaces; the internal mammary vessels descend in front of it; the pleura is immediately behind it. These relations are important during ligation of the internal mammary artery (p. 251).

The *innermost intercostal* part is incomplete and variable and passes from rib to rib deep to the internal intercostal. Its fibers pass in the same direction as those of the internal intercostal and can be distinguished from it only when separated by the intercostal nerves and vessels. Occasionally, some of the bundles skip over a rib and insert on the rib below. By its fascia it is connected to the sternocostal part anteriorly and the subcostal part posteriorly.

The *subcostal (part) muscle* is made up of slips that vary greatly in size and number. They lie on the internal surface of the lower ribs near their angles and may be looked upon as parts of the innermost intercostal which cover two intercostal spaces.

There are 11 intercostal spaces: the upper 9 are closed, but the lower 2 remain open anteriorly. They are all wider in front than behind; the widest is the 3rd, followed by the 2nd and then the 1st. The 7th, the 8th,

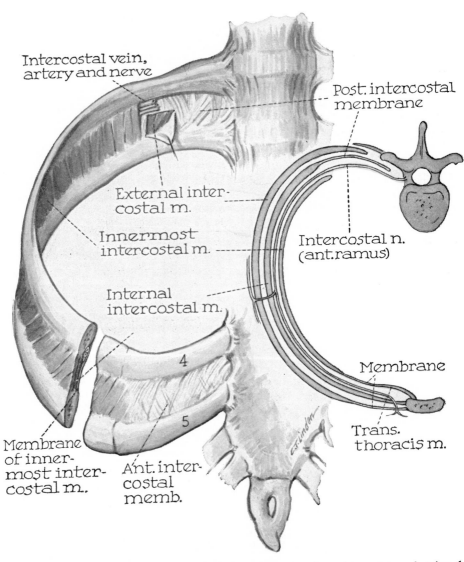

Intercostal vein, artery and nerve

Post. intercostal membrane

External inter-costal m.

Innermost intercostal m.

Intercostal n. (ant. ramus)

Internal intercostal m.

4

5

Membrane

Trans. thoracis m.

Membrane of inner-most inter-costal m.

Ant. inter-costal memb.

FIG. 181. An intercostal space; a diagrammatic presentation of two views, showing the relations of muscles, vessels and nerves. In the posterior part of the space, the nerve is situated almost between the ribs, but from the angles of the ribs forward, it lies in the sub-costal groove.

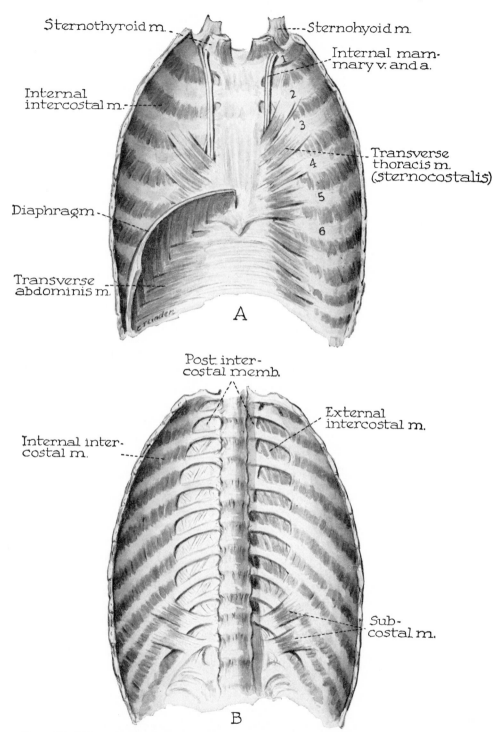

Sternothyroid m.

Sternohyoid m.

Internal mammary v. and a.

Internal intercostal m.

Transverse thoracis m. (sternocostalis)

Diaphragm

Transverse abdominis m.

A

Post. intercostal memb.

External intercostal m.

Internal intercostal m.

Subcostal m.

B

FIG. 182. The transversus thoracis muscle. This has 3 parts, namely, the sternocostalis, the innermost intercostal and the subcostal. The innermost intercostal is shown in Figure 181. The sternocostalis is the most constant in position, and the innermost intercostal the least constant. (A) Anterior wall viewed from within; (B) posterior wall viewed from within.

the 9th, and the 10th are very narrow. The spaces are wider in inspiration than in expiration, and their width can be increased by bending the body to the opposite side.

The subcostal groove in a typical rib is situated on the deep surface of its sharp lower border. It contains from above downward the respective intercostal vein, artery and nerve (V.A.N.). In the posterior part of the space the nerve is situated midway between the ribs, but from the angles of the ribs forward it lies in the subcostal groove.

BLOOD VESSELS

Intercostal Arteries. Since there are 11 intercostal spaces, there must be 11 intercostal arteries. These originate posteriorly and are designated as the posterior intercostal arteries. The anterior intercostal arteries arise from the internal mammary (Fig. 183). Not all 11 posterior arteries arise from the aorta, since only the lower 9 have this origin; the upper 2 are branches of the highest intercostal, a branch of the costocervical trunk of the subclavian. The right aortic intercostals are longer than the left because of the position of the aorta to the left of the vertebral column. Each vessel divides into anterior and posterior branches. The posterior supplies the spinal canal, the back musculature and the overlying skin. It is the anterior branch of the posterior intercostal artery which passes forward in the subcostal groove. The intercostal vessels and their corresponding nerves pass anteriorly in the plane between the innermost intercostal and the internal intercostal muscles. The lower intercostal vessels and nerves occupy a corresponding plane in the abdominal wall. Anteriorly, the vessel divides into superior and inferior (collateral) branches which unite with those from the internal mammary artery. Since the lowest two intercostal spaces remain open, the lowest two intercostal arteries continue on into the abdominal wall.

The subcostal artery is the same as any intercostal artery, but since there is no 12th space, it assumes a separate name.

The internal mammary artery arises from the undersurface of the first portion of the subclavian artery opposite the thyrocervical trunk (Fig. 184). It descends behind the innominate vein and the sternoclavicular articulation and then passes vertically downward on the deep surface of the thoracic wall about ¼ inch from the outer border of the sternum. It is covered by skin, fascia, pectoralis major muscle, anterior intercostal membrane, internal intercostal muscle and costal cartilage. In the region of the 6th intercostal space, it ends by dividing into superior epigastric and musculophrenic branches.

Opposite each of the upper 6 intercostal spaces the internal mammary gives off perforating branches which pass forward through the intercostal spaces. In females the 2nd and the 3rd perforating branches are much larger, since they supply not only the overlying muscles and skin but the mammary gland as well.

Corresponding to each perforating artery, the internal mammary also gives rise to 2 anterior intercostal arteries. These small vessels pass laterally, one lying near the lower border of the rib above, and the other lying near the upper margin of the rib below; they anastomose with the posterior intercostals. Therefore, each intercostal space has 3 intercostal arteries (1 posterior and 2 anterior); however, this is not true for the lowest 2 spaces, since they remain open and have no anterior branches.

Of surgical importance is the fact that the internal mammary artery lies directly on the pleura in the first 2 intercostal spaces. Below this level the transversus thoracis separates the vessel from the pleural membrane. Therefore, in order to avoid injury to the pleura, it is advisable to ligate the vessel below the first 2 interspaces. The vessel also supplies a slender branch, the pericardiophrenic, which accompanies the phrenic nerve. Because of its close relation to the nerve, the artery may be injured in the operation of phrenic avulsion and produce a hemorrhage large enough to necessitate ligation of the internal mammary artery.

The superior epigastric artery continues in the original direction of the internal mammary; it descends through the diaphragm and enters the rectus sheath to anastomose with the inferior epigastric (external iliac). The musculophrenic passes downward and laterally along the costal margin of the diaphragm which it perforates. It ends, much reduced in size, opposite the last intercostal space and supplies intercostal branches to spaces 7, 8 and 9.

Ligature of the internal mammary artery is performed through a transverse incision in the anterior end of the 3rd interspace. The pectoralis major is divided in the line of its fibers, and the anterior intercostal membrane is exposed. This is incised, exposing the internal intercostal muscle. The vessel and its veins are found lying between the internal intercostal and the transversus thoracis (sternocostal part) muscles.

The internal mammary veins (venae comitantes of the internal mammary artery) unite opposite the 3rd costal cartilage, or a little lower, to form a single venous trunk which ascends along the medial side of the artery and enters the innominate vein at the thoracic inlet. These veins possess numerous valves and receive branches from the anterior intercostal veins of the upper 6 spaces, perforating branches, muscular branches, mediastinal, pericardial and thymic veins as well as the superior epigastric and musculophrenic venae comitantes. The internal mammary vessels are covered in their lower portions posteriorly by the transversus thoracis muscle, but in the upper part are in direct contact with the parietal pleura. The internal mammary vessels are crossed anteriorly by the intercostal nerves and are associated with lymph glands.

ARRANGEMENT OF THE 12
SPINAL NERVES

The spinal nerves (Fig. 183) are arranged segmentally and are attached to the spinal cord by 2 roots: an anterior which is motor (efferent) and a posterior which is sensory (afferent). The posterior root has a *ganglion* on it. These roots leave the vertebral canal via the intervertebral foramina and immediately join to form a spinal nerve. Since this nerve has both sensory and motor fibers, it is spoken of as a mixed nerve; it divides into anterior and posterior rami. The *anterior rami* are larger and have a tendency to form plexuses (cervical, brachial, lumbar, sacral and pudendal), but the smaller *posterior rami* supply the muscles of the back and, in addition, the overlying skin.

An intercostal nerve is the anterior nerve ramus. There are 12 pairs of such thoracic or intercostal nerves, 11 of which are truly intercostal and 1 subcostal. The 12th is the *subcostal* since it has to run its course in the abdominal wall and not in an intercostal space. The 1st intercostal nerve also differs somewhat because the greater part of it goes into the formation of the brachial plexus. Each nerve sends a *white ramus communicans* to a corresponding sympathetic ganglion and receives a *gray ramus communicans* from it.

A typical intercostal nerve continues forward and supplies muscular and two cutaneous branches. The cutaneous branches are: (a) the *lateral cutaneous nerve,* which emerges in the midaxillary line, divides into anterior and posterior branches and supplies the side of the chest; (b) *the anterior cutaneous nerve,* which is the termination of the intercostal, appears at the inner end of an intercostal space, where it supplies the skin over the sternum and the front of the chest. Since the 1st thoracic nerve is mainly given to the formation of the brachial plexus, it is very small and supplies neither lateral nor anterior cutaneous branches. The 2nd intercostal nerve has lateral and anterior cutaneous branches, but its lateral branch does not divide in two, since it crosses the axilla as the *intercostobrachial nerve,* which supplies the skin of the posteromedial aspect of the arm as far as the elbow. The 7th supplies the region of the epigastrium; the 10th, the umbilical region; and the 12th innervates that region which is situated midway between the umbilicus and the pubis. Nerves 2, 3, 4, 5 and 6 run typically intercostal or thoracic courses, but 7, 8, 9, 10 and 11 travel partly in the thoracic and partly in the abdominal wall, thus taking a thoracico-abdominal course.

The typical thoracic nerves 2 to 6 are separated from the pleura by the innermost intercostal muscle and the transversus thoracis. After supplying the intercostal muscles, they cross in front of the internal mammary artery and in company with the perforating artery, pierce the internal intercostal muscle, the anterior intercostal membrane and the pectoralis major, terminating as an anterior cutaneous nerve of the thorax.

In the abdominal course, the thoracicoabdominal nerves (7th to 11th) leave their interspaces between the diaphragm and the transversus abdominis and pass between the internal oblique and the transversus abdominis to the back of the rectus sheath. After piercing the sheath they travel in front of the superior or inferior epigastric artery, supply and pierce the rectus abdominis muscle and continue to the anterior abdominal wall; finally, in company with a cutaneous branch of the epigastric artery they end as anterior cutaneous nerves of the abdominal wall.

The intercostal and subcostal nerves supply the following muscles: external and internal intercostals, subcostals, transversus thoracis, levator costarum, external and internal oblique, transversus abdominis, rectus abdominis, and pyramidalis. Dorsally, these nerves supply the serratus posterior superior and the serratus posterior inferior.

The upper 6 intercostal nerves do not reach the midline of the body but end at the inner side of the intercostal space. This is of some diagnostic importance, since a swelling

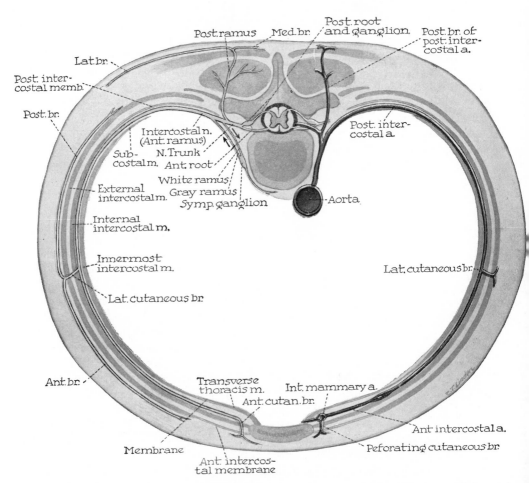

FIG. 183. An intercostal artery and a spinal nerve (diagrammatic). The intercostal vessels and nerves pass in an intermuscular plane between the transversus thoracis (innermost intercostal) and internal intercostal muscles.

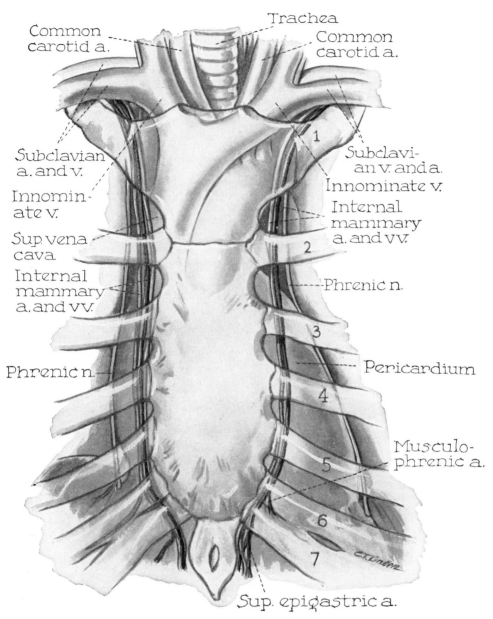

Common carotid a.

Trachea

Common carotid a.

Subclavian a. and v.

Innomin-ate v.

Sup. vena cava

Internal mammary a. and vv.

Phrenic n.

1

Subclavi-an v. and a.

Innominate v.

Internal mammary a. and vv.

2

------Phrenic n.

3

------- Pericardium

4

Musculo-phrenic a.

5

6

7

Sup. epigastric a.

FIG. 184. The internal mammary vessels.

over the center of the sternum could not be a cold abscess which has tracked around from the spine along the course of the inter-costal nerve, because such a collection could not extend beyond the lateral edge of the sternum. These intercostal nerves run an oblique course, but the area supplied by any one of them is horizontal. Head has shown that before anesthesia is evident in the region of their nerve distribution, at least 3 contigu-ous nerves must be divided since the over-lapping from the nerve above and the nerve below would compensate for any injury to a single nerve.

Breast (Mammary Gland)

EMBRYOLOGY AND EMBRYOLOGIC MALFORMATIONS

Although the mammary glands do not come into use until adult life, nevertheless, they are the first of all the glands which arise from the epidermis to appear during the development of the embryo. In a 6-weeks-old human embryo an ectodermal ridge, known as the milk line or primary ridge, is noted. This thickening extends along the body wall on either side from the axilla to the groin. In the human it atrophies, but a small portion remains in each pectoral region, which becomes the mammary gland. Since these ridges consist of tissue which is potentially mammary, failure of their normal disappearance will result in the persistence of accessory breast tissue. Such tissue remains along the line and can appear anywhere from the axilla to the inner aspect of Scarpa's triangle (Fig. 185). The rare presence of accessory breast tissue in locations such as the gluteal region and the shoulder can be explained only by an ectopic placement of the milk ridge. Normally, that portion of the ridge

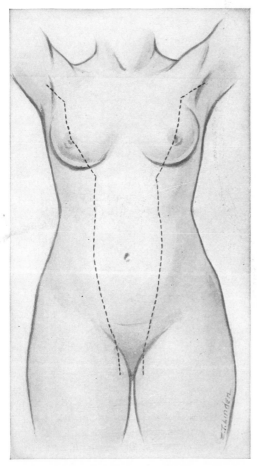

FIG. 185. The milk lines. These ridges consist of potential mammary tissue, and their failure to disappear would result in accessory breasts.

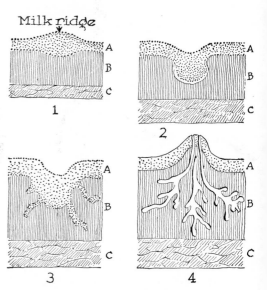

FIG. 186. The development of the mammary gland: (A) ectoderm, (B) mesoderm (subcutaneous tissue), (C) pectoralis major muscle. (1) At the second month, (2) at the third month, (3) at the fifth month, (4) at birth.

254

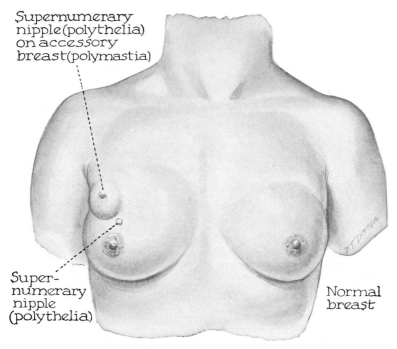

Supernumerary
nipple(polythelia)
on accessory
breast(polymastia)

Super-
numerary
nipple
(polythelia)

Normal
breast

Fig. 187. Congenital abnormalities of the breast.

which is located in the pectoral region starts
to grow inward in the shape of buds, which
form slender tubes and from them the ducts
and the secreting tissues of the breast eventually develop. The nipple is either flat or
depressed at birth and only later does it evert
so that it projects above the surrounding skin
(Fig. 186).

The congenital abnormalities which may
occur are (Fig. 187):

1. *Polymastia.* This condition presents
more than one breast on one or both sides
and is due to the persistence of part of the
milk ridge. The accessory breast may be well
developed or tiny, and instances have been
noted where these breasts have been used for
suckling. As many as 10 have been recorded
in one individual.

2. *Polythelia.* This condition is one in
which supernumerary nipples are found over
a given breast and not necessarily on the milk
ridge.

3. *Gynecomastia.* This is the presence of
a female breast or breasts in the male.

Congenital absence, amastia, either unilateral or bilateral, has also been recorded.
Unilateral amastia is believed to be due to

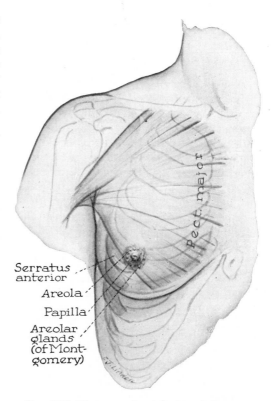

Serratus
anterior

Areola

Papilla

Areolar
glands
(of Mont-
gomery)

Pect. major

Fig. 188. The normal, adult, female breast.

the foramen or of longer in or opening in the axillary fascia thru which the tail of the breast passes through

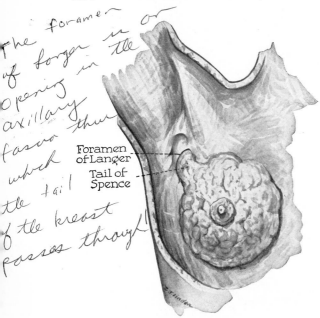

Foramen of Langer
Tail of Spence

FIG. 189. The axillary tail of Spence.

pressure of an arm in utero against the pectoral region. When this exists the pectoral muscles on the affected side are also atrophic or absent.

MAMMARY GLAND PROPER (STRUCTURE AND FORM)

The mammary gland extends vertically from the 2nd to the 6th rib inclusive and horizontally from the side of the sternum (parasternal) to the midaxillary line. The greater part of the breast, about two thirds, rests on the pectoralis major muscle; and the rest, about one third, on the serratus anterior (Fig. 188). The breast is hemispherical in shape, but tonguelike processes may extend upward, downward or medially from it; the most common of such processes is the so-called *axillary tail of Spence* (Fig. 189). This is a prolongation of breast tissue from the upper outer part of the breast, which passes through an opening in the axillary fascia, called the *foramen of Langer*. Therefore, although the breast proper is superficial to the axillary fascia, the axillary tail is deep to this fascia. Such a process is in direct contact with the axillary glands; therefore, if it is enlarged it may be mistaken for an axillary tumor or for axillary lymph adenopathy.

Since the breast is a modified sebaceous gland, it lies *in* the superficial fascia and not upon or deep to it. The deep surface rests on the fasciae which cover the pectoralis major and the serratus anterior muscles. The gland is made up of lobes (usually 12) which are subdivided into lobules, and these in turn are composed of acini. The lobes are arranged like the spokes of a wheel which converge on the nipple, and each lobe is drained by a lactiferous duct; from 12 to 20 such ducts open onto the nipple (Fig. 190 A). The organ is fixed to the overlying skin and the underlying pectoral fascia by fibrous bands known as *Cooper's ligaments* (Fig. 190 B). These are clinically important because cancer cells invade them and subsequently cause their contraction, which results in dimpling of the skin or fixation of the growth. By the same process, a malignant tumor may be fixed to the underlying pectoral fascia and then cannot be moved in the long axis of the muscle. The ducts open independently of each other on the surface of the nipple, and each has a dilated ampulla just before it ends. The *nipple* is conical in shape and usually is found in the 4th intercostal space. Its base is surrounded by a circular pigmented area called the *areola,* which has many small rounded elevations (cutaneous glands) known as the *areolar glands of Montgomery.* These are sebaceous glands for lubrication of the nipple during lactation.

VESSELS, NERVES AND LYMPHATICS

Arteries. The arterial supply is derived chiefly from two sources: namely, the anterior perforating branches of the internal mammary artery and mammary rami of the axillary or one of its main branches (Fig. 191). Anson, Wright and Wolfer are of the opinion that no mammary branches are derived from the anterior intercostal arteries.

The *anterior perforating arteries* are branches of the internal mammary. The first 4 or 5 of these supply the breast, but only 2, usually the 1st and the 4th (or the 2nd and the 3rd) are well developed; however, almost all of these vessels have a tendency to travel transversely and cephalad to the nipple.

The lateral thoracic artery, a branch of

the second part of the axillary, descends along the lateral margin of the breast and sends small branches into the gland, but its larger branches are distributed to the thoracic wall. Mammary branches of this latter vessel also have a tendency to travel transversely across the breast and in this way anastomose with the mammary rami of the perforating arteries. The thoraco-acromial artery, also a branch of part two of the axillary, is usually described as being one of the vessels which supply the breast tissue. This apparently is incorrect, since the pectoral branches of this

vessel remain on the deep aspect of the pectoralis major, supply it and do not enter the gland (Fig. 191 B).

Therefore, blood is supplied to the breast from *two* arterial sources: (1) the anterior perforating branches of the internal mammary and (2) the lateral thoracic arteries. Since these vessels pass cephalad to the nipple and in a transverse direction, the blood supply of the gland is located mainly at its superomedial and superolateral aspects. Therefore, an incision into the breast should be placed below the nipple to preserve the

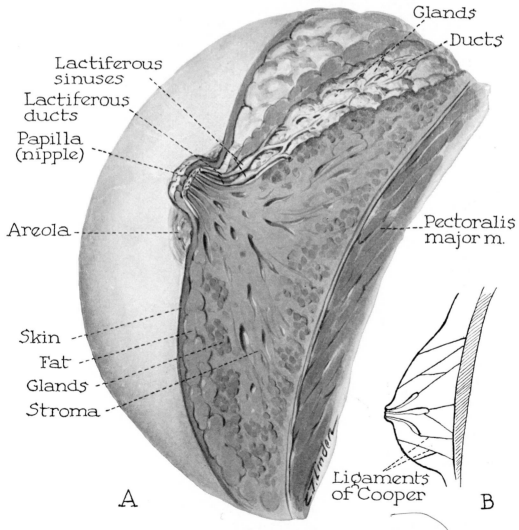

FIG. 190. Cross section of an adult female breast: (A) the breast has been dissected layer by layer, (B) attachments of Cooper's ligaments.

blood supply and to make the scar less visible. Since no major vessels reach the gland from its inferior aspect, plastic procedures on the pendulous breast as well as diagnostic incisions into the breast should be placed in the inferior quadrants.

Veins. Although the main veins follow the arterial pattern just described, many of

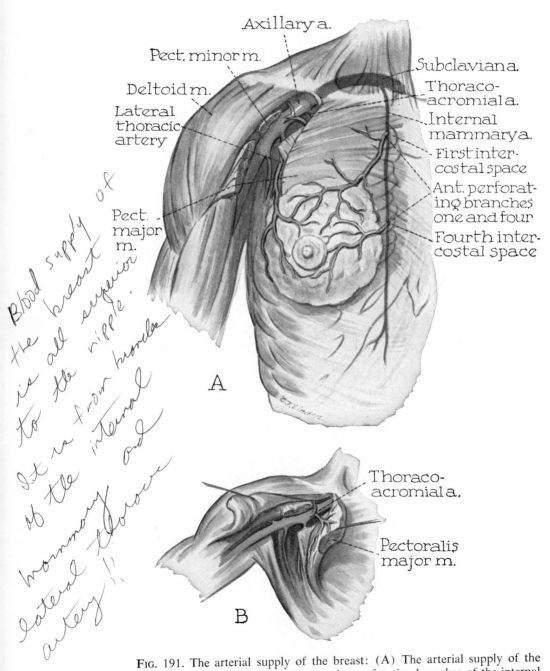

Blood supply of the breast is all superior to the nipple. It is from branches of the internal mammary and lateral thoracic artery !!

FIG. 191. The arterial supply of the breast: (A) The arterial supply of the breast is derived from two sources: anterior perforating branches of the internal mammary artery and the lateral thoracic artery. (B) The thoraco-acromial artery supplies the pectoralis major muscle and not the breast.

the smaller veins resemble the lymphatics and form a plexus beneath the areola. These are especially visible in the lactating breast. Large veins pass from the plexus toward the periphery and end in the axillary and the internal mammary veins.

Lymphatics. The lymph drainage consists of 3 parts: cutaneous, areolar and glandular (Fig. 192).

The cutaneous lymphatics carry the lymph from the integument of the breast, with the exception of the areola and the nipple, and converge in collecting trunks, which flow into the axillary glands of the same side. At the inner quadrants, and especially those near the sternum, lymphatics may cross and terminate in the breast or axillary glands of the opposite side.

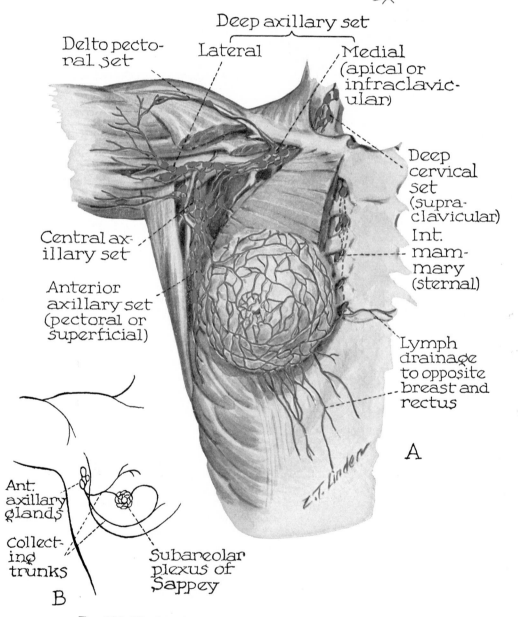

FIG. 192. The lymph drainage of the breast: (A) the cutaneous and glandular lymphatics, (B) the areolar lymphatics.

The areolar lymphatics drain the nipple and the areola and pass into the *subareolar plexus of Sappey* (Fig. 192 B). The plexus is drained by two main lymph channels: one for the inner part and one for the outer. They usually unite into one main trunk, which passes to the anterior group of axillary glands.

The anterior axillary (pectoral or superficial) *set* is really the main group and is placed under the anterior axillary fold, following the course of the lateral thoracic vein. These glands are found in the region of the 3rd rib. From this set the glands drain to the *central axillary set,* which is situated in the fat of the upper part of the axilla, under the axillary tuft of hair and along the inner border of the axillary vein. The intercostohumeral nerve passes outward between these glands, and enlargement of the latter may produce pressure on the nerve, resulting in pain along the axilla or inner border of the arm. From here the lymph vessels pass to the *deep axillary glands,* part of which form a lateral group which passes along the course of the axillary vein; the other part forms the *apical group* which has also been referred to as the infraclavicular glands. These glands lie behind the costocoracoid membrane. Therefore, it is impossible to free them adequately unless the whole region of the costocoracoid membrane is removed. The deep axillary glands become continuous with the *deep cervical glands* in the supraclavicular fossa.

Although the above path is the usual one taken, there are other lymphatic zones of cancer spread. Some of the lymphatics from the upper and the outer quadrants of the breast form a trunk that pierces the pectoralis major muscle and directly enters the gland along the axillary vein, thereby short-circuiting the axilla. Lymphatics also leave the inner quadrant of the breast and reach the glands inside of the chest cavity, lying on each side of the internal mammary artery (Fig. 193). Occasionally, a few vessels pass to the *cephalic gland* which lies in the deltopectoral groove. In some instances breast cancer may spread downward in the lymphatics to the epigastric region and there invade the abdominal wall. Development of metastases in the liver and in the pelvic cavity can be explained by such permeation. It is possible for cancer from one breast to spread across the midline to the other subpectoral plexus, then to the opposite axilla and finally to the opposite breast. The pectoral lymph plexuses should not be regarded as separate systems but rather as communicating networks.

Nerves. The nerve supply of the skin of breast is derived from the anterior and lateral branches of the 4th to the 6th intercostal nerves, which reach it by way of the 2nd to the 6th intercostals.

SURGICAL CONSIDERATIONS

BREAST ABSCESS

Breast abscesses may be subcutaneous, intramammary or submammary. The incision for a subcutaneous or inframammary abscess should be so placed that it radiates from the nipple but never transversely across the breast. If the abscess is deeper, submammary or retromammary, this incision is not utilized, but instead a thoracomammary approach in the inframammary fold is used. This is the same incision that is utilized for benign tumors of the breast, since practically any portion of the gland can be examined through it (Fig. 194). With the breast retracted upward and medially, the incision is placed in the pigmented line. Then it is carried down to the underlying muscle, and the breast is displaced upward. The necessary procedure is done, be it draining an abscess or removing a tumor. The breast is permitted to fall back into its normal position where it is sutured.

RADICAL MASTECTOMY

Radical mastectomy can be outlined in 6 anatomic steps, each having 3 substeps. This is only a plan and may be altered to fit any standard technic (Figs. 195, 196). The plan is outlined as follows:

1. **Incision:**
   a. Coraco-umbilical line
   b. Mobilization of skin medially to the midline of the sternum
   c. Mobilization of skin laterally to the latissimus dorsi (posterior axillary fold)

2. **Axillary Fascia Step:**
   a. Incision of axillary fascia along the lower border of pectoralis major
   b. Division of the pectoralis major near its insertion, leaving the clavicular part intact
   c. Division and ligation of the thoraco-acromial vessels and nerves
3. **Clavipectoral Fascia Step:**
   a. Incision into the clavipectoral fascia along the lower border of the pectoralis minor
   b. Division of the pectoralis minor muscle
   c. Insertion of the pectoralis minor utilized as an axillary vein splint
4. **Axillary Vein Dissection:**
   a. Clamp, cut and ligate all venous tributaries
   b. Axillary glands and fat dissected downward
   c. Subscapular vessels used as a guide to the thoracodorsal nerve
5. **Posterolateral Dissection:**
   a. Exposure of the subscapular muscle

b. Exposure of the latissimus dorsi
c. Exposure of rectus abdominis
6. **Medial Dissection:**
   a. Dissection of pectoralis major and minor muscles
   b. Clamp and ligate perforating vessels (especially Number 2)
   c. Remove mass en bloc and close

Incision. Many incisions have been advised; however, the one described extends from the coracoid process above, which is always palpable, to the umbilicus below, which is always visible (Fig. 195 A). Forceps are placed in the breast, which is elevated, and then traction is made laterally; the incision is placed along the coraco-umbilical line. Next, traction is made to the opposite side, and the incision is completed along the coraco-umbilical line. The lateral and medial skin flaps are formed; they extend medially past the midline of the sternum and laterally to the latissimus dorsi.

Axillary Fascia. The second step is the axillary fascia phase. This fascia provides a covering for the pectoralis major muscle. An

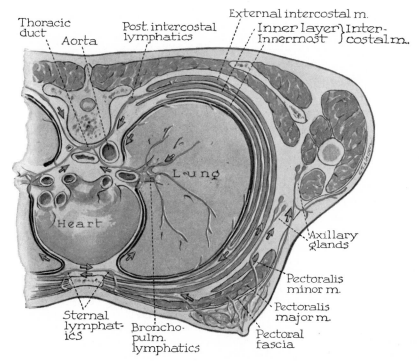

Fig. 193. Transverse section through the thorax, showing paths of lymph drainage from the breast.

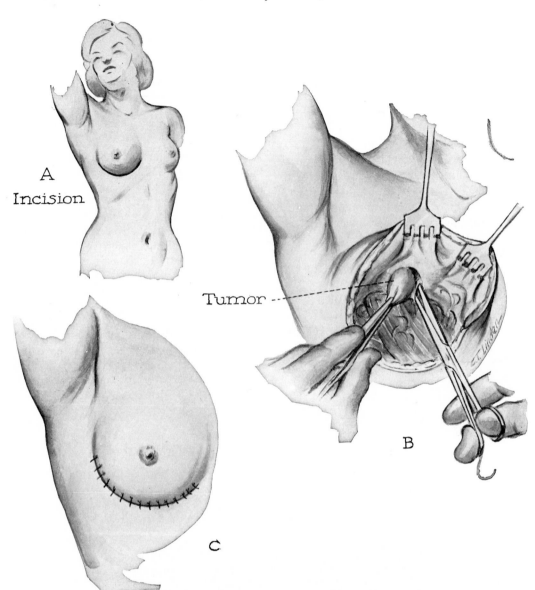

A
Incision

Tumor ---

B

C

FIG. 194. Inframammary approach to breast pathology: (A) incision in inframammary fold, (B) removal of small benign tumor, (C) closure.

FIG. 195 (*Facing page*). Radical mastectomy: (A) The incision extends around the breast from the coracoid process to the umbilicus. The musculature in this region is shown. (B) A finger is placed through an incision in the axillary fascia, it emerges at the claviculosternal groove of the pectoralis major and not at the deltopectoral groove. This permits the clavicular portion of the muscle to remain intact and in this way protects the cephalic vein. (C) A finger is placed through an incision in the clavipectoral fascia. The finger passes under the pectoralis minor muscle, which is severed close to the coracoid process. The thoraco-acromial vessels have been divided and tied.

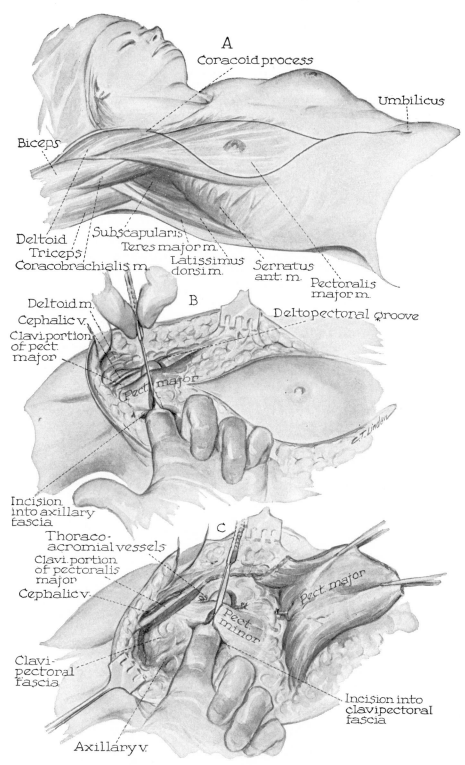

A

Coracoid process

Umbilicus

Biceps

Deltoid
Triceps
Coracobrachialis m.

Subscapularis
Teres major m.
Latissimus
dorsi m.
Serratus
ant. m.
Pectoralis
major m.

B

Deltoid m.
Cephalic v.
Clavi. portion
of pect.
major

Deltopectoral groove

Pect. major

E.T. Linden

Incision
into axillary
fascia

Thoraco-
acromial vessels
Clavi. portion
of pectoralis
major
Cephalic v.

C

Pect. major

Pect.
minor

Clavi-
pectoral
fascia

Incision into
clavipectoral
fascia

Axillary v.

FIGURE 195. (*Caption on facing page.*)

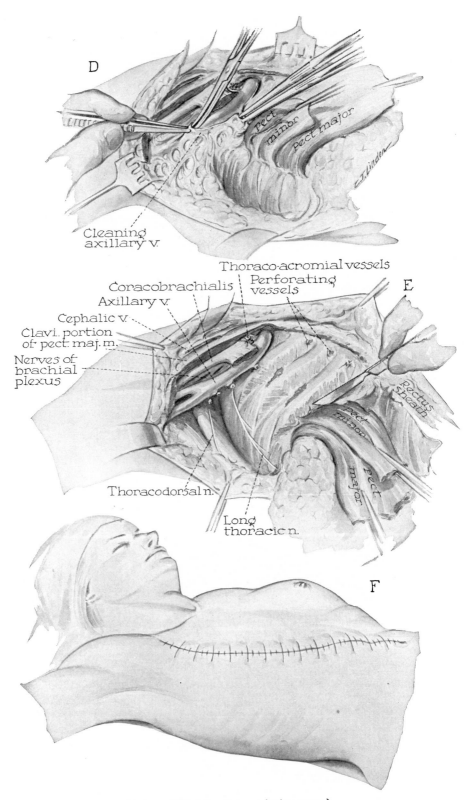

FIGURE 196. (*Caption on facing page.*)

incision is placed into the fascia along the lower border of the pectoralis major (Fig. 195 B). The index finger of the left hand is placed through the defect and is guided, not to the deltopectoral groove, which seems natural, but rather to the claviculosternal groove, which is not as well marked. If the clavicular portion of the pectoralis major muscle remains intact, it protects the cephalic vein, which runs in the deltopectoral groove. In the course of the operation it might become necessary to ligate or remove the axillary vein; if the cephalic vein is intact, the venous return of the superior extremity will not be impaired. The pectoralis major is cut near its insertion, and its sterno-abdominal part is reflected medially. As the pectoralis major is reflected medially, the thoraco-acromial vessels and the anterior thoracic nerves appear as a neurovascular bundle along the medial border of the pectoralis minor. These are clamped, severed and ligated.

Clavipectoral Fascia. The third step is the clavipectoral fascia phase. This fascia provides the covering for the pectoralis minor muscle. It is incised along the lower border of the pectoralis minor, so that the index finger of the left hand may be slipped under it and around the muscle (Fig. 195 C). The pectoralis minor is divided, but a small part is left attached to the coracoid process; this acts as a splint for the axillary vein. With both pectoral muscles divided and retracted medial and downward, the axilla is exposed and then is ready for dissection of its contents.

Axillary Vein Dissection. In the axillary vein phase, the axillary sheath which covers the vein is opened carefully, and the vascular branches below the vein are individually identified, cut and tied (Fig. 196 D). These usually include the short thoracic vein, the lateral thoracic artery, the long thoracic vein, the subscapular vein, the lateral thoracic vein and the subscapular artery. The axillary lymph glands and fat are dissected downward. The subscapular vessels act as a guide to the thoracordorsal nerve, and the lateral thoracic artery is the guide to the long thoracic nerve. If possible, these nerves should be saved, but if they are involved they must be sacrificed.

Posterolateral Dissection. This is carried out next. After the axillary cleansing has been accomplished, the subscapular muscle, the teres major and the latissimus dorsi come to view; the rectus sheath is also exposed.

Medial Dissection. This is the final stage. The origins of the pectoralis major and minor are severed, the mass is retracted laterally and downward, and the perforating vessels are sought in the intercostal spaces; they are found close to the lateral margin of the sternum (Fig. 196 E). These must be clamped, cut and ligated, with special emphasis being placed on perforating branch Number 2, which has been discussed thoroughly (p. 256). The entire mass is removed en bloc, and the wound is closed (Fig. 196 F). At times skin grafts may be necessary.

Currently, supraradical mastectomy is advocated by some surgeons for carcinoma of the breast. These procedures vary according to one's definition of "radical." Some surgeons advocate internal mammary artery (lymph node) dissection, removal of the clavicle, the ribs, and/or the superior extremity. This has become an individual problem and decision.

FIG. 196. (*Facing page*). Radical mastectomy (*Continued*). (D) The axillary vein is exposed by dividing the axillary sheath. The vessels below this vein are individually identified, severed and tied, and the axillary fat and lymph glands are dissected distally. (E) The entire mass is dissected downward. The attachments of the pectoral muscles are divided, and the perforating vessels are cut and ligated. If possible, the long thoracic and thoraco-dorsal nerves are saved. The rectus sheath is exposed and at times removed. (F) Closure.

Diaphragm

The word diaphragm is derived from the Greek "dia" (in-between) and "phragma" (fence). It is a dome-shaped, musculo-apo-neurotic partition which is located between the thorax and the abdomen.

EMBRYOLOGY

The embryology of the diaphragm is com-plicated because the diaphragmatic elements are derived from several sources. The ante-rior, lateral and central parts, which make up the greater portion, are formed from the transverse septum and the fused ventral mesentery. The posterolateral portion is formed by the fusion of the dorsal mesentery and the mesoderm derived from the receding

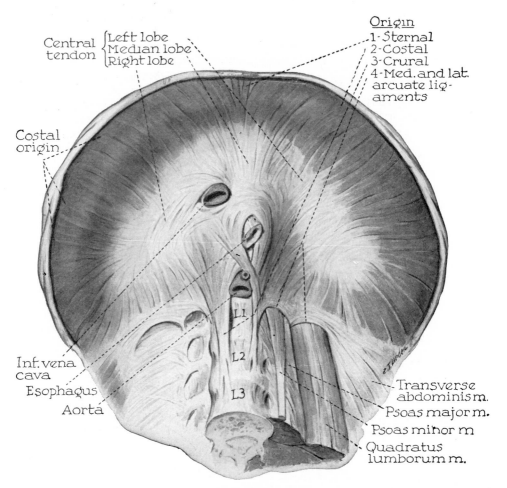

FIG. 197. The diaphragm viewed from below. The central tendon consists of 3 lobes and is the site of insertion of the diaphragm. The 4 points of origin have been identified.

266

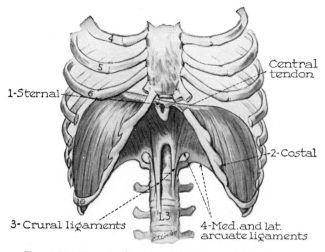

Central
tendon

1-Sternal

2-Costal

3- Crural ligaments

4-Med. and lat.
arcuate ligaments

FIG. 198. The diaphragm viewed from in front. The
lower costal cartilages have been removed to show the 4
points of origin.

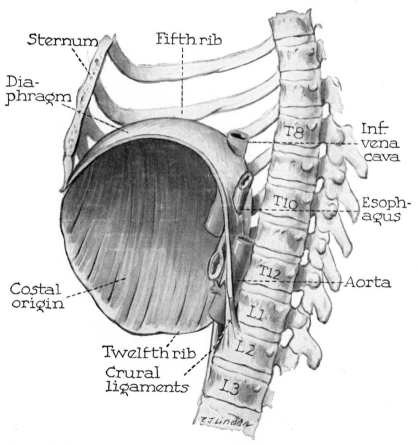

Sternum   Fifth rib

Dia-
phragm

T8

Inf.
vena
cava

T10

Esoph-
agus

T12

Aorta

Costal
origin

Twelfth rib

Crural
ligaments

L1

L2

L3

FIG. 199. The diaphragm viewed from the left. The 3 main apertures are
shown, and their thoracic levels are labeled.

wolffian body and the pleuroperitoneal membrane. Some embryologists divide diaphragmatic development into 3 stages.

In the first stage, the coelomic space is a continuous one until the growth of the organs divide it into pericardial, pleural and peritoneal cavities. The septum transversum forms the ventral part of the diaphragm; the pericardial cavity lies ventral to it. Since the septum is confined to the ventral half of the embryo, the pleural space remains continuous with the peritoneal cavity posteriorly. This resulting continuity is the pleuroperitoneal canal, and the developing esophagus, stomach and its mesentery pass through it. Should the development proceed only to this point, the abdominal organs would have a direct route into the thorax. A hernia formed during this stage would have no sac.

In the second stage, the pleuroperitoneal canal becomes obliterated by the proliferation of the primitive dorsal mesentery of the stomach and the esophagus. The pleural and peritoneal cavities are now fully formed and if a herniation should occur during this phase, a sac would be present.

During the third or final phase, the phrenic nerve with a muscle mass invades the diaphragm. This muscle replaces the membranous structures; the last area to be muscularized is the dorsal part. If the ingrowth of muscle is incomplete, the posterior part will be closed only by pleura and peritoneum. In these cases, the crura of the diaphragm, which form the back of the muscle, will be absent in whole or in part.

DIAPHRAGM PROPER

Adult Diaphragm. This musculotendinous partition is located between the pleurae and the pericardium above and the peritoneal cavity below. When relaxed and viewed from below, it forms a dome-shaped roof for the abdomen. Its circumferential part is fleshy, and these muscle fibers curve upward and inward from every side to join the edges of an aponeurotic sheath called the *central tendon* (Fig. 197). It is this tendon which acts as the site of insertion for the diaphragm. The central tendon is strong, its tendinous bundles passing in different directions and interlacing with one another, giving it a pleated appearance. At times it has a trilobate appearance. Its median part is wide and is

called the median lobe; the extremities or horns of the tendon are referred to as the right and the left lobes. The latter is the narrower. The tendon is inseparably blended above with the fibrous layer of the pericardium.

Origin. The origin of the diaphragm is quite extensive and takes place at the circumference of the thoracic outlet. It is best to consider it as originating at 4 points: sternal, costal, the crura, and the medial and lateral arcuate ligaments (Figs. 197, 198).

The *sternal origin* consists of short right and left slips from the posterior aspect of the xiphoid process which are separated from each other by a little areolar tissue. These fibers pass upward and backward to the anterior margin of the central tendon where they insert.

The *costal origin* is extensive and rises at a very steep angle. It usually consists of 6 fleshy muscle bundles which arise from the deep surface of the lower 6 costal cartilages, interdigitating with the costal origin of the transversus abdominis muscle. These fibers insert into the lateral and anterior borders of the central tendon.

The *crura* are long tapering bundles which are fleshy above and tendinous below. The right crus arises from the sides of the bodies of the upper 3 lumbar vertebrae and the intervertebral disks; the left arises from the upper 2 lumbar vertebrae. The medial fibers of the 2 crura decussate in front of the commencement of the abdominal aorta; the fibers of the right crus encircle the esophagus. Both crura ascend forward and reach the posterior border of the central tendon.

Ligaments. The *lateral* and *medial arcuate ligaments* (lumbocostal arches) are lateral to the crura. The medial arcuate ligament is the upper thickened border of the psoas fascia which stretches between the side of the body of the 2nd and the tip of the transverse process of the 1st lumbar vertebrae. The lateral arcuate ligament is the thickening of the anterior lamella of the lumbar fascia which extends from the tip of the first lumbar transverse process to the lower border of the last rib. From this origin, the muscle fibers arch upward to reach the posterior border of the lateral part of the central tendon.

Nerves. The nerve supply of the diaphragm

is derived from the right and the left phrenic nerves (C3, C4, C5).

Arteries. The arteries that supply it are the pericardiophrenic, the inferior phrenic, the musculophrenic and the intercostals.

Actions. The diaphragm is the chief muscle of respiration and it is in the abdominal type of breathing that it plays its greatest role. When its fibers contract, they straighten out, so that the domelike appearance is lost. In deep inspiration, the central tendon descends for a short distance.

FORAMINA (OPENINGS)

The continuity of the diaphragm is broken by 3 large apertures and several smaller ones. The large openings accommodate the aorta, the esophagus and the inferior vena cava (a, e, i) (Fig. 199). The thoracic levels at which these structures pass are: the inferior vena cava at the 8th thoracic, the esophagus at the 10th and the aorta at the 12th.

Aortic Opening. This is located in the median plane in front of the lower border of the 12th thoracic vertebra and between the crura. It is bounded anteriorly by a tendinous arch which connects the medial borders of the crura to each other. Through this orifice pass the aorta, the thoracic duct and the azygos vein (Fig. 200). The thoracic duct and the azygos vein are covered by the right crus.

Esophageal Opening. This oval aperture lies opposite the 10th thoracic vertebra in front, to the left of the aortic opening and behind the central tendon. The descussating fibers seem to act as a sphincter for the cardiac end of the stomach and prevent its contents from returning to the esophagus. In addition to the esophagus, it transmits the right and the left vagus nerves and the esophageal branches of the left gastric artery with its companion veins. In cirrhosis of the liver, when an obstruction to the portal system is present, these veins at the lower end of the esophagus become dilated and varicosed, and frequently rupture. The vagi do not run to either side of the esophagus but are situated so that the left vagus passes anteriorly and the right posteriorly. The left, being anterior, supplies the anterosuperior surface of the stomach, and the right innervates the postero-inferior. The position of this opening is somewhat variable, since it may be found in the median plane or even to the right of it and may be very close to the aortic opening.

Inferior Vena Cava Opening. This opening is wide, and about 1 inch to the right of the median line on a level with the 8th thoracic vertebra. It is in the central tendon between the right and the median lobes; as this tendon stretches when the diaphragm contracts, the flow of venous blood into the thorax is facilitated. The opening transmits the inferior vena cava, some branches of the right phrenic nerve and a few lymph vessels from the liver. The phrenic nerve first pierces the muscle and then supplies it on its abdominal surface.

The numerous smaller orifices transmitting vessels and nerves found in the diaphragm are: (1) the superior epigastric vessels between the sternal and the costal origins; (2) the musculophrenic vessels, which pass between the slips from the 7th and the 8th costal cartilages; (3) the lower 5 intercostal nerves accompanied by small vascular twigs, which pass between the slips from the 7th costal cartilage down; (4) the last thoracic (subcostal) nerve and the subcostal vessels, which pass behind the lateral arcuate ligament; (5) the sympathetic trunk, which passes behind the medial arcuate ligament; (6) each crus is pierced by the great, the lesser and the least splanchnic nerves; and (7) the inferior hemiazygos vein pierces the right crus.

Costophrenic Recess. The costophrenic recess is that portion of the pleural cavity which is unoccupied by lung except after full inspiration. Here the diaphragmatic pleura is in contact with the costal pleura. When in full inspiration, the inferior border of the lung insinuates itself into this recess, and retraction of the overlying intercostal spaces is seen externally as the diaphragm decends and opens the costophrenic recess.

SURGICAL CONSIDERATIONS

DIAPHRAGMATIC HERNIAS

Abnormal openings through the diaphragm which permit herniation of abdominal viscera into the thoracic cavity constitute the most common lesions of this structure which require surgery. Diaphragmatic hernias are classified as *congenital, acquired* and *traumatic*. All the traumatic, and many of the congenital hernias have no sacs. Therefore, they are not true hernias, but it is convenient to adhere to common usage and utilize the term. Most of the congenital hernias pass through the pleuroperitoneal canal (Bochdalek) and have no sacs. The majority of acquired (nontraumatic) hernias are located at the esophageal hiatus and have sacs. Since the liver affords protection to the right half of the diaphragm, hernias are rarely found here.

Diaphragmatic hernioplasty may be accomplished through abdominal, thoracic or combined abdominal and thoracic incisions (Fig. 201).

Interruption of the phrenic nerve on the involved side can be either temporary or permanent and is of value as a procedure performed preliminary to radical operative repair. It prevents spasm and movement of the muscle and causes relaxation of the hernial ring; hence, it is of value in the closure of the opening.

The transthoracic route rarely requires rib resection. The incision is usually placed in the 6th or the 7th intercostal space and extends from the costochondral junction backward to the posterior axillary line. The ribs are separated. At times reduction of the hernia may be impossible via this route, and then an abdominal incision becomes necessary for bimanual manipulation and replacement of the viscera. The opening in the diaphragm is closed by imbricating its margin. Usually, a double row of sutures is used, and then the individual incisions are closed in layers.

The abdominal route utilizes a long, left

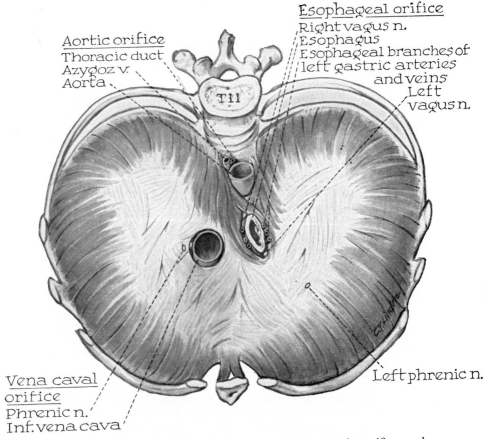

Fig. 200. The diaphragm seen from above. The 3 major orifices and the structures passing through them are shown.

rectus incision (Fig. 201 A). The left lateral ligament of the liver should be cut so that the left lobe of the liver can be retracted. This affords excellent exposure. The herniated viscera are freed of adhesions and reduced; at times it becomes necessary to enlarge the hernial ring for this reduction. The opening in the diaphragm is closed, usually by an imbrication method using interrupted sutures.

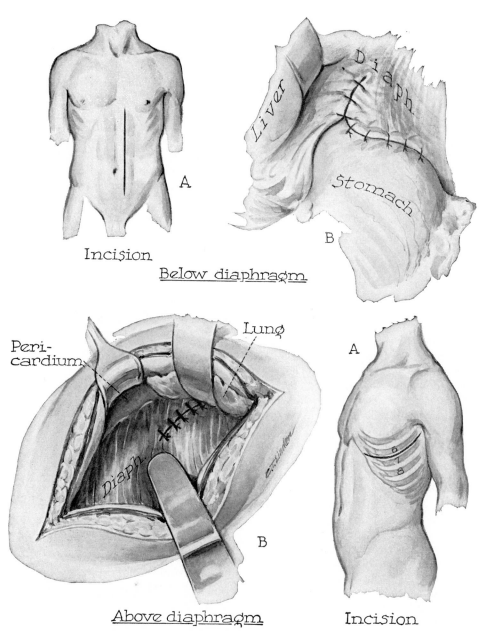

FIG. 201. Two approaches to a diaphragmatic hernia. Below the diaphragm: (A) long left rectus incision, (B) repair of hernial orifice. Above the diaphragm: (A) incision in 6th intercostal space, (B) repair of hernial orifice.

THORAX

Pleural Cavities and Pleurae

VISCERAL AND PARIETAL PLEURAE

The thoracic cavity is divided into right and left pleural cavities and a region situated between these called the mediastinum. The lung invaginates the pleural cavity so completely that only a potential space remains, and by this process the pleura becomes divided into *visceral* (lung) and *parietal* (*wall*) *layers* (Fig. 202 A).

The visceral pleura invests the lung, dips into its fissures and adheres so firmly that it is impossible to strip it from lung tissue.

The parietal pleura is subdivided, according to location, into 4 parts: costal, cervical, diaphragmatic and mediastinal (Fig. 202 B).

The costal pleura lines the ribs and their cartilages, the sides of the vertebral bodies and the back of the sternum. This is the thickest of all the parietal pleurae and is separated from the thoracic wall by the thin endothoracic fascia. It is directly continuous above with the *cervical pleura* (*cupola*) which covers the apex of the lung. This portion of the pleura extends upward into the root of the neck behind the interval between the two heads of the sternocleidomastoid muscle. Posteriorly, it reaches the level of the head of the 1st rib, but anteriorly it rises about 1½ inches above the sternal extremity of that rib. Hence, it is protected by the rib posteriorly but not so anteriorly. This is explained by the fact that ribs do not run horizontally but obliquely; there is a drop of about 1½ inches between the vertebral and the sternal attachments of the 1st rib. The upper aspect of the cervical pleura is covered by a layer of connective tissue called Sibson's fascia. This fascia forms the internal lining of the scalene muscles and spreads out, fan-like from the transverse process of the 7th cervical vertebra to the inner border of the 1st rib (Fig. 174). It separates the pleura from the first part of the subclavian artery, the phrenic nerve and the internal mammary artery.

The *diaphragmatic pleura* is thin and very adherent to the diaphragm; it covers that part of the diaphragm not covered by the diaphragmatic pericardium. It is continuous with the costal pleura laterally, but medially it becomes continuous with the *mediastinal pleura*. The diaphragmatic pleura meets the costal pleura in 2 places: behind the sternum (sternal reflection) and in front of the bodies of the thoracic vertebrae (vertebral reflection) (Fig. 202 C). At the point at which the visceral pleura meets the mediastinal layer of parietal pleura there forms a pleural passageway. The upper part of this passageway contains those structures constituting the *root* of the lung (pulmonary vessels and bronchus). The lower part is empty; hence, its walls approximate each other and form the *pulmonary ligament*.

Only after deep inspiration are the lungs and the parietal pleurae completely in contact with each other. In ordinary breathing the lungs are not completely expanded; therefore, the edges of the pleurae fall together, preventing the formation of a cavity. This touching of the pleurae takes place mainly along the anterior and lower borders. During quiet respiration the costal and the diaphragmatic pleurae remain in apposition below the lower border of the lung. The space thus formed is known as the costodiaphragmatic recess. It is about 2 inches deep behind, 3 inches deep in the midaxillary line and a little over 1 inch deep in front.

SURFACE MARKINGS

The surface markings of the lungs and the pleurae are of diagnostic value and can be constructed in the following way (Fig. 203): The junction of the costal and the mediastinal pleurae (costomediastinal line of pleural reflection) is not the same on both sides of the body. On the right, it starts about 1½ inches above the sternoclavicular joint and passes to the middle of the manubrium opposite the 2nd costal cartilage. From this point it drops vertically near the midline of the sternum to the xiphosternal joint, where it becomes continuous with the costodiaphragmatic line of reflection. On the left side, the line of pleural reflection is the same until the 4th interspace. Here it curves outward to the left border of the sternum along which it descends to the xiphosternal junction. It becomes continuous with the costodiaphragmatic line of reflection just as it does on the opposite side.

The junction of the costal and the diaphragmatic pleurae (costodiaphragmatic line of pleural reflection) may be marked by a line which starts at the xiphosternal joint and passes posteriorly to the 12th thoracic vertebra, the line being convex downward.

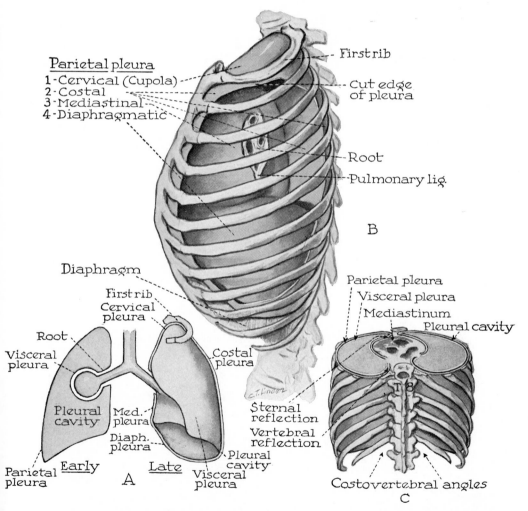

FIG. 202. The pleural cavities and the pleurae. (A) Diagrammatic presentation showing an early stage of development and the end result. The lung invades the pleural cavity so completely that only a potential pleural space remains. The process divides the pleura into visceral and parietal portions. (B) Side view seen from the left. The lung has been removed, and a window cut in the costal pleura. The 4 parts of the parietal pleura are identified, as are the pulmonary root and ligament. (C) The sternal and vertebral reflections.

It crosses the 10th rib in the midaxillary line, lies about 2 inches above the costal margin and marks the lowest level of the pleural sac (not lung). It ascends slightly after passing this point and terminates opposite the 12th thoracic vertebra.

Lungs. The lungs may also be marked on the surface of the body. The apices lie about ½ inch above the inner third of the clavicles, then descend behind the sternoclavicular joints toward the midline of the sternum (level of the 2nd rib). At this point the lungs almost touch each other. The anterior border of the right lung follows the line of its pleura

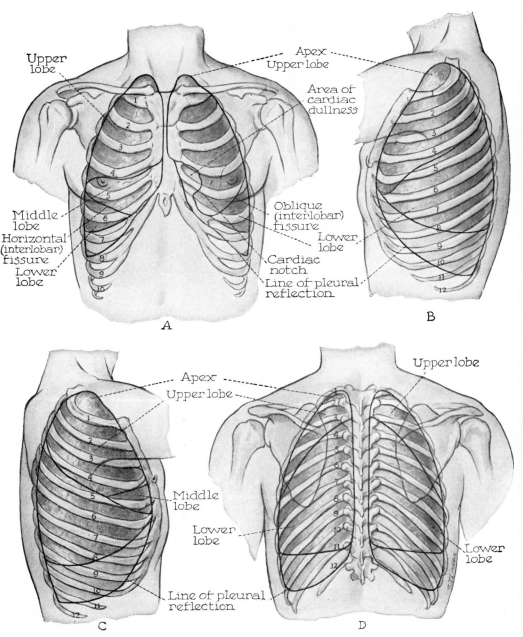

FIG. 203. The surface markings of the lungs and the pleurae: (A) anterior view, (B) left lateral view, (C) right lateral view, (D) posterior view.

directly downward to the 6th costal cartilage. The anterior border of the left lung descends as far as the 4th costal cartilage where it curves to the left, exposing an area of pericardium called the area of cardiac dullness. This curving line ends opposite the 6th costal cartilage about 1½ inches from the midline; the summit of this space is in the 4th interspace about 2 inches from the midline. The lower borders of the lungs are practically at the same level on both sides; they lie at a higher level (about 3 inches) than their corresponding pleural sacs (the costodiaphragmatic line). The lower border of each lung can be marked by a line which passes laterally behind the 7th rib in the midclavicular line, and the 8th rib in the midaxillary line; the latter is its lowest level. From here it terminates posteriorly opposite the 10th thoracic spine.

SURGICAL CONSIDERATIONS

FRACTURED RIBS

The ribs which are usually fractured are the 3rd to the 8th; ribs 1 and 2 and those below the 8th are infrequently involved (Fig. 204). The fracture of the bone proper is of no great importance with the exception of the local discomfort which it produces. However, complications such as puncture of the pleura, the lung, the liver or the spleen, as well as diaphragmatic hernia, secondary pleural effusion and surgical emphysema may result in serious sequelae. Little displacement or shortening occurs in rib fractures because of the attachment of the intercostal muscles and fixation of both rib extremities.

ASPIRATION OF THE CHEST

The chest is aspirated as either a diagnostic or a therapeutic procedure (Fig. 205). It is performed best with the patient seated and with the arm of the involved side placed on the opposite shoulder. If this is impossible, the aspiration may be done with the patient lying on the uninvolved side. The site of election is usually a little posterior to the posterior axillary line in the 6th, the 7th or 8th intercostal space. Some prefer the midaxillary line. The needle should be passed a

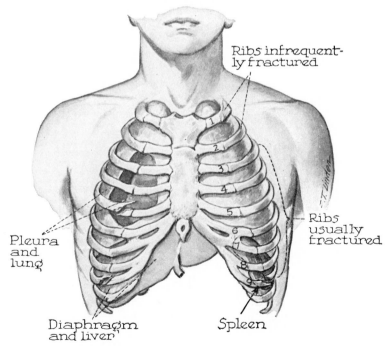

Ribs infrequently fractured

Ribs usually fractured

Pleura and lung

Diaphragm and liver

Spleen

FIG. 204. Fractured ribs and their complications. The sharp end of a broken rib may injure the pleura, the lung, the liver, the spleen or the diaphragm.

little toward the superior surface of the lower rib so that the intercostal artery and nerve are not injured.

THORACOSTOMY

Thoracostomy is an opening made through the chest wall for the purpose of drainage. It may be a *closed* (interspace) or an *open* (rib resection) drainage. The indication for such drainage is usually empyema.

Closed Method. This is usually made in the 7th or 8th interspace in the midaxillary line or in line with the angle of the scapula. Procaine is injected at the selected site, and

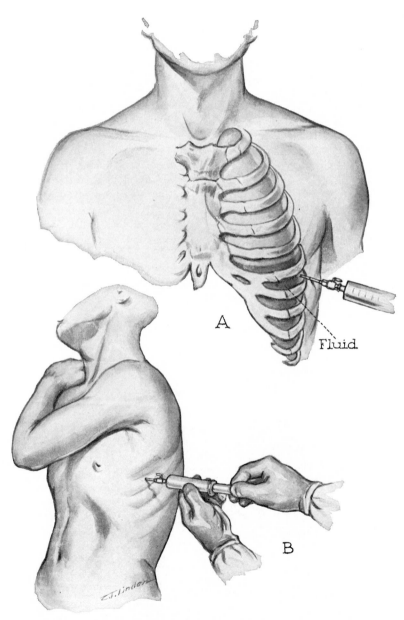

FIG. 205. Aspiration of the chest. (A) Diagrammatic presentation of the relation between the aspirating needle and the fluid level. (B) Aspiration in the midaxillary line.

a small stab incision is made (Fig. 206). A trocar is inserted just over the rib, thus avoiding the intercostal artery, vein and nerve which lie on the undersurface of the rib. This is advanced into the pleural space where the fluid is located. The obturator is withdrawn, and a catheter is inserted. Then the trocar is drawn over the catheter, which fits snugly and may be fixed by pins or a suture.

Open Method (Rib Resection) and Thoracoplasty. This method necessitates the resection of a piece of rib. The angle of the scapula is palpated, and then the patient's arm is elevated and placed to the opposite side. The rib immediately below this point is usually selected as the one suitable for resection (Fig. 207). If the rib above is chosen, the scapula may act as a shutter; if a rib much lower is selected, an inadvertent trans-

thoracic laparotomy may be performed. An incision is made directly over the rib selected, the soft tissues are divided to the periosteum, which is completely freed, and about 2 to 4 cm. of rib is removed. The pleural cavity is aspirated to make sure that pus is present. The aspirating needle may be left in place, and an incision is made adjacent to it. The cavity is explored, and then drainage is instituted.

In *chronic, nontuberculous empyema* the lung is compressed by intrapleural fluid. At times a draining sinus results. Radical surgical intervention is necessary. Even after evacuation of the pus, expansion of the lung is not possible, and a pleural dead space results which is difficult to obliterate. Two procedures have been advised which aim at approximating the lung surface and the chest wall, thus eliminating the dead space. The

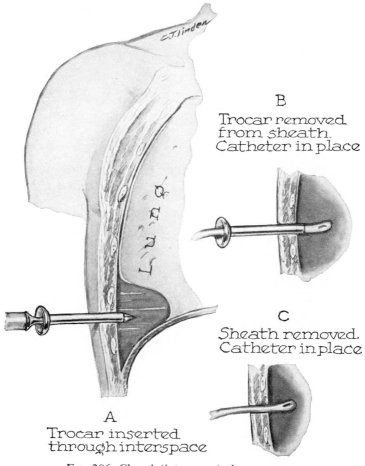

B
Trocar removed from sheath. Catheter in place

C
Sheath removed. Catheter in place

A
Trocar inserted through interspace

Fig. 206. Closed (interspace) thoracostomy.

first is *pulmonary decortication,* in which one attempts to mobilize the lung. If this is sufficiently accomplished, the lung gradually expands and fills the pleural cavity. The other procedure is *thoracoplasty,* which consists of subperiosteal removal of usually 6 ribs to permit the chest wall to fall in and meet the collapsed lung. This may be accomplished by either a posterior or an anterolateral approach (Fig. 208). Another method which has been utilized to obliterate such a cavity is the use of a muscle flap.

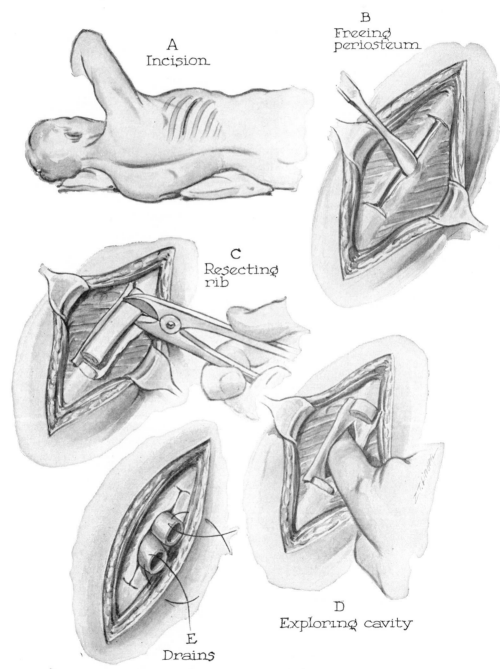

FIG. 207. Open (rib resection) thoracostomy.

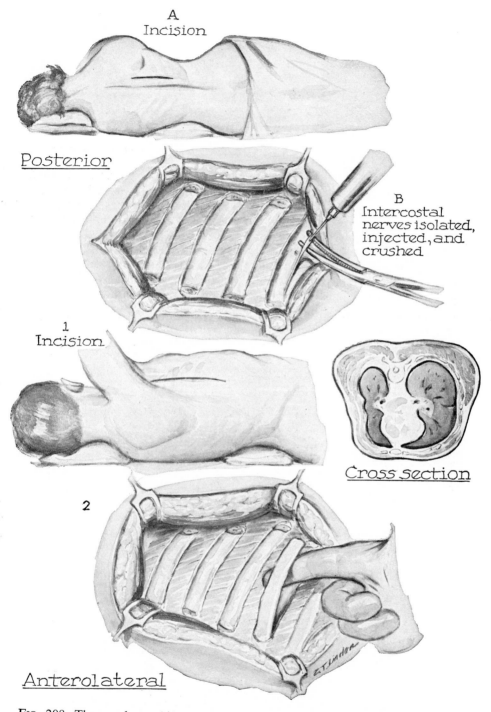

A
Incision

Posterior

B
Intercostal
nerves isolated,
injected, and
crushed

1
Incision

Cross section

2

Anterolateral

FIG. 208. Thoracoplasty. (A) and (B) show the posterior approach; (1) and (2) demonstrate the anterolateral approach. The cross section shows the effect of this procedure, which permits the chest wall to fall in and meet the collapsed lung.

Lungs (Pulmones)

EMBRYOLOGY

Embryologically, the pulmonary system arises as an outgrowth of the digestive tract. It begins as a small bud which grows from the ventral part of the pharynx (Fig. 209). The bud increases in length to form the trachea, which in turn divides into right and the left primary bronchi (Fig. 210). The ends of these bronchi continue to grow and divide until eventually a complex bronchial tree with the terminal alveoli is formed. At first, the pleural cavity is in direct communication with the abdominal cavity, the two together forming the celom. Later, these are separated by a transverse partition, the diaphragm.

THE LUNGS PROPER

The lungs are a pair of comparatively light organs which are conical in shape, each of which possesses an apex, a base, 2 surfaces, 3 borders (anterior, inferior and posterior) and a root. Although they lie within the pleural cavities, they do not fill all the available space during normal respiration. The weights of the ordinary, healthy adult lungs, containing the average amount of blood, are about 620 grams for the right lung and about 570 grams for the left. If the lungs are in a healthy state, they lie free in the pleural cavity and are attached at only 2 points: at their roots and at the pulmonary ligaments. However, healthy lungs are rarely found in dissecting rooms, since adhesions due to

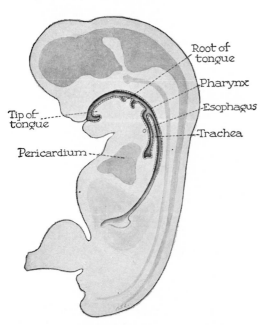

FIG. 209. Embryogenesis of the pulmonary system. This system arises as a bud from the ventral part of the digestive tract (pharynx).

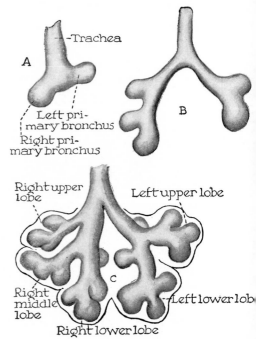

FIG. 210. Embryogenesis of the lungs.

pleurisy are usually present between the visceral and the parietal layers of pleura. The 2 lungs are not exactly symmetrical in shape because of the higher level of the diaphragm on the right, the projection of the heart to the left of the midline, and the impressions made by surrounding structures. At birth, the lungs are pinkish white, in adult life dark gray, and as age advances the mottling assumes a black color, due to carbonaceous deposits. As a rule the posterior border is darker than the anterior.

Apex. The apex of the lung is examined in the lower part of the neck because of the obliquity of the thoracic inlet (Fig. 211). It is rounded and rises into the root of the neck for about 1½ inches above the level of the anterior part of the 1st rib. It is situated behind and above the medial third of the clavicle and is crossed by the subclavian artery, which makes a groove on its anterior border slightly below its summit. The lung is separated from the artery by the pleura and a thin membrane known as Sibson's fascia (Fig. 174). The summit of the apex is in front of the neck of the 1st rib. The lung apex lies behind the clavicle, the anterior scalene muscle, the subclavian vessels and Sibson's fascia, which is attached along the inner border of the 1st rib and strengthens the pleura over the apex. The pleura in this region may be opened inadvertently during surgery near the subclavian vessels and also can be torn while removing deep-seated tumors from the depth of the neck. The pleura and the lungs may be injured in stab wounds of the neck or by fragments of bone in comminuted fractures of the clavicle.

Base. The base (diaphragmatic surface) is concave. The diaphragm separates it on the right side from the liver and on the left from the stomach, the liver and the spleen. Because the right dome of the diaphragm is higher and more convex than the left, the right lung is shorter, and its base is more concave. Laterally and behind, the base is

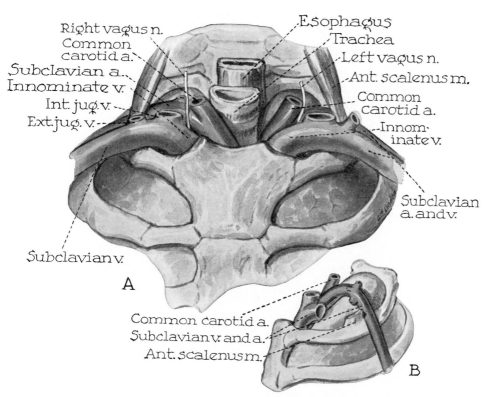

FIG. 211. The apex of the lung. This is associated with the root of the neck. The inset shows the subclavian artery crossing the apex.

bounded by a thin sharp margin which projects into the phrenocostal sinus of the pleura between the lower ribs and the costal attachments of the diaphragm.

SURFACES

The two surfaces of the lungs are the

costal surface and the medial (mediastinal).

The costal surface is smooth, convex and includes the bulky posterior part of the lung. It is related to the inner surfaces of the ribs, the costal cartilages, the intercostal spaces and, to a slight degree, the back of the sternum.

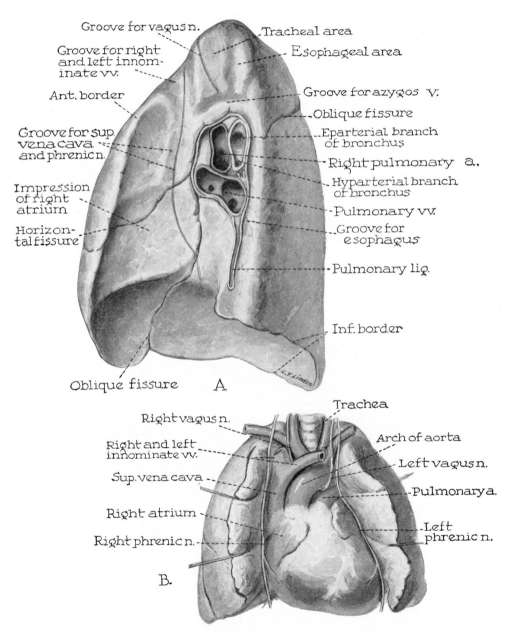

FIG. 212. The medial surface of the right lung. (A) Grooves and impressions made by structures in immediate contact with this surface, viewed from the left. (B) The lungs and the heart, seen from in front.

The medial surface of each lung is divided into anterior (mediastinal) and posterior (vertebral) parts. Both parts present different relationships on the 2 sides of the body and must be considered separately.

On the *right* side, the *hilum* is occupied by the eparterial and the hyparterial bronchi, the right pulmonary artery and the upper and the lower right pulmonary veins (Fig. 212 A). In the hilum, numerous lymph glands and nerves are also found. Below and in front of it, the mediastinal part presents a cardiac impression which is formed by the right atrium and a groove for the phrenic nerve. The superior vena cava is in contact with the right lung in front of the hilum, and

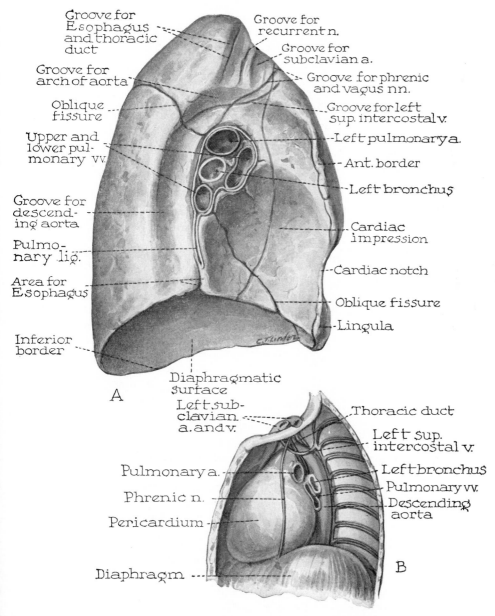

FIG. 213. The medial surface of the left lung. (A) Grooves made by structures in contact with the surface, viewed from the right. (B) The left thoracic cavity seen from the left.

the impression made by this vessel is continuous with the groove made by the right innominate vein above and the cardiac impression below (Fig. 212 B). Above the hilum a groove is sometimes visible which runs into the groove for the superior vena cava; it is produced by the vena azygos. The groove produced by the esophagus is found immediately behind this. The vertebral part of the medial surface of the right lung is in relation to the heads of the ribs, the sympathetic trunk, the vertebral bodies, the splanchnic nerve and the aortic intercostal arteries and veins.

On the *left* side, the hilum reveals a single left bronchus, the left pulmonary artery, upper and lower left pulmonary veins, numerous lymph glands and nerves. The ventricles of the heart produce a deep cardiac impression below and in front of the hilum (Fig. 213 A). The arch of the aorta passes backward above the root of the lung and is continuous behind the hilum, along with the groove produced by the descending thoracic aorta (Fig. 213 B). Above the groove for the aortic arch, the subclavian artery passes upward in contact with the lung and then turns laterally in front of the apex. The vertebral part of the medial surface of the left lung is grooved by the descending thoracic aorta which separates the lung from the bodies between the 4th to the 9th thoracic vertebrae. Other relationships in this area are the same as those described for the right lung.

BORDERS

The 3 borders of the lungs are the anterior, the inferior and the posterior (Figs. 212-213).

The anterior borders of the lungs are thin and sharp because they are squeezed between the body of the sternum and the pericardium. On the right side the border is straight and coincides with the costomediastinal line of pleural reflection. On the left side, however, the anterior border presents a deep notch opposite the 4th and the 5th intercostal spaces known as the *cardiac notch*. Here the border of the lung falls short of the sternum by about an inch, leaving part of the pericardium separated from the chest wall by pleura alone. This area which is unoccupied

by lung has been referred to as the "area of superficial cardiac dullness."

The inferior border separates the base of the lung from the costal and the medial surfaces. Laterally and behind, it is sharp and projects down to the upper part of the costodiaphragmatic recess. The inferior borders of both lungs are practically at the same level, and during quiet respiration they lie at a higher level than the costodiaphragmatic line of pleural reflection.

The posterior border is indistinct and rounded, due to the confluence of the medial and the costal surfaces which occupy the deep hollow of the thoracic cavity. It projects into the phrenocostal sinus.

FISSURES, LOBES, AND BRONCHOPULMONARY SEGMENTS

Oblique Fissure. Each lung presents a complete oblique fissure which passes through the costal, the diaphragmatic and the mediastinal surfaces as far as the root. This fissure crosses the posterior border about 2½ inches below the apex and the inferior border about 2 inches from the median plane.

Transverse Fissure. The right lung reveals a second fissure known as the transverse fissure. It runs horizontally at the level of the 4th costal cartilage and meets the oblique fissure in the midaxillary line. The left lung, therefore, is divided into two lobes, a superior and inferior, by the interlobar fissure (oblique); the right is divided into three lobes, superior, middle and inferior, by the two (oblique and transverse) interlobar fissures (Figs. 214-215).

The superior (upper) lobe lies above and in front of the oblique fissure and includes the apex, anterior border, a large part of the costal surface and the greater part of the mediastinal surface of the lung.

The inferior (lower) lobe is the larger of the two, and is situated below and behind the fissure. It includes almost all of the base, a large part of the costal surface, and the greater part of the posterior border.

Middle Lobe. In the right lung the middle lobe is the smallest. It is wedge-shaped and includes the lower part of the anterior border and the anterior part of the base of the lung. It lies in the front part of the thorax and is entirely anterior to the midaxillary line. The

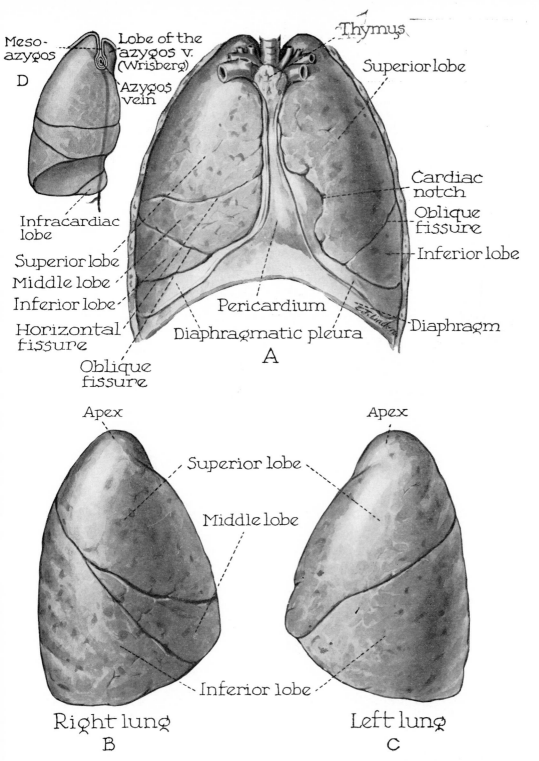

Meso-azygos

D

Lobe of the azygos v. (Wrisberg)

Azygos vein

Thymus

Superior lobe

Cardiac notch

Oblique fissure

Inferior lobe

Infracardiac lobe

Superior lobe

Middle lobe

Inferior lobe

Horizontal fissure

Pericardium

Diaphragmatic pleura

Diaphragm

Oblique fissure

A

Apex

Apex

Superior lobe

Middle lobe

Inferior lobe

Right lung

B

Left lung

C

FIG. 214. Lobes and fissures of the lungs. (A) Front view; the usual arrangement of 3 lobes on the right and 2 lobes on the left is shown. (B) The right lung seen from the right side. (C) The left lung seen from the left side. (D) The 2 accessory lobes which may be found associated with the right lung. The infracardiac lobe is constant in quadrupeds, but in man the pericardium fuses with the diaphragm and suppresses its development. The lobe of the azygos vein (Wrisberg) is also shown.

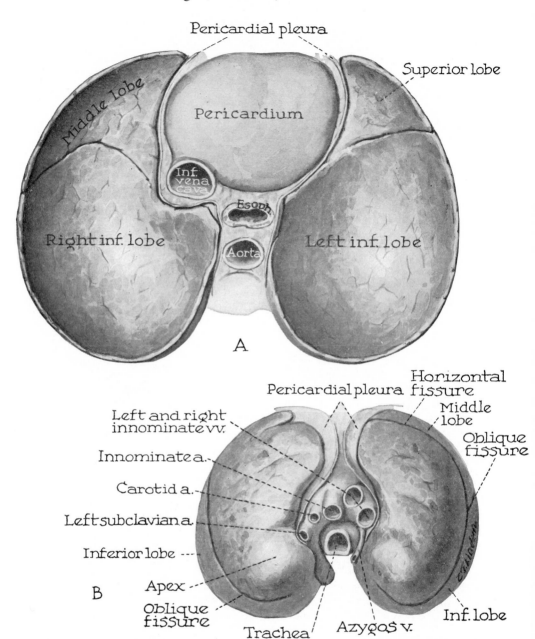

FIG. 215. Lobes and fissures of the lungs. (A) Seen from below. The relationship of the middle lobe on the right and the superior lobe on the left should be noted; (B) seen from above. The relationship of fissures to lobes is shown.

cardiac notch is formed by a deficiency of the upper lobe of the left lung.

Bronchopulmonary Segments. The lobes are subdivided into smaller units called bronchopulmonary segments which may be defined as the area of distribution of a bronchus. The various descriptions of the anatomy of the tracheobronchial tree have

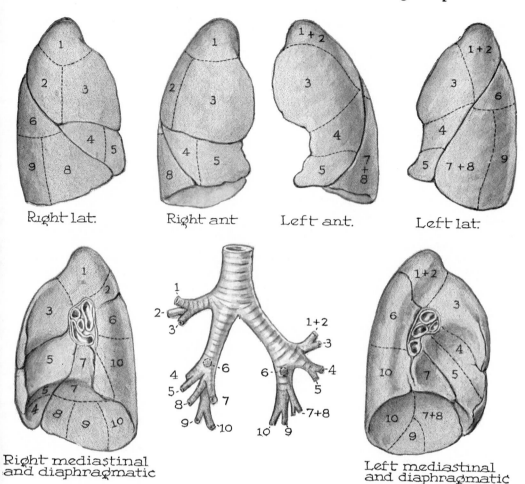

Right lat.   Right ant   Left ant.   Left lat.

Right mediastinal
and diaphragmatic

Left mediastinal
and diaphragmatic

FIG. 216. Nomenclature for the lungs and the bronchi (After Jackson and Huber). The numbers in parentheses relate to the numbers on the illustration. The lobes are divided into smaller units called bronchopulmonary segments, each of which is determined by the area of distribution of a bronchus. The *right lung* presents 3 lobes; upper, middle and lower. The upper has been colored blue, the middle yellow and the lower red. The upper lobe has 3 segments: (1) apical, (2) posterior and (3) anterior. The middle lobe has 2 segments: lateral (4) and medial (5). The lower lobe consists of 5 segments: superior (6), medial basal (7), anterior basal (8), lateral basal (9) and posterior basal (10). The *left lung* is divided into 2 lobes: an upper, colored blue, and a lower, colored red. The upper lobe is divided into 2 divisions: upper and lower (lingular). The upper division has 2 bronchopulmonary segments: they are known as the apical, which is also called the apical posterior (1 and 2) and an anterior (3). The lingular division also has 2 segments: superior (4) and inferior (5). The left lower lobe segments are similar to those on the right except that the medial basal is a branch of the anterior basal rather than a separate branch of the lower lobe bronchus. The term "anterior-medial basal" (7 and 8) is used to call attention to this fact. The other numerical representations are the same as those of the right side. The colors and the numbers which have been used on the bronchi correspond to the colors and the numbers of the individual bronchopulmonary segments.

resulted in much confusion; hence, we have chosen the nomenclature used by Jackson and Huber which seems to be acceptable to the surgeon, the bronchoscopist, the radiologist and the anatomist (Fig. 216). It may be listed as shown at the bottom of the page:

At times, 2 branches which generally constitute separate major segmental bronchi may have a common trunk. This would explain the variation in descriptions of the right upper lobe which is described as having 4 segments by some and by others as having only 3. Since fissures may be quite inconstant, it is far better to subdivide the lungs according to bronchial distribution.

The *right lung* usually presents 3 lobes: upper, middle and lower. The upper lobe consists of 3 segments: apical, posterior and anterior. The middle lobe has 2 segments: lateral and medial. The lower lobe has 5 segments which are known as the superior, the medial basal, the anterior basal, the lateral basal and the posterior basal.

The *left lung* usually consists of 2 lobes: upper and lower. Moreover, the upper lobe has 2 subdivisions which are known as the upper and the lower divisions. The lower division of the upper lobe is also called the *lingular division.* Two segments make up the upper division; these are known as the apical (apical-posterior) and the anterior. The lingular division is made up of 2 segments: superior and inferior. In the left lower lobe the segments are similar to those on the right, except that the medial basal is a branch of the anterior basal rather than a separate branch of the lower lobe bronchus. It has been suggested that the term anterior-medial basal be used to call attention to this fact.

VARIATIONS

Variations are found in the number of lobes of the lungs which may be either decreased or increased. The right upper and middle lobes may be fused, and the left lung may have 1 or even 3 lobes. The right lung sometimes has 5, since 2 accessory lobes may be associated with the 3 usual ones.

Infracardiac Lobe. One such accessory lobe is the infracardiac lobe, which is constant in quadrupeds; in these animals it separates the pericardium from the diaphragm (Fig. 214 D). In man, since the pericardium fuses with the diaphragm, the infracardiac lobe is completely suppressed.

Lobe of the Azygos Vein. The most important accessory lobe is the so-called lobe of the azygos vein (Wrisberg). The azygos vein travels upward in front of the vertebral column, arches forward above the root of the lung and ends in the superior vena cava before the latter pierces the pericardium. Therefore, the arch of the azygos vein crosses laterally in respect to the esophagus, the trachea and the right vagus nerve. During development, the right lung bud has to pass outward under the arch formed by the anterior end of the future azygos vein (right posterior cardinal vein). If the lung bud does not clear it, part of the lung remains lateral and part medial to it. Therefore, the vein becomes embedded in the developing lung tissue, and

RIGHT LUNG		LEFT LUNG	
LOBES	SEGMENTS	LOBES	SEGMENTS
Upper	{ Apical { Posterior { Anterior	*Upper* — Upper Division	{ Apical-posterior { Anterior
Middle	{ Lateral { Medial	*Upper* — Lower (Lingular) Division	{ Superior { Inferior
Lower	{ Superior { Medial Basal { Anterior Basal { Lateral Basal { Posterior Basal	*Lower*	{ Superior { Anterior-medial { Basal { Lateral Basal { Posterior Basal

the part medial to it becomes the lobe of the azygos vein (Fig. 214 D). This condition was first described by Wrisberg in 1717. When the apex of the right lung is split by the arch of the azygos vein, a bifid apex results. The vein is suspended by a pleural "mesentery" which is referred to as a double pleural septum or "meso-azygos." If this is seen on the roentgenogram, the meso-azygos appears as a fine line running from the apex of the lung downward with the convexity outward as it approaches the mediastinum at about the level of the 2nd costal cartilage. This line ends in a small, dense, pea-sized shadow, which represents the azygos vein (Fig. 217). Such an accessory lobe is important to identify, since it might cause confusion in the interpretation of a roentgenogram, in pulmonary surgery, or during postmortem examinations. It may form the entire apex of the lung, part of it, or may be entirely disassociated from it, depending on the location of the vein.

Root of the Lung
(Radix Pulmonis)

The root of the lung is a short but broad pedicle consisting of 3 essential structures, the pulmonary artery, pulmonary veins and bronchi. Associated with these are the bronchial vessels, nerves and lymph glands.

Pulmonary Ligament. This ligament (p. 272) is also considered with the root. Although there are some differences in the right and the left roots, it is well to remember that the bronchi lie posterior to the vessels, and the pulmonary veins usually lie below the corresponding right or left pulmonary arteries. Many anomalies in this region have been recorded.

The right root has the following boundaries (Fig. 212): anteriorly, the superior vena cava and the phrenic nerve; superiorly, the arch of the azygos vein; posteriorly, the azygos vein proper.

The left root is bounded in the following way (Fig. 213): anteriorly, by the phrenic nerve; superiorly, by the aortic arch; posteriorly, by the descending thoracic aorta. It might help to recall that on the right side, an inverted "U" is formed by the phrenic nerve and the azygos vein, while on the left side, a similar inverted "U" is formed by the phrenic nerve and aorta. The structures of each root are bound together by connective tissue and pleura which surround them like a cuff.

Blood Vessels

Much has been written about the variations of the bronchovascular patterns (Boyden *et al.*) and the variations of the origin, the course and the distribution of the bron-

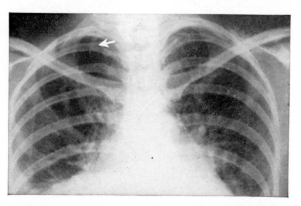

Fig. 217. Azygos lobe seen on a roentgenogram. The apex of the right lung is split by the arch of the azygos vein. Since the vein is suspended by pleural "mesentery," a meso-azygos results; this appears as a fine line running from the apex downward, with its convexity outward (see arrow). It ends in a small dense pea-sized shadow which represents the azygos vein.

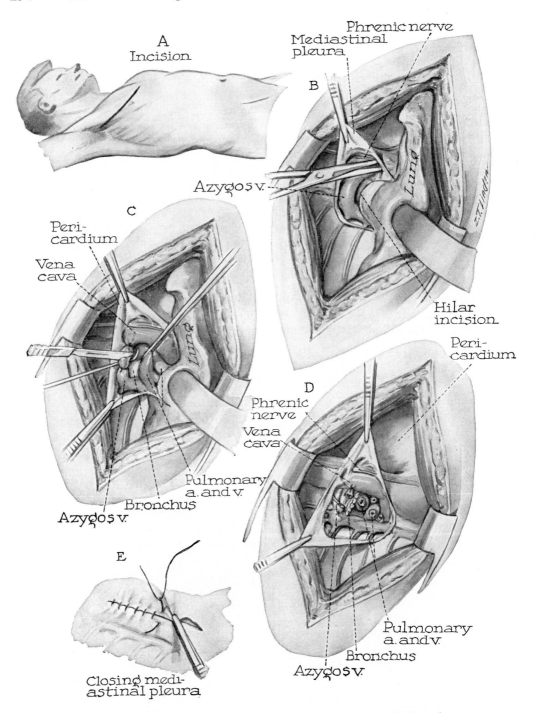

Fig. 218. Pneumonectomy (right side). (A) Anterior approach through a transverse incision over the 3rd intercostal space. (B) Exposure of hilar structures by incising the mediastinal pleura anteriorly and superiorly. (C) Ligation and division of the azygos vein. (D) Ligation and division of hilar structures followed by removal of the lung. (E) Pleuralization.

chial arteries (Cauldwell *et al.*). Such works may be consulted for detailed study; however, the following description presents the most commonly accepted basic concepts.

The pulmonary veins, usually 2 on each side consisting of an upper and a lower, return oxygenated blood to the heart. Two main venous trunks from each lung open into the left atrium on its lateral border.

The pulmonary artery, after leaving the right ventricle, passes superiorly for about 4 cm. and a little to the left of the ascending aorta. The right branch goes to the right lung behind the aorta, and the left branch to the left lung in the concavity of the aortic arch (Fig. 221). In the lung pedicle, the right divides into 2 branches, and the left remains single. These vessels end in a capillary network over the alveolar tissues carrying the impure venous blood from the right ventricle to the lung. A thrombus of the right side of the heart of systemic venous origin can release an embolism which blocks a branch of the pulmonary artery, causing a suppression of part of the lung. A pulmonary infarct may result which might degenerate and become a pulmonary abscess.

The bronchi are easily identified by the film, elastic, fibrocartilaginous plates. On the right side there is an additional bronchus

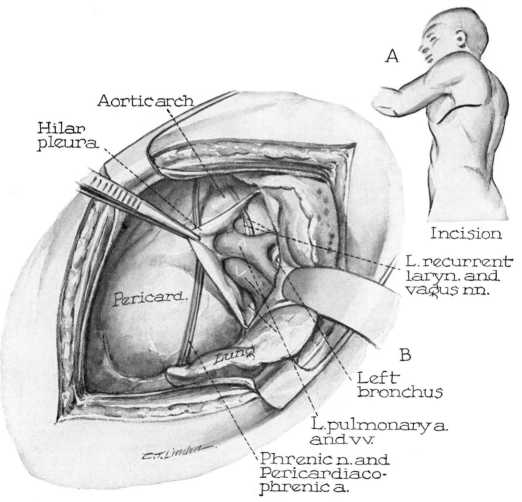

A

Aortic arch

Hilar pleura

Incision

L. recurrent laryn. and vagus nn.

Pericard.

Lung

B

Left bronchus

L. pulmonary a. and vv.

C.T.Linden

Phrenic n. and Pericardiaco- phrenic a.

Fig. 219. Pneumonectomy (left side): (A) incision, (B) isolation of hilar structures.

which receives the name of the *eparterial bronchus,* because it is at a higher level than the artery. This is in contradistinction to the hyparterial bronchi which are found on both sides below the pulmonary artery. The cuff or sleeve of pleura which surrounds these structures is quite narrow in its inferior or lower portion because it is traversed only by a few lymph vessels and, therefore, remains collapsed; its anterior and posterior walls are applied to each other and form the pulmonary ligament.

The bronchial arteries which supply the lung stroma are found on the posterior surfaces of the bronchi; they arise from the aorta or from an intercostal artery and pass behind the bronchi. Bronchial veins accompany them.

SURGICAL CONSIDERATIONS

PNEUMONECTOMY

Nissen, Overholt, Rienhoff, Graham and Alton Ochsner have pioneered in pneumonectomy and have shown the advisability of performing this operation for primary pulmonary malignancies. Several types of incisions may be employed, the choice depending upon the presence or the absence of adhesions, and the location of the pathology (Figs. 218-219). Some surgeons think that anatomic planes exist in the pulmonary hilus, and they state that a venous plane is found more superficially than an arterial plane or a bronchial plane. However, there are so many variations in the hilar structures that the method is not practical, especially since the inferior pulmonary vein may often be the most posterior structure.

The anterior approach usually consists of a transverse incision over the 3rd intercostal space extending from the lateral border of the sternum to the anterior axillary line (Fig. 218). The pectoral muscles are divided and the pleural cavity entered through the third intercostal space. Greater exposure can be gained by separating the 3rd and 4th ribs after disarticulating their costochondral junctions, and by ligating the internal mammary vessels both above and below. The pleural cavity is opened, and adhesions are divided by sharp dissection. The hilar structures are exposed in the mediastinum by incising the

mediastinal pleura, anteriorly and superiorly. The phrenic nerve may be crushed by an artery forceps. This facilitates surgery and also aids the early postoperative course. It is important to isolate and ligate the hilar structures individually and not by mass ligations. On the right side, the isolation, the ligation and the division of the azygos vein is the first structure to be dealt with; it extends over the right main bronchus. Then the pulmonary artery is isolated, doubly ligated and divided. The bronchus is usually ligated next, but it may be necessary to isolate, transfix, ligate and divide the superior pulmonary vein first. Then the bronchus is freed, ligated and divided; usually it is closed by interrupted sutures. The short inferior pulmonary vein is next found, transfixed, ligated and severed. The posterior mediastinal pleura is then incised, and the lung is removed. The edges of the divided mediastinal pleura are approximated, covering the stumps of the ligated hilar structures. When a large amount of mediastinal pleura has been extirpated, it might be necessary to utilize the adjacent pericardium to cover the ligated stump. The thoracic wall is closed in layers by passing heavy nonabsorbable sutures around the adjacent ribs. Following this, the pleura and the intercostal muscles are approximated, either with or without drainage. A posterolateral approach is preferred by some surgeons.

LOBECTOMY AND PULMONARY SEGMENTAL RESECTION

Both of these procedures have been used for such conditions as bronchiectasis, pulmonary tuberculosis, chronic lung abscesses and metastatic lesions. Clagett and Deterling have described a technic of lingulectomy in bronchiectasis. Churchill and Belsey, and Overholt and Langer have stressed the importance of pulmonary segmental resection. They state that bronchiectasis is a segmental disease and rarely involves an entire lobe. Nelson stressed the point that each bronchopulmonary segment possesses an independent bronchovascular structure and is separated from adjacent pulmonary tissue by an avascular cleavage plane. Therefore, segmental resection not only eradicates all of the diseased tissue, but also spares the uninvolved segment.

Lung Abscess

A nontuberculous lung abscess is a circumscribed pyogenic infection of the lung. It is usually associated with a history of tonsillectomy or aspiration of a foreign body such as teeth, peanuts, etc. Fusiform bacilli, Vincent's spirochetes and streptococci may be aspirated with the foreign body or blood. The right lower lobe is most commonly involved.

Treatment may be instituted in one of 3 ways: intercostal drainage, costectomy with drainage, or a 2-stage operation.

Intercostal drainage is accomplished by means of an incision made parallel with the overlying muscle fibers which are separated and retracted. The incision is extended through the intercostal muscles and to the parietal pleura. Evidence of motion of the lung is noted. If the pleura is thickened, and if normal gliding movements of the lung cannot be seen, one concludes that the visceral and parietal pleurae have become adherent by adhesions, and opening of the abscess is safe. If adhesions have not been formed between the pleural surfaces, the operation is interrupted, and the wound is packed with gauze to promote the formation of adhesions. After a week or 10 days, pleural adhesions are usually present in sufficient amount to protect the pleural cavity from contamination, and then the abscess opened. An aspirating needle usually locates the abscess first, and when pus is found, the needle is followed with a scalpel or a cautery into the abscess cavity. Then drainage is instituted.

Costectomy with drainage is usually the operation of choice, since it provides adequate drainage. The abscess is located by several roentgenograms, and the skin incision is placed as close to the pathology as possible. A section of rib is resected, usually from 5 to 8 cm. long, which overlies the abscess. The pleura is exposed, and if the pleurae are adherent, the abscess is entered; if not, a 2-stage operation is performed.

The 2-stage operation with rib resection is considered by many to be a safer procedure. The periosteum is stripped from 2 or 3 ribs for a distance of 8 or 10 cm. The middle one of these 3 ribs is resected. The periosteum is raised from the 2 adjacent ribs which will be resected later. Gauze is packed beneath the denuded rib to form adhesions between the visceral and the parietal pleurae. At the end of 7 to 10 days, the wound is reopened; the abscess is located with a needle and entered. Then drainage is instituted.

Trachea and Extrapulmonary Bronchi

THE TRACHEA PROPER

The trachea begins where the larynx ends, that is, at the lower border of the cricoid cartilage which is on a level with the 7th cervical vertebra (Fig. 220). It is from 4 to 5 inches long, half of which is in the neck (cervical portion), and the other half in the thorax (thoracic portion). The trachea enters the thoracic inlet opposite the upper border of the manubrium sterni and ends at its lower border (Fig. 220 A and 220 B); the latter point is situated on a level between the 3rd and the 4th thoracic spines, where it divides into right and left primary bronchi. Its thoracic portion is opposite the manubrium and wholly within the superior mediastinum. It occupies the median plane except at its lower end where the aortic arch pushes it slightly to the right. About 15 or 20 horseshoe-shaped rings of hyaline cartilage keep its lumen open and support the lateral and anterior aspects, but they are deficient posteriorly where the wall is flattened. The posterior portion is closed by the *trachealis muscle,* which is made up of transverse plain fibers supplied by the recurrent laryngeal nerve (Fig. 220 C). Anteriorly, the trachea is crossed by the isthmus of the thyroid (2nd to 4th ring), and below that structure it is related to the inferior thyroid veins which pass downward upon it, frequently communicating with each other and opening into the innominate veins. In young children, the left innominate vein may appear above the level of the manubrium sterni, forming an anterior relation of the trachea.

RELATIONS

Posteriorly, the trachea is in contact with the esophagus. *Anteriorly,* in the neck, the isthmus of the thyroid gland covers the 2nd, the 3rd and the 4th tracheal rings (Figs. 220-221). In its lower part, it is crossed by the arch of the aorta, with the deep cardiac plexus intervening. Also in front of the trachea are the roots of the innominate and the left common carotid arteries which separate it from the left innominate vein. As these 2 arteries travel upward they diverge, and in the interval which is made by this divergence, the remains of the thymus gland are found. More anteriorly, the manubrium sterni is situated with the lower part of the sternohyoid and the sternothyroid muscles which arise from the back of it.

On the *right side,* the trachea is in relation to the right pleura and lung, the right vagus nerve and the arch of the azygos vein. In the neck, it is related to the right lobe of the thyroid gland from the commencement of the trachea to the 6th ring. The right recurrent laryngeal nerve passes along its lateral posterior aspect.

On the *left side,* it is related to the left common carotid and the subclavian arteries, the phrenic and the vagus nerves, and the lower part of the arch of the aorta where it is separated from the left pleura and lung. The left recurrent laryngeal nerve has the same relationship as the right. Many tracheobronchial lymph glands are associated with the trachea at its bifurcation: the paratracheal glands lie on each side of it in the superior mediastinum.

RIGHT AND LEFT EXTRAPULMONARY BRONCHI

The bronchi diverge from each other on

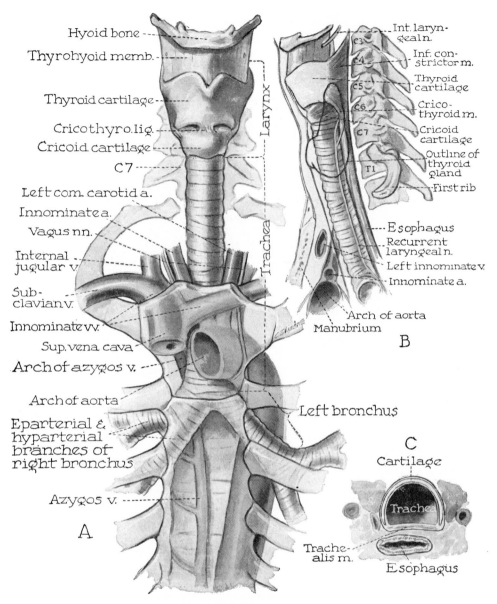

Hyoid bone

Thyrohyoid memb.

Thyroid cartilage

Cricothyro.lig.

Cricoid cartilage

C7

Left com. carotid a.

Innominate a.

Vagus nn.

Internal jugular v.

Sub-clavian v.

Innominate vv.

Sup. vena cava

Arch of azygos v.

Arch of aorta

Eparterial & hyparterial branches of right bronchus

Azygos v.

A

Larynx

Trachea

Int. laryn-geal n.

Inf. con-strictor m.

Thyroid cartilage

Crico-thyroid m.

Cricoid cartilage

Outline of thyroid gland

First rib

Esophagus

Recurrent laryngeal n.

Left innominate v.

Innominate a.

Arch of aorta

Manubrium

B

Left bronchus

C

Cartilage

Trachea

Trache-alis m.

Esophagus

FIG. 220. The trachea and the extrapulmonary bronchi: (A) relations as seen from in front; (B) viewed from the left side; (C) the trachealis muscle seen in cross section.

their way to the roots of the lungs, and differ in size, length and the direction in which they run.

The right bronchus is shorter, wider and more vertical. Because of this, foreign bodies from the trachea usually pass to the right side. It is about 1 inch long and, since it supplies the larger lung, is larger in size. Anterior to it are the right pulmonary artery,

the pericardium, the lower part of the superior vena cava and the ascending aorta. The arch of the azygos vein is placed above, and the bronchial vessels and the posterior pulmonary plexus are posterior. The upper pulmonary vein is anterior; the lower pulmonary vein is below. The right bronchus gives off a branch which is called the *eparterial branch,* so named because it arises above the

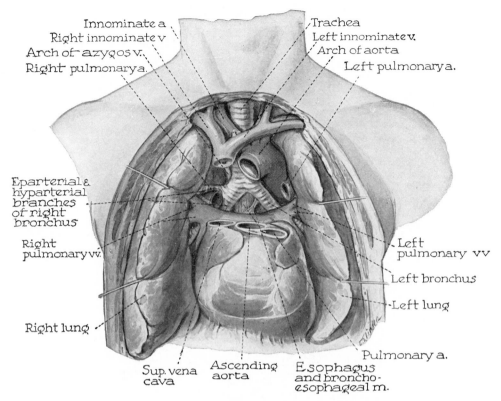

Innominate a
Right innominate v
Arch of azygos v.
Right pulmonary a.

Trachea
Left innominate v.
Arch of aorta
Left pulmonary a.

Eparterial &
hyparterial
branches
of right
bronchus

Right
pulmonary vv.

Left
pulmonary vv

Left bronchus

Left lung

Right lung

Pulmonary a.

Sup. vena
cava

Ascending
aorta

Esophagus
and broncho-
esophageal m.

FIG. 221. The relations of the trachea and primary bronchi. The eparterial and the hyparterial branches of the right bronchus have been identified. A broncho-esophageal muscle was present in this specimen.

right pulmonary artery; it passes to the upper lobe of the right lung. The bronchus continues as the *hyparterial branch* which passes below the artery and divides into two, one branch for the middle lobe and one for the lower (Fig. 221).

The left bronchus has farther to travel than the right, since the left lung hilum is farther from the median plane. Therefore, it is nearly twice as long as the right and less vertical. The arch of the aorta passes backward and over it, and the descending thoracic aorta runs downward and behind it. Anteriorly,

are the left pulmonary artery and the pericardium, which separate the bronchus from the left atrium. The posterior pulmonary plexus, the esophagus and the bronchial vessels are situated behind this bronchus. Occasionally, a muscle band exists between the esophagus and the left bronchus; this is called the *broncho-esophageal muscle.*

The carina is a sagittal spur located at the margin of the primary bronchus. It is easily seen through the bronchoscope as it passes upward into the lumen. It is employed as a landmark by the bronchoscopist.

Mediastinum
(Interpleural Space)

BOUNDARIES OF THE MEDIASTINA

The mediastinum is the middle compartment of the chest which is situated between the 2 pleural cavities. Its boundaries are (Fig. 222): anterior, the sternum; posterior,

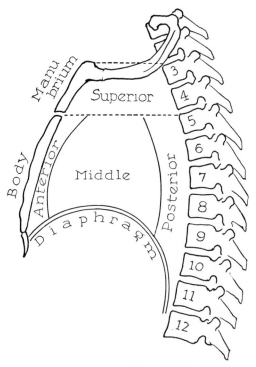

FIG. 222. Diagrammatic sagittal section of the mediastinum. An imaginary line which extends from the sternal angle to the disk between the 4th and the 5th thoracic vertebrae divides the mediastinum into superior and inferior mediastina. The inferior mediastinum is divided by the heart into anterior, middle and posterior mediastina.

the bodies of the 12 thoracic vertebrae; superior, the thoracic inlet; inferior, the diaphragm. The sides are formed by the mediastinal pleurae. It is divided into superior and inferior mediastina by an imaginary line which extends from the sternal angle (manubriosternal joint) to the disk between the 4th and the 5th thoracic vertebrae. The inferior mediastinum is subdivided into 3 mediastina by the heart, which acts as the key structure in this subdivision. That part of the inferior mediastinum which contains the heart is called the middle mediastinum; that part in front of it makes up the anterior, and the part situated behind the heart constitutes the posterior mediastinum.

Each of the 4 mediastina have their own boundaries.

Superior. The superior mediastinum boundaries are: superior, the thoracic inlet; inferior, an imaginary line extending from the sternal angle to the disk between the 4th and the 5th thoracic vertebrae; anterior, the manubrium sterni; posterior, the bodies of the upper 4 thoracic vertebrae.

Anterior. The anterior mediastinum boundaries are: superior, the imaginary line separating it from the superior mediastinum; inferior, the diaphragm; anterior, the body of the sternum; posterior, the anterior aspect of the pericardium.

Middle. The middle mediastinum boundaries are: superior and inferior, the same as the anterior mediastinum; anterior, the anterior part of the pericardium; posterior, the posterior part of the pericardium.

Posterior. The posterior mediastinum boundaries are: superior, same as the anterior and the middle mediastina; inferior, same as the anterior and the middle mediastina; anterior, the posterior aspect of the pericardium; posterior, the bodies of the lower 8th thoracic vertebrae.

CHIEF CONTENTS OF EACH MEDIASTINAL SPACE

The superior mediastinum contains: the arch of the aorta and its 3 branches (innominate, left common carotid and left subclavian arteries); the innominate veins; the upper half of the superior vena cava; the vagus, the phrenic and the left recurrent nerves; the esophagus, the trachea and the thoracic duct; the thymus or its remains in the adult with some lymph glands (Figs. 223 and 224).

The anterior mediastinum contains a few lymph glands (anterior mediastinal glands) and a little areolar tissue.

The middle mediastinum contains: the

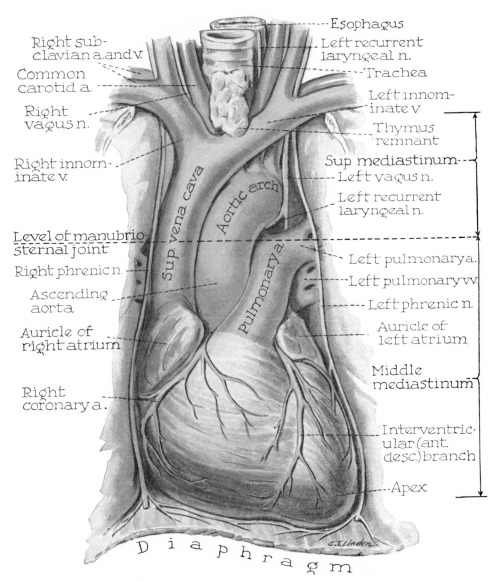

FIG. 223. Contents of the superior and the middle mediastina viewed from in front.

heart enclosed in the pericardium; the ascending aorta; the lower half of the superior vena cava (with the azygos vein entering it); the bifurcation of the trachea; the pulmonary artery dividing into right and left branches; the right and the left pulmonary veins; the

phrenic nerves; the bronchial lymph glands.

The posterior mediastinum contains: the esophagus; the descending thoracic aorta; the vagi; the thoracic duct; the azygos; the hemiazygos and the accessory hemiazygos veins (Fig. 225).

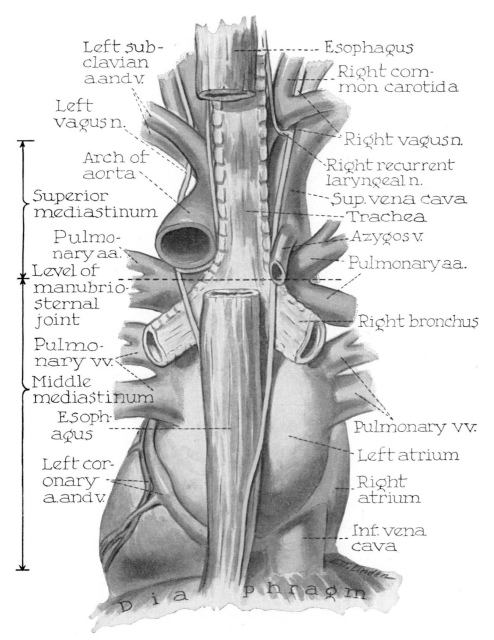

Left sub-clavian a.and v.

Left vagus n.

Arch of aorta

Superior mediastinum

Pulmonary aa.

Level of manubrio-sternal joint

Pulmonary vv.

Middle mediastinum

Esophagus

Left coronary a.and v.

Esophagus

Right common carotid a

Right vagus n.

Right recurrent laryngeal n.

Sup. vena cava

Trachea

Azygos v.

Pulmonary aa.

Right bronchus

Pulmonary vv.

Left atrium

Right atrium

Inf. vena cava

Diaphragm

FIG. 224. Contents of the superior and the middle mediastina viewed from behind.

SURGICAL CONSIDERATIONS

DRAINAGE OF MEDIASTINAL ABSCESS

Most mediastinal abscesses (mediastinitis) are drained through a right supraclavicular incision which is made in a transverse direction (Fig. 226 A). This is deepened between the thyroid gland and the trachea medially, and the carotid sheath and the sterno-cleidomastoid muscle laterally. A finger is in-

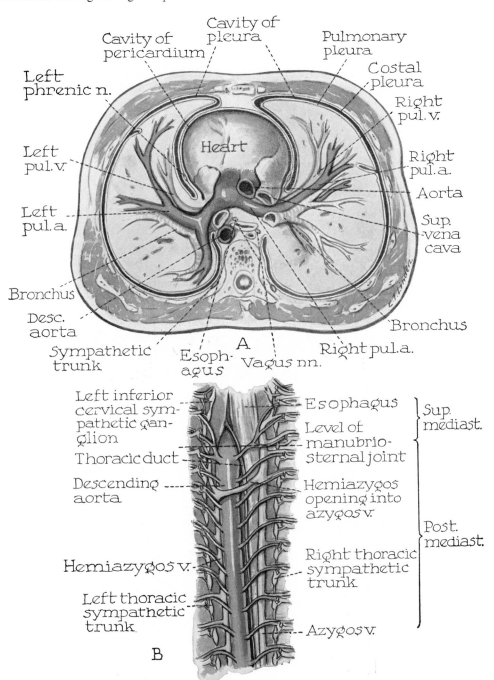

FIG. 225. Contents of the posterior mediastinum: (A) cross section; (B) seen from behind.

troduced along the right side of the esophagus and follows this downward until the abscess is reached and opened (Fig. 226 B). Rarely is it necessary to perform an anterior or posterior mediastinotomy.

CARCINOMA OF THE ESOPHAGUS

Carcinoma of the midthoracic esophagus has been treated quite successfully by Churchill, Garlock, Sweet and others. The lesion has been eradicated successfully by radical resection with high intrathoracic esophagogastrostomy. The essential steps in the operation are as follows (Fig. 227):

The usual incision is placed at the left costal margin anteriorly; it extends posteriorly over the 8th or the 9th rib and then curves upward for a short distance between the spine and the left scapula. The 8th or the

9th rib is resected. If greater exposure is necessary, the 5th, the 6th, or the 7th ribs are divided posteriorly.

The left thoracic cavity is entered, the mediastinal pleura is incised, and dissection is begun anterior to the esophagus. Resectability depends on whether or not the growth has invaded the left main bronchus, the aortic arch or the inferior pulmonary vein. If these structures can be mobilized safely, dissection posterior to the esophagus is begun.

The posterior dissection is left until last, to avoid interfering with the blood supply, resulting from the division of the esophageal arteries arising from the aorta. When the posterior dissection is completed, the tumor is freed from the right mediastinal pleura.

The esophagus is mobilized from the aortic

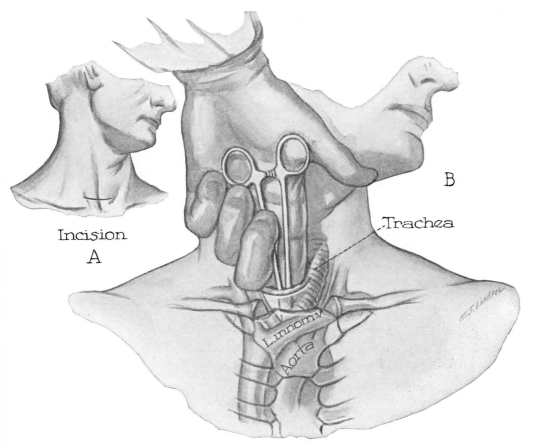

FIG. 226. Drainage of a mediastinal abscess: (A) right supraclavicular transverse incision; (B) the abscess is sought in a space between the trachea medially and the carotid sheath laterally.

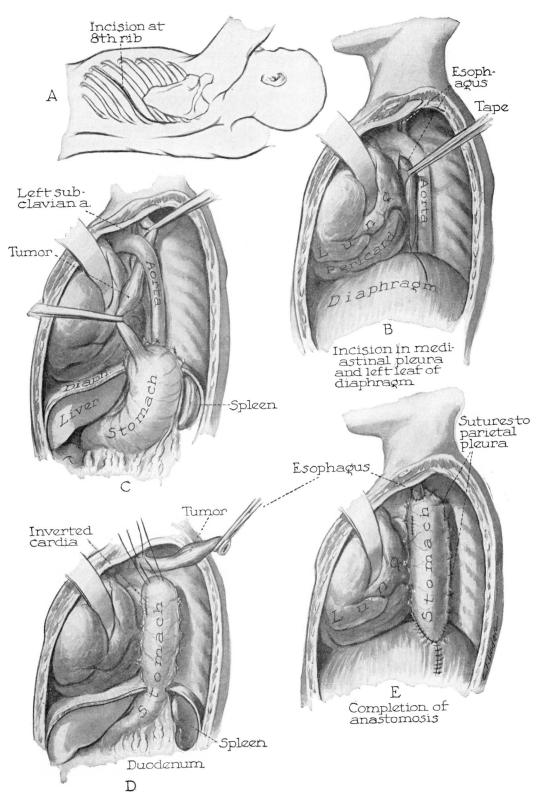

A — Incision at 8th rib

B — Esophagus / Tape / Aorta / Lung / Pericard / Diaphragm
Incision in mediastinal pleura and left leaf of diaphragm

C — Left subclavian a. / Tumor / Aorta / Diaph. / Liver / Stomach / Spleen

D — Inverted cardia / Tumor / Esophagus / Stomach / Spleen / Duodenum

E — Esophagus / Sutures to parietal pleura / Lung / Stomach
Completion of anastomosis

FIGURE 227. (*Caption on facing page.*)

arch downward, and the abdomen is entered through an incision in the diaphragm which extends from the esophageal hiatus to the insertion at the costal margin. Phrenic nerve crushing immobilizes the diaphragm. The greater curvature of the stomach is mobilized by dividing the gastrolienal ligament and ligating the left gastroepiploic vessels and vasa brevia. The gastrocolic omentum is divided as far as the pylorus, but the right gastric and gastroepiploic vessels are protected. In the region of the lower esophagus and cardia, it may be necessary to ligate branches of the superior suprarenal, inferior phrenic and pericardiophrenic vessels.

Next, the gastrohepatic ligament is severed and occasionally a hepatic branch of the right inferior phrenic artery is found in this structure. The left gastric vessels are ligated. The stomach is divided distal to the cardia, and the distal portion is inverted with sutures. An incision is made in the mediastinal pleura above the aortic arch, and the attachments of the esophagus behind the arch are freed. These are usually small vessels which arise from the aorta and the bronchial arteries.

When the esophagus has been fully mobilized, it may be pulled up from behind the aortic arch and prepared for the anastomosis. The esophagus and the tumor are resected, and the anastomosis is completed. To relieve tension on the anastomotic suture line, interrupted sutures fix the stomach to the parietal pleura and the diaphragm, which is closed. The stomach now receives its blood supply from the right gastric and the right gastroepiploic arteries.

If the anastomosis is placed below the aortic arch, an adequate blood supply to the esophagus is maintained by the small arteries from the aorta and the bronchial vessels. However, if it is necessary to dissect the esophagus above the aortic arch, the blood supply is entirely dependent on the descending branches from the inferior thyroid artery. The thoracic duct may be encountered or injured in these high dissections; it is important to ligate this structure to prevent a leakage of chyle.

Ivor Lewis states that carcinoma in the middle third of the esophagus should be approached through a *right* transpleural route. His reasons for this are the following:

This offers easier accessibility; only the vena azygos major requires ligating; and the aortic arch, instead of being an obstacle, becomes a safety barrier between the surgeon and the opposite pleural cavity. Therefore, he concludes that to operate on this part of the esophagus through the left side is unanatomic.

His operation is usually performed in 2 stages. The first stage is done through an upper left paramedian incision, the abdomen being carefully explored. If there are no metastases on the greater curvature of the stomach, this structure is mobilized as has been described above. A jejunostomy is done to improve the patient's nutrition. From 10 to 15 days later, the second stage is accomplished by removing the right 6th rib and entering the chest. The vena azygos major is divided, and the procedure progresses much in the same way as has been described. Lewis claims that the cardia of the stomach can be delivered readily into the right thoracic cavity.

TRANSTHORACIC SUPRADIAPHRAGMATIC SECTION OF THE VAGUS NERVES (VAGECTOMY, VAGOTOMY)

Dragstedt and others have advocated this procedure (Fig. 228) as a therapeutic measure for duodenal ulcers in the absence of pyloric stenosis, gastrojejunal ulcers and gastric ulcers where the diagnosis is certain.

The incision is placed over the 8th rib on the left side, and the rib is resected widely.

FIG. 227 (*Facing page*). Resection for carcinoma of the midthoracic portion of the esophagus. (A) The incision is placed at the left costal margin anteriorly, extends posteriorly over the 8th or the 9th rib and curves upward between the spine and the left scapula. (B) Anterior dissection of the esophagus. (C) The esophagus and the stomach have been mobilized and prepared for resection. (D) The anastomosis between the esophagus and the stomach is made high in the thoracic cavity. (E) To relieve tension on the anastomotic suture line, interrupted sutures fix the stomach to the parietal pleura and the diaphragm.

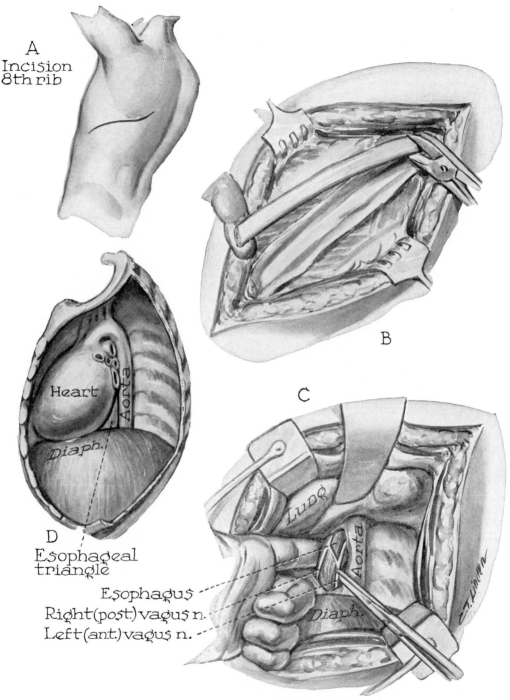

FIG. 228. Transthoracic vagus nerve section (vagotomy). (A) Incision over the left 8th rib. (B) Removal of a section of the left 8th rib. (C) Mobilization of the esophagus and exposure of the vagus nerves. A communicating nerve branch which is quite constant is noted in this subject. (D) The esophageal triangle. The esophagus can be found readily in a triangle bounded in front by the heart, behind by the descending aorta and below by the diaphragm.

Greater exposure may require the additional removal or fracture of adjacent ribs. The left pleural cavity is entered through the rib bed, and the collapsed lung is retracted upward. The inferior pulmonary ligament is identified and severed. The lower end of the esophagus will be found in an *anatomic triangle* which is bounded in front by the heart, behind by the descending aorta and below by the diaphragm (Fig. 228 D). Cutting the inferior pulmonary ligament exposes this triangle and the esophagus.

The vagus nerves are identified by palpation, since they have no elastic fibers and feel like taut cords. In most cases, they appear as 2 main trunks, but recent work on vagal anatomy reveals that considerable variation in the arrangement of the nerves takes place. The *left* vagus appears anterior to the esophagus and extends to the lesser curvature of the stomach. The *right* vagus is situated posteriorly. A large communicating branch between the vagi is a rather constant finding. Additional small fibers may be found on the esophagus. All the nerves and fibers are severed, and the large ones are ligated. The esophagus is returned to its bed, and the pleura is closed.

Pericardium

PERICARDIAL SAC

The pericardium is a fibroserous sac which is located in the middle mediastinum and encloses the heart and the roots of the great vessels. It has the appearance of a truncated cone with its base resting on and fused with the central portion of the diaphragm. Its blunt apex reaches the level of the second costal cartilage (Figs. 229-230). The outline of the pericardium corresponds to that of the heart except that it reaches the 2nd costal cartilage on both sides, whereas the heart extends only to the 3rd cartilage on the right.

PERICARDIAL LAYERS

The pericardium has 3 layers so arranged that the fibrous pericardium is entirely parietal, but the serous has both visceral and parietal layers.

FIBROUS PERICARDIUM

The fibrous pericardium is applied to and is firmly fused with the outer surface of the parietal layer of serous pericardium. It is a sheet of considerable strength which fuses with the central tendon of the diaphragm inferiorly and can be separated from it only by sharp dissection. Superiorly and posteriorly, it blends with the outer coats of the great vessels as they enter or leave the pericardial sac. It is by means of the outer fibrous coat of the arch of the aorta that the fibrous pericardium blends with the pretracheal layer of deep cervical fascia.

Relations. The fibrous pericardium lies behind the body of the sternum and the costal cartilages from the 2nd to the 6th inclusive. Its anterior surface is separated from these structures by the lungs and the pleura except at 2 places. One point of contact is in the median plane, where the fibrous sac is attached to the upper and the lower parts of the body of the sternum. This is brought about by two condensations of mediastinal areolar tissue which are called the upper and the lower *sternopericardial* ligaments; these are of clinical importance in adhesive pericarditis.

The other point of contact is in the region of the *bare area of the pericardium,* which has no covering of lung. This is located at the sternal end of the left 5th costal cartilage (Fig. 230). Here the cardiac notch leaves a deficient area of left pleura, and the pericardium comes in direct relation to the left sternocostalis muscle and the sternum. This area is of importance to the surgeon, since he may tap the pericardial sac at this point without injury to the pleura. Both side walls of the pericardium are in relation to the mediastinal pleura.

VISCERAL AND PARIETAL LAYERS

The *visceral* layer of *serous pericardium* is usually called the *epicardium.* It is exceedingly thin and is so closely adherent to the outer surface of the heart that any attempt to detach it results in injury to the superficial layers of cardiac musculature. However, over the right side and the anterior surface of the ventricular portion of the heart, a certain amount of fat, even in thin individuals, occurs between the muscular tissues and the epicardium. The visceral layer covers the anterior and inferior surfaces of the heart and ascends on the back of the left atrium, where it is reflected downward as the *parietal layer* of serous pericardium. This reflection forms the upper limit of a cul-de-sac, known as the oblique sinus of the pericardium (p. 310). The parietal layer follows and adheres to the fibrous pericardium.

The pericardial sac can be marked on the surface of the thorax as extending from the

2nd costal cartilage above to the 6th below. On the right, it extends for ½ inch beyond the right margin of the sternum, and to the left it forms a line which passes upward and medial from the cardiac apex to the 2nd left costal cartilage about 1½ inches from the midline. The latter is convex upward and to the left.

When the anterior wall of the pericardium is opened, it is noticed that its outer wall appears to be fibrous (fibrous pericardium), but its inner wall is lined with a thin, glisten-

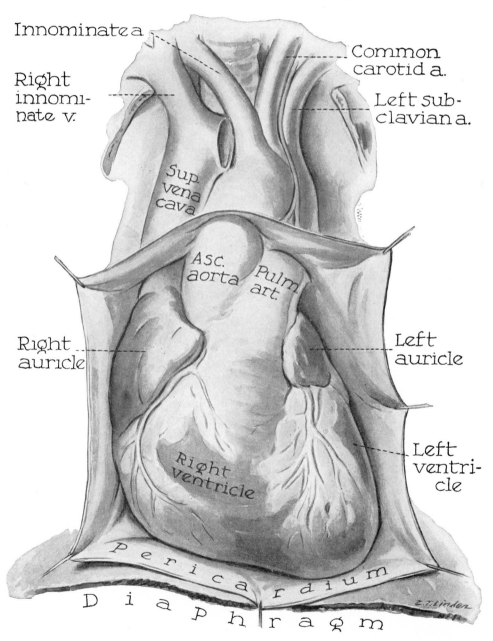

FIG. 229. The pericardium. This fibroserous sac encloses the heart and the roots of the great vessels. The pericardium has been cut open to reveal these structures.

ing serous membrane (parietal layer of serous pericardium). The parietal and the visceral layers of pericardium are continuous with each other anteriorly where the great arteries leave the heart, and posteriorly where the great veins enter it. That space which exists between the 2 layers of serous pericardium is a potential cavity called the pericardial cavity. It contains sufficient serous fluid to minimize friction between its 2 surfaces during heart action.

SURGICAL CONSIDERATIONS

PERICARDIOCENTESIS

Aspiration of the pericardial cavity is done for diagnostic purposes or to release pressure in the pericardial cavity. Even with large effusions, the heart remains anterior and may be injured during this procedure. The aspirating needle should be placed to the left of the xiphoid, thus avoiding the internal mammary artery. Then it should be directed upward, backward and to the left, so that the heart is avoided and the left lateral pouch of dilated pericardium entered. If the needle is passed straight back, the left coronary artery may be injured (Fig. 231).

PERICARDIOSTOMY (PERICARDIOTOMY)

C. S. Beck and others have emphasized the importance of the subatmospheric pressure which exists in the mediastinum. When the pericardium is opened, this is raised to atmospheric pressure, and the resultant compression on the heart causes a rise in venous pressure and a slight transient fall in arterial pressure. A normal heart may tolerate these changes, but should the heart be damaged, the patient might succumb.

Many incisions and approaches for the purposes of draining the pericardial cavity have been described. One of the more common extends from the junction of the left 5th costal cartilage and sternum downward over the cartilages of the 5th, the 6th and the 7th ribs. About an inch of cartilage of the 5th, the 6th and the 7th ribs is removed, and the internal mammary vessels are ligated. The pericardium lies beneath, and the pleural space is to the left. An incision is made into the pericardium, and the fluid is aspirated from each lateral pericardial recess and from the oblique sinus. The pericardium is left open to drain. Soft rubber tubes are introduced into the opening; however, this is to be avoided in tuberculous pericarditis.

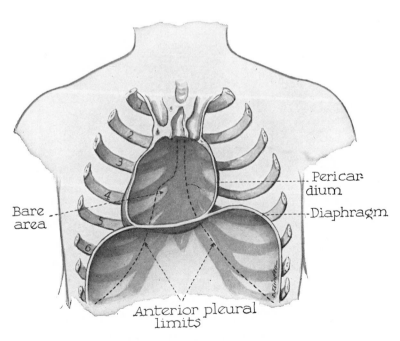

FIG. 230. The pericardium seen from within and behind.

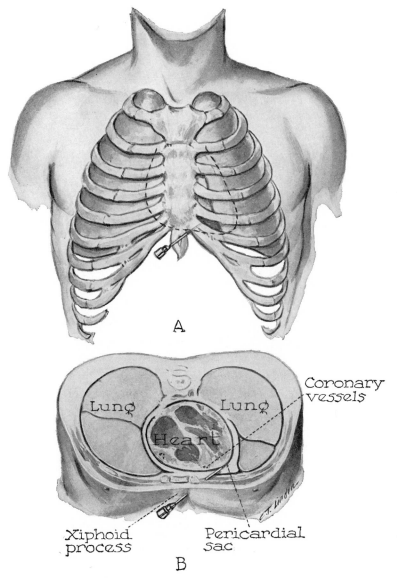

A

Coronary
vessels

Lung   Lung

Heart

Xiphoid   Pericardial
process   sac

B

FIG. 231. Aspiration of the pericardial cavity (pericardiocentesis).
(A) The aspirating needle is placed to the left of the xiphoid, thus
avoiding the internal mammary vessels. (B) The needle is directed
upward, backward and to the left, so that the left coronary vessels are
not injured.

Heart

THE HEART PROPER

With the pericardium opened, the heart (Fig. 232) presents a *fixed* posterosuperior portion—the atria (auricles); and a free antero-inferior portion—the ventricles. A groove containing fat, the auriculoventricular groove (coronary sulcus), marks the line of separation between atria and ventricles; it contains the right coronary artery. Passing downward and to the left, a similar groove is found which divides the ventricular portion of the heart, as seen in front, into a larger right and a smaller left ventricle. This groove corresponds to the attachments of the anterior margin of the septum between the right and the left ventricles and is known as the *anterior interventricular groove* (anterior longitudinal sulcus); it contains the anterior descending branch of the left coronary artery. All 4 chambers of the heart are visible from the "front" view; however, only a very small portion of the left atrium is visible: the auricle of the left atrium.

The right border of the heart, which is convex, is formed by the right atrium; the left border is formed, almost entirely, by the left ventricle. The auricle of the left atrium aids in the formation of the left border at its uppermost part. Between the 2 auricles, the lower part of the pulmonary trunk covers the ascending aorta. That part of the right ventricle which is immediately below the pulmonary trunk is called the *infundibulum*.

If the left index finger is passed in front of the superior vena cava, it can be directed from right to left behind the aorta and the pulmonary artery. The finger now lies in the *transverse sinus of the pericardium* (Figs. 233 and 234). If the thumb is brought into contact with this index finger, the *arterial end* (aorta and pulmonary artery) of the heart lies between the 2 digits. All large vessels below the transverse pericardial sinus constitute veins (superior and inferior venae cavae and pulmonary veins). The sinus is bounded in front by the aorta and the pulmonary artery, and behind by the superior vena cava and the left atrium. It is possible to pass a finger through the sinus because the aorta and the pulmonary artery are enclosed in a complete sheath of visceral pericardium; the superior and the inferior venae cavae and the pulmonary veins are only partially covered (front and sides) by this layer. The transverse sinus connects the right and the left upper portions of the pericardial cavity. It is through this sinus that a rubber catheter is placed in the Trendelenburg operation for pulmonary embolus.

If the fingers of the right hand are placed behind the apex of the heart and passed upward and to the right, they are stopped in a cul-de-sac of pericardium which lies behind the heart, between the left atrium and the pericardium. This is known as the *oblique sinus of the pericardium*. It is really an inverted "U" bounded below and on the right by the inferior vena cava and the right pulmonary veins, and above and on the left by the pulmonary veins. The sinus lies in front of the esophagus and the descending thoracic aorta (Fig. 234). Fingers placed in the transverse and the oblique sinuses cannot touch each other because they are separated by 2 layers of serous pericardium surrounding the veins as they enter the left atrium.

SUPERIOR AND INFERIOR VENAE CAVAE

The superior vena cava measures about 7 cm. in length and is formed by the junction of the 2 innominate veins, draining the blood from the upper half of the body (Figs. 229, 232 and 234). It begins immediately below the cartilage of the 2nd right rib, close to the sternum; it descends vertically behind the 1st and the 2nd intercostal spaces and

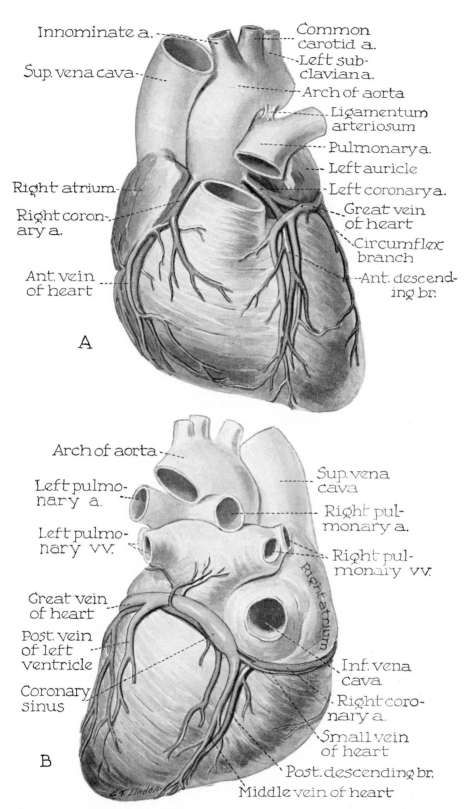

Innominate a.

Sup. vena cava

Right atrium

Right coron-
ary a.

Ant. vein
of heart

A

Common
carotid a.

Left sub-
clavian a.

Arch of aorta

Ligamentum
arteriosum

Pulmonary a.

Left auricle

Left coronary a.

Great vein
of heart

Circumflex
branch

Ant. descend-
ing. br.

Arch of aorta

Left pulmo-
nary a.

Left pulmo-
nary vv.

Great vein
of heart

Post. vein
of left
ventricle

Coronary
sinus

B

Sup. vena
cava

Right pul-
monary a.

Right pul-
monary vv.

Right atrium

Inf. vena
cava

Right coro-
nary a.

Small vein
of heart

Post. descending br.

Middle vein of heart

FIG. 232. Heart and great vessels: (A) seen from in front, (B) seen from behind.

ends in the upper part of the right atrium opposite the upper border of the 3rd right costal cartilage. The lower half of the vessel lies within the pericardium and is devoid of valves at its orifice. The intrapericardial portion lies entirely within the fibrous pericardium and is covered in front and on either side by the serous pericardium which binds it to the fibrous layer. On its right side, it is separated from the right phrenic nerve and its companion vessels by the pericardium; on its left, and overlapping it slightly anteriorly, is the ascending aorta. Because of its close relationship to the ascending aorta, it may be compressed by aortic aneurysms. The transverse sinus intervenes between the superior vena cava and the ascending part of the aorta. In front of the vein, at its termination, is the right auricular appendix, and higher it is separated from the right lung and the pleura by the pericardial wall. Behind the vein is the fibrous pericardium which separates it from the root of the right lung. The vena azygos enters the back of the superior vena cava immediately before it pierces the fibrous pericardium (Fig. 220).

The inferior vena cava (Figs. 232 and 234) is formed by the junction of the 2 common iliac veins on the right side of the 5th lumbar vertebra and returns the blood from

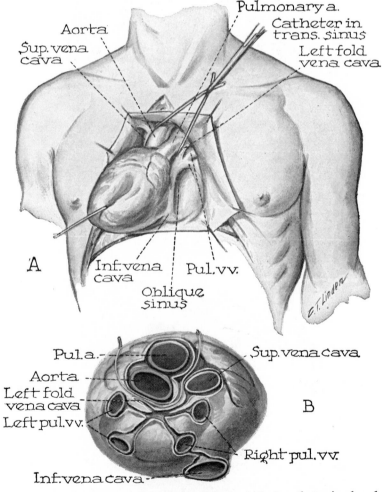

FIG. 233. Transverse and oblique sinuses. (A) A catheter is placed in the transverse sinus. (B) The transverse sinus (in green) seen from above. The structures in front of the green line constitute the arterial flow of the heart (aorta and pulmonary artery); those behind the green line are veins (venae cavae and pulmonary veins).

the parts below the diaphragm to the heart. This vessel ascends along the front of the vertebral column to the right side of the aorta, passes in a groove on the posterior surface of the liver and then perforates the diaphragm between the median and the right portions of its central tendon. It pierces the fibrous pericardium, passes behind the serous pericardium and opens into the lower posterior part of the right atrium. Therefore, only a small part of this vessel, about ¾ inch, is intrathoracic.

Near its atrial orifice is a semilunar valve which has been called the *valve of the inferior vena cava* (Fig. 235). This is usually rudimentary in the adult but may be large in the fetus, where it performs an important function. In the fetus this valve serves to direct the blood from the inferior vena cava through the foramen ovale into the left atrium. In its intrathoracic portion the following relationships are noticed: the diaphragm is in front of it; the vena azygos and the greater splanchnic nerve are behind it; the phrenic nerve, the right pleura and the lungs are lateral. The latter 2 structures also lie behind it.

COMPARTMENTS OF THE HEART

The compartments of the heart may be studied in the order in which they are traversed by the blood (Fig. 237).

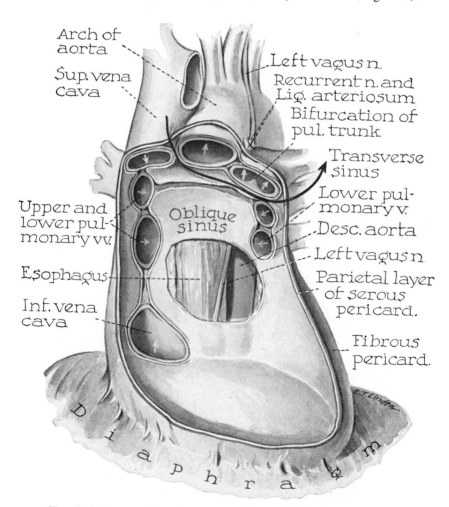

FIG. 234. Transverse and oblique sinuses. A window has been cut in the pericardium to show the posterior relation of the esophagus, the aorta and the left vagus nerve. The small arrows represent the flow of blood to and from the heart.

Right Atrium. If the heart is pulled to the left, a good view is obtained of the right side of the auricular portion and of the superior and the inferior venae cavae. The right atrium (Figs. 235 and 237) begins at the orifice of the inferior vena cava behind the 6th right cartilage.

Immediately in front of the opening of the superior and the inferior venae cavae, an indistinct line might be seen which is called the *sulcus terminalis*. This line is of interest because it indicates the junction between the sinus venosus and the right auricle and marks a ridge which is on the inside of the right auricle called the *crista terminalis*. The sinus venosus is represented in the adult human heart by that part of the right auricle which

lies behind the sulcus and receives the superior and the inferior venae cavae. If a window is cut in the right auricle, the crista terminalis is seen extending from the front of the orifice of the superior vena cava to the front of the orifice of the inferior vena cava. The atrium behind the crista is smooth, and in front it is trabeculated. The rugose appearance of the auricle in front of the crista is brought about by muscle bands which resemble the teeth of a comb; hence, the name *musculi pectinati*.

The posterior wall of the atrium represents the *atrial septum,* which separates the right atrium in front from the left behind. Near its center is noted a shallow oval depression, which is bounded by a thickened ridge every-

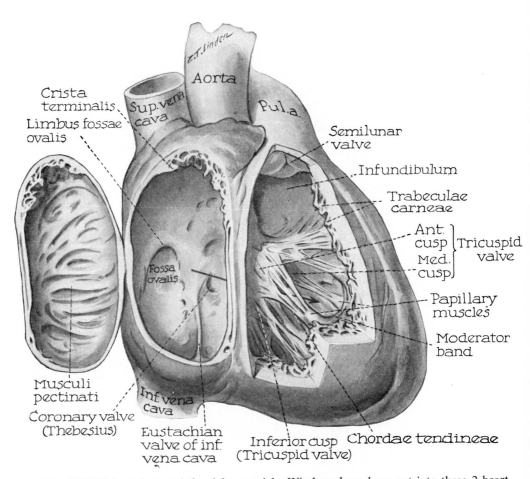

FIG. 235. Right atrium and the right ventricle. Windows have been cut into these 2 heart chambers to show their internal structure. The arrow passes through the right atrioventricular orifice.

where except below. This depression is the *fossa ovalis,* and the ridge surrounding it is the *annulus ovalis* (limbus fossae ovalis).

From the anterior horn of the annulus, there will usually be seen a crescentric membrane which passes forward and to the right, reaching the anterior wall of the auricle immediately in front of and to the right of the opening of the inferior vena cava. It is called the *eustachian valve* (valve of the inferior vena cava), which directed blood in the fetus from the inferior vena cava to the fossa ovalis, and was known as the foramen ovale.

The *tricuspid orifice* (right atrioventricular orifice) occupies the lower portion of the anterior wall of the right atrium. It is large enough to admit the tips of 3 fingers; it opens into the lower and posterior part of the right ventricle and is bounded by the tricuspid valve. The surface projection of this aperture lies obliquely behind the sternum close to the midline and extends from the level of the 4th left costal cartilage to the level of the 6th right cartilage.

Medial to the opening of the inferior vena cava, the coronary sinus may be found. The opening of the sinus points to the left and is guarded by a small pocketlike valve called the *coronary valve (Thebesius),* which turns the blood of the coronary sinus forward into the atrioventricular orifice.

Right Ventricle. This chamber (Fig. 235) has a thick muscle wall and is somewhat triangular in outline. The *infundibulum* (conus arteriosus) is the uppermost part of the right ventricle, the walls of which are smooth and have no projecting muscular bundles; it leads into the pulmonary artery. The inner surface of the right ventricle is extremely irregular because of a lacework of muscular ridges which are called the *trabeculae carnea.* Some of these are attached to the wall only at each extremity, but they are free elsewhere.

A number of conical muscular projections are also found; these are the *papillary muscles.* They are attached at their bases to the wall of the ventricle, and their apices are connected to the cusps of the tricuspid valve by a number of tendinous strands called the *chordae tendinae.* There is usually a large inferior papillary muscle which is attached to the anterior wall. One of these trabeculae,

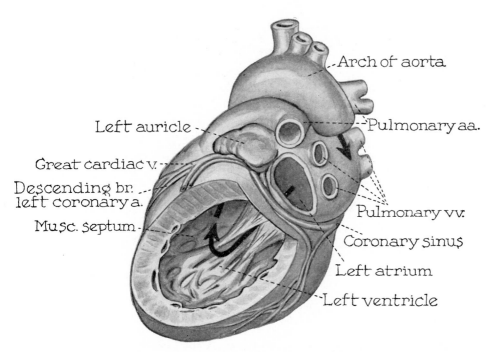

FIG. 236. Left atrium and the left ventricle. Windows have been cut into these chambers, and arrows indicate the course of the blood stream.

which is unusually strong and well marked, passes across the right ventricle from the septum to the base of the anterior papillary muscle; it is called the *moderator band*.

The entrance to the right ventricle is by way of the right atrioventricular orifice, and the exit is the pulmonary orifice. The right atrioventricular orifice is situated at the lower and posterior part of the ventricle; it is about 1 inch in diameter and is surrounded by a fibrous ring. It usually admits the tips of 3 fingers and is guarded by a valve which possesses 3 cusps; hence, the name tricuspid valve. One of the cusps is anterior; another, medial; and the third, inferior. They are semilunar in shape. The atrial surfaces of the cusps are smooth, but their ventricular surfaces are roughened by the attachments of the chordae tendinae. The pulmonary orifice, in the upper posterior part of the ventricle at the apex of the infundibulum, is surrounded by a thin fibrous ring to which the bases of the 3 cusps of the pulmonary valve are attached.

Left Atrium. Only the auricle of the left atrium (Figs. 236-237) can be seen in front, and to view the remainder of this chamber, one must lift the apex of the heart upward and examine the posterior surface of the organ. The left atrium is quadrilateral in shape, and its interior reveals the openings of the 4 pulmonary veins, usually 2 on either side. These veins are unguarded by valves. The interior of the chamber is quite smooth except in its auricular portion, where musculi pectinati are present. In a fresh heart the interior of the left atrium looks much paler than that of the other chambers, because of the greater thickness of the endocardium, which can be stripped off easily, though it is quite difficult to do this in any other cardiac chamber. Blood leaves the left atrium and enters the left ventricle via the left atrioventricular orifice. This is smaller than the one on the right and admits only 2 fingers.

Left Ventricle. The cavity of the left ventricle (Fig. 236) is longer and narrower than that of the right, and the walls are much thicker. Its interior reveals a dense meshwork of trabeculae carneae which are finer but

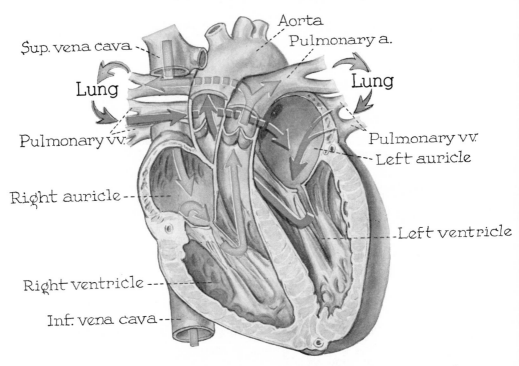

FIG. 237. Diagram of heart chambers, valves and vessels. The arrows indicate the direction of blood flow, and the colors designate oxygenated and nonoxygenated blood.

more numerous than those of the right. However, the papillary muscles of this ventricle are less numerous and much stronger; the chordae tendinae from each papillary muscle pass to both cusps of the mitral valve. The left atrioventricular orifice is surrounded by the bicuspid (mitral) valve, which consists of a larger anterior cusp and a smaller posterior one. Blood leaves the left ventricle via the aortic orifice, which is at the upper right and posterior part, and (like the pulmonary orifice) is surrounded by a fibrous ring to which the bases of the cusps of the aortic valve are attached. The aortic valve, like the pulmonary, has 3 semilunar cusps (Fig. 238).

BLOOD VESSELS AND NERVES

The *trunk* of the *pulmonary artery* (Figs. 229 and 232) arises from the infundibulum of the right ventricle, passes upward and backward and carries the blood from the right ventricle to the lung. It is about 2 inches long and nearly 1 inch in diameter. It lies within the fibrous pericardium, being enclosed with the ascending aorta in a sheath of serous pericardium. As it passes upward, it lies between the right and the left auricles which embrace it; being in front of the aorta, it conceals the roof of this vessel. It is behind the sternal extremity of the 3rd left costal cartilage, and as it travels upward and backward, it bifurcates below the arch of the aorta like the letter "T" into right and left pulmonary arteries. This bifurcation takes place opposite the sternal end of the second left costal cartilage.

The *ligamentum arteriosum* is a fibrous band which extends from the bifurcation of the pulmonary trunk to the lower aspect of the aortic arch. It represents the remains of the ductus arteriosus of the fetus, a vessel which short-circuits the blood from the pulmonary circulation into the aorta. The left recurrent laryngeal nerve hooks around the left side of the ligament.

The *pulmonary artery* has the following *relations:* anterior, the pericardium and the left pleura and lungs; posterior, the ascending aorta and the left atrium; superior, the

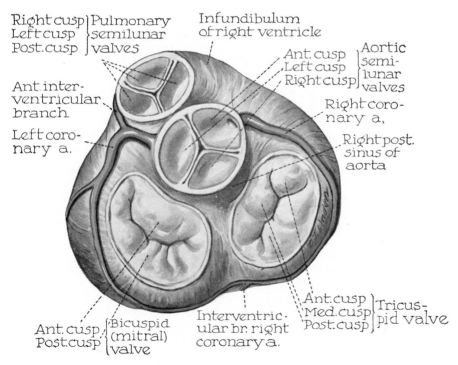

FIG. 238. The heart valves seen from above. The origins of the coronary arteries are shown.

arch of the aorta and the ligamentum arteriosum; laterally, the corresponding coronary arteries and auricles; on the right side, the ascending aorta.

The *right pulmonary artery* is longer than the left; it commences below the arch of the aorta and passes to the hilum of the right lung. In its course, it travels behind the ascending aorta and the superior vena cava, and in front of the esophagus and the stem of the right bronchus. It divides into 3 primary branches, one for each lobe.

The *left pulmonary artery* passes directly to the left in front of the descending aorta and the left bronchus. At the root of the left lung it divides into 2 primary branches, one for each lobe.

The *aorta* is the great arterial trunk of the body. It is situated partly in the thorax and partly in the abdomen. It commences at the left ventricle, arches over the root of the left lung, descends in front of the vertebral column through the diaphragm and enters the abdomen. It ends opposite the left side of the body of the 4th lumbar vertebra by bifurcating into 2 common iliac arteries. It is conveniently divided into 4 parts: the ascending aorta, the arch of the aorta, the descending aorta and the abdominal aorta. The ascending aorta springs from the left ventricle at the aortic orifice and travels upward and to the right. It is about 2 inches long and extends from the lower border of the 3rd left costal cartilage to the level of the 2nd right cartilage. At the 2nd right costal interspace it is covered only by a thin layer of right lung; therefore, the aortic sounds can be heard best at this point. The superior vena cava lies to its right, and the pulmonary artery to its left; its branches are the right and the left coronary arteries (p. 320). The arch of the aorta is directed to the left, but the principal inclination is backward. It begins at the level of the 2nd costal cartilage at the right border of the sternum and extends to the left of the body of the 4th thoracic vertebra. Since aneurysms may involve this part of the vessel, its relations become clinically important.

Relations of the arch to the aorta. *Five* structures lie posterior and to the right: (1) the trachea, (2) the esophagus, (3) the left recurrent laryngeal nerve, (4) the thoracic

duct and (5) the vertebral column. *Five* structures lie anterior and to the left: (1) the lung and the pleura, (2) the left phrenic nerve, (3) the left vagus nerve, (4) the cardiac nerve and (5) the superior intercostal vein. *Five* structures lie below: (1) the left bronchus, (2) the right pulmonary artery, (3) the ligamentum arteriosum, (4) the left recurrent laryngeal nerve and (5) the superficial cardiac plexus. *Five* structures lie above: (1) the left common carotid artery, (2) the left subclavian artery, (3) the innominate artery, (4) the thymus and (5) the left innominate vein.

The arch of the aorta supplies 3 branches in the order named: the innominate, the left common carotid and the left subclavian arteries (Fig. 232).

The *innominate artery* arises from the aorta in front of the trachea and then passes upward, backward and to the right. At the posterior aspect of the sternoclavicular joint, it divides into the right subclavian and the right common carotid arteries. Anteriorly, it is separated from the manubrium sterni by the remains of the thymus and the left innominate vein; the vein crosses the artery near the origin of the latter. To the right side of the artery lie the right innominate vein and the superior vena cava, which intervenes between the artery and the right pleura and lung. To its left side, it is related to the left common carotid artery and the trachea. Posteriorly, it lies on the trachea below and the longus cervicis muscle above.

The *left common carotid artery* arises from the aortic arch immediately to the left of the innominate artery. It passes upward and to the left and enters the neck behind the left sternoclavicular joint. At their origins, the left common carotid and the innominate arteries lie side by side, but they diverge as they ascend. Anteriorly, the artery is crossed by the left innominate vein, and the remains of the thymus intervene between it and the manubrium. Posteriorly, it is in contact with the trachea, the left recurrent laryngeal nerve and the esophagus. On its left side it is related to the left phrenic and vagus nerves, the left subclavian artery and the left lung and pleura. On its right side is the innominate artery.

The *left subclavian artery* arises from the

aortic arch behind and to the left of the common carotid. It arches upward and laterally and enters the neck. Except at its origin, where it is crossed by the left innominate vein, this artery lies in a groove on the left lung.

The *descending aorta* is continuous with the arch at the lower border of the left side of the 4th thoracic vertebra. Its length varies with the length of the thorax, but it averages from 7 to 8 inches. It travels on the left side of the body of the upper posterior mediastinal

vertebrae (the 5th, the 6th and the 7th) into which it usually forms a groove. It then inclines to the median plane and, at this level, passes through the diaphragm and enters the abdomen. Throughout its course it is in close contact with the left mediastinal pleura and the left lung and, as it descends, it passes behind the root of the left lung and the pericardium. It is crossed obliquely by the esophagus, which passes from its right to its left side (Fig. 153). Throughout its course, the thoracic duct and the azygos vein lie on its

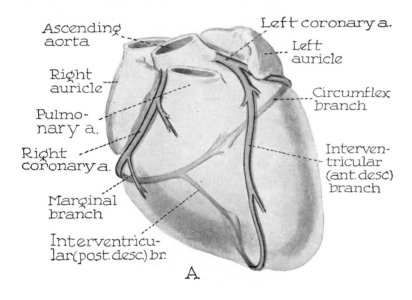

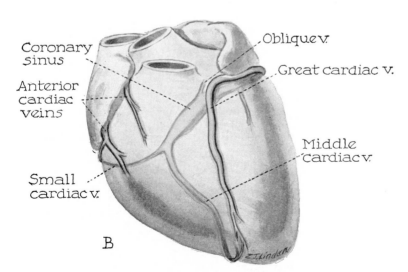

FIG. 239. Arteries and veins of the heart: (A) coronary arteries; (B) the venous drainage.

right posterolateral side, and these structures pass with it through the aortic orifice in the diaphragm at a level between the 12th thoracic and 1st lumbar vertebrae. The hemiazygos vein is on its left posterolateral side. Branches arise from both the front and the back of the descending aorta. The posterior branches consist of 9 pairs of posterior intercostal arteries of the lower 9 intercostal spaces, and one pair of subcostal arteries (p. 300). Those branches which arise from the front of the vessel are 2 left bronchial arteries, 4 esophageal and some small mediastinal, phrenic and pericardial branches.

The *coronary arteries* are the nutrient vessels of the heart (Figs. 238-239 A). They arise from dilatations of the root of the aorta, which are called the sinuses of the aorta. There are 3 such sinuses—1 anterior and 2 posterior—but only 2 coronary arteries—a right and a left. The right coronary arises from the anterior sinus, and the left from the left posterior sinus. The origins of these vessels are hidden anteriorly by the right auricular appendix and the pulmonary artery. The vessels pass forward, one on

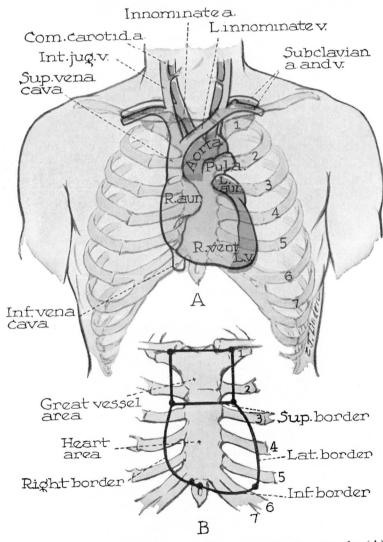

FIG. 240. Thoracic projection of the heart and the great vessels: (A) the structures in situ, (B) the heart and the great vessel areas are projected by marking 6 points on the anterior chest wall.

either side of the pulmonary artery, and have the corresponding auricular appendage to their lateral sides.

The right artery travels in the right atrioventricular sulcus to the back of the heart until it reaches the beginning of the posterior interventricular groove, where it gives rise to a well-developed *posterior descending interventricular branch.*

The left coronary artery reaches the anterior interventricular sulcus, into which it sends an *anterior descending interventricular branch,* and the main trunk of the artery (circumflex artery) continues around the left side of the heart to reach its posterior aspect. The course of this vessel may be obscured by fat in the left auriculoventricular sulcus.

The *cardiac veins* accompany the arteries in the sulci and usually are superficial to the arteries (Fig. 239 B). The companion of the left coronary artery is the *great cardiac vein.* It follows the course of the interventricular branch of the left coronary artery and the circumflex branch. The companion of the interventricular branch of the right coronary artery is the *middle cardiac vein.* Most of the venous blood of the heart enters the *coronary sinus,* which lies in the atrioventricular sulcus at the lower end of the oblique pericardial sinus. It is about 1½ inches long and opens into the right atrium at the left of the orifice of the inferior vena cava.

The *nerves* which supply the heart are derived from the vagus and the cervical ganglionated chain (p. 63). They spread over the aortic arch and the heart and are distributed with the branches of the coronary vessels.

THORACIC PROJECTION OF THE HEART AND THE GREAT VESSELS

The heart and the great vessels may be projected onto the anterior chest wall in the following way (Fig. 240). Four points are marked on the thorax. Two of these are placed in the middle of each 2nd intercostal space, and 1 inch lateral to either sternal margin. If a line joins these 2 points, it identifies the clinical base of the heart (superior border) and demarcates it from the great vessels. The 3rd point is placed just below and medial to the nipple in the left

5th intercostal space, and the 4th mark is located at the junction of the upper and the middle thirds of the xiphoid. If these 4 points are joined, the heart area is outlined quite accurately. The great vessel area is outlined by drawing a horizontal line across the manubrium about ½ inch below the suprasternal notch. This line extends a little less than 1 inch lateral to either sternal margin. Two vertical lines connect these points to the cardiac area.

The internal jugular and the subclavian veins unite behind the sternoclavicular articulation to form the innominate vein. The left innominate vein is longer because it must pass obliquely behind the upper half of the manubrium to join the right innominate vein, thus forming the superior vena cava. This junction takes place behind the middle of the right border of the manubrium. The superior vena cava is thus formed in the region of the angle of Louis and continues as far as the right 3rd costal cartilage. At this point the right atrium begins and continues from the 3rd costal cartilage to the 6th, making a slight convex bulge outward; this represents the right border of the heart. The inferior vena cava enters the right atrium approximately at the level of the 6th costal cartilage. Therefore, a straight line can be drawn 1 or 2 cm. laterally to the right border of the sternum which connects the right internal jugular vein with the inferior vena cava. This line would mark the right internal jugular vein, the superior vena cava, the right atrium and the inferior vena cava. The inferior margin of the heart extends from the 6th costal cartilage on the right, near the entrance of the inferior vena cava, to the apex of the heart. It is convex and lies on the diaphragm. The cardiac apex is located in the 5th left intercostal space, approximately 3½ inches from the median plane. However, this is a variable point, since it lies higher in children (4th interspace), lower in older people and is changed in pathologic conditions of the heart. The line indicating the division of the right atrium from the right ventricle (atrioventricular sulcus) is drawn from the 3rd left to the 6th right sternocostal joints. The left auricle can be indicated by drawing a small circle approximately the size of a dime at the sternal margin of the

2nd left intercostal space. The left ventricle is marked as a small strip which extends between the 3rd and the 6th left costal cartilages to the apex. Therefore, all 4 chambers of the heart may be mapped out over the sternocostal surface.

The veins in this area usually lie superficial to the arteries. The ascending aorta overlaps the superior vena cava as it passes upward and to the right. The arch of the aorta passes backward and to the left, behind the lower half of the manubrium; it is below the left innominate vein. The latter crosses in front of the vein, the left common carotid and left subclavian arteries. The pulmonary artery passes upward and to the left, between the auricles. It lies in front of and hides the root of the aorta, and below the aortic arch it divides into a right and left pulmonary artery.

The *veins* of the sternocostal area consist of the right and the left innominates.

The *right innominate* vein passes almost vertically downward for about 1 inch, but the left, which is nearly 3 times as long, runs almost horizontally behind the upper half of the manubrium. It joins the right vein behind the lower part of the 1st right costal cartilage near its junction with the manubrium. At times the left innominate vein may appear above the suprasternal notch. This happens more frequently in children. If this should be the case, the vein is in danger in operations about the root of the neck. To the left side of the vein is the innominate artery, but the vein somewhat overlaps the artery. It is separated from the sternoclavicular joint by the sternohyoid and the sternothyroid muscles.

The *left innominate* vein begins behind the

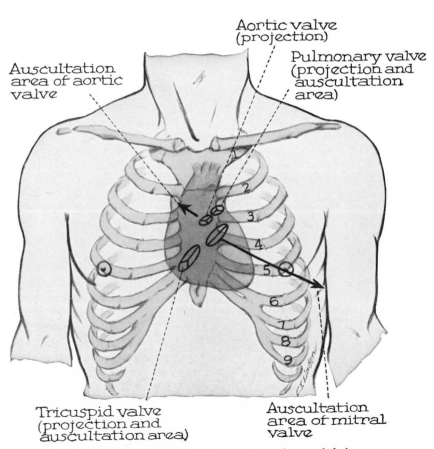

Aortic valve (projection)

Pulmonary valve (projection and auscultation area)

Auscultation area of aortic valve

Tricuspid valve (projection and auscultation area)

Auscultation area of mitral valve

FIG. 241. Surface projection of the heart valves and their areas of maximum audibility.

left sternoclavicular joint and ends by joining the right innominate to form the superior vena cava. In its oblique course it passes behind the remains of the thymus and in front of the left subclavian, the left common carotid and the innominate arteries.

AREAS OF MAXIMUM AUDIBILITY OF HEART VALVE SOUNDS AND THEIR THORACIC PROJECTION

The audibility of the heart valves (Fig. 241) depends on the depth of the valves from the surface of the chest, the sound-

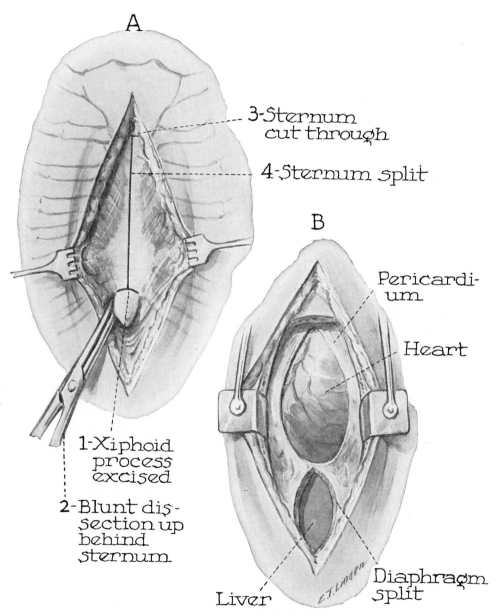

A

3-Sternum cut through

4-Sternum split

B

Pericardi- um

Heart

1-Xiphoid process excised

2-Blunt dis- section up behind sternum

Liver

Diaphragm split

FIG. 242. The Duval-Barasty incision. This provides excellent exposure of the heart and protects the pleural cavities.

transmitting quality of tissue and the direction of blood flow in the heart chambers.

The *tricuspid* valve is heard best at the lower left quarter of the body of the sternum. This is where the right ventricle is nearest the surface. Authors disagree on this point.

The *pulmonary* valve is heard best at the 3rd left costal cartilage close to the sternum. This is opposite the valve proper, since the pulmonary trunk recedes from the surface as it travels upward.

The *mitral* valve is placed deeper than the valves of the right side of the heart; it is located posterior to the left half of the sternum on a level with the 4th costal cartilage. Its auscultatory area is in the direction of the blood flow as it passes from auricle to ventricle and is over the cardiac apex.

The *aortic* valve sound is heard best in the second right intercostal space at the sternal margin and is projected along the course of the blood stream. The ascending aorta passes forward, upward and to the right.

SURGICAL CONSIDERATIONS
EXPOSURE OF THE HEART

Many incisions have been described, but only the more popular ones are considered.

The Duval-Barasty incision to the pericardium and the heart gives excellent exposure and protects the pleural cavities (Fig. 242). Its only drawback is that it takes time to open and close and may be associated with shock. The incision is made in the midline from the 2nd rib to the midepigastrium. The xiphoid is removed, and the sternum is split to the 2nd interspace where it is cut transversely. The split halves of the sternum are retracted, the pleurae pushed aside, and the pericardium opened anteriorly. The diaphragm and the anterior pericardium are incised, making the incision a thoraco-abdominal one.

Spangaro's incision is really an intercostochondral thoracotomy which provides a rapid approach to the heart but not as good exposure as does the Duval-Barasty (Fig. 243). The incision is made through the 4th intercostal space from the margin of the sternum to the anterior axillary line. The internal mammary vessels are ligated and divided. The 4th and the 5th ribs and cartilages are

separated, and the left lung is retracted. The pericardium is incised in the long axis of the heart, and the pathologic areas are exposed and treated.

Parasternal and semicircular incisions which utilize flaps have also been advocated.

WOUNDS OF THE HEART

The immediate dangers in heart wounds are tamponade and hemorrhage. Aspiration while preparations for the operation are being made may be lifesaving. D. C. Elkin has reviewed this subject and emphasizes that, if time permits, all efforts should be made to avoid entering the pleural cavity, since a pneumothorax adds to the shock. One of the above-mentioned incisions is utilized, and the wound in the pericardium is located and enlarged. If this is not found, the pericardium is opened between stay sutures. When the intrapericardial pressure is released, the bleeding becomes profuse, and the contractions of the heart increase in force.

The greatest difficulty is encountered in placing the first stitch. When the cardiac wound is located, the index finger of the left hand is placed over it, and the surrounding blood is removed by suction. The first suture is placed directly beneath the finger and may be used for traction and hemostasis. Then the wound is closed with unabsorbable suture material, the sutures passing into the muscle but not into the heart chambers.

Claude Beck has emphasized the fact that wounds located in the edges of the heart, on its posterior surface, or behind the sternum are reached best by placing an apex suture. By this method the heart may be rotated so that the injury can be exposed properly. Beck's control suture steadies the heart while the other sutures are being placed. The pericardium should be closed loosely with interrupted sutures so that space is allowed for drainage of the intrapericardial fluid which will accumulate. Muscle, fascia and skin are closed in layers.

PERICARDIECTOMY

Warren Cole, Weber and Keeton have described a technic of pericardiectomy for constrictive pericarditis. They state that the excision of the scar should be started over the

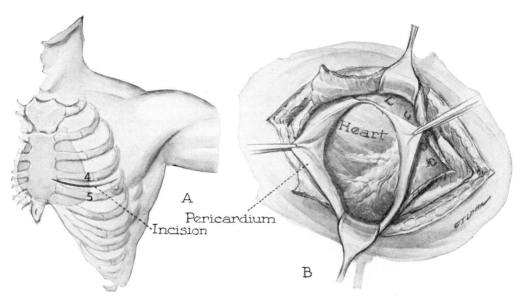

FIG. 243. Spangaro's incision. This approach provides rapid access
to the heart, but at times inadequate exposure.

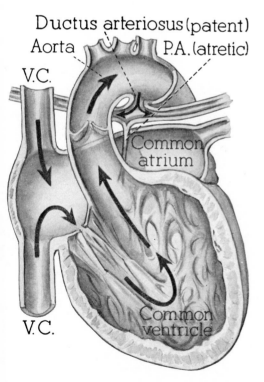

FIG. 244. Cor biloculare—the primitive
2-chambered heart.

left ventricle, and an attempt should be made
to find a cleavage plane between the scar and
the cardiac musculature. Dissection continues in this plane. Since all landmarks are
usually obliterated, the coronary vessels may
be difficult to find, and injury to these vessels
is dangerous. Harrington has stressed the importance of epicardiolysis as well.

CONGENITAL DEFECTS

Congenital defects of the heart and the
great vessels were described as early as 1777
by the eminent Dutch physician Sandifort,
who gave a remarkably clear description of
what is known today as the "tetralogy of
Fallot." One of the most prolific contribu-
tors to the knowledge of these anomalies was
Maude E. Abbott. To her goes the credit in
a large measure for being responsible for
today's diagnostic precision which resulted in
a new and gratifying field of surgery. When
one discusses these dramatic events, the
names of Bailey, Blalock, Crafoord, Gross
and Taussig must be mentioned also. In a
book of this type the many cardiac anomalies
are too numerous to be mentioned. Some of
the more common ones will be described so

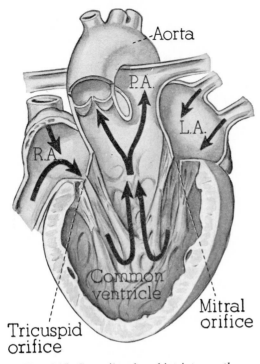

as to give the student of surgical anatomy a mere taste of this intriguing field of study.

Cor Biloculare (2-Chambered Heart). This is a most primitive type of cardiac defect (Fig. 244). It has a single atrium, a single ventricle and a common atrioventricular valve. It must be remembered that many anomalies may appear in a given specimen. Therefore, in the diagram herein presented it will be noted that the pulmonary artery lies behind the aorta and is atretic. Pulmonary circulation takes place via a patent ductus arteriosus. Death ensues in these patients in infancy or early childhood.

Cor Triloculare Biatriatum (3-Chambered Heart) consists of 2 atria and a single ventricle (Fig. 245). No ventricular septum exists, and in the diagram shown here there is an associated transposition of the aorta and the pulmonary artery. It resembles the 2-chambered heart in that there is a free admixture of venous and aerated blood in the single ventricle. The chances of survival are somewhat greater than in the 2-chambered heart, although death occurs commonly during infancy.

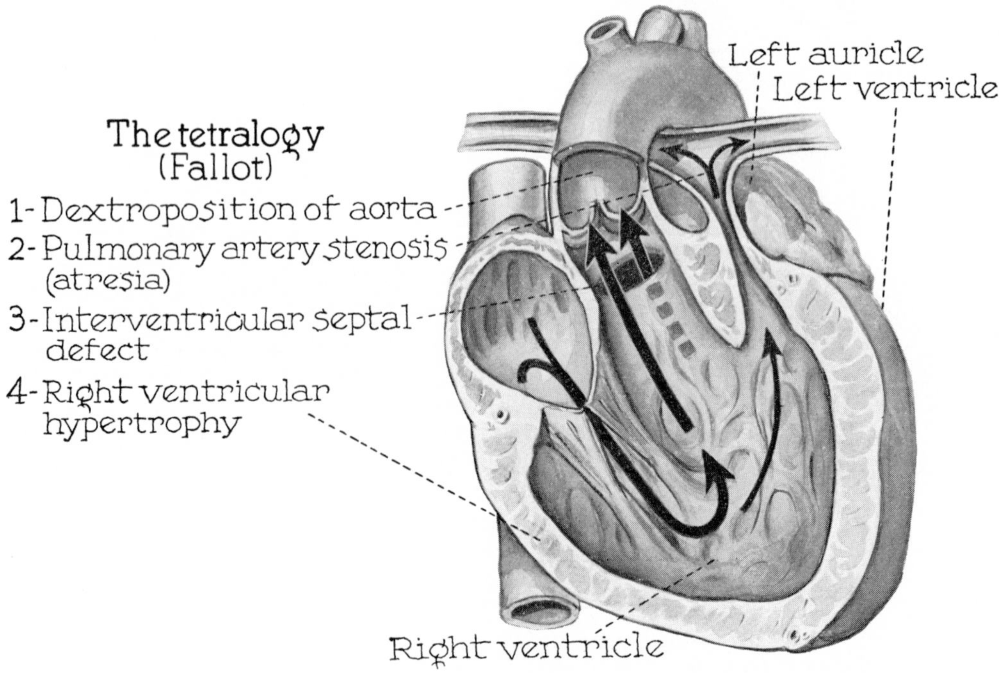

Fig. 245. Cor triloculare biatriatum—the 3-chambered heart.

Fig. 246. The tetralogy of Fallot.

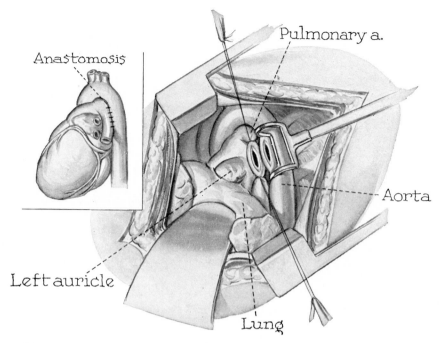

FIG. 247. The Potts operation for tetralogy of Fallot. This illustration depicts a left-sided approach and a Potts clamp applied to the mobilized aorta. This clamp allows flow of blood through part of the aortic lumen. The pulmonary artery is temporarily obstructed proximally and distally to the site of anastomosis.

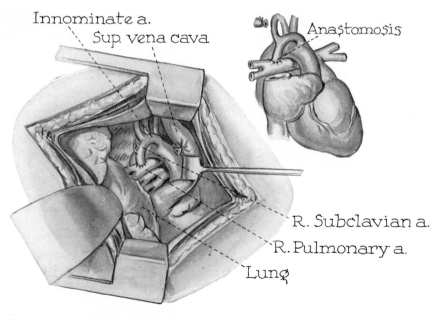

FIG. 248. The Blalock-Taussig anastomosis of the right subclavian branch of the innominate artery to the right pulmonary artery for tetralogy of Fallot.

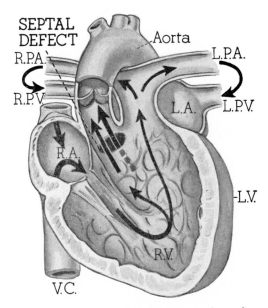

FIG. 249. Diagrammatic presentation of the Eisenmenger complex.

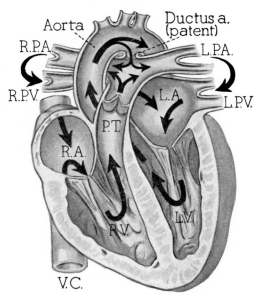

FIG. 250. A patent ductus arteriosus.

The tetralogy of Fallot as originally described consisted of (Fig. 246):

1. Pulmonary stenosis (atresia)
2. Dextraposition of the aorta
3. Interventricular septal defect
4. Hypertrophy of the right ventricle

This is the most common malformation associated with cyanosis which permits the patients to survive beyond 2 years of age. Potts and Blalock have attempted to correct the pulmonary stenosis by creating an artificial ductus arteriosus. Potts accomplished this by performing a side-to-side anastomosis between the pulmonary artery and the aorta (Fig. 247). The Blalock procedure consists of an end-to-side anastomosis between a systemic branch of the aorta (subclavian) and one of the 2 pulmonary arteries (Fig. 248). Numerous modifications of these procedures have been described.

The Eisenmenger complex reveals a heart that has a ventricular septal defect with biventricular origin of the aorta (Fig. 249). The aorta straddles a defect in the membranous portion of the ventricular septum. Because of this the right and the left ventricles share in the propelling of blood into the aorta; the pressure in the 2 ventricles is similar, being at systemic levels. In the Eisen-

menger complex the small arteries in the lungs closely resemble those of the normal fetus in which there is increased resistance to pulmonary blood flow.

Patent ductus arteriosus permits blood to flow from the aorta into the pulmonary artery (Fig. 250). It should be recalled that during fetal life the ductus arteriosus is a normally functioning channel which short-circuits blood from the pulmonary artery to the aorta. This should become obliterated at or shortly after birth. If the ductus remains open, great volumes of blood reach the pulmonary artery via the aorta and are reflected in a left ventricular dilatation and hypertrophy. Two types of patent ductus arteriosus have been described: one in which it is cylindrical and one in which it is stubby, the latter being known as the window type. Evidence of progressive cardiac failure in an acyanotic infant strongly suggests the possibility of this condition. The patient frequently lives to adult life; however, life expectancy is reduced materially. Among the chief causes of death in untreated cases are bacterial infection and left ventricular failure. The closure of a patent ductus arteriosus is now a standard surgical procedure (Fig. 251).

A patent ductus should be ligated or di-

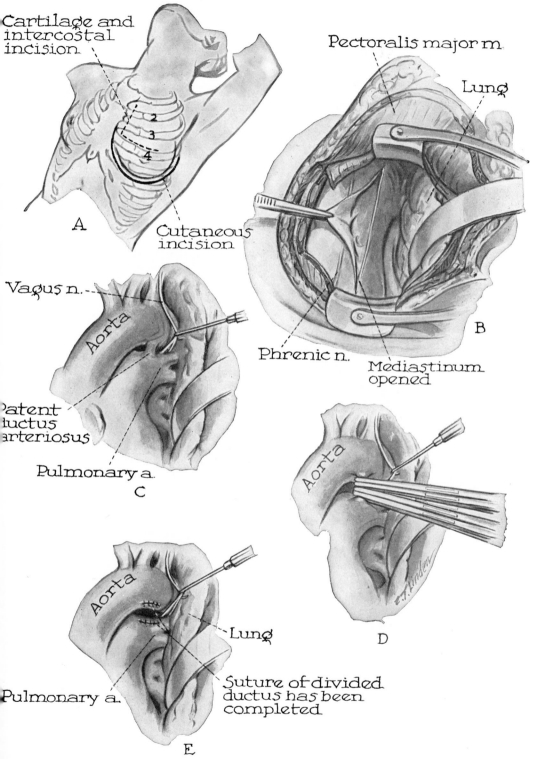

Fig. 251. Operation for patent ductus arteriosus.

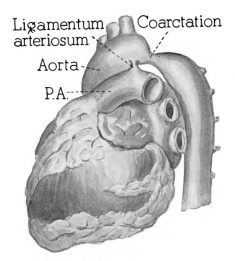

Ligamentum arteriosum

Coarctation

Aorta

P.A.

FIG. 252. Coarctation of the aorta.

vided to improve circulatory function and to diminish the hazards of blood stream infection. The operation is performed usually through an incision in the left mammary fold as advocated by Gross (Fig. 251). This extends from the sternum to the anterior axillary line. The breast is reflected cephalad, and the soft tissues are divided so that the 3rd and the 4th costal cartilages are exposed. The pleural cavity is entered through the 3rd intercostal space, the 3rd and 4th cartilages are divided, and the ribs retracted. The lung is retracted, the mediastinal pleura incised, and the arch of the aorta and the pulmonary artery exposed. The phrenic and the vagus nerves are identified and mobilized, and the patent ductus is completely exposed. The latter is divided between clamps and carefully sutured. Harrington has expressed the belief that the older an individual grows the shorter the ductus becomes, so that in adults the duct has really become an arteriovenous fistula. The parietal pleura of the mediastinum is sutured, and closure of the chest wall is accomplished in layers.

Coarctation of the Aorta. This narrowing or constriction can occur anywhere in this vessel from the midpoint of the arch down to its bifurcation. However, very few are found in the abdomen or the lower thorax. But 98 per cent of coarctations are located in the first part of the descending aorta just beyond the arch (Fig. 252).

There has been a tendency to divide this condition into two distinct forms. In the first, the so-called "infantile type," there is a long segment of constriction, and it is associated with severe intracardiac abnormalities, commonly leading to death within the first few years of life. The second, the so-called "adult type," was supposed to have a blockage of a short segment and be prone to involve the aorta beyond the origin of the left subclavian artery. Hence, it is not accompanied by marked intracardiac malformations, and the prognosis is better for life into adult years.

Modern authorities in this field believe that there is little point in classifying coarctations of the aorta into these two artificial groups because of the tremendous amount of overlapping, thus making the classification useless. Some authors are of the opinion that the relationship of coarctation to the ligamentum arteriosum (obliterated ductus arteriosus) is important.

Probably more important than this relationship is the advisability of determining whether or not the ductus arteriosus is patent. Collateral arterial circulation is rarely seen in children but may be detected after the 1st decade, particularly in thin subjects (Fig. 253). Pulsations may be seen and felt above and below the clavicles, in the axillae, in the intercostal spaces, particularly in the forward half of the chest, in the epigastrium and over the upper half of the back. When collateral circulation is marked, these pulsations may appear in the anterior abdominal wall; at times they have been traced down as far as the inguinal regions. Some of the causes of death from coarctation of the aorta are left ventricular failure, rupture of the aorta, bacterial endocarditis and rupture of an aneurysm of the Circle of Willis.

Surgical correction of the condition is accomplished in one of three ways: (1) the ideal correction is removal of the narrow segment with an end-to-end anastomosis between the proximal and the distal ends of the aorta; (2) a bypass procedure has been advocated in which the left subclavian artery has been anastomosed to the distal end of the aorta; (3) resection of the constricted

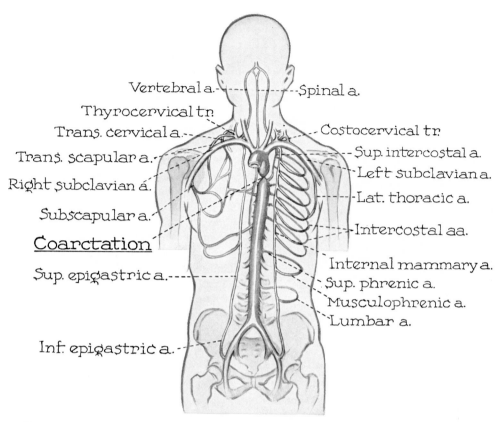

Fig. 253. Diagrammatic representation of the collateral circulation in coarctation.

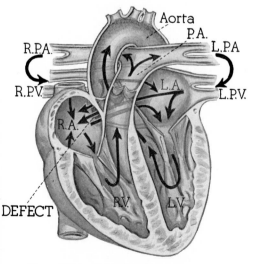

Fig. 254A. Diagrammatic representation of an atrial septal defect. The arrows indicate the possible flow of blood.

segment with the insertion of a graft between proximal and distal ends of the aorta.

Atrial septal defect is among the commoner types of congenital cardiac anomalies, particularly those seen in adult life. The usual form of this defect is a valvular incompetence of the foramen ovale (Fig. 254A). This defect allows oxygenated blood to flow from the left atrium to the right atrium, thus resulting in a recirculation of oxygenated blood through the lungs. Such defects, if appreciable, cause dilatation and hypertrophy of the right ventricle, enlargement of the right atrium, and enlargement of the pulmonary trunk and its branches. There is no cyanosis so long as the shunt is arteriovenous. Symptoms may be absent or minimal, and in the extreme instances congestive heart failure and sudden death may occur. On occasion an embolus may escape through an

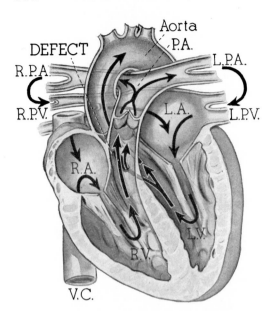

DEFECT

R.P.A.

R.P.V.

Aorta

P.A.

L.P.A.

L.A.

L.P.V.

R.A.

L.V.

R.V.

V.C.

FIG. 254B. Ventricular septal defect. The arrows indicate the possible flow of blood.

atrial septal defect, resulting in a phenomenon known as "paradoxical embolism."

Ventricular septal defects may occur in either the membranous or the muscular portions of the ventricular septum (Fig. 254B). This defect permits the shunt of blood from the left ventricle to the right ventricle, producing an increased load of work on both ventricles. Patients who survive the 1st year of life with such defects may live many years without disability and reach adulthood with few signs, if any, and no cardiac enlargement. Bacterial endocarditis is a common complication in patients who survive infancy.

Alexander and Byron have reported a case of aortectomy. The problem of collateral circulation is interesting.

Gitlow and Sommer have reported a case of complete coarctation in which the collateral circulation took place chiefly by way of the internal mammary, the superior intercostal and the subscapular arteries.

Bramwell and Jones studied the collateral circulation in a case of complete aortic coarctation which occurred just distal to the left subclavian artery. They conclude that the main anastomoses were: (1) the musculophrenic branches of the internal mammary to the inferior phrenic branches of the abdominal aorta, and the superior phrenic branches of the thoracic aorta which formed a network above and below the diaphragm; (2) via the scapular and the cervical branches of the subclavian and the axillary arteries, to the lateral dorsal branches of the aortic intercostal; (3) via the superior intercostals through the upper two, to the next lower intercostals. However, Alexander and Byron have stressed that in their case much of the collateral circulation took place through the superior and the inferior epigastric arteries.

Ochsner and Dixon have reviewed cases of *superior vena cava thrombosis* rather extensively and have reported on personal experiences with this condition. They have advised exploratory superior mediastinotomy, which is also used as a decompressive measure.

THORAX

Azygos System of Veins and Superior Vena Cava

The azygos system (Fig. 255) consists of 3 veins which form longitudinal collecting trunks into which the intercostal veins drain: the azygos (vena azygos major), the hemiazygos (vena azygos minor inferior) and the accessory hemiazygos (vena azygos

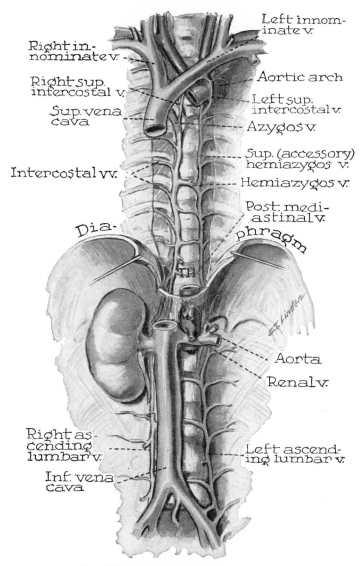

Left innom-
inate v.

Right in-
nominate v.

Aortic arch

Right sup.
intercostal v.

Left sup.
intercostal v.

Sup. vena
cava

Azygos v.

Sup. (accessory)
hemiazygos v.

Intercostal vv.

Hemiazygos v.

Post. medi-
astinal v.

Dia-

phragm

TH

Aorta

Renal v.

Right as-
cending
lumbar v.

Left ascend-
ing lumbar v.

Inf. vena
cava

FIG. 255. The azygos system of veins.

minor superior). The azygos is located on the right side, and the hemiazygos and the accessory hemiazygos on the left. The right and the left ascending lumbar veins constitute the most caudal portion of the system and drain into the azygos and the hemiazygos, respectively. These veins, because they link together the superior and the inferior venae cavae, constitute important anastomosing channels.

The azygos vein begins in the abdomen, approximately where the renal vein enters the inferior vena cava. Its origin is variable, but most anatomists are of the opinion that it arises from the posterior aspect of the inferior vena cava; however, others have described its origin as being formed by the union of the right ascending lumbar and subcostal veins, whereas still others consider it as a branch of the right renal vein. It enters the thorax on the right side of the thoracic duct and the descending aorta, passes upward in front of the vertebral bodies and is overlapped by the right edge of the esophagus. It passes into the thorax through the aortic opening of the diaphragm. At the upper border of the root of the right lung, it emerges from under cover of the esophagus, arches forward above the right bronchus and terminates in the superior vena cava. Therefore, this vein has vertical and horizontal portions and is related to the mediastinal aspect of the right lung and the pleura. Although it has imperfect valves, its tributaries have complete ones. The tributaries are formed by numerous small veins such as the esophageal, the pericardial, the bronchial and the mediastinal; in addition to these, it receives the 2 hemiazygos veins, the lower 8 posterior intercostals (subcostal) of the right side, and the right superior intercostal vein. The last is the common trunk formed by the union of the veins from the 2nd and the 3rd intercostal spaces.

The hemiazygos vein (vena azygos minor inferior) begins in the left ascending lumbar or renal vein. It enters the thorax through the left crus of the diaphragm, ascending on the left side of the vertebral column as high as

the 9th thoracic vertebra, where it passes across the column and behind the aorta, the esophagus and the thoracic duct to end in the azygos vein. In its course, it crosses 3 or 4 of the lower left intercostal arteries and is covered by the pleura. It receives the lower 4 or 5 left intercostal veins, at times the lower end of the accessory hemiazygos, the small left mediastinal and the lower left esophageal veins.

The accessory hemiazygos vein (vena azygos minor superior) varies much in size, position and arrangement, since it is often continuous with or drained by the left superior intercostal vein. Therefore, it varies inversely in size with the left superior intercostal. It descends on the left side of the vertebral column and receives veins from the 3 or 4 intercostal spaces between the superior left intercostal and the highest tributary of the hemiazygos; it either crosses the body of the 8th thoracic vertebra, emptying into the azygos, or ends in the hemiazygos. If it is very small or entirely absent, the left superior intercostal extends as low as the 5th or the 6th intercostal space.

If the inferior vena cava is obstructed, the azygos and the hemiazygos veins are one of the principal means by which collateral venous circulation is carried out, since they connect the venae cavae and communicate with the common iliac veins via the ascending lumbar and with many tributaries of the inferior vena cava.

For additional study of the azygos system of veins and its variations and anomalies, one can refer to the works of Seib, Huseby and Boyden and of H. Neuberger.

The superior vena cava is about 2 inches long and commences at the lower border of the right first costal cartilage, where it is formed by the union of the 2 innominate veins. It pierces the pericardium opposite the 2nd right costal cartilage and ends in the upper and back part of the right atrium behind the 3rd right cartilage. It has no valves, and its tributaries are the 2 innominate veins, the vena azygos and a few small mediastinal and pericardial veins.

Thoracic Duct

EMBRYOLOGY

In the fetus, the thoracic ducts are a pair of vessels which ascend through the posterior mediastinum on each side of the descending thoracic aorta (Figs. 256B and C). They continue through the superior mediastinum, on each side of the esophagus, to the root of the neck where each arches laterally, immediately behind the carotid sheath, and opens into the angle between the subclavian and the internal jugular veins. Because of pressure from the aorta, the left duct atrophies; the right persists, crosses to the left side and empties into the left subclavian vein. The disappearance and the persistence of the ductus is subject to great variation, so that any arrangement of anastomoses may result. Jossifow described some of these variations and the level of formation.

THE ADULT DUCT

The adult duct (Fig. 256A) is approximately the same length as the spinal cord, about 18 inches. It begins in the abdomen at the upper end of the *cisterna chyli,* which is an elongated sac placed under the right crus of the diaphragm.

Three major lymph trunks drain into the cisterna: the right and the left lumbars and the intestinal. The 2 lumbar trunks are short vessels which convey the lymph from the lower limbs, the pelvis (viscera included), the kidneys, the suprarenals and the deep lymphatics of the abdominal walls. The left lumbar trunk reaches the cisterna by passing behind the aorta. The intestinal trunk carries lymph from the stomach, the spleen, most of the liver and the intestines.

The thoracic duct has abdominal, thoracic and cervical parts. The abdominal part leaves the cisterna, passes to the aortic orifice of the diaphragm and, with the vena azygos on its right, enters the thorax. In the thorax, it passes up in the posterior mediastinum with the azygos vein on the right and the aorta on the left. Behind it are the vertebrae, the right intercostal vessels, the hemiazygos and the accessory hemiazygos veins. In front are the diaphragm, the esophagus and the pericardium. At the level of the 7th thoracic vertebra, the duct begins to cross obliquely to the left until it reaches the left side of the body about at the level of the 5th thoracic vertebra. It then continues up along the left border of the esophagus, medial to the pleura and behind the left subclavian artery into the neck. The cervical part forms an arch which reaches as high as the 7th cervical vertebra; it arches behind the carotid system (internal jugular vein, vagus nerve and common carotid artery). As it travels to the left, it crosses the scalenus anterior muscle, the phrenic nerve and the transverse scapular vessels. The so-called vertebral system (vertebral artery, vein and sympathetic trunk) lies behind.

The duct ends medially, usually as a single vessel which enters the junction of the left internal jugular and subclavian veins; this opening is guarded by valves which prevent the regurgitation of blood. Kampmeier reported that although many valves are present in the early development of the thoracic duct, most of them disappear later. In the adult the duct is usually provided with valves at or near its opening into the subclavian vein. It sometimes divides into two, but these usually re-form into a single duct again. This is important to recognize in wounds of the neck. In its course, the duct returns lymph from both lower limbs, the abdomen (except the upper surface of the right lobe of the liver), the left side of the thorax, the left side of the head and the neck, and the left upper limb.

The right lymph duct is a short vessel,

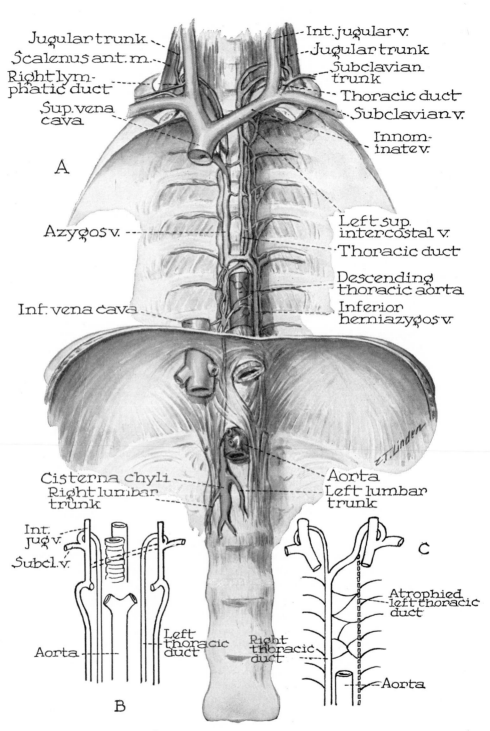

Jugular trunk

Scalenus ant. m.

Right lymphatic duct

Sup. vena cava

A

Azygos v.

Inf. vena cava

Int. jugular v.

Jugular trunk

Subclavian trunk

Thoracic duct

Subclavian v.

Innominate v.

Left sup. intercostal v.

Thoracic duct

Descending thoracic aorta

Inferior hemiazygos v.

Cisterna chyli

Right lumbar trunk

Aorta

Left lumbar trunk

Int. jug. v.

Subcl. v.

Aorta

Left thoracic duct

B

Right thoracic duct

C

Atrophied left thoracic duct

Aorta

FIG. 256. Thoracic duct: (A) adult duct; (B) and (C) embryology of the thoracic duct.

about 1 inch long, which passes down on the scalenus anterior muscle and enters the junction of the right internal jugular and the subclavian veins. It is formed by the union of the right jugular, the subclavian and the bronchomediastinal trunks; however, these may open separately. The right duct returns lymph from the upper surface of the right lobe of the liver, from the right lung and the pleura, and also from the right side of the heart.

Chylothorax and/or chylous ascites usually results from pressure on the thoracic duct or from trauma. It has been stated that the flow through this duct can amount to as much as 60 to 190 ml. per hour. Hence, following trauma, a tremendous loss of lymph may take place over a relatively short period of time. The duct is usually injured in operations such as thoracic sympathectomy or in surgery in the region of the posterior mediastinum or the neck. A moot question among surgeons is whether one should ligate the duct or attempt an end-to-end anastomosis following injury. Thoracic ductography has been reported by Lowman and also by Stranahan. Such studies reveal marked variations in thoracic duct patterns which should be compared with the usual textbook descriptions.

Sympathetic Chain

The term "autonomic" implies autonomous or self-controlling. It suggests automatic regulation without cerebral control, in this instance, of visceral functions. Therefore, the autonomic nervous system controls the motor functions of the viscera, since it controls all smooth (involuntary) muscle, cardiac muscle and glands.

In general, most viscera are supplied by two opposing sets of nerves which are antagonistic to each other; when one stimulates, the other inhibits activity. Both the stimulating and the inhibiting mechanisms require a 2-neuron chain between the nucleus of origin in the central nervous system and the peripheral organ which is to be innervated.

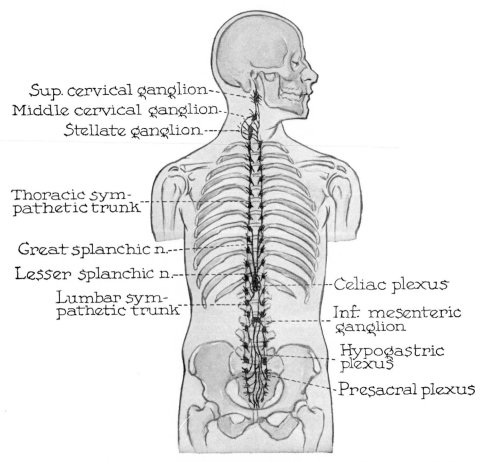

Sup. cervical ganglion

Middle cervical ganglion

Stellate ganglion

Thoracic sympathetic trunk

Great splanchic n.

Lesser splanchic n.

Lumbar sympathetic trunk

Celiac plexus

Inf. mesenteric ganglion

Hypogastric plexus

Presacral plexus

FIG. 257. The sympathetic ganglionated chain, the splanchnic nerves and the communicating rami.

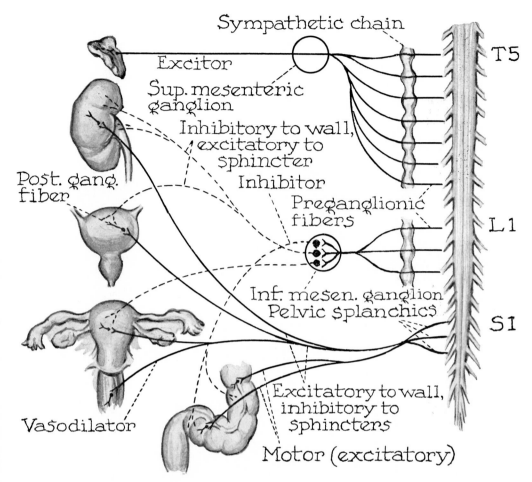

Sympathetic chain

Excitor

Sup. mesenteric ganglion

Inhibitory to wall, excitatory to sphincter

Inhibitor

Post. gang. fiber

Preganglionic fibers

T5

L1

Inf. mesen. ganglion
Pelvic splanchics

S1

Excitatory to wall, inhibitory to sphincters

Vasodilator

Motor (excitatory)

FIG. 258. Diagrammatic representation of the autonomic nerve supply to the viscera of the lower abdomen and the pelvis. The dotted lines represent postganglionic fibers of the thoracolumbar outflow. The postganglionic fibers of the craniosacral outflow are represented as short solid lines in or on the walls of the structures innervated.

Such a system requires a synapse between the 2 neurons which occurs in ganglia outside of the central nervous system. The ganglion may be used as a point of reference, since the fibers lying closest to the brain or the spinal cord are called preganglionic (presynaptic) fibers. The second fiber, the cell of origin of which lies in one of the ganglia and carries impulses to an organ, is known as a postganglionic (postsynaptic) fiber. Hence, the autonomic nervous system resembles the somatic in that it consists of central and peripheral parts. The central elements of the autonomic system are intrinsic parts of the central nervous system, being located in the cerebral cortex, the hypothalmus, the brain stem, the cerebellum and the spinal cord. Many authorities believe that there is no actual nerve tissue contact between autonomic nerves and the structures supplied by them, but that the resultant action comes from a liberation of chemical substances resembling epinephrine (Adrenalin) and acetylcholine, and the divergent effects produced thereby are often referred to as adrenergic and cholinergic, respectively. Such a concept presupposes the existence of definite nerve endings with junctional zones between them and the viscera innervated.

It has become customary to divide the

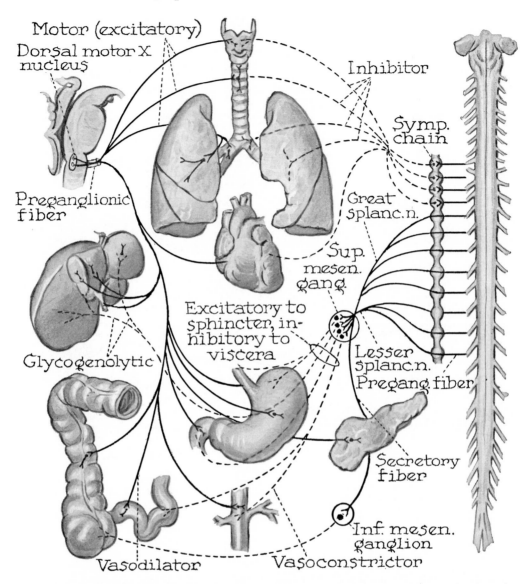

Motor (excitatory)
Dorsal motor X nucleus
Inhibitor
Symp. chain
Preganglionic fiber
Great Splanc. n.
Sup. mesen. gang.
Excitatory to sphincter, inhibitory to viscera
Glycogenolytic
Lesser Splanc. n.
Pregang. fiber
Secretory fiber
Inf. mesen. ganglion
Vasodilator
Vasoconstrictor

FIG. 259. A diagrammatic presentation of the autonomic nerve supply to the thoracic and the abdominal viscera. The dotted lines represent postganglionic fibers of the thoracolumbar outflow. The craniosacral outflow (postganglionic fibers) are shown as short solid lines in or on the walls of the structures innervated.

autonomic nervous system into 2 major portions based on the origin of the preganglionic fibers from the central nervous system. The preganglionic fibers which arise from the thoracic and the lumbar spinal cord are referred to as the thoracolumbar (sympathetic) part. The preganglionic fibers which originate either in certain cranial nerve nuclei or the sacral part of the spinal cord are referred to as the craniosacral (parasympathetic) part. The sympathetic trunks enter the thorax from the neck and descend in front of the heads of the ribs and in front of the posterior intercostal vessels and nerves (Fig. 257).

The thoracic trunks usually have 10 or 11

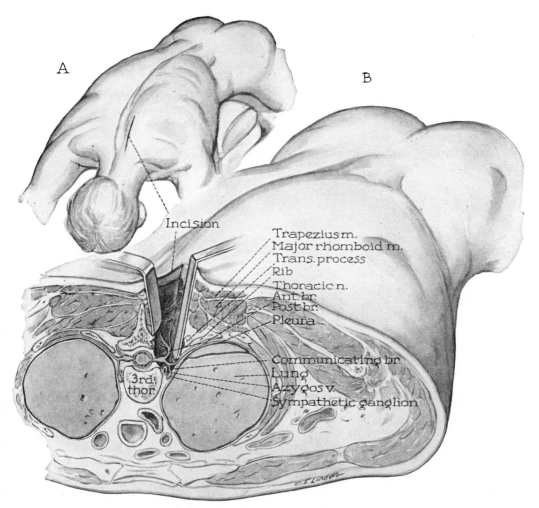

A

B

Incision

Trapezius m.
Major rhomboid m.
Trans. process
Rib
Thoracic n.
Ant. br.
Post. br.
Pleura

Communicating br.
Lung
Azygos v.
Sympathetic ganglion

3rd
thor.

FIG. 260. Thoracic sympathectomy (posterior approach).

separate ganglia which vary in size; occasionally, there may be 12. The 1st thoracic ganglion is frequently fused with the inferior cervical sympathetic ganglion to form the stellate (cervicothoracic) ganglion. The 2nd thoracic ganglion may be fused with the first. The remaining thoracic ganglia frequently lie at the levels of the corresponding intervertebral disks. The portion of the sympathetic trunk between two adjacent ganglia may be double and at other times may appear very slender. The sympathetic trunks enter the abdomen via the diaphragm by passing behind the medial lumbocostal arches. The trunks and the ganglia are connected with the ventral rami of the thoracic

nerve by means of rami communicantes which supply branches to adjacent viscera and blood vessels and then send splanchnic nerves into the abdomen (Figs. 258 and 259).

Each ganglion has from 1 to 4 rami communicantes which connect it with the corresponding nerves; connections may also be made with the nerve above or the nerve below. Three ganglionic sympathetic fibers in the spinal nerves reach the sympathetic trunk by way of these rami communicantes. Postganglionic fibers from the trunk and the ganglia to these nerves also course in these rami. Sensory (pain) fibers from the thoracic and the abdominal organs pass through the rami and thus reach the spinal nerves and the dorsal routes (see Fig. 183).

Although one cannot be too dogmatic in teaching, it may be safe to state that the thoracolumbar outflow is a mechanism associated with emergency situations in contrast with the conservatism of the craniosacral outflow. On the basis of this concept, we may now enumerate specific reactions which result from activation of the thoracolumbar system:

1. The pupil of the eye dilates because of excitation of the dilator pupillae muscle.

2. The blood pressure becomes elevated because of vasoconstriction, both peripheral and visceral.

3. The cardiac rate is increased.

4. Visceral musculature is inhibited.

5. External sphincters are activated, thus resulting in spasms.

6. The salivary and the digestive glands are inhibited in their activities.

7. The adrenal medulla is activated and pours out epinephrine, enhancing and reinforcing all of the above-mentioned responses.

SURGICAL CONSIDERATIONS

SYMPATHECTOMY

Sympathectomy may be helpful in dealing with causalgia, painful post-traumatic arthritis, painful amputation stump and the phenomenon of phantom limb. In these conditions the upper thoracic ganglia can be blocked temporarily with procaine, and the effect recorded. When pain recurs within a few hours after such injections, the sympathetic connections should be destroyed permanently. It is best to employ the preganglionic type of sympathectomy, as the effect of this operation is believed to be due to the elimination of vasomotor impulses and not to interruption of sensory fibers. The physiologic reasons for this have been well described by White and Smithwick. Sympathectomy as a form of treatment for hypertension will be discussed presently.

Whether it is desired to resect the upper thoracic sympathetic ganglia or to sever their central connections, the exposure is the same (Fig. 260). The patient is placed on the operating table face down, with several pillows under the chest. The incision is made 5 cm. lateral and parallel with the spinous processes; it is 10 cm. in length and centered over the ribs to be resected. The trapezius, the rhomboid minor and major, and the serratus posterior superior muscles are divided. The lateral border of the erector spinae and the overlying muscles are retracted. This exposes the rib and the transverse process to be resected. The rib is separated from the intercostal muscles and the underlying pleura and is cut off 4 cm. lateral to its articulation. The pleura is stripped away, and the sympathetic chain is located. It is best to divide the trunk below the 3rd thoracic ganglion first and then work upward, freeing it from the sides of the vertebrae and cutting its rami.

Abdominal Walls

Transverse incisions heal better

ANTERIOR ABDOMINAL WALL

BOUNDARIES

The anterior abdominal wall is bounded above by the costal margins and the xiphoid process of the sternum; only the costal cartilages of ribs 7, 8, 9 and 10 take part in this boundary, for the 11th and the 12th ribs do not reach the margin. It is bounded below and on each side by the portion of the iliac crest lying between the iliac tubercle and the anterior superior iliac spine, by the inguinal ligament, the pubic crests and the upper end of the pubic symphysis. The xiphoid process lies at the bottom of the depression between the two 7th costal cartilages; its edges and

tip afford attachment for the aponeurosis of the transversus abdominis muscle. Since it is painful and at times difficult to palpate the xiphoid, the lower end of the body of the sternum serves as a preferable landmark.

SURFACE ANATOMY

The lines of tension of the abdominal skin are nearly transverse; therefore, vertical scars tend to stretch, but transverse incisions become less conspicuous with time.

The skin of the abdomen is loosely attached to the underlying structures except at the umbilicus where it is normally firmly adherent.

The linea alba extends in the midline from

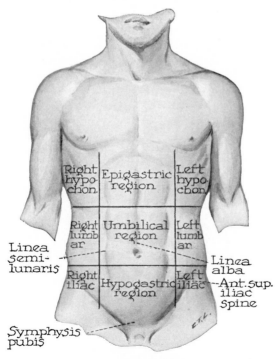

FIG. 261. The 9 regions of the anterolateral abdominal wall.

343

The recti almost touch in the midline inferior to the umbilicus!!

Above the umbilicus the linea alba is a broad

the xiphoid to the symphysis pubis; it is divided by the umbilicus into a supra-umbilical portion, which is a band about ½-inch wide, and an infra-umbilical part, which is so narrow that the recti almost touch. This is important surgically, since a midline incision placed above the umbilicus comes directly onto this broad band, but in an infra-umbilical midline incision it is difficult to find the threadlike midline. The linea alba is a fibrous raphe formed by the decussation of the 3 lateral abdominal muscles; since it contains few or no blood vessels, it can be incised with very little bleeding.

Clinically, the anterolateral abdominal wall has been divided into 9 regions created by 2 horizontal and 2 vertical lines (Fig. 261). The 2 horizontal lines are constructed in the following way: the upper line is placed at the level of the 9th costal cartilages, and the lower at the top of the iliac crests. The 2 vertical lines extend upward from the middle of the inguinal (Poupart's) ligament to the cartilage of the 8th rib. The 9 regions thus constructed are: 3 upper regions—left hypochondriac, epigastric and right hypochondriac; 3 middle regions—left lumbar, umbilical and right lumbar; 3 lower regions —left iliac, hypogastric and right iliac. Identifying the regions in this way aids in the description and the location of the viscera and the abdominal masses.

The umbilicus, or navel, is located in the linea alba, a little nearer the symphysis than the xiphoid. Usually its level is between the disks of the 3rd and the 4th lumbar vertebrae, but since it may vary in position, it is not too reliable a landmark.

It is a puckered scar which marks the site of the umbilical cord, through which 4 tubes

The linea alba is formed by the decussation of the 3 lateral abdominal muscles.

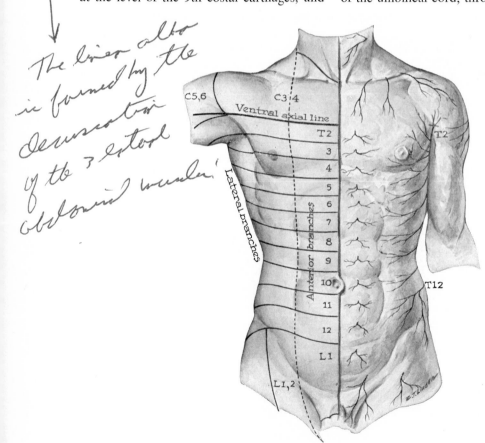

Fig. 262. The superficial nerve distribution of the anterolateral abdominal wall.

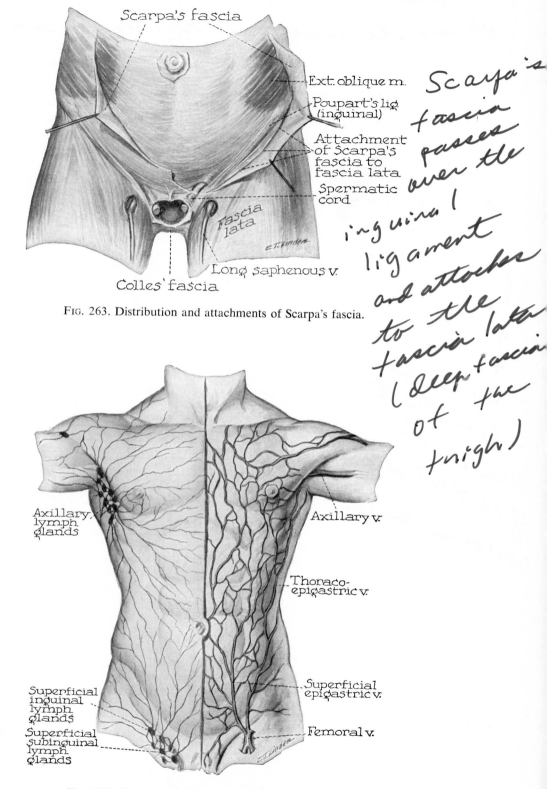

FIG. 263. Distribution and attachments of Scarpa's fascia.

FIG. 264. The superficial veins and lymphatics of the anterolateral abdominal wall.

Scarpa's fascia passes over the inguinal ligament and attaches to the fascia lata (deep fascia of the thigh)

passed in fetal life; they are the urachus, the right and the left umbilical arteries and the left umbilical vein (Fig. 290). They are situated in the properitoneal fat layer of the anterior abdominal wall and produce peritoneal folds. When the peritoneal aspect is studied in the adult, these 4 tubes are present as 4 atrophic fibrous cords. In the embryo, a structure called the vitello-intestinal duct is present; this connects the small bowel with the umbilicus.

If this structure is not obliterated at the time of birth, feces will discharge at the umbilicus; if the urachus is not completely obliterated at birth, urine will be noted at the same site. The hypogastric arteries of the fetus become the obliterated hypogastric arteries of the adult and pass over the lower abdominal wall as they proceed from the internal iliac arteries to the umbilicus; they may remain open and supply superior vesical branches to the urinary bladder.

The umbilical vein becomes the round ligament, or ligamentum teres, of the liver. The physiologic communication between the peritoneal cavity and the umbilical cord may persist, resulting in umbilical hernias (p. 375). The umbilicus may be the site for the collection and the discharge of bile and pus and may be the location of new growths such as papillomas or metastases from gastrointestinal carcinomas. The well-known but infrequently seen caput medusae is located in this region and is the result of the communication between the portal and the systemic circulations when the former is impaired.

The rectus abdominis muscle (p. 347) stands out on each side of the median line in the well-developed individual and forms a longitudinal prominence which is broader above than below; its lateral margin, which is slightly convex, is indicated by a groove on the skin known as the *linea semilunaris*. This line extends from the pubic tubercle to the costal margin of the 9th costal cartilage.

NERVES AND SUPERFICIAL FASCIA

Nerves. The skin of the anterior abdominal wall is supplied by the lower 6 thoracic and 1st lumbar nerves (Fig. 262). The lower 6 thoracic nerves give off anterior and lateral branches, but the lateral branch of the last thoracic nerve crosses the iliac crest to supply the skin of the buttocks.

The first lumbar nerve becomes the *ilio-hypogastric nerve*, which pierces the external oblique aponeurosis about 1 inch above the superficial inguinal ring, and the *ilio-inguinal nerve*, which passes directly through the superficial inguinal ring. The level of the umbilicus marks the 10th thoracic nerve.

The superficial fascia appears as a single layer in the upper part of the anterior abdominal wall, but in the lower region, especially between the umbilicus and the symphysis pubis, it is easily divided into 2 distinct layers: (1) a superficial layer of superficial fascia, which is a fatty stratum known as *Camper's fascia*, and (2) a deeper membranous layer called *Scarpa's fascia*, which is in contact with the deep fascia. The superficial layer contains small blood vessels and nerves. This fatty connective tissue gives roundness to the body, thus preventing unsightly angularity. The deep layer of superficial fascia is quite devoid of fat and blood vessels and descends on each side in front of the inguinal ligament to blend with the fascia lata of the thigh immediately below and nearly parallel with the ligament (Fig. 263). In the region of the pubic bone it is carried downward over the spermatic cords, the penis and the scrotum into the perineum, where it is known as *Colles' fascia*.

Tobin and Benjamin are of the opinion that the subcutaneous tissue is made up of only one layer and that the concept of an outer fatty and inner membranous layer is not justified.

ARTERIES, VEINS AND LYMPHATICS

The superficial arteries accompany the cutaneous nerves; those which accompany the lateral cutaneous nerves are branches of the posterior intercostal arteries, while those which travel with the anterior cutaneous nerves are derived from the superior and the inferior epigastric vessels. In addition to these, 3 small branches of the femoral artery are found in the superficial fascia of the groin. They are the superficial external

Below the umbilicus, the linea alba is small.

pudendal, the superficial epigastric and the superficial circumflex iliac arteries p. 359).

The superficial veins on each side of the anterior abdominal wall are divided into 2 groups: an upper and a lower. The upper group returns the blood via the lateral thoracic and the internal mammary veins to the superior vena cava; the lower group returns its blood via the femoral vein to the inferior vena cava. Both groups anastomose freely through the thoraco-epigastric vein; the superficial veins may dilate and compensate for an obstruction of either the superior or the inferior vena cava or for an obstruction of the external or the common iliac veins. The para-umbilical veins communicate with both of these groups and constitute an important connection between the portal and the systemic venous systems.

The superficial lymph vessels are divided into supra-umbilical and infra-umbilical groups. The supra-umbilical vessels drain into the pectoral lymph glands, and the infra-umbilical into the superficial inguinal glands (Fig. 264).

MUSCLES

In addition to the 3 lateral flat muscles of the anterior abdominal wall (external and internal obliques and transversus abdominis), there are the recti and the pyramidalis. The 3 lateral muscles have been discussed elsewhere (p. 359).

Rectus Abdominis Muscle. This appears as a long, broad, muscular band, which stretches between the pubis and the thorax on each side of the linea alba (Fig. 265). It originates by tendinous fibers from the pubic crest and the anterior pubic ligament. As it ascends it widens and becomes thinner; it inserts on the thorax as fleshy muscular fibers.

This insertion takes place along the anterior surfaces of the 5th, the 6th and the 7th costal cartilages and the xiphoid process (Fig. 265B). The insertion which is onto the front of the chest can be visualized along a horizontal line that extends from the xiphoid process to the end of the 5th rib; it is approximately 3 times as broad (3 inches) as the origin from the front of the symphysis. Its medial border is separated from that of

its fellow by the linea alba. Below the umbilicus, where the linea alba is a fine line, the 2 recti are practically in contact with each other, but above the umbilicus they are about ½ inch apart.

The anterior surface of the muscle is crossed by 3 tendinous intersections: one at the costal margin, one at the umbilicus and one between these two. A 4th may be present below the umbilicus, but it is not constant. The muscle is adherent to the anterior wall of the rectus sheath where these intersections appear, but since they do not penetrate the entire muscular depth, the rectus is nowhere adherent posteriorly. By this arrangement a long muscle is divided into a number of shorter ones, thus increasing its strength and efficiency.

The actions of the recti are shared with the abdominal obliqui and the transversus. These muscles act as efficient protectors of the abdominal viscera, and by their tonicity they maintain intra-abdominal pressure and help keep the viscera in place. They are also muscles of respiration, since their contraction causes them to press on the abdominal viscera, forcing them upward and thus elevating the diaphragm. They also play a part in defecation, since their contraction increases intra-abdominal pressure and helps the rectum to evacuate its contents. The rectus is a flexor of the vertebral column, pulling the thorax downward toward the symphysis; in this action its antagonist is the sacrospinalis. The rectus receives its nerve supply from the lower 6 intercostal nerves.

Rectus Sheath. This may be divided into 3 parts, each having a different construction: (1) above the costal margin, (2) from the rib margin to midway between the umbilicus and the pubis and (3) from midway between the umbilicus and the pubis to the pubis (Fig. 266).

1. *Above the Rib Margin.* This part of the sheath is incomplete. The anterior wall is made up of the aponeurosis of the external oblique, since this is the only one of the lateral abdominal muscles which extends above the costal margin. The posterior wall is absent and as a result of this, the rectus muscle lies directly on the cartilages.

2. *From the Rib Margin Down to Mid-*

The line of Douglas marks the pt above which the internal oblique aponeurosi splits into 2/ea

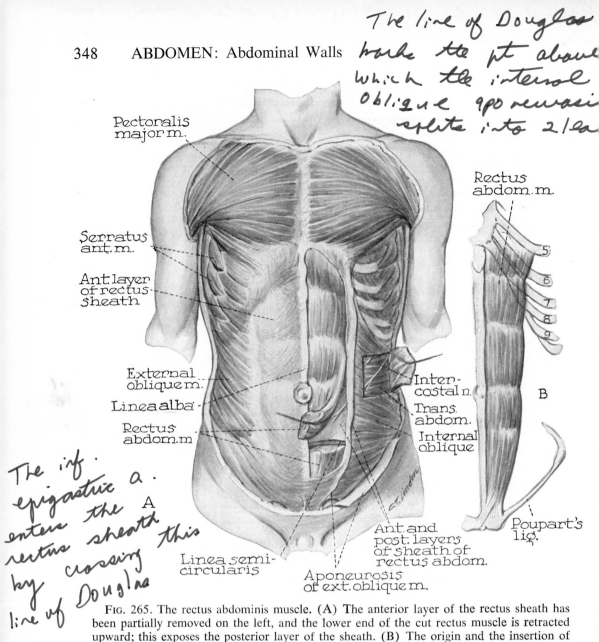

Pectoralis major m.

Rectus abdom. m.

Serratus ant. m.

Ant. layer of rectus sheath

5
6
7
8
9

External oblique m.

Linea alba

Rectus abdom. m

Inter-costal n.

Trans. abdom.

Internal oblique

B

The inf. epigastric a. enters the rectus sheath by crossing this line of Douglas

A

Linea semi-circularis

Ant. and post. layers of sheath of rectus abdom.

Poupart's lig.

Aponeurosis of ext. oblique m.

FIG. 265. The rectus abdominis muscle. (A) The anterior layer of the rectus sheath has been partially removed on the left, and the lower end of the cut rectus muscle is retracted upward; this exposes the posterior layer of the sheath. (B) The origin and the insertion of the muscle.

way Between the Umbilicus and the Pubis. This part of the sheath is complete. The internal oblique aponeurosis divides at the lateral border of the rectus muscle into an anterior layer and a posterior layer. The anterior wall of the sheath consists of the aponeurosis of the external oblique plus the anterior layer of the aponeurosis of the internal oblique. The posterior wall consists of the posterior layer of aponeurosis of the internal oblique, the aponeurosis of the transversus abdominis and the transversalis fascia. The transversus, where it extends behind the rectus, is muscular almost to the midline. Where the posterior sheath ends, midway between the umbilicus and the pubis, an arched lower border, which is called the *linea semicircularis* (Douglas), is formed (Fig. 265A). This line is an important dividing point, since cephalad to it the internal oblique aponeurosis splits into its 2 leaves, but below this point no such division takes place. The in-

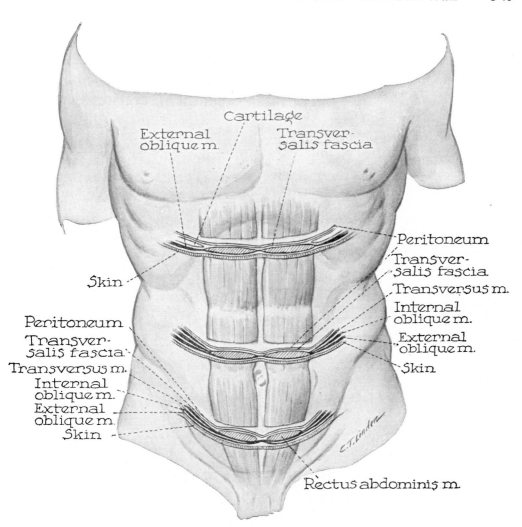

Cartilage

External   Transver-
oblique m.   salis fascia

Peritoneum
Transver-
salis fascia
Transversus m.
Internal
oblique m.

Skin

External
oblique m.

Skin

Peritoneum
Transver-
salis fascia
Transversus m.
Internal
oblique m.
External
oblique m.
Skin

Rectus abdominis m.

FIG. 266. The rectus sheath. Above the rib margin the anterior wall of the sheath is made up of the aponeurosis of the external abdominal oblique muscle; the posterior wall is absent, since the rectus muscle lies directly on cartilage. From the rib margin to midway between the umbilicus and the pubis, the anterior wall of the sheath consists of the aponeurosis of the external oblique plus the anterior layer of the aponeurosis of the internal oblique; the posterior wall consists of the posterior layer of the aponeurosis of the internal oblique, the aponeurosis of the transversus abdominis muscle and the transversalis fascia. From midway between the umbilicus and the pubis to the pubis, the anterior wall is formed by the aponeuroses of the external and the internal obliques and the transversus; the posterior wall is formed by the transversalis fascia.

ferior epigastric artery enters the sheath by crossing this edge.

3. *From Midway Between the Umbilicus and the Pubis to the Pubis.* The anterior wall is formed by the aponeuroses of the external and the internal obliqui and the transversus; here all the aponeuroses pass in front of the rectus. The transversus and the internal oblique are fused, but the external oblique does not fuse until it nearly reaches the midline. The posterior wall is formed by the transversalis fascia.

The contents of the rectus sheath are: (1) the rectus and the pyramidalis muscles, (2)

The rectus lies right on transversalis fascia

the superior and the inferior epigastric vessels, (3) the termination of the lower 5 intercostals and the 12th thoracic nerves with their accompanying vessels.

The nerves enter the sheath by piercing the posterior wall near the lateral margin and then run for a short distance between the posterior sheath and the rectus before entering the muscle proper.

The superior epigastric artery enters the rectus sheath behind the 7th costal cartilage and anastomoses with the inferior epigastric artery, which enters in front of the arcuate line. In this way the vessels of the upper and the lower limbs are brought into communication. Their branches are cutaneous, muscular and anastomotic.

Pyramidalis Muscle. This triangular muscle lies in front of the rectus; it is frequently absent. It arises from the front of the pubis and is inserted into the lower part of the linea alba between the rectus and the anterior wall of its sheath. It is supplied by the last thoracic nerve and acts as a tensor of the linea alba.

SURGICAL CONSIDERATIONS

ABDOMINAL INCISIONS

Numerous abdominal incisions have been described, but only those which are commonly used will be discussed. They may conveniently be divided in the following way (Fig. 267).

1. Rectus
   - A. Paramedian
   - B. Pararectus
   - C. Transrectus (muscle-splitting)
2. Oblique
   - A. McBurney
   - B. Kocher's subcostal
   - C. Iliac

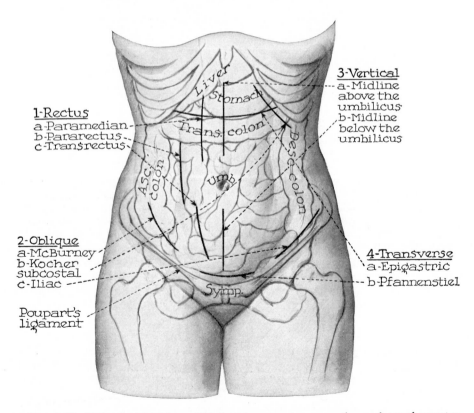

FIG. 267. Abdominal incisions. The incisions most commonly used are the rectus, the oblique, the vertical and the transverse. Examples of each are depicted in the illustration.

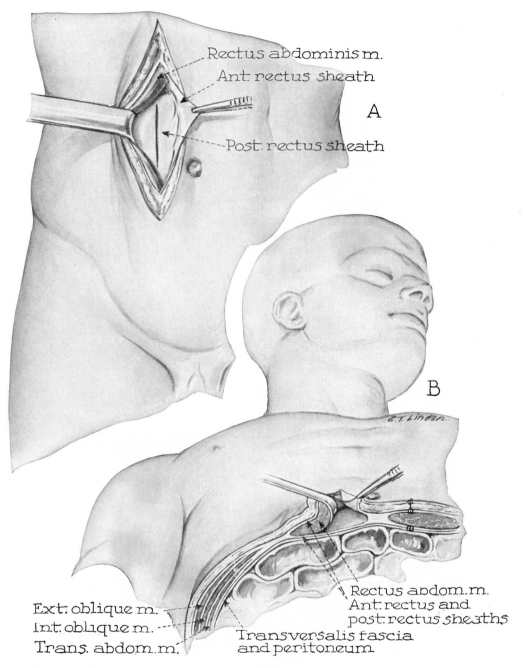

Rectus abdominis m.
Ant. rectus sheath

A

Post. rectus sheath

B

Ext. oblique m.
Int. oblique m.
Trans. abdom. m.

Rectus abdom. m.
Ant. rectus and
post. rectus sheaths
Transversalis fascia
and peritoneum

FIG. 268. The paramedian incision. This incision may be made in the upper or the lower abdomen and either on the right or the left side. (A) The incision in longitudinal section with the medial border of the right rectus muscle retracted laterally. (B) Cross section, showing the repair on the left side.

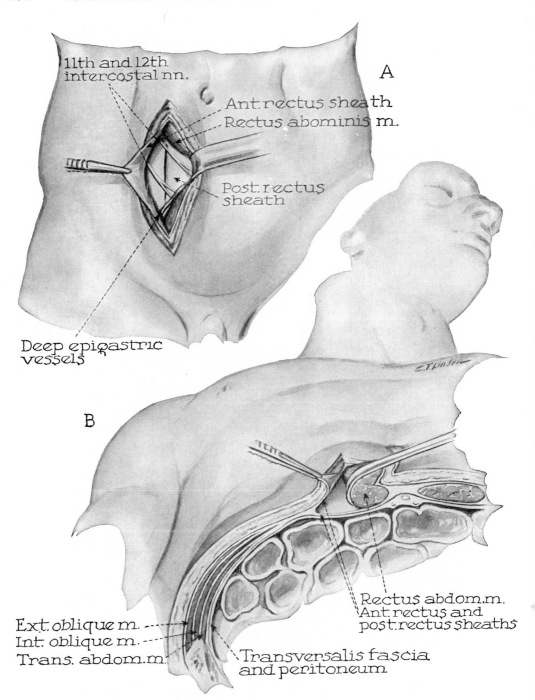

FIG. 269. The pararectus incision. (A) The 11th and the 12th intercostal nerves are shown passing along the retracted lateral border of the rectus muscle. (B) Cross section, showing the lateral border of the rectus muscle retracted medially.

3. Vertical: Midline
    A. Above the umbilicus
    B. Below the umbilicus
4. Transverse
    A. Epigastric
    B. Pfannenstiel

Rectus Incisions. Incisions through the rectus sheath and muscle may be used either above or below the umbilicus.

The *paramedian incision* is made about 1 inch to the right or the left of the midline (Fig. 268). The skin and the fascia are divided to the rectus sheath; the opening of the sheath exposes the rectus muscle. The medial border of the rectus is retracted laterally, exposing the posterior rectus sheath and the peritoneum; these are divided in the same line as the skin. The wound is sutured in 3 layers: (1) the peritoneum and the posterior rectus sheath, (2) the anterior rectus sheath and (3) the skin. The muscle returns of its own accord (trap-door action) over the posterior suture line. Injury to vessels and nerves is minimal, and the exposure of pelvic structures is excellent. *line a semilunaris*

The *pararectus incision* is similar to the paramedian, except that the approach to the abdominal cavity is along the lateral border instead of the medial border of the rectus muscle (Fig. 269). This incision has the disadvantage of encroaching on the nerves which enter and supply the rectus muscle laterally. The closure is accomplished in 3 layers, as described above. If the incision must be enlarged downward toward the pubis, the deep epigastric vessels may be encountered. Should this be the case, the artery and its 2 accompanying veins can be ligated and divided.

A *transrectus (muscle-splitting) incision* is performed in the same manner as the other 2 rectus incisions but differs in that the muscle is divided longitudinally through its medial third. The medial third is chosen in order to minimize injury to the nerve fibers. The muscle is divided in the line of its fibers, the tendinous inscriptions are clamped and ligated, and the posterior sheath and the peritoneum are incised. The incision is closed in layers.

Oblique Incisions. These have been uti-

lized, especially in surgery on the appendix and the gallbladder.

The *McBurney incision* (Fig. 270) is an oblique muscle-splitting incision which passes through the lateral abdominal musculature and is supposed to minimize postoperative weakness of the abdominal wall by incising the individual muscles in the direction of their fibers. The level and the length of this incision will vary according to the position of the appendix and the size of the patient. In a general way, however, it may be stated that it is made at the junction of the middle and the outer thirds and at right angles to an imaginary line joining the anterior superior iliac spine with the umbilicus. One third of the incision is placed above this line, and two thirds below it; the incision is usually about 3 inches long. The skin is incised in the direction of the fibers of the external abdominal oblique; this incision is carried through the superficial fascia until the fibers of the external oblique aponeurosis are seen. The latter is divided and separated from the underlying internal oblique; a distinct cleavage plane exists between these 2 muscles. The freed edges of the external oblique aponeurosis are retracted, and the horizontal fibers of the internal oblique muscle are exposed. The transversus abdominis muscle and the internal oblique have fibers which run in almost the same direction in this area; the cleavage between these 2 muscles is not too distinct. As soon as the transversalis fascia is exposed it is incised in the direction of the internal oblique opening. This exposes the preperitoneal fat and the peritoneum; these are incised. Various methods of enlarging the incision have been described, but since these do not adhere to the McBurney or gridiron principle, and since they encroach on the weak semilunar lines, such descriptions have been avoided intentionally. Usually this incision is closed in 3 layers: the first including the peritoneum and transversalis fascia; the second, the aponeurosis of the external oblique, and the third closes the skin. Some surgeons prefer to put a few approximating sutures in the internal oblique and the transversus muscles.

The *Kocher's subcostal incision* is used for operations on the biliary tract, but a similar

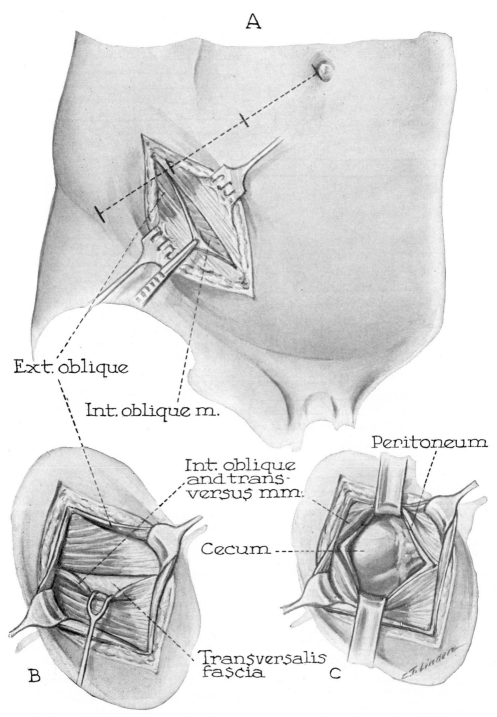

FIG. 270. The McBurney incision. (A) The skin incision is placed at the junction of the outer and middle thirds of a trisected line extending from the umbilicus to the anterior superior iliac spine; the aponeurosis of the external abdominal oblique muscle is incised in the line of its fibers. (B) The internal oblique and the transversus abdominis muscles are incised. (C) The peritoneum is incised, and the cecum is exposed.

incision may be placed on the left side for operations on the spleen or the cardiac end of the stomach. The incision is made parallel with and about 1 inch from the costal margin; it commences at the base of the xiphoid and is carried into the flank as far as is deemed necessary. The rectus muscle and the external abdominal oblique are divided. The posterior rectus sheath and the internal oblique are exposed and are divided in the line of the incision; the peritoneal cavity is entered. The incision is closed in layers.

The *iliac incision* is utilized in exposure of the ureter or the larger pelvic vessels. It is made parallel with and directly in front of the anterior portion of the iliac crest; it aims to reach the extraperitoneal structures below the brim of the pelvis. It is carried directly through the musculature and the transversalis fascia. The peritoneum is not opened but is mobilized and retracted medially. The necessary procedures are carried out extraperitoneally.

Vertical Incisions. The *midline incision above the umbilicus* is made directly in the linea alba, which can be located easily by the depression or pigmentation present. It begins just below the xiphoid cartilage, extends to the umbilicus and is usually 4 to 5 inches long. The skin and the superficial

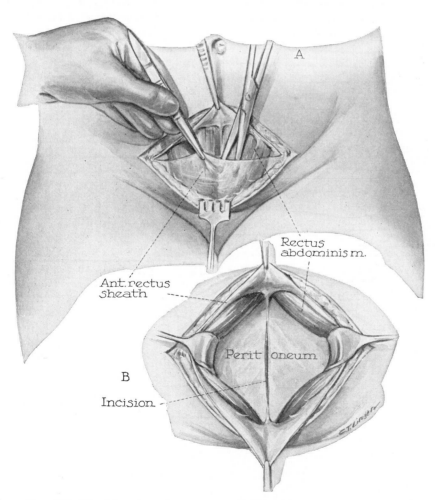

Ant. rectus sheath

Rectus abdominis m.

Perit|oneum

B

Incision

FIG. 271. The Pfannenstiel incision. (A) The skin and the anterior layer of the rectus sheath have been divided transversely. (B) The recti are drawn laterally, and the transversalis fascia, the extraperitoneal fat and the peritoneum (the only structure labeled) are incised vertically.

fascia are incised to the aponeurosis. The advantages of this incision are that it is almost bloodless, no muscle fibers are encountered, no nerves are injured, and it gives access to both sides of the abdomen. However, it has a disadvantage in that only one layer is available for repair because of the fusion of the aponeuroses in the midline; therefore, it cannot be relied upon and may result in weakness and herniation.

The *midline incision below the umbilicus* is employed almost routinely in gynecologic operations. Since the recti below the umbilicus are so close together, and because the linea alba is only a fine line, the right or the left rectus sheath is entered routinely, and the muscle is retracted laterally. Because of this, it is not exactly in the midline, and the repair is made in layers. Such a repair will result in a strong abdominal wall and does not have the disadvantage of weakness that a midline incision above the umbilicus would have.

Transverse Incisions. These abdominal incisions give excellent exposure but entail more time in execution and repair. They result in nicer-looking scars and produce less injury to the nerves and the blood vessels, since they run parallel with them.

The *transverse epigastic incision* extends from the lateral edge of one rectus to the lateral edge of the other. The underlying anterior rectus sheath, the rectus muscles, the posterior rectus sheath and the peritoneum are divided transversely on each side. If further exposure is required, the incision may be extended laterally beyond the lateral edge of the recti by splitting the oblique muscles. The individual layers of the abdominal wall are sutured separately, but it is to be recalled that only one fused layer is found in the region of the linea alba. This same incision has been modified by Sanders, who utilizes lateral retraction of the recti rather than division of these muscles.

The *Pfannenstiel incision* is a suprapubic transverse incision which is placed at or in the upper pubic hair line and in this way becomes concealed (Fig. 271). The skin, the subcutaneous tissue and the right and the left anterior rectus sheaths are divided transversely. The cut edges of the sheaths are dissected upward and downward for a short

distance; this exposes the recti and the pyramidalis when the latter is present. The exposed recti are freed from the underlying transversalis fascia and then are retracted laterally. The transversalis fascia, the properitoneal fat and the peritoneum are incised longitudinally. In closing the wound, the layers are sutured separately in the line of their division.

INCISIONAL HERNIAS

Cattell has described a method which results in a 5-layer repair in which the various components of the abdominal wall are not separated at the hernial ring. It has the advantage that no dissection is carried out at a point where it is most difficult to identify the layers, and its repair results in great strength at the point of greatest potential weakness (Fig. 272).

The old scar is excised by an elliptical incision, and the sac which usually lies immediately subcutaneous is identified; this is freed down to the hernial ring. The fascia is exposed. The sac is opened, and the contents are freed carefully and reduced; frequently, resection of the omentum is necessary. The first suture line includes the hernial ring and the inner side of the peritoneum. By everting the peritoneum, a smooth peritoneal surface remains in the peritoneal cavity. The redundant part of the sac is resected, but about 1 inch is left; this constitutes the second layer of repair. Then an elliptical incision is placed through the rectus sheath fascia; this extends to the muscle. These fascial flaps are dissected free on either side, and a third layer of sutures is placed; the sutures approximate the inner side of the 2 edges of cut fascia, thereby covering the peritoneal suture line. Suture line Number 4 approximates the muscles, and Number 5 the lateral edges of the incised fascial flaps. Then the skin is approximated.

INGUINAL REGION

The 9 Abdominal Layers. This region has been called the inguino-abdominal region and the inguinal trigone, the trigone being bounded by the inguinal ligament, the lateral margin of the rectus muscle and a horizontal line drawn from the anterior superior iliac spine to the rectus margin. Nine abdominal

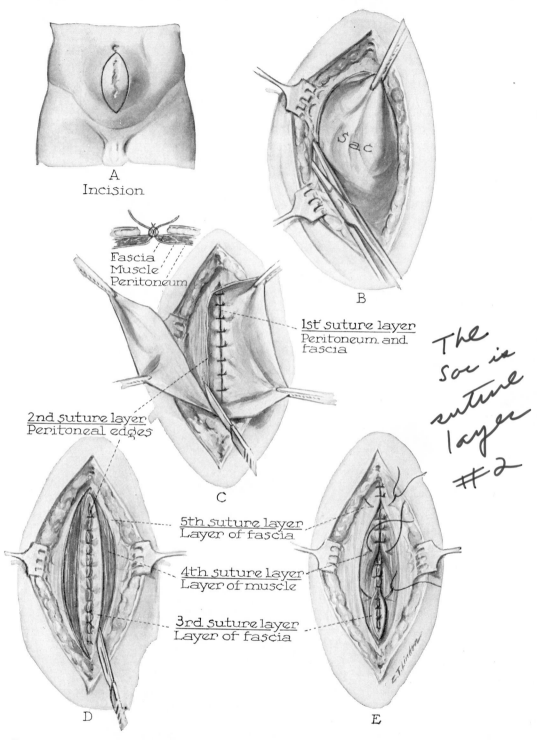

A
Incision

B

Fascia
Muscle
Peritoneum

1st suture layer
Peritoneum and
fascia

The sac is suture layer #2

2nd suture layer
Peritoneal edges

C

5th suture layer
Layer of fascia

4th suture layer
Layer of muscle

3rd suture layer
Layer of fascia

D

E

FIG. 272. Repair of incisional hernia. This method results in a 5-layer repair (Cattell).
(A) Excision of old scar by means of an elliptical incision. (B) Identification and freeing of sac. (C) The sac has been opened, and the first suture line placed, which includes
the hernial ring and the inner surface of peritoneum. All but an inch of redundant sac
is removed; this constitutes suture layer Number 2. (D) and (E) show the utilization of
the rectus sheath and muscle in layers 3, 4 and 5.

layers make up this region; these layers appear and are discussed in the following order (Fig. 273):

1. Skin
2. Superficial fascia (Camper's layer)
3. Superficial fascia (Scarpa's layer)
4. External oblique muscle
5. Internal oblique muscle
6. Transversus abdominis muscle
7. Transversalis fascia
8. Properitoneal fat
9. Peritoneum

The skin of this region is smooth and mov-

able and presents 3 particular landmarks for surface anatomy. They are: the anterior superior iliac spine, which is readily palpable; the pubic tubercle, which is less easily palpated, especially in the obese; and the umbilicus.

The superficial fascia is divided into 2 layers: a superficial layer of superficial fascia and a deep layer of superficial fascia. The superficial layer is known as Camper's fascia, and the deep layer as Scarpa's fascia. They usually are separable below the umbilicus but are fused above this point (Fig. 273).

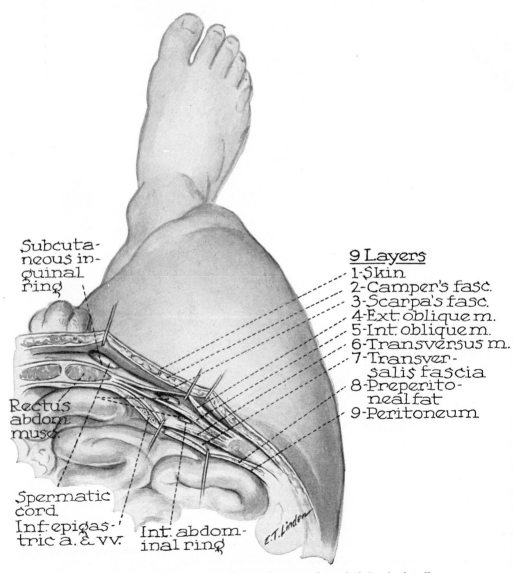

Subcutaneous inguinal ring

9 Layers
1-Skin
2-Camper's fasc.
3-Scarpa's fasc.
4-Ext. oblique m.
5-Int. oblique m.
6-Transversus m.
7-Transversalis fascia
8-Preperitoneal fat
9-Peritoneum

Rectus abdom. musc.

Spermatic cord
Inf. epigastric a. & vv.   Int. abdominal ring

C.T.Linden

FIG. 273. The 9 layers that make up the anterolateral abdominal wall.

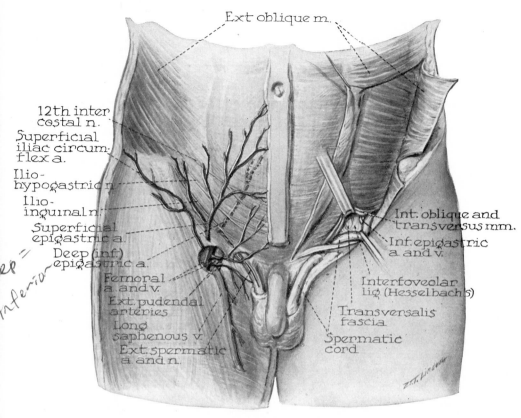

Fig. 274. The inguino-abdominal region. On the right side the superficial vessels and nerves are shown; on the left, the deeper structures (musculature) are depicted in their relations to the inguinal canal.

Camper's fascia is the fatty layer which is continuous with the adipose tissue covering the body generally. It is also called the *panniculus adiposus,* its thickness depending on the amount of fat present; the cutaneous vessels and nerves run in this layer (Fig. 274). The arteries found here are derived from the femoral artery and ascend from the thigh. They are: the superficial epigastric, which bisects the inguinal ligament and runs toward the navel; the superficial external pudendal, which runs medially across the spermatic cord and supplies the scrotum; the superficial circumflex iliac artery, which passes laterally below the inguinal ligament.

Scarpa's fascia is the membranous layer of superficial fascia; it contains no fat. The attachments of this fascia are clinically important because it is under this layer that extravasations of urine and blood take place. Scarpa's fascia passes over the inguinal ligament and attaches to the deep fascia of the thigh (fascia lata). This attachment takes place about a finger's breadth below and parallel with the inguinal ligament (Fig. 263). Medially, it attaches along a line that passes with, but lateral to, the spermatic cord; this line extends from the pubic tubercle to the pubic arch. The fixation occurs lateral to the pubic tubercle. Urine, blood or an exploring finger cannot extend beyond this attachment. Medial to the tubercle, Scarpa's fascia does not attach but continues over the penis and the scrotum; it continues as *Colles' fascia,* which covers the superficial compartment of the perineum.

The external abdominal oblique muscle arises from the lower 8 ribs (5 to 12); its

The external oblique aponeurosis forms all the ligaments.

The lacunar ligament is a portion of the ext. O. apo. if crus Klot rolls under the spermatic cord to attach to the pectineal line on the superior pubic ramus lateral to the pubic tubercle

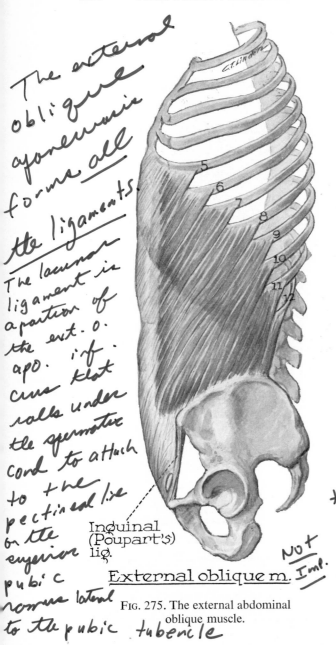

Inguinal (Poupart's) lig.

Not Imp.

External oblique m.

FIG. 275. The external abdominal oblique muscle.

muscle fibers become tendinous below the line joining the anterior superior iliac spine to the umbilicus. From the anterior superior iliac spine to the pubic spine the aponeurosis forms a free border which is called the inguinal (Poupart's) ligament, under which vessels, nerves and muscles pass from the abdomen to the thigh.

The **external oblique aponeurosis** forms the inguinal, the lacunar, Cooper's and the reflected inguinal ligaments (Figs. 276 and 277).

The **inguinal ligament (Poupart's)** is a tendinous part of the external oblique aponeurosis which extends from the anterior superior iliac spine to the pubic tubercle. The muscles which lie below it are the iliac, the psoas major and the pectineus. The ligament folds back on itself, forming a groove; the lateral half of this is not seen because it is obscured by the origin of the internal oblique and the transversus muscles. However, the medial half forms the gutterlike floor of the inguinal canal.

The **lacunar ligament (Gimbernat's)** is that part of the inguinal ligament which is reflected downward, backward and lateral. It attaches to the pectineal line, and its free crescentic margin forms the medial boundary of the femoral ring. It is the pectineal part of the inguinal ligament.

Cooper's ligament is the lateral continuation of the lacunar ligament. It extends from the base of the lacunar ligament laterally along the pectineal line to which it is attached.

The **reflected inguinal ligament (triangular ligament)** consists of reflected fibers which take their origin from the inferior crus of the superficial inguinal ring and the lacunar ligament (Fig. 276 B). They pass medially behind the spermatic cord and continue medially between the superior crus of the superficial inguinal ring and the conjoined tendon; they insert into the linea alba. Because of its triangular shape, this ligament has been called the triangular fascia. Arson and McVay found it unilaterally in only 3 per cent of bodies and bilaterally in less than 1 per cent.

The **superficial inguinal "ring" (subcutaneous inguinal "ring," external abdominal "ring")** (Fig. 278) has had the term "ring"

fibers are directed downward, forward and medial (Fig. 275). It interdigitates with the serratus anterior above; a continuous sheet of fascia covers both muscles. The most posterior fibers run vertically downward and insert into the anterior half of the iliac crest. Between the last ribs and the iliac crest a free border forms the lateral boundary of the lumbar (Petit's) triangle (p. 378). The

The pectineal ligament is the lateral continua. of the lacunar ligament.

The ring is not an open defect since + is covered by intercrural fibers.

applied to it, but this is unfortunate. In reality, it is a triangular thinned-out part of the aponeurosis of the external oblique muscle through which the spermatic cord in the male and the round ligament in the female pass. The apex of the triangle lies lateral to the pubic tubercle; its base, formed by the lateral half of the pubic crest, lies medial to the tubercle. The 2 sides are called the crura. The inferior crus (external pillar) is the medial end of the inguinal ligament; it attaches to the pubic tubercle. The superior crus (internal pillar) is that part of the aponeurosis which attaches to the pubic crest and the symphysis. The "ring" is not an open defect, since it is covered by the intercrural (intercolumnar) fibers which pass from one crus to the other. As the testicle made its descent, it encountered these intercrural fibers at the external "ring." The fibers were

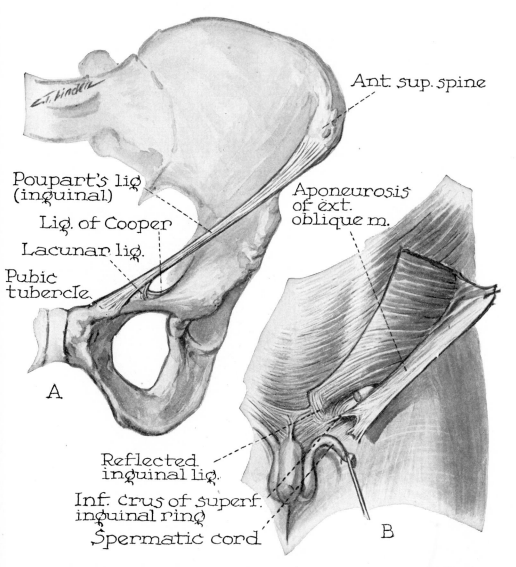

Ant. sup. spine

Poupart's lig. (inguinal)

Lig. of Cooper

Lacunar lig.

Pubic tubercle

Aponeurosis of ext. oblique m.

A

Reflected inguinal lig.

Inf. crus of superf. inguinal ring

Spermatic cord

B

FIG. 276. The ligaments in the inguinal region. (A) Poupart's ligament and its relations to Cooper's ligament and the lacunar ligaments. (B) The reflected inguinal ligament. The aponeurosis of the external oblique has been reflected laterally.

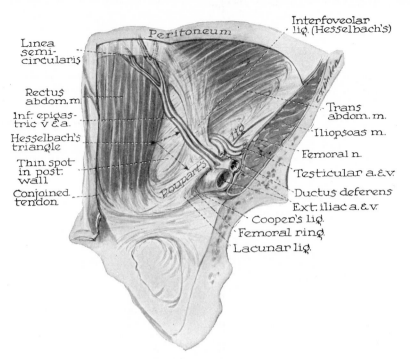

FIG. 277. Posterior view of the inguino-abdominal and the inguino-femoral regions. The peritoneum and the transversalis fascia have been removed.

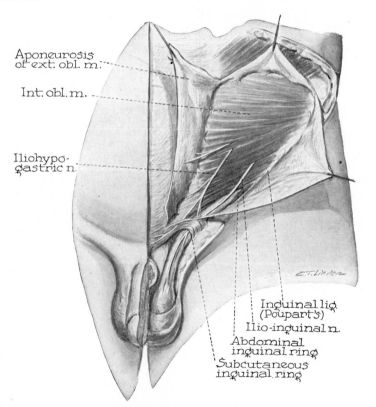

FIG. 278. The superficial inguinal "ring." The external oblique aponeurosis has been severed and retracted, but the "ring" remains intact.

pushed ahead by the descending testicle and formed a covering for the cord which is known as the *external spermatic fascia*.

The internal abdominal oblique muscle (Fig. 279) lies between the external oblique and the transversus abdominis muscles. This fan-shaped muscle has a narrow origin and a broad insertion. It originates from the outer half of the inguinal ligament, from the intermediate line on the iliac crest and from the posterior lamella of the lumbodorsal fascia through which it gains attachment to the lumbar spines. Because of this last fact, the muscle has no free posterior border.

The uppermost fibers run almost vertically upward and are inserted into the lower 4 ribs and their cartilages. The intermediate fibers form an aponeurosis which divides above the semicircular line (of Douglas) into 2 lamellae at the lateral border of the rectus muscle (Fig. 265). The anterior lamella accompanies the external oblique aponeurosis to form the anterior rectus sheath, and the posterior lamella accompanies the aponeurosis of the transversus abdominis to form the posterior rectus sheath. Below the semicircular line the combined aponeuroses of all 3 lateral abdominal muscles fuse and pass in front of the rectus muscle as the anterior rectus sheath.

Those fibers which originate from the inguinal ligament arch above the spermatic cord in the male and the round ligament in the female and become tendinous. They insert conjointly with those of the transversus abdominis into the crest of the pubis. It is this fusion of the tendinous portions of the internal oblique and transversus muscles that results in the structure known as the *conjoined tendon* (inguinal aponeurotic falx). However, in recent publications, Zieman, Zimmerman, Anson, McVay and Blake have emphasized the numerous structural variations present in this region. In 20 cadavers, Zieman could find only 2 in which the conjoined tendon appeared as a definite structure. The author also has been impressed with the rarity with which the conjoined tendon can be demonstrated at the operating table.

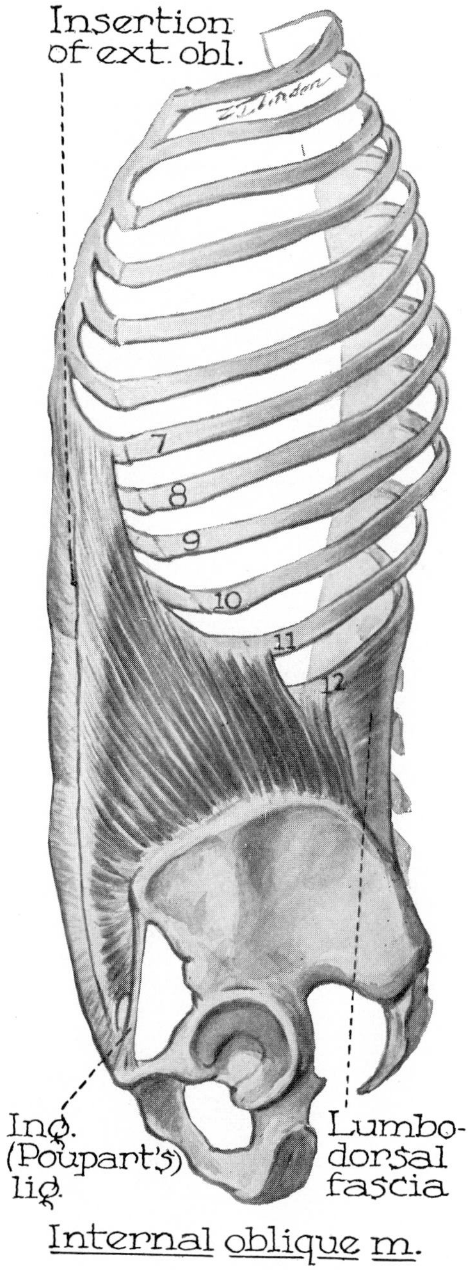

If one wishes to delve into the literature of this structure one will find many conflicting descriptions and opinions. Thus it

Insertion of ext. obl.

7
8
9
10
11
12

Inġ. (Poupart's) liġ.

Lumbo-dorsal fascia

Internal oblique m.

FIG. 279. The internal abdominal oblique muscle.

seems that the terms "conjoined tendon" and "falx inguinalis" have lost greatly the value they once had as descriptive terms. Many who have studied this particular structure and region feel that the terms should be

It is doubtful that the conjoined tendon even exists.

Nerves + vessels to the anterolat abd wall come between the internal oblique + transversus abdominis

Rectus
sheath

7
8
9
10
11
12

Ing.
(Poupart's)
lig.

Transversus
abdominis m.

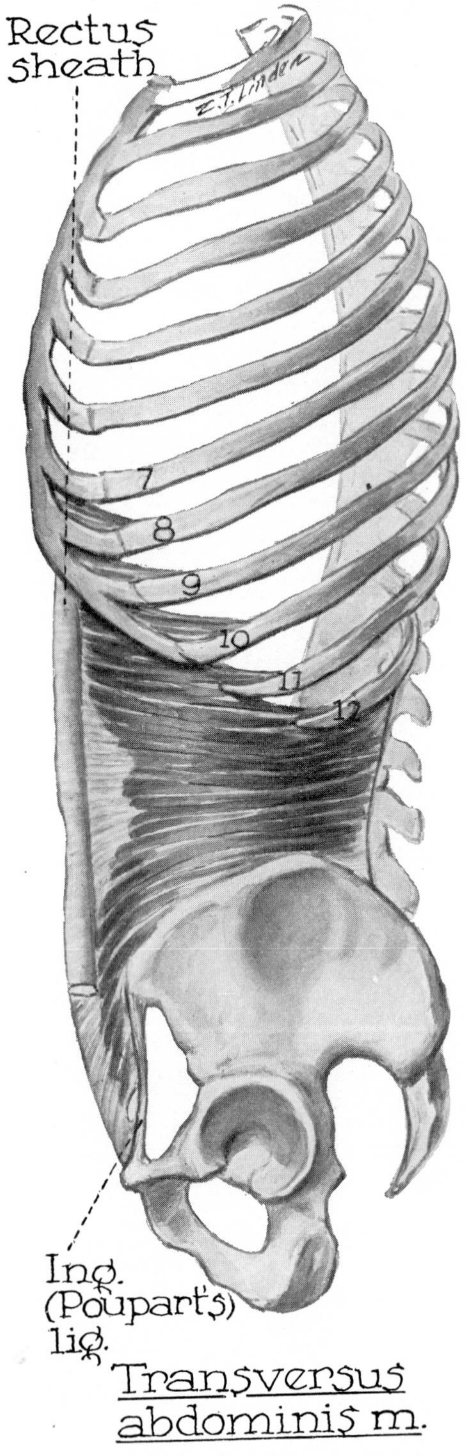

FIG. 280. The transversus abdominis
muscle.

abandoned. In place of this the transversalis fascia is considered to be a more important structure. It is interesting to ask various surgeons to demonstrate the so-called "conjoined tendon." Invariably, they have great trouble in identifying a true tendon and almost always point to a part of the rectus fascia in the region of the symphysis pubis. It should be emphasized that, although the fibers of the internal oblique arch over the spermatic cord, they insert behind it.

The transversus abdominis (transversalis) muscle (Fig. 280) is the deepest of the 3 lateral abdominal muscles. Only a little areolar tissue exists between it and the internal oblique muscle. It arises from the outer third of the inguinal ligament, from the inner lip of the iliac crest, from the middle layer of the lumbodorsal fascia and from the inner surface of the lower 6 costal cartilages where it interdigitates with the fleshy slips of the diaphragm. It is inserted into the linea alba and through the conjoined tendon into the pubic crest. Its aponeurosis passes behind the rectus muscle to the level of the linea semicircularis, but from this level downward it passes in front of that muscle. Most of the fibers pass in a horizontal direction; hence, its name transversus.

Since the internal oblique originates from the lateral half of the inguinal ligament and the transversus abdominis originates from the lateral third of the ligament, the testicle in its descent misses the transversus fibers but comes in contact with the internal oblique fibers, dragging some of the latter downward. These form muscle loops along the spermatic cord which are known as the *cremaster muscle*. The action of this muscle is to draw the testicles upward.

The *nerves* in this region are found in the interval between the internal oblique and the transversus abdominis muscles and then enter the rectus sheath (Fig. 265). The 7th and 8th thoracic nerves pierce the posterior lamella of the internal oblique aponeurosis at the costal margin and then pass upward and medially. The 9th nerve passes medially and slightly downward. The 10th, the 11th and the 12th nerves take a more downward course as they travel medially. The last 4 nerves pierce the posterior layer of the internal oblique aponeurosis at the lateral edge of the rectus sheath, continue medially behind the rectus muscle and then pierce its substance. All these nerves supply the 3 lateral muscles as well as the rectus abdominis. They finally pass through the anterior rectus sheath and end by supplying the overlying skin.

The 3 flat abdominal muscles form an elastic muscular corset which helps to maintain intra-abdominal pressure; this is of importance in retaining the viscera in place. By contracting simultaneously with the diaphragm they aid in urination, defecation, vomiting and parturition. By contracting alternately with the diaphragm (as an antagonist) they aid in exhalation. In the inguinal region these muscles form an arcade traversed by the spermatic cord. Grant has used the phrase "inguinal arcade" to describe this. When the inguinal portions of the internal oblique and transversus muscles contract, their arched fleshy fibers become straighter; this results in the lowering of the roof of the arcade and the constriction of the passage. The contraction of the external oblique approximates the anterior wall to the posterior wall, and a sphincterlike action results (Fig. 281).

The transversalis fascia, also called the endo-abdominal fascia, is a connective tissue layer which covers the entire internal surface of the abdomen. This fascia covers certain muscles and in each case assumes the name of the muscle which it accompanies, such as the diaphragmatic fascia, the iliac fascia, etc. Its thickness is variable, but that part which is below the inferior margins of the internal oblique and transversus abdominis muscles usually is well developed. It is in this unprotected area that it forms the floor of Hesselbach's triangle and, when torn or weakened, predisposes to the development of a direct inguinal hernia. The fascia lies between the transversus abdominis muscle and the pro-peritoneal fat layer. In certain areas, especially in those people where the fat layer is wanting, a fusion may result between the transversalis fascia and the peritoneum. In a situation such as this the two layers cannot be separated, and the peritoneal cavity must be entered as if through one layer. This fascia is applied to the posterior surface of

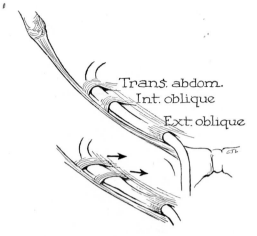

FIG. 281. The inguinal arcade. Grant has used this phrase to describe the muscular arcade traversed by the spermatic cord. Note the lowering of the roof of this arcade when the transversus abdominis and the internal oblique muscles contract.

the rectus sheath, and where the latter terminates at the semicircular line, it lies in direct contact with the posterior surface of the rectus muscle. Inferiorly, it is attached to the outer half of the inguinal ligament and to the iliac crest, where it becomes continuous with the iliac fascia. Over the inner half of the inguinal ligament it covers the femoral vessels upon which it passes, behind the ligament and downward into the thigh, forming part of the anterior wall of the femoral sheath. Medial to the femoral vessels it is attached to the pectineal line and the pubic crest.

Anson and Daseler have suggested that the abdominal fasciae in the adult be divided into three layers: an internal layer for the gastrointestinal tract with its vessels and nerves; an intermediate layer for the urogenital system, the adrenals and their associated vessels and nerves, together with the aorta and the vena cava; and an external layer for the parietal musculature (body wall) with its nerves and vessels. The last-mentioned outer stratum is what the majority of modern textbooks refer to as the transversalis fascia. Tobin verified this work and states that these strata are clinically important as surgical guides and as barriers to or pathways for the spread of infection or extravasations of blood or urine.

Descent of the Testicle. The factors responsible for this descent are not understood. In the early months of intra-uterine life the scrotum is undeveloped, and the testis is located in the abdomen (lumbar region) (Figs. 282 and 283). The testicle develops between the transversalis fascia and the peritoneum in the stratum of the properitoneal fat. In the 3rd month of intra-uterine life it descends from the loin to the iliac fossa and from the 4th to the 7th months it rests at the site of the internal (abdominal) inguinal ring. During the 7th month it passes through the inguinal canal into the scrotum, preceded by a peritoneal diverticulum called the *processus*

vaginalis; its vessels, nerves and duct are dragged after it.

The *gubernaculum testis* is a triangular structure, the base of which is attached to the testis (epididymis), and the apex to the bottom of the scrotum. Some authors have suggested the theory that the testicle passes through the inguinal canal as a result of its being pulled into the scrotum by the contraction (or atrophy) of the musculature of the gubernaculum. Others are of the opinion that this is fallacious. Wells believes the gubernaculum to be associated with an "inguinal bursa," thereby guiding the testis in its descent.

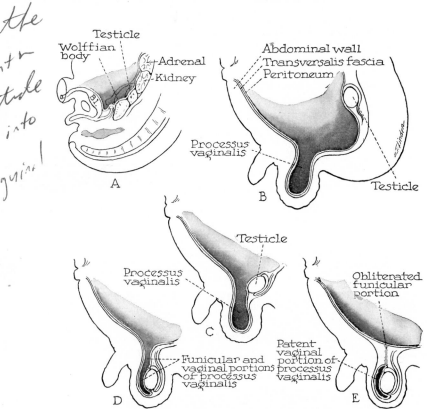

Fig. 282. The descent of the testicle. (A) Early development in the lumbar region. (B) The testicle at a later stage of development in the lumbar region; it lies between the transversalis fascia and the peritoneum. The vaginal process has formed. (C) At the end of the 3rd month of intra-uterine life the testicle reaches the pelvic brim. (D) As the testicle descends in the scrotum, the vaginal process becomes differentiated into a funicular portion which is applied to the spermatic cord and a vaginal portion which is applied to the testicle. (E) The testicle has reached the base of the scrotum. Normally, the funicular portion becomes obliterated, and the vaginal portion remains patent.

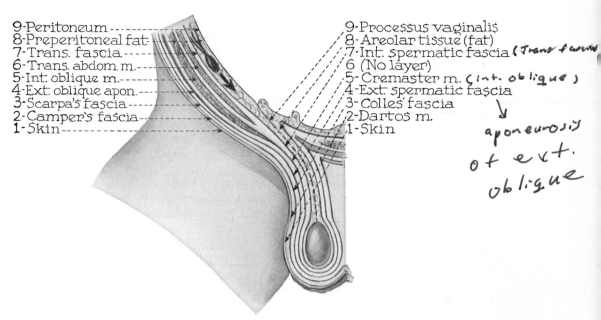

9-Peritoneum
8-Preperitoneal fat
7-Trans. fascia
6-Trans. abdom. m.
5-Int. oblique m.
4-Ext. oblique apon.
3-Scarpa's fascia
2-Camper's fascia
1-Skin

9-Processus vaginalis
8-Areolar tissue (fat)
7-Int. spermatic fascia (Trans. fascia)
6 (No layer)
5-Cremaster m. (int. oblique)
4-Ext. spermatic fascia
3-Colles' fascia
2-Dartos m.
1-Skin

↓
aponeurosis
of ext.
oblique

FIG. 283. Schematic drawing of the descent of the testicle. The relations between the abdominal wall, the inguinal canal, the spermatic cord and the scrotum have been stressed. As the testicle descends, it encounters certain layers of the anterior abdominal wall which it pushes ahead of it. This results in certain coverings of the spermatic cord and layers of the scrotum. The numbers indicating the layers in the scrotum and the coverings of the cord correspond to the same numbers which identify the layers of the anterior abdominal wall.

The remnants of the gubernaculum become the *scrotal ligament;* this is a short band which connects the inferior pole of the testicle to the bottom of the scrotum. Prior to the descent of the testicle, the vaginal process of peritoneum extends into the scrotum. This applies itself to the cord and the testicle; it forms an incomplete covering, but at no point does the processus vaginalis completely surround them.

That part of the vaginal process which is applied to the testicle is the *tunica vaginalis testis* (vaginal portion); it remains patent. That part of the vaginal process which is applied to the spermatic cord, between the tunica vaginalis testis and the abdominal (deep) inguinal ring, becomes the *funicular process;* it loses its patency and becomes a fibrous cord known as the vaginal ligament (p. 269).

As the testicle descends, it contacts the transversalis fascia; it does not force a hole through it, but instead pushes or evaginates this fascia. In this way it acquires a tubular covering called the *internal spermatic fascia (infundibuliform fascia).* Therefore, the internal spermatic fascia is that evaginated portion of the transversalis fascia which supplies a covering for the spermatic cord. At that point where the testicle meets the transversalis fascia and pushes it forward, the internal inguinal ring is formed. Hence, the internal ring is a thinned-out part of the transversalis fascia.

As the descent of the testicle continues, it passes below the curved border of the internal oblique muscle. It does not come in contact with the transversus abdominis muscle, since this structure lies on a higher level and therefore offers no resistance to the descent of the gland. As the testicle touches the lower border of the internal oblique muscle it drags some of its lowermost muscle fibers with it, thus forming a series of loops; in this way a second covering of the cord, the *cremaster muscle,* is acquired.

The next layer that the gland comes in contact with is the aponeurosis of the external abdominal oblique muscle; it arrives at this point at the 8th month. It evaginates this aponeurosis and acquires another covering of the spermatic cord called the *external spermatic fascia*. Thus the testis and the cord have acquired 3 coverings: (1) the internal spermatic fascia from the transversalis fascia, (2) the cremaster muscle from the internal oblique and (3) the external spermatic fascia from the aponeurosis of the external abdominal oblique aponeurosis. The so-called "rings" are not true rings or defects. The internal "ring" is a thinned-out portion of transversalis fascia, and the external "ring" is a thinned-out portion of the aponeurosis of the external abdominal oblique aponeurosis. The testicle pushes Scarpa's fascia ahead of it; it becomes the Colles' fascia of the perineum. Camper's fascia (panniculus adiposus) is a fatty layer and, since there is no fat in the scrotum, it is replaced by the dartos muscle. At the 9th month the testicle reaches the scrotum.

The Inguinal Canal. The fully developed inguinal canal (Fig. 284) is not a canal in the true sense of the word but is a cleft which takes an oblique course through the inguino-abdominal region. In the adult its length is about 4 to 5 cm.

The entrance to the canal is through the *abdominal (deep) inguinal ring,* which is located a little above the center of the inguinal ligament. The exit is through the *subcutaneous (superficial) inguinal ring* (p. 360).

The *interior wall* of the canal is formed by the aponeurosis of the external abdominal oblique in its entire length, and the fleshy fibers of the internal oblique in the lateral half. The *posterior wall* is formed by the transversalis fascia in the entire length of the canal, and the conjoined tendon in the medial half; the latter structure lies in front of the transversalis fascia and behind the cord.

The *roof* is formed by the arched lower border of the internal oblique and to a lesser degree by the transversus abdominis. The *floor* is represented by a groove which is formed by a fusion of the upper grooved surface of the inguinal ligament, the lacunar

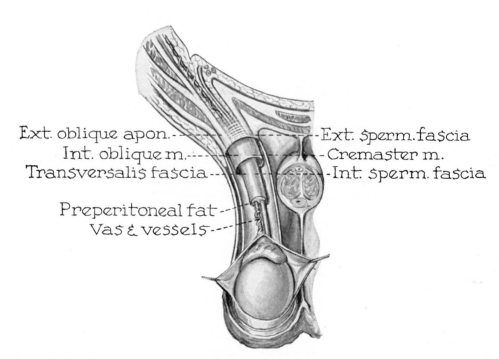

Ext. oblique apon.----
Int. oblique m.----
Transversalis fascia---

Preperitoneal fat---
Vas & vessels---

-Ext. sperm. fascia
-Cremaster m.
-Int. sperm. fascia

FIG. 284. The formation of the external spermatic fascia, cremaster muscle and the internal spermatic fascia.

ligament and the transversalis fascia. The cord rests on this groove.

Types of Indirect Inguinal Hernias (Fig. 285). Soon after birth, the *processus vaginalis*, a peritoneal diverticulum, becomes occluded at two points. First, at the internal abdominal ring and, second, directly above the testis. That part of the vaginal process which is situated between these two points, the *funicular process,* becomes obliterated.

If the vaginal process remains patent throughout its entire course and the opening above is wide enough, bowel or omentum may enter this process and pass into the scrotum. This condition is known as a *vaginal (congenital) indirect inguinal hernia.* When only the proximal or funicular portion of the vaginal process remains open, a *funicular indirect hernia* results.

An *encysted hernia* is the same as a vaginal type plus a process of peritoneum which lies in front of the sac and extends up to the external ring. This is due to the catching of a diverticulum of the processus vaginalis at the external ring during development.

In the *infantile* type, the conditions are exactly the same as are found in the funicular type, plus a process of peritoneum which is found in front of the hernia as high as the external ring. Therefore, at operation a peritoneal sac is found in front of the hernial sac; this may be very confusing unless they are identified properly.

The *interstitial* types of hernias are due to a diverticulum of the processus vaginalis which becomes caught between the layers of the developing abdominal wall (Fig. 286). These types of hernias are rare and usually are found associated with imperfectly descended testicles. The sac may be:

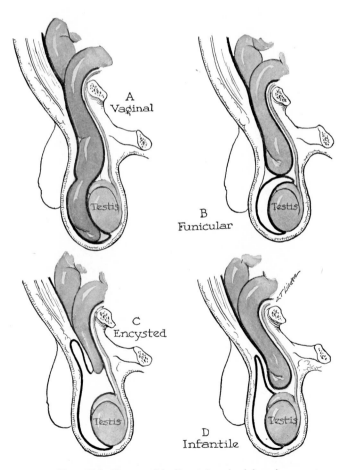

FIG. 285. Types of indirect inguinal hernias.

[handwritten top margin: In a true hydrocele, there is a collection of fluid in some part of the process vaginalis.]

1. Proparietal (extraparietal), between the superficial fascia and the external oblique muscle.

2. Interparietal (intramuscular), between the internal and the external oblique muscles.

3. Retroparietal (intraparietal) between the transversalis fascia and the peritoneum.

Types of Hydroceles (Fig. 287). In the true hydrocele there is a collection of fluid in some part of the processus vaginalis; the types may be vaginal, congenital, infantile and hydroceles of the cord.

The *vaginal* type presents a collection of fluid, not due to any fault of development, in the tunica vaginalis. Since it is acquired, it becomes important to determine whether

it is the so-called common "idiopathic" variety or secondary to some disease of the testis or the epididymis, such as a malignancy or tuberculosis.

The *congenital* type is also known as an intermittent hydrocele; it is due to a tiny communication between the processus vaginalis and the peritoneal cavity which permits the escape of fluid. It may be confused with a congenital hernia.

In the *infantile* type, the processus vaginalis is occluded only at the internal abdominal ring.

In *hydrocele of the cord,* the funicular process fails to shrink to a fibrous cord so that a tubular cavity results. This is shut off

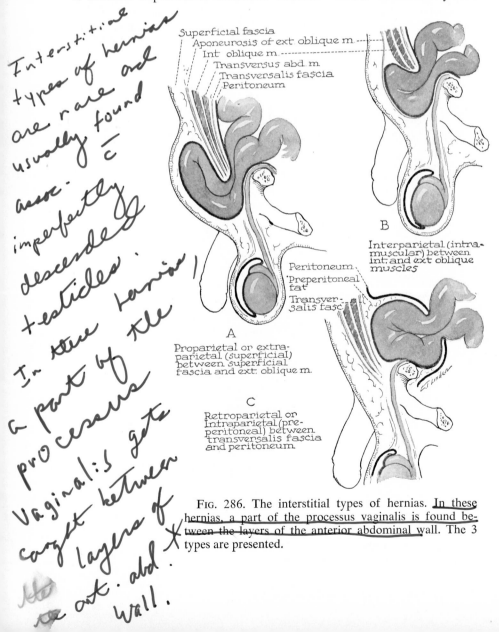

Superficial fascia
Aponeurosis of ext oblique m.
Int oblique m.
Transversus abd. m.
Transversalis fascia
Peritoneum

A
Proparietal or extra-parietal (superficial) between superficial fascia and ext. oblique m.

Peritoneum
Preperitoneal fat
Transversalis fascia

B
Interparietal (intra-muscular) between int. and ext oblique muscles

C
Retroparietal or Intraparietal (pre-peritoneal) between transversalis fascia and peritoneum.

FIG. 286. The interstitial types of hernias. In these hernias, a part of the processus vaginalis is found between the layers of the anterior abdominal wall. The 3 types are presented.

[handwritten left margin: Interstitial types of hernias are rare and usually found c̄ assoc. imperfectly descended testicles. In these hernias a part of the processus vaginalis gets caught between layers of the ant. abd. wall.]

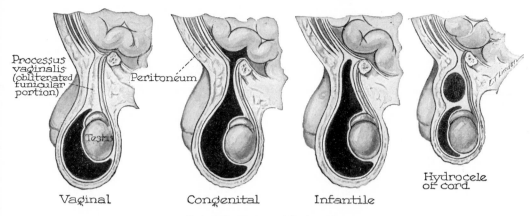

Processus vaginalis (obliterated funicular portion)

Peritoneum

Testis

Hydrocele of cord

Vaginal   Congenital   Infantile

FIG. 287. Types of hydroceles.

from the peritoneum above and the tunica vaginalis below. As it becomes distended with fluid it forms one or more swellings which are separated from the testicle.

SURGICAL CONSIDERATIONS

INGUINAL HERNIAS, INDIRECT AND DIRECT

Indirect Hernias. Many methods exist for the repair of an *indirect inguinal hernia*. An exhaustive and exhausting literature is accessible to any one interested in special studies of this problem. However, in considering herniorrhaphies, certain points should be stressed, such as the modern concept of the conjoined tendon (doubting the existence of such a structure), the importance of the transversalis fascia, and the management of the sac. A method which emphasizes these points will be described (Fig. 288).

The *incision* is made from a point which joins the middle and the outer thirds of a line between the anterior superior iliac spine and the umbilicus to a point which marks the pubic tubercle. It is difficult actually to feel this tubercle, since the spermatic cord passes over it; hence, the pubic bulge which is produced by the spermatic cord is the landmark used. The incision is deepened through Camper's and Scarpa's fascia until the aponeurosis of the external abdominal oblique is exposed. The external inguinal ring is identified, and the continuation of the external abdominal oblique over this ring, namely, the external spermatic fascia, is incised. Then the external oblique aponeurosis is incised, and its edges are held apart and dissected

free from the underlying internal oblique muscle.

The iliohypogastric and the ilio-inguinal nerves usually can be demonstrated at this point. The lower border of the internal oblique becomes visible, and its continuation, the cremaster muscle loops, should be elevated. These are severed, and the internal oblique is freed from the underlying transversalis fascia. The transversus abdominis muscle is not seen because it is not situated this low.

A small blunt retractor is placed under the dissected free edge of the internal oblique, and this muscle is retracted cephalad. The lateral cut edge of the external oblique aponeurosis is retracted outward, thus exposing Poupart's ligament. The finger or a blunt instrument is placed on this ligament and passed downward to the pubic spine. This elevates the spermatic cord, which then is retracted laterally.

Since the hernial sac is found at the *upper inner quadrant* of the cord, lateral traction on the cord tenses the transversalis fascia which overlies the sac. It is at this quadrant that the transversalis fascia should be opened. Then the properitoneal fat layer is identified; it serves as an excellent guide, since the peritoneum (sac) lies immediately subjacent to this fat. However, the transversalis fascia, the properitoneal fat and the peritoneum may be fused into one layer, especially in thin individuals, so that the sac is entered immediately when an attempt is made to dissect the transversalis fascia.

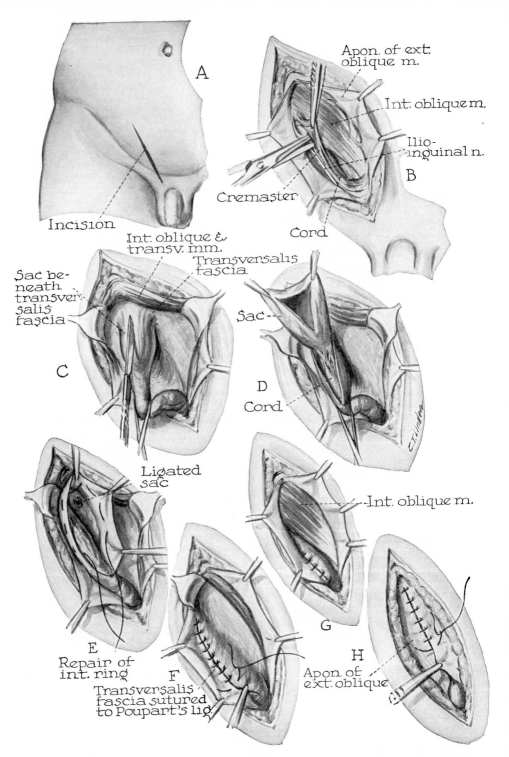

A

Incision

Apon. of ext. oblique m.

Int. oblique m.

Ilio-inguinal n.

B

Cremaster

Cord

Int. oblique & transv. mm.

Transversalis fascia

Sac beneath transversalis fascia

Sac

C

D

Cord

Ligated sac

Int. oblique m.

E
Repair of int. ring

F
Transversalis fascia sutured to Poupart's lig.

G

H
Apon. of ext. oblique

FIG. 288. The repair of an indirect inguinal hernia. (A) The incision extends from a point which joins the middle and the outer thirds of an imaginary line between the antero-superior iliac spine and the umbilicus to the pubic tubercle. (B) The cremaster fibers are cut, and the lower border of the internal oblique muscle is freed. (C) The internal oblique

(*Continued on facing page*)

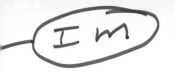
The sac is dissected free from the surrounding structures, it is opened, and its contents are reduced. Its neck should be freed as high as possible, which anatomically implies on a level with the deep epigastric vessels. In indirect inguinal hernias these vessels lie medial to the neck of the sac. With downward traction on the sac and upward traction on the internal oblique and the transversalis fascia, a high ligation becomes possible. The sac is transfixed and ligated, and the redundant tissue distal to the ligature is cut away.

The defect in the transversalis fascia, which the surgeon has created, must be repaired properly to prevent the development of a *direct* hernia. This closure is accomplished by means of a purse-string suture which incorporates the fascia overlying the spermatic cord. Then the free edge of transversalis fascia is sutured to Poupart's ligament. No sutures are placed in the internal oblique muscle, since this would interfere with its sphincteric or shutterlike action. The cut edges of the aponeurosis of the external abdominal oblique are sutured, thus reconstructing the roof of the inguinal canal. Scarpa's fascia and the skin are closed as separate layers.

Direct Hernias. Since the underlying cause of a *direct inguinal hernia* is a weakness of or defect in the transversalis fascia, the method of repair becomes the most important feature. The operation is essentially the same as that described for an indirect hernia. When the bulge of a direct hernia has been located, the thinned transversalis fascia is opened and the underlying properitoneal fat and the hernial sac are freed. The sac usually is not opened but is reduced by means of a purse-string suture. One attempts to repair the defect in the thin transversalis fascia by means of mattress sutures which imbricate it. The resulting free edge of trans-

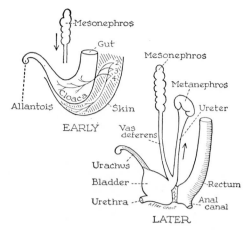

FIG. 289. Embryology of the umbilical region. The cloaca, a part of the hindgut, separates into a dorsal part (rectum) and a ventral part. The ventral part divides into a cranial part (the urachus), a middle part (the bladder) and a caudal part (the urethra).

versalis fascia then is sutured to Poupart's ligament. If the fascia is too thin and will not hold the sutures, a flap of the anterior rectus sheath (internal oblique aponeurosis) is freed and sewed to Poupart's ligament. Numerous modifications, including cutis grafts, wire mesh and fascia lata have been used to strengthen this defect.

Jennings, Anson and Wright have described a method for the repair of indirect inguinal hernias; they utilize a midline incision, retract the rectus muscle and grasp the sac abdominally. The sac is freed from the cord and is ligated high; the abdominal incision is closed. The method has found favor with some surgeons.

UMBILICAL REGION

The umbilical region occupies the central part of the anterolateral abdominal wall.

---

muscle is retracted upward, and the transversalis fascia is incised at the upper, inner quadrant of the cord. (D) The sac is elevated and opened. (E) The sac has been ligated high; the transversalis fascia is repaired by means of a purse-string suture which incorporates the fascia overlying the cord. (F) The free edge of transversalis fascia is sutured to Poupart's ligament. (G) No sutures are placed in the internal oblique muscle. (H) The aponeurosis of the external abdominal oblique is sutured.

You don't open the sac in a direct hernia → you simply imbricate it !!

omph. duct (meckel's) → the way by which the yolks
communicates c̄ the fetal intestinal tract.
N.; it disappears when the embryo is 6-12 mm. in
length.

374   ABDOMEN: Abdominal Walls

Embryology. The cloaca is a part of the hindgut which ultimately separates into a dorsal part (rectum) and a ventral part. The ventral section divides into 3 components: (1) a cranial component which becomes the urachus (*allantois*), (2) a middle part which becomes the bladder and (3) a caudal part which becomes the urethra and, in the female, part of the vagina (Fig. 289). The upper part of the allantois is continued into the umbilicus and the umbilical cord; the intra-abdominal portion of the allantois is called the urachus. The urachus and the allantois become a solid cord, which may develop cystlike dilatations. These dilatations are characteristic of this cord and may be found at any period in the development of the embryo. They persist in many adults and account for the small cysts found at operation. If the urachus remains patent at birth, a urinary umbilical fistula results.

If the peritoneal surface of the umbilical region is examined, 4 fibrous cords are seen radiating from it (Fig. 290). These are the remains of 4 tubes which pass through the umbilical cord in fetal life; they are the urachus, the right and the left umbilical arteries and the left umbilical vein. They are situated in the extraperitoneal fatty layer of the anterior abdominal wall and produce peritoneal folds.

In the early human embryo the alimentary tract communicates with the yolk sac by means of a *vitello-intestinal* (omphalomesenteric) duct. This structure usually disappears when the embryo is between 6 and 12 mm. in length; it does not leave a residual peritoneal fold. However, its vessels persist long after the duct has disappeared. Although the duct normally disappears, a part of it may remain or it may be found patent. If patent, an umbilical fecal fistula develops. If only the inner end remains patent, a Meckel's diverticulum develops which may or may not be adherent to the umbilicus. Rarely, the median portion persists, and the duct becomes obliterated at both ends; in such cases an intestinal cyst results. At times the omphalomesenteric vessels persist as fibrous cords which may give rise to intestinal obstruction.

Vessels. Originally, there were 2 arteries and 2 veins. The left vein is the larger and persists, but the smaller right vein disappears before the embryo is 10 mm. long.

The 2 umbilical arteries pass from the internal iliac artery to the umbilicus. They run to either side of the urachus but soon become obliterated and are then known as the obliterated hypogastric (umbilical) arteries. In adults they appear as fibrous cords, but they may remain patent and then constitute the superior vesical branches to the urinary bladder.

The umbilical vein (*left*) passes upward and backward from the umbilicus to the liver, occupying the free border of the falciform ligament; in this way the falciform ligament forms a "mesentery" for this vessel. At birth, when the umbilical cord is cut, the left umbilical vein becomes obliterated and thereafter is known as the round ligament or ligamentum teres of the liver.

Umbilicus. Under normal conditions all the umbilical structures (duct, vessels and urachus) atrophy, and the umbilical ring becomes reduced to a small orifice. It heals rapidly, fibrous changes take place, and a puckered scar called the umbilicus (navel) results. The retraction of the umbilical vein usually draws the scar against the uppermost circumferences of the umbilical ring; this is the weak spot where umbilical hernias may occur.

The umbilical papilla is usually circular; it may bulge in the newborn, but in the adult it becomes retracted. At the umbilical ring, a thin layer of skin becomes fused directly to the ring margin, and there is no fat. Ascites or multiple pregnancies may dilate and enlarge the ring.

The umbilical fascia, when it exists, is derived from the transversalis fascia.

The superficial lymphatics of the umbilical region pass in the subcutaneous fat and drain in 4 directions. The upper set passes to the axillary lymph glands, and the lower ones to the superficial inguinal group. These channels dip a little deeper and may rest on the muscular aponeurosis. Those from the upper umbilical region pass to either side of the falciform ligament of the liver, pierce the diaphragm and drain into the anterior mediastinal glands. Small lymph channels are found along the course of the round ligament of the liver; along this channel carcinoma of

Ca of the stomach + g.b. can go to the
umbilical lymph . node thru the lymph channels fou
along the round ligament,

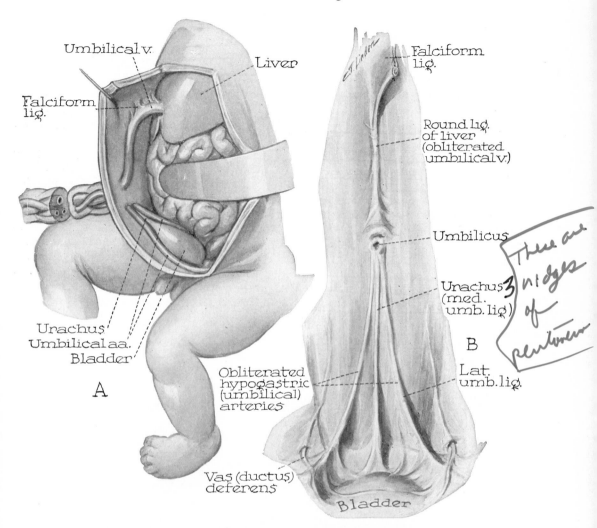

Umbilical v.

Liver

Falciform lig.

Falciform lig.

Round lig. of liver (obliterated umbilical v.)

Umbilicus

These are ridges of peritoneum

Urachus (med. umb. lig)

B

Urachus
Umbilical aa.
Bladder

A

Obliterated hypogastric (umbilical) arteries

Lat. umb. lig.

Vas (ductus) deferens

Bladder

Fig. 290. The umbilicus. (A) In the fetus, 4 structures radiate from the umbilicus: the umbilical vein above and the 2 umbilical arteries and the urachus below. (B) The umbilicus seen from within, in the adult. The obliterated umbilical vein becomes the round ligament of the liver. The urachus becomes the median umbilical ligament, and the 2 obliterated umbilical arteries become the lateral umbilical ligaments.

the gastrointestinal tract (stomach and gall-bladder) reaches the telltale umbilical lymph node. The lateral channels at first pass later-ally, then curve downward to reach the deep inguinal glands. Thus, the lymph channels from the lower portion of the umbilicus may pass directly downward to the deep inguinal set. Therefore, it is possible to find carcino-matous metastases at the umbilicus; a pri-mary malignant tumor from the ovaries and the adnexae spreads by means of the lower set, and carcinoma from the gastrointestinal tract from the upper set.

Types of Umbilical Hernias. Hernias may occur in this region, and, owing to the per-sistence of the embryologic communication between the peritoneal cavity and the um-bilical cord, a congenital umbilical hernia may develop. Umbilical hernias have been classified as follows: (1) hernia of the um-bilical cord, (2) umbilical hernia in adults and (3) umbilical hernia in children.

Hernias of the umbilical cord may contain a considerable portion of the abdominal vis-cera. The coverings of such a hernia are amnion, Wharton's jelly and peritoneum.

These coverings are so thin that the hernial contents may be seen through these diaphanous coverings. There is no skin over such a protrusion except at its edges. The condition has also been referred to as *exomphalos* and may be subdivided into complete or partial.

The umbilical hernia of adults is the acquired umbilical hernia. The umbilical cicatrix becomes greatly stretched, allowing a process of peritoneum with coils of gut or omentum to escape through it. It is usually large and requires surgical repair. It should be recalled that the fibers of the rectus sheath run transversely; hence, Mayo has devised a procedure in which the incision follows the course of these transverse fibers.

The congenital hernia of children usually is due to one of two causes, namely, the persistence of a small peritoneal process into the umbilical cord or an imperfect closure in the linea alba immediately above the umbilicus. Straining at stool and coughing may be additional predisposing factors.

Repair of Umbilical Hernias

An umbilical hernia rarely protrudes directly through the umbilical ring, but rather appears above or below it. A wide, elliptical, transverse incision is made, including the umbilicus at its central point. The incision is deepened to the rectus sheaths, and the neck of the sac is defined and freed from all adjacent tissues. Horizontal incisions are made at each end of the rectus sheaths; these enlarge the neck of the sac and aid in the reduction of its contents. The sac is opened at its neck; the contents are freed and returned to the peritoneal cavity. Some surgeons prefer to close the peritoneum as a separate layer

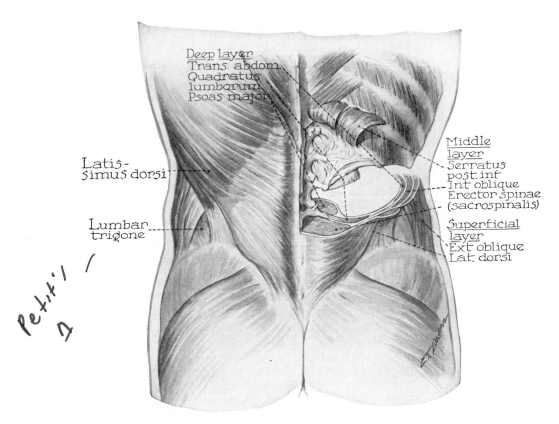

Fig. 291. The muscles of the lumbar region. A posterior view showing the musculature divided into 3 groups: superficial, middle and deep. The serratus posterior inferior has been reflected upward.

but since this is usually very difficult to define, because of the great amount of scarring, a repair is effected which includes fascia, scar and peritoneum together. The repair is made by imbricating the upper flap over the lower with interrupted mattress sutures. This is followed by interrupted sutures placed between the free margin of the overlapping sheath and the lower flap.

POSTEROLATERAL WALL (LUMBAR OR ILIOCOSTAL REGION)

The lumbar region also has been referred to as the iliocostal and posterolateral region of the abdominal wall. It is a quadrilateral area situated between the lowest rib, the iliac crest, the vertebral column and a vertical line erected at the anterior superior iliac spine. The superficial fascia is arranged in two layers between which a large amount of fat usually is deposited.

To understand the arrangement of the musculature in this region, reference should be made to the lumbodorsal (lumbar) fascia (p. 378).

MUSCULATURE
(SUPERFICIAL, MIDDLE AND DEEP LAYERS)

The muscles of the lumbar region can be divided conveniently into 3 groups: superficial, middle and deep (Figs. 291 and 292).

The *superficial* musculature consists of:
1. Latissimus dorsi
2. External abdominal oblique

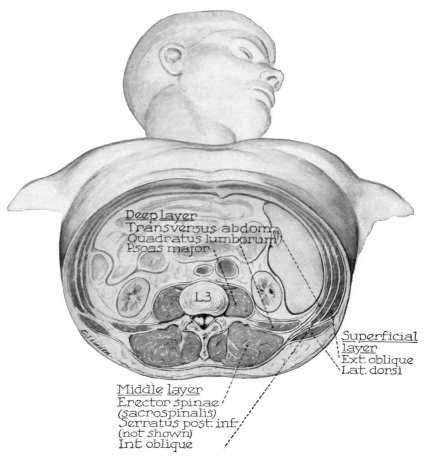

Deep layer
Transversus abdom.
Quadratus lumborum
Psoas major

L3

Superficial layer
Ext. oblique
Lat. dorsi

Middle layer
Erector spinae
(sacrospinalis)
Serratus post. inf.
(not shown)
Int. oblique

FIG. 292. The muscles of the lumbar region in cross section at the level of the 3rd lumbar vertebra. The serratus posterior inferior muscle is not shown in this view.

The *middle* layer consists of:
1. Serratus posterior inferior
2. Sacrospinalis (erector spinae)
3. Internal oblique muscle

The *deep* group consists of:
1. Quadratus lumborum
2. Psoas major
3. Transversus abdominis

The Superficial Muscles. The *latissimus dorsi* arises from the lower 6 thoracic vertebrae, from all the lumbar and upper sacral spines and from the supraspinous ligament through the posterior layer of the lumbodorsal fascia. It also has an origin by means of fleshy fibers from the outer lip of the iliac crest (posterior part), the last 3 or 4 ribs, and at times an additional origin from the inferior angle of the scapula. From this very extensive origin the muscle inserts by means of a tendon, which is 1 inch broad, into the floor of the intertubercular sulcus of the humerus (p. 668).

As the muscle passes upward and laterally to its insertion, it twists around the lower border of the teres major in such a way that its surfaces and borders become reversed. The upper border of the muscle passes across the inferior angle of the scapula, forming a muscular pocket for this scapular angle; in this way the scapula is held against the chest wall. Paralysis of this muscle is one of the causes of "winging" of the scapula.

The muscle takes part in the formation of the *lumbar triangle of Petit,* which is bounded in front by the posterior border of the external oblique, behind by the anterior border of the latissimus dorsi and below by the iliac crest (Fig. 291). The actions of the muscle are: adduction of the humerus, extension of the arm at the shoulder and medial rotation. The muscle is supplied by the subscapular artery and the thoracodorsal nerve. Its action can be tested by grasping the posterior axillary fold and asking the patient to cough vigorously; as this is done, the muscle will be felt to contract.

The *external abdominal oblique* (p. 359) descends obliquely downward and forward and presents a free posterior border. It arises from the 9th, the 10th and the 11th ribs. During kidney operations these posterior fibers may be retracted ventrally, or they may be incised. Such incisions should be placed parallel with the lower ribs to avoid cutting the nerves. The free posterior border of the external oblique usually is located at the midpoint of the iliac crest.

The Middle Group of Muscles. Phylogenetically, the serratus muscles form a continuous muscular sheet. This becomes divided into superior and inferior parts.

The *serratus posterior inferior* appears in this region, blends with the lumbar fascia and through it gains attachment to the upper lumbar and the lower thoracic spines. It is under the latissimus dorsi and passes upward and transversely to ribs 9, 10, 11 and 12. (The *serratus posterior superior* is a flat muscle which lies under the rhomboids. It arises from the lower cervical and the upper thoracic spines, passes downward and laterally and inserts into ribs 2, 3, 4 and 5.) The muscles are supplied by corresponding intercostal nerves. The serratus posterior superior elevates and the serratus posterior inferior depresses the ribs into which they insert. The serratus posterior inferior is an important surgical landmark in kidney operations, since its lowermost fibers lie superficial to the posterior lumbocostal ligament and mark this ligament (Fig. 294). Since the pleura is on a level with the lumbocostal ligament or slightly above it, incisions which encroach upon the muscle and the ligament should be avoided if the pleura is to escape injury.

The *sacrospinalis (erector spinae)* muscle is really an elongated group of muscles which extends upward from the dorsum of the sacrum and the posterior part of the iliac crest (Fig. 293). It corresponds to a muscle mass approximately as broad as the hand and is situated in the aponeurotic compartment formed by the posterior and the middle layers of the lumbodorsal fascia (Fig. 296 B). Laterally, it extends from the spines of the vertebrae to the angles of the ribs; vertically, it passes from the 4th piece of the sacrum to the mastoid process of the occipital bone. It is best to consider this group as 3 subdivisions.

1. The *iliocostalis* consists of lumbar, the thoracic and the cervical portions and is the most lateral group.
2. The *longissimus* is intermediate in posi-

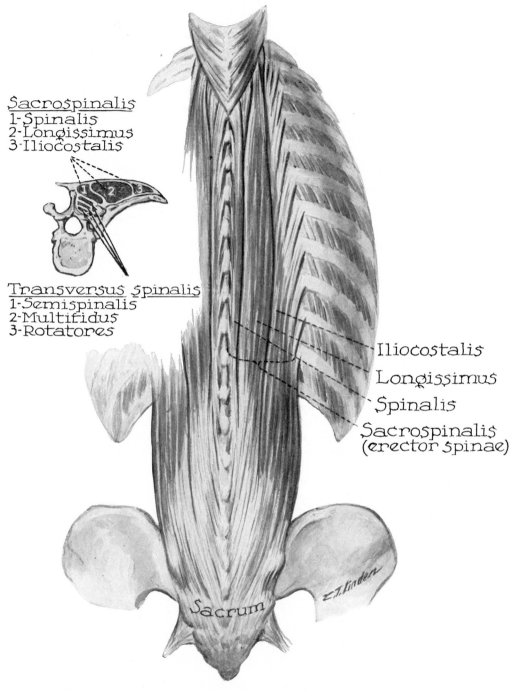

Sacrospinalis
1-Spinalis
2-Longissimus
3-Iliocostalis

Transversus spinalis
1-Semispinalis
2-Multifidus
3-Rotatores

Iliocostalis

Longissimus

Spinalis

Sacrospinalis
(erector spinae)

Sacrum

Fig. 293. The sacrospinalis (erector spinae) muscle. This muscle mass is conveniently divided into 3 muscles (iliocostalis, longissimus and spinalis) from lateral to medial. The inset shows a cross section of this group and also of the muscles which constitute the transversus spinalis group.

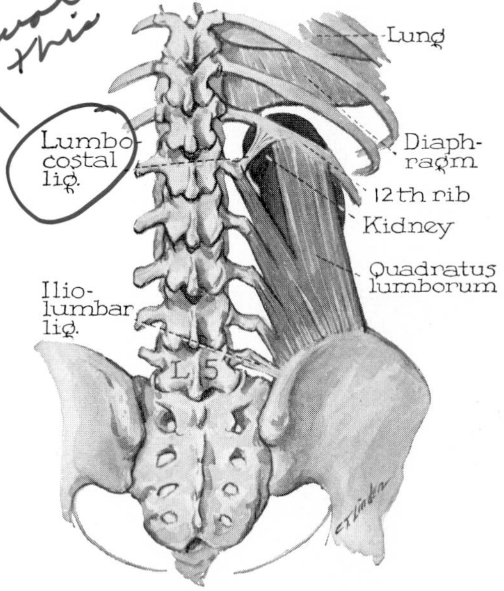

Fibers of lower 6 or 7 ribs serratus post: if superficial to this

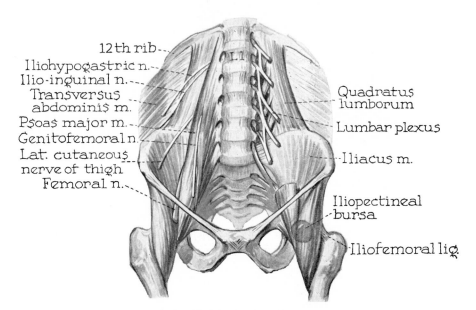

Lung

Diaph-
ragm

12th rib

Kidney

Quadratus
lumborum

Lumbo
costal
lig.

Ilio-
lumbar
lig.

L 5

FIG. 294. The quadratus lumborum muscle. The relations of this muscle to the iliolumbar ligament, the lumbocostal ligament and the kidney are shown.

tion and is the widest and bulkiest of the 3 subdivisions; its uppermost part is the longissimus capitis.

3. The *spinalis* constitutes the most medial subdivision and is the shortest of the three.

In kidney incisions only the lateral bundles (iliocostalis) of the sacrospinalis muscle are encountered. If they must be cut, the incision should be made transversely to the fibers, slightly below and parallel with the 12th rib, so that the lateral and the ventral branches of the last thoracic and the 1st lumbar nerves, and the dorsal branches of the 10th and the 11th thoracic nerves and their accompanying vessels may be avoided.

The *internal oblique* muscle, which arises from the iliac crest and the inferior part of the lumbodorsal fascia, extends posteriorly to the external oblique and forms the floor of Petit's triangle (lumbar trigone). If this muscle is traced upward as it extends onto the lumbar fascia, it presents a free superior border.

Another group, the *transversus spinalis,* is made up of 3 muscle masses which lie deep to the sacrospinalis (Fig. 293) and extend from the 4th piece of sacrum to the skull. They fill the groove which exists between the spines of the vertebrae and their transverse processes. These 3 muscles lie one on top of each other. From superficial to deep they are: the semispinalis, the multifidus and the rotatores.

The Deep Group of Muscles. The *quadratus lumborum* is a flat muscle which lies lateral to the psoas (Fig. 294). It arises from

12th rib

Iliohypogastric n.

Ilio-inguinal n.

Transversus
abdominis m.

Psoas major m.

Genitofemoral n.

Lat. cutaneous
nerve of thigh

Femoral n.

Quadratus
lumborum

Lumbar plexus

Iliacus m.

Iliopectineal
bursa

Iliofemoral lig.

FIG. 295. The lumbar plexus.

the iliolumbar ligament (which extends from the 5th lumbar transverse process to the posterior part of the iliac crest), from the adjoining part of the iliac crest and from the tips of the lower lumbar transverse processes. It takes an upward and medial course and becomes inserted into the lower border of the 12th rib. It fixes the last rib so that it assists the action of the diaphragm in inspiration and bends the vertebral column to the side. The anterior and the middle layers of lumbar fascia surround this muscle. Its nerve supply is derived from lumbar nerves 1, 2, 3 and 4. The anterior layer of lumbodorsal fascia separates it from the transversalis fascia. Its upper portion is strengthened anteriorly by the lateral lumbocostal ligament. Normally, the kidney extends about 1 inch lateral to the lateral margin of this muscle; since the muscle can be drawn medially, only rarely is it necessary to sacrifice its lateral bundles for exposure in kidney operations.

The psoas major muscle may be considered as part of the iliacus muscle which has migrated above the iliac crest. (The psoas minor is present in approximately 50 per cent of individuals.) It occupies the bony trough which is situated between the bodies

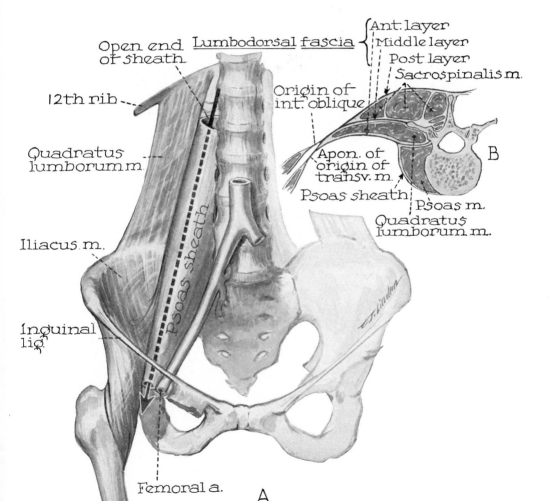

FIG. 296. The psoas muscle and sheath. (A) The psoas sheath and the course taken by a psoas abscess. (B) Transverse section of the psoas mucle and sheath. The layers of the lumbodorsal fascia are shown.

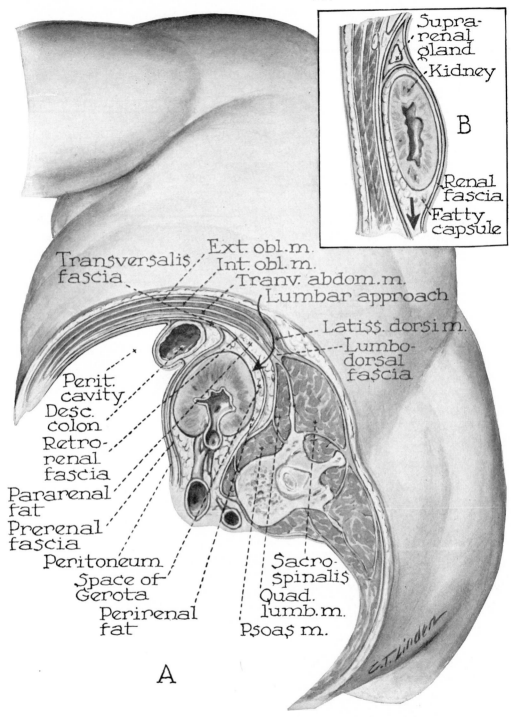

FIG. 297. Fascial relations of the kidney. (A) Cross section through the hilus of the kidney. The renal fascia is derived from the transversalis fascia. At the lateral border of the kidney the transversalis fascia splits into an anterior prerenal and a posterior retrorenal layer. The fat surrounding the kidney is arranged in 2 layers: (1) pararenal (retrorenal) fat and (2) perirenal fat. The latter fills the space of Gerota. The arrow indicates the lumbar approach. (B) Longitudinal section through the kidney. The 2 layers of renal fascia fuse at the upper pole of the kidney but remain open at the lower pole. This explains the downward path (indicated by the arrow) of a ptotic kidney and also explains why the suprarenal remains in situ during the course of a nephrectomy.

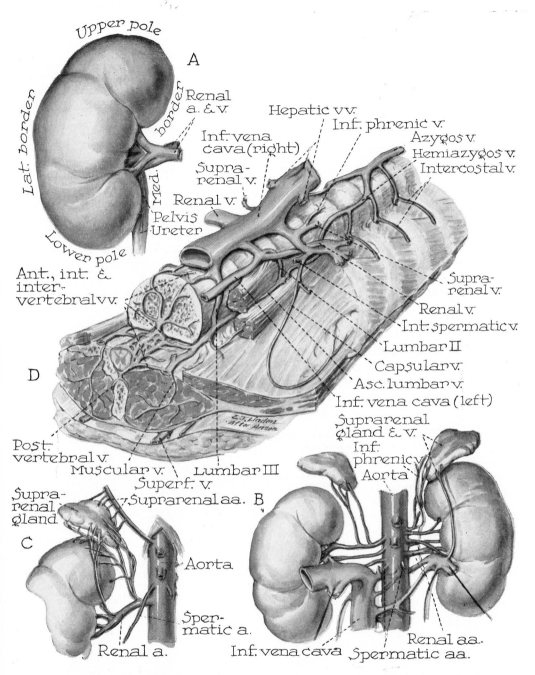

Upper pole

A

Lat. border

Med. border

Renal a. & v.

Inf. vena cava (right)

Supra-renal v.

Renal v.

Pelvis

Ureter

Lower pole

Ant., int. & inter-vertebral vv.

Hepatic vv.

Inf. phrenic v.

Azygos v.

Hemiazygos v.

Intercostal v.

D

Supra-renal v.

Renal v.

Int. spermatic v.

Lumbar II

Capsular v.

Asc. lumbar v.

Inf. vena cava (left)

Suprarenal gland & v.

Inf. phrenic v.

Aorta

Post. vertebral v.

Muscular v.

Superf. v.

Lumbar III

Suprarenal aa.

B

Supra-renal gland

C

Aorta

Sper-matic a.

Renal a.

Inf. vena cava

Spermatic aa.

Renal aa.

Fig. 298. The kidney and its blood vessels. (A) Front view of the right kidney. (B) When the accessory renal arteries arise from the main renal, the phrenic or the suprarenal arteries, they are small and go to the upper pole of the kidney. (C) When the accessory renal arteries are large, they usually are arranged serially and go to both poles and the hilus of the kidney. (D) The venous drainage of the dorsum of the trunk at the renal level. On the right, the pattern is a simple one: the renal and the suprarenal veins empty directly into the inferior vena cava. On the left the pattern is a complicated one in which the left renal vein is the center of an extensive venous network: the inferior phrenic and suprarenal veins enter from above. The spermatic (ovarian), lumbar, capsular and anomalous vena cava enter from below and to the side. Other veins which make communications are the azygos and the hemiazygos (via the lumbars) and the internal and the external vertebral plexuses (via the intervertebrals and the lumbars).

and the transverse processes of the lumbar vertebrae (Fig. 295). It arises from the 12th thoracic and all of the lumbar vertebrae and passes downward and laterally along the margin of the pelvic brim; it continues beneath the inguinal ligament, enters the thigh and inserts onto a traction epiphysis of the lesser trochanter of the femur. Since this muscle is placed deeply and medially, it does not come directly into view in kidney surgery. It is supplied by lumbar nerves 2, 3 and 4 and is a powerful flexor of the thigh. It also assists in medial rotation of the thigh and flexes the trunk on the lower limb.

The sheath of the psoas is a stout membranous covering which is situated around the muscle (Fig. 296). This sheath is attached medially to the bodies of the lumbar vertebrae, and laterally it blends with the anterior layer of the lumbodorsal fascia. It extends behind the femoral artery into the thigh where it blends with the psoas tendon; above it is kept open by its upper attachment to the body of the 2nd lumbar vertebra medially and the 1st lumbar transverse process laterally. Pus from a tuberculous thoracic vertebra may enter the sheath and become directed into the thigh where a puffy swelling may appear behind and on each side of the femoral vessels. Such collections may rupture higher up into the anterior compartment of the lumbodorsal fascia or under the iliac fascia.

The transversus abdominis muscle also appears in this region. It arises from the fusion of the 3 aponeurotic layers of lumbodorsal fascia and extends over the anterolateral wall toward the linea alba, where it becomes muscular. The upper part of the transversus aponeurosis is strengthened by the posterior lumbocostal ligament. The peritoneum is separated from this muscle by extraperitoneal fat and transversalis fascia.

The nerves which are encountered in this regions are the 12th thoracic and the 1st lumbar. The *first lumbar nerve* gives rise to the larger iliohypogastric and the smaller ilio-inguinal nerves. These travel between the psoas major and the quadratus lumborum muscles. The iliohypogastric nerve pierces the transversus abdominis aponeurosis and then continues between it and the internal oblique. The ilio-inguinal nerve travels along the inner surface of the transversus aponeurosis until it perforates that muscle near the anterior part of the iliac crest. It then pierces the internal oblique and continues through the inguinal canal (Fig. 278).

The vessels found here are the 12th intercostal artery (subcostal) and the lumbar artery and vein. The 12th intercostal artery is the last parietal branch of the thoracic aorta. It passes behind the lateral arcuate ligament above the subcostal nerve and accompanies that nerve across the quadratus lumborum and through the transversus muscle. It ends in twigs to the transversus and the internal oblique muscles.

The subcostal vein lies above the artery, close to the last rib. Therefore, the order of these structures is: vein, artery and nerve. The vein passes behind the lateral arcuate ligament to join the azygos vein or the inferior hemiazygos (Fig. 255).

KIDNEYS

Fascial Relations. The surgical anatomy of the kidneys is closely related to the lumbodorsal and the renal fasciae.

The lumbodorsal fascia consists of 3 layers —anterior, middle and posterior—which fill the gap between the 12th rib and the iliac crest (Fig. 296). The posterior and the middle layers are very dense and are stronger than the anterior. The *posterior layer* arises from the tips of the spines of the lumbar, the sacral and the thoracic vertebrae; the *middle layer* arises from the tips of the transverse processes of the lumbar vertebrae; and the *anterior layer* arises from the anterior surfaces of the lumbar transverse processes near their roots. The psoas fascia springs from this layer.

As these 3 layers pass laterally they fuse near the outer border of the quadratus lumborum muscle; the fusion results in the formation of a dense tendinous structure known as the *aponeurosis of origin of the transversus abdominis muscle*. It is from this structure that the internal oblique muscle partly arises. Between the posterior and the middle layers of lumbodorsal fascia the sacrospinalis muscle group (erector spinae) is found, and between the middle and the anterior layer the quadratus lumborum is situated.

The renal fascia is derived from the transversalis fascia. Tobin is of the opinion that the renal fascia is derived from "retroperitoneal tissue." At the lateral border of the kidney the transversalis fascia splits into an anterior (prerenal) and a posterior (retrorenal) layer; in this way the perirenal fascial space of Gerota is formed (Fig. 297 A). The anterior layer is carried medially in front of the kidney and its vessels, the aorta and the vena cava, and becomes continuous with its corresponding layer of the opposite side. The posterior layer extends medially behind the kidney and blends with the fascia of the quadratus lumborum and the psoas major muscles. Through this layer it gains attachment to the vertebral column.

The two layers of renal fascia fuse at the upper pole of the kidney but remain separated at the lower pole (Fig. 297 B). This structural arrangement explains two facts: (1) it is possible to shell out the kidney within its capsule, leaving the suprarenal gland in situ, because this fascia forms a separate chamber for the suprarenal gland, and (2) diminution of the perirenal fat predisposes to mobility (floating) of the kidney; since the renal fascia does not fuse at the lower pole the kidney drops caudad but does not carry the suprarenal gland with it. The renal fascial envelope is poorly defined in the cadaver; however, like many other fascial layers, it is quite definite in the living. G. A. G. Mitchell is of the opinion that the anterior and the posterior layers of renal fascia fuse superiorly and laterally. Contrary to the accepted view, he states that they are also united medially and inferiorly.

The fat surrounding the kidney is arranged in two separate fat planes, which are: (1) the pararenal fat (retrorenal fat) and (2) the perirenal fat (Fig. 297 A).

The pararenal fat is that layer of fat which lies behind the kidney and is located between the aponeurosis of origin of the transversus abdominis muscle and the posterior layer of renal fascia. It varies from a small layer 5 mm. thick to a cushion of enormous size. As soon as the aponeurosis of origin of the transversus muscle is incised, the first fat layer is reached.

The perirenal fat, the second fat layer, is a specialized layer which lies in the fascial space of Gerota and fills this space. Before this fat can be seen, the posterior layer of renal fascia must be incised. It forms the fatty capsule of the kidney and runs completely around it, passing medially into the hilum and insinuating itself between the renal vessels. Its consistency is almost semiliquid; because of this property, it gives the kidney a certain amount of movement transmitted to it by the diaphragm.

The Kidney Proper (Vessels and Nerves). The kidney has 3 capsules: (1) the renal fascia (transversalis fascia), (2) the adipose capsule (perirenal fat) and (3) the capsule proper, a fibrous membrane which normally strips easily from the kidney (in inflammatory conditions it strips with difficulty and tears kidney tissue).

The kidney is reddish-brown in color and is soft in consistency. It is from 4 to 5 inches long, 2½ inches wide and 1 inch in thickness at its middle. It is usually referred to as "bean-shaped," having upper and lower poles, anterior and posterior surfaces, and medial and lateral borders (Fig. 298 A). The hilum is a vertical slit on the medial border which is bounded by thick lips of renal substance. Through it the branches of the renal artery enter the gland, and the veins and the ureter leave.

The hilum leads into a wide space inside the kidney called the *sinus of the kidney.* A number of structures lie in the sinus: branches of the renal artery; tributaries of the renal veins; short funnel-shaped tubes called calyces, which unite to form the ureter; the dilated proximal end of the ureter called the pelvis of the ureter; and the lymph vessels, nerves and fat.

The renal artery may divide into many branches before entering the gland, and it also sends a branch behind the ureter, the retro-ureteric branch of the renal artery. Anson, Cauldwell, Pick and Beaton conducted a comprehensive study of the blood vessels in the dorsal portion of the trunk. They state that supernumerary renal arteries are more likely to be present than absent and that the arrangement of these vessels varies greatly. Commonly, the main artery is accompanied by lesser accessory renals which may give off an internal spermatic. When the accessory renals arise from the main renal, phrenic or suprarenal arteries, they are small and go to the upper pole of the kidney (Fig. 298 B); if they are large, they usually are arranged in a serial manner and affect both poles as well as the hilus of the kidney (Fig. 298 C). These vessels pass to the kidney either in front of or behind the inferior vena cava or may clasp the renal vein. Therefore, our concept of the so-called kidney "pedicle" may better be looked upon as a "ladder" of vessels which arise from the aorta over an area which might correspond to the entire height of the kidney.

The veins emerge through the walls of the sinus and are quite small; they unite to form larger veins, which for the greater part lie in front of the arteries but may come to lie between the arteries and even behind the ureter. Anson *et al.* state that the pattern of the renal veins does not follow that of the renal arteries in number or in course. They believe that the right renal vein may be single, double or triple; however, duplication of the left renal vein is very rare. However, division

of a single renal vein en route to the inferior vena cava is common, and in such instances, the divisions surround the aorta and form a circumaortic venous ring. Accessory renal veins are infrequent, but the complexity of the venous pattern is due to the continuity of the renal veins with veins which drain the surrounding structures. The left renal vein appears to be at the center of a huge venous network (Fig. 298 D). This makes nephrectomy hazardous and permits the spread of infectious materials and neoplasms. The left renal vein is longer than the right; it has a greater distance to travel to the inferior vena cava, which lies to the right of the midline. The lymph vessels follow the veins and drain into nearby glands in the region of the inferior vena cava and the aorta.

The *nerves* are derived from the 12th thoracic (subcostal nerve) and the 1st lumbar (iliohypogastric and ilio-inguinal nerves); they run more or less parallel with the last rib. The subcostal nerve is accompanied by the subcostal vessels. The 3 nerves lie in the

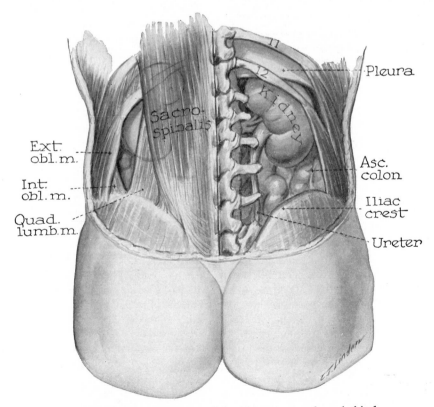

FIG. 299. Posterior relations of the kidneys, seen from behind.
The deep musculature has been removed on the right side.

pararenal fat; as they run forward, they come to lie between the transversus abdominis and the internal oblique muscles.

Both kidneys lie above the level of the umbilicus; the right kidney reaches the upper border of the 12th rib, the left reaches the lower border of the 11th rib and can be placed approximately opposite the last thoracic and upper 2 lumbar vertebrae (Fig. 299). The right organ, as a rule, lies somewhat lower than the left because of the volume of the right lobe of the liver. Occasionally, the kidneys occupy the same level, and in rare instances their relations are reversed. The long axes of the organs are not parallel but are oblique to the spine; therefore, the upper poles are closer to each other than are the lower. The lower poles are about 1 inch above the highest point of the iliac crest; the outer border of the organ lies about ½ inch lateral to the outer border of the sacrospinalis muscle.

The kidneys rest on 4 muscles: the diaphragm above, the transversus muscle laterally, the psoas muscle medially and the quadratus lumborum muscle (between the preceding two).

The 12th rib is an important landmark in the kidney anatomy and is separated from the kidney by the pleura and the diaphragm. The 12th rib takes an oblique course downward, while the lower border of the pleura is horizontal; therefore, these 2 lines cross like the letter "X." This rib may be very short so that the sacrospinalis muscle covers it completely, and in such cases the 11th rib is often mistaken for the 12th, and an incision is placed too high; in such cases, the pleura may be opened inadvertently. The 12th rib and the outer border of the sacrospinalis muscle form an angle which is known as the *kidney angle*. Pressure over this angle usually elicits tenderness in kidney lesions; lumbar incisions for kidney operations commence here.

The *relations* of the anterior surface of the kidneys differ (Fig. 300). They are both capped by the suprarenal glands, but the right kidney's anterior surface is related to the liver above, the hepatic flexure of the colon below and the second part of the duodenum near the kidney hilum. Its lower pole is crossed by the ascending branch of the right colic artery. It is covered with peritoneum except at its extreme upper, inner and lower parts. At times a coil of small intestine may come into relation with the inferior

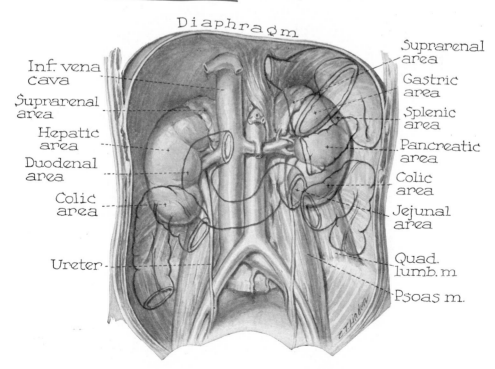

FIG. 300. Anterior relations of the kidneys.

pole. The left kidney has in front of it the stomach above, the spleen laterally, the pancreas transversely across it from the hilum to the splenic area, and the transverse colon below; the lower pole is in contact anteriorly and medially with coils of jejunum. It is crossed by the ascending branch of the left colic artery. Only gastric, splenic and jejunal surfaces are covered by peritoneum.

The diaphragm separates the upper pole of the kidney from the pleura. Dorsal to the pleura are the 12th rib and the muscles of the back. In some individuals weak spots are left in the diaphragm above the 12th rib near its free end. The triangle is more marked on the left side because the liver covers it on the right. If such triangles are well developed, the lateral aspect of the kidney is in close relation with the pleura and the last rib, being separated from them by only a little adipose tissue.

The kidneys are kept in place by attached vessels, by the pressure of surrounding organs and by their fat and fascia. The kidneys move downward with respiration for an excursion of about 2 cm.

At times the lower poles of the kidneys are fused across the midline by a thick bridge of kidney tissue which crosses in front of the inferior vena cava and the aorta. This is called a "horseshoe kidney."

SURGICAL CONSIDERATIONS

NEPHRECTOMY

No single incision accomplishes the desired exposure for all conditions affecting the kidney (Fig. 301). Furcolo described a transfascial approach which gives excellent exposure and produces minimal tissue damage. Another useful incision is the one herein described for nephrectomy.

The incision begins about 1 inch above the junction of the last rib and the erector spinae muscle group. This passes almost vertically downward, with a slight inclination forward, to a point about halfway be-

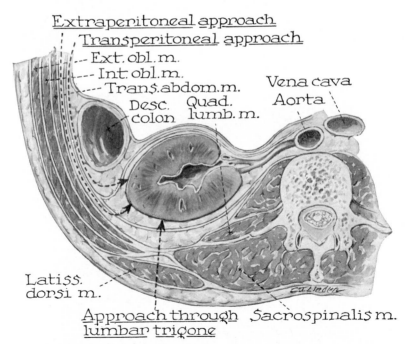

Extraperitoneal approach
Transperitoneal approach
Ext. obl. m.
Int. obl. m.
Trans. abdom. m.
Desc. colon
Quad. lumb. m.
Vena cava
Aorta
Latiss. dorsi m.
Approach through lumbar trigone
Sacrospinalis m.

FIG. 301. Various approaches to the kidney must be utilized, since no single approach admits sufficient exposure for all surgical procedures on this organ. The illustration shows the extraperitoneal and the transperitoneal approaches, as well as the approach through the lumbar trigone.

tween the 12th rib and the iliac crest (Figs. 302 and 303 A). From this point it curves inward and forward and runs parallel with the iliac crest about 2 inches from it. The incision is carried through the skin and the subcutaneous tissue until the musculature is exposed. The muscle layer consists of the latissimus dorsi and the serratus posterior inferior at the posterior end of the wound and the external oblique at the anterior extremity. The muscles (latissimus dorsi, serratus posterior inferior, external oblique, internal oblique and transversus abdominis) are divided until the lumbar fascia is exposed. Deep to this fascia are the 12th dorsal nerve and vessels which cross from above downward and forward. If possible, they should be spared. Usually a well-developed layer of pararenal (retrorenal) fat will be found between the lumbar aponeurosis and the retrorenal leaf of perinephric fascia. The retrorenal leaf of renal fascia is opened and another fat layer, the perirenal layer, comes into view. This is the surgeon's cleavage plane, since it is this fat which immediately surrounds the kidney. This fat continues around the pelvis, the great vessels and the ureter (Fig. 302). The peritoneum is pushed forward as the fat is wiped away, both poles are mobilized, and the kidney is delivered into the wound. Nephrectomy (Fig. 303) can be accomplished after exposing and delivering the pedicle with its contained vessels and ureter. These are clamped and divided, the kidney is removed, and the pedicle is ligated.

NEPHROPEXY

In nephropexy, Zieman has pointed out the importance of anchoring a movable kid-

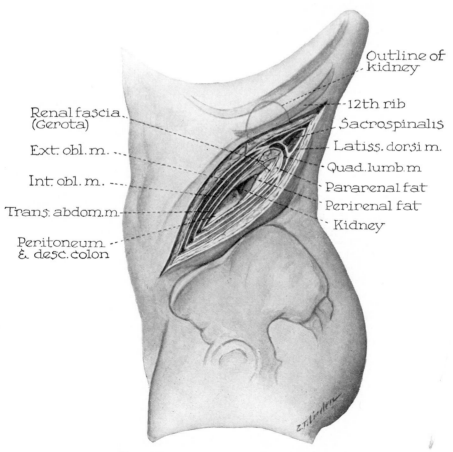

Renal fascia
(Gerota)

Ext. obl. m.

Int. obl. m.

Trans. abdom. m.

Peritoneum
& desc. colon

Outline of
kidney

12th rib

Sacrospinalis

Latiss. dorsi m.

Quad. lumb. m.

Pararenal fat

Perirenal fat

Kidney

FIG. 302. Exposure of the left kidney.

Kidneys + adrenals have separate fascial capsules

ney along its anatomic plane. In this way nature's own confining fascial covering (transversalis fascia) is utilized.

THE SUPRARENAL GLANDS

These are two in number and are situated, one on each side, in the epigastric region (Fig. 298). They are flattened from before backward, broad from side to side and set upon the superior extremity of the corresponding kidney. They have separate fascial capsules; this permits the removal of a kidney without removal of the suprarenal (Fig. 297 B). For the same reason, a suprarenal

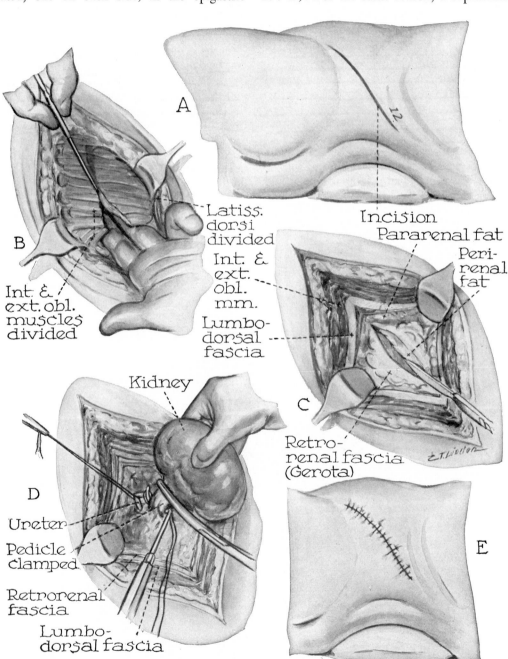

A

B

Int. & ext. obl. muscles divided

Latiss. dorsi divided

Int. & ext. obl. mm.

Lumbo- dorsal fascia

Incision

Pararenal fat

Peri- renal fat

C

Retro- renal fascia (Gerota)

Kidney

D

Ureter

Pedicle clamped

Retrorenal fascia

Lumbo- dorsal fascia

E

FIG. 303. Nephrectomy through a lumbar approach.

does not move with a so-called floating kidney. However, Davie found that in 6 out of 1,500 postmortem examinations the suprarenal and the kidney were fused so intimately that nephrectomy in these cases would have resulted also in a suprarenalectomy. If this thought is kept in mind, careful exploration will reveal a small space (cleavage plane) filled with connective tissue between the inferomedial angle of the suprarenal and the kidney, where the two structures may be separated.

The right suprarenal is pyramidal in shape and smaller than the left. It is situated between the diaphragm and the right lobe of the liver. Its anterior surface is related to the inferior vena cava medially and the bare area of the liver laterally. The posterior surface is related to the kidney inferiorly and the crus of the diaphragm superiorly. The right celiac ganglion lies on the medial side of the right suprarenal gland.

The left suprarenal is semilunar in shape and seems to have slipped down on the medial border of the kidney as far as the renal vessels. Therefore, its lower pole is in contact with the renal vessels and its upper pole is in contact with the spleen. Its anterior surface is related to the stomach superiorly and to the pancreas inferiorly. The posterior surface is related to the crus of the diaphragm medially and the kidney laterally.

The blood supply has been carefully described by Anson *et al.* (Fig. 298).

ABDOMEN

Esophagogastrointestinal Tract

EMBRYOLOGY

ROTATION AND FIXATION

In the earliest days of its development, the gastrointestinal tract is represented as a straight tube of uniform caliber which is suspended in the midline of the abdominal cavity by a ventral and a dorsal mesentery (Fig. 304). The dorsal mesentery extends along the entire length of this tube; it may be subdivided into mesogastrium, mesoduodenum, mesojejunum, meso-ileum and the various mesocola. However, the ventral mesentery extends only as far as the first inch of the duodenum or, in other words, as far as the umbilicus; it is referred to as the ventral mesogastrium. The straight gastrointestinal tube lies between 2 layers of mesentery and therefore has right and left surfaces. The aorta supplies the entire tube by means of 3 branches: the celiac axis and the superior and the inferior mesenteric arteries. The celiac axis supplies the foregut (stomach and duodenum as far as the entrance of the bile duct). The superior mesenteric artery supplies the midgut (from the entrance of the bile duct to the junction of the middle and the left thirds of the transverse colon). The inferior mesenteric artery supplies the hindgut (from the left third of the transverse colon to the rectum).

Since the adult intestinal tract is well over 20 feet in length, and since the abdominal cavity is only 2 feet long, many changes must take place to accommodate the one to the other.

The initial short segment of the straight tube is the abdominal esophagus; distal to this, the upper part of the foregut bulges to form the stomach. The lower inch of foregut and the entire midgut lengthen to form the redundant umbilical loop, which has a descending proximal limb and an ascending distal limb (Fig. 304). The small intestine eventually develops from the descending limb and part (about one half) of the ascending limb; the remaining half of the ascending limb bulges into a cecal bud. The segment at the terminal portion of the umbilical loop (initial colic segment) is directly continuous with the hindgut (terminal colic segment). Elongation of the initial colic segment (midgut) forms the ascending colon and the greater part of the transverse colon. The terminal colic segment (hindgut) forms the remainder of the transverse colon, the descending, the sigmoid and the pelvic portions of the colon. The rectum develops from the primitive cloaca.

The upper end of the hindgut is fixed to the posterior abdominal wall by the mesentery of the terminal colic segment. Where the midgut meets the hindgut or, in other words, where the initial colic segment meets the terminal colic segment, an angle is formed known as the "colic angle." The extremities of the midgut are anchored by the fixed upper duodenum above and the fixed "colic angle" below. These two fixed points are quite close together, and the mesentery-filled space between them is known as the duodenocolic isthmus.

Part of the umbilical loop (descending limb and first half of ascending limb) grows so rapidly that the embryonic peritoneal cavity is unable to contain it; as a result of this, part of the loop grows into the umbilical cord (extra-embryonic celom). This results in an umbilical hernia which is temporary and physiologic.

The superior mesenteric artery supplies the umbilical loop (midgut). It starts as a branch of the abdominal aorta, passes through the duodenocolic isthmus, sends branches to the umbilical loop and ends as the vitelline artery which supplies the vitello-

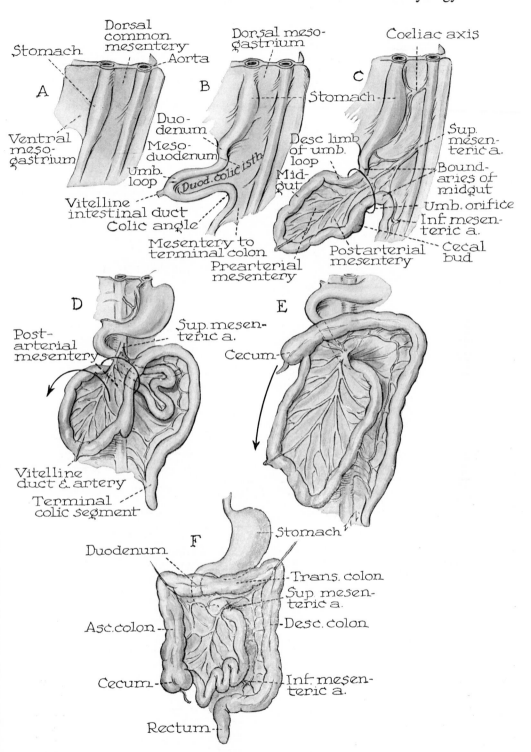

FIG. 304. Rotation and fixation of the gastrointestinal tract.

intestinal duct. This duct, also called the omphalomesenteric duct, is the communication between the midgut and the yolk sac; normally, it disappears. It will be discussed in detail under the heading of Meckel's diverticulum (p. 435). As the artery runs in the mesentery of the umbilical loop it sends branches upward to the descending limb and downward to the ascending limb of the loop. Some authors prefer to refer to the limb and the mesentery supplied by the upward running branches as the prearterial limb and the prearterial mesentery; the limb and the mesentery supplied by the branches which run downward are referred to as the postarterial limb and the postarterial mesentery (Fig. 304 C).

At the beginning of the 5th week, rotation takes place. It starts while the midgut loop is still in the umbilical cord. The growth of the right lobe of the liver starts rotation by pressing on the prearterial segment so that this segment is pushed to the right and downward. This in turn forces the postarterial segment up and to the left. The growth of the liver has thereby succeeded in rotating or pushing the umbilical loop 90° counterclockwise so that the primitive left surface of the mesentery of the loop now faces upward, and the primitive right surface faces downward (Fig. 304 D). If rotation is arrested at this stage, the appendix and the cecum are found on the left side of the body.

About the beginning of the 10th week the umbilical loop, which now lies transversely, starts to return from the umbilical cord to the abdominal cavity. This return takes place in a definite and orderly manner. The proximal part of the prearterial segment returns first. At this stage, the superior mesenteric artery is fixed firmly from its origin at the aorta to its termination at the umbilicus so that it forms a taut cord. The return of the small gut starts to the right of this artery, but since the intra-abdominal space to the right of the artery is small, the coils which have been reduced first are pushed to the left and behind the artery. As these coils pass to the left they encounter the dorsal mesentery of the hindgut which occupies the midline. This in turn is also pushed to the left ahead of the small gut so that the descending colon comes to occupy the left flank, and what was the

"colic angle" is pushed upward and to the left to form the splenic flexure. As the last coil of ileum enters the abdominal cavity it carries the superior mesenteric artery with it. The cecum and the right half of the colon now follow, crossing in front of the origin of the superior mesenteric artery. At this stage, the following has been accomplished (Fig. 304 E):

1. The duodenum lies behind the superior mesenteric artery.

2. The transverse colon is in front of the superior mesenteric artery.

3. The small gut travels from the left upper to the right lower quadrant of the abdomen.

4. The descending colon has been pushed to the left.

5. The cecum and the appendix are under the liver.

6. There is no ascending colon.

As rotation continues, descent of the cecum and fixation of the gut to the posterior abdominal wall takes place. The cecum descends until it reaches the right iliac fossa; as a result of this, an ascending colon is formed. The ascending, the transverse and the descending portions of the colon now have reached their ultimate positions, thus forming an inverted "U" which embraces the jejunum and the ileum. The cecum, the ascending colon and the ascending mesocolon (postarterial) fuse with the right parietal peritoneum. The upper limit of ascending mesocolon overlies a part of the loop of the duodenum and the head of the pancreas, which aids in fixing these structures to the posterior abdominal wall.

The transverse colon and the mesocolon do not fuse with the posterior abdominal wall; hence, part of the colon hangs free in the peritoneal cavity by its unfused mesentery. The two transverse "colic angles" (hepatic and splenic flexures) are fixed. The jejunal and the ileal loops with their mesentery acquire no posterior fixation so that they hang free by a common jejuno-ileal mesentery which passes obliquely from the duodenojejunal flexure to the ileocecal angle.

The descending colon, with its mesocolon, normally fuses with the left parietal peritoneum. A peculiar characteristic of the mesentery of the sigmoid is that it does not fuse

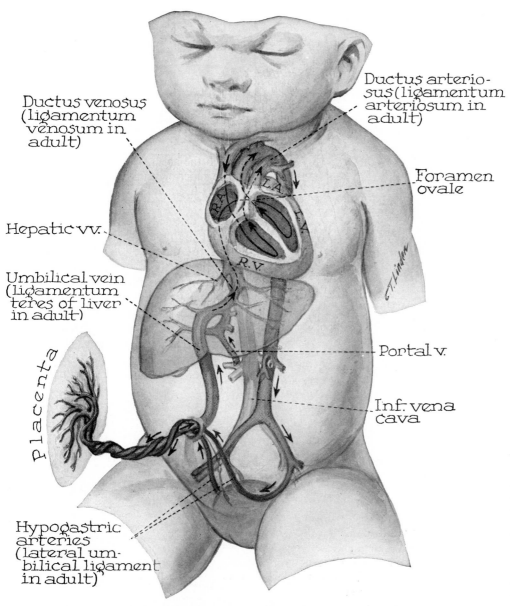

Ductus venosus (ligamentum venosum in adult)

Ductus arterio- sus(ligamentum arteriosum in adult)

Foramen ovale

Hepatic vv.

Umbilical vein (ligamentum teres of liver in adult)

Placenta

Portal v.

Inf. vena cava

Hypogastric arteries (lateral um- bilical ligament in adult)

Fig. 305. Normal fetal circulation. Red indicates arterial blood; blue indicates venous blood; and purple indicates an admixture of both.

with the left pelvic peritoneum, and because of its redundancy it forms an intersigmoid recess or fossa of variable depth (p. 451).

If the surgeon bears in mind the facts just described, he will recall that cohesion has taken place between the two surfaces of peritoneum, but that these layers are not firmly fixed. They may be restored to their embryologic state by opening and separating them.

No vessels, nerves or other vital structures pass between them; hence, the surgeon refers to such spaces as "cleavage planes."

Fixation along the entire alimentary tract has taken place by lateral fixation, either right or left. Therefore, when one wishes to restore a segment of gut to its embryologic state, one must incise lateral to the segment, enter the cleavage plane and free the gut in

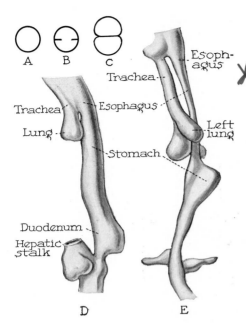

FIG. 306. Embryology of the esophagus. (A), (B) and (C) represent the medial growth of two lateral septa which divide the early single tubular structure into an anterior (ventral) trachea and a posterior (dorsal) esophagus. (D) The trachea and the esophagus as a single structure. (E) Later development and separation of the esophagus and the trachea.

a medial direction. In this way, the primitive dorsal mesentery is reconstructed.

It is unnecessary to free the transverse colon or the sigmoid because they do not fuse. However, fusions and fixations are variable so that at times fusion does not take place, and the ascending colon hangs free by its original mesentery; on the other hand, the sigmoid, which normally does not fuse with the parietal peritoneum, may do so, either partially or completely, and may require separation.

FETAL CIRCULATION

Since the lungs do not function in fetal life, the fetus receives oxygenated blood from the placenta by way of the umbilical vein (Fig. 305). This vein passes through the liver and enters the inferior vena cava via the ductus venosus. Some of the blood may circulate through the liver and enter the in-

ferior vena cava through the hepatic veins. As the inferior vena cava enters the right auricle it contains a mixture of oxygenated blood from the placenta and unoxygenated blood from the fetus. Most of the blood from the inferior vena cava passes through the foramen ovale and into the left auricle, where it mixes with the venous blood returning from the lungs. This blood passes from the left auricle to the left ventricle and out through the aorta.

The superior vena cava conveys the blood from the head and the superior extremities to the right auricle. The greater part of this blood is directed to the right ventricle and then out the pulmonary artery.

Most of the blood from the pulmonary artery passes through the ductus arteriosus to the aorta, the trunk and the inferior extremities. Part of this blood is returned to the right auricle via the inferior vena cava, and part flows through the hypogastric arteries to the umbilical arteries and out to the placenta for removal of waste products and oxygenation. The blood in the pulmonary artery which does not pass through the ductus arteriosus passes through the main branches of the pulmonary artery to the lungs, through which it circulates but receives no oxygen; it returns to the left auricle by way of the pulmonary veins.

In the fetus, the work of the right ventricle is increased because it not only pumps blood through the ductus arteriosus but also against the high pressure of the collapsed lungs. Hence, during intra-uterine life the right ventricle does more work, so that at birth the thickness of both ventricles is approximately the same.

The fetal structures as compared with those in adult life may be outlined in the following manner:

FETUS	ADULT
Umbilical vein	Ligamentum teres of liver
Ductus venosus	Ligamentum venosum
Ductus arteriosus	Ligamentum arteriosum
Hypogastric arteries	Lateral umbilical ligaments

he trachea
esophagus start
ff at 1 structure,

ESOPHAGUS

EMBRYOLOGY

At a very early period in fetal development the stomach is separated from the primitive pharynx by a constriction which is the future esophagus (Fig. 306). Owing to the development of the lungs, the constriction becomes lengthened, but previous to this elongation the trachea and the esophagus form a single tubular structure. The latter becomes divided by the growth of 2 lateral septa which fuse and form the trachea anteriorly and the esophagus posteriorly. The esophagus becomes converted into a solid cord of cells, losing its tubular nature; this cord later becomes canalized to form a tube again. The embryology of the esophagus explains the development of an esophagotracheal fistula which would be due to a lack of fusion of the 2 lateral septa. If there is imperfect canalization of the solid cord stage, a congenital stricture may result.

ADULT ESOPHAGUS

The fully developed esophagus is a muscular tube lined with mucous membrane; it is about 10 inches long (Fig. 307). It commences at the lower margin of the pharynx, which is opposite the 6th cervical vertebra,

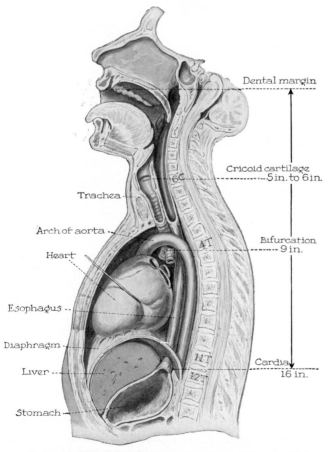

FIG. 307. The esophagus seen from the left side. The distance from the upper incisor teeth to the beginning of the esophagus (cricoid cartilage) is about 6 inches; from the upper incisors to the level of the bronchi, 9 inches; to the cardia, 16 inches. Therefore, the esophagus itself is about 10 inches long.

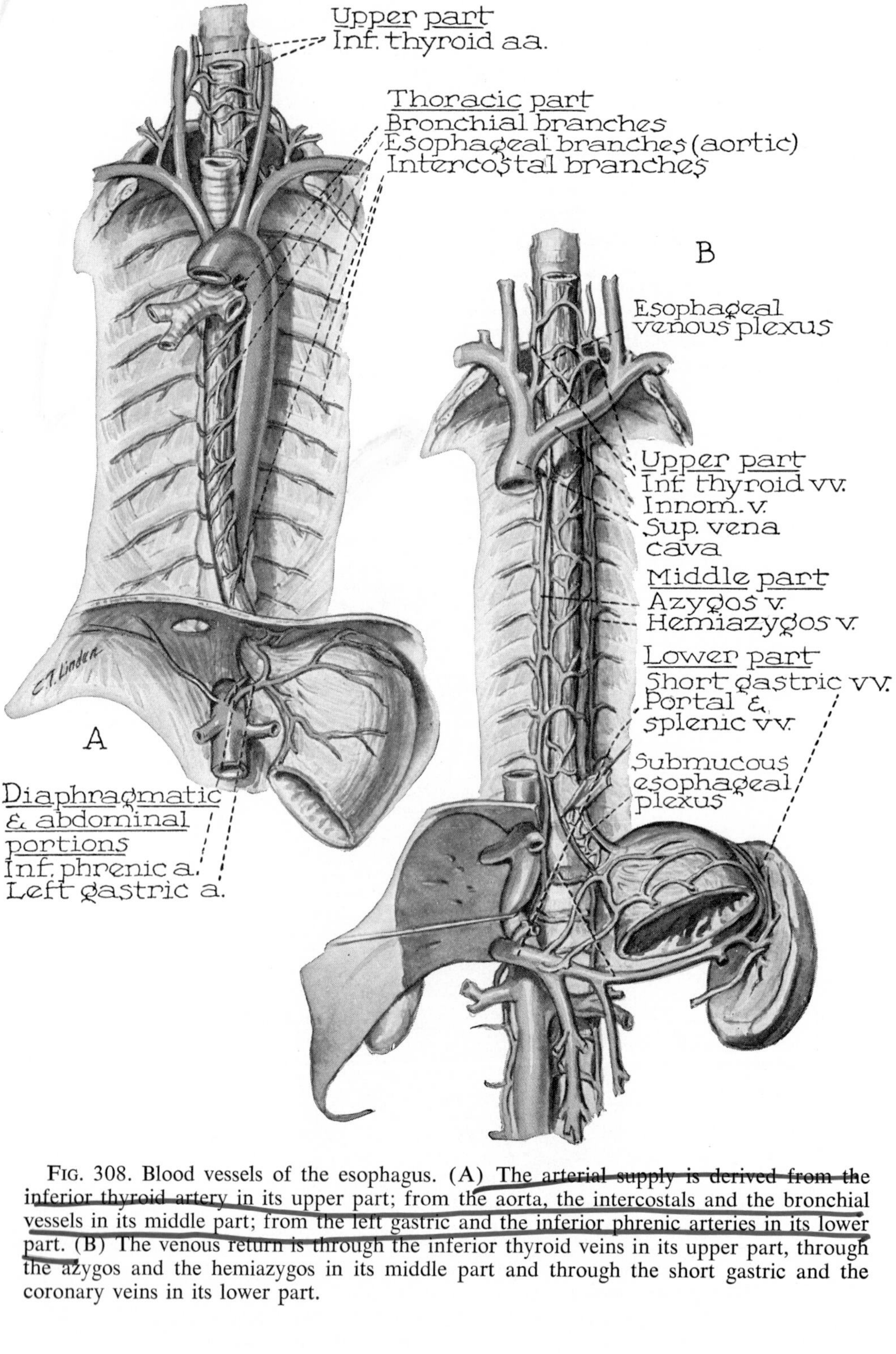

Upper part
Inf. thyroid aa.

Thoracic part
Bronchial branches
Esophageal branches (aortic)
Intercostal branches

B

Esophageal
venous plexus

Upper part
Inf. thyroid vv.
Innom. v.
Sup. vena
cava

Middle part
Azygos v.
Hemiazygos v.

Lower part
Short gastric vv.
Portal &
splenic vv.

Submucous
esophageal
plexus

A

Diaphragmatic
& abdominal
portions
Inf. phrenic a.
Left gastric a.

Fig. 308. Blood vessels of the esophagus. (A) The arterial supply is derived from the inferior thyroid artery in its upper part; from the aorta, the intercostals and the bronchial vessels in its middle part; from the left gastric and the inferior phrenic arteries in its lower part. (B) The venous return is through the inferior thyroid veins in its upper part, through the azygos and the hemiazygos in its middle part and through the short gastric and the coronary veins in its lower part.

and at the lower border of the cricoid cartilage. Its termination is at the cardiac orifice of the stomach opposite the 11th thoracic vertebra. In its course it passes through the lower part of the neck, the superior mediastinum, the posterior mediastinum and the diaphragm; its terminal inch or inch and a half is within the abdomen. The distance from the front teeth to the junction of the esophagus and the stomach is about 16 inches.

Three constant constrictions are found in the esophagus. The first is at its beginning on a level with the cricoid cartilage. The second is behind the bifurcation of the trachea (broncho-aortic constriction) on a level with the 4th thoracic vertebra. The third is at its passage through the esophageal hiatus in the diaphragm. The last is not a narrowing of the tube itself but is due to the muscular fibers of the diaphragm which surround the esophagus. Its relations in the neck, the thorax and the abdomen are surgically important (Fig. 153).

In the neck it lies in front of the vertebral column and the longus cervicis (colli) muscle. On each side it is related to the thyroid lobe, and its left border is in close contact with the thoracic duct (Fig. 153). Anteriorly, it is in direct contact with the trachea and the recurrent laryngeal nerves. To the left side of the esophagus the left inferior thyroid, the left carotid and the left subclavian arteries are found; on its right side, the right carotid artery is found. As it descends it inclines to the left side of the midline; hence, the surgical approach usually should be from the left.

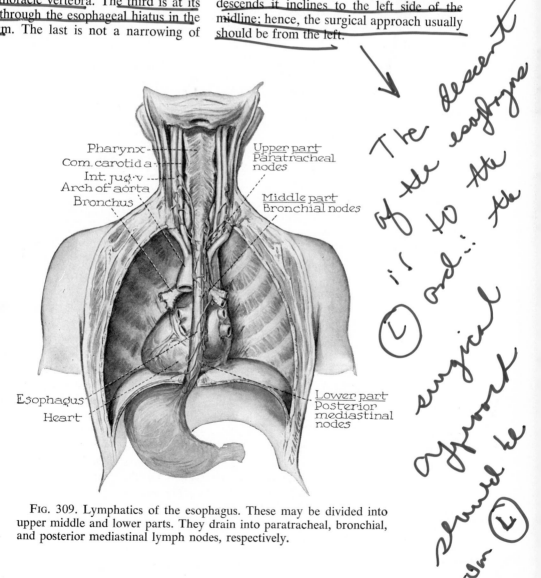

FIG. 309. Lymphatics of the esophagus. These may be divided into upper middle and lower parts. They drain into paratracheal, bronchial, and posterior mediastinal lymph nodes, respectively.

In the thorax the esophagus does not remain directly in the midline, but opposite the 5th, the 6th, the 7th and the 8th thoracic vertebrae it returns to its midline position. In the lower part of the thorax it again inclines to the left, passes forward from the vertebral column and pierces the muscular part of the diaphragm at the level of the 10th thoracic vertebra. Therefore, it passes through the superior and the posterior mediastina. Posteriorly, the esophagus is closely related to the bodies of the vertebrae in the upper two thirds of its course, but the longus colli, the thoracic duct, the azygos and the hemiazygos veins and the right posterior (aortic) intercostal artery intervene. In the lower third the esophagus is separated from the vertebral column by the descending thoracic aorta and projections of the pleural sacs. Anteriorly, in the upper part of the thorax, the esophagus is in close relation to the trachea and its bifurcation and to the left recurrent laryngeal nerve. Opposite the 5th thoracic vertebra it is crossed by the left bronchus, the bifurcation of the trachea being situated a little to the right of the median plane. Below this level the pericardium separates the esophagus from the left atrium. The right edge of the esophagus is closely related to the mediastinal aspect of the right lung; the left edge is related to the thoracic duct and to the left subclavian artery in the superior mediastinum. On a level with the 4th thoracic vertebra it is crossed by the aortic arch, and below that level is related to the descending thoracic aorta; still lower it is related to the mediastinal surface of the left lung. Below the roots of the lung, the 2 vagi emerge from the posterior pulmonary plexus and come in contact with the esophagus. From this point, the right vagus descends on the posterior surface of the esophagus, and the left descends on its anterior surface. Because of the close relationship of the pleura to the esophagus an empyema may be a late finding in esophageal carcinoma.

In the abdomen, the esophagus passes through the esophageal opening in the diaphragm, opposite the 10th thoracic vertebra, and ends at the cardiac opening of the stomach, opposite the 11th thoracic vertebra. Its entire abdominal part is about 1 inch long and is covered by peritoneum in front and over its left side. Posteriorly, it is in contact with the diaphragm and the left phrenic artery between it and the diaphragm.

VESSELS AND NERVES

The arterial supply (Fig. 308 A) is derived from the esophageal branches of the inferior thyroid artery in its upper part; in the thorax, from the esophageal branches of the descending aorta, the right intercostal and bronchial arteries. The diaphragmatic and abdominal portions are supplied by the left gastric and the left inferior phrenic arteries.

The venous return of the esophagus (Fig. 308 B) passes through the esophageal venous plexus which is located in the submucosa and from which branches pass through the musculature to an intercommunicating venous plexus on the external surface. From the upper part of this latter plexus the blood drains to the inferior thyroid veins, then to the innominate veins and finally to the superior vena cava. From the middle portion of the esophagus, the veins drain to the azygos and the hemiazygos. The lower part of the esophageal plexus drains into the coronary and the short gastric veins. In such conditions as cirrhosis of the liver there is an obstruction to the venous flow in the portal vein, and the blood is shunted to the superior vena cava via the coronary vein, the esophageal plexus and the azygos vein; this leads to the formation of esophageal varices.

The lymphatic drainage of the esophagus also may be subdivided into upper, middle and lower parts (Fig. 309). Lymph from the upper part drains into the paratracheal and the inferior deep cervical nodes. The middle of the esophagus is drained by lymphatics which pass to bronchial nodes. The lower part is drained by vessels which travel to the posterior mediastinal glands and then to the celiac and the suprapancreatic nodes.

The nerves of the esophagus are derived from both the sympathetic and the parasympathetic systems (Fig. 310). The sympathetic innervation is derived from the cervical and the thoracic chains. In the neck, these fibers arise from the superior and the inferior cervical ganglia; there may be a communication between the inferior ganglion and the recurrent laryngeal nerve. The ansa subclavia loops over the front of the subclavian artery and connects the middle and the inferior cervical ganglia. The superior ganglion connects with the ganglia of the vagus. In the thorax, the esophagus receives its sympathetic fibers from the upper thoracic ganglia and the greater and the lesser splanchnic nerves. In the abdomen, a few fibers from the celiac plexus supply it.

The parasympathetic supply of the esophagus is received via the vagus nerves. The upper part is supplied through the recurrent laryngeal nerve. The midportion of the esophagus receives its vagus fibers from the pulmonary plexuses, which are located on the posterior part of each bronchus. Esophageal nerves also are derived from the vagi which supply the lower part.

STOMACH
(VENTRICULUS OR GASTER)

EMBRYOLOGY

To understand thoroughly the surgical anatomy of the stomach and the maneuvers necessary for good surgical exposure, the embryology must be understood (Fig. 311). The stomach is developed from that part of the foregut which is situated between the esophagus and the pharynx in front and the liver bud and the yolk sac behind. During the 4th week, the stomach is located in the neck; at that time, the heart, the lungs and the stomach all lie near the exit of the vagal

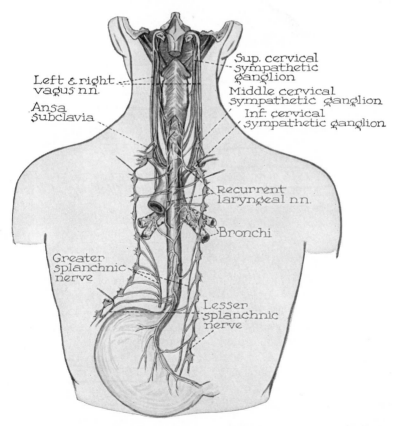

FIG. 310. Nerve supply of the esophagus, seen from behind. The sympathetic nerves are presented in green, and the parasympathetic (vagus) fibers in yellow.

fibers from the central nervous system. During the 6th and the 7th week the growth of the lung buds causes an elongation of the esophagus and a backward migration of the stomach so that it changes from a cervical structure to one which is located in the lower thorax. This organ, whose embryologic position has its long axis in the median plane and its greater curvature facing dorsally, changes its position so that in the fully developed stage it becomes almost transversely placed with its greater curvature facing downward and to the left and its lesser curvature facing upward and to the right. This change is brought about by two combined axial rotations: the first takes place about the long axis of the stomach and the second about the anteroposterior axis. The first rotation (longitudinal axis) swings through an arc of 90°; as a result of this, the primitive left gastric surface is directed forward; the primitive right gastric surface, backward; the greater curvature with its attached dorsal mesogastrium, to the left; and the lesser curvature with its attached ventral mesogastrium, to the right. The lesser peritoneal cavity (omental bursa) now forms a retrogastric pouch; the spleen and the splenic artery are on the left; and the meso-esophagus has become so shortened that the esophagus lies almost against the posterior wall. The second rotation (anteroposterior axis) draws the pyloric end of the stomach to the right and the cardiac end to the left. The opening into the lesser sac is formed and is known as the epiploic foramen (of Winslow).

ADULT STOMACH

The stomach is the most dilated part of the digestive tube. It is approximately 10 inches long, 5 inches wide and has a normal capacity of about 2 pints. It is capable of great dilatation and may shrink into a more-or-less tubular form when empty. At its upper part it is approximated to the diaphragm by the esophagus; at its lower end it is more-or-less fixed because of its connection with the duodenum; however, it should be recalled that the first inch of duodenum has some degree of mobility. The position and the shape of the stomach are not fixed, since they vary considerably and are dependent upon the posture of the body, the amount of the gastric contents, the stage of gastric digestion, the degree of contraction of both abdominal and gastric musculature, the pressure of surrounding viscera, respiration and gastric tonus. The long axis of the viscus passes downward, forward, to the right and finally backward and slightly upward. Its shape has been likened to a "horn of plenty" as it lies in the upper left part of the abdomen. It is largely under shelter of the ribs, from which it is separated by the diaphragm; the lower part of the left pleura and the left lung overlap it. Therefore, it lies in the epigastric and the left hypochondriac regions in such a manner that only one sixth of this viscus is to the right of the midline. The stomach has 2 orifices, 2 curvatures, 2 surfaces and 2 incisurae. It is further subdivided into a fundus, a body and a pyloric portion.

The 2 incisurae, or "notches," are the incisura angularis and the incisura cardiaca (cardiac notch) (Fig. 312). The left border of the esophagus is not continuous with the greater curvature as a straight line but meets it at an acute angle and forms the *cardiac notch* (incisura cardiaca). The *incisura angularis* (angular notch) is the deepest part of the concavity formed by the lesser curvature; therefore, it is the angle formed by the junction of the vertical and the horizontal parts of the lesser curvature; it is an important landmark in surgery of the stomach. If we locate the cardiac notch and draw a horizontal line across it and then drop an oblique line from the incisura angularis to the greater curvature, we shall have constructed the subdivisions of the stomach, namely:

1. The fundus is above the level of and to the left of the cardiac notch.

2. The body is that part which lies between the cardiac notch and the incisura angularis.

3. The pyloric portion, the remainder, is further subdivided into pyloric antrum and pyloric canal.

The 2 orifices are the cardiac and the pyloric.

The cardiac orifice (cardia) is the point of junction between the esophagus and the stomach; it marks that point at which the

2 curvatures begin. The esophageal end, which has been referred to as the cardia, is fixed to the diaphragm. It is about 1 inch to the left of the midline, about 4 inches be-

hind the 7th left costal cartilage and is located at the level of the 9th thoracic spine. It presents the following boundaries: in front, the left lobe of the liver; behind, the diaphragm;

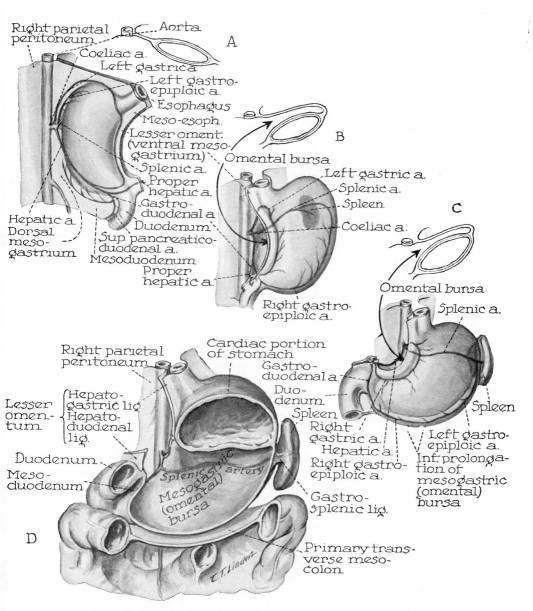

FIG. 311. Embryology of the stomach. (A) Early development of the stomach as it is situated between the two leaves of peritoneum which form the dorsal and the ventral mesogastria. (B) After the first rotation (longitudinal axis) in which the stomach swings through an arc of 90°. The omental bursa is formed. (C) After the second rotation (anteroposterior axis); this draws the pyloric end of the stomach to the right and the cardiac end to the left. (D) After rotation is completed, and with the distal portion of the stomach removed to show the peritoneal relations.

to its right, the esophageal branches of the left gastric vessels.

The pyloric orifice is the communication between the stomach and the duodenum (duodenopyloric junction). This opening lies 1 inch to the right of the midline at the level of the 1st lumbar vertebra.

The 2 surfaces are anterior and posterior.

The anterior surface is more convex than the posterior and is directed upward and forward. It lies below the lesser curvature and is covered by the left and also by a part of the right lobe of the liver; therefore, in the epigastrium and below the xiphoid, the stomach is not in immediate contact with the anterior abdominal wall. Downward and to the left, however, there is a gastric triangle formed where this surface rests against the inner surface of the abdominal wall. It is bounded on the left by the 8th and the 9th costal cartilages, on the right by the free margin of the liver and below by the transverse colon. It represents the most accessible portion of the stomach through an abdominal incision. In the left hypochondriac region,

the stomach is covered not only by the ribs and the intercostal muscles but also by the left lung, the left pleural cavity and by the diaphragm. Thus, penetrating wounds in this region may injure the pleura, the lung and the stomach; therefore, gastric contents may escape into the pleural cavity. The so-called space of Traube is situated in the left hypochondriac region and represents that portion of the stomach which is not covered by the neighboring viscera. It is bounded above and to the right by the inferior margin of the left lung; below and to the right by the costal margin; and posteriorly and to the left by the spleen. When the stomach is empty, the transverse colon is displaced upward and comes to lie in front of the contracted viscus.

The posterior surface runs downward and backward and forms a large part of the anterior wall of the lesser peritoneal sac (omental bursa). This sac separates the posterior surface from the so-called "stomach bed." The greater curvature is in relation to the transverse colon below and behind; the adjoining part of the posterior surface rests on

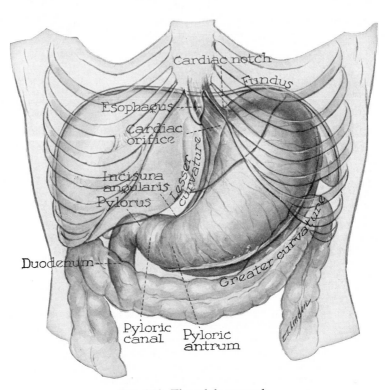

FIG. 312. The adult stomach.

the transverse mesocolon. Above the transverse mesocolon, the stomach is in contact with the anterior surface of the pancreas; above the pancreas, the stomach lies to the left of the median plane and rests on the upper part of the left kidney and the left suprarenal gland. At a still higher level, the stomach (fundus) occupies the concave gastric area of the spleen and comes into relationship with the left half of the diaphragm. The normal stomach is separated anteriorly and posteriorly from the neighboring organs only by capillary spaces; this separation is effected in such a manner that direct contact is made.

The 2 curvatures are the lesser on the right and the greater on the left.

The lesser curvature extends between the cardiac and the pyloric orifices. It has vertical and horizontal parts which join at the incisura angularis and form a concave border in the form of a letter "J." This curvature is continuous with the right margin of the esophagus and normally is overlapped by the liver. It affords attachment for the lesser omentum (gastrohepatic part) and contains the arterial circle formed by the right and the left gastric arteries.

The greater curvature is convex and is 4 or 5 times as long as the lesser. Its upper third is directed toward the left; the middle third, downward and to the left; and the lower third, downward and to the right. It starts at the incisura cardiaca, passes upward as high as the 6th left costal cartilage and ends at the pylorus. Along the lower part of the greater curvature, the 2 layers of peritoneum which envelop the stomach pass downward as the greater omentum; on the left, they pass backward toward the spleen as the gastrosplenic ligament. Although the lesser curvature is comparatively fixed owing to its attachments, the greater curvature is freely movable, and its position alters as the stomach becomes full or empty, contracted or relaxed. When an individual is standing, the greater curvature may descend to the umbilicus or below it, but when lying down, it is an inch or more above the umbilicus. In ptosis, the curvatures become more nearly vertical in position, and both curvatures descend; but in gastric dilatation the greater curvature is lower, without altering the position of the somewhat fixed lesser curvature. The right and the left gastroepiploic vessels form an arterial circle as they separate the 2 layers of peritoneum which are attached here.

The *fundus* is the rounded uppermost part of the stomach which is situated above the level of the esophageal junction; during life, it probably always contains gas. It bulges upward into the left cupola of the diaphragm as high as the level of the 5th costal cartilage and, therefore, is related to the heart, the pericardium and the left lung. This partly explains the increased cardiac activity and the accelerated respirations which are produced by the upward pressure of a full or distended stomach. The top of the fundus is almost on a level with the left male nipple.

The *body* of the stomach is the main portion which lies between the incisura angularis and the incisura cardiaca (between the fundus and the pylorus). Its general direction is oblique and to the left.

The *pylorus* is the point of junction between the stomach and the duodenum. The outer surface of the pylorus is marked by a circular constriction (duodenopyloric constriction). It lies in the transpyloric plane, about 1 inch to the right of the midline, behind the quadrate lobe of the liver and in front of the neck of the pancreas. Its position usually is marked by a prepyloric vein (vein of Mayo) which descends over its anterior surface from the right gastric vein to the right gastroepiploic vein. However, this vein may be ill-defined.

The pyloric portion of the stomach is divided into proximal and distal parts. The proximal part represents a slight dilatation and is known as the *pyloric antrum*. The distal part is more tubular and is called the *pyloric canal*. The pylorus usually is considered as that terminal half-inch of stomach which is in contact with and covered by the liver. Since the liver hides it from view and since most perforated peptic ulcers occur in this area, it becomes an area of great surgical importance.

The pylorus has thicker walls than the

KNOW

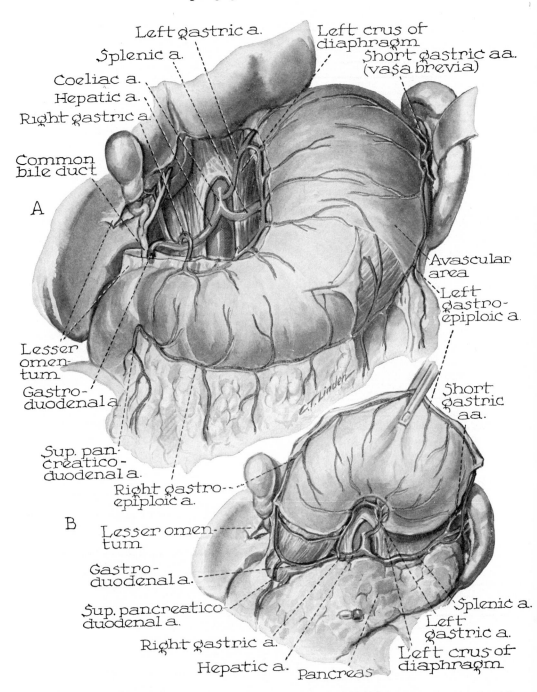

Left gastric a.

Splenic a.

Coeliac a.

Hepatic a.

Right gastric a.

Common bile duct

A

Left crus of diaphragm

Short gastric aa. (vasa brevia)

Avascular area

Left gastro-epiploic a.

Lesser omentum

Gastro-duodenal a.

Short gastric aa.

Sup. pancreatico-duodenal a.

Right gastro-epiploic a.

B   Lesser omentum

Gastro-duodenal a.

Sup. pancreatico-duodenal a.

Right gastric a.

Hepatic a.   Pancreas

Splenic a.

Left gastric a.

Left crus of diaphragm

FIG. 313. Arterial supply of the stomach. (A) The lesser omentum has been removed, and a wedge of greater omentum has been lifted to show the relations of the vessels. (B) The stomach has been elevated so that the posterior gastric surface is viewed.

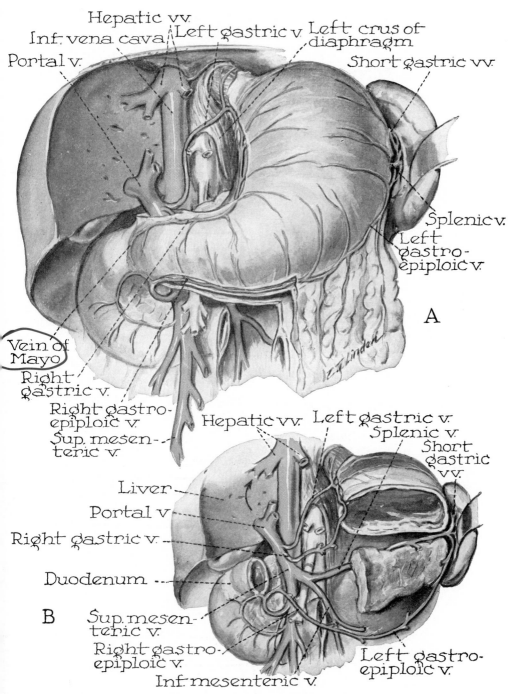

FIG. 314. Veins of the stomach. (A) The liver has been sectioned to show the venous relations. (B) The distal four fifths of the stomach and part of the pancreas have been removed.

Pyloric sphincter is ↑ thickness of the circular muscle fiber.

rest of the stomach because of an increase in the circular muscle fibers. This thick muscular ring closes and relaxes the pyloric orifice and forms the *pyloric sphincter.*

Normally, the pylorus is in a closed state, but when open it is capable of admitting a fingertip. Despite its narrowness, many cases are reported in which foreign bodies as large as pencils, forks, keys, etc. have been passed through it. Behind, it is related to the portal vein, the hepatic artery and the common duct.

Two layers of peritoneum envelop the stomach; at the lesser curvature these meet and pass upward as the *lesser omentum,* which becomes attached to the liver and the diaphragm. This omentum has 2 parts: the gastrohepatic and the duodenohepatic. The gastrohepatic part is avascular, thin, transparent and contains no important structures. The duodenohepatic part of the lesser omentum is thick and contains 3 vital structures: the common duct, the portal vein and the hepatic artery. The 2 layers of peritoneum which clothe the stomach meet at the greater curvature and pass downward as one great fold. Different parts of this fold receive different names according to their attachments: the gastrohepatic ligament is attached to the diaphragm; the gastrosplenic ligament, to the spleen; and the greater omentum, to the transverse colon. That portion of greater omentum which is situated between the stomach and the transverse colon is known as the gastrocolic ligament (see Peritoneum, p. 412).

VESSELS AND NERVES

The arterial supply to the stomach (Fig. 313) is derived from the celiac axis (p. 406). The lesser curvature is supplied by the *left gastric (coronary) artery* which reaches the cardiac end of the curvature along the left edge of the gastrohepatic omentum. It passes upward and to the left on the left crus of the diaphragm, and then it turns over the upper border of the lesser sac to reach the stomach. It continues downward, forward and to the right, and passes along the curvature to anastomose with the *right gastric (pyloric) artery,* a branch of the hepatic.

The greater curvature is supplied by the following arteries:

The *vasa brevia* (short gastric), which are usually 4 or 5 in number arise from the splenic artery or from one of its terminal branches. These pass between the layers of the gastrosplenic ligament to the left end of the greater curvature and anastomose with esophageal, gastric branches, and the left gastroepiploic artery.

The *left gastroepiploic artery* arises from the splenic near its termination, passes in the gastrosplenic ligament to the stomach and then runs from left to right along the greater curvature between the layers of the gastrocolic ligament. It anastomoses with the right gastroepiploic artery after sending branches to both surfaces of the stomach.

The *gastroduodenal artery* takes origin from the hepatic above the duodenum, passes behind it between the neck of the pancreas and the duodenum and ends at the lower border of the first part of the duodenum by dividing into a *superior pancreaticoduodenal* and a *right gastroepiploic.* The latter artery passes from right to left between the layers of the gastroepiploic omentum, sending gastric branches upward to both walls of the stomach, and ends by anastomosing with the left gastroepiploic

The veins of the stomach (Fig. 314) correspond to the arteries; they terminate in the portal vein or the 2 large vessels which form it (superior mesenteric and splenic veins). They form 2 great loops: the one along the lesser curvature and the other along the greater. Associated with these are some short gastric veins at the fundus. The loop on the lesser curvature is made up of the left gastric (coronary) and the right gastric veins.

The left gastric vein accompanies the left gastric artery along the lesser curvature and receives tributaries from both surfaces of that organ and also from the esophagus. It continues backward in the left gastropancreatic fold to the posterior wall of the abdomen, then it turns downward and to the right and empties into the portal vein.

The right gastric vein passes to the right along the lesser curvature of the stomach and

↓ KNOW

at the pylorus turns backward and enters the portal vein. It receives venous blood from both surfaces of the stomach and from a vein which travels upward in front of the pylorus, the prepyloric vein of Mayo. The latter vessel usually connects the right gastric and the gastroepiploic veins. The venous loop along the greater curvature lies between the layers of the greater omentum and is made up of the left and the right gastro-epiploic veins.

The left gastroepiploic vein passes upward and to the left and empties into the splenic vein.

The right gastroepiploic vein runs to the right, arches backward at the pylorus and usually enters the superior mesenteric. The left gastric vein (portal system) anastomoses with the lower esophageal vein; the latter in turn anastomoses with the upper esophageal veins which drain through the azygos into the caval venous system. On this way, an important communication is formed between the portal and the caval systems (portacaval anastomosis). The veins at the inferior end of the esophagus may become distended and varicosed in such conditions as cirrhosis of the liver (portal obstruction); their rupture results in severe hematemesis which may be fatal (see Esophagus).

The lymph drainage of the stomach (Fig. 315) follows the 3 branches of the celiac axis (hepatic, gastric and splenic). Hence, here are 3 sets of lymph glands and ducts: (1) hepatic, (2) gastric and (3) pancreatcosplenic.

The hepatic glands lie in the lesser omentum along the course of the bile ducts; part of them follow the course of the cystic and the hepatic arteries and are known as the cystic (hepatic) glands. They receive lymph from the liver and the gallbladder. Since this set of glands follows the course of the hepatic artery or its branches, they give rise to a group of glands (subpyloric) which are located on the head of the pancreas and in the angle between the first and the second parts of the duodenum. They receive lymph from the right two thirds of the greater curvature of the stomach; this lymph travels via the inferior gastric glands. Therefore, the hepatic group of glands has 3 separate sets associated with it: a hepatic proper, following the duct; a cystic, following the cystic artery; and a subpyloric, following the gastroduodenal artery.

Gastric Glands. The second group of glands is the gastric. It is divided into superior and inferior subgroups. The superior glands follow the course of the left gastric artery along the lesser curvature of the stomach and between the layers of the lesser omentum. The inferior glands follow the right gastroepiploic vessels between the layers of the greater omentum; they are found mainly along the pyloric half of the greater curvature.

Pancreaticolienal Glands. The third group is the pancreaticolienal (splenic set). These follow the course of the splenic artery along the upper border of the pancreas. Some are found in the gastrosplenic ligament in relation to the short gastric branches of the splenic artery.

Preaortic (Celiac) Glands. The efferent lymphatics from all of these glands pass to glands which surround the celiac axis in front of the aorta; these are known as the celiac group or preaortic glands. The lymph drainage of the stomach can be represented diagrammatically in the following way: the stomach is divided by an imaginary line in its long axis, two thirds being to the right of this line and one third to the left. A line is now constructed dividing the left third into two at the junction of its upper third and the lower two thirds. In this way 3 areas of lymph drainage are marked out. Area 1 represents that part of the stomach which drains into the superior gastric glands; Area 2 drains into the inferior gastric; and Area 3 drains via the pancreaticolienal glands. The celiac group empties into the receptaculum chyli after receiving lymph from all these areas.

Nerves. The stomach is innervated by both the parasympathetic and the sympathetic nervous systems (Fig. 316).

The parasympathetic nerve supply is derived from the *vagus nerves* which originate in the medulla, descend in the carotid sheath and into the thorax. On the posterior surface of the root of each lung each vagus aids in the formation of the so-called posterior pulmonary plexus, and from these, branches continue to the esophagus and the stomach. The nerves then pass through the esophageal orifice of the diaphragm and reach the respective surfaces of the stomach, where the right vagus is known as the *posterior gastric nerve* and the left vagus as the *anterior;* they pass along the lesser curvature of the stomach.

Much recent work has been done on the anatomy and the distribution of the vagi. Probably our most reliable information comes from E. Perman, who, in 1935, performed a series of painstaking and accurate dissections dealing with this subject. His conclusions are interesting, instructive and apparently accurate. He concludes that both vagi reach the stomach through the lesser omentum and that they divide into branches without the formation of a plexus of intertwining fibers. He states that anastomoses exist between the various branches, but that they do not lose their individuality as would be the case in a nerve plexus.

The left vagus nerve sends branches to the liver and to the anterior wall of the stomach. Those branches traveling to the liver turn to the right, pass through the lesser omentum and to the porta hepatis. The gastric branches divide into several smaller nerves which spread over the anterior wall and can be followed to the greater curvature.

The right vagus nerve is arranged in a similar manner: one part goes to the celiac plexus and the remainder supplies the posterior wall of the stomach. Perman was unable to follow branches of either the left or the right vagus into the greater omentum.

Recently, papers have appeared dealing with the subject of the nerve supply to the stomach, but they too are quite contradictory. Bradley, Small, Wilson and Walters examined 111 cadavers; they concluded that there was a great variation in nerve pattern from the cardiopulmonary plexus to the stomach, but the nerves were very constant in course and distribution after reaching the stomach. They divided the nerve patterns into 4 groups. Miller and Davis studied the vagus nerves below the level of the pulmonary plexus in 13 cadavers. They state

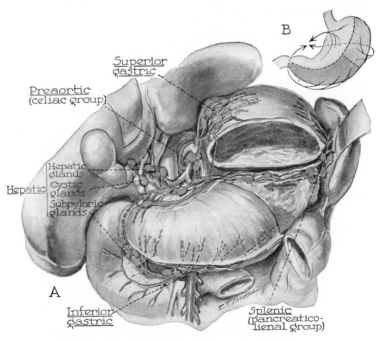

FIG. 315. Lymphatics of the stomach. (A) The arrows indicate the lymph drainage. (B) Diagram of lymph zones and flow.

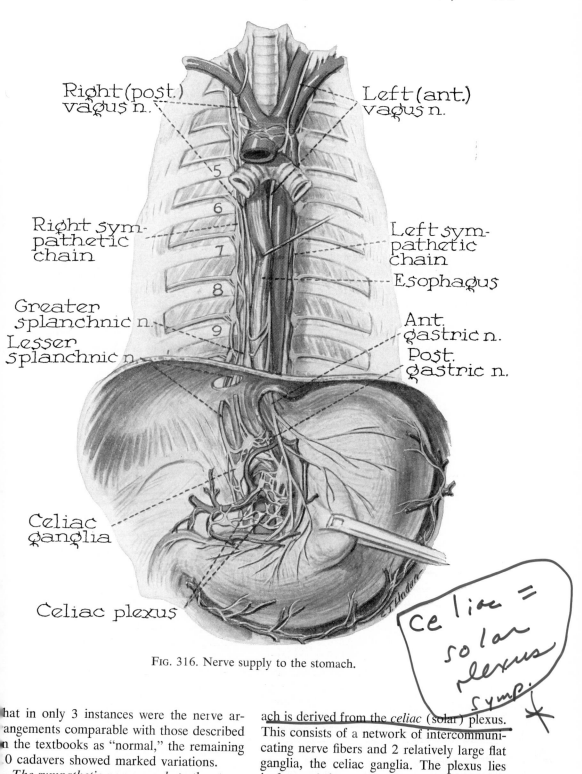

Right (post.) vagus n.

Left (ant.) vagus n.

5

6

Right sympathetic chain

7

Left sympathetic chain

Esophagus

8

Greater splanchnic n.

9

Lesser splanchnic n.

Ant. gastric n.

Post. gastric n.

Celiac ganglia

Celiac plexus

Celiac = solar plexus symp.

FIG. 316. Nerve supply to the stomach.

hat in only 3 instances were the nerve arrangements comparable with those described in the textbooks as "normal," the remaining 0 cadavers showed marked variations.

The sympathetic nerve supply to the stomach is derived from the *celiac* (solar) plexus. This consists of a network of intercommunicating nerve fibers and 2 relatively large flat ganglia, the celiac ganglia. The plexus lies in front of the upper part of the abdominal portion of the aorta around the celiac-artery. The right and the left celiac ganglia lie on corresponding crura of the diaphragm, the right being situated behind the inferior vena cava. The fibers to the plexus reach it from the greater and the lesser splanchnic nerves. The *greater splanchnic nerve* on either side arises from the right sympathetic chain between the 5th and the 10th thoracic ganglia. The *lesser splanchnic nerve* also arises from the sympathetic chain in the region of the 9th and the 10th thoracic ganglia. The greater splanchnic nerve usually terminates in the upper end of the ganglion; the lesser splanchnic reaches the lower end.

The celiac plexus supplies nerves which travel along the branches of the celiac artery; these fibers continue along the subdivisions of the 3 vessels and terminate in the stomach wall. In the gastric wall, a plexus is situated between the muscle layers (myenteric plexus) and another in the submucosa (submucous plexus). They contain both sympathetic and parasympathetic fibers, and from them terminal nerve fibers are supplied to the musculature and the glands of the stomach.

The stomach has 4 coats: serous, muscular, submucous and mucous. The serous coat is an investment of peritoneum which completely covers the anterior and the posterior surfaces of the stomach; the only uncovered parts are the greater and the lesser curvatures and a small area to the left of the cardia which is in direct contact with the diaphragm. The muscular coat consists of 3 layers of involuntary muscle: an outer longitudinal, a middle circular and an incomplete inner oblique. The longitudinal muscle is continuous with that of the esophagus; the circular layer becomes thickest in the region of the pylorus and forms the pyloric sphincter. In infants, excessive thickening of this circular layer at the pylorus may give rise to the condition known as *congenital pyloric stenosis*. The submucosa consists of an abundant, loosely arranged connective tissue layer which contains vessels of considerable size. The toughness of this layer explains its ability to hold sutures. The mucosa is freely movable upon its underlying lax submucosa and, in the undistended state, presents numerous folds giving it a rugose appearance. These folds are arranged chiefly in longitudinal directions.

ATTACHMENTS OF THE STOMACH (OMENTA)

Peritoneal folds attach the stomach to the liver, the transverse colon, the spleen, the biliary ducts, the pancreas and the diaphragm. These folds are indicated by such names as omenta or gastric ligaments (Fig. 317). Omenta are defined as compound peritoneal folds which pass from the stomach to other intra-abdominal organs. These attachments are found only along the curvatures of the stomach. The 2 gastric surfaces—the anterior belonging to the general peritoneal cavity and the posterior belonging to the lesser cavity (omental bursa)—are free and unattached. All omenta and gastric ligaments of the adult stomach originate from the midline mesenteries of embryonic life, and the only way to gain a clear picture of these connections is through a visualization of the succeeding steps in gastric development.

The lesser omentum is a wide fold of peritoneum which is hidden by the left lobe of the liver. It is attached to the first inch of duodenum, the lesser curvature of the stomach, the diaphragm for ½ inch between the esophagus and the upper end of the fissure for the ligamentum venosum, the bottom of that fissure and to the lips and the right end of the porta hepatis. Its right border is a free edge at which the 2 layers are continuous with each other (Fig. 313 A). It forms the anterior boundary of the opening (foramen of Winslow) into the lesser sac which separates it from the inferior vena cava. Between its layers and at its right border are the common duct, the portal vein and the hepatic artery; the right and the left gastric arteries are found along the lesser curvature.

The greater omentum is formed by the elongation of the primitive dorsal mesogastrium which does not cease growing with the completion of gastric rotation but con

submucosa of the st onward is very tough —holds sutures well

tinues until a broad sheet of peritoneum (floor of omental bursa) hangs down from the greater curvature of the stomach, ventral to the coils of small intestine (Fig. 317 A). After passing downward and being reflected upward, it again reaches the dorsal wall of the abdomen at a point slightly above the line of attachment of the transverse mesocolon. It is thereby brought into contact with the upper layer of the transverse mesocolon, with which it ultimately fuses (Fig. 317 B). This brings the floor of the omental burst into union with the transverse mesocolon. The dorsal mesogastrium and the transverse mesocolon fuse to form a common supporting membrane; the layers composing the dependent part of the bursa fuse with each other to obliterate the distal part of the lumen of the bursa. Fat is laid down in this omental apron which provides an insulating layer for the protection of the abdominal viscera.

The reflections of the gastric and the omental surfaces of the peritoneum as encountered by the surgeon can be traced easily both with regard to the greater and the lesser peritoneal cavities (Fig. 317 C). Beginning at the porta hepatis, a peritoneal surface extends downward as the anterior leaf of the gastrohepatic (lesser) omentum, passes over the ventral surface of the stomach and then downward as the anterior leaf of greater omentum; it then turns back and upward as the posterior leaf of the greater omentum until the transverse colon is reached.

Starting at the porta hepatis again, another peritoneal surface, the dorsal leaf of lesser omentum passes downward, covers the dorsal gastric wall and continues downward from the greater curvature of the stomach; it turns back and upward to the transverse colon as the innermost leaf of the greater omentum. It then passes over the anterior and upper walls of the transverse colon and backward to the posterior parietes as the uppermost layer of the transverse mesocolon. When illustrations of the ascending double layer are studied in the adult, the 2 layers seem to diverge and enclose the transverse colon and continue as the mesocolon. How-

ever, this is a wrong impression, since the ascending double layer in the fetus passes up in front of the transverse colon to the posterior wall and to the lower border of the pancreas. On gaining the latter, the anterior or inner serous layer of ascending omentum passes in front of the pancreas as the posterior wall of the omental bursa and then continues over the undersurface of the liver to its starting point. The outer or posterior serous layer of ascending omentum passes behind the pancreas to reach the body wall; it is reflected from this to become continuous with the upper layer of the transverse mesocolon. The original fetal relations become the surgeon's cleavage planes, which detach the greater omentum from the transverse colon and its mesentery.

These peritoneal reflections are related to the wall of the omental bursa in the following way: the pouch extends behind and below the liver and the stomach, above the transverse mesocolon, within the greater omentum (when not fused) and behind the lesser omentum.

SURGICAL CONSIDERATIONS

Gastrojejunostomy

Gastrojejunostomy is indicated in the patient who has a pyloric obstruction and low gastric acidity. It is used also as a palliative measure to provide relief for an obstructed pylorus (inoperable carcinoma) or as a preliminary procedure for future surgery. The operation may be done anterior or posterior to the transverse colon.

A posterior gastrojejunostomy (Fig. 318) is accomplished by passing the posterior wall of the stomach through a rent in the transverse mesocolon and performing an anastomosis between the stomach and a proximal loop of jejunum. The gastric site for the stoma should be placed at the most available and dependent part near the greater curvature and in line with the esophagus. The details and the structural orientation may be found in the description of gastric resection which follows. Following the anastomosis, the rent in the transverse mesocolon is

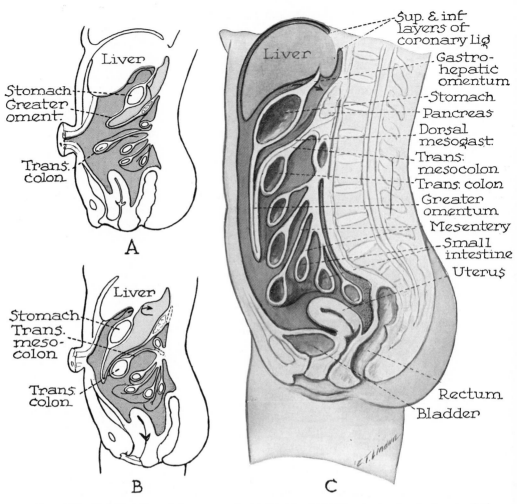

FIG. 317. Attachments of the stomach (omenta). (A) The early development of the greater omentum from the primitive dorsal mesogastrium. (B) Later development, showing beginning fusion of dorsal mesogastrium and transverse mesocolon. (C) Adult lesser and greater omenta. The arrow indicates the foramen of Winslow.

sutured to the posterior wall of the stomach to prevent internal herniation.

Anterior gastrojejunostomy (Fig. 319) is preferred by many surgeons; it is technically simpler, does not endanger the middle colic artery and does away with many of the hazards if reoperation becomes necessary. The anastomosis is placed on the anterior surface of the stomach and anterior to the transverse colon. In an anterior gastro-jejunostomy it is preferable to suture the greater curvature to the proximal end of the jejunum.

GASTRECTOMY

Subtotal gastrectomy is done for carcinoma of the stomach and for peptic ulcer. It is difficult to standardize such a procedure, since every clinic has a technic of its own; however, a standardized subtotal gastrectomy utilizing an end-to-side antecolic anastomosis will be described here (Figs. 320 and 321). Many men's names and modifications are associated with gastric operations, but space does not permit a review of such procedures; these can be found in any standard surgical text.

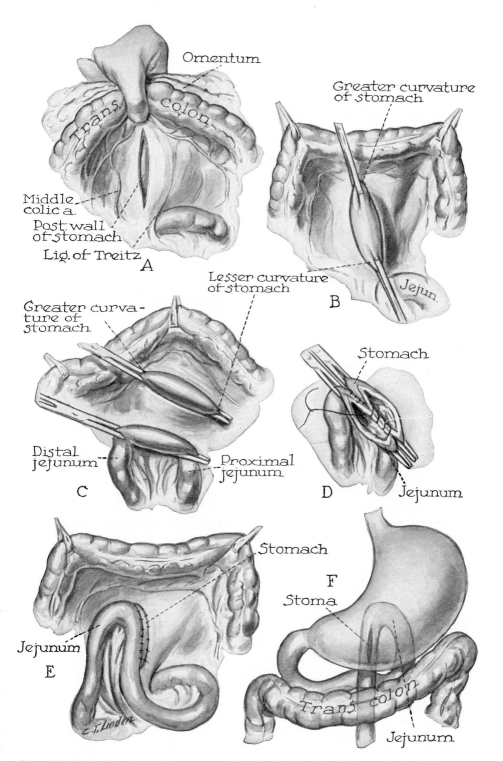

Omentum

Greater curvature of stomach

Trans. colon

Middle colic a.
Post wall of stomach
Lig. of Treitz
A

Jejun
B

Lesser curvature of stomach

Greater curvature of stomach

Distal jejunum

Proximal jejunum

Stomach

C

D

Jejunum

Stomach

F

Stoma

Jejunum

E

Trans colon

Jejunum

Fig. 318. Posterior gastrojejunostomy. (A) An incision has been made in the transverse mesocolon to the left of the middle colic artery. (B) The posterior wall of the stomach is delivered through the rent in the mesocolon. (C) The lesser curvature is approximated to the proximal jejunum and the greater curvature to the distal end of the jejunal loop. (D) The anastomosis. (E) The stomach is sutured to the mesocolon. (F) The completed anastomosis.

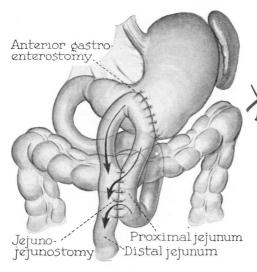

Anterior gastro-
enterostomy.

Jejuno-
jejunostomy   Proximal jejunum
                 Distal jejunum

FIG. 319. Anterior gastrojejunostomy with
entero-anastomosis.

The incision is usually one of the upper
rectus incisions, either placed to the right or
the left of the midline, depending on the
surgeon's preference and the site of the lesion.
Operability must be determined first. This
can be done by opening the hepatogastric
part of the lesser omentum and placing a
finger into the lesser peritoneal cavity. The
index finger of the left hand serves admirably
for this purpose; it makes its exit through an
avascular point in the gastrocolic part of the
greater omentum. A strip of gauze replaces
the finger and is used for traction. This too
greatly simplifies exposure of the duodenum
and also protects the transverse mesocolon
with its middle colic artery which will lie behind the gauze traction tape. Mobilization of
the greater curvature is accomplished next;
it extends to the "avascular triangle" (p.
428) on the left, and an inch distal to the
pylorus on the right. After freeing the greater
curvature of its vascular attachments and
ligating the left and the right gastro-epiploic
arteries, the lesser curvature is mobilized.

Mobilization of the lesser curvature already has been partially accomplished by the
opening made in the hepatogastric part of
the lesser omentum; this is continued by cutting and ligating the right gastric artery. After
mobilization of the curvatures, upward traction is maintained on the gauze tape so that
the stomach may be separated from its at-

tachments posteriorly to the pancreas (pan-
creaticogastric folds). In patients who have
an adherent ulcer which is situated in the
duodenum, it is safer to expose and thus
protect the common duct.

Division of the duodenum is accomplished
next; the distal end is closed. Ligation of the
left gastric artery is simpler and safer after
the stomach has been severed from its duodenal attachment. Then the stomach can be
retracted to the patient's left side; this enables
the surgeon to visualize the left gastric artery
as it approaches the lesser curvature posteriorly.

Location of the ligament of Treitz is accomplished by making upward traction on
the transverse colon, thus stretching its mesocolon; the duodenojejunal angle and the ligament of Treitz will be found immediately to
the left of the midline. To perform the antecolic operation, a long jejunal loop is required; this usually measures from 10 to 12
inches from Treitz's ligament. The jejunal
loop is approximated to the posterior wall of
the stomach near the line of resection. An
anastomosis is performed which places the
greater curvature of the stomach to the proximal end of jejunum and the lesser curvature
to the proximal end of the jejunal loop.

TRANSABDOMINAL VAGUS NERVE SECTION
(VAGOTOMY) (Fig. 322)

The abdominal approach to the gastric
nerves (vagi) allows exploration of the abdominal contents and the lesion; it also facilitates the performance of a gastro-enteros-
tomy if pyloric obstruction is present or is
likely to occur.

A long incision is necessary for proper exposure. A left muscle-splitting rectus incision
which commences in the angle between the
xiphoid and the left costal cartilage and extends 1 or 2 inches below the umbilicus is
utilized. The peritoneal cavity is entered, and
the left triangular ligament of the liver is exposed. This bloodless fold is severed, and
then becomes possible to retract the left lobe
of the liver to the right. The peritoneum covering the lower end of the esophagus is incised, the posterior mediastinum is entered
and the lower 3 or 4 inches of the esophagus
are mobilized and exposed. The vagus nerves
are identified by palpation; they feel like taut

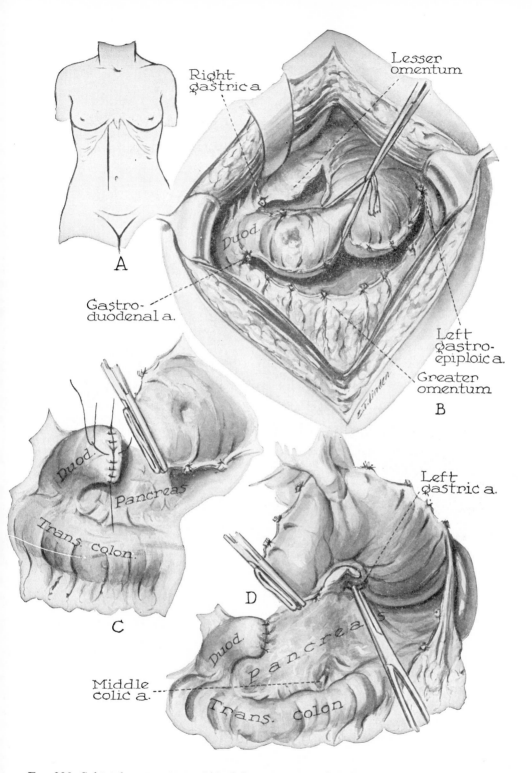

Fig. 320. Subtotal gastrectomy: (A) right upper rectus incision; (B) the lesser and the greater curvatures have been mobilized, and the right gastric, the gastroduodenal and the left gastroepiploic arteries have been ligated; (C) closure of the duodenal stump; (D) isolation of the left gastric artery.

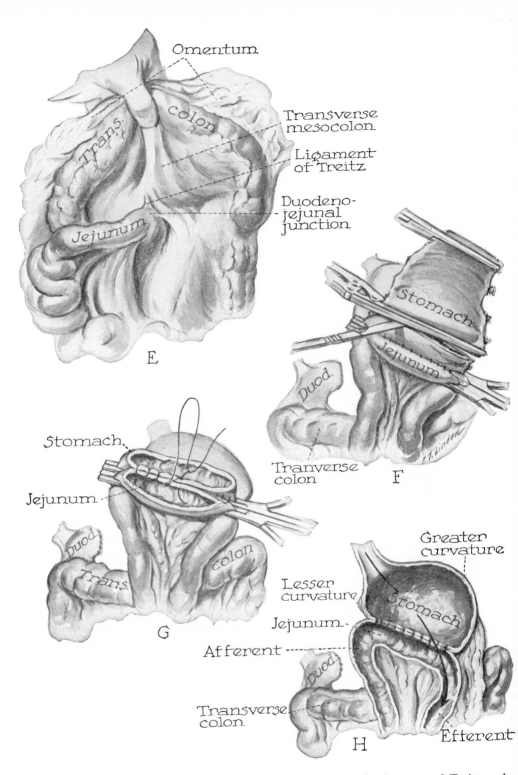

Fig. 321. Subtotal gastrectomy (*Continued*): (E) locating the ligament of Treitz and the duodenojejunal junction; (F) the jejunum has been brought over the front of the transverse colon and approximated to the posterior wall of the stomach; (G) the anastomosis; (H) the completed antecolic, end-to-side gastrojejunostomy following resection of the involved stomach.

cords which can be differentiated readily from the more yielding muscle of the esophagus. The left (anterior) vagus has a tendency to hug the esophagus, but the right (posterior) vagus travels a slight distance away from it.

By finger dissection the fibers are assembled into 2 main trunks comprising the right and the left vagi; these are ligated and divided. The position of the right and the left trunks below the esophageal hiatus is found to be

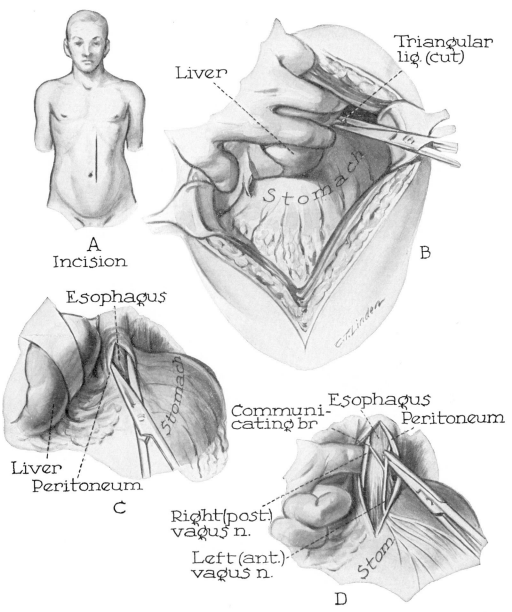

FIG. 322. Transabdominal vagus nerve section (vagotomy). (A) The incision commences in the angle between the xiphoid process and the left costal arch and ends an inch below the umbilicus. (B) The left triangular ligament is exposed and made taut by gently pulling the left lobe of the liver to the right. It is severed. (C) The left lobe of the liver is retracted to the right, and the peritoneum covering the lower end of the esophagus is incised. (D) The esophagus is delivered, and the vagi are cut.

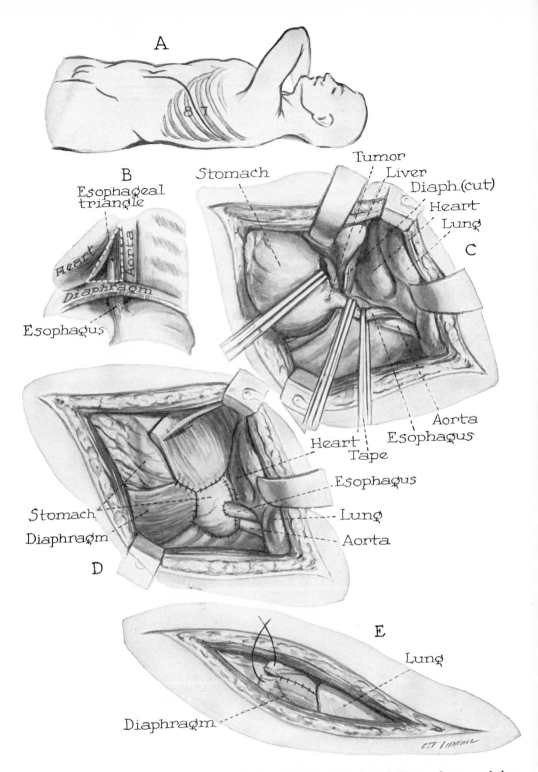

A

B

Esophageal
triangle

Heart

Aorta

Diaphragm

Esophagus

Stomach

Tumor

Liver

Diaph.(cut)

Heart

Lung

C

Aorta

Esophagus

Heart

Tape

Esophagus

Lung

Aorta

Stomach

Diaphragm

D

E

Lung

Diaphragm

FIG. 323. Surgical treatment for carcinoma of the lower third of the esophagus and the cardiac end of the stomach: (A) The incision; (B) the esophageal triangle is bounded in front by the heart, behind by the descending aorta and below by the diaphragm; (C) the lower end of the esophagus and the upper end of the stomach are mobilized and removed; (D) anastomosis and repair of the diaphragm; (E) closure.

remarkably constant; however, many times these nerves are numerous and communicating, and their distribution does not follow a uniform pattern. At the conclusion of the operation, the left lobe of the liver is permitted to fall into place; it has been found unnecessary to resuture the severed left triangular ligament.

Carcinoma of the Lower Third of the Esophagus and the Cardiac End of the Stomach (Fig. 323)

Most lesions involving the lower part of the esophagus and the cardiac end of the stomach can be removed through a combined thoracico-abdominal approach. The incision affords an excellent exposure of the upper abdomen and the thoracic cavity, thus enabling more extensive resections. Humphreys, Garlock, Adams and Phemister, Marshall, Churchill and Sweet—all have applied some form of this approach for such lesions.

A left upper rectus incision is made; this extends from or below the umbilicus to the left costal arch. The peritoneal cavity is entered, and a thorough exploration is carried out to determine the extent of the growth, fixation to vital structures and the presence or the absence of metastases (liver, peripancreatic, pelvic and diaphragmatic). Should the tumor prove to be operable, the incision is extended over the costal arch and then upward and outward into the 7th intercostal interspace. The costal arch is divided, and the pleural cavity is entered. The intercostal muscles and the pleura are incised well past the inferior angle of the scapula, and the left leaf of the diaphragm is severed. The diaphragm is divided radially from the esophageal hiatus to its peripheral attachment. Large phrenic vessels are encountered; these should be properly isolated, divided and tied. The inferior pulmonary ligament is severed; this exposes an esophageal triangle which is

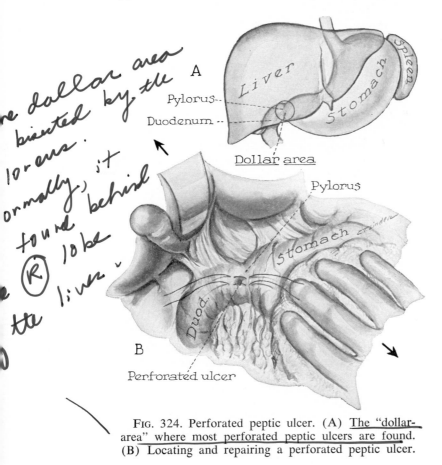

FIG. 324. Perforated peptic ulcer. (A) The "dollar-area" where most perforated peptic ulcers are found. (B) Locating and repairing a perforated peptic ulcer.

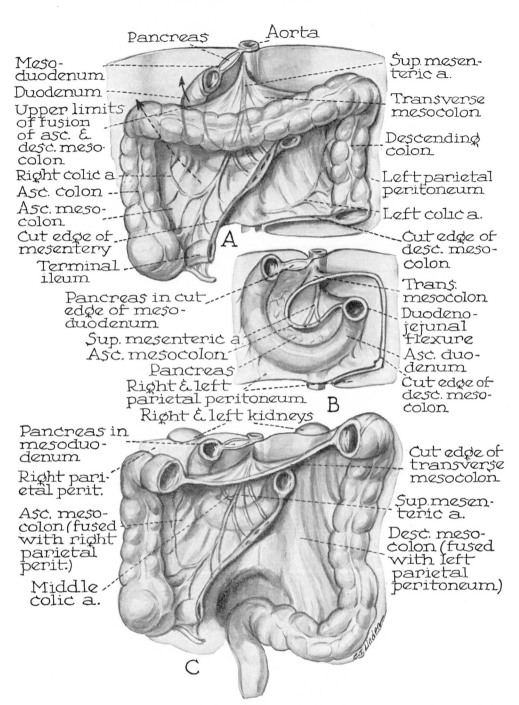

Pancreas   Aorta

Meso-
duodenum

Duodenum

Upper limits
of fusion
of asc. &
desc. meso-
colon

Right colic a

Asc. colon

Asc. meso-
colon

Cut edge of
mesentery

Terminal
ileum

Sup. mesen-
teric a.

Transverse
mesocolon

Descending
colon

Left parietal
peritoneum

Left colic a.

Cut edge of
desc. meso-
colon

A

Pancreas in cut
edge of meso-
duodenum

Sup. mesenteric a

Asc. mesocolon

Pancreas

Right & left
parietal peritoneum

Right & left kidneys

Trans.
mesocolon

Duodeno-
jejunal
flexure

Asc. duo-
denum

Cut edge of
desc. meso-
colon

B

Pancreas in
mesoduo-
denum

Right pari-
etal perit.

Asc. meso-
colon (fused
with right
parietal
perit.)

Middle
colic a.

Cut edge of
transverse
mesocolon

Sup. mesen-
teric a.

Desc. meso-
colon (fused
with left
parietal
peritoneum)

C

Fig. 325. Embryology. (A) Rotation of the umbilical loop has been completed, and the ascending and the transverse colon segments have been formed. The right portion of the transverse mesocolon is the upper limit of fusion between the ascending mesocolon and the right primitive parietal peritoneum; the left portion of the transverse mesocolon is the upward limit of fusion between the descending mesocolon and the left primitive parietal peritoneum. The duodenojejunal angle is to the left of the midline and rests against the mesentery of the transverse colon. (B) The descending duodenum and part of the transverse duodenum fuse with the right parietal peritoneum; the remainder of the transverse duodenum and the ascending duodenum fuse with the descending mesocolon. (C) Final stage, following posterior peritoneal fixation and fusion.

bounded in front by the heart, behind by the descending aorta and below by the diaphragm (Fig. 323 B). In this triangle the esophagus can be identified easily. The technic for the resection and the anastomosis is essentially the same as that described under lesions of the midthoracic esophagus (Fig. 227). The diaphragm is repaired, and the now somewhat enlarged esophageal hiatus is sutured to the stomach. The pleura, the intercostal muscles and the overlying soft tissues are approximated, and the abdominal incision is closed in layers.

CLOSURE OF A PERFORATED PEPTIC ULCER
(Fig. 324)

Most perforations of a peptic ulcer occur at the so-called "dollar-area." This circular area, about the size of a silver dollar, is bisected by the pylorus. Normally, the right lobe of the liver covers this region and attempts to seal the perforation. Therefore, to locate most perforated peptic ulcers, the right lobe of the liver should be retracted upward, and the stomach should be pulled gently in a downward direction and to the left (Fig.

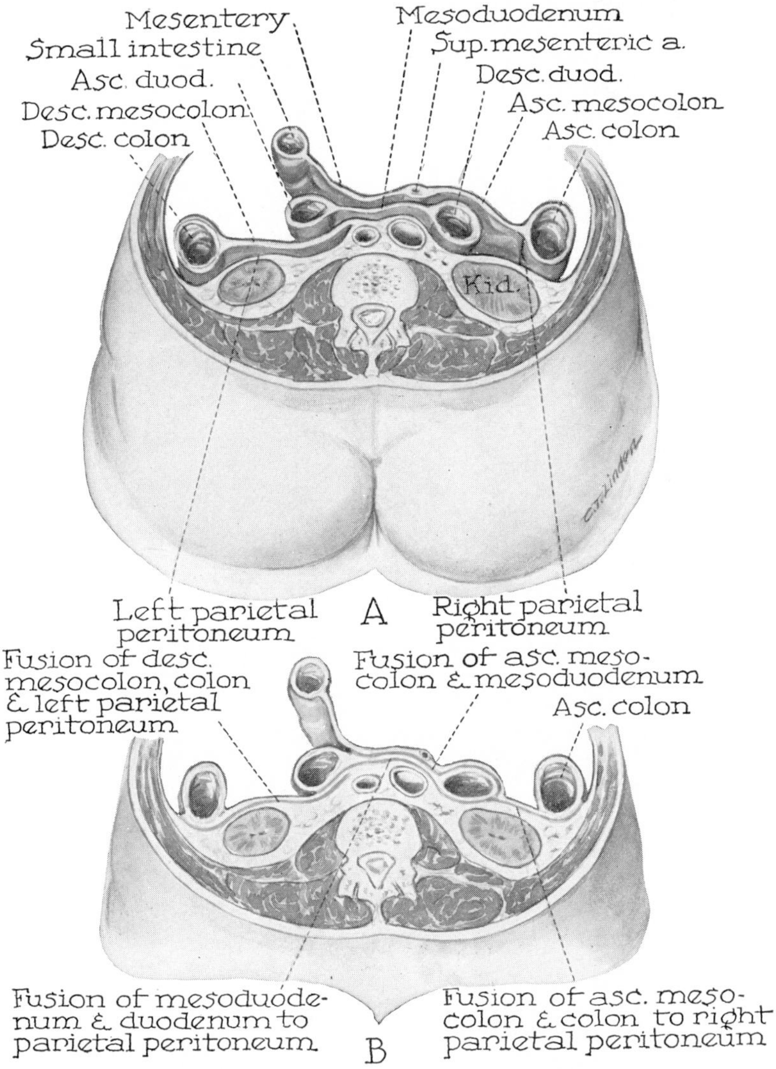

KNOW

Mesentery,
Small intestine
Asc. duod.
Desc. mesocolon
Desc. colon

Mesoduodenum
Sup. mesenteric a.
Desc. duod.
Asc. mesocolon
Asc. colon

Kid.

Left parietal
peritoneum   A   Right parietal
peritoneum

Fusion of desc.
mesocolon, colon
& left parietal
peritoneum

Fusion of asc. meso-
colon & mesoduodenum.
Asc. colon

Fusion of mesoduode-
num & duodenum to
parietal peritoneum   B

Fusion of asc. meso-
colon & colon to right
parietal peritoneum

FIG. 326. Embryology. (A) Early stage of development before fusion has taken place. (B) After fusion of the ascending mesocolon with mesoduodenum; posterior fixation of the colon is also shown.

324 B). If the perforation is not found with this maneuver, then the lesser and the greater curvatures should be examined; still failing to find the ulcer, the gastrocolic ligament must be severed and the posterior wall of the stomach inspected. Many methods of repair have been advocated; these vary from a simple graft of omentum placed over the perforation to excision and closure.

SMALL INTESTINE

The small intestine (duodenum, jejunum and ileum) has an average length of 22 feet,

the extremes being 30 and 15 feet. The division into jejunum and ileum is arbitrary, since there is no one point at which it may be said that the jejunum ends and the ileum begins. The lumen of the small intestine is widest in the duodenum and narrowest near the ileocecal valve; for this reason a foreign body tends to become impacted in the region of the latter. The upper jejunum may be differentiated from the lower ileum by the fact that the number of arterial arcades and the amount of fat in the mesentery increases distally. Clear spaces (lunettes) between the

More fat & more B.V. in the ileum than in the jejunum!!

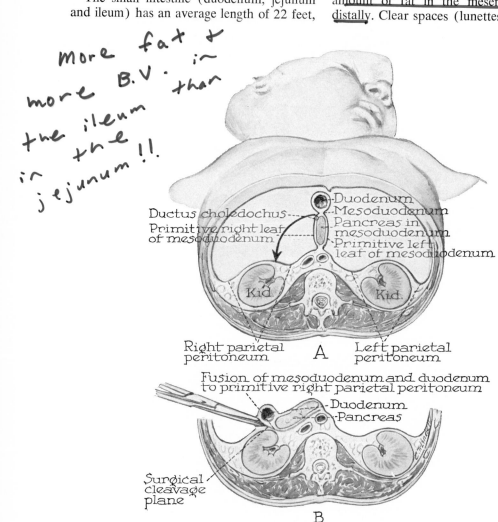

FIG. 327. Embryology of the duodenum. (A) Cross section through the duodenum and the mesoduodenum before rotation of the gastroduodenal segment. The arrow presents the direction of rotation against the right primitive parietal peritoneum. (B) The same as "A," after fusion has taken place. The surgical cleavage plane for mobilization of the duodenum and the head of the pancreas is indicated.

vessels approaching the bowel are present in the more proximal part of small bowel but are absent in the distal portion. The jejuno-ileum fills the space below the transverse colon and the mesocolon and more or less overlies the ascending and the descending colons; it rests on the iliac fossae and is related to the pelvic viscera. The great omentum hangs down from the transverse colon and, depending on its degree of development, separates the intestines from the anterior abdominal wall. No small intestines occupy the fetal pelvis, but in the adult pelvis the amount depends on the state of distention of the bladder and the rectum and upon the position of the pelvic colon.

DUODENUM

Embryology. The early development of the duodenum (Figs. 325, 326 and 327) has been described on p. 403. The rotation of the intestines to their ultimate abdominal positions is produced by drawing the initial colic segment to the right so that the duo-

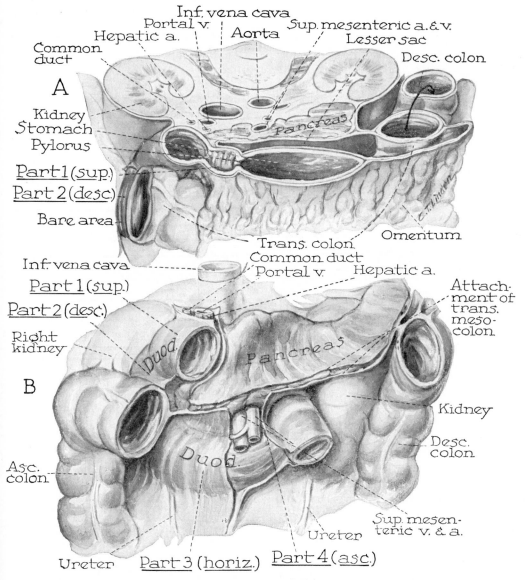

FIG. 328. The duodenum. (A) The relations of Parts 1 and 2 of the duodenum. (B) The 4 parts of the duodenum are shown, and the peritoneal relations of each are presented.

denojejunal junction and the small intestines lie toward the left (Fig. 325). This places the duodenojejunal angle against the mesentery of the terminal intestine, with which it fuses. The degree of fusion accounts for the fossae and the peritoneal folds which are found in this region. These fossae and folds are of surgical interest, since deficient fixation of the angle increases the depth and the capacity of the fossae, and loops of intestines may herniate into them and become strangulated. Hyperfixation of the duodenojejunal angle may fix the duodenum so firmly that it becomes kinked and does not empty properly. The descending duodenum and part of the transverse duodenum fuse with the primitive right parietal peritoneum. The remainder of the transverse duodenum and the ascending duodenum fuse with the descending mesocolon, and the duodenojejunal angle fuses with the transverse mesocolon. The superior part of the ascending mesocolon forms a fusion fascia with the anterior part of the mesoduodenum (p. 423). Proper cleavage planes can be found easily, and surgical mobilization can be accomplished readily if these embryologic details are kept in mind.

Adult Duodenum. The duodenum (Fig. 328) receives its name because at first it was thought to be 12 inches long; in reality, it is closer to 10 or 11 inches in length. Not only is it the first and shortest part of the small bowel, but also it is the lightest, thickest and most fixed of the three parts. It extends from the pylorus to the duodenojejunal, making a C-shaped curve; the concavity of the curve is directed upward and to the left and is occupied by the head of the pancreas. The duodenum may be traced upward, backward and to the right, then downward until it is crossed by the transverse colon. The portion which comprises the entire first and upper half of the second part lies in the supracolic compartment.

To visualize further the duodenum it is necessary to turn the greater omentum upward and displace the coils of jejunum and ileum downward and to the left. Then the duodenum can be traced downward and horizontally to the left on the upper part of the posterior wall of the right infracolic compartment. It disappears behind the root of the mesentery; this portion is difficult to demonstrate because it lies behind the peritoneum of the posterior abdominal wall. Anteriorly, it is related to coils of the small intestine which separate it from the transverse mesocolon. To its right side the lower pole of the right kidney is found.

The rest of the duodenum lies in the left infracolic compartment, and to visualize it the coils of jejuno-ileum must be drawn upward and to the right. This portion is identified easily and can be traced upward, close to the root of the mesentery and to the duodenojejunal flexure. Here it bends forward and downward and becomes continuous with the jejunum. The flexure usually lies to the left and on a level with the second lumbar vertebra. Therefore, the duodenum is found in the supracolic and both infracolic compartments.

The "C" which the duodenum forms is covered anteriorly and on its convexity by peritoneum except where the transverse colon crosses the second part and holds the peritoneum away. The posterior surface and concavity of the "C" are devoid of peritoneum. Approximately the first inch of the first part is almost entirely covered by peritoneum. In the region where the bile duct enters the second part of the duodenum, diverticula, devoid of a peritoneal covering, may occur. This is of surgical importance, since the removal of such a diverticulum is associated with the risk of peritonitis because of infection in the retroperitoneal tissues. Because of the C-shaped curve which it makes, its beginning and end are close together. It lies on the posterior wall of the abdomen above the level of the umbilicus and is almost entirely in the right half of the abdomen.

For convenience of description the duodenum is divided into the following 4 parts:

1. Superior part—about 2 inches long
2. Descending part—about 3 inches long
3. Horizontal part—about 4 inches long
4. Ascending part—about 1 inch long

The first (superior) part begins at the pylorus on a level with the body of the first lumbar vertebra and passes backward, upward and to the right. Here it is in close relation with the liver; it ends at the neck of the gallbladder by bending sharply to become the second part. After death, this area usually is stained green by bile that leaks through the walls of the gallbladder. Since its 1st inch is clotted on the front and the back with peritoneum, it is connected with the omenta both above and below. The lesser omentum passes from its superior border to the liver, and the greater omentum hangs from its lower border. Posteriorly, it is separated from the neck of the pancreas by the lesser peritoneal sac; anteriorly, it is related to the quadrate lobe of the liver. The 1st inch of part one of the duodenum can be moved with the stomach. The 2nd inch is covered with peritoneum only above and in front where it is related to the liver and the neck of the gallbladder; posteriorly, it is directly related to the gastroduodenal artery, the bile ducts, the portal vein and part of the neck of the pancreas (Fig. 330). Inferiorly, it is related directly to the head of the pancreas. The portal vein and the common duct separate it posteriorly from the inferior vena cava (Fig. 328). Since this part of the duodenum takes a backward rather than a sideward course, the structures related to it lie medial rather than behind it. The intimate relation between the first part of the duodenum and the gallbladder explains the adhesions which exist between them when either is diseased, and also explains the spontaneous passage of gallstones into the duodenum (autocholecystoduodenostomy). The term "duodenal bulb" applies to the 1st inch of duodenum.

The second (descending) part passes vertically downward in front of the hilum and the adjoining part of the anterior surface of the right kidney. It descends to the level of the 3rd lumbar vertebra, bends sharply to the left and becomes the third part. Part two of the duodenum is crossed by the transverse colon; the colon at this point may or may not have a mesentery. Only parts of the anterior surface above and below the transverse colon are covered by peritoneum (Fig. 328 B).

Above the attachment of the transverse colon, the descending duodenum lies in the supramesocolic compartment; below this attachment, it lies in the inframesocolic compartment where it is related to the ascending colon. Above the transverse colon it is related to the ascending colon, and anteriorly it is related to the gallbladder and the right lobe of the liver.

Below the transverse colon it is related anteriorly to the jejunum; the head of the pancreas lies to its medial side, and the ascending colon, the hepatic flexure and the right lobe

of the liver to its lateral side, in that order from below upward. Posteriorly, it rests on the psoas major muscle, being partly separated from it by the renal vessels and the ureter. The bile duct and the pancreatic ducts enter this part on the posteromedial surface a little below its middle (Fig. 398). The accessory pancreatic duct opens about ¾ inch above (cephalad) the openings of the common bile and the main pancreatic ducts. Because of its peritoneal attachments, this part of the duodenum is quite firmly fixed in its position.

The third (horizontal) part of the duodenum is about 4 inches long and passes horizontally and to the left. Since it is crossed by the root of the mesentery, it is found in the right and the left infracolic compartments. From right to left it crosses in front of the right psoas muscle, the ureter, the inferior vena cava and the abdominal aorta; it ends to the left side of the body of the 3rd lumbar vertebra. Its upper border is related to the head of the pancreas, and its lower border to the jejunum. Anteriorly, it is crossed about its middle by the superior mesenteric vessels as they pass to the root of the mesentery. Therefore, it crosses through a vascular angle which is formed by the superior mesenteric vessels in front and the aorta behind. The superior mesenteric vessels may compress the duodenum so that a dilatation of the stomach or a duodenal ileus may result. The peritoneum covers it anteriorly except where the root of the mesentery crosses it (Fig. 328 B). To the right of the mesentery it is covered by loops of jejunum which separate it from the transverse colon. It finally bends upward to become the fourth part.

The fourth (ascending) part is a little more than 1 inch long and represents the shortest part of the duodenum. It turns upward along the left side of the aorta on the left psoas muscle and ends about 1 inch to the left of the median plane at the level of the 2nd lumbar vertebra. At this point it bends sharply forward to form the duodenojejunal flexure; here it becomes continuous with the jejunum. Anteriorly, it is related to the root of the mesentery and the coils of the jejunum; posteriorly, to the medial border of the left psoas muscle, the left renal and the spermatic (ovarian) vessels; on its right, to the vertebral column and on its left side to

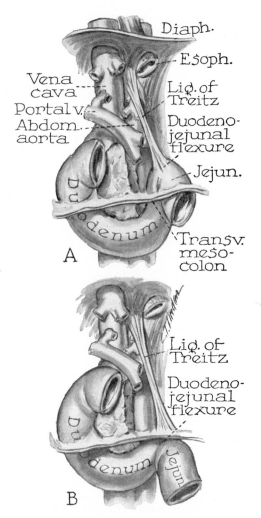

FIG. 329. The ligament of Treitz. (A) The short type of ligament which pulls the duodenojejunal flexure above the transverse mesocolon and results in a "U"-shaped duodenum. (B) The long type of ligament which allows the duodenojejunal flexure to lie below the transverse mesocolon and results in a "C"-shaped duodenum.

the proximal coils of jejunum. This part of the duodenum sometimes overlaps the pelvis of the left kidney. Internally, it lies along the aorta and is adherent to the pancreas; externally, it is found on the inner side of the left kidney.

A vascular arch is found in the space which separates the duodenum from the kidney; it has been called the *vascular arch of Treitz.* This arch is formed by the left colic

artery and the inferior mesenteric vein as they ascend together near the left border of the duodenum to the root of the transverse mesocolon.

The duodenojejunal flexure, although usually retroperitoneal, may penetrate into the root of the transverse mesocolon (Fig. 329). It usually lies to the left of the disk between the 1st and the 2nd lumbar vertebrae but may approach the midline or begin at the middle of the 2nd or even the 3rd lumbar vertebra. Its relation to the transverse mesocolon depends on the length of the ligament of Treitz (Fig. 329). Posteriorly, it is in relation to the lumbar portion of the diaphragm; above, it is related to the inferior border of the pancreas, and it is embraced by the concavity of the arch formed by the inferior mesenteric vein before it terminates below and behind the pancreas (Figs. 328 B, 331 A and B).

The flexure is related to the internal border of the left kidney on its left and, anteriorly, to the posterior wall of the stomach, from which it is separated by the transverse mesocolon. It is overlapped somewhat by the pancreas. The duodenojejunal flexure is fixed by the so-called muscle or ligament of Treitz.

The suspensory ligament (muscle) of Treitz is a band of fibrous muscular tissue which extends from the duodenojejunal angle and the ascending portion of the duodenum to the right pillar of the diaphragm. It is triangular in shape and originates from a broad base upon the superior border of the duodenojejunal angle. It passes upward behind the pancreas and in front of the aorta. It is better developed in the more muscular individuals and fixes the duodenojejunal angle to the posterior abdominal wall. The length of the ligament of Treitz determines whether the duodenum will be "U"-shaped or "C"-shaped (Fig. 329). If the ligament is long, the duodenojejunal flexure lies below the transverse mesocolon, and the "C"-shaped duodenum results. If the ligament is short, the duodenojejunal flexure lies above the transverse mesocolon, and the "U"-shaped duodenum is found.

The surgeon should be able to locate this ligament rapidly and in this way orient himself and "run" the intestinal tract (jejunoileum) in search of pathology; he is also able to select that segment of small bowel which he wishes to utilize in a gastrointestinal anastomosis.

The ligament and the angle are found in the following way: the surgeon's left hand grasps the greater omentum and the transverse colon, and, maintaining upward traction on these structures, the transverse mesocolon is made taut. Then the right hand is placed on the lower surface of the stretched transverse mesocolon and follows it posteriorly to its attachment in the region of the first lumbar vertebra; the hand is placed to the left and immediately encounters the duodenojejunal angle with the ligament of Treitz immediately above it.

Arteries. Since the relationship of the duodenum to the head of the pancreas is so intimate, their blood supplies naturally overlap. Many vascular patterns and anomalies have been described; nevertheless the most constant vascular patterns and those of greatest surgical significance are described herein. Pierson has made an accurate study of this region, and much of his material is of practical value.

The gastroduodenal artery is a branch of the hepatic artery and arises dorsal and superior to the pyloroduodenal junction (Fig. 330). It courses downward, medial to the common duct, and terminates at the lower border of the first part of the duodenum by dividing into the *right gastroepiploic* and the

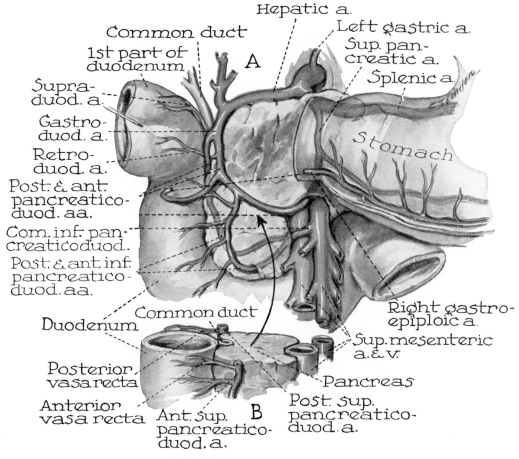

FIG. 330. Arterial blood supply of the duodenum. (A) The formation of the anterior and the posterior arterial arcades is shown. The arrow and the horizontal line indicate the level at which the cross section shown as "B" was taken. (B) Cross section showing the intimate relation between the duodenum, the pancreas and the common ducts. Anterior and posterior vasa recta are shown.

anterior superior pancreaticoduodenal arteries.

The gastroduodenal artery gives off a *posterior superior pancreaticoduodenal artery* as it passes dorsally to the superior margin of the duodenum.

The first part of the duodenum receives 2 smaller branches, namely, the *supraduodenal artery* to the superior wall and the anterior surface, and the *retroduodenal artery* which arises about ½ inch above the bifurcation of the gastroduodenal and supplies the lower two thirds of the posterior wall; it sometimes extends as far as the second part.

The remainder of the first part of the duodenum is supplied by branches from the right gastroepiploic and the superior pancreaticoduodenal arteries. The superior anterior and posterior pancreaticoduodenal arteries anastomose with corresponding *anterior* and *posterior inferior pancreaticoduodenal arteries* from the superior mesenteric. In this way two arterial arcades are formed, one on the posterior surface of the head of the pancreas and the other on the anterior surface. They are called respectively, the *posterior* and the *anterior arcades* of the pancreas.

The 2 inferior pancreaticoduodenal arteries arise from a common trunk from the superior mesenteric called the *common inferior pancreaticoduodenal artery.* From the 2 arterial arcades the duodenum receives anterior and posterior sets of vasa recta (Fig. 330 B). Shapiro and Robillard have stressed the possible dangers ("blowouts" and leakage) which might result from injury and ligation of

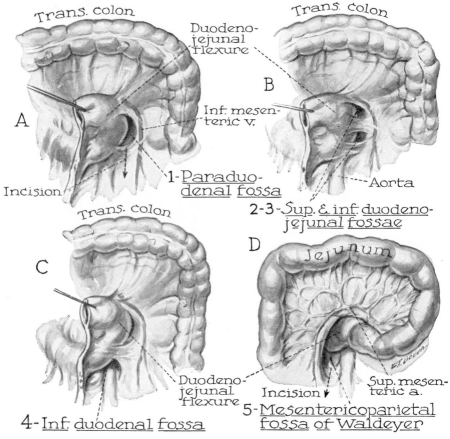

FIG. 331. The 5 duodenal fossae. (A) The paraduodenal fossa. Enlargement of this fossa must be made in a downward direction to avoid the inferior mesenteric vein. (B) The superior and the inferior duodenojejunal fossae formed by 2 peritoneal folds. (C) The inferior duodenal fossa extends behind the third part of the duodenum. (D) The mesentericoparietal fossa is located behind the first part of mesojejunum.

the vasa recta during a too radical mobilization of the duodenal stump from the pancreas in the course of a gastric resection. They further stress the futility of thorough ligation for the control of hemorrhage from a duodenal ulcer, stating that such a procedure is tantamount to complete devascularization of the duodenum and the head of the pancreas.

The nerves are derived from the celiac and the superior mesenteric plexuses and follow the course of the arteries.

The lymphatics of the duodenum are closely related to those of the pancreas. There are anterior and posterior sets of glands which drain into the superior pancreatic and pancreaticoduodenal lymph glands on the anterior and the posterior aspects of the groove between the duodenum and the pancreas. The efferent vessels from these glands pass in two directions: upward to the hepatic lymph glands and downward to the preaortic lymph glands around the superior mesenteric artery. There are also some communications with the lymphatics of the ascending colon and the appendix.

Duodenal Fossae. There are 5 *duodenal fossae* which may be encountered (Fig. 331).

1. *The paraduodenal fossa* lies to the left of the duodenojejunal flexure and opens to the right and upward. It occurs in about 20

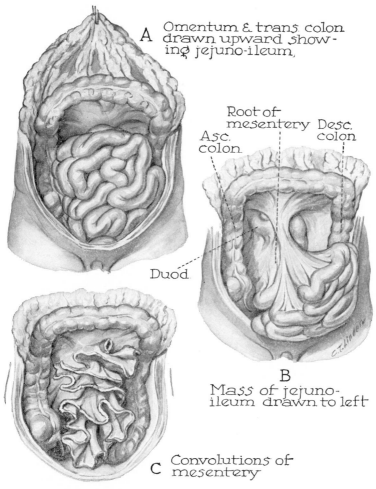

Fig. 332. The jejuno-ileum. (A) The normally placed coils of jejuno-ileum: the jejunum is above and to the left, and the ileum is below and to the right. (B) The stretched root of mesentery. (C) The jejuno-ileum has been removed, and the convolutions of the mesentery are shown.

per cent of people and rarely, if ever, exists with any other type of duodenal fossa. It is bounded on the right by the aorta, on the left by the kidney, above by the pancreas and the renal vessels and anteriorly by the inferior mesenteric vein which runs in the anterior wall of the fossa. This anterior relationship is of surgical importance, since a hernia into this fossa may press upon the inferior mesenteric vein and produce hemorrhoids. In case this fossa is the site of a strangulated hernia, its surgical enlargement should be brought about in a downward direction; in this way injury to the inferior mesenteric vein is avoided (Fig. 331 A).

2. *The superior duodenojejunal fossa* faces downward, is about 1 inch in depth and is in front of the 2nd lumbar vertebra.

3. *The inferior duodenojejunal fossa* is directed upward and is in front of the 3rd lumbar vertebra. The last two mentioned fossae are formed by two peritoneal folds which pass to the left from the terminal portion of the duodenum. The inferior mesenteric vein passes along their left extremities.

4. *The inferior duodenal fossa* is rarely seen; if present, it extends behind the 3rd part of the duodenum.

5. *The mesentericoparietal fossa (Waldeyer)* is located behind the first part of the mesojejunum; it lies immediately behind the superior mesenteric artery and below the duodenum. Its orifice faces to the left. In front, it is bounded by the superior mesenteric artery and behind, by the lumbar vertebrae. A swelling produced by a herniation of small bowel into it would occupy the right half of the abdominal cavity. The orifice of this fossa is so large that small gut may enter or leave it without causing symptoms or strangulation. The bowel can be withdrawn from this fossa without much difficulty. Should enlargement become necessary, the relationship of the superior mesenteric vessels must be kept in mind, and the fossa should be incised only in a downward direction.

THE JEJUNO-ILEUM

The jejunum and the ileum together measure about 20 feet in length (Fig. 332). They comprise the second and the third portions of the small intestine; they also make up about two fifths of the total length which is the jejunum, and three fifths the ileum. There is no sharp dividing line between these two parts of bowel; they differ from the duodenum in that they are not fixed but are suspended from the posterior wall by a fold of peritoneum, the mesentery (Fig. 332 B). The caliber of the lumen of the small bowel is not uniform but diminishes from above downward, being narrowest at its termination. This is of practical importance, since foreign bodies are usually stopped at this narrowest part, which consists of the last 6 to 12 inches of ileum. The jejuno-ileum is completely covered with peritoneum except along its line of attachment to the anterior border of the posterior mensentery. To accommodate the great length of small intestine, the mesentery is thrown into extensive series of convolutions (Fig. 332 C). The posterior line of attachment of the mesentery begins around the descending aorta opposite the body of the 2nd lumbar vertebra, deviates obliquely to the right at an angle of about 45° and terminates in the region of the right sacro-iliac joint. Since the coils of the small intestine are movable, their position is variable; the jejunum tends to be above and to the left, and the ileum below and to the right. The coils are hemmed in on the right, above and to the left by the colon, and are related posteriorly to the posterior abdominal wall and the retroperitoneal structures; also, they are in relation anteriorly to the anterior abdominal wall and the greater omentum, the latter as a rule being spread over them. The 2 parts of the small bowel which lie in the pelvis are:

1. The terminal ileum (except the last 2 inches) which is fixed in the right iliac fossa.

2. The 5 feet of small gut which begin at a point 6 feet from the duodenojejunal flexure and continue to a point 11 feet from that flexure; this is due to the great length of the mesentery to this part of bowel. These are the parts of the small bowel which are most likely to be affected in pelvic peritonitis and become adherent to pathologic adnexae; they are the most probable sites for small bowel intestinal obstructions.

From the pylorus to the ileocecal valve the small intestine has a complete external muscular coat of longitudinal fibers and an internal muscular coat of circular fibers. However, the mucous membrane differs in different parts of the gut. In the first part of the duodenum, the inner lining is smooth, but the branched tubular duodenal glands are numerous, especially near the pylorus. The plicae circulares are true infoldings of mucous membrane which are set at right angles to the long axis of the gut; they begin in the second part of the duodenum and become closely packed below the duodenal papilla. They are equally close in the upper part of the jejunum, but toward its lower end they diminish. In the ileum they become more widely separated and finally in the terminal portion are entirely absent. These plicae increase the area of absorptive surface without increasing the length of the gut. Small collections of lymphoid tissue form tiny elevations in the mucous membrane. They are known as solitary lymphatic nodules; however, larger collections of lymphoid tissue constitute the aggregated lymphoid nodules (Peyer's patches) which are most numerous toward the terminal portion of ileum, where they form elongated oval areas on the antimesenteric border of the bowel. They are absent in the upper two thirds of the jejunum; they are marked best in younger individuals and tend to disappear as one grows older.

Is it jejunum or ileum? This question may be answered if a few differential anatomic points are observed. The upper part of the small intestine is thicker, and its diameter becomes diminished from above downward. The blood vessels of the small bowel are larger proximally; therefore, they are only primary vascular loops which are associated with vasa recta some 3 to 5 cm. long (Fig. 333). Distally, secondary vascular loops or arcades are seen; these produce smaller windows, "lunettes," and shorter vasa recta, the latter being approximately 1 cm. in length. The more distally small bowel is observed, the greater is the amount of fat; proximally, it is quite easy to see through the windows formed by the vascular loops, whereas the fat prevents these windows from being transparent in the distal ileum.

Mesentery. A fold of peritoneum which

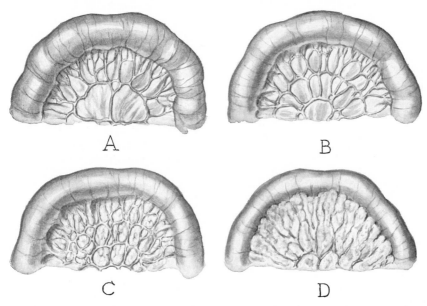

FIG. 333. Localization of the jejuno-ileum. (A) About 3 feet from the duodenojejunal flexure, primary loops with long vasa recta are shown. (B) About 7 feet from the duodenojejunal flexure, secondary vascular loops are present with "lunette" formation. (C) Ten to 12 feet from the duodenojejunal flexure, tertiary vascular loops are present, and increased mesenterial fat is seen. (D) In the terminal ileum the vascular arches and "lunettes" are obscured by fat.

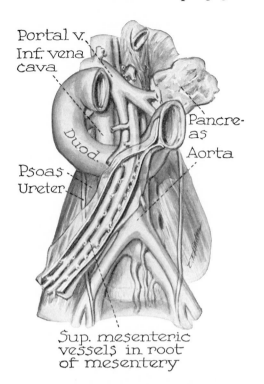

Portal v.
Inf. vena cava
Duod.
Pancreas
Aorta
Psoas
Ureter
Sup. mesenteric
vessels in root
of mesentery

FIG. 334. The root of the mesentery. In its oblique course downward the root of the mesentery crosses the third part of the duodenum, the abdominal aorta and the right psoas muscle.

connects the intestines to the posterior abdominal wall and conveys vessels and nerves to and from it is called a mesentery. The *mesentery proper* connects the coils of jejunoileum to the posterior abdominal wall below the line of attachment of the transverse mesocolon. Its *root* or radix (parietal attachment) extends from the left side of the 2nd lumbar vertebra downward and to the right to the right sacro-iliac joint, a distance of about 6 inches. In its oblique course downward and to the right the root of the mesentery crosses in front of the third part of the duodenum, the abdominal aorta and the right psoas muscle (Fig. 334). Although the root of the mesentery measures only 6 inches in length, it accommodates 20 feet of small bowel; this is accomplished by its folding and ruffling. The small intestine is so mobile and convoluted that the surgeon may explore many

feet without being able to determine whether he is progressing toward the duodenum or toward the ileum. By the simple procedure of placing a hand on each side of the mesentery and drawing the hands forward from the root to the intestinal border, the convolutions are untwisted, and the direction in which the gut is traveling becomes obvious. The first coil of jejunum and the last coil of ileum run parallel with each other despite the 20 intervening feet of jejuno-ileum. The first coil of jejunum passes downward and to the left, in front of the left kidney, and the last coil of ileum passes upward and to the right out of the pelvic cavity and across the external iliac vessels. The intestinal branches of the superior mesenteric vessels, the mesenteric lymph glands and vessels, and the fat lie between the 2 layers of the mesentery proper. Removal of a cyst or a solid tumor of the mesentery endangers the blood supply to the intestine.

In traversing the inframesocolic compartment, the mesentery converts it into 2 parts: the one to the right is smaller and terminates in the right iliac fossa; the other to the left is larger and passes into the true pelvis.

Arteries. The *arteries* which supply the jejuno-ileum arise from the left side of the *superior mesenteric artery* (Fig. 335). The latter arises behind the neck of the pancreas and passes in front of the uncinate process; in this way it reaches the third part of the duodenum in front of which it crosses and enters the root of the mesentery. It continues downward into the root of the mesentery and passes in front of the inferior vena cava, the right psoas muscle and the right ureter; it ends by anastomosing with one of its own branches, the *ileocolic artery.*

Close to the origin of the superior mesenteric artery the *inferior pancreaticoduodenal artery* is given off. It divides into anterior and posterior branches which connect with similar branches of the *superior pancreaticoduodenal artery,* thus forming two arches, one in front of and the other behind the head of the pancreas (Fig. 330). Each arch supplies branches to the head of the pancreas and sends a row of straight vessels (vasa recta) to the second and the third parts of the duodenum. Between the two rows, the common bile duct descends. Therefore, these arches constitute the anastomosis which exists between the superior mesenteric artery and the celiac axis.

The *jejunal* and the *ileal arteries* constitute 12 or more branches which spread out from the left side of the superior mesenteric artery and pass between the layers of mesentery to reach the jejuno-ileum. They unite and form loops or arches from which the straight terminal branches (vasa recta) alternately pass to opposite sides of the jejunum and the ileum. In the intestinal wall the vessels run parallel with the circular muscle coat, traversing the serous, muscle and submucous layers successively. The vasa recta do not anastomose themselves but pass to the submucous plexus where their ramifications anastomose freely. They are believed to be end-arteries.

Veins. The *superior mesenteric vein* returns blood from the small intestines and the ascending and the transverse colon. Behind the neck of the pancreas this vein unites with the splenic vein to form the portal vein (Fig. 362).

Lymphatics. The lymphatics of the jejuno-ileum drain into the superior mesenteric glands within the mesentery; here they are closely related to the arterial arches. These glands may be involved in mesenteric lymphadenitis, tuberculosis and other inflammatory as well as neoplastic conditions.

Nerves. The nerve supply to the small intestine is derived from the celiac plexus of the sympathetic system and from the vagus nerve. In small bowel lesions referred pain is experienced in areas of the 9th, 10th and the 11th thoracic nerves. Pain usually is about the umbilical region and may spread to the lumbar region and the back.

Meckel's Diverticulum

This outpouching resembles the finger of a rubber glove extending at right angles from the terminal ileum opposite its mesenteric attachment (Fig. 336). Such a diverticulum usually occurs within the terminal *two* feet of ileum, is usually *two* inches long, is pres-

ent in *two* per cent of all people and occurs *two* to one in favor of males.

In the human embryo, the convexity of the umbilical loop of the primitive gut communicates with the yolk sac by the omphalo (vitello) intestinal duct. This duct normally becomes occluded and should disappear entirely; however, all or part of it may persist. If the duct remains completely patent, a congenital fecal fistula results at the umbilicus. The commonest anomaly of this duct is a blind diverticulum which is attached to the ileum; this has been described as a Meckel's diverticulum. As a rule, it has the same diameter as the gut from which it arises; its end may be free or attached to the umbilicus by a fibrous cord. The vessel which accompanies such a diverticulum is the terminal part of the superior mesenteric artery; therefore, a Meckel's diverticulum has an artery of its own. It is important to remember that such diverticula may have ectopic pancreatic or gastric tissue contained within. These islands of digestive tissue appear at two sites, namely, at the blind end of the diverticulum or at its base where it attaches to the ileum. Therefore, it is important that a wide excision of the base or even a resection of the attached ileum be done. When a simple diverticulectomy is performed, the enzymes may be activated by the surgery, and the sutures (catgut) are digested; this may result in a fatal peritonitis.

SURGICAL CONSIDERATIONS

Open and Closed Anastomoses

Open Method of Small Bowel Anastomosis (Fig. 337). Removal of part of the small intestine (enterectomy) is done for tumors, trauma and gangrene of the bowel. Clamps are applied in such a way that the tissue to be removed is placed in crushing clamps, and the tissue which remains for the anastomosis is held by nontraumatizing clamps. Following removal of the mass, the intestinal clamps are placed side by side, and a posterior seroserous suture line, either interrupted or continuous, is placed (Fig. 337 B). A Maunsell mesenteric stitch is placed, and a traction suture is utilized on the antimesenteric borders of the bowel. The Maunsell stitch is important, since it protects the mesenteric triangle which is deficient of peritoneum and also ligates the vessels along the mesenteric border. Then a posterior layer of through-and-through sutures is placed (Fig. 337 C). This is followed by an anterior through-and-through suture (Fig. 337 D), the clamps are removed, and the anterior seroserous suture completes the anastomosis (Fig. 337 E). The rent in the mesentery is closed.

Closed "Aseptic" Method of Anastomosis. Four crushing clamps are placed on the

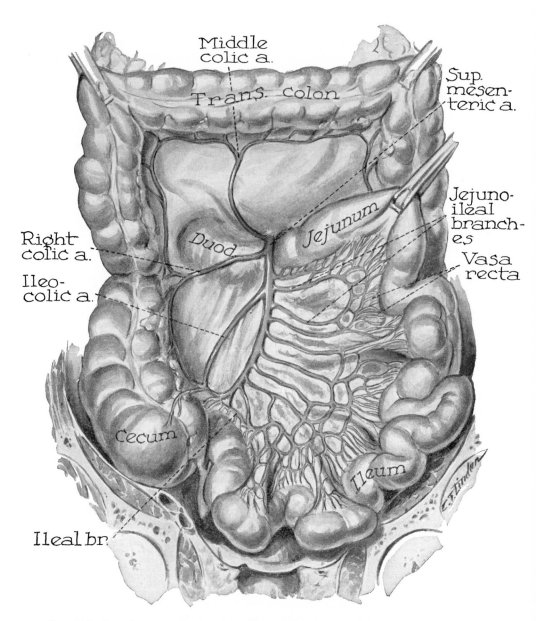

Fig. 335. Superior mesenteric artery. This vessel passes in front of the third part of the duodenum and supplies the distal part of the duodenum, the jejuno-ileum and the right half of the colon.

bowel, and the diseased mass is resected (Fig. 338). A continuous or interrupted suture method may be used; the former will be described. The suture starts on the side opposite the surgeon and passes at right angles to the clamp; following this, the suture passes parallel with the clamps and ends on the opposite side to which it started. The handles are reversed, and the same type of suture is placed again. The forceps are removed, and the sutures are tied. The lumen is opened by finger pressure to either side of the invaginated tissue. The operation is completed by a layer of interrupted or continuous seroserous sutures, and the margins of the mesentery are sutured.

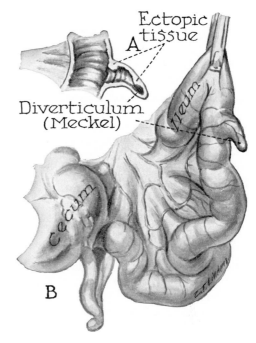

FIG. 336. Meckel's diverticulum: (A) view of the interior of the diverticulum with possible locations of ectopic gastric or pancreatic tissue, (B) external view.

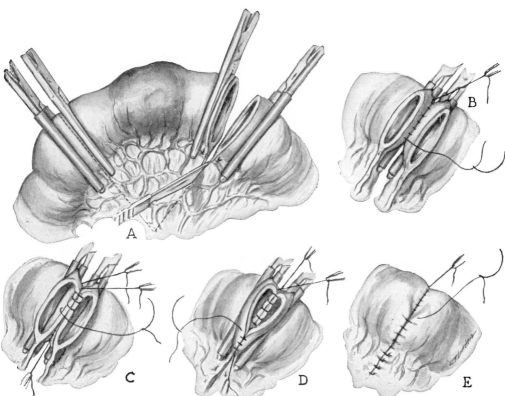

FIG. 337. Open method of small bowel anastomosis: (A) clamps placed and bowel resected, (B) posterior seroserous layer, (C) posterior through-and-through layer, (D) anterior through-and-through layer, (E) anterior seroserous layer.

In this operation an artificial fistulous opening is created between the lumen of the small bowel and the body surface. It may be temporary or permanent. If jejunum is used, the operation is known as a jejunostomy; if the ileum is used, it is called an ileostomy. Many methods and modifications have been described, but they all utilize the principles of opening the bowel, transfixing the tube and peritonizing with some method of invagination or tunneling.

LARGE INTESTINE (COLON)

EMBRYOLOGY

Following the stage of the formation of a distinct intestinal loop, a torsion takes place about the superior mesenteric artery (p. 393, Fig. 304). Following this primary torsion, the small intestine begins to lengthen so rapidly that the abdominal cavity cannot retain it; hence, a temporary but "normal" umbilical hernia results. By contrast, the large intestine and its associated mesentery grow relatively little at this period. In embryos of 10 weeks the abdominal cavity has increased sufficiently in size to permit the intestines to return. Probably because of the cecal swelling, the large intestine is the last to leave the umbilical cord and re-enter the abdominal cavity.

The cecum, the ascending colon and approximately half of the transverse colon are derived from the midgut, the remainder of the large bowel being derived from the hindgut. The cecum becomes fixed on the right side close to the crest of the ileum.

At this stage, however, the colon passes obliquely upward to the left of the stomach, where it curves sharply to form the splenic flexure and continues as the future descending colon.

As the liver decreases in relative size, a hepatic flexure appears in the originally oblique proximal colon; this flexure demarcates ascending from transverse colon.

Posterior peritoneal fixations of the colon

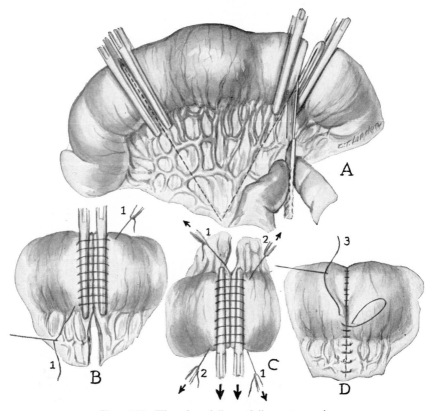

FIG. 338. The closed "aseptic" anastomosis.

take place so that the ascending mesocolon and the colon fuse with the right parietal peritoneum and the anterior surface of the descending duodenum and its mesentery; the descending colon fuses with the left parietal peritoneum (Figs. 339 and 340). The mesentery to the remainder of small bowel remains free and unfused (Fig. 332).

These various fusions may be complete or incomplete; they form surgical cleavage

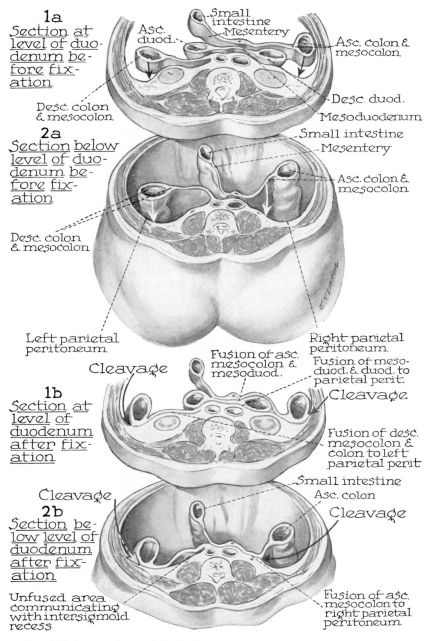

1a
Section at level of duodenum before fixation

Asc. duod.

Small intestine
Mesentery

Asc. colon & mesocolon

Desc. colon & mesocolon

Desc. duod.

Mesoduodenum

2a
Section below level of duodenum before fixation

Small intestine
Mesentery

Asc. colon & mesocolon

Desc. colon & mesocolon

Left parietal peritoneum

Cleavage

Right parietal peritoneum

Fusion of asc. mesocolon & mesoduod.

Fusion of meso-duod. & duod. to parietal perit.

Cleavage

1b
Section at level of duodenum after fixation

Fusion of desc. mesocolon & colon to left parietal perit.

Small intestine
Asc. colon

Cleavage

2b
Section below level of duodenum after fixation

Cleavage

Unfused area communicating with intersigmoid recess

Fusion of asc. mesocolon to right parietal peritoneum

Fig. 339. Embryology of the large bowel. Sections 1a and 2a are cross sections before posterior fixations have taken place. Sections 1b and 2b are corresponding cross sections after posterior fixations have taken place.

planes which permit proper bloodless mobilization of a given segment of bowel. The transverse colon and the mesocolon do not fuse with the posterior parietal peritoneum but hang suspended from the posterior abdominal wall and remain fixed at the two colic angles. The redundant sigmoid loop does not fuse with the left pelvic peritoneum. The upper boundary of the mesosigmoid is the retrosigmoid or intersigmoid recess (fossa), the depth of which depends on the inferior limit of fusion of the descending

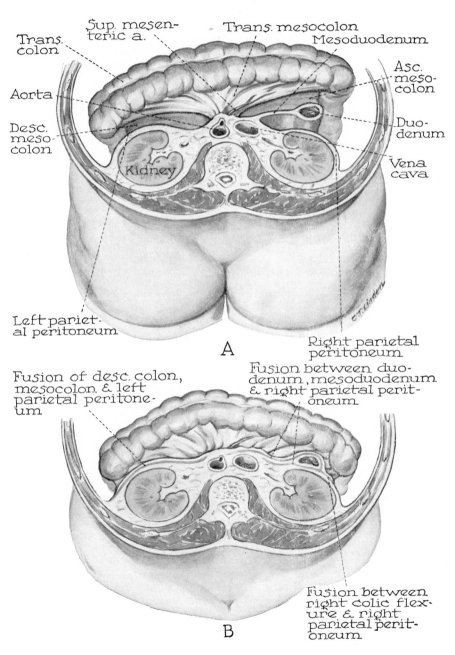

FIG. 340. Embryology of the large bowel: (A) before posterior fixation; (B) after posterior fixation.

mesocolon. Into this recess a loop of small bowel may herniate and strangulate (Fig. 352).

The rectum is the only part of the entire alimentary tube which maintains its primitive sagittal position; it has no mesentery.

LARGE INTESTINE PROPER

The differences between the small and the large intestines may be listed as follows:

1. The large bowel is sacculated; the small bowel is smooth.

2. The large bowel has *taeniae coli;* the small bowel has none. One of the taeniae lies along the line of the mesenteric attachment, and the other 2 are equidistant from it and from each other. All 3 converge on the cecum to the base of the vermiform appendix. These taeniae are explained by the fact that the outer longitudinal muscle of the large bowel does not form a complete coat as it does in the small intestine. It is arranged in 3 narrow longitudinal bands which are shorter than the gut itself, thereby causing a puckering and forming sacculations. If the taeniae are cut, the sacculated form is lost.

3. The large bowel has *appendices epiploicae;* the small bowel has none. These are little fatty tags which project from the serous coat of the large intestine. Those in the region of the appendix, the cecum and the rectum generally contain little fat; they may even be absent in these areas. Most of them are attached to the colon between its internal margin and the anterior taenia. In the iliac and the pelvic regions the appendices appear in two rows, one on each side of the anterior taenia.

4. The largest intestine has a greater caliber than the small bowel. The size of the colon diminishes from its cecal extremity, the diameter of which is usually 6 cm.; at the sigmoid colon, its narrowest part, the diameter is usually 2½ cm.

5. Internally, the large intestine has no aggregated lymph nodules, villi or circular folds, all of which are present in the small intestine. The mucous membrane of the large bowel is thrown into folds opposite the constrictions between its sacculations. These folds are not permanent as in the small bowel; hence, the former can be smoothed when the longitudinal muscle bands are cut.

The large bowel begins in the right iliac fossa as a blind head, called the cecum, to which the vermiform appendix is attached. The cecum continues upward into the ascending colon, which lies on the right half of the posterior wall of the abdomen. At the inferior surface of the liver, the ascending colon makes a sharp bend medially to form the right colic (hepatic) flexure, which lies on the anterior surface of the right kidney; it continues as the transverse colon. The latter crosses the abdomen transversely to the lower part of the spleen and on the front of the left kidney; it makes a sharp bend to form the left colic (splenic) flexure, which passes into the descending colon. This continues down the left side of the posterior abdominal wall to the iliac crest, then downward and medially in the left iliac fossa to end at the medial margin of the psoas major muscle as the pelvic (sigmoid) colon. This part of the colon hangs into the pelvis as a loop and ends at the middle of the middle piece of sacrum; it continues as the rectum. The primitive mesentery possessed by the large bowel in fetal life is retained by only two parts of the large intestine, namely, the transverse and the pelvic colons. The extent to which the ascending and the descending colons are surrounded by peritoneum is variable. They usually are surrounded on 3 sides and remain bare posteriorly. However, it may be completely surrounded by peritoneum but have no mesentery; finally, the mesentery may persist wholly or in part. Because of its usual method of fixation, the position of the large bowel is more constant than that of the small bowel. The large bowel is 5 or 6 feet long (one quarter that of the small bowel) and forms a 3-sided frame around the small gut, leaving the most inferior part open to communicate with the pelvis.

Because all parts of the colon are capable of greater distention than the small intestine, the adjective "large" has been used.

CECUM

The ileocecal region and the attached appendix form an important surgical and structural unit (Fig. 341). During early development the cecal segment forms a tube of uniform dimension. However, the lower part of the cecal segment lags in growth, while the upper part continues to increase with the rest of the colon. This difference in size becomes greater, and finally the lower tapering extremity becomes the vermiform appendix, and the larger part situated directly above it becomes the cecum (Fig. 342).

At birth, the cecum has a conical smooth external appearance, but by the 3rd year longitudinal bands or taeniae with sacculi between them are present. The sacculus between the anterior and the lateral bands develops more rapidly and out of proportion to the others. This large sacculus forms the most dependent part (fundus) and constitutes the greater part of the anterior wall of the cecum. The appendix is attached medially and posteriorly; it is not associated with this large cecal sacculus.

The cecum, or head of the colon, as it has sometimes been referred to, is a blind pouch which normally is found in the right iliac fossa. It is that portion of large intestine which is below the ileocecal valve and is usually 2½ inches long and 2½ inches wide. It has a more-or-less complete peritoneal in-

vestment, which accounts for its having a certain degree of mobility, but it is held in place because of its continuity with the ascending colon.

From its anterior surface the peritoneum is continuous upward over the ascending colon, but from the upper part of its posterior surface the peritoneum is reflected backward and downward over the iliac muscle, thereby forming a small cul-de-sac behind the cecum; this is known as the *retrocecal recess*. When such a recess or fossa is well developed, it frequently contains the vermiform appendix.

Posteriorly, the cecum rests on the iliopsoas muscle, the lateral cutaneous nerve of the thigh (femoral nerve) and very often the external iliac artery. When distended it is in contact with the greater omentum and the anterior abdominal wall, but when collapsed it is covered by a few coils of small intestine. The ileocecal orifice and valve are located internally in its upper half, and the opening of the vermiform appendix is in the posteromedial aspect (Fig. 341). The ileocecal valve is a shelflike projection of mucous

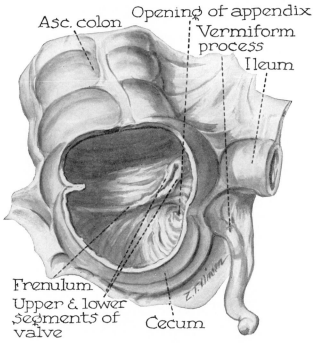

Fig. 341. Cecum. A window has been cut in the anterior cecal wall to show the valve and the opening of the appendix.

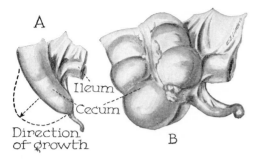

FIG. 342. Embryology of the cecum.

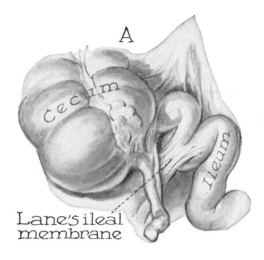

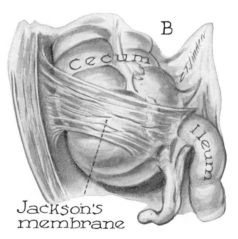

FIG. 343. Accessory peritoneal bands.

membrane where the wall of the ileum has become invaginated into the lumen of the cecum.

The cecum is not only the widest part of the large bowel, but it is also the thinnest. Because of this, almost all spontaneous perforations of the large intestine occur in this region.

The taeniae coli of the cecum are anterior, posterior and medial. They converge on the base of the vermiform appendix, for which they provide a complete longitudinal muscle coat.

The position of the cecum may vary. In its low position it may lie in the depth of the pelvis and in its high position, due to incomplete development of the colon, it may occupy a position below the liver and on the right kidney. In the fetus and the infant it lies high; this should be kept in mind when an incision is being contemplated for an appendectomy in children. It usually elongates and descends with advancing age and may be present in the sac of an inguinal hernia. Occasionally, the cecum and the colon retain their posterior fetal peritoneal connections and then are suspended from the posterior abdominal wall by a mesentery which permits a large range of mobility. This makes it possible for the ileocecal segment to become twisted (volvulus) and may also be an etiologic factor in the occurrence of intussusception. Appendices eplipoicae frequently are absent over this portion of the large intestine.

Membranes. Accessory peritoneal bands or membranes which are of surgical importance are found in this region (Fig. 343). Two in particular warrant mentioning: Lane's and Jackson's membranes.

Lane's ileal membrane is a thickening of parietal peritoneum in the region of the right iliac fossa. It extends from this fossa to the antimesenteric border of the last 2 or 3 inches of ileum. It was thought by Lane that a shortening of this band would produce a kink (Lane's kink) of the small gut; however, it is unusual to find any obstruction caused by it. Therefore, it may pull the ileum to the right and make locating the appendix more difficult. It is an avascular membrane and may be cut with impunity.

Jackson's membrane is a fold of peritoneum that is thin and transparent and extends from the posterior abdominal wall to the region of the ascending colon. It then continues downward and inward and attaches

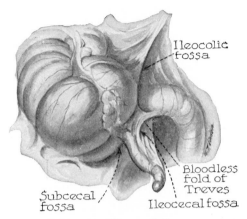

FIG. 344. The cecal fossae.

to the anterior longitudinal band of the ascending colon or cecum. A characteristic feature of this membrane is the presence of fine parallel vessels which are seen through it; they rarely, if ever, require ligation.

Fossae. The *cecal (pericecal) fossae* are pouches which are formed in the ileocecal region by peritoneal folds. They are of importance to the surgeon because the appendix may occupy any one of them; herniations into these fossae also have been recorded. The 3 main cecal fossae are the following (Fig. 344): (1) The ileocolic (superior ileocecal), (2) the ileocecal and (3) the subcecal (retrocecal).

The ileocolic or *superior ileocecal fossa* lies above the ileocolic junction and is formed by a peritoneal fold which passes across the ileocolic angle. It is bounded anteriorly by the ileocolic fold, which contains the *ileocolic artery* and *vein,* and posteriorly by the ascending colon; it opens toward the left.

The ileocecal fossa is formed by the so-called ileocecal or bloodless fold of *Treves.* This fold extends from the terminal ileum to the cecum and the mesentery of the appendix. The fossa is quite constant and large enough to admit 2 fingers. Deaver has noted that the depth of this fossa varies and at times may extend upward behind the ascending colon as far as the right kidney and the duodenum. If the appendix cannot be found, this fossa should be the first to be investigated. It is bounded anteriorly by the ileocecal fold; superiorly, by the posterior surface of the ileum and its mesentery; and posteriorly, by the mesentery of the appendix.

The subcecal (retrocecal) fossa is situated behind the cecum and at times extends behind the ascending colon. It is bounded anteriorly by the posterior surface of the cecum; posteriorly, by the iliac fossa, which is covered by parietal peritoneum—to the right by the peritoneum of the right colic gutter, and to the left by the mesentery. It has been the experience of the author to find the most common site for the appendix in this fossa.

VERMIFORM APPENDIX

Position. In fetal life the appendix opens into the apex of the cecum, but in the adult the opening is an inch below the ileocolic junction (Fig. 345). It may occupy any position, depending on its length and its mesentery. Wakeley, in 10,000 cases, found it either to be postcecal or retrocolic in 65.28 per cent of the cases. It has been the impression of the author that the vermiform appendix is found in a retrocecal position in at least 70 per cent of those cases seen at the operating table and in the cadaver. Although the relation of the base of the appendix to the cecum is quite constant, it may occupy one of many positions.

The so-called *paracolic position* is one in which the appendix is located on the outer side of the ascending colon.

In the *splenic position,* the appendix is entirely intraperitoneal but passes up in the direction of the spleen, either in front of or behind the terminal ileum.

The *promontoric position* is one in which the appendix is directed transversely inward toward the promontory of the sacrum.

At times the appendix is *pelvic;* it then hangs over the pelvic brim and is in the true pelvis.

It has also been described as assuming a *midinguinal position* when it passes down toward the middle of the inguinal ligament.

Length. The appendix is usually from 3 to 4 inches in length, but extremes varying from 1 to 9 inches have been recorded. It is entirely covered by peritoneum and has a mesentery (meso-appendix) which is derived from the left side of the mesentery proper.

Blood Supply. The *appendicular artery* is a branch of the ileocolic, which reaches the appendix along the mesentery; if the mesentery is incomplete, the artery lies on the wall of the appendix proper. It does not pass retrocecally but rather retro-ileally.

A large amount of lymphoid tissue is present in the appendix; hence its name the "abdominal tonsil"; this tissue diminishes with age.

Mesentery. The appendicular mesentery represents a triangular fold of peritoneum which is continuous with the lower or left layer of small bowel mesentery and reaches the appendix by passing downward behind the termination of the ileum. As a rule, the mesentery does not extend to the upper half of the appendix.

McBurney's Point. When inflamed and in its usual position, a point of tenderness known as McBurney's point is located at the junction of the middle and the outer thirds of a line joining the umbilicus and the anterior superior iliac spine.

Abscess. The site of an appendix determines the site of an abscess which may form as a result of appendicitis. When situated in front of the cecum, the abscess is walled off in front by coils of small intestine and omentum. An abscess behind the cecum may be intraperitoneal or extraperitoneal. In the latter case it ascends upward to the perinephric or even the subphrenic regions, usually causing some tenderness and edema in the loin. Such abscesses should be approached posteriorly, while those which are intraperitoneal should be approached along the outer side of the cecum (Fig. 346). When situated on the inner side of the cecum and in front of the mesentery of the small intestine, the abscess may be bounded again in front by the anterior abdominal wall; but when situated behind the mesentery, the peritoneal cavity must be transversed before such an abscess can be evacuated. A *pelvic abscess* is accompanied by rectal or vesical irritation, depend-

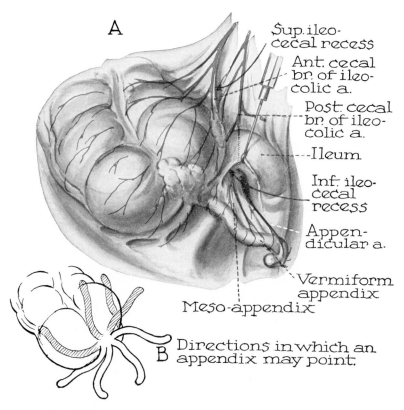

FIG. 345. The vermiform appendix and the ileocecal region. (A) The appendix is shown lying over the pelvic brim; this is not its most frequent position (see text). (B) Various positions in which the appendix may be found.

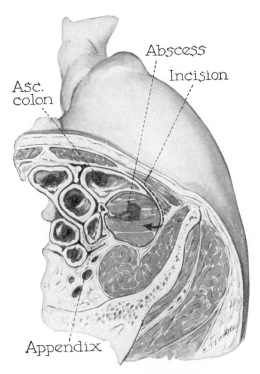

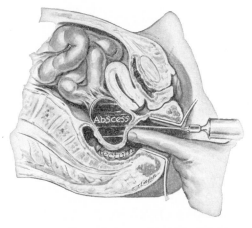

FIG. 347. Drainage of a pelvic abscess. An aspirating needle is placed through the anterior rectal wall, where the abscess points, and into the abscess. The bowel floats above the abscess and therefore is protected. An incision is placed where the pus is aspirated, and the abscess is drained.

FIG. 346. Extraperitoneal drainage of an appendiceal abscess. The incision is placed laterally, the peritoneum is peeled away from the abdominal wall, and the abscess is entered. In this way the peritoneal cavity is not soiled.

ing upon which of these two structures is involved. Such an abscess may discharge into the bladder, the cecum, the colon or the rectum. Abscesses in the pelvis may be evacuated vaginally or rectally (Fig. 347).

APPENDECTOMY

Since the appendix is a mobile part, and since it may be found almost anywhere in the abdomen, a variety of incisions have been described for its removal. However, this still remains a personal problem with the surgeon.

The appendix is located by first making upward traction on the cecum; the ileal fat pad is located and turned to the left (Fig. 348). This usually uncovers the appendix which, in most instances, is found retrocecally. If the appendix is not located after dislocating the cecum and the ileal fat pad, one assumes that it is retroperitoneal, and

mobilization of the cecum becomes necessary. This is accomplished by incising along the paracecal gutter and dislocating the cecum and the ascending colon to the patient's left. When the appendix is delivered, the meso-appendix is clamped and cut; the base of the appendix is ligated with or without clamping. The hemostats on the meso-appendix are replaced by ligatures; if a purse-string is used, this is placed now. A hemostat is placed above the ligated base, and the appendix is removed between this ligature and the clamp. There are many modifications of this procedure.

ASCENDING COLON

This part of the colon lies between the cecum and the right colic (hepatic) flexure. It varies in length, depending on the location of the cecum, its average length being between 5 and 8 inches. It is covered anteriorly, medially and laterally by peritoneum (Fig. 349); in exceptional cases an ascending mesocolon may be present.

Posteriorly, it is related to the iliacus muscle and its fascia, to the fascia covering

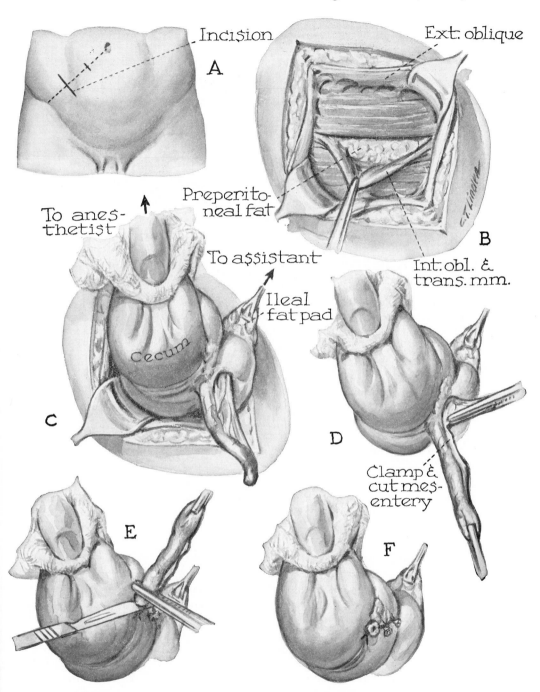

FIG. 348. Appendectomy: (A) McBurney incision; (B) the external oblique, the internal oblique and the transversus abdominis muscles have been incised in line with their fibers; (C) the appendix is located by displacing the cecum upward and the ileal fat pad to the left (assistant); (D) the meso-appendix is clamped and cut; (E) the appendix is amputated between the clamp and the ligature; (F) no inversion technic.

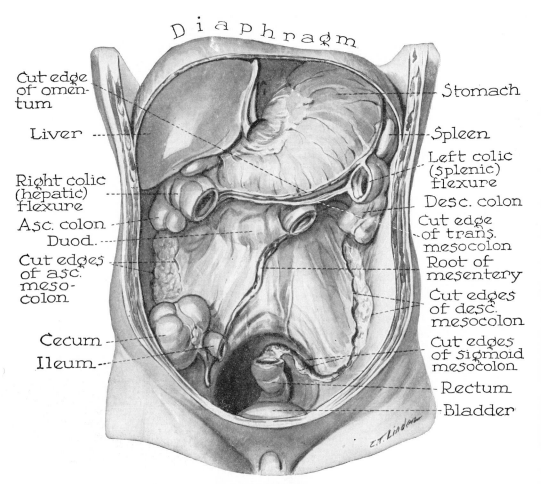

FIG. 349. The mesenteries and their attachments. The jejuno-ileum, the ascending, the transverse, the descending and the sigmoid colons have been removed.

the quadratus lumborum and to the lower part of the right kidney (Fig. 350).

Medially, it is related to the psoas muscle and the descending duodenum. To the right of the ascending colon is the so-called right paracolic gutter. If an ascending colon mesentery exists, it permits the bowel to fall away from the loin, thus dragging the cecum and the hepatic flexure with it. Though no symptoms may result, this at times may account for such conditions as duodenal ileus, cecal stasis, volvulus, ileocecal intussusception and movable right kidney. The ascending colon has to support and propel a column of liquid feces against gravity and to do this it should be firmly fixed to the posterior abdominal wall.

Anteriorly, the ascending colon is either in direct contact with the anterior abdominal wall or separated from it by the greater omentum and part of the small bowel. The ascending colon is very short, and it occupies only that space which exists between the iliac crest and the undersurface of the liver. Since it passes directly in front of the right kidney, an abscess of this kidney may discharge into this portion of bowel.

RIGHT COLIC (HEPATIC) FLEXURE

This is an angle or bend which forms at the junction of the ascending and the transverse colons. It lies in front of the right kidney and under the liver and the gallbladder (Fig. 349). It may form an obtuse or an acute angle but is not as sharp as the angle of the splenic flexure. Medial to it is the second part of the duodenum, and lateral to it is the edge of the liver or the lateral abdominal wall; above, it touches the liver; posteriorly, it lies on the right kidney. It is clothed with peritoneum except on its posterior surface. A peritoneal band from the lesser omentum sometimes passes downward to the flexure; it is called the *hepatocolic ligament*.

TRANSVERSE COLON

The transverse colon measures from 18 to 20 inches in length and is the longest section of the large intestine. It runs across the abdomen from right to left in front of the duodenum and the pancreas; above, it is in relation to the stomach; below, to the coils of the small intestine (Figs. 349 and 350). At its beginning, where the mesocolon is short or absent, it crosses the second part of the duodenum, but past this point the increased length of its mesentery allows a sagging of the colon over the small bowel. This sagging may be so marked that the transverse colon reaches the symphysis pubis. To the left, the mesentery is shortened again, and the colon is held close to the pancreatic tail, which it follows under the stomach and to the lower pole of the spleen.

The right side of the transverse colon is in close contact with the gallbladder and is commonly found to be bile-stained after death. In some cases, gallstones may ulcerate through the wall of the gallbladder and into the transverse colon (autocholecystotransversocolostomy). Hepatic abscesses may drain into the transverse colon. Since this

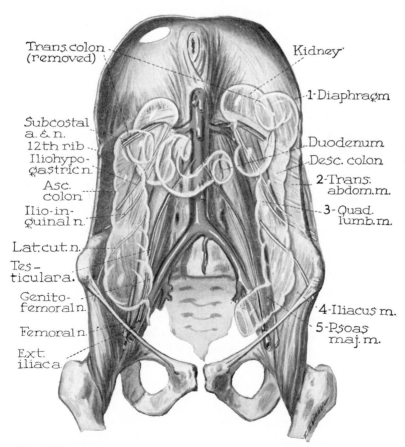

Fig. 350. Relations of the ascending, the transverse and the descending colons. The numerals indicate the 5 muscles over which the descending colon passes.

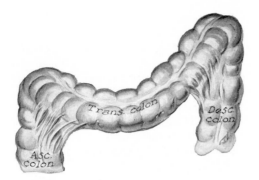

FIG. 351. The intercolic membranes.

part of the colon possesses a mesentery (transverse mesocolon), a wide range of movement is possible.

It is related anteriorly to the anterior 2 layers of the greater omentum and the anterior abdominal wall; posteriorly, it lies in contact with the second part of the duodenum and the head of the pancreas. In the rest of its extent it is separated from the posterior abdominal wall by coils of jejuno-ileum. The upper border of the transverse colon is separated from the greater curvature of the stomach by the lesser peritoneal sac and the anterior 2 layers of the greater omentum (Fig. 349).

The transverse mesocolon connects the transverse colon to the posterior abdominal wall. As it suspends the colon, it forms a horizontal partition which separates the cavity of the omental bursa and the supramesocolic structures from the inframesocolic compartment. In this way it acts as a barrier to infection between these areas. The posterior attachment of the transverse mesocolon extends to the anterior surface of the head, the neck and the body of the pancreas but may continue to the right and cross the anterior surface of the second part of the duodenum (Fig. 349).

The middle colic artery passes between the 2 layers of the transverse mesocolon; although it is called the "middle" colic artery, it should be noted that it passes well to the right (Fig. 358). To the left of this vessel is a wide area (avascular area of Riolan) which contains no blood vessels; when incised, it allows the fingers to be introduced into the lesser peritoneal cavity. The great variations in the position of the transverse

colon result in the formation of a "V"-shaped or "U"-shaped bend. Within the female pelvis a pendulous transverse colon may acquire adhesions which attach to the uterus, the ovaries and the fallopian tubes, thus causing a kink sufficient to produce an obstruction. Abnormally long transverse colons have been found not only in ventral and umbilical hernias but also in inguinal and femoral hernias. As the transverse colon passes from right to left it ascends; thus the splenic flexure is placed at a higher level than the hepatic. The transverse colon is covered on its posterior surface with the peritoneum of the general peritoneal cavity, but on its anterior surface it has acquired a covering of peritoneum of the omental bursa. Peritoneal bands may produce "normal" kinking of the transverse colon. Two such bands which are found most commonly associated with this part of the colon are the mesocolicojejunal membrane and the intercolic membrane.

The *mesocolicojejunal membrane* is a band which extends from the undersurface of the transverse mesocolon to the antimesenteric border of the first part of the jejunum.

The *intercolic membranes* are peritoneal folds which bind together the ascending colon and the proximal part of the transverse colon, and the descending colon and the distal part of the transverse colon (Fig. 351). If these intercolic membranes are present, they cause the so-called "double-barreled" colon and have been considered a cause of partial large bowel obstruction.

LEFT COLIC (SPLENIC) FLEXURE

This lies at a higher level and on a deeper plane than the right; it also forms a sharper bend (Figs. 349 and 350). It is limited above by the tail of the pancreas and the base of the spleen; it rests on the outer border of the left kidney, the diaphragm and the transversus muscle.

The *phrenicocolic ligament* is a fold of peritoneum which connects the splenic flexure to the diaphragm opposite the 10th or the 11th rib. It is bloodless and may be cut with impunity in mobilizing the splenic flexure or during splenectomy. This peritoneal fold aids in the fixation of the left colic flexure and also forms a floor upon which the spleen rests. The posterior surface of the splenic flexure is bare as a rule, but the entire flexure may be enclosed in peritoneum and then is connected with the end of the pancreas by a short fold of transverse mesocolon. Because of the situation and the fixation of this flexure its exposure and mobilization are more difficult than any other part of the large intestine.

DESCENDING COLON

This part of the large bowel includes what was formerly called the iliac colon; however, it is not considered as a separate part but rather an integral part of the descending colon. The latter and its associated iliac colon are 10 or 11 inches long and extend from the left colic flexure above to the pelvic inlet below. (Some authors still prefer to state that the descending colon ends at the iliac crest and that the portion below the iliac crest is known as the iliac colon.)

The descending colon is more deeply placed than the ascending colon; it rarely possesses a mesentery. It starts in an angle which is situated between the left kidney and the transversus abdominis muscle; it descends in front of the lateral border of this kidney and curves medially along its lower pole. It then passes vertically downward in front of the quadratus lumborum muscle, crosses the iliac crest and continues downward on the iliacus muscle, almost reaching the inguinal ligament. It turns medially across the left psoas muscle and becomes continuous with the pelvic colon in front of the external iliac artery. This colon separates the left infracolic compartment from the left paracolic gutter. The greater omentum and the coils of the jejuno-ileum intervene between it and the anterior and lateral abdominal walls. Medially, it is related to the left kidney and the psoas major muscle; posteriorly, it crosses 5 muscles (Fig. 350). They are, in succession: the diaphragm, the transversus abdominis, the quadratus lumborum, the iliacus and the psoas major.

A number of vessels and nerves separate the descending colon from some of these muscles. Thus the iliohypogastric and the ilio-inguinal nerves separate it from the quadratus lumborum; the lateral cutaneous nerve of the thigh and the iliac branches of the iliolumbar

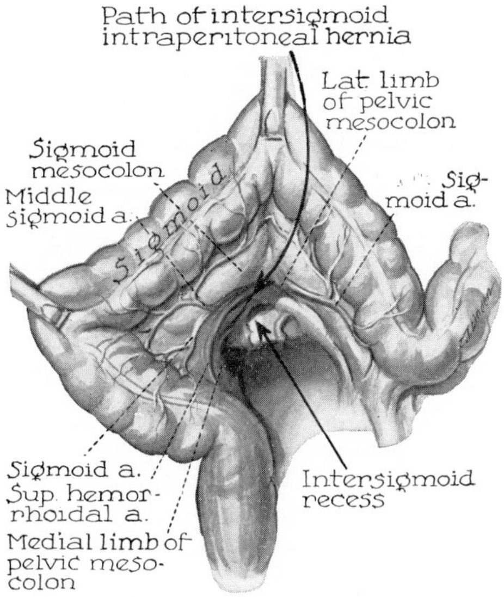

FIG. 352. The pelvic mesocolon. The attachment of this mesocolon is placed obliquely and forms an inverted "V." The intersigmoid recess and the path of an intraperitoneal hernia are identified by arrows.

vessels separate it from the iliacus; the femoral nerve, from the iliacus and psoas; and the external iliac vessels, from the psoas. The testicular (ovarian) vessels and the branches of the genitofemoral nerve are in close relation to the external iliac artery. Although it is stated that the nerves lie between the muscles and the descending colon, this is not correct, because the nerves lie beneath the fascia which covers the muscles. Therefore, the iliohypogastric and the ilio-inguinal nerves are separated from the colon by the fascia covering the quadratus lumborum and the lateral cutaneous nerve of the thigh, and the femoral nerve is separated from the bowel by the iliac fascia; this fascia must be incised before the nerves can be demonstrated.

PELVIC (SIGMOID) COLON

The external iliac artery can be considered as the dividing line between the iliac and the pelvic colons, the latter commencing in front of the artery about 2 inches above the inguinal ligament (Fig. 358). The average length of this part of the colon is between 10 and 15 inches but may vary from 5 to 35 inches. It ends in the midline at the level of the 3rd sacral vertebra, where it becomes continuous with the rectum.

The differentiation between the sigmoid and the rectum is marked by the facts that: the diameter of the rectum is diminished, the peritoneum ceases to enclose the rectum, and the rectum has no appendices epiploicae.

In the pelvis, the colon is related to the urinary bladder anteriorly, to the sacrum posteriorly and to the terminal coils of ileum on its right side. It is suspended from the posterior wall of the pelvis by a mesentery which

is known as the *pelvic mesocolon*. Although this mesocolon varies with the length of the sigmoid, nevertheless, the attachment of its root is quite constant.

This obliquely placed mesocolon has an inverted V-shaped course (Fig. 352). Its line of attachment reveals the following: a lateral limb which extends along the iliac arteries from the middle of the external iliac artery to the middle of the left common iliac artery; the medial limb extends from the middle of the left common iliac to the middle of

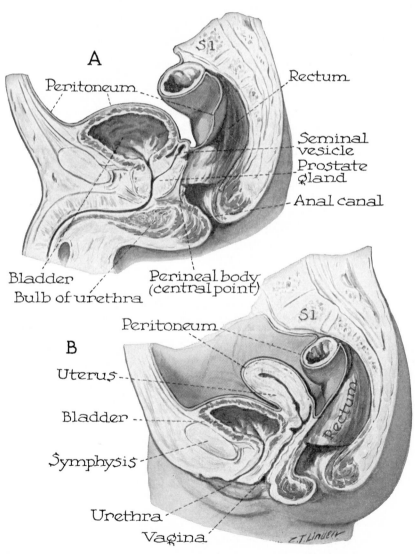

FIG. 353. The rectum and its peritoneal relations: (A) sagittal section of rectal relations in the male, (B) sagittal section of rectal relations in the female.

the third sacral vertebra. At the apex of this "V" there is a small peritoneal recess, the opening of which looks downward; it is known as the intersigmoid recess (fossa intersigmoidea). It may be deep or merely represented by a dimple; it acts as a guide

to the left ureter. If a finger is placed in this fossa, the ureter can be rolled on the underlying common iliac artery; if the peritoneum over it is divided, the left ureter is exposed. Internal herniations with strangulations of small bowel may take place into this fossa.

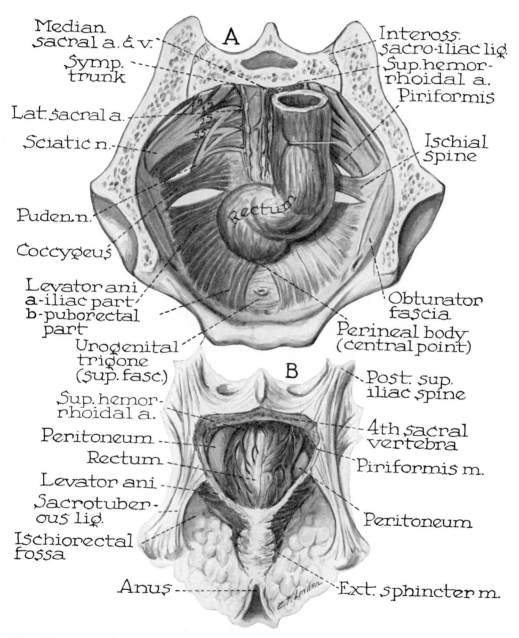

Median sacral a. & v.
Symp. trunk
Lat. sacral a.
Sciatic n.
Puden. n.
Coccygeus
Levator ani
a-iliac part
b-puborectal part
Urogenital trigone (sup. fasc.)
Sup. hemorrhoidal a.
Peritoneum
Rectum
Levator ani
Sacrotuberous lig.
Ischiorectal fossa
Anus

A

Inteross. sacro-iliac lig.
Sup. hemorrhoidal a.
Piriformis
Ischial Spine
Obturator fascia
Perineal body (central point)
Post. sup. iliac spine
4th sacral vertebra
Piriformis m.
Peritoneum
Ext. sphincter m.

B

Rectum

FIG. 354. Anterior and posterior relations of the rectum: (A) seen from above and in front; (B) seen from behind; part of the sacrum and the coccyx have been removed.

The superior hemorrhoidal artery runs downward and medially to the rectum in the medial limb of the pelvic mesocolon.

The length of the mesocolon determines the length, the location and the mobility of the pelvic colon proper; therefore, there is a wide variation. Usually, the pelvic colon is situated partly in the abdomen and partly in the pelvis. However, if the mesocolon is long, it may cross past the midline and appear in the right lower abdominal quadrant; it may be exposed in the course of an appendectomy. Such a mobile pelvic colon may twist upon itself, producing a volvulus.

The *mesosigmoid membrane* is a thickening and a shortening of the peritoneum of the left iliac fossa; it binds the junction of the iliac and the pelvic colons to the pelvic brim. This band has been referred to as Lane's first and last kink. The reason for this is that Lane thought this band was the first to appear but involved the last part of bowel. If present, it must be cut when this portion of the colon is to be mobilized; it is avascular.

Rectum

The rectum (Figs. 353 and 354) begins at the point where the colon ceases to have a mesentery; this usually occurs in front of the 3rd sacral vertebra. It not only loses its mesentery but also differs from the colon in that it is not sacculated, has no taeniae coli or appendices epiploicae. Its upper third is covered anteriorly and at the sides by peritoneum; the middle third is covered only anteriorly by peritoneum; and the lowest third is entirely devoid of peritoneum (Fig. 353). The rectum is about 5 inches long and occupies the posterior part of the pelvis. It follows the curve of the sacrum and the coccyx and ends 1 inch in front of the tip of the coccyx by bending sharply downward and backward into the anal canal.

It derives its name "rectum" from the fact that in lower animals this part of the intestinal tract is straight; however, the human rectum is not straight. It has an anteroposterior curve where it follows the concavity of the sacrum and the coccyx; it also has 3 lateral curves or flexures. The upper and the lower of these are concave toward the left, and the middle is concave toward the right.

Corresponding to the concavity of these flexures are the *valves of Houston*. These rectal valves appear as crescentric horizontal folds which arise transversely from the lateral aspects of the bowel; with the exception of the outer longitudinal muscular coat, all the coats of the rectum take part in their formation. Three such valves are usually present: the middle one is on the right side, and the superior and the inferior are on the left. Toward the lower portion of the rectum, the lumen expands to form the ampulla; therefore, the lumen of the rectum, is narrower at its upper and lower ends.

Relations. The rectum has the following relations (Fig. 354).

Posteriorly is the superior hemorrhoidal artery which is so intimately associated with it that the artery is removed with the rectum in cases of carcinoma involving this part. The sacrum, the coccyx and the anococcygeal body are also situated here, and the periformis, the coccygeus and the levator ani form a smooth curved bed in which the rectum is situated posterolaterally. The median sacral vessels lie between it and the sacrum and the coccyx. Separating the rectum from its muscular bed are the sympathetic trunk, the lower lateral sacral vessels and nerves and the coccygeal nerve.

Anteriorly, so long as it is covered by peritoneum, the rectum is related to the terminal part of the pelvic colon. Below the peritoneal reflection, however, it is related to the posterior surface of the bladder in the median plane and to the end of the vas deferens and the seminal vesicles on each side of this plane. The anterior wall of the rectal ampulla is related to the posterior surface of the prostate. It is separated from these structures by loose areolar tissue and the rectovesical fascia. In the female the only differences in the anterior relations are that the upper two thirds are related to intestines which separate the rectum from the uterus and the upper third of the vagina. The lower third of the rectum is directly related to the middle third of the vagina. On each side are the so-called *rectal stalks* (lateral or suspensory ligaments). These are situated in the lower two thirds and are condensations of areolar tissue around the middle hemorrhoidal artery and veins (Fig. 358). J. W. Smith is of the opinion that they are situated 1 inch above the levator and extend from the third piece of the sacrum to the rectal wall. This areolar tissue then has a backward as well as a lateral prolongation and contains the nervi erigentes (sacral 2nd and 3rd), as well as the middle hemorrhoidal vessels.

Blood Supply. Five arteries supply the rectum: the superior hemorrhoidal artery, which is a continuation of the inferior mesenteric; the 2 middle hemorrhoidals derived from the internal iliac; and the 2 inferior hemorrhoidals, which are branches of the internal pudendals.

The superior hemorrhoidal (rectal) artery is a continuation of the inferior mesenteric and begins at the middle of the left common iliac artery. It enters the root of the medial limb of the pelvic mesocolon and descends in it to the 3rd sacral vertebra. Here it divides into 2 diverging branches which pass downward, first on the back and then on the sides of the rectum. These divide into smaller branches which are disposed around the rectum; they pierce the muscular coat about its middle and descend in the submucosal to the anal canal.

The middle hemorrhoidal (rectal) arteries are small and inconstant branches of the internal iliac. They pass to the sides of the rectum and are enclosed within the condensations of the visceral pelvic fascia which forms the so-called rectal stalks or lateral ligaments of the rectum.

The inferior hemorrhoidal (rectal) artery arises on each side from the internal pudendal (pudic) artery, which is situated in Alcock's canal. It supplies the anal canal and the lower part of the rectum, chiefly its posterior part. The superior hemorrhoidal artery supplies the entire internal surface and the upper half of the external surface of the rectum, but the middle and the inferior hemorrhoidal arteries are confined chiefly to the external surface of the lower half. The middle sacral artery also contributes slightly to the blood supply of the posterior rectal wall.

ANAL CANAL

The anal canal represents the terminal portion of the large intestine and is about 1½ inches long. It runs downward and backward at right angles to the rectum, through the fascia and between the 2 levators into the perineum, where it opens on the exterior at the anus.

Relations. Anteriorly, in the male, the perineal body (central point of the perineum) separates it from the transverse perineal muscles, the membranous urethra and the bulb of the penis; in the female, it is separated from the lower third of the vagina.

Posteriorly, it is related to the anococcygeal body, a collection of dense fibrous tissue which is situated between the anal canal and the coccyx, and blends above with the median raphe of the levator ani.

On each side the puborectal (levator ani)

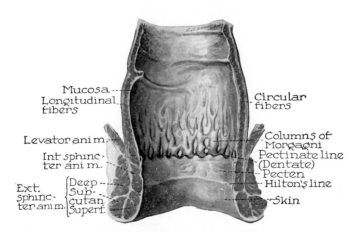

Mucosa
Longitudinal fibers
Levator ani m.
Int sphincter ani m.
Ext. sphincter ani m. {Deep, Sub-cutan, Superf.

Circular fibers
Columns of Morgagni
Pectinate line (Dentate)
Pecten
Hilton's line
Skin

FIG. 355. The anal canal. The pecten is situated between Hilton's line and the pectinate line. The 3 parts of the external sphincter ani muscle are identified.

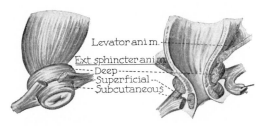

FIG. 356. The external sphincter muscle and its "three layers."

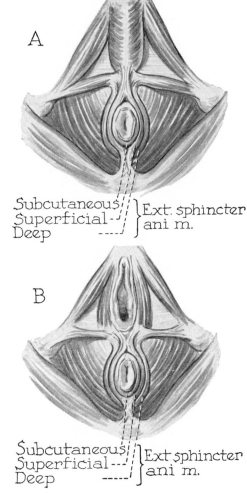

FIG. 357. The external sphincter ani muscle: (A) in the male; (B) in the female.

muscles separate the anal canal from the ischiorectal fossa.

Landmarks. A view of the anal canal through the anoscope presents 4 rather definite landmarks: (1) the anocutaneous line, (2) Hilton's line, (3) the pectinate line and (4) the anorectal line (Fig. 355).

The anocutaneous line also has been referred to as the anal verge. Normally, it is in a state of apposition, the epithelium surrounding it being thrown into folds by the involuntary action of a muscle which has been called the "corrugator of the anal skin."

Hilton's (intersphincteric) white line is really more blue in color than white and is more palpable than visible. It marks the sharp nonmuscular interval which exists between the internal and the external sphincters and feels like a depression. It lies halfway between the anal verge and the more superior pectinate line. Directly above Hilton's line is an area about one eighth to one third of an inch in width; Stroud has called this "the pecten." It has been given this name because, arising from its upper edge, there is a serrated margin that resembles the teeth of a comb. Miles has stressed the importance of this area because of the heavy deposits of fibrous tissue underlying it; he believes that it is necessary to cut this stenosing fibrous ring to cure anal fissures. It is an important anatomic landmark, since it is the line over which prolapsing masses of mucosa fall through the sphincteric region. Some authors believe that Hilton's white line is identical with the pecten.

The pectinate line also has been referred to as the dentate line; it is the upper border of the area just described as the pecten. It has received its name because of its comblike arrangement brought about by the anal papillae

which are continuous above with the columns of Morgagni. The bases of the anal papillae are connected by irregular folds which are known as anal valves. This arrangement forms small pockets between the vertical columns; these are known as the *crypts of Morgagni*.

The area which has been described as the pecten, or that area which exists between Hilton's line below and the pectinate line above, is an important surgical landmark. Pennington has stated that 85 per cent of all proctologic diseases occur in this area. There are structural as well as clinical differences which result at this line:

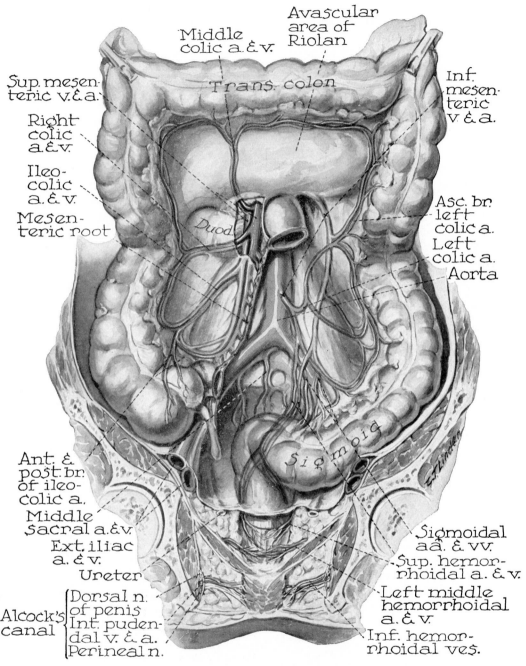

FIG. 358. Blood supply of the large bowel. The branching vessels which pass along the inner margin of the colon form the so-called marginal "artery" of Drummond.

1. Stratified squamous epithelium is found below this line, and above it is columnar epithelium. The line itself is said to be covered by transitional epithelium.

2. At this line the external sphincter replaces the internal.

3. The sympathetic and the cerebrospinal nerves meet here. The skin distal to the

line is supplied by the inferior hemorrhoidal nerve, which carries pain fibers, but the mucous membrane proximal to the line is supplied by sympathetic fibers which do not contain pain fibers. Therefore, any anorectal condition which is associated with pain must be situated below the pecten. For this reason a carcinoma of the rectum is "silent," but a fissure-in-ano produces severe pain.

4. Internal hemorrhoids occur above this line, and external hemorrhoids occur below it.

5. The line divides the lymphatic drainage. The intestine above the line drains into the pelvic lymph glands (sacral and hypogastric), but the rectum below it drains into the superficial inguinal glands by lymphatics which pass around the inner side of the root of the thigh. This explains the reason that lesions below the pecten may be associated with inguinal lymphadenopathy, but lesions above this line do not show such adenopathy.

6. The pecten marks the dividing line between the superior and the inferior hemorrhoidal vessels (p. 462). Therefore, the small veins in the submucosa of the pecten communicate the portal with the systemic circulation at this point (portacaval communication).

7. Focal infections take place at this line because this is the location of the crypts of Morgagni; hence, cryptitis, papillitis and fistulae-in-ano are located here.

8. Developmental defects may be found here. Since the anal canal is formed by a fusion of an ingrowth of skin from below, known as the proctodeum, and a downgrowth of hindgut from above, the anal membrane which forms a partition between these two is located at the pecten. The septum disappears, as a rule, leaving only the dentate line, but should it remain intact, the membrane then is visible and separates the hindgut from the proctodeum.

The anorectal line should not be confused with the anocutaneous line. The anorectal line lies about 1½ cm. above the pectinate line. The anorectal junction lies 1½ inches above the anocutaneous line when the canal is empty. It can be identified when the posterior wall appears while withdrawing the proctoscope.

Sphincters. The anal sphincters are 2 in number, namely, the external and the internal sphincters ani (Figs. 355-357).

The internal sphincter is the lower, thickened portion of the circular muscle of the bowel; it is about 1 inch long and can be felt on digital examination. It encloses the upper two thirds of the canal. The *external sphincter* is a subcutaneous muscle which is mainly placed superficial to the internal sphincter. The fibers of this muscle are arranged in 3 layers: subcutaneous, superficial and deep. The subcutaneous fibers are without bony attachment; they surround the anal orifice, and some decussate anteriorly. This part bears the same relation to the anal canal as does the internal sphincter. Its upper edge is separated from the lower edge of the internal sphincter by the intersphincteric groove The superficial fibers arise from the anococcygeal body, pass around the sides of the anus and are inserted into the perineal body (central point of the perineum). These fibers lie lateral to the subcutaneous portion and, therefore, are less in direct contact with the anal canal. Instead of being flattened and tubelike, it is broad horizontally to the plane of the skin. The deep fibers resemble the subcutaneous layer in that they have no direct bony attachment but encircle the lower half of the anal canal and form a true sphincteric muscle. This deep layer is intimately associated with the puborectal portion of the levator ani. The external sphincter is supplied by the perineal branch of the 4th sacral and also by the inferior hemorrhoidal nerves.

VASCULAR SUPPLY OF COLON, RECTUM AND ANAL CANAL

Arteries. The colon receives its blood from the superior and the inferior mesenteric arteries (Fig. 358).

The superior mesenteric artery supplies that part of the intestinal tract which extends from the second part of the duodenum to the right half of the transverse colon. The vessel crosses in front of the third part of the duodenum and then enters the mesentery proper. It passes between the head and the body of the pancreas and may be followed upward to the aorta, whence it arises. Since the body of the pancreas is associated with the transverse mesocolon anteriorly and the splenic vein posteriorly, the superior mesenteric artery has 3 anterior relations, namely, the transverse mesocolon, the pancreas and the splenic vein; the left renal vein is posterior to it and, therefore, is clamped between the artery and the aorta.

The superior mesenteric artery passes downward and to the right, where it ends by forming an arch with one of its own branches (the ileal branch of the ileocolic artery). Throughout its course it is surrounded by the superior mesenteric plexus of sympathetic nerves from the celiac plexus. It is accompanied by its vein which lies to its right side, either in front of the right colic and the ileocolic branches or behind them. As it descends in the mesentery, it passes the following structures, from left to right: the third part of the duodenum, the aorta, the inferior vena cava, the right ureter and the testicular (or ovarian) vessels.

The branches of the superior mesenteric artery are numerous and are accompanied by veins. The jejuno-ileal branches arise from its convex border, and the usual 3 colic branches arise from its concave right border. The colic branches, from above downward, are: the middle colic, the right colic and the ileocolic. Although the inferior pancreatico-duodenalis is not a colic branch, nevertheless it arises from the right side of the vessel. Many variations of the above arrangement are possible; these must be kept in mind during surgery of the colon.

The middle colic artery arises below the pancreas, enters the transverse mesocolon and passes downward, forward and to the right; it is the first branch of the superior mesenteric artery. It divides into left and right branches. The left branch anastomoses near the splenic end of the transverse colon with the left colic artery; the right branch anastomoses on the inner side of the ascending colon with the right colic artery. Since the middle colic artery lies in the transverse mesocolon, it is situated posterior to the stomach; therefore, it is in danger of being caught when the right gastro-epiploic vessels are clamped, since only 2 layers of peritoneum separate the 2 vessels. The main trunk of the middle colic artery does not lie directly in the midline but rather to the right; hence, any surgical opening which is made through the transverse mesocolon should be made to the left of this vessel where the large so-called avascular area of Riolan is found. When the transverse colon and the greater omentum are pulled upward, the artery is seen to curve upward in the right half of the transverse mesocolon.

The right colic artery arises a little below the middle colic and passes to the right behind the peritoneum and on the posterior wall of the right infracolic compartment. It crosses in front of the inferior vena cava, the right testicular (or ovarian) vessels and the right ureter. On reaching the upper part of the ascending colon, it divides into a superior branch which anastomoses with the middle colic artery and an inferior branch which anastomoses with the ileocolic artery. At times it does not arise as an independent branch but springs from the ileocolic or from the middle colic artery. It supplies the ascending colon.

The ileocolic artery is the lowest branch which is given off from the concavity of the superior mesenteric artery. It supplies the last 6 inches of ileum, cecum, appendix and part of the ascending colon. As it descends subperitoneally it crosses the inferior vena cava, the ureter, the genitofemoral nerve and the testicular (or ovarian) vessels, which lie on the psoas fascia. It terminates by dividing into ascending and descending branches. The descending (ileocecal) branch divides into anterior and posterior cecal, appendicular and ileal branches. The anterior cecal branch runs in the superior ileocecal fold of peritoneum in front of the cecum and supplies this area; the posterior cecal branch supplies the posterior cecal surface. The ileal branch anastomoses in the mesentery with the end of the superior mesenteric artery, thus forming a single, or sometimes a double, tier of arches from which vasa recta pass to the last 6 inches of ileum.

The appendicular artery usually arises from the posterior cecal branch, descends behind the ileum and runs in the free border of the mesentery of the appendix (Fig. 345). Therefore, bleeding from the appendicular artery is retro-ileal and not retrocecal. The ascending branch of the ileocolic artery anastomoses with the right colic.

The inferior mesenteric artery supplies the descending and the sigmoid colons and the proximal part of the rectum. It does this by means of its left colic, sigmoid and superior hemorrhoidal branches. It arises from the front of the aorta about 1½ inches above its bifurcation. This origin is located approximately ¾ inch above the umbilicus and in front of the third lumbar vertebra. It is smaller than the superior mesenteric artery, has a more limited distribution and is surrounded by the inferior mesenteric plexus of nerves which is derived from the aortic plexus. Its veins lie to its lateral side but is not in close contact with it. (The 2 mesenteric arteries are situated between the 2 mesenteric veins.) As it passes downward it inclines somewhat to the left, lying on the aorta and the psoas fascia, then crosses the left common iliac artery and enters the pelvis as the superior hemorrhoidal (superior rectal) artery. As it descends it gives off the left colic, sigmoid and superior hemorrhoidal branches.

The left colic artery (Fig. 359) arises about 1½ inches along the stem of the inferior mesenteric artery below the duodenum, passes subperitoneally to the left and crosses the testicular vessels, the ureter and the inferior mesenteric vein. It divides into ascending and descending branches.

The sigmoid artery also has been referred to as the inferior (lower) left colic artery. The sigmoid branches are usually 3 or 4 in number and supply the descending and the pelvic colons. As they pass to the left side

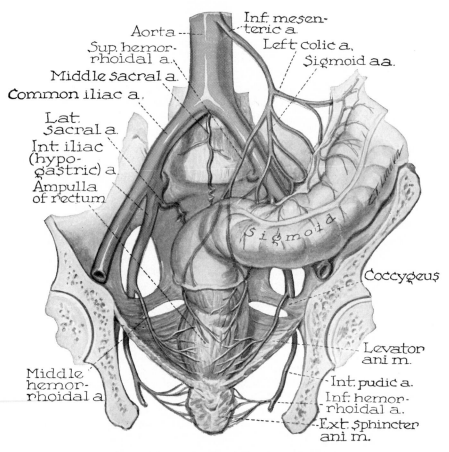

Fig. 359. Arterial blood supply of the sigmoid and the rectum.

they divide and anastomose with each other. The lowest sigmoidal branch is connected to the superior hemorrhoidal vessel by a very small branch.

Because of this supposed weak link, there was thought to be little or no anastomotic connection between the superior hemorrhoidal and the sigmoidal vessels. This "weak spot" has been called the "critical point of Sudeck."

Formerly, it was believed that ligation of the superior hemorrhoidal artery below the origin of the lowest sigmoidal artery would produce a necrosis of the rectosigmoid and the upper part of the rectum. The "critical point of Sudeck" was discussed in connection with this. It was thought that the marginal artery, which runs parallel with the colon, ends abruptly in the region of the lower sigmoid and does not anastomose with the blood supply from below. Dixon is of the opinion that although this might appear to be true, it actually is not; hence, he definitely states that the superior hemorrhoidal artery can be ligated and even some of the marginal artery resected without damaging the blood supply to the remaining portion of the descending colon, the rectosigmoid or the rectum. He further states that all of the colon which lies below the brim of the true pelvis remains

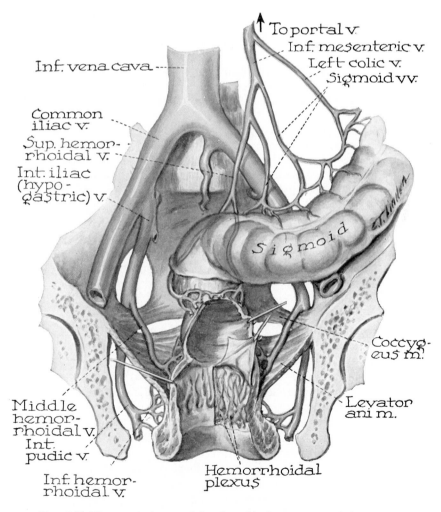

FIG. 360. Venous drainage of the sigmoid, the rectum and the anus.

viable without the superior hemorrhoidal or marginal arteries. Dixon is of the opinion that the distal part of the bowel is adequately supplied by the middle and the inferior hemorrhoidal arteries. Based on this, he has described a radical anterior resection of the lower part of the sigmoid colon and the rectosigmoid in which he re-establishes the continuity of the large bowel. In this way sphincteric action is preserved.

The inferior mesenteric artery continues beyond the origin of the lowest sigmoid artery as the *superior hemorrhoidal artery* (Fig. 359). The latter continues downward into the pelvis behind the rectum; it divides into right and left branches which subsequently anastomose with the middle and the inferior hemorrhoidal vessels in the submucous layer of the anal canal.

The so-called *marginal "artery" of Drummond* is formed from the vessels which supply the large intestines. These are the following: the end of the superior mesenteric and the adjacent branches of the ileocolic, the right colic, the middle colic. the upper left colic and the lower left colic (sigmoid). By anastomosing with each other, these vessels form an "artery" which passes along the margin of the large intestine and is known as the marginal "artery" of Drummond; it extends from the end of the ileum to the end of the pelvic colon. It is situated about a ½ inch from the margin of the large bowel, is closest to the descending and the pelvic colons and is capable of supplying the gut by means of its anastomoses even though one of the large feeding trunks may be ligated.

The *arteries* which supply the *rectum and the anal canal* are the superior, the middle and the inferior hemorrhoidals and the middle sacral arteries. These vessels form rich anastomoses around the anorectal region.

The superior hemorrhoidal artery is a direct continuation of the inferior mesenteric and is the largest and most important of the rectal vessels. After leaving the pelvic mesocolon, it reaches the posterior wall of the rectum, at the upper part of which it divides into 2 lateral branches; these enter the muscular coat and divide into numerous smaller branches. The latter anastomose freely with the inferior and the middle hemorrhoidal arteries and supply the entire length of the anal canal and the rectum.

The middle hemorrhoidal arteries arise, one on each side, from the anterior division of the internal iliac (hypogastric) artery. They reach the lateral surface of the rectum enclosed within the visceral pelvic fascia, thereby forming the lateral ligaments of the rectum (Fig. 359). They are distributed chiefly to the lower and the anterior parts of the rectum, and they also supply the base of the bladder and the upper part of the vagina.

The inferior hemorrhoidal arteries arise, one on each side, from the internal pudic (pudendal) arteries which travel in Alcock's canal (Fig. 358). They supply the anus and the lower part of the rectum, mainly at its posterior aspect.

The middle sacral artery arises from the abdominal aorta near its termination and continues downward in the median plane on the posterior surface of the rectum, which it supplies by means of a few small twigs. The superior hemorrhoidal artery supplies the entire internal surface and the upper half of the external surface of the rectum, and the middle and the inferior hemorrhoidal arteries supply the external surface of the lower half.

Veins. The rectal veins are arranged in a similar manner to the arteries but differ from those of the other divisions of the large bowel in that they form a *hemorrhoidal plexus* within the thickness of the bowel (Fig. 360). This plexus is developed best in the anal region; it begins inferiorly at the internal margin in a number of small veins which increase in size and number as they ascend. In the anal canal the plexus chiefly occupies the columns of Morgagni.

In the upper part of the rectum the venous trunks traverse the muscular layer and end exteriorly where they unite to form *the superior hemorrhoidal vein*. This vein drains into the inferior mesenteric vein and finally into the portal vein; hence, the greater part of blood from the rectum and the anal canal joins the portal circulation.

The middle hemorrhoidal vein chiefly drains the external surface of the rectum in its lower half. It accompanies the artery of the same name and terminates in the internal iliac vein.

The inferior hemorrhoidal vein drains the lower part of the anal canal and joins the internal pudic (pudendal) vein, which empties into the internal iliac vein.

Certain structural factors are important in the development of varicosities of these veins which are known as hemorrhoids. They are the absence of valves and the oblique passage of the veins through the muscular wall; since the greater part of the venous blood of the rectum returns to the portal circulation, any portal obstruction alters the return flow.

The superior mesenteric vein lies on the right side of its artery (Fig. 358). It begins at the lower end of the root of the mesentery, passes upward and to the left and receives tributaries which correspond to the branches of the superior mesenteric artery. The right gastro-epiploic vein from the greater curvature of the stomach also empties into it. It leaves the root of the mesentery, crosses in front of the third part of the duodenum and the uncinate process of the pancreas and terminates behind the neck of the pancreas by joining the splenic vein to form the portal vein.

The inferior mesenteric vein is a continuation of the superior rectal (hemorrhoidal); it passes upward on the posterior abdominal wall to the left side of the inferior mesenteric artery. It receives tributaries which correspond to the branches of the artery, then curves to the right above the duodenojejunal flexure, passes behind the body of the pancreas and joins the splenic vein. The branches of the lower and the upper left colic artery cross either in front or behind it (Fig. 361), but the testicular artery and the genitofemoral nerve always cross behind it.

The portal vein is formed behind the neck of the pancreas by the union of the superior and the inferior mesenteric veins and the splenic veins (Fig. 362). It passes upward and to the right behind the first part of the duodenum, and at the upper border of the duodenum it enters and ascends in the lesser omentum; it then divides into right and left branches. In its course it receives the left and the right gastric veins from the lesser curvature of the stomach, as well as the pancreaticoduodenal vein.

Although this pattern of the formation of the portal vein is described frequently, it

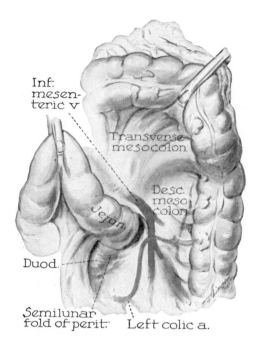

Inf. mesenteric v.

Transverse mesocolon

Jejun.

Desc. meso colon

Duod.

Semilunar fold of perit.   Left colic a.

FIG. 361. The upper end of the inferior mesenteric vein.

must be emphasized that many other patterns are possible (Fig. 363). Rousselot has emphasized the importance of such variations in the clinical behavior of patients suffering with congestive splenomegaly (Banti's syndrome).

The portal vein delivers to the liver blood which has circulated through the spleen, the pancreas and through the whole length of the alimentary tract from the lower end of the esophagus to the upper end of the anal canal. The *hepatic veins* carry blood from the liver to the inferior vena cava, which lies in a groove on the posterior aspect of that organ. When the liver becomes diseased, the portal vein may become obstructed, as in cirrhosis of the liver. Communications exist between the portal vein and the inferior vena cava (portacaval communications) (Figs. 362 and 364). These anastomoses exist but do not function unless obstruction to the portal vein, either in its intraperitoneal or intrahepatic course, is present. Such communications have been referred to as the accessory portal system, and are found at the following places.

1. *At the lower end of the esophagus* the esophageal branches of the left gastric veins (portal) anastomose with the esophageal

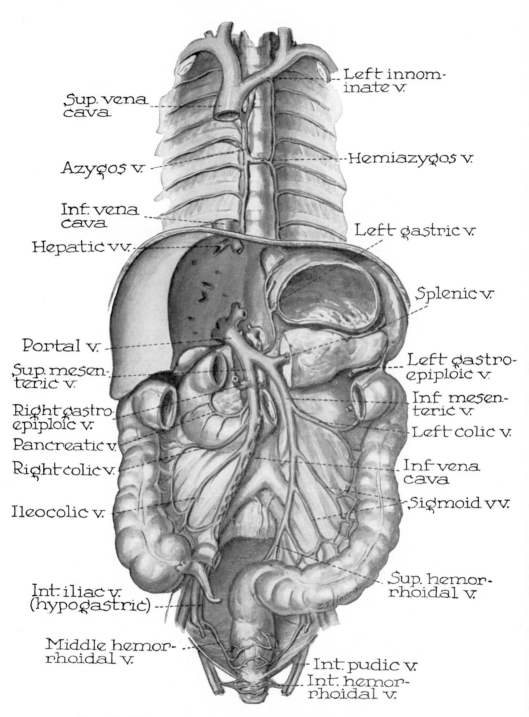

Sup. vena cava

Azygos v.

Inf. vena cava

Hepatic vv.

Portal v.

Sup. mesenteric v.

Right gastroepiploic v.

Pancreatic v.

Right colic v.

Ileocolic v.

Int. iliac v. (hypogastric)

Middle hemorrhoidal v.

Left innominate v.

Hemiazygos v.

Left gastric v.

Splenic v.

Left gastroepiploic v.

Inf. mesenteric v.

Left colic v.

Inf. vena cava

Sigmoid vv.

Sup. hemorrhoidal v.

Int. pudic v.

Int. hemorrhoidal v.

FIG. 362. The portal system of veins. The usual pattern of this system is presented; however, many variations are possible.

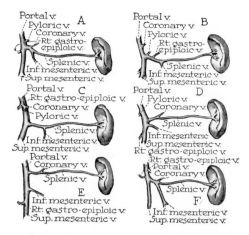

FIG. 363. Variations in the pattern of the portal system. These variations have been taken from some of the standard textbooks in anatomy.

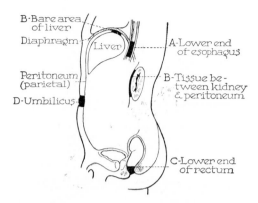

FIG. 364. Sites of anastomoses between the portal and the caval systems: (A) at the lower end of the esophagus; (B) at the bare area of the liver and the retroperitoneal structures; (C) at the lower end of the rectum; (D) at the umbilicus.

branches of the azygos veins (caval). In portal obstruction these esophageal veins may become varicosed and dilated and produce large varices which project into the esophageal mucosa. Since they are unsupported, they may rupture when the patient is in apparently good health; this results in an exsanguinating hemorrhage; they have been referred to as "esophageal piles."

2. *In the bare area of the liver* small veins, known as the veins of Retzius, unite the diaphragmatic veins (caval) with the hepatic veins (portal). To this group belong the retroperitoneal veins which lie about the abdominal viscera (liver, suprarenals, duodenum, pancreas, ascending and descending colons, etc.). They divert the blood into such caval veins as the lower intercostals, diaphragmatic, lumbar, epigastric and iliolumbar.

3. *At the lower end of the rectum* the superior hemorrhoidal (rectal) vein becomes the inferior mesenteric which drains into the portal vein. The inferior and the middle hemorrhoidal veins empty into the hypogastric (caval) vein. In obstructions of the portal system the veins in the rectum become dilated, and the blood passes into the caval channels. These dilated vessels form hemorrhoids (piles).

4. *Around the umbilicus,* veins passing along the falciform ligament to the umbilicus connect the veins of the liver (portal) with the epigastric veins around the umbilicus (caval). Enlargement of these veins produces the so-called caput Medusae.

Although connections exist between these two venous systems, they seldom suffice to produce a portal compensation when the portal system is obstructed. In an attempt

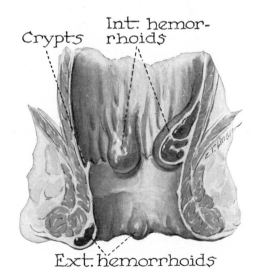

FIG. 365. Internal and external hemorrhoids.

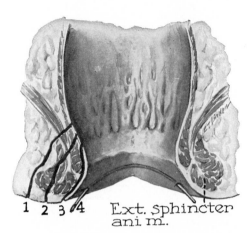

FIG. 366. Types of fistulae-in-ano. The fistula may burrow above, below or through the sphincter ani muscle. Number 4 represents the horseshoe type of fistula.

to communicate the portal and the caval systems, surgical procedures which result in portacaval and splenorenal shunts are now being done. At present the results of these operations are quite encouraging.

RECTAL SURGERY

HEMORRHOIDECTOMY

Hemorrhoids or piles are varicosities of the hemorrhoidal veins. Internal hemorrhoids, or varices of the superior and the middle hemorrhoidal veins, are covered by mucous membrane and are above the pectinate line. External hemorrhoids are dilatations of the inferior hemorrhoidal veins, are covered by skin and appear below the pectinate (dentate) line (Fig. 365). An external

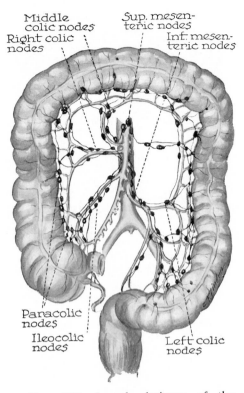

FIG. 367. Lymph drainage of the colon. These lymphatics mainly follow the course of the chief blood vessels. Most of the lymph drainage is to the group of glands located around the upper part of the superior mesenteric artery; from here the efferent vessels drain to the main intestinal lymph trunk.

pile is usually associated with each of the 3 primary internal hemorrhoids (3, 7 and 11 o'clock). Therefore, in doing a hemorrhoidectomy a hemostat is placed on the

FIG. 368. Extent of resection necessary in malignant lesions involving portions of the large bowel. (A) Carcinoma of the cecum or the ascending colon requires removal of the terminal 6 or 8 inches of the ileum, the cecum, the ascending colon and the transverse colon up to the middle colic artery. (B) Carcinoma of the transverse colon requires removal of enough bowel to incorporate from 3 to 4 inches of normal tissue to either side of the growth. (C) Carcinoma of the splenic flexure requires removal of the colon from the junction of the middle and the left thirds of the transverse colon to the middle of the descending colon. (D) Carcinoma of the descending colon requires resection similar to that used for splenic flexure carcinoma, plus the removal of the upper half of the pelvic colon. (E) Carcinoma of the pelvic colon requires removal of the middle of the descending colon to the region of the pelvirectal junction. (F) Carcinoma of the rectum requires removal of the bowel distal to the lower part of the sigmoid.

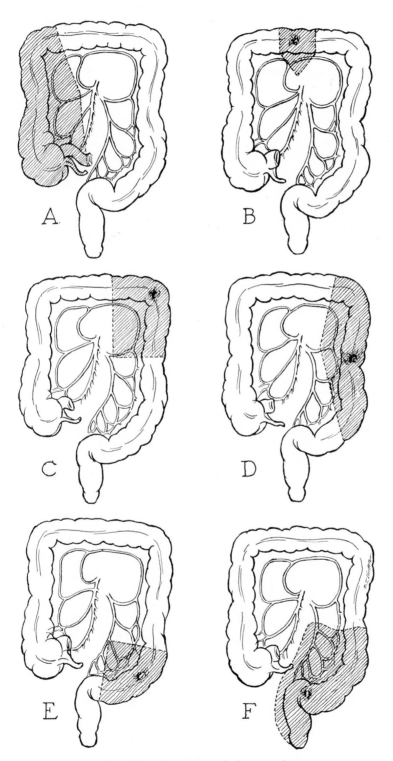

FIG. 368. (*Caption on facing page.*)

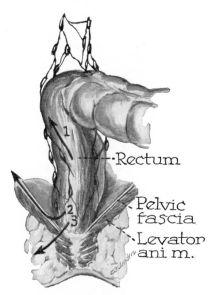

FIG. 369. Lymphatic drainage of the rectum. The arrows indicate the 3 zones of lymphatic spread. Zone 1 travels upward; Zone 2 laterad, between the pelvic fascia and the levator ani muscle; Zone 3 spreads downward.

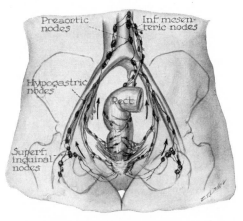

FIG. 370. Lymph drainage of the anal canal and the lower rectum. The arrows indicate the two main courses of lymph flow. Lymph from the lower part of the anal canal passes across the perineum to the superficial inguinal nodes. Lymph from the upper part of the anal canal passes upward to the inferior mesenteric nodes.

external hemorrhoid; this is elevated, and an incision is made in the skin. This dissection is carried to the mucocutaneous junction, and a clamp is placed on the entire internal pile. A suture is passed beneath the tip of the clamp and tied; this ligates the nutrient artery. The pile above the clamp is removed, and an over-and-over suture replaces the hemostat. The suture is made taut, and the 2 ends are tied together.

ISCHIORECTAL ABSCESS AND FISTULAS

Many authorities are of the opinion that an *ischiorectal abscess* and a *fistula-in-ano* result from an infected crypt of Morgagni. The infection may burrow above, below or through the sphincter ani muscle (Fig. 366). As a result of this burrowing, the ischiorectal fossa is reached, and here an ischiorectal abscess develops. This may open spontaneously or is opened surgically, but in either event a fistula-in-ano with its external opening results. The internal opening corresponds to the infected crypt. Successful treatment of such fistulas depends on the eradication of the internal opening as a primary focus of infection and removal of the fistulous tract. If the tract is subcutaneous, a fistulectomy can be done. However, if the tract lies deeper and has many ramifications, a wide excision with healing by secondary intention becomes the method of choice.

LYMPHATICS OF THE COLON

G. Gordon Taylor has remarked that the surgery of cancer is the surgery of the lymphatic system; therefore, a thorough understanding of the regional lymph drainage aids the surgeon when operative intervention is contemplated. In the case of the colon, the involved bowel should be resected well to either side of the malignant growth, together with the lymphatic channels which drain the affected parts (Fig. 367). Since the removal of the main artery to a segment of bowel may devitalize that portion of the intestine, it becomes necessary to resect a considerable length of colon. Therefore, typical lesions result in typical resection patterns (Fig. 368):

1. *Cancer of the cecum and the ascending colon.* The blood vessel which supplies this part of the colon is the ileocolic branch of the superior mesenteric artery; it supplies the

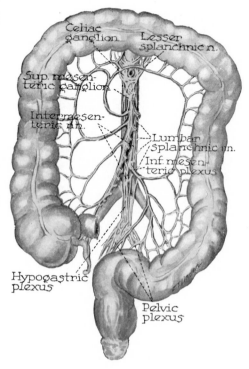

FIG. 371. Nerve supply of the large bowel.

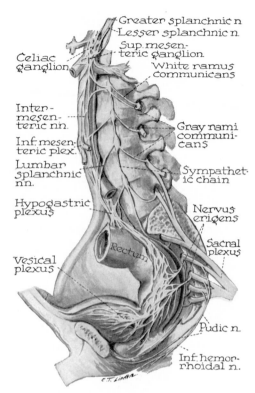

FIG. 372. Side view of the nerve supply to the lower part of the large bowel and to the anal canal.

last 6 to 8 inches of the ileum, the cecum, the ascending colon and the hepatic flexure. Therefore, in this resection it becomes necessary to remove the terminal 6 inches of ileum, the cecum, the ascending colon and the hepatic flexure, since these associated lymphatics should be included.

2. *Cancer of the hepatic flexure.* This flexure is supplied by the right colic and the middle colic arteries. As for cancer of the ascending colon and the cecum, the amount to be removed is essentially the same as that previously described, since the lymph drainage and the blood supply are the same.

3. *Cancer of the transverse colon.* This part of the large intestine is supplied by the middle colic branch of the superior mesenteric artery. It is necessary to remove from 3 to 4 inches to either side of the growth, thereby removing the lymph-draining area.

4. *Cancer of the splenic flexure.* The splenic flexure is supplied by the left colic branch of the inferior mesenteric artery. The area supplied by the left colic includes the colon from the junction of the middle and

the left thirds of the transverse colon to the middle of the descending colon; therefore, this area must be removed.

5. *Cancer of the descending colon.* This portion of the colon is supplied by the left colic and the upper sigmoid branch of the inferior mesenteric artery. Resection which is necessary here is the same as for the splenic flexure plus the upper half of the pelvic colon.

6. *Cancer of the iliac colon.* The iliac colon is supplied by the upper and the lower sigmoid arteries. Resection involves the removal of the lower half of the descending colon, the iliac colon and the upper half of the pelvic colon.

7. *Cancer of the pelvic colon.* This portion of the colon is supplied by the sigmoid and the superior hemorrhoidal branches of the inferior mesenteric artery. In carcinoma of this portion of the bowel it is desirable to resect the middle of the descending colon where the left colic area begins. The lower

extent of this resection naturally varies with the situation of the growth. If the growth is situated fairly high in the pelvic colon, the resection is accomplished near the pelvirectal junction with an anastomosis of the divided ends of bowel; however, if the lesion is low in the pelvic colon, the rectum also may require excision.

8. *Cancer of the rectum.* This part of the large bowel is involved in half of all cases of carcinoma of the colon. W. E. Miles has described 3 zones of lymphatic spread in carcinoma of the rectum: downward, lateral and upward (Fig. 369).

The downward spread involves the perineal skin, the ischiorectal fat and the external sphincter ani muscle. This set of lymph vessels constitutes the lowest of the 3 sets and is situated between the white line and the anal orifice.

The lateral spread of lymph vessels constitutes the middle zone, which is situated between the levator ani and the pelvic fascia. It includes the levator ani muscle, the sacral and the internal iliac glands, the base of the bladder and the seminal vesicles. In the female, the posterior vaginal wall, the cervix and the base of the broad ligaments also are involved. Occasionally, there is a lymph gland which is situated on the uterine artery where it crosses the ureter (Toirier's gland).

The upward flow of lymphatics involves the pelvic peritoneum, the pelvic mesocolon and the glands at the bifurcation of the left common iliac artery. These vessels follow the course of the superior hemorrhoidal arteries. Although the 3 systems drain in different directions, they communicate freely.

Lymph from the anal canal and the adjoining part of the rectum in general follows two courses (Fig. 370). The lymph vessels from the lower part of the anal canal pass downward and forward across the perineum and then travel along the vulva or the scrotum to the inner margin of the thigh and in this way reach the superficial inguinal lymph nodes. Lymph from the upper part of the anal canal and the rectum passes upward to the preaortic nodes, which are associated with the inferior mesenteric group of nodes. If this is kept in mind, it can be understood readily that involvement of the superficial inguinal glands could be associated only with

a lesion extremely far down in the terminal part of the anal canal.

Gilchrist and David found retrograde metastases to the level of 4 cm. below the primary lesion in 2 cases out of 22. However, in both of these cases the lymph nodes above the lesion were completely blocked with carcinomatous cells.

If a rectal lesion as well as its associated lymphatics is to be removed, the extent of the operation is great. It would be necessary to remove most of the pelvic colon and the mesocolon, the rectum, the anus, the surrounding skin, the fat of the ischiorectal fossae and the levator ani muscles.

NERVE SUPPLY OF THE COLON

The nerve supply to the large bowel is derived from the autonomic nervous system, except for the lower end of the anal canal, which is supplied by the inferior hemorrhoidal nerve (Figs. 371 and 372). Therefore, the colon has both sympathetic and parasympathetic fibers.

The sympathetic fibers are derived from the lower thoracic and the upper lumbar segments of the spinal cord. They reach the sympathetic chain via corresponding white rami communicantes. The thoracic fibers then proceed to the celiac plexus by way of the lesser splanchnic and possibly the lowest splanchnic nerves. From here they proceed to the superior mesenteric plexus by way of communicating nerves. The fibers which supply the cecum, the appendix, the ascending and the transverse colons originate in the superior mesenteric ganglia, from which nerves pass along the superior mesenteric artery to reach the bowel. Some of the other nerve fibers which leave the superior mesenteric ganglion join the intermesenteric nerves anterior to the aorta. The lumbar sympathetic nerves leave the sympathetic chain via the lumbar splanchnic nerves and join the intermesenteric nerves. The fibers to the descending colon, the sigmoid colon and the upper rectum originate in the inferior mesenteric plexus and follow the course of the inferior mesenteric artery to the bowel wall. The intermesenteric nerves pass downward, anterior to the bifurcation of the aorta, as the hypogastric plexus. This plexus divides into right and left pelvic plexuses, each lying to one side of the rectum; these fibers supply the bladder, the prostate, the pelvic organs and also form the so-called rectal plexus.

The parasympathetic fibers arise from both the vagus and the pelvic nerves; these are distributed to the large bowel with the sympathetic fibers. The nervi erigentes are the sacral autonomic nerves which arise from the 2nd, the 3rd and the 4th sacral nerves. They join the pelvic plexuses on each side and are distributed to the bowel with the sympathetic fibers. Some fibers follow the course of the left common iliac artery to the inferior mesenteric artery and are distributed to the descending colon and the sigmoid.

The pudendal nerve originates from the 2nd, the 3rd and the 4th sacral nerves; it accompanies the internal pudendal artery. It enters the perineum, runs in Alcock's canal and gives off the inferior hemorrhoidal nerve, which reaches the external sphincter and the lower cutaneous part of the anal canal.

LARGE BOWEL SURGERY

CECOSTOMY

A cecostomy may be performed either as an emergency procedure for large bowel obstruction or as an elective procedure preliminary to operations on the colon. The so-called "blind" type of cecostomy is a simple and efficient method for decompression. A modified McBurney incision is made close to the anterior superior iliac spine, and the cecum is identified and delivered. Two noncrushing clamps are placed on a longitudinal band, and a piece of gauze is placed between the cecum and the parietal peritoneum. The clamps are taped in place. At least 3 hours are permitted to elapse for walling-off, and then an incision is made between the clamps and into the cecum; a mushroom catheter is sewed into the cecal lumen.

COLOSTOMY

The Devine colostomy has been called a "defunctioning" operation because the contents of the proximal colon are prevented from entering the distal colon. Devine has resected successfully segments of the left half of the colon with primary suture of the sigmoid to a short rectal stump.

In performing a *loop colostomy,* the portion of bowel selected is brought out through the incision, and a small opening is made in its mesentery near the bowel wall. Through this opening a tape or a rubber tube is passed for traction. The peritoneum is closed beneath the loop with 2 or 3 sutures; the anterior fascia and the skin also are sutured beneath the loop in the same manner. The closure of the wound is completed with interrupted sutures placed above and below the loop. A glass rod or a rubber tube is placed beneath the loop to prevent retraction.

RESECTION OF THE COLON

In malignant diseases involving the right side of the colon, a segment should be removed which includes the terminal 6 or 8 inches of the ileum, the cecum, the ascending colon, the hepatic flexure and part of the transverse colon. Lesions which involve the colon in that part of bowel which is situated between the middle colic and the superior hemorrhoidal artery can be resected and anastomosed or exteriorized by means of the Mikulicz procedure. Lesions which involve the lower sigmoid, the rectosigmoid and the rectum usually require an abdominoperineal operation, but some (Dixon and Devine) prefer to remove the malignancy and attempt an anastomosis (Fig. 368).

Resection of the right side of the colon is done for lesions which involve the terminal ileum, the cecum, the ascending colon, the hepatic flexure and the proximal third of the transverse colon (Fig. 373). A long right rectus incision is made, the ascending colon is pulled toward the midline, and the posterior parietal peritoneum is incised along the lateral paracolic gutter; an avascular, retrocolic cleavage plane is entered. This mobilizes the right colon so that it hangs by its original mesentery. As the medial dissection is continued, the spermatic (ovarian) vessels first come into view, and then the ureter, which usually remains adherent to the peritoneum; the retroperitoneal portion of the duodenum must be separated from the mesentery of the upper part of the ascending colon (Fig. 373 B). The mesentery which holds the ileum, the ascending colon and that part of the transverse colon which is to be removed is then clamped, cut and

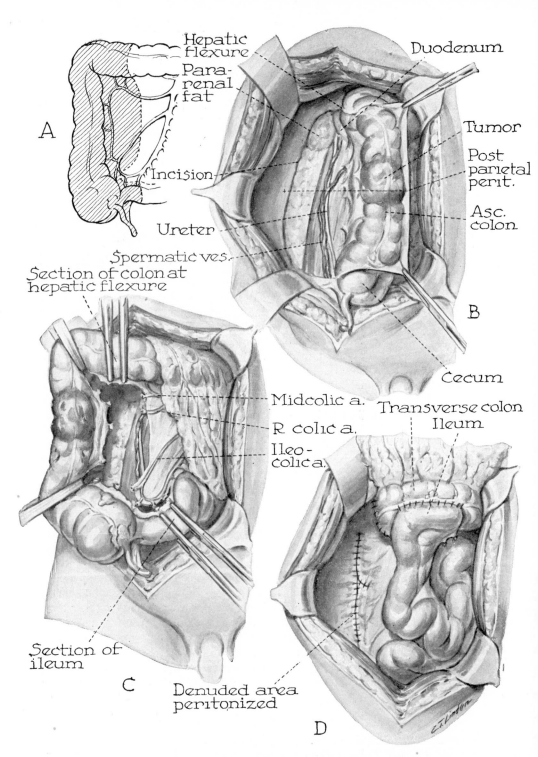

FIG. 373. Right hemicolectomy. This resection includes the last 6 to 8 inches of ileum and is usually done for malignant neoplasms. (A) The amount of tissue to be removed. (B) Mobilization of the ascending colon reveals the spermatic (ovarian) vessels, the ureter and the duodenum. (C) Clamps applied prior to the resection of the bowel. The major blood vessels have been divided and tied. (D) Lateral anastomosis between the terminal ileum and the transverse colon has been completed.

ligated; 2 clamps are placed on the ileum at the point where it is to be transected, and 2 more clamps are placed on the transverse colon at the point where it is to be removed. The bowel between these clamps is severed. The anastomosis is accomplished by closure of the blind ends of the ileum and the colon, followed by a lateral anastomosis; closure of only the end of the colon with an end-to-side ileotransverse colostomy is preferred by some.

Most neoplasms which are situated between the *middle colic* and the *superior hemorrhoidal arteries* and involve the transverse colon, the splenic flexure, the descending colon, the sigmoid and at times the rec-

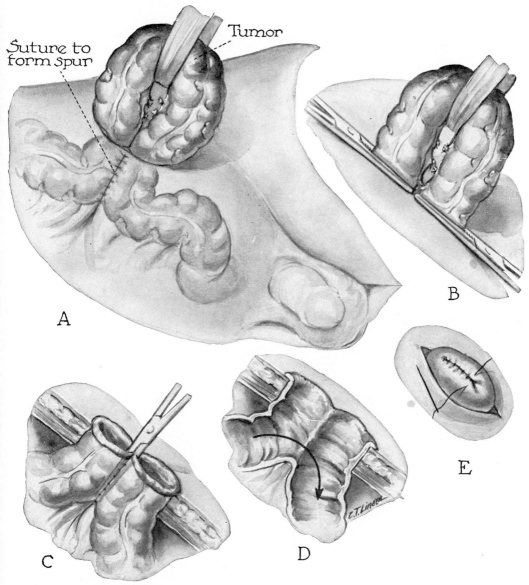

Fig. 374. The Mikulicz (exteriorization) procedure. (A) The involved bowel (sigmoid in this case) is mobilized and exteriorized. A spur has been formed by suturing together the bowel that is proximal and distal to the lesion. (B) The involved segment is removed. (C) The spur is crushed. (D) The resulting single-barreled colostomy. (E) Closure of the bowel.

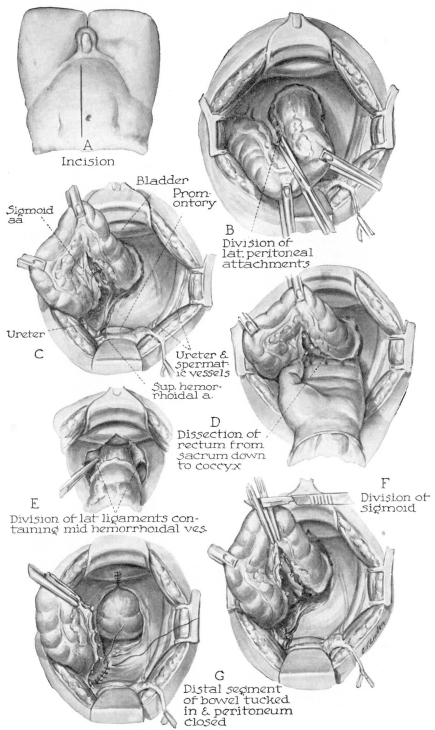

A
Incision

Sigmoid
aa

Bladder
Prom-
ontory

B
Division of
lat. peritoneal
attachments

Ureter

C

Ureter &
spermat-
ic vessels

Sup. hemor-
rhoidal a.

D
Dissection of
rectum from
sacrum down
to coccyx

E
Division of lat ligaments containing mid hemorrhoidal ves.

F
Division of
sigmoid

G
Distal segment
of bowel tucked
in & peritoneum
closed

FIG. 375. Abdominoperineal resection: (A) long, lower left rectus incision; (B) both right and left leaves of peritoneum have been divided and then joined in the midline; (C) isolation of ureters, spermatic vessels and superior hemorrhoidal artery; (D) the superior hemorrhoidal artery has been ligated and divided, and the rectum is freed posteriorly to the tip of the coccyx; (E) mobilization of the rectum from its lateral attachments; (F) the sigmoid is divided between clamps; (G) the distal end of the divided sigmoid is placed deep into the pelvis. The sutured peritoneum forms the new pelvic floor.

tosigmoid may be removed by the Mikulicz exteriorization procedure or by resection with primary anastomosis. Both open and closed anastomoses have their advocates.

MIKULICZ AND MILES PROCEDURES

Mikulicz Procedure. This involves exteriorization of the bowel; some surgeons believe this is safer than a primary anastomosis (Fig. 374). The involved segment of

bowel, with wide margins of normal tissue to either side of it, is brought out of the wound and is exteriorized. A spur is formed by suturing the afferent and the efferent loops of bowel together. The exteriorized bowel is removed, and at a later date the spur is crushed. The latter maneuver converts a double-barreled colostomy into a single-barreled colostomy. Some weeks later, this colostomy is closed, and the segment of

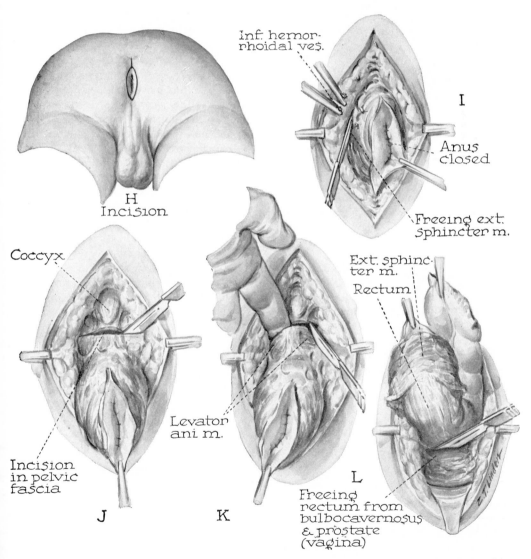

FIG. 376. Abdominoperineal resection (*Continued*): (H) circular incision around the anus; (I) dissection carried through the sphincter ani muscle; (J) the pelvic fascia is incised immediately below the tip of the coccyx; (K) the levator ani muscles on both sides are divided; (L) dissection is completed, and the involved segment is removed.

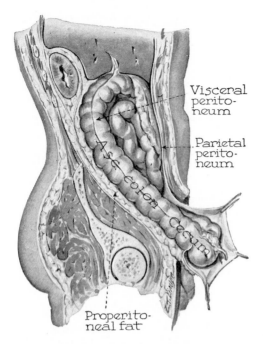

FIG. 377. A sliding hernia seen through a sagittal section on the right side. Both visceral and parietal peritoneum form the sac. The blood vessels are in the properitoneal fat layer.

bowel is replaced into the peritoneal cavity; in this way, bowel continuity is re-established.

Miles Procedure. Many operations have been devised for carcinoma of the rectosigmoid and the more distal lesions. A *one-stage abdominoperineal resection (Miles)* will be described (Figs. 375 and 376).

A lower left rectus incision is made; this is carried well above the level of the umbilicus. The posterior parietal peritoneum lateral to the sigmoid is divided, and the sigmoid, the mesosigmoid and the descending colon are mobilized. Once this cleavage plane is entered, the mesosigmoid is freed almost to the midline, and 3 structures are identified. From left to right they are: the left spermatic (ovarian) vessels, the left ureter and the superior hemorrhoidal vessels. At this stage the left ureter is in danger of being ligated when the superior hemorrhoidal vessels are tied; for this reason, the ureter should be identified and retracted.

Then the left colic artery, the first and the second sigmoidal arteries and the superior hemorrhoidal artery are isolated; a point of division which ensures viability to the remaining sigmoid is selected. The sigmoid is reflected to the left side, and the posterior parietal peritoneum is incised in a fashion similar to that used on the right side until this incision connects with the one made on the left. The right ureter is identified. A usual good guide for the level of ligation of the superior hemorrhoidal artery is the promontory of the sacrum; this permits preservation of the remaining sigmoidal blood supply. When the superior hemorrhoidal vessels have been divided, a cleavage plane is easily found between the posterior surface of the bowel and the sacrum. With the hand kept as close to the sacrum as possible, a loose areolar space is entered, and the rectum is freed as low as the tip of the coccyx; this mobilizes the rectum posteriorly.

Next the operation is directed toward freeing the rectum anteriorly. In the male, a cleavage plane is found between the prostate and the bowel; in the female, between the uterus and the bowel. This dissection is carried downward until the seminal vesicles are seen in the male or until the *tip* of the cervix can be felt in the female. With the bowel freed anteriorly and posteriorly, only its lateral attachments remain, namely, the so-called lateral or suspensory ligaments. These contain the middle hemorrhoidal vessels as they pass to the lateral bowel wall on each side. Some surgeons believe it unnecessary to ligate these vessels; however, it makes for cleaner and safer surgery to clamp, cut and place a ligature around them. Following these maneuvers, the bowel is detached completely from its anterior, posterior and lateral attachments. Once the bowel is freed completely, 2 clamps are placed on the sigmoid, and the bowel is divided between these. The proximal clamp remains on the permanent colostomy. The distal bowel is folded on itself and is turned down into the true pelvis so that it comes to lie in the hollow of the sacrum. The peritoneum is freed from the bladder, and a new pelvic floor is made by suturing this mobilized peritoneum. In the

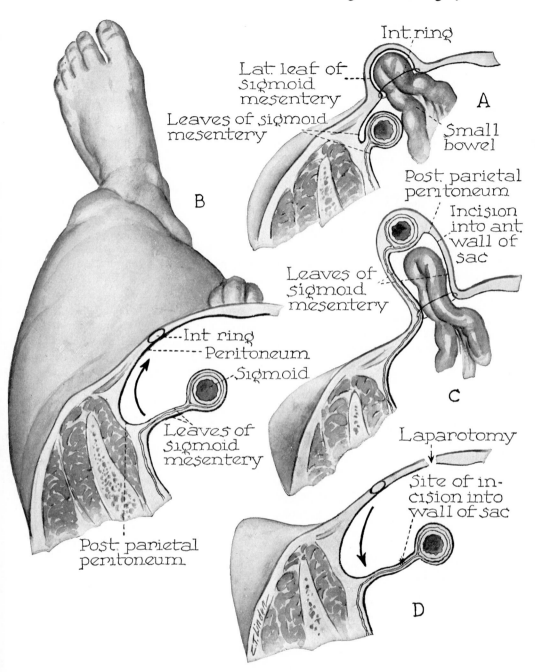

Lat. leaf of Sigmoid mesentery

Int. ring

Leaves of sigmoid mesentery

A

Small bowel

B

Post. parietal peritoneum

Incision into ant. wall of sac

Leaves of sigmoid mesentery

C

····Int. ring

········Peritoneum

····Sigmoid

Leaves of Sigmoid mesentery

Laparotomy

Site of incision into wall of sac

Post. parietal peritoneum

D

FIG. 378. Sliding hernia. (A) This figure is used for comparison to show the formation of a typical inguinal hernia sac. (B) The posterior parietal peritoneum lateral to the sigmoid will pass through the internal inguinal ring; this results in an unfolding of the peritoneal leaves which form the mesosigmoid. (C) On opening the peritoneum, one finds the colon occupying the apex of the sac. The continuity of the peritoneum is over the colon and continues along the posterior wall of the sac. (D) If a laparotomy is performed and the sigmoid is drawn into the peritoneal cavity, the opening which previously has been made in the "sac" becomes a defect in the lateral leaf of the mesosigmoid.

female, instead of dissecting the peritoneum off of the bladder, the uterus and the adnexae may be used as the anterior flap and the peritoneum as a posterior one. The wound is closed around the permanent colostomy. The patient is placed on his left side, back or abdomen for the perineal part of the operation.

An incision is made around the anus so that it passes over the sacrococcygeal joint and meets in the perineum (Fig. 376 H). This incision is deepened, and the inferior hemorrhoidal vessels are ligated. A transverse incision is made just below the tip of the coccyx, and the deep pelvic fascia (fascia propria) is identified and incised. This enters the presacral space which has been dissected previously. A finger is placed laterally so that the upper surface of the levator ani muscle is felt and divided at its posterior two thirds. The same is done on the opposite side. The entire distal bowel segment can then be withdrawn easily, the transverse perinei muscles are severed, and the anterior portion of the levators is divided. This leaves the bowel attached anteriorly for a short distance either to the muscles over the membranous urethra or the vagina. A cleavage plane is found, the bowel is removed, and all bleeding points are controlled. The wound may be drained or closed tightly.

SLIDING HERNIA

Sliding hernia has been defined as the extrusion of an organ (ascending, descending or sigmoid colons) in such a way that the visceral peritoneum forms part of the sac (Fig. 377). Therefore, attempts to isolate the sac as in indirect inguinal hernia are impossible. R. R. Graham is of the opinion that the formation of such a hernia is the result of a pushing mechanism which shoves the posterior parietal peritoneum lateral to the sigmoid so that it appears at the internal ring. As a result of this, the mesosigmoid unfolds, and the sigmoid comes to lie at the apex of the hernia (Fig. 378). The vessels then lie behind the colonic segment and are exposed to injury if they are mistaken for adhesions and if dissection is carried in this plane. If one attempts to separate such "adhesions," encroachment on the blood supply of the colon may result in devitalization of the bowel. Since complete reduction of the contents, high ligation of the sac and proper repair are impossible in this type of hernia, another method must be sought. Moschowitz suggested that the peritoneal cavity also be opened and the sigmoid be drawn back into it through the abdominal incision. It then is noted that the opening which has been made in the hernial sac through the inguinal incision is truly an incision in the anterior (lateral) layer of mesosigmoid. This defect is closed. Following this, no hernial sac is present. The abdominal wound is closed, and the inguinal canal is repaired by one of the routine methods.

Liver (Hepar)

EMBRYOLOGY

The hepatic diverticulum is the primordial outgrowth of cells destined to form the secretory tubules of the liver, its duct system and the gallbladder. It arises ventrally during the 4th week from the entodermal lining of the gut, and when it is first recognizable, it lies just caudad to the heart. A maze of anastomosing and branching cell cords grows ventrad and cephalad. The distal portions of these cords give rise to the secretory tubules of the liver, and their proximal portions form

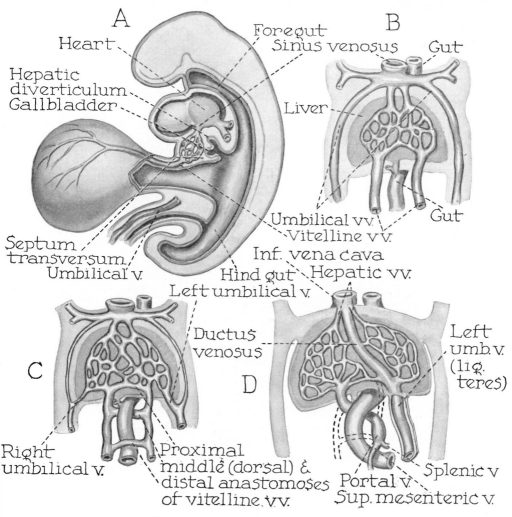

FIG. 379. The embryology of the liver.

479

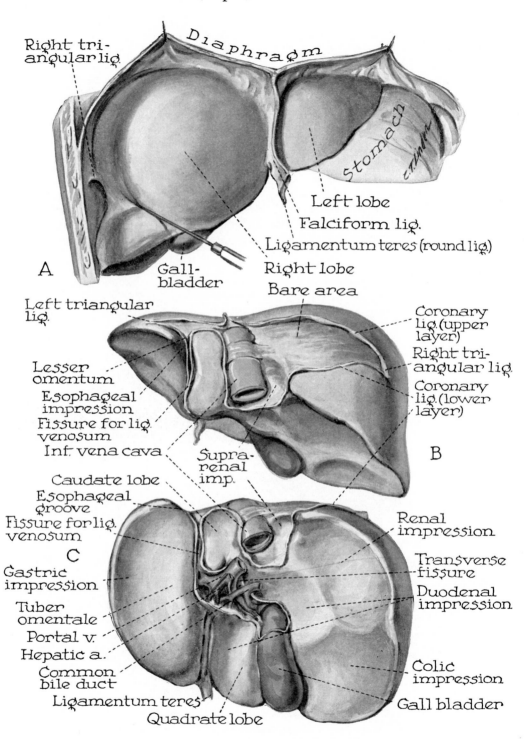

Right tri-
angular lig.

Diaphragm

Stomach

Left lobe

Falciform lig.

Ligamentum teres (round lig.)

Right lobe

Bare area

A

Gall-
bladder

Left triangular
lig.

Coronary
lig.(upper
layer)

Right tri-
angular lig.

Lesser
omentum

Esophageal
impression

Fissure for lig.
venosum

Inf. vena cava

Coronary
lig.(lower
layer)

Supra-
renal
imp.

B

Caudate lobe

Esophageal
groove

Fissure for lig.
venosum

C

Renal
impression

Gastric
impression

Transverse
fissure

Tuber
omentale

Duodenal
impression

Portal v.

Hepatic a.

Common
bile duct

Ligamentum teres

Quadrate lobe

Colic
impression

Gall bladder

FIG. 380. The liver: (A) seen from in front, the right lobe is pulled toward the midline
to place the right triangular ligament on a stretch; (B) seen from behind; (C) the inferior
surface.

the hepatic ducts. The growing hepatic tubules push between the 2 layers of splanchnic mesoderm which form the ventral mesentery and spread these 2 layers apart. The investing mesodermal layers form the fibrous connective tissue capsule of the liver and the interstitial connective tissue of the liver lobules.

At about the 3rd week the vitelline veins of the yolk sac pass through the septum transversum to the sinus venosus. The vitelline veins divide and intermingle with the liver cords to form an irregular mass of sinusoids. The terminal ends of these veins project out of the liver and enter the sinus venosus. A series of anastomoses take place between the vitelline veins. In the liver the 2 veins communicate ventral to the duodenum. Near the liver there is another anastomosis which is located dorsal to the duodenum, and below this there is a third which is again ventral to the duodenum (Fig. 379).

As a result of partial atrophy of the vitelline veins an "S"-shaped vessel results which passes around the gut and toward the liver. By this time the yolk sac and part of the vitelline veins atrophy. The remainder of these veins persists as the superior mesenteric vein; with the splenic vein it enters into one of the ventral anastomoses, thus forming the portal vein. The right vitelline vein distal to the anastomosis disappears.

The umbilical veins on their way to the sinus venosus contact the growing right and left lobes of the liver. The liver taps the blood from these veins which now mixes freely with the blood from the vitelline veins of the sinusoids. As a result of this the original connections of the umbilical veins to the sinus venosus atrophy. By the 6th week the right umbilical vein becomes smaller and gradually disappears. Therefore, placental blood is drained by only the left umbilical vein into the liver. Simultaneously, the opening of the sinus venosus is shifted to the right side. The large amount of blood entering the liver via the right umbilical vein takes a diagonal passage across the sinusoids and toward the right side of the sinus venosus. This new channel is known as the ductus venosus.

The part of the right vitelline vein which is situated between the liver and the sinus venosus becomes the main passageway of the veins entering the heart. It forms the terminal part of the inferior vena cava. The corresponding proximal part of the left vitelline vein disappears. After birth, the umbilical vein obliterates, and its remnant, the ligamentum teres, remains as a fibrous cord between the umbilicus and the liver. The ductus venosus becomes the solid ligamentum venosum.

THE LIVER PROPER

The liver is the largest gland in the body; it is extremely vascular and has many functions to perform (Fig. 380). It receives its arterial blood supply from the hepatic artery, and the portal vein conveys blood to it from the intestinal tract. The blood of the liver is drained by the hepatic veins, which open into the inferior vena cava.

This organ resembles the shape of a pyramid, the base being to the right and the apex to the left; the sides of the pyramid are formed by the superior, the inferior, the anterior and the posterior surfaces. In the adult it constitutes approximately 1/50th of the body weight; it occupies the uppermost part of the abdomen, chiefly on the right side. The organ is in close relation with the diaphragm and is covered by the ribs, which afford it some protection.

At birth the liver is relatively larger. This is especially true of the left lobe; the prominent bulging of an infant's abdomen is mainly due to the large size of the gland.

The falciform ligament of the liver is a wide fold of peritoneum which lies obliquely between the liver and the anterior abdominal wall. The right surface of this ligament is in close contact with the abdominal wall, and the left surface is in contact with the liver. The ligament has 3 borders: an upper border which is attached to the diaphragm and to the anterior abdominal wall as far as the umbilicus; the second border is attached to the upper and the anterior surfaces of the liver, dividing it into right and left lobes; the third border is a free edge where the 2 layers of the ligament become continuous with each other. The round ligament (ligamentum teres) passes in this free edge.

If the left lobe of the liver is pulled away from the diaphragm, a fold of peritoneum,

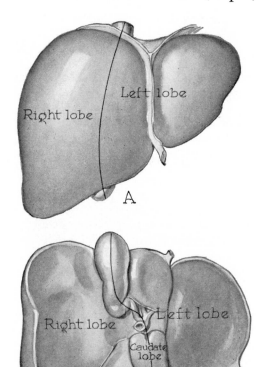

FIG. 381. The so-called "true" lobation of the liver. The heavy line divides the liver into right and left lobes. This division corresponds to the distribution of the right and the left hepatic ducts, the right and the left hepatic arteries and the right and the left branches of the portal vein. It should be noted that the caudate lobe belongs to both right and left liver lobes.

the *left triangular ligament,* is placed on the stretch. It connects the left hepatic lobe to the diaphragm and presents 3 borders. One border is attached to the back of the upper surface of the left lobe; the second is attached to the central tendon of the diaphragm and the third is a free edge which is directed toward the left where the 2 layers of the ligament are continuous with each other (Figs. 384 and 385).

If the fingers of the right hand are passed backward over the top of the right lobe, they are stopped by a layer of peritoneum which

is known as the *upper layer of the triangular (coronary) ligament* (Fig. 384). This is reflected from the back of the right lobe onto the diaphragm.

If the fingers of the left hand are passed upward behind the right part of the right lobe and pressed backward, they will be stopped by the *lower layer of the triangular (coronary) ligament.* The lower layer is reflected from the inferior surface of the liver onto the right kidney, the adrenal gland and the inferior vena cava; it also is referred to as the hepatorenal ligament. Below this ligament is a peritoneal space known as the hepatorenal pouch (Morison's).

The upper and the lower layers of the coronary ligament approximate each other at the right extremity of the liver, and where they fuse they form the *right triangular ligament.* This ligament is not as well marked as the left, because its 2 layers diverge so rapidly.

Between the 2 layers of the coronary ligament there is a fairly large triangular area of liver which is devoid of peritoneum and is known as the *bare area*; it is attached directly to the diaphragm by areolar tissue. The apex of this bare triangular area corresponds to the meeting point of the 2 layers of the coronary ligament on the right where they form the right triangular ligament. The base of the triangle is formed by the fossa for the inferior vena cava. The bare area is in contact with the inferior vena cava, the upper part of the right suprarenal gland and the diaphragm. It is connected to the liver by connective tissue in which are found the veins of Retzius, which form a portasystemic anastomosis (Fig. 364).

The student's "crutch," the time-honored letter "H," is formed by structures which lie on the inferior surface of the liver (Fig. 380 C). The left limb of the letter "H" divides this surface into right and left lobes. It contains embryonic structures, namely, the fissure for the ligamentum teres (left umbilical vein) in front and the fissure for the ductus venosus behind. Fetal blood is returned from the placenta to the fetus by means of the umbilical vein, which enters the abdomen at the umbilicus, passes upward along the free margin of the falciform ligament to the undersurface of the liver. At the transverse fissure of the liver (porta hepatis) it divides into 2 branches; one of these joins the portal vein and enters the right lobe, the other joins the ductus venosus, thereby short-circuiting the blood to the inferior vena cava (Fig. 386). Therefore, since the umbilical vein and the ductus venosus were continuous with each other in fetal life, it is quite natural that their adult landmarks (ligamentum teres and ligamentum venosum) should also be continuous, thereby forming the left limb of the "H."

The right limb of the "H" contains visceral structures, the fossa for the gallbladder in front and the inferior vena cava behind. The transverse part of the "H" is formed by the porta hepatis (the transverse fissure) and this contains, from before backward, the hepatic duct, the hepatic artery and branches of the portal vein. The porta is deep and wide and is about 2 inches long; a portion of the lesser omentum is attached to it. The nerves of the liver and most of its lymph vessels also are found here. Besides these structures it also contains fatty tissue and some lymph glands which, when enlarged, may obstruct the flow of bile in the hepatic ducts, thereby causing jaundice. The hepatic duct is formed on the right side of the porta by the union of the right and the left hepatic ducts. The branches of the hepatic artery enter on the left side of the common duct and then pass behind the right and the left ducts; the portal vein lies behind the artery. The porta hepatis is bounded anteriorly by the quadrate lobe and posteriorly by the caudate lobe of the liver.

LOBES AND SURFACES

Lobes. It has long been taught that the

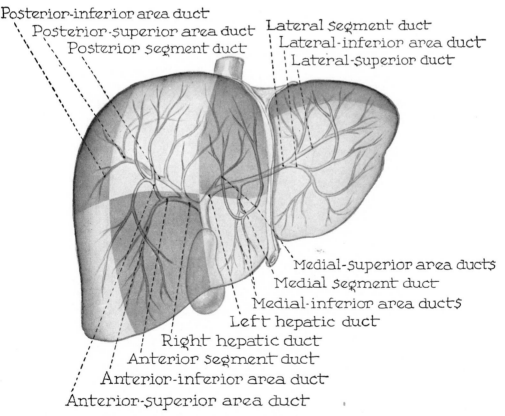

FIG. 382A. Complete drawing of the prevailing pattern of the bile ducts and the liver segments as seen from above. (After Healey and Schroy)

liver consists of 2 lobes—a larger right and a smaller left lobe. The proportion between the 2 is as 6 is to 1. They are divided by the fissure for the ligamentum venosum on the posterior surface, the fissure for the ligamentum teres on the inferior surface and the attachment of the falciform ligament on the superior and the anterior surfaces. Two circumscribed areas which are found over the medial part of the right lobe are also referred to as "lobes"; they are the quadrate lobe on the inferior surface, situated between the gallbladder and the fissure for the ligamentum teres, and the caudate lobe on the posterior surface, situated between the inferior vena cava and the fissure for the ligamentum venosum.

McNee and others believe that the true anatomic and physiologic division of the liver into right and left lobes is by a plane that passes through the fossa of the gallbladder and the fossa of the vena cava (Fig. 381). The two parts thus separated are approximately equal in size, with each lobe having its own arterial supply, portal supply and biliary drainage. Therefore, we must differentiate between an anatomic (surgical) division of the lobes and a true (functional) division.

Bilaterality of the liver has been studied for many years. Healey and Schroy have reported on an analysis of the prevailing patterns of branchings of the biliary ducts. They have also included in their study the major variations of such branchings. Their description of a prevailing pattern of bile ducts is presented in Figures 382 and 383. It should be noted that such branching is associated with divisions of the liver into various segments. The liver is divided into a right and a left lobe by a lobar fissure that is roughly in line with the gallbladder bed and the inferior vena cava on the visceral surface. The right lobe of the liver is divided by the right segmental fissure into anterior and posterior segments. The left lobe is divided by the left

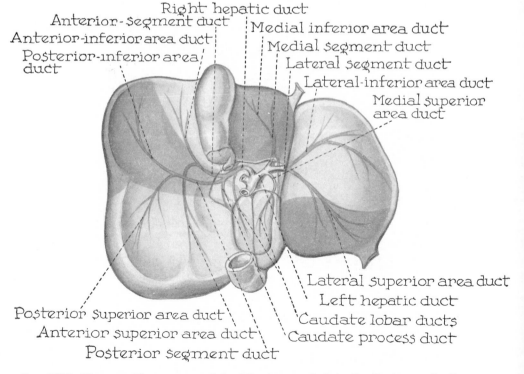

FIG. 382B. The prevailing pattern of the bile ducts and their distribution to the liver segments as seen from below. (After Healey and Schroy)

segmental fissure (fossa for the ligamentum venosum) into medial and lateral segments. In turn, each segment is divided according to its biliary drainage into superior and inferior areas. It is the opinion of these authors that the quadrate lobe should be regarded as pertaining to liver tissue that is associated with the medial segment. Intrahepatic anatomy of the bile ducts becomes increasingly important surgically, since various methods are now described for corrective procedures on previously involved or injured common ducts. This is true particularly in intrahepatic cholangiojejunostomy with partial hepatectomy (Longmire). Partial hepatectomies are also being performed for tumors of the liver.

Surfaces. The base of the pyramidal-shaped liver is the *right lateral surface*; it is somewhat quadrilateral and convex. It is related to the diaphragm opposite the 7th to the 11th ribs in the midaxillary line. The pleura and the right lung are important relations to this surface; they are separated by the diaphragm. In the midaxillary line the pleura overlaps the liver as low as the 10th rib and the lung to the 8th. The 12th rib, as a rule, does not reach sufficiently far forward to come into relationship to this hepatic surface. Therefore, a puncture wound over the lower part of the right side of the thorax may pass through the pleura, the lung, the diaphragm, the peritoneum and the liver (Fig. 362).

The anterior surface of the liver is of considerable clinical importance, since it is the surface which is most readily accessible for examination as far as the 10th costal cartilage on the right side. The median portion, which lies against the anterior abdominal wall, is palpated easily and thus yields valuable information. If inspiration is forced, almost the entire inferior border of the liver can be felt.

The superior surface is related to the diaphragm, which separates it from the 2 pleural sacs and the pericardium. On the right side it rises into a convexity that reaches almost to the level of the right nipple. On the left, the surface ends as a thin edge which is opposite the 5th rib in a line dropped from the left nipple.

The posterior surface cannot be seen until

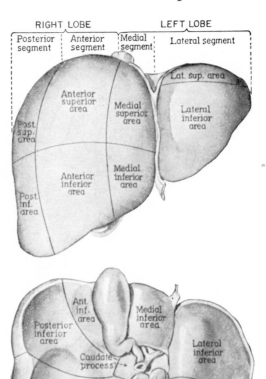

FIG. 383. Two views of the segmental area of the liver.

the liver has been removed from the body (Fig. 380 B). On the left this surface is covered with peritoneum of the greater sac, and a groove made by the esophagus is formed here. In the median plane is the caudate lobe, which is covered with peritoneum of the lesser sac. This lobe lies between the fossa for the vena cava and the fossa for the ductus venosus. To the right of this the bare area is found. The inferior vena cava occupies the leftmost portion of the area, and the kidney and the adrenal gland encroach upon it from below.

The inferior surface also has been called the visceral surface of the liver (Fig. 380 C). It faces downward, to the left and backward. It is covered with the peritoneum of the greater sac and everywhere shows the im-

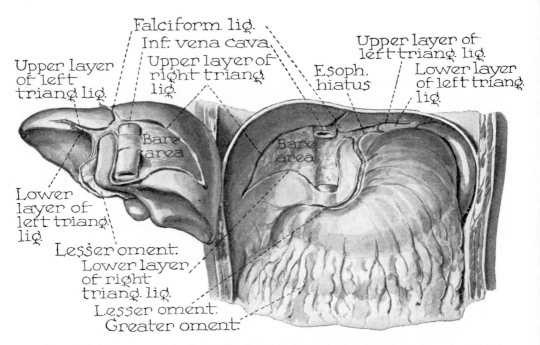

Upper layer
of left
triang. lig.

Falciform lig.

Inf: vena cava.

Upper layer of
right triang.
lig.

Upper layer of
left triang. lig.

Esoph.
hiatus

Lower layer
of left triang.
lig.

Bare
area

Bare
area

Lower
layer of
left triang
lig.

Lesser oment.
Lower layer,
of right
triang. lig.
Lesser oment.
Greater oment.

FIG. 384. Ligaments of the liver. The liver has been displaced to the right and out of the peritoneal cavity so that its ligamentous attachments may be seen. Therefore, this illustration shows the posterior aspect of the liver and the anterior aspect of the posterior abdominal wall to which the liver is normally attached.

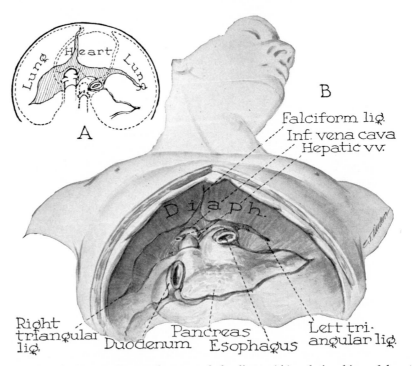

Lung   Heart   Lung

A

B

Falciform lig.
Inf: vena cava
Hepatic vv.

Diaph.

Right
triangular
lig.

Pancreas
Duodenum   Esophagus

Left tri-
angular lig.

FIG. 385. Diaphragmatic attachments of the liver; (A) relationships of heart and lungs; (B) seen from below the diaphragm, with the liver removed.

prints of viscera with which it is in contact. It is only distinctly separated from the inferior surface, and the "H" which has been described occupies this surface. The part of this surface which belongs to the left lobe is related to the stomach and to the lesser omentum. The gastric impression appears as a wide, shallow, concave area to the left. The omental part is a bulging prominence to the right and behind; it is called the *tuber omentale*.

The quadrate lobe lies between the fissure for the ligamentum teres and the fossa for the gallbladder. This lobe is related to the pyloric part of the stomach and the first part of the duodenum below, and to the right part of the lesser omentum above. It is the quadrate lobe which attempts to seal over perforated peptic ulcers, the vast majority of which occur in this portion of the stomach or in the duodenum. The gallbladder lies in front of the first and the second parts of the duodenum, but the latter extends beyond it and is in relation to the adjoining part of the right lobe. Directly to the right of the duodenal area the right colic flexure leaves its imprint, and behind this the undersurface of the right lobe is related to the right kidney, which leaves its renal impression.

The liver is completely covered with peritoneum except in 3 locations, namely, the bare area, the groove for the inferior vena cava and the gallbladder fossa. The lesser omentum is attached to the margins of the porta hepatis and around its right extremity; its 2 layers are continued from the left extremity of the porta hepatis to the fissure for the ligamentum venosum. At the upper end of this fissure these 2 layers separate.

The ligaments mentioned in connection with the liver should not be regarded as supporting the entire weight of the organ, since it, like other abdominal and pelvic organs, is kept in place by intra-abdominal pressure which is attributed mainly to the tonus of the muscles of the anterior and the lateral abdominal walls. Therefore, it is of little or no consequence when one of the so-called "supporting" ligaments of the liver is severed during surgical procedures, since the liver will not become ptotic.

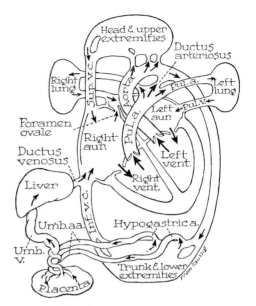

Fig. 386. Diagrammatic representation of fetal circulation.

VESSELS, NERVES AND LYMPHATICS

Arteries. The liver has 3 vessels associated with it: the hepatic artery, the portal vein and the hepatic veins.

The hepatic artery, one of the trifurcating branches of the celiac axis, supplies arterial blood to the substance of the liver.

Daseler, Anson *et al.* reported on investigations made in 500 laboratory specimens. They observed that the *common hepatic artery* arose as a branch of the celiac axis in 416 of the 500 (83.20%). This vessel was absent in 61 cases (12.20%). When the common hepatic artery was absent, the right and the left hepatic lobes derived their arterial supply from separate branches. These anatomists found that in 358 of 439 cases studies (81.54%) the common hepatic artery was a rather long trunk which divided into its hepatic branches within 4 cm. of the liver surface; in 81 cases (18.46%) the artery was short and divided into hepatic branches which ascended for a distance of more than 4 cm.

A normal *right hepatic artery* (one which supplies the right lobe of the liver after originating from a normal common hepatic artery) was present in 416 of 500 cases

(83.2%). Replacing and accessory right hepatic arteries are also encountered. In 15 cases (3%) the accessory right hepatic artery arose from the superior mesenteric artery; in 13 cases (2.6%) it arose as a branch of the left hepatic artery; in 5 cases (1%) from the gastroduodenal artery; in 2 cases (0.4%) from the celiac axis; and in only 1 case (0.2%) it arose directly from the aorta.

A normal *left hepatic artery* was found in 410 of the 500 specimens (82%). A replacing type of left hepatic artery occurred in 90 of the 500 cases (18%). These replacing vessels may originate from the celiac axis, the left gastric artery, the superior mesenteric artery, the gastroduodenal artery or directly from the aorta. In 175 of the 500 specimens (35%), an accessory left hepatic artery was encountered.

N. A. Michels noted that, in 100 bodies investigated, no two patterns of the arterial

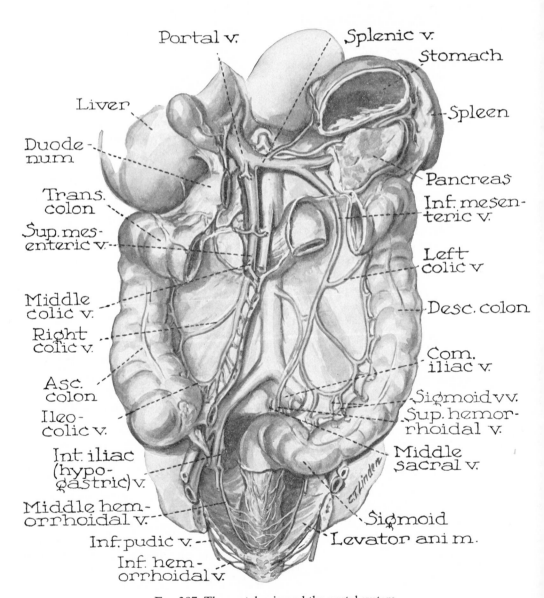

FIG. 387. The portal vein and the portal system.

supply to the liver were the same. The hepatic artery varied in the origin, the caliber, number and the distribution of its main branches. The typical common hepatic artery divides into a right, a middle (to the quadrate lobe) and a left branch.

To shut off completely the arterial blood supply to the liver would be fatal, but a collateral anastomosis exists. In recent years opinions have been divided as to whether or not necrosis will result in man from ligation of a common, a right or a left hepatic artery. Viability of the liver may be explained by the following: (1) If the common hepatic artery is ligated, hepatic circulation is maintained in a ratio of 1 to 8 because the right artery may arise from the superior mesenteric artery. (2) If the right or the left hepatic artery is ligated, the corresponding lobe does not of necessity necrose. This is explained by the fact that the larger branches of the right and the left hepatic arteries (precapillaries) anastomose with each other in the fissure of the liver. (3) If the hepatic artery is obstructed gradually on the aortic side of the right gastric artery, circulation may be maintained by the anastomosis of the right and the left gastric arteries. Hence, it must be accepted that the effects of ligation of the so-called "normal" hepatic artery would differ at various levels (Fig. 388).

Veins. *The portal vein* also brings a great quantity of blood to the liver (Fig. 387). This vessel is formed between the head and the neck of the pancreas by the union of the splenic, the superior mesenteric and the inferior mesenteric veins (Fig. 362). It forms a rather thick vessel, which measures about 7½ cm. in length. At the porta hepatis it divides into right and left branches. If the portal vein is obstructed by either intrahepatic or extrahepatic causes, the portal blood is shunted to the systemic veins where the 2 systems meet (Fig. 364). This collateral circulation has been referred to as the accessory portal system.

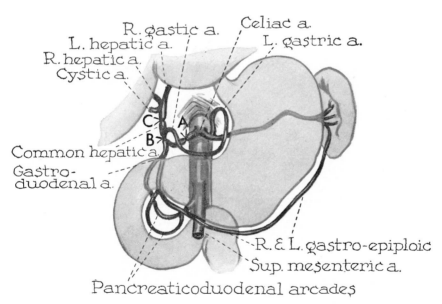

FIG. 388. Ligation of the common hepatic artery at A would spare the entire collateral circulation; it should be noted that in this instance the gastroduodenal and the right gastric arteries are distal to the point of ligation. At B the ligation is placed distal to the gastroduodenal but proximal to the right gastric artery; this could markedly reduce the collateral circulation. A ligature at C or beyond this point abolishes the collateral channels, thus depriving the liver of arterial blood. Accessory vessels may be present, and some authors believe that these could prevent necrosis.

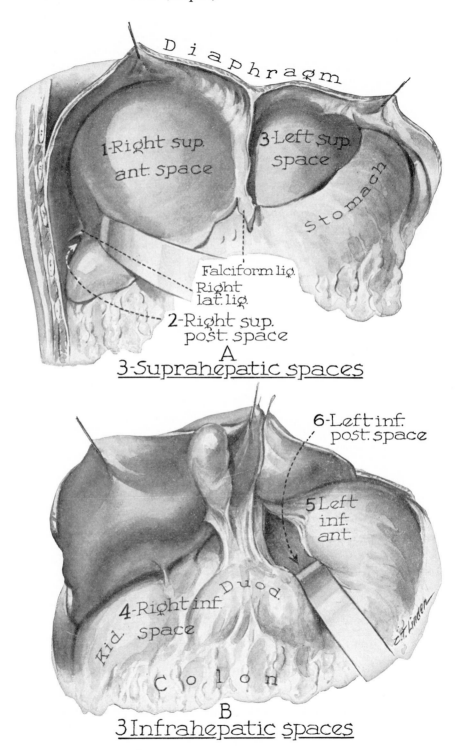

FIG. 389. The 6 subphrenic spaces: (A) the 3 suprahepatic spaces; (B) the 3 infrahepatic spaces.

The hepatic veins carry blood from the liver to the inferior vena cava. Some of these veins are small and open into the vena cava at various points; however, the chief hepatic veins are a left and a right, coming respectively from the right and the left liver lobes. They enter the inferior vena cava immediately before it leaves the liver.

Nerves. The nerves of the liver are derived from the left vagus and the sympathetic. They enter at the porta hepatis and accompany the vessels and the ducts to the interlobular spaces.

Lymphatics. The lymph vessels of the liver terminate largely in a small group of lymph glands in and around the porta hepatis. The efferent vessels from these glands pass to the celiac lymph glands. Some of the superficial lymph vessels in the anterior surface of the liver pass to the diaphragm in the falciform ligament and finally reach the mediastinal glands. There is another group which accompanies the inferior vena cava into the thorax and ends in a few small glands which are related to the intrathoracic part of the vessel.

SURFACE ANATOMY

The limits of the liver are determined by palpation and percussion. Only an approximation of the size of the gland can be obtained; the exact location of these limits is difficult to obtain because the lower edge of the lung overlaps the liver above, and the lower edge of the liver overlaps the stomach and the intestine below. The upper limit of the right lobe (highest point of the liver) lies beneath the right dome of the diaphragm; it is on a level with the upper margin of the 5th rib about 1 inch medial to the mammary line and about 1 cm. below the right nipple. The upper limit of the left lobe corresponds to the upper border of the 6th rib in the mammary line, about 1 inch below the left nipple. At this point, the left tip of the liver is separated from the apex of the heart only by the diaphragm. The lower border of the liver can be traced best from right to left. It follows the costal arch as far as the tip of the 9th costal cartilage; however, in the erect position it may descend an additional inch below the ribs. From the 9th costal cartilage,

it crosses obliquely until it reaches the tip of the 8th costal cartilage on the left side. From this point on it continues laterally until it meets the upper and the lateral limits of the left lobe. In the midline, the lower border of the liver lies midway between the xiphoid and the umbilicus.

PRACTICAL AND SURGICAL CONSIDERATIONS

THE 6 SUBPHRENIC SPACES

The one large subphrenic area is divided into 6 subphrenic spaces (Fig. 389). The "subphrenic space" is a region situated between the diaphragm above and the transverse colon and its mesocolon below. The liver divides this space into suprahepatic and infrahepatic spaces. The suprahepatic space is bounded above by the diaphragm and below by the superior surface of the liver; the infrahepatic space is bounded above by the inferior surface of the liver and below by the transverse colon and its mesocolon.

Suprahepatic Spaces. The suprahepatic space is divided into 3 smaller suprahepatic (subphrenic) spaces in the following way: the suprahepatic area is divided into right and left portions by the falciform ligament, which extends between the superior surface of the liver and the diaphragm. From the back of the right lobe of the liver and running upward to be reflected onto the diaphragm, is the upper layer of the coronary ligament (Fig. 384).

A space is now formed which lies above the liver, to the right of the falciform ligament and in front of the upper layer of the coronary ligament. Therefore this space is called the *right superior anterior subphrenic space*. It is bounded above by the diaphragm, below by the superior border of the liver, behind by the upper layer of the coronary ligament and medially by the right surface of the falciform ligament. The lower layer of the coronary ligament on the right forms the roof of a space which is limited by the liver in front and the posterior parietal peritoneum behind. This is smaller than the anterior space just described; since it still is associated with the superior surface of the liver and since it lies to the right of the falciform ligament but behind the lower layer of the coronary ligament, it is called the *right superior posterior subphrenic space.*

To the left of the falciform ligament but still in the suprahepatic area, the left triangular (coronary) ligament courses along the posterior border of the left lobe of the liver and separates the superior surface from the inferior surface of the liver. In this respect it differs from the ligament on the right, which has 2 diverging layers, thus dividing the superior surface on the right into anterior and posterior spaces. Since the layers of the left ligament do not diverge, and since they run directly at the junction of the superior and the inferior borders, the left suprahepatic space constitutes only one space and is not divided into two. It is called the *left superior subphrenic space* and is bounded by the diaphragm above, the superior surface of the left lobe of the liver below and the left side of the falciform ligament medially.

Infrahepatic Spaces. The infrahepatic area also is divided into 3 subphrenic spaces. In addition, this area is divided into right and left sides by the round ligament and the ligament of the ductus venosus. To the right of these structures is a large space known as the *right inferior subphrenic space.* It is bounded above by the inferior surface of the liver and below by the transverse mesocolon and the colon; medially, it extends to the round ligament.

To the left are 2 spaces separated from each other by the stomach and the lesser omentum. The space anterior to the stomach is known as the *left anterior inferior subphrenic space,* and the space posterior to the stomach is known as the *left inferior posterior subphrenic space.* The left anterior inferior space also has been referred to as the perigastric space; in this space a perigastric abscess may form following the perforation of a peptic ulcer. The right inferior space is bounded above by the inferior surface of the liver, below by the transverse colon and the mesocolon and anteriorly by the anterior abdominal wall. The left inferior posterior subphrenic space is better known as the lesser peritoneal cavity. It is bounded above by the inferior surface of the liver; below, by the transverse mesocolon; anteriorly, by the

stomach and the lesser omentum; and, posteriorly, by the posterior parietal peritoneum of the lesser sac.

The bare area, which is really the space within the confines of the coronary ligament, has not been included as one of the 6 subphrenic spaces but is considered as an *extraperitoneal space.* The space most frequently involved in infection and abscess formation is the right posterior superior space. The reason for this is that the most frequent causes of peritoneal contamination are on the right side (suppurative appendicitis, cholecystitis or perforated peptic ulcer). The right posterior superior space is the earliest space involved because inflammatory exudate travels upward from the right iliac fossa and along the paracolic gutter.

DRAINAGE OF SUBPHRENIC ABSCESSES

Alton Ochsner and Amos Graves have done much to standardize the treatment of subphrenic abscesses. They conclude that adequate drainage of such an abscess should consist of early and proper evacuation in such a way that contamination of the peritoneal and the pleural cavities is avoided. The various spaces are approached through different routes (Fig. 390).

The right superior posterior space, which is the most frequent to be involved, is drained through a "retroperitoneal operation." The right inferior space frequently is associated with it and may be drained simultaneously through the same incision. This approach does not enter the pleural or the peritoneal cavities.

The technic is as follows. The patient is placed upon the unaffected side and on a kidney rest. The incision is made directly over the 12th rib, which is resected subperiosteally; the erector spinae muscle mass is retracted medially. A transverse incision is made at right angles to the spine, which passes across the rib bed at the level of the spinous process of the 1st lumbar vertebra. The incision through the 12th rib bed is made transversely and not parallel with the skin incision; only in this way can one be sure that the pleural cavity will not be entered. The costophrenic angle of the pleura has not been found to pass caudally as far as the

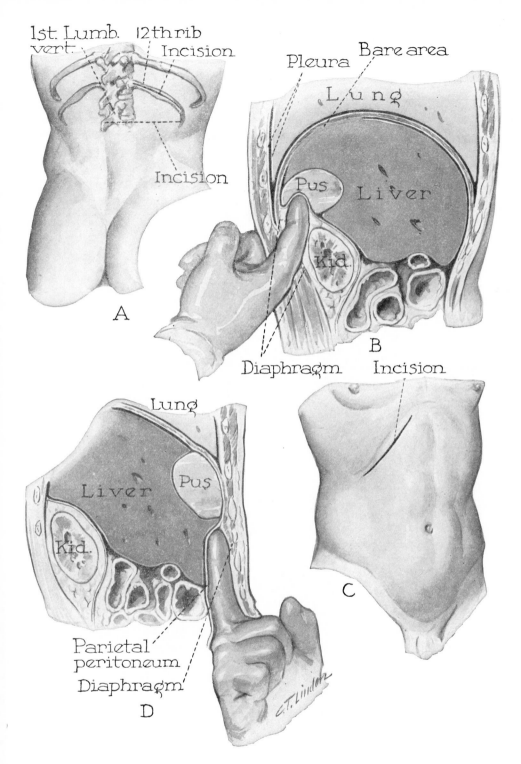

FIG. 390. Drainage of subphrenic abscesses: (A) line of incision over the 12th rib and deeper transverse incision at the level of the 1st lumbar spinous process; (B) approach to an abscess in the right superior posterior subphrenic space; (C) incision for drainage of an abscess in the right superior anterior subphrenic space; (D) drainage of a right superior anterior subphrenic space abscess.

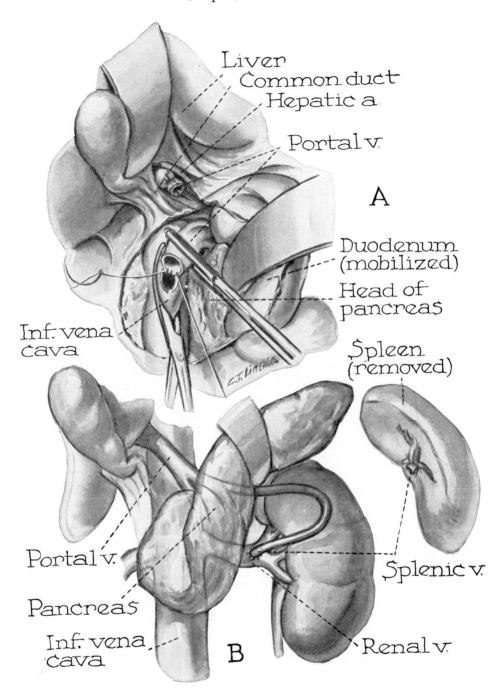

Fig. 391. Portacaval shunts. (A) This depicts an end-to-side anastomosis between the portal vein and the inferior vena cava. The remaining cut end of the portal vein has been ligated close to the liver. (B) The end of the splenic vein has been anastomosed to the side of the left renal vein. The spleen has been removed.

spinous process of the 1st lumbar vertebra. The transverse incision passes through the bed of the 12th rib and the attachment of the diaphragm, the latter appearing usually as a few muscle fibers. Directly beneath this, the renal fascia is identified; it is continuous above and anteriorly with the posterior parietal peritoneum. The peritoneum is separated from the undersurface of the diaphragm, and the right superior posterior subphrenic space

is entered (Fig. 390 B). The abscess cavity is entered and drained.

Abscesses which involve the right superior anterior, the right inferior, the left anterior inferior and the left superior spaces can be drained extraperitoneally through an anterior approach (Figs. 390 C and D). If the retroperitoneal approach can be employed for the right inferior space, this is preferable. However, in those cases which require anterior

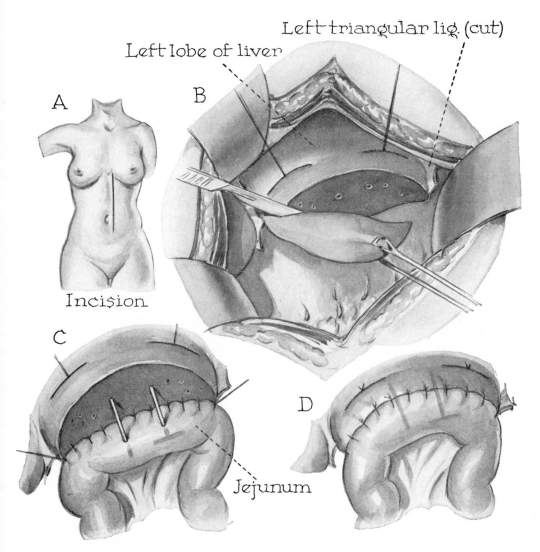

Fig. 392. The author's modification of the Longmire operation for irreparable damage to the common and/or the hepatic ducts. It should be noted that 2 anastomoses are performed. In addition to the usual catheter the author has added a T-tube.

approaches (right superior anterior and left superior), one attempts to follow the suggestion of Clairmont and drain these both extraperitoneally and extrapleurally. The incision is made just beneath and parallel with the costal margin through the oblique abdominal muscles and the transversalis fascia to the peritoneum. The parietal peritoneum is separated from the undersurface of the diaphragm, and the peritoneum is mobilized upward until the abscess is reached. The cavity is opened extraperitoneally and drained.

PORTACAVAL SHUNTS

Recent favorable reports by Whipple, Blakemore, Linton and others have stimulated interest in various types of portacaval shunts (Fig. 391). These procedures are being done at present for cases of portal hypertension which have tendencies toward esophagogastrointestinal bleeding. Various types of shunts have been used, the most common of which is an anastomosis between the portal vein and the inferior vena cava (Fig. 391 A). This anastomosis has been done in the form of an end-to-side portacaval shunt; this is done wholly as an abdominal procedure and requires the dissection and the isolation of the structures in the hepatoduodenal part of the lesser omentum (portal vein, common duct and hepatic artery). More recently, Blakemore has described a right thoracicoabdominal approach which provides excellent exposure of both the inferior vena cava and the portal vein. With this incision, a lateral anastomosis between the vessels is possible, and the dissection of the common duct and the hepatic artery is unnecessary. Other types of shunts which have been used are the divided superior mesenteric vein to the side of the inferior vena cava distal to the renal veins, the proximal end of the divided inferior mesenteric vein to the side of the left ovarian vein and end-to-side splenorenal anastomosis (Fig. 391 B). Rienhoff has advocated hepatic artery ligation for portal hypertension.

LIVER RESECTION

Resective lesions have increased during recent years, particularly neoplastic and traumatic lesions of the liver. Major hepatic resections with lowered morbidity and mortality are being accomplished by strict adherence to surgical principles and anatomic knowledge. The works of Healey and Schroy and of Goldsmith and Woodburne can be referred to for their views regarding "planes" of resection. The caudate lobe is usually treated as an area unto itself. The Longmire operation (intrahepatic cholangiojejunostomy) and its modifications should be in the armamentarium of every surgeon interested in biliary tract surgery. This may be a last resort whereby a life can be saved following injury to and reparative processes of the common duct. The author's modification of the Longmire procedure is shown in Figure 392.

ABDOMEN

Gallbladder and Bile Ducts

EMBRYOLOGY

The hepatic diverticulum arises from the foregut, and from it the gallbladder and the extrahepatic biliary ducts develop. At first the gallbladder lies in the ventral mesentery; at the 2nd month it becomes embedded in hepatic tissue; and at a later date it assumes its superficial position. The lumina of the gallbladder and also of the ducts is occluded by an epithelial proliferation during the 2nd month. Occasionally, the bud for the gallbladder divides, giving rise to a double or bifid organ.

ADULT GALLBLADDER AND BILE DUCTS (VESSELS)

The gallbladder (vesica fellea) is a pear-shaped hollow viscus which is closely connected to the inferior surface of the right lobe of the liver (Figs. 393, 394 and 395). Usually, it is from 3 to 4 inches long, holds 1½ ounces of bile and forms the right boundary of the quadrate lobe of the liver. The peritoneum which is reflected from its sides attaches it to the liver. It consists of a fundus, a body, an infundibulum and a neck (Fig. 393).

Fundus. The fundus usually projects beyond the liver and at times may be kinked or notched, forming a so-called Phrygian cap; if this cap is well developed, the fundus becomes fixed and folded. When the fundus protrudes beyond the liver margin it is cov-

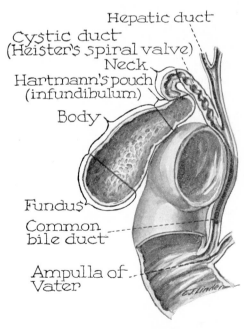

FIG. 393. The gallbladder. This is divided into a fundus, a body, an infundibulum (Hartmann's pouch) and a neck.

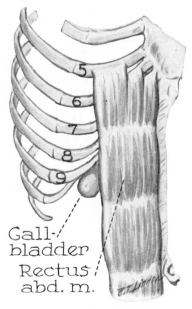

FIG. 394. Surface anatomy of the gallbladder. The fundus of the normal gallbladder usually is found in an angle formed by the right rectus muscle and the costal margin.

ered on all sides with peritoneum. It is in contact with the anterior abdominal wall opposite the 9th costal cartilage in an angle formed between the right rectus muscle and the costal margin (Fig. 394).

Body. The body is the main part of the gallbladder; it lies in the fossa on the inferior surface of the liver. It is covered with peritoneum at the side and below, but its superior (anterior) surface is in direct contact with the liver; its inferior (posterior) surface is related to the second part of the duodenum and to the transverse colon (Fig. 395 A). Usually, no peritoneum is found between the posterior part of the body of the gallbladder and the liver; however, occasionally the gallbladder may be loosely attached and mobile by a fold of peritoneum which

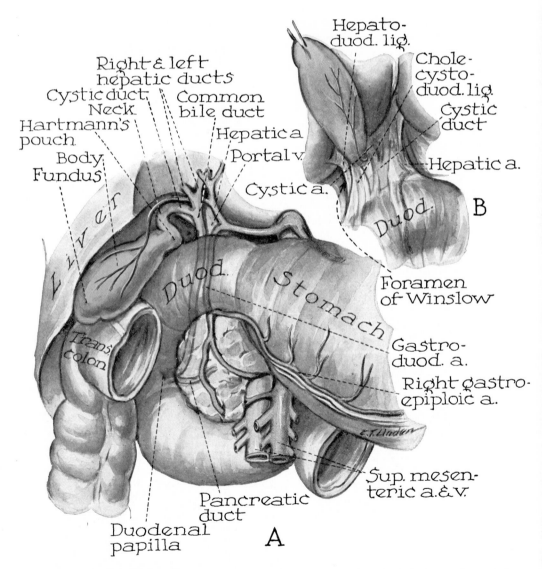

Fig. 395. The gallbladder and its surrounding relations. (A) The inferior surface of the body of the gallbladder is related to the second part of the duodenum and the transverse colon. (B) Hartmann's pouch is bound down toward the first part of the duodenum by the cholecystoduodenal ligament.

surrounds the entire organ and forms a mesentery.

Infundibulum. *The infundibulum (Hartmann's pouch)* is that part of the organ which is situated between its body and its neck; it appears as an overhanging pouch which runs parallel with the cystic duct and thereby hides it. Hartmann's pouch is one of the most important surgical guides for proper identification and exposure of the cystic duct. The pouch is bound down toward the first part of the duodenum by the right edge of the lesser omentum, preferably referred to as the *cholecystoduodenal ligament* (Fig. 395 B). This ligament is also a most important anatomic landmark in surgery; only by serving it can Hartmann's pouch be mobilized properly and the cystic duct identified clearly. The cholecystoduodenal ligament, which is present in almost all cases as a normal structure, has been referred to erroneously as "adhesions."

Neck. The neck of the gallbladder continues from the upper part of the infundibulum and narrows to become the cystic duct. It is closely applied to the liver and is in relation inferiorly with the end of the first part of the duodenum. M. Lichtenstein is of the opinion that the *spiral valve of Heister* is an infolding of the wall of the cystic duct which

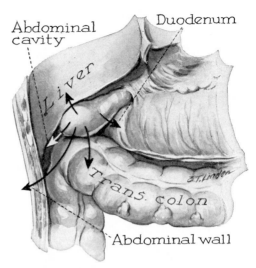

Fig. 396. Possible paths of spontaneous rupture or auto-anastomoses between the gallbladder and the surrounding viscera.

is found only in bipeds. He believes that its function is to maintain the patency of the cystic duct. It is the presence of this valve that makes catheterization or probing of the duct difficult.

Since the gallbladder is so closely related to the duodenum, the jejunum, the transverse colon, the liver and the abdominal wall, spon-

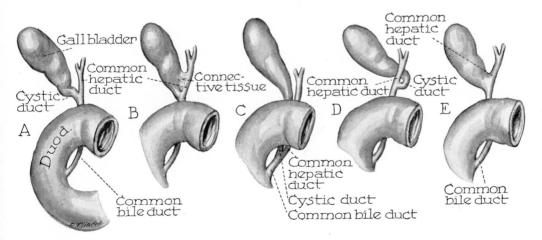

Fig. 397. Variations of the cystic duct (Flint). (A) The so-called normal cystic duct. (B) The cystic duct lies parallel with the hepatic duct, both being joined by connective tissue. (C) The cystic and the hepatic ducts do not join until their entrance into the duodenum. (D) The cystic duct joins the hepatic duct on its left side. (E) Absence of the cystic duct.

taneous rupture or auto-anastomoses between it and these organs might occur (Fig. 396).

Ducts. *The cystic duct* is usually about 1 inch long and extends from the neck of the gallbladder to the porta hepatis; here it joins the hepatic duct to form the common bile duct. It is the only extrahepatic bile duct that is tortuous in appearance, the tortuosity being due to the presence of Heister's spiral valve. It usually passes downward for a short distance with the common hepatic duct before joining it, but the cystic duct may present many variations or anomalies, the more common of which are seen in Figure 397. Be-

cause of these variations perfect exposure is necessary before a ligature is placed on any structure in this region.

The common hepatic duct is about 1 inch or less in length and is formed in the porta hepatis by the union of the right and the left hepatic ducts, which emerge from the right and the left lobes of the liver, respectively. It is joined by the cystic duct to form the common bile duct.

The common bile duct (*ductus choledochus*) is from 3 to 4 inches long and ¼ inch wide. At times it is considered a direct continuation of the hepatic duct but is more conveniently thought of as being formed by the

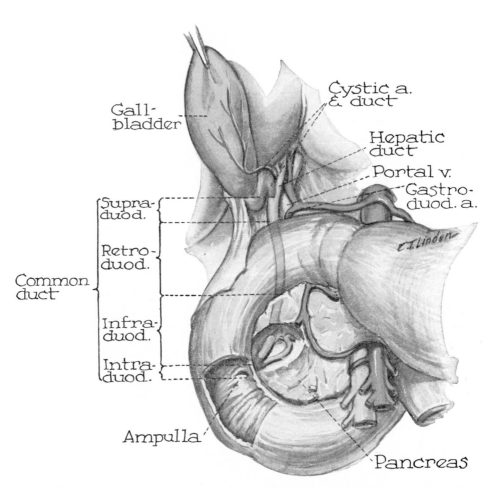

FIG. 398. The 4 parts of the common duct in relation to the duodenum. Part 1 is above the duodenum (supraduodenal); part 2 is behind the duodenum (retroduodenal); part 3 is below the duodenum (infraduodenal); part 4 is within the wall of the duodenum (intraduodenal).

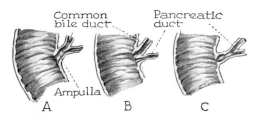

FIG. 399. Types of union of the common bile duct and the pancreatic duct: (A) both ducts open independently into the ampulla; (B) both ducts open independently into the bowel; (C) both ducts join and open into the ampulla by a common channel.

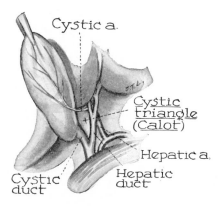

FIG. 400. The so-called "normal" cystic artery and the triangle of Calot. The triangle is formed by the cystic artery (base) and the junction of the cystic and the hepatic ducts (apex).

union of the cystic and the hepatic ducts. It begins near the porta hepatis and descends in the free margin of the lesser omentum; it then continues behind the first part of the duodenum and enters a groove in the back of the head of the pancreas. It passes *through* the pancreas, downward and slightly to the right, and ends in the second part of the duodenum a little below its middle and on its posteromedial surface. It is convenient to divide the common duct into the following 4 parts, each being related surgically to the duodenum (Fig. 398):

1. *The supraduodenal portion* of the common duct is that part which is situated above the duodenum; it is about 1 inch long. It descends in the right margin of the lesser omentum (cholecystoduodenal ligament), to the right of the hepatic artery and anterior to the portal vein. This part of the common duct is felt by a finger placed in the foramen of Winslow.

2. *The retroduodenal part* is situated behind the duodenum, with the right edge of the portal vein behind it and the gastroduodenal artery to its medial or left side. Since the first part of the duodenum is usually quite mobile, this part may be exposed with ease.

3. *The infraduodenal part* is located below the duodenum. Since the head of the pancreas is in this region, it has also been referred to as the pancreatic portion of the common duct. This part of the duct does not pass between the duodenum and the pancreas but usually forms a groove, or at times a tunnel, in the upper and lateral parts of the posterior surface of the pancreas through which it passes. Because of its intrapancreatic position, this part of the duct is difficult to expose. It is closely related to the right edge of the inferior vena cava, which lies behind it (Fig. 402). The portal vein approaches it obliquely from below and from the left, and the gastroduodenal artery is on its left side. This part of the duct is placed in a cage of vessels formed by the vasa recti which arise from the arcades formed by the superior and the inferior pancreaticoduodenal arteries (Fig. 330).

4. *The intraduodenal portion* is that part of the common duct which passes obliquely through the wall of the duodenum and enters it in its second part. This section of the duct is joined on its left side by the main pancreatic duct. A reservoir usually is formed by this junction within the duodenal wall; it is known as the *ampulla of Vater*. The latter opens into the duodenum on the summit of an elevation known as the *duodenal papilla*. Various types of union of the pancreatic duct and the common bile duct are possible (Fig. 399). Both ducts may open independently into the ampulla, they may open independently into the bowel, or they may even join together and open into the ampulla by a common channel. Therefore, a stone blocking the papilla will not always have the same effect; the effect depends on the type of union which is present.

The intrinsic and proximate blood vessels of the common and the hepatic ducts have been studied and described by Shapiro and Robillard. The important arterial branches to these ducts primarily arise from the cystic and the posterosuperior pancreaticoduodenal arteries, rather than from the hepatic artery, as has been thought previously. Therefore, it is important to do minimal stripping for exposure along the medial side of the duct to reduce the danger of devascularization and ischemic necrosis in common duct surgery. The venous drainage of the extrahepatic biliary passages is upward into the hepatic veins without major anastomoses with the portal system.

Cystic Artery. This is one of the most anomalous structures in the body. The so-called "normal" cystic artery is found in about 60 per cent of the cases and arises as a branch of the right hepatic artery. When the artery arises in this manner, a cystic triangle

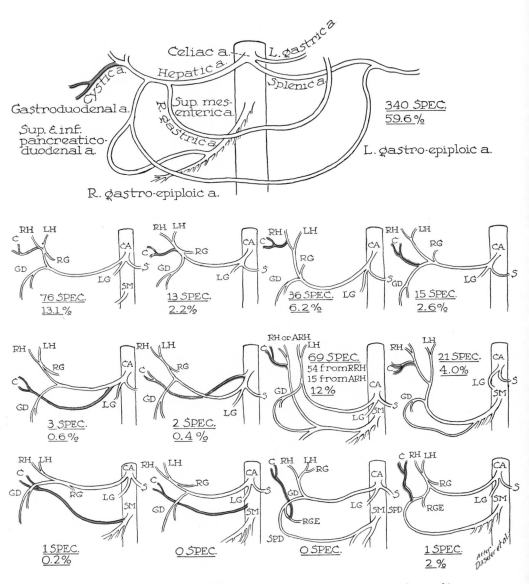

FIG. 401. Variations in the origin of the cystic artery (after Daseler *et al.*).

of Calot is formed; the base of this is the cystic artery; the apex is formed by an angle which results from the junction of the cystic and the hepatic ducts (Fig. 400). As a rule, the cystic artery divides into a superficial and a deep branch, the latter being distributed to the medioposterior, nonperitoneal surface of the gallbladder. Daseler, *et al.* reported on a study of 500 cadavers and have classified the sites of origin of the cystic artery into 12 different types (Fig. 401). Duplications and triplications of the vessel have been reported. Since most cases of duct injury are due to hemorrhage from a divided cystic artery or an anomalous arterial branch, the surgeon must acquaint himself with the possible arterial patterns and attempts to identify them. The course of the cystic artery is so variable, and the occurrence of duplicate and triplicate branches so common, that perfect exposure and separate ligation of the cystic duct and artery always must be attempted. It is true that under most unusual circumstances the cystic artery and the duct must be ligated with a single tie; however, this is the exception and not the rule.

The foramen of Winslow and its boundaries are surgical guides which aid in the performance of safe gallbladder and common duct surgery. The foramen is found readily by placing a finger along the free margin (right side) of the lesser omentum; this locates the foramen and permits the finger to enter the lesser peritoneal cavity (Fig. 402). The boundaries around a finger so placed in the foramen are: cephalad to the finger, the gallbladder is found; caudad, is the superior margin of the first part of the duodenum; on the palpating finger is the lesser omentum which contains 3 structures, namely, the common duct, the portal vein and the hepatic artery (the duct and the artery lie on the vein); behind the finger is the inferior vena cava. If the cystic artery retracts or if there is bleeding during the course of biliary surgery, it is wise to place the index finger in the foramen of Winslow and grasp the hepatic artery between the index finger and the thumb. Pressure so made will control the bleeding, since the cystic artery arises from the hepatic. It is wise also to place a gauze sponge in the foramen of Winslow during biliary surgery to

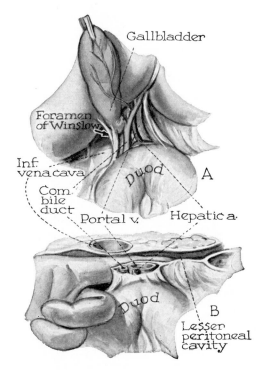

FIG. 402. The foramen of Winslow and its boundaries. (A) The finger (probe) is placed in the foramen which is bounded above (cephalad) by the gallbladder, below (caudad) by the duodenum, anteriorly by the common duct, the portal vein and the hepatic artery, and posteriorly by the inferior vena cava. (B) The foramen seen in cross section from above.

prevent injury to the inferior vena cava, and also for immediate orientation.

The lymphatics of the gallbladder drain into the lymph glands at the hilus of the liver and into the liver substance.

GALLBLADDER SURGERY

CHOLECYSTOSTOMY

This operation is reserved for the poor-risk patient with acute progressive infections of the gallbladder or in those cases where removal of the organ would be technically difficult or too dangerous (Fig. 403).

The gallbladder is exposed, and a trochar is inserted into its lumen; its liquid contents are aspirated; and any stones which are present are removed. After aspiration, the organ can be grasped with noncrushing forceps. The opening is enlarged; a rubber tube is inserted into the lumen and is held there by a transfixing suture. A purse-string suture or interrupted inverting sutures are placed about the opening in the gallbladder and tightened around the tube. Some surgeons advocate additional drains.

CHOLECYSTECTOMY

A right rectus incision which divides the muscle at its inner third usually is used (Fig. 404). The fundus of the gallbladder is grasped and lifted upward. A hemostat is placed on Hartmann's pouch, and lateral and upward traction is maintained so that the cholecystoduodenal ligament is placed on a stretch. It will be remembered that these two structures, Hartmann's pouch and the cholecystoduodenal ligament, are the surgeon's two most important guides. The left index finger is placed in the foramen of Winslow, and the boundaries around this foramen are reviewed quickly. The cholecystoduodenal ligament is snipped carefully and spread so that the proper cleavage plane is entered. This permits mobilization of Hartmann's pouch; the cystic duct then comes into view. The cystic artery usually is found medial and cephalad to the cystic duct. The cystic duct and the cystic artery are ligated individually. Ligation of the cystic duct should be done about 1 to 2 cm. proximal to its junction with the common duct. This prevents "tenting" of the common duct. A cleavage plane which permits easy removal of the gallbladder is found between the gallbladder and the liver bed. By peeling the gallbladder in this fashion, peritoneal flaps are made automatically; these are incised, the gallbladder is removed, and the flaps are permitted to fall into place or are sutured together.

CHOLEDOCHOSTOMY

Any one of the 4 parts of the common duct may require exploration. This usually can be accomplished through its first or supraduodenal portion. A longitudinal incision about 2 cm. long is placed in this portion of the

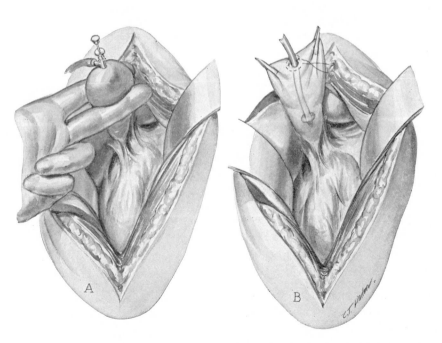

FIG. 403. Cholecystostomy. (A) The distended gallbladder is steadied by the hand of the surgeon as an aspirating trocar is placed into the lumen of the organ. (B) A Pezzer catheter is sutured into the gallbladder for purposes of drainage.

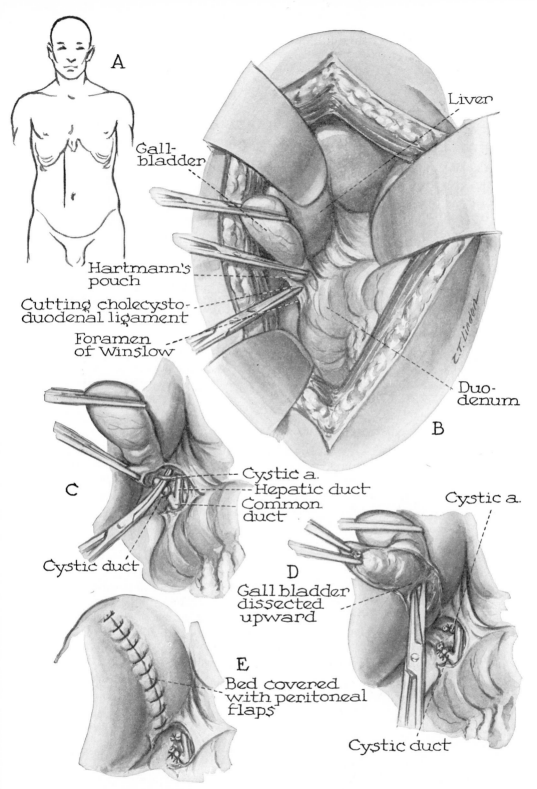

FIG. 404. Cholecystectomy. (A) Incision. (B) Upward and lateral traction is made on Hartmann's pouch; this stretches the cholecystoduodenal ligament, which is incised. (C) The extrahepatic biliary ducts and the cystic artery are exposed. (D) The cystic artery and the cystic duct are ligated and divided; the gallbladder is removed from below upward. (E) The gallbladder has been removed, and the liver has been peritonized.

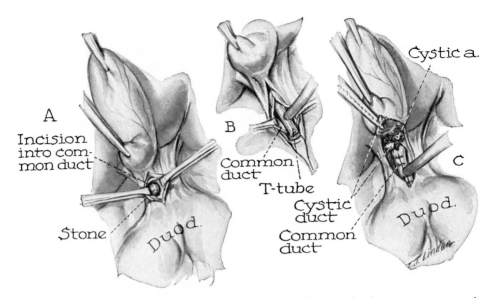

FIG. 405. Choledochostomy. (A) An incision is made into the lesser omentum and the supraduodenal part of the common duct. (B) The stone is removed, and a "T"-tube is inserted into the common duct. (C) The "T"-tube is in place, and the gallbladder is removed from below upward.

common duct between the cystic duct and the duodenum (Fig. 405). The cut edges of the duct are grasped, a blunt curved probe is passed downward to the ampulla of Vater and, if possible, into the duodenum. The hepatic duct is explored. After determining the patency of the ampulla of Vater, a "T"-tube is inserted into the common duct; it is fixed there and the duct is sutured around the

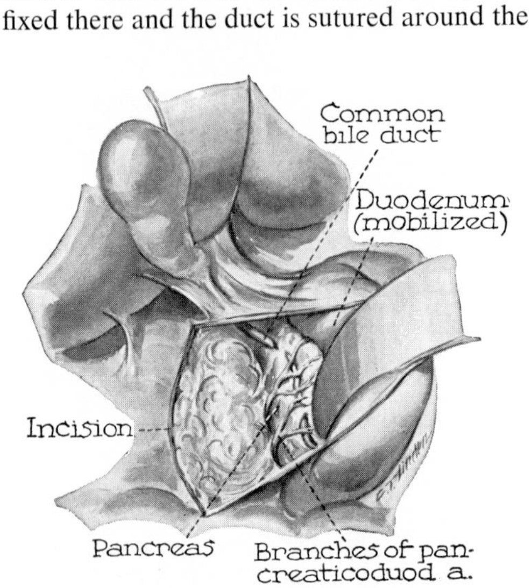

FIG. 406. Approach to the pancreatic portion of the common bile duct.

neck of the tube. This is reinforced further by a few sutures placed in the lesser omentum. For exploration of the third part of the common duct (infraduodenal or pancreatic portion), it becomes necessary to mobilize the descending part of the duodenum (Fig. 406). This is accomplished by incising the parietal peritoneum along the lateral border of the descending duodenum, permitting medial rotation of the latter. Although some authors state that this renders the intrapancreatic portion of the common duct accessible, this is usually not true, because the duct lies within pancreatic tissue and is surrounded by blood vessels. If a stone is impacted in part 4 (intraduodenal portion) of the common duct, it can be approached transduodenally (Fig. 407).

CHOLECYSTO-ENTEROSTOMY

In certain types of obstructive jaundice it may be necessary to perform an anastomosis between the gallbladder and some part of the small bowel, namely, duodenum or jejunum; cholecystogastrostomies also have been done (Fig. 408). These procedures are discussed under surgery of the pancreas (p. 518).

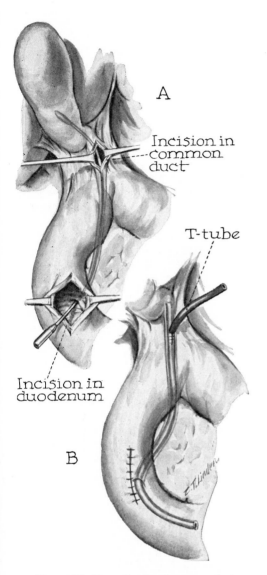

A

Incision in common duct

T-tube

Incision in duodenum

B

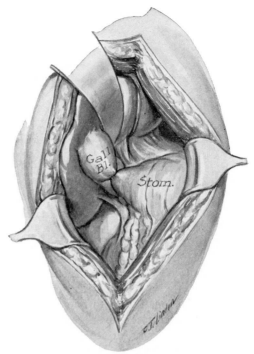

Fig. 408. Cholecystogastrostomy. Although the fundus of the gallbladder usually is depicted as the site selected for the anastomosis, the illustration reveals that the body of the gallbladder may be used if the latter is small.

Fig. 407. Transduodenal approach to the intraduodenal part of the common duct. (A) The 4th part of the common duct (intraduodenal portion) is explored through an incision in the duodenum. An additional incision is made into the supra-duodenal part of the common duct. A probe determines the patency of the duct. (B) A long "T"-tube (Cattell) is placed through the common duct and into the duodenum.

Spleen

EMBRYOLOGY

To understand the peritoneal attachments of the spleen and their surgical applications, the embryologic changes which take place must be understood. The stomach (before rotation) is attached posteriorly by a dorsal mesogastrium and anteriorly by a ventral mesogastrium (Fig. 409 A). The spleen originates as a localized cellular collection in the left layer of the dorsal mesogastrium. These cellular collections fuse with one another to form a lobulated spleen, the notch or notches of which are the only surface traces of lobulation in the adult organ.

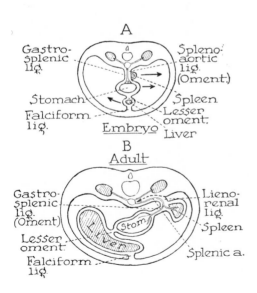

FIG. 409. Embryology of the spleen. (A) Before rotation the dorsal mesogastrium is divided by the spleen into gastrosplenic and spleno-aortic ligaments. (B) After rotation the spleno-aortic ligament becomes the splenorenal (lienorenal) ligament. Fusion to the posterior abdominal wall has taken place.

The spleen divides the dorsal mesogastrium into: (1) a gastrosplenic part and (2) a spleno-aortic part (lienorenal ligament). As growth takes place, the spleen and the stomach shift to the left, and the liver shifts to the right. The spleno-aortic ligament is pushed against the posterior abdominal wall, and a fusion takes place between the two opposed surfaces (Fig. 409 B). The spleno-aortic ligament, having been pulled to the left, comes in contact with the left kidney; because of its new position, it is referred to as the linenorenal (splenorenal) ligament. The splenic artery runs in the lienorenal ligament.

To mobilize the spleen it becomes necessary to incise the left leaf of the lienorenal ligament and to enter the fusion (cleavage) plane behind the splenic artery. This converts the lienorenal ligament back to its early form, namely, the spleno-aortic ligament. It is a bloodless maneuver and will be discussed under the heading of "Splenectomy."

That part of the dorsal mesogastrium which is located between the greater curvature of the stomach and the spleen is the gastrosplenic omentum; it contains continuations of the splenic artery known as the vasa brevia. The lienorenal ligament and the gastrosplenic omentum form the *splenic pedicle,* which connects the spleen to the kidney and the stomach; this pedicle consists of 4 layers (Figs. 410 B and 411).

ADULT SPLEEN

The spleen is covered completely by peritoneum except at the hilum (Fig. 410). It presents 4 surfaces: (1) a posterior surface which is convex and lies in contact with the diaphragm, (2) an anterior surface toward the stomach, (3) an inferior surface, which is small and rests on the splenic flexure of the colon and (4) an internal, which is in contact with the left kidney. The hilum is on the anterior or gastric surface, and posterior to it is a depression which lodges the tail of the pancreas. Vessels and nerves enter and leave at the hilum, and the lienorenal and the gastrosplenic ligaments attach here.

A phrenicocolic (costocolic) ligament runs from the splenic flexure of the colon to the diaphragm opposite the 10th and the 11th ribs (Fig. 410 A). This ligament is usually avascular and forms a floor on which the spleen rests, thus giving it additional support; it is of surgical importance in the mobilization of the spleen and the splenic flexure.

The adult spleen is placed high in the left

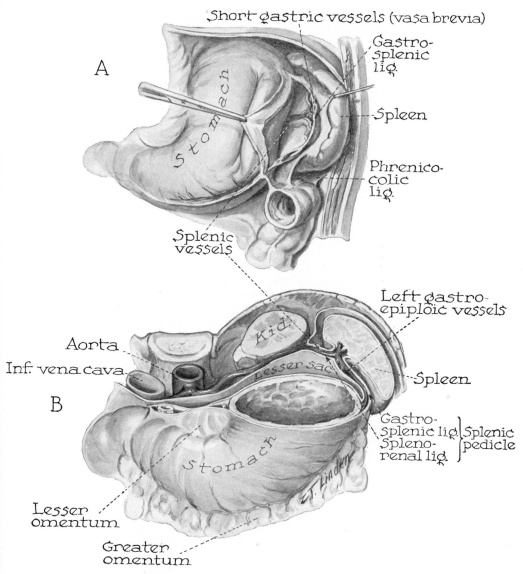

FIG. 410. The spleen. (A) The gastrosplenic ligament (part of the greater omentum) has been divided; the short gastric and the splenic vessels can be seen. (B) Cross section seen from above. The splenic pedicle consists of 4 layers: 2 derived from the splenorenal ligament and 2 derived from the gastrosplenic ligament.

posterior corner of the abdomen and lies deep to the 9th, the 10th and the 11th left ribs; its long axis corresponds to that of the 10th rib (Fig. 411). The peritoneal cavity, the diaphragm and the pleural cavity separate it from the ribs; the left lung intervenes in its upper third.

If the surgeon stands to the right of the patient and passes his right hand above the phrenicocolic ligament, he will be able to follow the diaphragm posteriorly, and the spleen will fall into his hand. At times, adhesion of variable density attach the spleen to the diaphragm; these must be severed before the organ can be mobilized properly. The exploring hand is stopped by the left layer of the lienorenal ligament

Vessels

The splenic artery passes to the left, along the upper border of the body and the tail of the pancreas and across the left kidney to reach the spleen (Fig. 410). The artery does not enter the spleen as a single large vessel but breaks up into from 5 to 8 terminal splenic branches.

The splenic vein is formed at the hilum of the spleen and is joined by the left gastroepiploic and other veins from the greater curvature of the stomach. It passes to the right in the lienorenal ligament behind the pancreas and lies below the splenic artery (Fig. 387). Behind the neck of the pancreas it joins the superior mesenteric vein to form the *portal vein;* in its course it receives the *inferior mesenteric vein.*

Accessory splenic tissue has been found in 11 per cent of autopsy material (Adami); the most common sites are near the hilum, the mesentery or the omentum, the tail of the pancreas and the bowel wall (Gray).

SPLENECTOMY

This operation has been performed for injuries to the spleen, hemolytic jaundice, Gaucher's disease, splenic anemia, tumors, cysts, hypersplenism and splenomegaly which produces pressure symptoms.

Many incisions have been described, including a thoracico-abdominal approach. The one preferred by Warren Cole is a curved oblique incision which starts high in the epigastrium about ¾ inch to the left of the midline and extends downward for a distance of 2 inches or more, then curves to the left and runs parallel with the costal margin; it sacrifices only the 11th nerve. Both the rectus sheath and the lateral oblique muscles are severed. Another incision frequently used is a straight paramedian one (Fig. 412 A). The right hand of the surgeon should be passed between the diaphragm and the spleen to determine its size and degree of mobility. If it is freely mobile and not anchored to the diaphragm by adhesions, the fingers of the right hand can be swept around its inferior border, and the organ brought through the abdominal incision and delivered onto the anterior abdominal wall. However, this usually is not the case, and mobilization becomes necessary. The gastrocolic and the gastrosplenic attachments are clamped and cut so that the anterior attachments of the spleen, or the anterior part of the pedicle, are

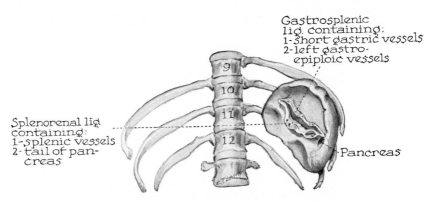

Fig. 411. The spleen in relation to the 10th rib. The cut splenic pedicle and its contents also are shown.

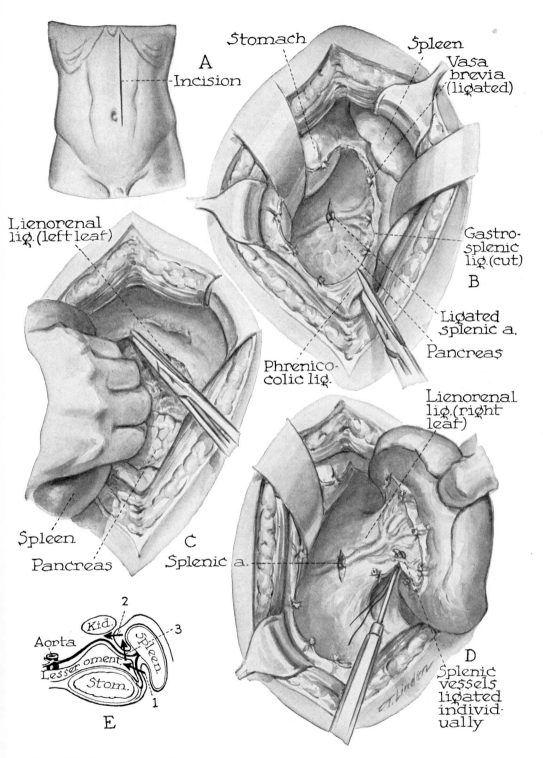

FIG. 412. Splenectomy. (A) Long left rectus incision. (B) The gastrosplenic ligament has been divided, and the vasa brevia have been ligated. An incision is made in the posterior parietal peritoneum, and the splenic artery is ligated. (C) The left leaf of the lienorenal ligament is cut. (D) The spleen is delivered, and individual ligation of the splenic vessels is accomplished. (E) Mobilization and removal of the spleen by dividing (1) the gastrosplenic ligament, (2) the left leaf of lienorenal ligament and (3) the right leaf of lienorenal ligament.

severed. The vessels which run in the gastro-splenic ligament (vasa brevia) are ligated (Figs. 412 B and E).

Cole is of the opinion that preliminary ligation of the splenic artery makes for better surgery. The posterior parietal peritoneum is incised over the upper border of the pancreas where the splenic artery is found. Since the artery runs a tortuous course, it humps over the upper border of the pancreas and can be seen, felt and ligated here.

The incision into the left leaf of the lienorenal ligament is next accomplished to permit further mobilization of the spleen (Fig. 412 C). This is divided, and the cleavage plane which permits delivery of the spleen and the splenic vessels is entered. If it is im-possible to see this leaf of peritoneum, it can be divided blindly over the upper pole of the kidney.

This step has been considered by many as a key to the operation, since this left leaf of lienorenal ligament anchors the spleen. When this ligament is cut, the spleen becomes mobile and can be drawn out through the abdominal incision. Following delivery, the vessels are ligated individually as they pass under cover of the right leaf of the lienorenal ligament.

The tail of the pancreas and the stomach should be carefully retracted and visualized before the clamps are applied to the remainder of the splenic pedicle so that these structures are not injured.

Pancreas

EMBRYOLOGY

The single adult pancreas is developed from two primitive pancreatic buds which are called the dorsal (proximal) pancreatic bud

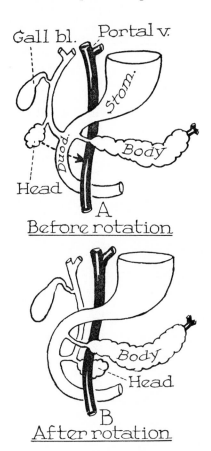

Before rotation

After rotation

FIG. 413. Embryology of the pancreas. (A) The 2 primitive pancreatic buds, dorsal and ventral, before rotation has taken place. The arrow indicates the path of rotation. (B) After rotation and before fusion of the pancreatic buds. The superior mesenteric vessels (portal vein) are "sandwiched in" between the primitive buds.

and the ventral (distal) pancreatic bud (Fig. 413).

The dorsal bud springs from the posterior border of the duodenum and grows between the leaves of the dorsal mesoduodenum; its duct system empties directly into the duodenum. The ventral bud arises from the anterior border of the duodenum and invades the ventral mesoduodenum; it originates with the primitive bile duct system; hence, its duct system communicates with that of the bile (Fig. 413 A).

The ventral bud rotates backward behind the duodenum, around its right side, and grows back into the dorsal mesoduodenum.

The two buds fuse; the ventral bud gives rise to the posterior portion of the lower part of the head and the uncinate process of the pancreas; the dorsal bud becomes the upper and the anterior part of the head, the neck, the body and the tail of the pancreas (Fig. 413 B). The right side of the pancreas is directed backward, and the left side forward; the right surface is applied to the posterior abdominal wall. The peritoneum which originally covered its right side is absorbed; therefore, in the adult, the pancreas appears to be retroperitoneal, being covered by the parietal peritoneum. At the time of fusion between the ventral and the dorsal buds, a communication is established between their ducts. The duct of the dorsal bud becomes the accessory pancreatic duct of Santorini, and the duct of the ventral bud becomes the main pancreatic duct of Wirsung. In about 20 per cent of individuals the accessory duct of Santorini becomes occluded and cannot compensate for trauma inflicted on the duct of Wirsung.

After rotation, the portal vein becomes "sandwiched in" between the dorsal bud which lies ventral to the vein and the ventral bud which now lies dorsal to the vein.

513

The last statement may appear confusing at first but if it is visualized it explains the ultimate positions of the superior mesenteric and the portal veins, between the head and the neck of the pancreas. It also explains how the accessory duct, which was formerly posterior, now enters on the anterior surface of the duodenum, and the main duct, which was originally anterior, now lies posteromedial.

ADULT PANCREAS

The adult pancreas is pistol-shaped (Figs. 414 and 415). Its length, which is variable, averages from 4 to 6 inches; it is divided indistinctly into a head, a neck, a body and a tail (Fig. 414). The head lies within the concavity of the duodenum and slightly overflows it. The neck is that portion which presents a slight constriction and lies in front of the portal vein.

The body of the pancreas continues to the left and upward; it presents a triangular shape on cross section, resulting in anterosuperior and anteroinferior surfaces. The transverse mesocolon attaches along the ridgelike junction of these 2 surfaces. The anterosuperior surface is covered by peritoneum of the lesser peritoneal cavity; the antero-inferior surface is covered by peritoneum of the greater peritoneal cavity. The right end of the transverse colon has no mesocolon; therefore, the head of the pancreas is directly attached to it, being separated from it only by a little areolar tissue.

The tail of the pancreas continues to the left and upward from the body until it abuts the spleen. Since it travels in the lienorenal ligament, this part of the pancreas loses its retroperitoneal characteristics and is more movable. The transverse mesocolon continues from the body to the tail of the pancreas so that the transverse colon hangs by a mesentery from only two parts of the pancreas, namely, the body and the tail. Pos-

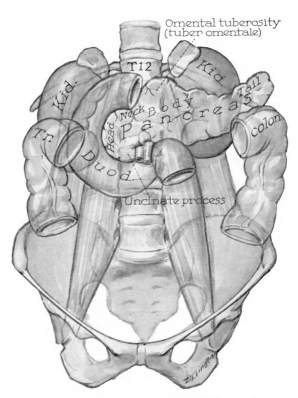

Fig. 414. Relations and divisions of the pancreas. The 2 projections of the pancreas, the uncinate process and the omental tuberosity, are identified.

teriorly, the head of the pancreas is in contact with the renal vessels and the inferior vena cava; behind the pancreatic neck lies the portal vein. Behind the body of the pancreas, from right to left, is the aorta (with the origin of the superior mesenteric and the renal arteries), the left suprarenal gland, the left kidney and the spleen.

The uncinate process (uncus hook) is a downward projection from the lower part of the head which hooks behind the superior mesenteric vessels.

The omental tuberosity (tuber omentale) is another pancreatic projection which projects upward from the body. It fits into the lesser curvature of the stomach, where it comes in contact with the lesser omentum, and separates it from the downward projecting tuber omentale of the liver (left lobe).

VESSELS

Arteries. The upper border of the pancreas is a good landmark for the arteries which supply it and other organs in this region (Fig. 415). The *splenic artery* passes to the left along the upper border of the body and the tail, and the *hepatic artery* passes to the right along the upper border of the head of the pancreas. Opposite the lower border of the duodenum the *gastroduodenal artery*

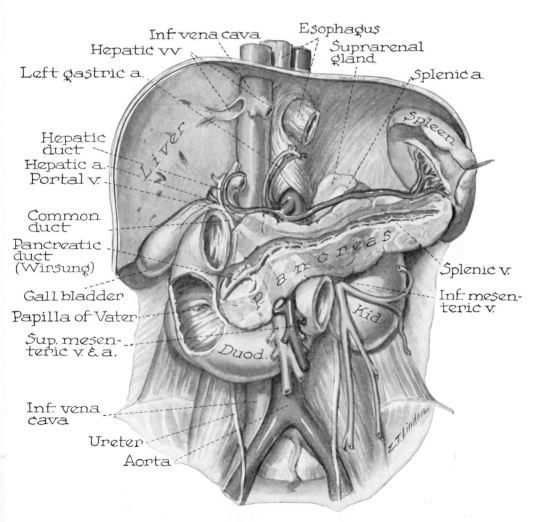

FIG. 415. The pancreas. The splenic artery passes to the left along the upper border of the body and the tail of the pancreas, and the hepatic artery passes to the right along the upper border of the neck and the head of the gland. The splenic vein lies behind the pancreas.

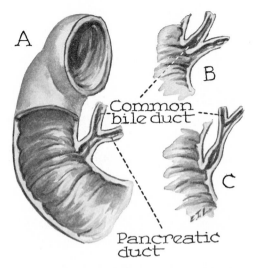

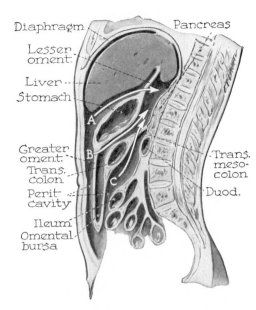

FIG. 416. Variations in the termination of the pancreatic duct. (A) Both ducts enter the ampulla of Vater independently. (B) The ducts enter the bowel independently. (C) The ducts join and enter the ampulla by a common channel.

FIG. 417. The 3 approaches to the pancreas: (A) through the lesser omentum; (B) through the greater omentum; (C) through the transverse mesocolon.

(*hepatic*) divides into a *superior pancreaticoduodenal* and *right gastroepiploic arteries* (Fig. 330). The *superior pancreaticoduodenal artery* divides and continues downward between the head of the pancreas and the duodenum as 2 parallel vessels, not as a single vessel, as is usually depicted. The *inferior pancreaticoduodenal* (*superior mesenteric*) *artery* also divides into 2 parallel vessels which anastomose with the 2 branches of the superior pancreaticoduodenal artery. In this way 2 arterial arches are formed: one in front of the head of the pancreas and another behind it. By means of these two arches the medial aspect of the duodenum receives an anterior and posterior set of vasa recta (Fig. 330). The head of the gland is supplied by the superior and the inferior pancreaticoduodenal arteries, and the body and the tail by the splenic artery.

Veins. Pancreatic veins issue from the pancreas and end in the *splenic vein*. The latter passes behind the body of the pancreas and below the splenic artery. It ends behind the neck of the pancreas by joining with the *superior mesenteric vein* to form the *portal vein*.

The lymphatics of the pancreas drain either directly or indirectly into the celiac glands around the root of the celiac artery.

DUCTS

The pancreatic duct of Wirsung forms the chief excretory channel of the gland. It begins in the tail and passes through the middle of the gland toward its head; its termination is quite variable (Fig. 416). In most instances, the duct opens independently into the ampulla of Vater, which then presents one opening common to both the pancreatic and the common bile ducts. In other instances, the pancreatic duct may join the common bile duct and both enter the ampulla by a common channel in another variation presents the common bile duct and the pancreatic duct enter the duodenum by entirely separate orifices.

The accessory pancreatic duct of Santorini represents the original duct of the dorsal bud. In the adult it passes to the right and in front of the common bile duct. It remains patent in most instances and opens into the duodenum about ¾ inch above the ampulla of Vater. In most individuals it anastomoses

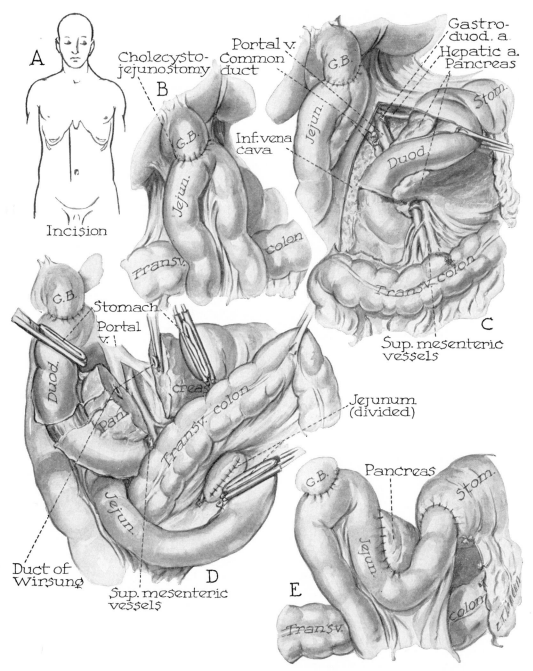

FIG. 418. Pancreatoduodenectomy. (A) A long right rectus incision gives ample exposure. (B) Cholecystojejunostomy may be done as a 1-stage operation or else combined with a radical 1-stage procedure. (C) The duodenum has been mobilized, and the gastroduodenal artery and the common duct have been severed and ligated. (D) The pylorus has been severed, and the pancreas has been incised over the superior mesenteric vessels. The jejunum has been divided immediately distal to the ligament of Treitz. (E) Following removal of the duodenum and the head of the pancreas, pancreaticojejunostomy and gastrojejunostomy complete the operation. In the 1-stage procedure it is thought preferable to anastomose the common duct to the jejunum.

with the chief pancreatic duct (Wirsung) within the head of the pancreas.

SURGICAL CONSIDERATIONS

The pancreas can be considered no longer as the "hermit" organ, since it now comes within the realm of modern surgery.

The approaches to the pancreas are along 3 anterior transperitoneal routes, namely, through the lesser omentum (gastrohepatic portion), the transverse mesocolon and the gastrocolic part of the greater omentum (Fig. 417). The last-named approach is preferred, since it affords greatest exposure and does not endanger the middle colic artery; however the site and the extent of the pathology determine which route is most applicable. If, for example, a pancreatic cyst points through the lesser omentum or the transverse mesocolon, these paths are taken.

PANCREATODUODENECTOMY

Pancreatoduodenectomy is done for carcinoma of the head of the pancreas, carcinoma of the ampulla of Vater and carcinoma of the lower end of the common bile duct (Fig. 418). It may be performed in 1 or 2 stages. Whipple has done much of the pioneer work in this field. Many types of operative procedures have been described, and a typical one will be discussed here.

The scope of this operation calls for a block resection of the head of the pancreas, the lower end of the common duct, the pylorus of the stomach and the entire duodenum. Hence, the gastrointestinal tract, the biliary tract and the pancreas are interrupted. The gastrointestinal tract can be restored by an end-to-side or end-to-end gastrojejunostomy. The biliary tract can be restored by an anastomosis of the common bile duct or the common hepatic duct to a portion of the gastrointestinal tract; in the 2-stage operation the gallbladder can be used for the anastomosis. Some surgeons advocate closure of the cut end of the pancreas; others prefer to anastomose it to the jejunum.

Surgery is contraindicated if the portal vein or the superior mesenteric vessels are involved, if there are multiple distant metastases, or if there is invasion beyond the limits of resection. Involvement of the portal vein can be discerned by division of the gastroduodenal artery and displacement of the common duct downward. Involvement of the superior mesenteric vessels is determined by division of the gastrocolic omentum and incision of the peritoneum along the inferior border of the pancreas.

If a 2-stage procedure is utilized, a cholecystojejunostomy is done first, and at the second stage this is displaced downward. The peritoneum over the right kidney is incised to the right of the duodenum, and the duodenum and the head of the pancreas are mobilized to the left. The gastrocolic omentum is divided, and the third part of the duodenum, the head of the pancreas and the superior mesenteric vessels are exposed. The gastroduodenal artery is divided and ligated; the common duct is divided, and the proximal end is invaginated. The stomach, the body of the pancreas and the jejunum are divided; the ligament of Treitz is freed. The block of tissue is removed, and the operation is completed by performing the following anastomoses: end-to-side or end-to-end gastrojejunostomy, pancreaticojejunostomy and cholecystojejunostomy (previously done in the 2-stage procedure).

SURGERY FOR PANCREATITIS

Pancreatitis is still a rather obscure lesion, but the surgical procedures which have been utilized, if the case is operated on, are in the form of cholecystostomy and incision of the pancreatic capsule. This capsule is the posterior parietal peritoneum which covers the organ.

ABDOMEN

Blood Supply of the Gut

The primitive gut is divisible into 3 parts: foregut, midgut and hindgut. The foregut ends and the midgut begins where the bile duct enters the duodenum; the midgut ends, and the hindgut begins at the junction of the right and the middle thirds of the transverse colon. Each of the above 3 portions has its own blood vessel, as follows: (1) the foregut is supplied by the celiac artery, (2) the midgut is supplied by the superior mesenteric artery, (3) the hindgut is supplied by the inferior mesenteric artery (Fig. 419).

The celiac artery supplies the stomach and the duodenum to the entrance of the bile duct and its associated glands, the liver, the pancreas and the spleen; the superior mesenteric artery supplies the duodenum distal to the entrance of the bile duct, the jejunum, the ileum and the colon almost as far as the left colic flexure; the inferior mesenteric artery supplies the descending colon, the sigmoid and the rectum. Only the more common vascular patterns will be described; the student must always remember that anatomic variations must continually be kept in mind.

CELIAC ARTERY (CELIAC AXIS)

The celiac artery (celiac axis) is the first branch of the abdominal aorta; it is short, about ½ inch long, and thick. The artery originally arose at the level of the 7th cervical vertebra, but during development, the lungs pushed the diaphragm caudally, and the diaphragm in turn forced the stomach and the celiac vessel downward. Therefore, in its final position the median arcuate ligament, which unites the two crura of the diaphragm, lies immediately above the artery, and the crura are on each side of it.

The vessel cannot be seen until the lesser omentum is incised, and then it is found immediately above the pancreas and behind the posterior parietal peritoneum. It is found at the level between the last thoracic and the 1st lumbar vertebrae. After passing almost horizontally forward for ½ inch it trifurcates into (1) the left gastric artery, (2) the splenic artery and (3) the hepatic artery.

Left Gastric Artery (Coronary Artery). This is the smallest of the 3 branches. It runs

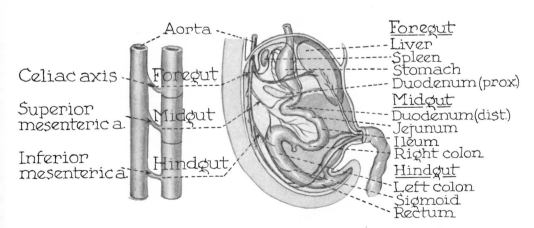

FIG. 419. A diagrammatic representation of the embryology of the foregut, the midgut and the hindgut, and the blood supply to each of these and their derivatives.

obliquely upward and to the left until it nearly reaches the esophagus; it then arches sharply forward to reach the lesser curvature of the stomach. In so doing it drags a fold of peritoneum with it; this forms a "mesentery" for the vessel, known as the left gastro-pancreatic fold. In its course it first lies on the left crus of the diaphragm behind the lesser sac; it then passes into the gastro-pancreatic fold and finally continues between the layers of the lesser omentum. When it reaches the stomach, it supplies esophageal branches which pass upward and anastomose with esophageal branches of the thoracic aorta. Its branches are distributed to both surfaces of the stomach; these anastomose with the short gastric branches of the splenic and the gastroepiploic arteries.

Splenic Artery (Lineal Artery). This is the largest branch of the celiac artery and is remarkable for its tortuosity. It travels to the left along the upper border of the pancreas, into which it sends branches. It crosses the left crus of the diaphragm, the left adrenal gland and the upper part of the left kidney. It then enters the lienorenal ligament, through which it gains entrance to the hilum of the spleen by means of 5 to 8 terminal splenic branches. Short gastric arteries (vasa brevia), from 4 to 6 in number, reach the fundus and the greater curvature of the stomach via the gastroepiploic vessels. The left gastro-epiploic artery arises from the front of the splenic artery close to its termination, passes forward between the layers of the gastro-splenic omentum into the greater omentum and then continues from left to right along

the greater curvature, about one finger's breadth from it. It anastomoses with the right gastroepiploic artery. In its course it supplies branches to both surfaces of the stomach and long slender omental branches.

Hepatic Artery. This artery passes to the right along the upper border of the pancreas, turns upward in the lesser omentum and runs in front of the portal vein and to the left of the common bile duct. Its gastroduodenal branch arises above the upper border of the first part of the duodenum, passes downward behind the duodenum and in its downward course lies between the duodenum and the pancreas. Opposite the lower border of the duodenum, the gastroduodenal artery divides into a right gastroepiploic and a superior pancreaticoduodenal artery. The *right gastroepiploic artery* travels from right to left between the layers of greater omentum, supplying the stomach, as does the left gastro-epiploic with which it anastomoses. The *superior pancreaticoduodenal artery* continues between the duodenum and the head of the pancreas. It forms a double arch by dividing into anterior and posterior branches and anastomoses with similar branches from the inferior pancreaticoduodenal branch of the superior mesenteric artery. The anterior arch runs in front of the head of the pancreas, and the posterior arch passes behind it (Fig. 330).

Right Gastric Artery. This artery arises opposite or near (usually distal to) the gastroduodenal artery, makes a sharp turn backward on itself and passes between the layers of the lesser omentum to the pylorus; it then

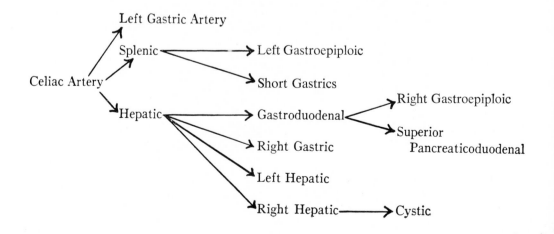

passes along the lesser curvature of the stomach and anastomoses with the left gastric artery. The hepatic artery continues upward to the porta hepatis, where it divides into right and left hepatic arteries which are distributed to corresponding lobes of the liver. The cystic artery is usually a branch of the right hepatic artery.

MESENTERIC VESSELS

Superior Mesenteric Artery. This vessel constitutes a vascular axis around which early rotation takes place. After rotation, those branches which originally arose from the right side of the vessel now arise from the left, and vice versa. This vessel originates from the front of the aorta about ½ inch below the origin of the celiac artery and opposite the first lumbar vertebra. At its origin it lies behind the pancreas and the splenic vein. Where it passes in front of the duodenum it is crossed anteriorly by the transverse colon; in the lower part of its course it lies behind the coils of the small intestine. Although the superior mesenteric artery and vein lie behind the body of the pancreas, they pass anterior to the uncinate process of the head of the pancreas. The vessel takes a downward and forward course, descending between the layers of the mesentery to the right iliac fossa where, considerably diminished in size, it anastomoses with one of its own branches, the ileocolic artery. As it travels in the root of the mesentery it crosses the third part of the duodenum, the aorta, the inferior vena cava, the right ureter and the psoas major muscle in the order named. Its branches are: the inferior pancreaticoduodenal, the intestinal (jejunal and ileal), the ileocolic, the right colic and the middle colic arteries; although mentioned last, the middle colic artery is really the first branch.

Inferior Pancreaticoduodenal Artery. This artery arises opposite the upper border of the transverse (third) portion of the duodenum. It courses to the right between the head of the pancreas and the duodenum, passing behind the superior mesenteric vein. The vessel divides into anterior and posterior branches which anastomose with corresponding anterior and posterior branches of the superior pancreaticoduodenal artery and in

this way forms 2 vascular arches: one in front of the right margin of the head of the pancreas and the other behind it. These arches supply the head of the pancreas and, by means of the straight vasa recta, supply the corresponding part of the duodenum. Of surgical importance is the fact that the pancreatic part of the common duct descends between these arches (Fig. 330).

Jejunal and Ileal Arteries. From 10 to 15 in number, these arteries spring from the left (convex) side of the superior mesenteric artery and pass obliquely forward and downward between the layers of the mesentery; each divides into 2 branches which anastomose with adjacent arteries to form a series of arcades, the convexities of which are directed toward the intestines. From these arcades, straight terminal vessels, the vasa recta, pass to the wall of the gut, some going to one side, and some to the other. Occasionally, one of these will divide and supply both sides of the gut wall. Distally, from jejunum to ileum the upper jejunal branches form only 1 or 2 arches, but the process of division and union is repeated 3 or 4 times in the region of the ileal branches; thus 4 or 5 tiers of arches are formed in the longer lower part of the mesentery. This latter fact may aid the surgeon in distinguishing between the upper and the lower coils of small intestine. The vasa recta themselves do not anastomose but pass to the submucous plexus, where they ramify and then anastomose.

In severing the bowel, it is advisable to remove less of the mesenteric than of the antimesenteric border so that the retained cut margin may have an adequate blood supply.

Colic Branches. The 3 colic branches are: the ileocolic, the right colic and the middle colic. They arise from the right side of the superior mesenteric artery. They travel behind the peritoneum, bifurcate and anastomose with the artery on each side of it; in this way the loops form a continuous vessel which runs along the mesenteric margin of the large bowel. This same arrangement continues in the branches of the left colic and the sigmoid branches (inferior mesenteric artery). The result is a continuous "vessel" known as the *"marginal artery of Drummond."* This "artery" extends from the ascending colon to the end of the pelvic colon; its distance from the margin of the bowel varies from almost hugging the bowel wall to 8 cm. away from it. It lies closest to the bowel along the descending and the pelvic colons.

Ileocolic Artery. This artery arises from the superior mesenteric artery about halfway down its right side; it descends subperitoneally toward the ileocolic region. In its course it crosses the inferior vena cava, the ureter and the testicular vessels (the latter two structures lie on the psoas fascia). It divides into ascending and descending branches. The ascending branch supplies the proximal part of the ascending colon and anastomoses with the right colic artery. The descending branch may be a very short trunk and is better referred to as the ileocecal artery. The latter also supplies the ileal branch, which anastomoses with the end of the superior mesenteric artery; therefore, it anastomoses with itself. The ileocecal artery also supplies anterior and posterior cecal branches.

The all-important and sometimes troublesome appendicular artery is a branch of the posterior cecal branch of the ileocecal artery. It passes behind the ileum and not behind the cecum. The artery enters the free border of the mesentery of the appendix and sends a few straight branches to the vermiform appendix. It does not anastomose with any other artery; hence, if it is obstructed or kinked, early gangrene of the appendix results.

Right Colic Artery. This vessel arises a little below the duodenum and runs to the right and behind the peritoneum. It crosses the same structures as the ileocolic artery and divides into an ascending branch which anastomoses with the middle colic and a descending branch which anastomoses with the ileocolic. Not infrequently, the right colic artery fails to arise as a separate branch but springs from the ileocolic or the middle colic artery.

Middle Colic Artery. This is the first branch of the superior mesenteric artery. The term "middle" should not be misleading, since the vessel actually passes to the right side of the transverse colon. Because of this fact the openings in the transverse mesocolon should be made in its left half. The vessel arises at the lower border of the pancreas and enters the root of the transverse mesocolon. It then passes downward and to the right between the 2 layers of the transverse mesocolon. It divides into a right branch, which supplies the right third of the transverse colon and anastomoses with the ascending branch of the right colic artery, and a left branch which supplies the left two thirds of the transverse colon and anastomoses with the superior left colic artery. Students erroneously picture the vessel as passing upward because of the many illustrations in which the transverse colon has been pulled up. In reality its course is distinctly downward. The middle colic artery may be injured while incising the transverse mesocolon in a posterior gastrojejunostomy, or it may be ligated accidentally with the gastrocolic ligament (greater omentum) in performing a gastrectomy. If the vessel has a free anastomosis with the left colic artery, necrosis will be avoided, but should the anastomosis be imperfect, the colon in the region of the splenic flexure becomes gangrenous and resection becomes imperative.

For *inferior mesenteric artery* see p. 460.

Pelvic Bones

The complete bony ring which forms the pelvis, so named because of its resemblance to a basin, is composed of 2 hip bones, anteriorly and laterally, and the sacrum and the coccyx, posteriorly. The cavity thus created is divided into a smaller inferior portion called the *true pelvis* and a larger superior one, the *false pelvis*. The line of separation between these two is the *iliopectineal line* (Fig. 420). The side walls of the true pelvis are formed largely by the pubes and the ischia; the side walls of the false pelvis are formed by the ilia.

Distinct differences exist between the male and the female pelves. The female pelvis is distinguished from the male pelvis by the following features: its bones are more delicate, its depth less, the entire pelvis is less massive, its muscular impressions are less marked, the anterior iliac spines are more widely separated, the superior aperture of the lesser pelvis is larger and more circular, the obturator foramina are triangular, the coccyx is more movable, and the pubic arch is wider and more rounded, forming an angle rather than an arch. In brief, the female pelvis appears to be wider, more shallow and more graceful.

HIP BONE

Galen wrote that since the hip bone resembles no commonplace object, no name had been given to the bone; therefore, it became known as the *innominate* or unnamed bone. It consists of 3 parts: the ilium, the ischium and the pubis. These meet at the acetabulum. Up to the age of 12 the connecting piece is a triradiate segment of cartilage which begins to ossify at about this period; ossification usually is complete by the age of 16 (Figs. 421 and 422).

ILIUM

The ilium (L. flank) is the largest of the 3 bones and forms the larger upper expanded area of the hip bone. It is fan-shaped, the

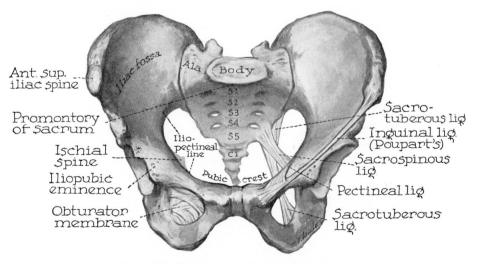

FIG. 420. The bony pelvis, seen from above.

handle of the fan being placed downward where the ilium joins the ischium and the pubis.

The iliac crest is the arched upper border which is easily felt in the living subject at the lower limit of the waist. Its margins are called the outer and the inner lips, and the interval between them is called the intermediate area. The highest point of the crest is at its middle and toward the back; this marks the level of the body of the 4th lumbar vertebra.

The iliac crest is crossed by cutaneous nerves; since no muscles cross it, the deep fascia attaches here. It terminates anteriorly in a small tubercle called the *anterior superior iliac spine,* which is an important surgical landmark and can be felt easily at the upper end of the fold of the groin.

The crest terminates behind in a sharp *posterior superior iliac spine* which can be felt on a level with the 2nd sacral spine, at the bottom of the small dimple which is visible in the upper and the medial part of the buttock.

The tubercle of the crest is a tiny projection on the external lip; it is palpable about 2 inches above and behind the anterior superior spine; in the living, it forms the highest point when viewed from in front. It is

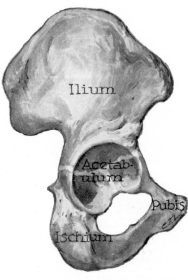

Fig. 421. The innominate (hip) bone. It consists of 3 parts (the ilium, the ischium and the pubis), which meet at the acetabulum.

approximately at the level of the body of the 5th lumbar vertebra.

Borders. *The anterior border* of the ilium is concave and extends from the anterior superior spine to the iliopubic eminence, which marks the junction between the ilium and the pubis. This border is subdivided into 2 equal concavities by the anterior inferior iliac spine, the latter being too deeply situated to be palpable through the skin; the iliopsoas leaves the abdomen through the notch between it and the iliopubic eminence.

The posterior border extends from the posterior superior iliac spine toward the ischial spine through a point on the margin of the greater sciatic notch opposite the middle of the acetabulum. It is subdivided into 2 unequal concavities by the *posterior inferior iliac spine,* which lies at the posterior limit of the sacro-iliac joint about 1 inch below the posterior superior iliac spine. The upper concavity is slight; the lower concavity forms the upper part of the *greater sciatic notch.*

Surfaces. The ilium has 2 surfaces, an inner and an outer.

The inner surface is subdivided into the iliac fossa, the tuberosity, the auricular surface and an area within the true pelvis (Fig. 422 B). The *iliac fossa* is the large, smooth, medial surface which is limited posteriorly by a roughened area, through which the hip bone articulates with the sacrum at the sacroiliac joint, and is limited inferiorly by a prominent ridge, the *iliopectineal line.* The *iliac tuberosity* is the rough part of the inner surface, and the *auricular surface* articulates with the sacrum. The *area within the true pelvis* is the lowest part which is smooth and helps to form the side wall of the true pelvis.

The outer (gluteal) surface, also known as the *dorsum ilii,* presents a wavy appearance and is crossed by 3 rough lines: the inferior, the middle and the posterior gluteal lines, which converge on the greater sciatic notch and divide the surface into 4 areas for the gluteal muscles (Fig. 422 A). The areas for the gluteus medius and minimus muscles are extensive; however, a small and restricted area is present between the gluteus minimus and the acetabular margin for the iliofemoral ligament and the reflected head of the rectus femoris. The *posterior gluteal line* passes upward and slightly forward from the posterior inferior iliac spine to the iliac crest. The *middle (anterior) gluteal line* runs from the middle of the upper border of the greater sciatic notch forward to the iliac crest, just in front of its tubercle. The *inferior gluteal line* is quite indistinct and passes from the apex of the greater sciatic notch to the notch which exists between the anterior superior and the anterior inferior iliac spines.

ISCHIUM

The ischium (G. buttock) consists of 3 parts: a body which adjoins the ilium, a tuberosity projecting downward from the body and a ramus (inferior) which passes from the tuberosity upward below the obturator foramen.

The body is triangular on cross section and therefore presents 3 surfaces which are separated by 3 borders. The borders are parts of the margin of the obturator foramen, the acetabulum and the greater sciatic notch. The surfaces are pelvic (medial), acetabular (lateral) and gluteal (posterior).

The tuberosity (tuber ischii) is an oval mass of bone which caps the posterior aspect of the lower part of the body of the bone. The upper part of the medial border is crossed by the tendon of the obturator in-

ternus; it is smooth, is covered by a bursa, and it forms part of the lesser sciatic notch. The lower part of the medial border is a rough crest for the attachment of the sacro-tuberous ligament. The lateral border gives origin to the quadratus femoris, and between this and the acetabulum the groove for the obturator externus is located. Its chief function is to support the body weight when sitting.

The ramus of the ischium is a flattened bar of bone that projects forward and medially from the tuberosity. It joins the inferior ramus of the pubis, and together these "conjoined rami" form the sides of the *pubic arch*.

Sciatic Notches. The *greater sciatic notch* is a wide gap which is situated between the posterior inferior iliac spine and the ischial spine; it is bounded by the posterior borders of the ilium and the ischium. The *lesser sciatic notch* is the small gap situated between the ischial spine and the ischial tuberosity. These notches are converted into sciatic foramina (greater and lesser) by the sacrospinous and the sacrotuberous ligaments. The floor of the cartilage-covered surface of the lesser sciatic notch is grooved by the tendon of the obturator internus.

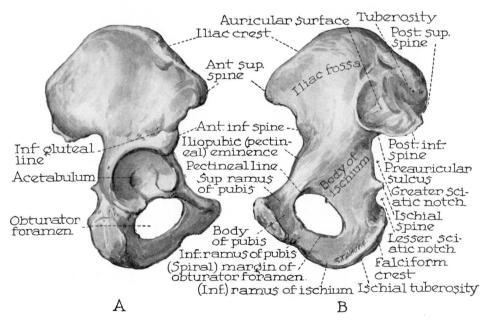

FIG. 422. The right hip bone: (A) seen from without; (B) seen from within.

Pubis

The pubic bone (L. pubis, adult) has received its name from that region where the hair develops during adulthood. It consists of a body and 2 rami (superior and inferior).

Body. The body is the wide, flattened, medial part of the bone, the pelvic surface of which looks upward and is smooth; it is in relation to the retropubic fat pad and the bladder. The femoral surface is rough, and the symphysial surface is joined to the opposite pubic bone by the fibrocartilage and the ligaments of the symphysis pubis; the lateral border bounds the obturator foramen.

Crest. The pubic crest forms the upper border of the body of the bone and is easily felt at the lower limit of the abdomen and at the side of the midline.

Tubercle. The crest terminates laterally in the pubic tubercle to which the medial end of the inguinal ligament is attached. If the hip bone is held in the erect position, the tubercle and the anterior superior iliac spine are in the same vertical plane.

Rami. *The superior ramus* has 2 ends, 3 surfaces and 3 borders. The medial end is expanded and becomes the body, and the lateral end expands and fuses with the ilium and the ischium to form part of the acetabulum. The upper border is sharp and is called the *pectineal line;* it extends from the pubic tubercle to the iliopubic eminence. The anterior border is a ridge known as the obturator crest; it extends from the pubic tubercle to the acetabular notch. The inferior border forms the upper margin of the obturator foramen. The pectineal surface is triangular in shape and is situated between the pubic crest and the iliopubic eminence; it gives origin to the pectineus muscle. The pelvic surface is smooth and continuous with

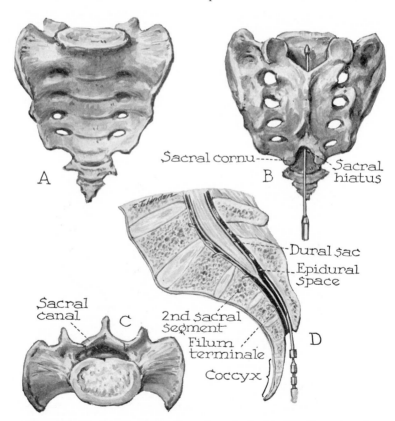

Fig. 423. The sacrum. (A) Seen from in front. (B) Posterior view, a probe has been placed through the sacral hiatus and into the sacral canal. (C) Seen from above. (D) Sagittal section showing a needle placed in the epidural space.

the body of the bone; the obturator surface is the upper boundary of the obturator foramen.

The inferior ramus passes downward and laterally from the body to meet the ramus of the ischium.

ACETABULUM

The acetabulum (L. little cup for vinegar) forms the socket for the head of the femur (Fig. 421). The ilium, the pubis and the ischium meet in the center of this cavity, and their lines of fusion radiate from the center like the spokes of a wheel. These lines are visible in the child, but in the adult they are no longer evident. The acetabulum is directed laterally and downward. It presents a horseshoe-shaped area which is covered with cartilage, but it leaves a rough acetabular fossa in the floor which adjoins the *acetabular notch* (the gap in the lower part of the cup above the obturator foramen). The transverse ligament completes the rim and converts the notch into a foramen (Fig. 648). The articular branches of the obturator and the medial circumflex arteries enter the joint through this notch.

The obturator foramen is below the acetabulum and is closed by the obturator membrane, which is attached to its margins except above at the obturator groove; through this groove the obturator vessels and nerves pass out of the pelvis.

SACRUM AND COCCYX

SACRUM

The sacrum is triangular in shape, possessing an upper surface which forms its base and a lower end which corresponds to the apex; it has pelvic, dorsal and 2 lateral surfaces (Fig. 423). The bone is formed by 5 fused vertebrae. The female sacrum is broader than the male sacrum and is more abruptly curved below. It is inserted like a wedge between the 2 hip bones; its base articulates with the last lumbar vertebra and its apex with the coccyx. The pelvic surface is marked by 4 transverse ridges at the ends of which are the anterior sacral foramina. There are 4 foramina on each side; they diminish in size from above downward and give exit to the anterior divisions of the sacral nerves and entrance to the lateral sacral arteries. Lateral to these foramina are the so-called lateral parts of the sacrum.

A sagittal section through the center of the bone shows that the bone is united at the circumference, but that a centrally placed interval is filled by fibrocartilage. The dorsal surface is convex and reveals the posterior sacral foramina which are smaller in size than the anterior and transmit the posterior divisions of the sacral nerves. The inferior articular processes of the 5th sacral vertebra are prolonged downward as the sacral cornua, which connect with the cornua of the coccyx.

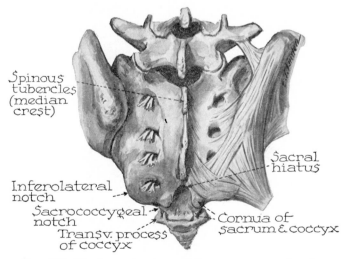

FIG. 424. The bony structure of the sacrococcygeal region.

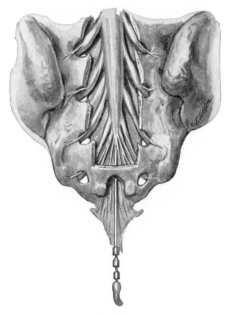

FIG. 425. Sacral anesthesia. A needle
has been placed through the sacral hiatus
and into the sacral canal. The bony roof
of the sacral canal has been removed.

The anterior projecting upper surface of the
body of the 1st sacral vertebra is the promontory. The posterior wall of the sacral canal
is formed by the superficial posterior sacrococcygeal ligament where the laminae of the
5th sacral vertebra are absent. The sacral

hiatus transmits the 5th sacral nerve, the
coccygeal nerves and the filum terminale.

Coccyx

The coccyx is formed from the rudimentary vertebrae which tend to fuse. The bone
has a base, an apex, dorsal and pelvic surfaces and lateral borders. Its apex points
downward.

Sacrococcygeal Region

Toward the base of the coccyx, where it
articulates with the sacrum, 2 lateral bony
prominences can be palpated; these are the
coccygeal and the sacral cornua which bound
the sacral hiatus (Fig. 424). The hiatus is
the external opening of the sacrococcygeal
canal. The termination of the subarachnoid
space can be indicated by a line which joins
the posterior superior spines of the 1st and
the 2nd sacral foramina.

The skin over the sacrococcygeal region
is resistant and thick; it is loose and movable
over the convexity of the sacrum but is bound
down in the region of the anal crease. The
inferior portion of the dorsal layer of lumbodorsal fascia forms a musculo-aponeurotic
layer over the sacrum. This fuses with the
tendinous origin of the spinal muscles.

Sacral anesthesia is an extradural type
which reaches the nerves within the sacral

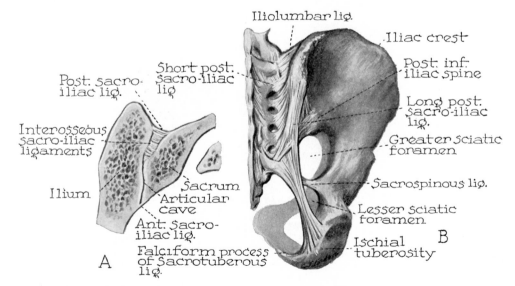

FIG. 426. The sacro-iliac region: (A) cross section; (B) seen from behind.

canal (Fig. 425). This produces anesthesia in the perineum and the external genitalia. In the caudad type of sacral anesthesia the needle is placed through the sacrococcygeal ligament, into the sacral hiatus and then upward along the sacral canal for from 3 to 4 cm.

SACRO-ILIAC REGION

Transsacral anesthesia is produced by direct injection of the anesthetizing agent into the sacral canal and around the sacral nerves via each of the posterior sacral foramina.

The sacro-iliac joints include the 3 upper sacral segments and the articular surfaces of the ilia (Fig. 426). The joints act as shock absorbers between the spinal column and the lower extremities. Although the sacro-iliac articulation is synovial in type, it permits very little movement. The articular surfaces of the joint are mainly smooth, but several projections and depressions help to lock and stabilize it. Union is maintained by anterior, interosseous, short and long posterior sacro-iliac ligaments. The sacrotuberous and the sacrospinous ligaments further stabilize the joint; these arise over the whole area of the posterior sacro-iliac ligaments and attach at the ischial tuberosity and the spine. The interosseous sacro-iliac ligament, the short and the long posterior sacro-iliac ligaments, and the iliolumbar ligament resist forward rotation of the upper end of the sacrum. The sacrotuberous and the sacrospinous ligaments resist backward rotation of the lower end of the sacrum (Fig. 427).

Surgical approaches to the sacro-iliac joint have been described by Smith-Petersen and Picque.

MUSCULAR AND LIGAMENTOUS ATTACHMENTS

The attachments to the hip bone can be outlined in the following way (Fig. 428):

Ilium:

To the anterosuperior iliac spine: the inguinal ligament, the sartorius and the tensor fasciae latae muscles.

To the outer lip: the external abdominal oblique muscle, the latissimus dorsi and the fascia lata.

To the intermediate area: the internal oblique muscle.

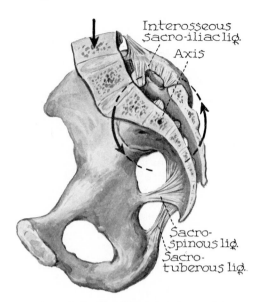

FIG. 427. The ligaments that resist sacral rotation.

To the inner lip: the transversus abdominis muscle, the quadratus lumborum muscle and the iliolumbar ligament. At the inner lip the transversalis fascia becomes continuous with the iliac fascia.

To the posterosuperior iliac spine: the long posterior sacro-iliac ligament.

To the posterosuperior and the posteroinferior iliac spines: the piriformis muscle.

To the antero-inferior iliac spine: the straight head of the rectus femoris muscle and the iliofemoral ligament.

To the gluteal surface: the reflected head of the rectus femoris muscle, the gluteus minimus, the gluteus medius and the gluteus maximus muscles.

To the upper part of the iliac fossa: the iliacus.

To the iliac tuberosity: the sacrospinalis muscle and the posterior and the interosseous sacro-iliac ligaments.

To the auricular surface: the anterior sacro-iliac ligament.

Ischium and Pubis:

To the ischial tuberosity: the quadratus femoris, the sacrotuberous ligament, the semitendinosus, the long head of the biceps and the adductor magnus.

To the ischial spine: the gemellus superior and the gemellus inferior muscles, the levator

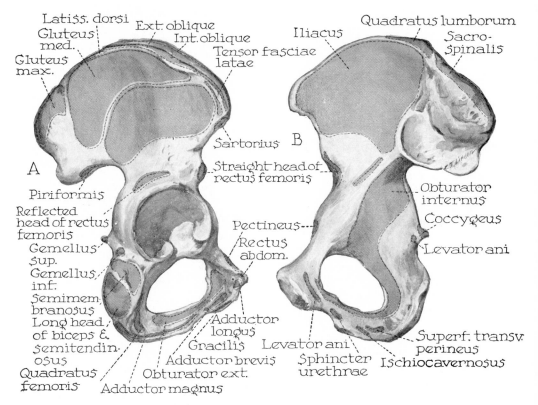

Latiss. dorsi   Ext. oblique   Quadratus lumborum
  Gluteus   Int. oblique   Iliacus   Sacro-
   med.   Tensor fasciae   Spinalis
Gluteus   latae
max.

                                          Sartorius   B
A   Straight head of
                                 rectus femoris
Piriformis   Obturator
Reflected   internus
head of rectus   Coccygeus
femoris   Pectineus
Gemellus   Rectus   Levator ani
sup.   abdom.
Gemellus
inf.
Semimem
branosus
Long head   Adductor
of biceps &   longus   Superf. transv.
semitendin   Gracilis Levator ani   perineus
osus   Adductor brevis Sphincter Ischiocavernosus
Quadratus   Obturator ext.   urethrae
femoris   Adductor magnus

FIG. 428. Muscular attachments to the iliac bone: (A) seen from without;
(B) seen from within.

ani, the coccygeus and the sacrospinous ligament.

To the pelvic surface of the ischium and the ilium: the obturator internus.

To the body of the pubis (pelvic surface): the levator ani, the puboprostatic ligament and the adductor longus.

From the region of the symphysis and the inferior ramus: the gracilis, the adductor brevis and the obturator externus. The adductor magnus originates at the lower end of the ischium medial to the gracilis. The crus penis, the ischiocavernosus, the superficial transverse perinei, the perineal membrane, the sphincter urethrae, the deep transverse perinei, the falciform process of the sacrotuberous ligament and the inferior pubic ligament are also attached here.

To the symphysial surface: the fibrocartilage of the symphysis and the anterior, posterior, superior and inferior pubic ligaments.

To the crest: the aponeurosis of the external abdominal oblique, the fascia lata, the conjoined tendon, the pyramidalis and the rectus abdominis muscles and the transversalis fascia.

To the pectineal line: the pectineus muscle, the pectineal fascia, the reflected part of the inguinal ligament, the conjoined tendon, the transversalis fascia and the psoas minor muscles.

To the antero-inferior iliac spine: the iliofemoral ligament.

To the obturator crest: the pubofemoral ligament.

Pelvic Diaphragm

MUSCLES

The muscles within the true pelvis may be considered in two groups: (1) two muscles which together form the pelvic diaphragm and are associated with the pelvic viscera (levator ani and coccygeus) and (2) two muscles which are associated with the lower extremity but arise in the pelvis (obturator internus and piriformis).

The walls of the pelvis minor are covered on each side by the obturator internus and posterior to this by the piriformis; these are referred to as the pelvifemoral group of muscles (Fig. 429). Therefore, the walls of the pelvis are padded by muscles of the thigh, since both the obturator internus and the piriformis insert into the femur. They are covered by fascia, which will be discussed subsequently (p. 535).

Obturator Internus Muscle. This muscle covers the inner aspect of the pelvis. It arises from the pelvic surface of the obturator membrane and from the pelvic surface of the hip bone behind the obturator foramen. In its posterior part the muscle extends up to the iliopectineal line. Its upper border recedes and falls short of the upper margin of the obturator foramen; thus, the obturator vessels and nerves can leave the pelvis without having to pierce it. The muscle bundles converge toward and almost fill the lesser sciatic foramen; the converging tendon bends sharply at the margin of the foramen and inserts on the medial surface of the greater trochanter just above the trochanteric fossa. It acts as an external rotator of the thigh. The nerve supply of the obturator internus muscle has been referred to as a "special nerve" which arises from L 5 and S 1 and 2.

Piriformis muscle (S 1 and 2). Like the obturator internus, this muscle arises from the osseoligamentous framework of the in-

terior of the pelvis. It lies on the posterior wall of the pelvis and arises from the 2nd, the 3rd and the 4th pieces of the sacrum. Its fibers travel outward and converge to form a musculo-aponeurotic tendon which leaves the pelvis through the greater sciatic foramen. It inserts into the top of the greater trochanter and, although it belongs, with the obturator internus, to the pelvifemoral group, nevertheless it serves a diaphragmatic function, since

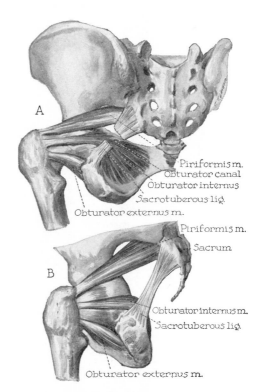

FIG. 429. Muscles of the true pelvis (obturator internus and piriformis). (A) Seen from behind; a section of the sacrotuberous ligament has been removed. (B) Posterolateral view.

531

it is continuous in the same plane with the coccygeus (Fig. 430 B). In the standing position, the muscle is on the wall rather than on the floor of the pelvic cavity. It abducts the flexed thigh and laterally rotates the extended thigh.

The pelvic diaphragm is composed of 2 muscles on each side: the levator ani and the coccygeus (Figs. 430, 431 and 432).

The levator ani may be divided into 2 parts: the *pubococcygeus* and the *iliococcygeus*. The 3 muscles (pubococcygeus, iliococcygeus and coccygeus) are the original "tail" muscles which take this origin from the pelvic bone and together form the whole of the pelvic diaphragm. A distinct space of cleft separates them, but this is apparent only when the fascia is removed. The levator ani

arises from the inner side of the pubis for a short distance lateral to the symphysis and from the tendinous arch (white line).

The pubococcygeal portion of the levator ani is placed more medially; its fibers pass in an anteroposterior direction and insert into a dense ligament behind the rectum. This ligament is known as the anterior sacrococcygeal ligament and is inserted into the lower two pieces of sacrum and the upper segment of coccyx. The pubococcygeus muscle has been termed the "visceral" part of the pelvic diaphragm, since this muscle fixes the terminal portions of the visceral tubes. There is no hiatus in the levator surrounding the visceral tubes. Therefore, the implantation of the medial fibers of the pubococcygeus firmly fixes the viscera and constitutes a firm attach-

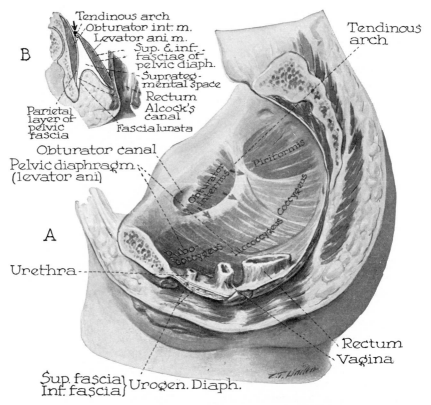

FIG. 430. The pelvic diaphragm and its fascia. (A) Sagittal section showing the origin of the levator ani from the arcus tendineum; the arrows indicate the space which may exist (hiatus of Schwalbe) if the obturator fascia forms a tendinous sling between the pubic bone and the ischial spine. A hernia could occur through such a gap. (B) Formation of Alcock's canal; the arrow indicates the hiatus of Schwalbe. The parietal and the diaphragmatic pelvic fasciae are shown.

ment. This intimate relationship between the pubococcygeus and the viscera is of surgical importance in the proper understanding of the mechanics of surgical repair.

The iliococcygeal portion of the levator ani is placed more laterally and posteriorly than the pubococcygeus, and its fibers take a more transverse course. It is inserted into the

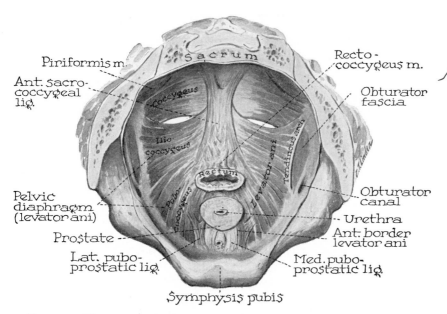

FIG. 431. The pelvic diaphragm (levatores ani and coccygei) seen from above. The pubococcygeus and the iliococcygeus muscles form the levator ani; the pubococcygeus is the stronger of the two.

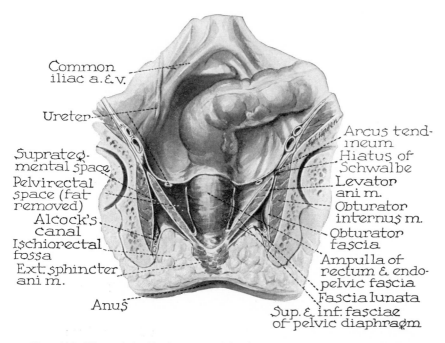

FIG. 432. The pelvic diaphragm and its fascia, seen in a frontal section.

sides of the sacrum and into the anococcygeal raphe. The iliococcygeus has no relation to the organs as they pass from the pelvis to the exterior; even its most anterior fibers do not reach the anal canal. In crossing the midline in front of the coccyx, the muscle forms part of the floor and the wall against which the terminal part of the rectum rests. It also offers indirect support to the sigmoid and to the jejuno-ileum when the body is in the standing position. It is of obstetric importance as a support but of no great importance in gynecologic repairs.

Coccygeus muscle. This fills the space between the coccyx and the ischial spine. It is of little importance as a diaphragmatic support but helps to complete or fill in the formation of the pelvic diaphragm. It is of major importance as a support in pregnancy but does not suffer in the course of a normal delivery.

The obturator internus, the piriformis and the coccygeus assist the associated ligaments in maintaining fixation of the sacro-iliac joint by holding the posterior wall of the pelvis together. Therefore, they are of importance in relation to backache and so-called sacro-iliac strain.

FASCIA

The pelvic fascia, which is distributed in the basin-shaped pelvis, may be divided into 3 main divisions: (1) the parietal fascia, which covers the muscles of the pelvic cavity, (2) the diaphragmatic fascia, which forms a covering for the pelvic diaphragm and (3) the endopelvic or visceral fascia, which covers the pelvic viscera.

The parietal layer of the pelvic fascia lines the sides, the back and the front of the pelvic cavity and covers the muscles which form a padding for this cavity (Fig. 430 B). It forms a rather firm layer over the muscles but a very thin layer over the periosteum. It is a downward continuation of the transversalis fascia, and as it enters the pelvis it attaches on each side to the bone at the linea terminalis (iliopectineal line). It then continues downward over the obturator internus muscle, forming a fascial covering for this muscle; it attaches to the bone about the margin of the muscle.

That portion of fascia which overlies the obturator internus muscle is known as the *obturator fascia*.

Over the upper portion of this fascia a

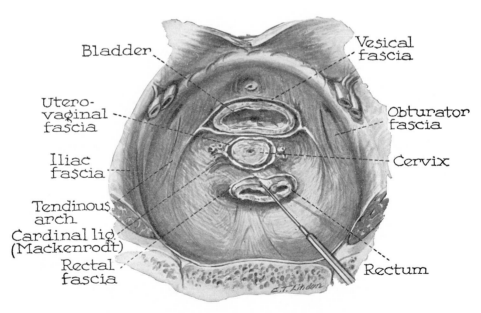

Fig. 433. The visceral part of the pelvic fascia. This layer of connective tissue envelopes the pelvic viscera.

curved line forms as a result of a thickening of the fascia; this thickened portion has been referred to as the *white line* or the *arcus tendineum* (Figs. 431 and 432). It is a linear thickening which extends from the symphysis pubis in front to the ischial spine posteriorly. It does not travel as a straight line but has a downward directed curvature. From this line the levator ani muscle and its pelvic fascia covering (diaphragmatic pelvic fascia) take origin (Figs. 430, 431 and 432).

It is true that in most instances the levator ani arises from the pubic bone anteriorly, the ischial spine posteriorly and the obturator fascia between these two points; however, at times the fascia forms a tendinous sling which attaches to bone only in front and behind. This results in a space which exists between the sling and the obturator fascia; such a space is known as the *hiatus of Schwalbe*. At times an elongation of pelvic peritoneum may enter the hiatus and into the so-called suprategmental space (Fig. 432). If this exists, a hernia into the ischiorectal fossa may result.

Diaphragmatic Pelvic Fascia. This fascia forms a sheath or envelope for the levator ani and the coccygeus muscles. Therefore, it has 2 layers, referred to as superior (internal) and inferior (external) layers (Figs. 430 A and 432).

The superior layer of diaphragmatic fascia is strong and thick, but the inferior layer is much thinner; the superior layer is strong enough to give additional support to the structures which rest upon the diaphragm.

The inferior layer is known as the anal fascia; caudally, it becomes continuous with the superior fascia of the urogenital diaphragm and with the fascia of the sphincter ani muscle (Fig. 430 B). The levator ani muscles and their fascial coverings divide the extraperitoneal space on each side of the rectum into an upper pelvirectal and a lower ischiorectal space, both of which are filled with fat and areolar tissue.

Along the lateral wall of each ischiorectal space *Alcock's canal* is found. This canal is formed by a split in the obturator internus fascia; it carries the pudendal vessels and nerves as they course horizontally backward.

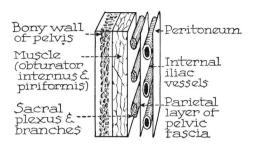

FIG. 434. Arrangement of structures on the side wall of the pelvis. The muscles (obturator internus and piriformis) and the sacral nerves are beneath the parietal layer of pelvic fascia; the internal iliac vessels are above it.

The visceral part of the pelvic fascia is that layer of connective tissue which envelopes the pelvic viscera (Fig. 433). On each side it is continuous with the fascia on the pelvic surface of the levator ani muscles and so indirectly becomes continuous with the parietal pelvic fascia along the origin of that muscle. It forms 3 tubes of fascia which encase in succession the urethra and the bladder, the vagina and the lower part of the uterus and the rectum. In each instance, the fascial sheath is in intimate contact with the musculature of the corresponding viscus and is believed to receive muscle fibers from it. These fascial tubes are connected by thickened portions of the visceral fascia ("ligaments").

On either side of the vagina and the lower uterus the *cardinal ligaments* extend laterally to the parietal pelvic fascia. These are the bases of the broad ligaments and are important in gynecologic surgery; they have also been referred to as Mackenrodt's ligaments.

On each side of the rectum its lateral ligaments extend backward to the sacrum; they are known as the *rectal stalks*. The front of the sacrum also is covered by fascia which passes behind the rectum and forms a fascia-enclosed space called the retrorectal space. This space is bounded in front by the fascia on the back of the rectum, behind by the presacral fascia, and on each side by the lateral rectal stalks. In the male it forms the important rectovesical fascia and the sheath of the prostate (p. 549).

The obturator internus and the piriformis

muscles are located outside of (beneath) the pelvic fascia, since they both ultimately leave the pelvis (Fig. 434). The sacral nerves are also beneath this fascia, since the majority of them leave the pelvis through the sacral foramina. Therefore, it is unnecessary for these muscles and nerves to pierce the fascia. On the other hand, the blood vessels of the pelvis (branches of the internal iliac vessels) are destined to remain in the pelvis and are located inside of (above) the pelvic fascia, between it and the peritoneum.

Pelvic Viscera

THE BLADDER (VESCIA URINARIS)

EMBRYOLOGY

The allantois is an evagination from the primitive hindgut (Fig. 435 A). Shortly after this forms, the gut caudad to the point of origin of the allantois enlarges to form the cloaca. The cloaca is divided into a ventral and a dorsal part by an ingrowing urorectal fold; the ventral part becomes the urogenital sinus, and the dorsal part becomes the rectum (Fig. 435 B). The urorectal fold cuts into the cephalic part of the cloaca, where the allantois and the hindgut meet, and then grows caudad to the cloacal membrane.

The entire upper part of the bladder (except the base) is derived from the cephalic or upper end of the anterior division of the cloaca, and the base and the prostatic urethra are formed from the lower end of the wolffian duct. These two portions fuse along a line marked by a bar of muscle, the interureteric bar, which is situated between the ureters (Fig. 436). Organs which have a double origin may develop congenital abnormalities at the site of fusion of the two parts; hence, when congenital diverticula of the bladder occur, they are found somewhere along the line of the interureteric bar and are in close proximity to the ureteric orifice. The urachus (the allantois of the embryo) is a fibrous cord which connects the apex of the

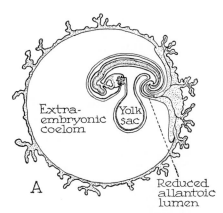

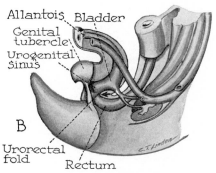

FIG. 435. Embryology of the urinary bladder. (A) The formation of the allantois, an evagination of the primitive hindgut. (B) The arrow indicates the downgrowth of the urorectal fold which divides the cloaca into a ventral part (the urogenital sinus) and a dorsal part (the rectum).

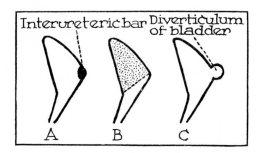

FIG. 436. Embryology of the urinary bladder. (A) The bladder is divided into upper and lower parts. (B) The parts meet at the interureteric bar. (C) Formation of a bladder diverticulum at the interureteric bar.

bladder to the umbilicus. If it remains patent throughout its entire length, urine will be discharged at the umbilicus (Fig. 437 B). It is believed that if this condition exists, an obstruction to the outflow of urine from the bladder is also present. The urachus may remain open only in localized areas, forming small lacunae which are known as the lacunae of Luschka. They are usually symptomless and are found at postmortem. If such a lacuna enlarges, there results a urachal cyst which is situated below the umbilicus in the midline (Fig. 437 B).

At birth, the true pelvis is underdeveloped; hence, little room is available for either intestines or bladder. During infancy the bladder is an abdominal organ, whether full or empty, and is in contact with the anterior abdominal wall (Fig. 438). The peritoneum is reflected off of the uterus and onto the vesical neck; in the male the reflection is even lower, off the rectum and onto the prostate. As the pelvis enlarges the bladder gradually sinks into it so that the larger part of the empty bladder is accommodated by the pelvis at the 6th year. Shortly after puberty, the bladder becomes a pelvic organ exclusively.

THE ADULT BLADDER

The empty and contracted urinary bladder has 4 angles, 4 surfaces and 4 ducts, a duct being attached to each angle. The spelling of each duct starts with the letter "U": 1 urachus, 1 urethra and 2 ureters (Fig. 437 A). The urachus attaches to the anterior angle (apex), the right and the left ureters attach to the posterolateral angles, and the urethra attaches to the inferior angle.

Surfaces. The 4 surfaces are the superior, the 2 inferolaterals and the posterior. They are somewhat triangular in shape and are bounded by the 3 angles which connect around the borders. The superior surface and about a ½ inch of the posterior surface are the only parts covered with peritoneum.

The superior surface is directed upward and is related to the coils of the ileum and the pelvic colon (Fig. 439). In the female, the uterus lies on this surface and tends to indent it. At its anterior end, this surface becomes somewhat pointed and forms the *apex* of the bladder. This is situated immediately behind the upper margin of the pubic symphysis and is continuous with a strong fibrous cord (median umbilical ligament) which passes upward in the midline between the transversalis fascia and the peritoneum (p. 541).

The inferolateral surfaces are in contact in front with the retropubic fat pad which fills the space of Retzius. More posteriorly, the surfaces are related to the obturator internus muscle and the lateral umbilical ligament (obliterated umbilical artery) above and to the levator ani muscles below. The numerous

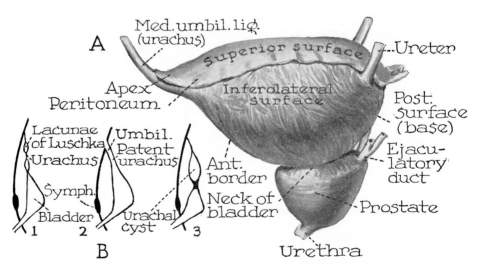

FIG. 437. The urinary bladder. (A) Side view showing the surfaces, the angles and the "ducts." (B) Malformations of the urachus.

veins of the vesical venous plexus pass backward and are in intimate relationship with these surfaces.

The posterior surface of the bladder faces as much downward as backward and has been referred to as the *base* or fundus of the urinary bladder. It lies in front of the rectum, and it can be palpated through the rectum. No peritoneum exists between the rectum and the posterior surface of the bladder, except to a very slight degree above; however, they are separated from each other by the vasa deferentia, the seminal vesicles and the rectovesical fascia (Denonvilliers').

The two vasa deferentia lie side by side on the posterior surface of the bladder and intervene between the seminal vesicles. The ureters enter at the superolateral angles.

Neck. The neck of the bladder is that part which is continuous with the urethra. In the male it is embraced by the prostate and in the female it lies on the upper layer of the urogenital diaphragm (triangular ligament). It is the lowest part of the bladder and is connected with the lower part of the back of the pubis by the pubovesical or puboprostatic ligaments. Because of the obliquity of the pubis in the erect posture, the bladder neck in the male lies a little below the level of the upper margin of the symphysis and

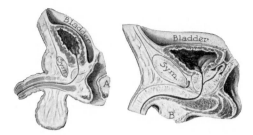

FIG. 438. The position of the empty bladder. (A) In infancy, as an abdominal organ. (B) In the adult, as a pelvic organ.

about 2½ inches behind it (Fig. 440). The bladder neck rests on the base of the prostate, and its muscle fibers are uninterruptedly continuous with those of the prostate. The union of the bladder and the prostate is marked on the outside by a groove in which lie the veins of the prostatic and the vesical plexuses. These veins extend above the groove onto the inferolateral surface of the bladder and below it onto the lateral aspect of the prostate gland.

As the bladder fills, the neck remains fixed, the upper wall rises and, with the other surfaces, increases in area and becomes more convex. The inferolateral surfaces approximate themselves to a greater area of the side

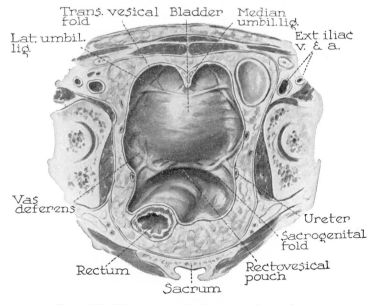

FIG. 439. The urinary bladder seen from above.

walls of the pelvis, the greater vessels and nerves, and the vasa deferentia. The borders become rounded and obliterated. The bladder continues to rise out of the pelvis, stripping the peritoneum from the anterior abdominal wall so that it is in direct contact with the transversalis fascia for about 1½ inches above the pubic bone. When contracted and emptied, the bladder lies in the lower and the anterior part of the pelvis immediately below the peritoneum in the extraperitoneal fatty tissue, the areolar element of which becomes condensed to form a sheath around it. A distended bladder pushes the prostate backward, making it more prominent on rectal examination; hence, the true size of the prostate can best be estimated through the rectum only when the bladder is empty.

The prevesical or retropubic space of Retzius is that space which is behind the pubic bone and in front of the urinary bladder (Fig. 440). The space is bounded anteriorly by the posterior sheath of the rectus muscle and the posterior surface of the pubis. It is limited below by the puboprostatic (pubovesical) ligaments in the fascia covering the levator ani. On each side it extends as far back as the internal iliac artery and its visceral branches. Superiorly, it is continuous with the interval that exists between the peritoneum and the transversalis fascia which extends up to the umbilicus; here it is limited on each side by the lateral umbili-

cal ligaments. The median umbilical ligament (urachus) bisects it. This extraperitoneal space is filled with fatty and areolar tissue which separates the bladder from the ventral pelvic wall. Inflammatory involvement of it may follow bladder infections and urinary extravasation as seen in extraperitoneal rupture of the bladder; an effusion into this space may extend into the extraperitoneal tissue of the abdominal wall or the pelvis. The surgeon may enter the bladder extraperitoneally through the space of Retzius.

Ligaments. The bladder is anchored at its base where it is fixed by continuity with the prostate and the urethra. The latter in turn is fixed to the urogenital diaphragm (triangular ligament). The neck of the bladder is fused by the *puboprostatic* (pubovesical in the female) *ligaments* (Fig. 441). In the female, the visceral attachments of these ligaments are to the neck of the bladder; therefore, they have been called the pubovesical ligaments. However, their anatomy is essentially the same.

The medial puboprostatic (pubovesical) ligaments are thickenings of the pelvic fascia which form a pair of strong thick bands that fix the prostate and the neck of the bladder. They arise from the lower part of the back of the pubis at the sides of the symphysis, pass backward and fuse with the strong fascia that surrounds the base of the prostate and the neck of the bladder. They form the resisting

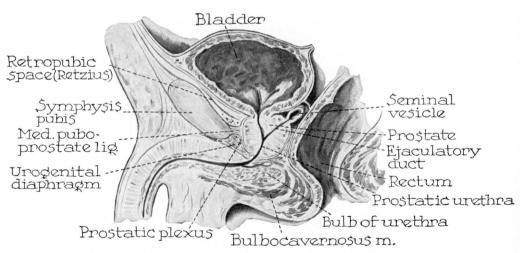

FIG. 440. Midsagittal section through the distended bladder. As the bladder fills, the neck remains fixed; the peritoneum is stripped from the anterior abdominal wall.

membrane that interrupts the fingers when pushed down between the bladder and the pubis when one examines the space of Retzius. A narrow fascial sheath unites each ligament with its fellow of the other side, and the two form a roof over the anterior part of the gap between the anterior borders of the levatores ani.

The medial puboprostatic ligaments constitute the strongest, most definite and most important part of the pelvic fascia. They are continuous laterally with the *lateral puboprostatic ligament,* which is that part of pelvic fascia covering the anterior part of the levator ani; it is connected with the fascial sheath of the prostate and the bladder at the side of the bladder neck.

The bladder is retained in position anteriorly by the *median umbilical ligament* (urachus); the *lateral umbilical ligaments* (atrophied fetal umbilical arteries) also stabilize the bladder anteriorly. The lateral and the median umbilical ligaments maintain the bladder against the anterior abdominal wall when it fills and rises out of the pelvis. Posteriorly, the bladder is supported by the rectovesical fascia (Denonvilliers') (p. 550).

Coats. The structure of the bladder reveals 5 coats: serous, fascial, muscular, submucous and mucous.

1. *The serous coat* is peritoneum which is restricted to the upper surface and also to a small part of the base in the male.

2. *The fascial coat* is extraperitoneal tissue which sheathes the bladder. It is loose except on the upper surface where it becomes an exceedingly thin layer which binds the serous to the muscular coat.

3. *The muscular coat* is a thick, strong, nonstriated muscle which is arranged in interesting bundles traveling in different directions. This is difficult to display in the dissecting room, but it is arranged in close bundles which pass both obliquely and circularly around the bladder. At the neck of the bladder these bundles become massed together to form a ring called the *sphincter of the bladder;* the sphincter is continuous inferiorly with the muscular wall of the urethra in the female and with the muscular substance of the prostate in the male.

4. *The submucous coat* is a layer of areolar tissue which forms a loose connection be-

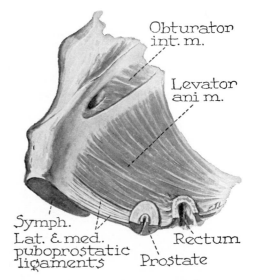

FIG. 441. The puboprostatic (pubovesical) ligaments.

tween the muscular and the mucous coats. The blood vessels and the nerves ramify in this coat before entering the mucosa.

5. *The mucous coat* is of the usual type.

The Interior of the Bladder. If the bladder is contracted and empty, the mucosa is thrown into folds and presents a wrinkled or rugose appearance; in the distended bladder, however, the mucosa becomes smooth.

The trigone (trigonum vesicae) is a triangular area which occupies most of the inner surface of the posterior bladder wall and remains smooth even when the bladder is empty (Fig. 442). It is elastic and tightly bound by areolar tissue to the muscular coat; therefore, it does not alter its appearance as does the rest of the mucous membrane. It is thinner than the rest of the mucosa. When a cystoscopic examination is made in a living subject, the trigone appears pink because this thinness permits the vessels to be seen through it. The rest of the mucous membrane of the bladder presents a straw-colored appearance. The apex of the trigone is formed by the internal urethral orifice, the base corresponding to a line which passes between the 2 ureteral orifices; it is known as the *interureteric ridge.* This ridge is mucous membrane which has been raised by an underlying bar of muscle. The sides of the trigone are about 1 inch wide when the bladder

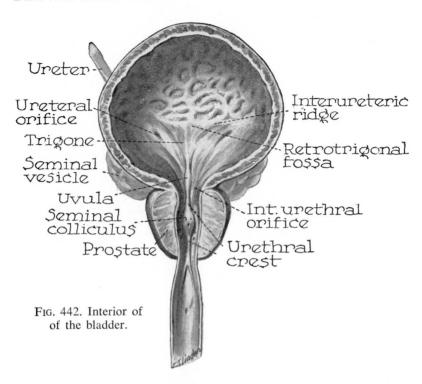

Ureter

Ureteral orifice

Trigone

Seminal vesicle

Uvula

Seminal colliculus

Prostate

Interureteric ridge

Retrotrigonal fossa

Int. urethral orifice

Urethral crest

FIG. 442. Interior of of the bladder.

is empty and about 1½ inches wide when it is full.

There are 3 openings into the bladder: 2 inlets and 1 outlet. These are situated at the angles of the trigone. The 2 orifices of the ureters constitute the inlets; they appear as a pair of semilunar slits which are placed at the extremities of the trigone and are sepa-

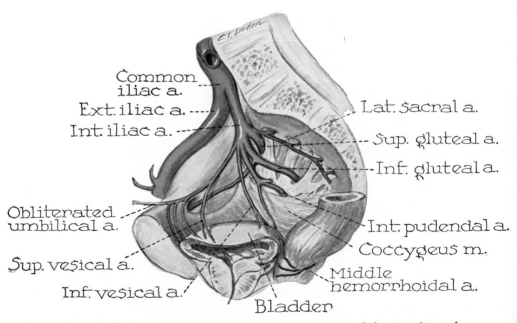

Common iliac a.

Ext. iliac a.

Int. iliac a.

Lat. sacral a.

Sup. gluteal a.

Inf. gluteal a.

Obliterated umbilical a.

Int. pudendal a.

Coccygeus m.

Sup. vesical a.

Inf. vesical a.

Middle hemorrhoidal a.

Bladder

FIG. 443. Arterial supply to the bladder. The relations of the superior and the inferior vesical arteries are shown.

rated by the interureteric redge. If a probe or a catheter is passed into these openings, it is noted that the ureter takes an oblique course through the bladder wall for about ¾ inch. This obliquity forms a valve which allows urine to pass into the bladder but prevents regurgitation as the bladder fills.

The internal urethral orifice is at the apex of the trigone. It is not completely circular because behind it an elevation known as the *uvula* or vesical crest pushes its posterior margin slightly forward. This uvula presents a bulging which results from the middle lobe of the prostate; if this lobe becomes enlarged, it may block the orifice partially or completely.

The retrotrigonal fossa is the interior of the fundus of the bladder. When it is deepened by increased intravesical pressure (prostatic hypertrophy), urine may accumulate here and stagnate. Foreign bodies may gravitate into this fossa, and bladder ruptures can occur through it.

VESSELS AND NERVES

Arteries. The arterial supply to the bladder is derived mainly from the internal iliac artery; small branches from the obturator and the internal pudendal arteries are supplied to the anterior part of the bladder (Fig. 443). The *superior vesical artery,* which is the unobliterated part of the umbilical artery, supplies the superolateral wall. The *inferior vesical artery* is distributed between the floor of the bladder, the prostate and the prostatic urethra. The *middle hemorrhoidal artery* supplies a branch to the posterior surface of the bladder.

Veins. The veins form perivesical plexuses which are most dense around the neck and the ends of the ureters; these drain into the inferior vesical veins. In the male, the larger veins lie in the groove between the bladder and the prostate and form the vesicoprostatic plexus.

Lymphatics. The lymph vessels of the anterior part of the bladder pass to the external iliac glands. From the posterior part, a few may pass to the external iliac glands, but the major portion of these drain into the internal iliac glands.

Nerves. The nerve supply accompanies the arteries and involves not only a complex co-

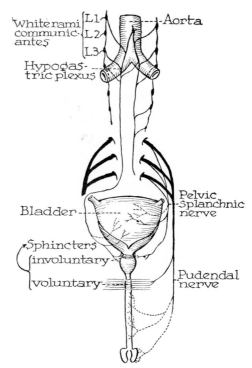

FIG. 444. Nerve supply to the bladder (diagrammatic).

ordination of sympathetic and parasympathetic nerves but also the voluntary control of the sphincter via the pudendal nerve (Fig. 444). The sympathetic nerves (hypogastric plexus) are the "filling" nerves of the bladder, since they inhibit the detrusor muscle which makes up the bladder wall; they cause increased tone in the internal sphincter, thereby permitting the bladder to retain its contents. On the other hand, the parasympathetic nerves (pelvic splanchnic nerves) are the "emptying" nerves of the bladder because they stimulate the contraction of the detrusor muscle, the elevation of the trigone and the relaxation of the internal sphincter. This is accompanied by voluntary relaxation of the external sphincter by means of cerebral control via the pudendal nerve.

SURGICAL CONSIDERATIONS

INJURIES TO THE BLADDER

Bladder wounds would occur far more frequently if the organ were not so well protected within the pelvic cavity. These injuries may occur in various ways: as a result of

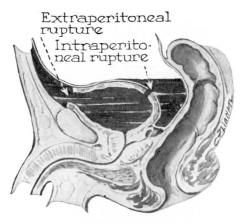

FIG. 445. Bladder injuries. A bladder injury may be either intraperitoneal or extraperitoneal.

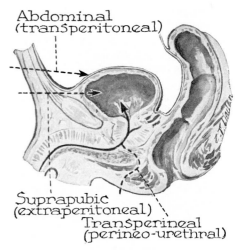

FIG. 446. Surgical approaches to the bladder.

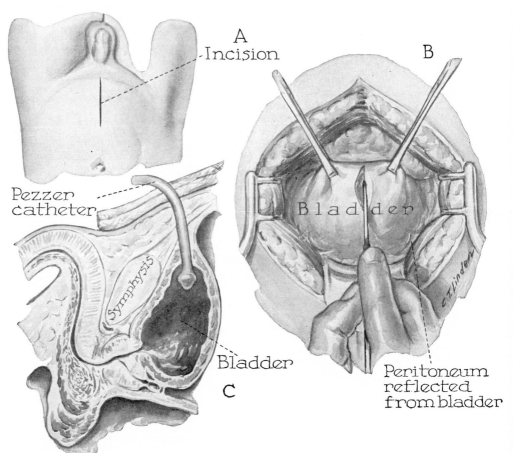

FIG. 447. Suprapubic cystostomy. (A) A vertical midline incision is made in the suprapubic region. (B) The muscles and the transversalis fascia are incised and retracted. The peritoneum is reflected upward, and the bladder is incised. (C) The completed cystostomy in sagittal section.

laceration by sharp bony fragments in fractures of the pelvis; from direct blows over the hypogastrium, especially if the bladder is distended; penetrating wounds account for a certain number of bladder injuries, as does violence exerted through the rectum, the vagina or the perineum. The injury may be intraperitoneal or extraperitoneal (Fig. 445). Intraperitoneal rupture occurs in the part of the bladder covered by peritoneum; extraperitoneal rupture involves only the mucomuscular coats of the viscus, since these are not covered by peritoneum. In the latter case, the lesion is subperitoneal, and the urine extravasates beneath the peritoneum. The most frequent site for rupture of the bladder is the posterosuperior aspect. Whether the rupture is intraperitoneal or extraperitoneal, immediate surgery must be employed.

Approaches to the Bladder

For diagnostic purposes, the urethral (cystoscopic) approach is employed. The 3 most common other approaches usually described are the suprapubic (extraperitoneal), the abdominal (transperitoneal) and a transperineal (perineo-urethral) (Fig. 446).

The suprapubic approach affords excellent access to the extraperitoneally placed bladder. It is particularly applicable in prostatectomy and in the removal of calculi and neoplasms.

The abdominal and the *transperineal approaches* are more of didactic than practical interest.

Suprapubic Cystostomy

This operation is accomplished through a vertical midline incision that is placed in the suprapubic region (Fig. 447). It is preferable to have the organ fully distended as a preliminary step. The incision is deepened to an interval between the rectus abdominis and the pyramidalis muscles. Behind these muscles and at the upper border of the symphysis lies the transversalis fascia. The prevesical space is exposed by dividing this fascia. If the bladder is distended, it can be felt by inserting a finger into the lower angle of the incision. The peritoneum is reflected upward; since the connection between the peritoneum and the bladder is loose, this maneuver is accomplished readily. The prevesical fat and the visceral layer of pelvic fascia are incised. Vesical veins may be found in this stratum. Now the bladder can be elevated and entered. A Pezzer type of catheter is introduced into the bladder for drainage.

PELVIC VISCERA IN THE MALE

The upper part of the pelvic colon usually can be lifted out of the male pelvis, but the lower part remains attached to the dorsal wall by the medial limb of the pelvic meso-

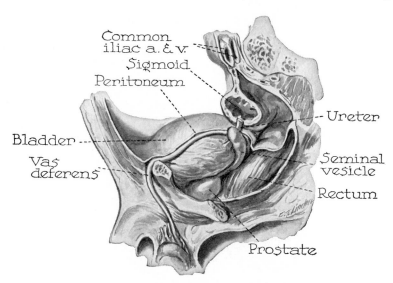

Fig. 448. The pelvic viscera in the male. The left wall of the pelvis has been removed, and the bladder is partly filled.

colon (Figs. 448 and 449). The rectum occupies the lower portion of the dorsal part of this cavity and follows the concavity of the sacrum and the coccyx. The urinary bladder lies in the lower and anterior part of the cavity behind the pubic bone. Both ureters usually can be seen shining through the peritoneum posteriorly at the side walls of the pelvis. The seminal vesicles lie on the back of the bladder between it and the rectum, and on each side the vas deferens can be seen through the peritoneum as it passes from the deep inguinal ring toward the bladder. Having crossed the pelvic brim, the vas first passes downward and backward and then medially across the ureter to reach the back of the bladder, where it descends along the medial side of the seminal vesicle close to the vesicle of the opposite side. The prostate lies below the bladder, directly in front of the lower part of the rectum, and encloses the prostatic urethra.

The pelvic peritoneum covers the dorsal wall of the pelvis and is reflected off as the medial limb of the pelvic mesocolon. At the 3rd piece of sacrum, the peritoneum reaches the rectum, to which it gives a partial covering, and then covers the front of the upper third of the rectum and its sides. At the middle third it covers only the anterior surface and the lower end of the middle third as it passes from the rectum to the bladder. It covers the upper surface of the bladder, from which it passes forward onto the anterior abdominal wall and the sides of the pelvic wall. From the sides of the upper third of the rectum it extends to the side walls of the pelvis, forming the floor of a pair of depressions called the *pararectal fossae*. As it continues forward from the rectum to the bladder it forms the floor of the depression known as the *rectovesical pouch*. When the peritoneum reaches the bladder it is tucked behind it to cover a small portion of its posterior surface in the median plane between the two vasa deferentia.

DEFERENT DUCTS

The vas (ductus) deferens has a scrotal, an inguinal and a pelvic course (Fig. 448). It begins at the lower end of the epididymis, passes upward over the back of the testis on the medial side of the epididymis and ascends to the superficial inguinal ring. It traverses the inguinal canal as a constituent of the spermatic cord; in the posterior part of the cord it is readily palpable because of its firmness. It leaves the other constituents of the spermatic cord at the deep inguinal ring.

The intrapelvic portion of each vas extends from the internal inguinal ring to the base of the prostate. It hooks around the origin of the inferior epigastric artery and passes backward with a slight downward bend on the side wall of the pelvis until it reaches the region of the ischial spines (Fig. 450). Here it makes a right angle bend which carries it medially, forward and downward across the terminal part of the ureter and down the posterior surface of the bladder. After hooking around the inferior epigastric artery, it crosses the external iliac artery and vein, the superior ramus of the pubis, and the obturator internus muscle, but it is separated from the latter by the lateral umbilical liga-

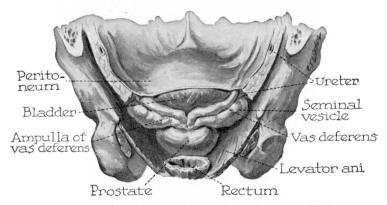

FIG. 449. Pelvic viscera in the male, seen from behind.

ment (obliterated umbilical artery) and the obturator artery, nerve and vein.

At the ischial spine, where it turns medially, it crosses the ureter and then passes downward on the posterior aspect of the bladder. In this part of its course it lies behind and in front of the rectum with the seminal vesicle on its inferolateral side and the vas of the opposite side in close contact with it. Until the vas reaches the posterior surface of the bladder it is in direct contact on its medial side with the peritoneum, but thereafter it lies below the peritoneal floor of the pelvis.

In its terminal part each vas is enclosed within the thickness of the frontally disposed rectovesical fascia (Denonvilliers') and becomes widened into an ampulla. The ampullae appear as elongated bags which are reservoirs for the semen; it is in the ampullae that a secretion of the mucous membrane of the vas is added. The vasa deferentia converge and unite with the excretory ducts of the seminal vesicles to form the ejaculatory ducts; these traverse the prostate and open into the prostatic urethra. The artery to the vas deferens arises either from the superior or the inferior vesical artery, runs in close relationship with the wall of the vas from the base of the bladder to the epididymis and anastomoses with the testicular artery.

SEMINAL VESICLES

The seminal vesicles are offshoots of the deferent ducts (Figs. 449 and 450). They appear as lobulated sacs, about 2 inches long and ½ inch in diameter and present the same histologic picture as the ampullated end of the vas. The bladder is in front, the rectum behind. The vas is medial and is capped above by peritoneum; laterally, it is separated from the levator ani by numerous vesical vessels. Each seminal vesicle lies obliquely so that its lateral surface faces downward as well as sideward, and it is related to the fat on the levator ani muscle. If the vesicle is teased apart, it is found to be a sacculated tube about 6 inches long which is folded and coiled into its baglike form (Fig. 451). The seminal vesicle is not to be considered simply a reservoir for spermatozoa; its function is to produce a secretion which forms a large part of the seminal fluid.

The ejaculatory duct is that duct which is common to both the vas and the vesicle. Its diameter is approximately that of a pencil. It is easily torn away from the prostate, the upper half of which it pierces obliquely to open beside the prostatic utricle. The arteries to the seminal vesicle and the ampulla of the vas are tiny branches which are derived from the vesical and the middle hemorrhoidal ar-

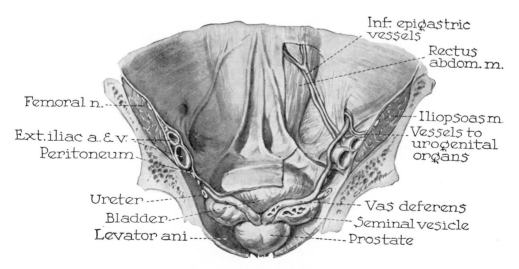

FIG. 450. The intrapelvic portion of the vas deferens (seen from behind). The left seminal vesicle and the ampulla of the vas have been sectioned, and part of the prostate has been removed in order to expose the ejaculatory duct.

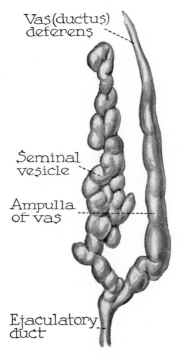

Vas (ductus) deferens

Seminal vesicle

Ampulla of vas

Ejaculatory duct

FIG. 451. The seminal vesicle. The vesicle has been unravelled. It is a tortuous tube with many outpouchings.

teries. The veins correspond to the arteries and the lymph vessels of the vesicle and the ampulla of the vas, and end in the internal and the external iliac glands.

PROSTATE GLAND

The prostate gland is a solid organ which surrounds the urethra between the bladder and the urogenital diaphragm (Fig. 440). It consists of fibrous tissue, plain muscle and glandular elements. It is broader than it is long, being about 1¼ inches long and 1½ inches broad. Its exact functions are not known. It adds a secretion which is concerned with the vitality of the spermatozoa. It has an apex (lower end), a base (upper surface), an anterior surface, a posterior surface and a pair of lateral surfaces. It is the size and the shape of a chestnut, surrounds the first 1¼ inches of the urethra and is traversed by the ejaculatory ducts.

The base or superior surface, although structurally continuous with the superimposed bladder (neither the fibers nor the muscular part shows any interruption as they pass from one organ to another), nevertheless shows a circular groove in which fat and veins are lodged. Its apex points downward and rests upon the superior fascia of the urogenital diaphragm (Fig. 452). Its anterior border or surface is blunt and rounded and is separated from the retropubic space (Retzius) by the puboprostatic ligaments and from the lower part of the symphysis by fibro-adipose tissue and a plexus of veins. The posterior surface is flattened and rests

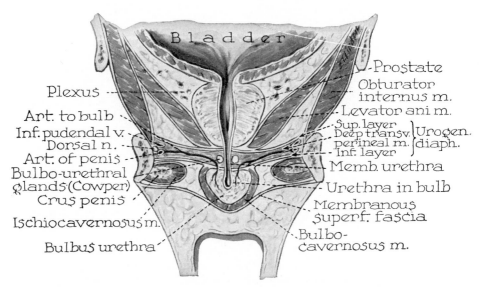

Bladder

Plexus
Art. to bulb
Inf. pudendal v.
Dorsal n.
Art. of penis
Bulbo-urethral glands (Cowper)
Crus penis
Ischiocavernosus m.
Bulbus urethra

Prostate
Obturator internus m.
Levator ani m.
Sup. layer
Deep transv. perineal m. } Urogen. diaph.
Inf. layer
Memb. urethra
Urethra in bulb
Membranous superf. fascia
Bulbo-cavernosus m.

FIG. 452. Diagrammatic presentation of relations of the prostate (coronal section).

against the lower inch of rectum. This is the portion of the prostate which is felt by digital examination, only the rectovesical fascia intervening. This surface is pierced on each side of the median plane by the ejaculatory ducts. The 2 lateral surfaces (inferolateral) are convex and are supported by the anterior fibers of the levator ani; the 2 anterior borders of the levators clasp the lower part of the prostate between them.

Lobes of the Prostate. In uterine life, longitudinal depressions appear on the walls of the urethra immediately inferior to the bladder. These depressions become buds which grow and penetrate the surrounding muscle and the connective tissue to form the ultimate 5 lobes of the prostate gland: an anterior, a posterior, a medial and 2 lateral lobes (Fig. 453).

The anterior lobe buds from the anterior wall of the urethra; its glandular elements gradually disappear so that at birth a few or no glandular elements remain. Therefore, adenomas rarely, if ever, occur in this lobe, and there is no encroachment on the lumen of the urethra from this direction.

The posterior lobe arises from the posterior wall of the urethra, inferior to the orifice of the ejaculatory ducts, and grows superiorly to occupy a plane behind these ducts. As it grows toward the base of the bladder it becomes both posturethral and postspermatic. This lobe lies behind the middle lobe, forms the entire posterior surface of the gland and is the lobe encountered during digital examination. Adenomas rarely, if ever, occur here, but primary carcinoma may. The 2 lateral lobes arise as tubular outgrowths from the lateral walls of the urethra. They grow laterally, anteriorly, posteriorly and upward until they occupy almost the entire base (upper portion) of the gland. As they grow anteriorly, they almost approximate one another in the anterior region of the urethra. Hypertrophy of these lobes causes urinary obstruction by lateral encroachment on the prostatic portion of the urethra, and if one lobe greatly exceeds the other in size, the urethra may be pushed laterally and be increased in length.

Clinically, the *median (middle) lobe* is the most important. It originates on the posterior

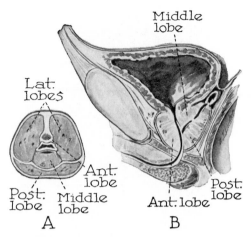

FIG. 453. The 5 lobes of the prostate: (A) a cross section at the neck of the bladder of an embryo; (B) sagittal section of the bladder and the prostate.

surface of the floor of the ejaculatory ducts. It is posturethral as is the posterior lobe; but, unlike the posterior lobe, it is prespermatic; it is below the neck of the bladder and contains much glandular tissue. In this region the subtrigonal and the subcervical glands (Albarran) are found. These mucous glands are entirely separate and distinct from the prostate and are important because of their intimate relationship to the bladder neck. Slight degrees of enlargement of these glands may lead to obstruction of the outflow of urine. The middle lobe normally projects into the urethra, causing a prominence on its floor; this prominence is known as the verumontanum (crista urethralis, seminal colliculus). This lobe is clinically important because it is the one in which adenomas frequently grow. The line of least resistance is inward into the urethra. As it enlarges it pushes the mucous membrane of the urethra ahead of it, extends into the bladder and may entirely block the internal urinary meatus. The effort of straining to urinate pushes it onto the internal meatus, thus further blocking the outlet.

Fascial Relations and Capsules. The prostate has 2 capsules: a true and a false (Fig. 454). The true capsule is formed by a condensation of tissue at the periphery of the gland. The false capsule is formed by the visceral layer of the pelvic fascia which pro-

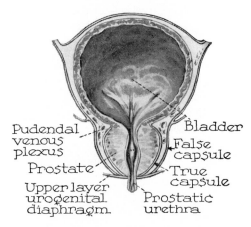

FIG. 454. The capsules of the prostate; diagrammatic presentation of the true and the false capsules in coronal section.

vides a sheath common to both the bladder and the prostate but is absent where these 2 organs are in contact. For this reason, adenomas of the prostate grow upward into the bladder, this being the line of least resistance.

A pudendal (prostatic) plexus of veins lies between the 2 capsules; it receives the deep dorsal vein of the penis in front. During suprapubic prostatectomy the surgeon enucleates the prostate from within both of its capsules and in this way leaves the prostatic plexus of veins undisturbed. During this operation the prostatic urethra is removed with the gland, and the ejaculatory ducts are torn. As a result of this, the patient, although not impotent, is sterile.

In the fetus the peritoneum of the pelvic floor extends down as a pouch behind the prostate gland; normally, this pouch is shut off from the peritoneal cavity and then exists as 2 layers with a potential space between them. These 2 layers are attached above to the peritoneum (cul-de-sac of Douglas) and below to the urogenital diaphragm and the perineal body. It is a prostatoperitoneal layer which is known as *Denonvilliers' fascia* (Fig. 455). The anterior layer of this fascia is attached firmly to the prostate, but the posterior layer is attached loosely to the pelvic fascia around the rectum. The potential space between these layers is called the *retroprostatic space of Proust.*

This space should not be confused with the misnamed prerectal space which is supposed to exist between the rectum and the fascia of Denonvilliers. In the performance of a perineal prostatectomy the surgeon must find the space of Proust, which exists between the 2 fascial layers, if he wishes to avoid difficulties such as excessive bleeding and entrance into the rectum. It may be difficult at times to find this space, which has been so aptly described as passing "between wind and water."

Roux has described a so-called recto-urethralis muscle. It consists of 2 muscle bundles, superior and inferior, both of which are derived from the longitudinal muscle coat of the bowel wall; it holds the recto-anal angle forward. These muscle bundles are attached to the upper part of the perineal body and must be divided in perineal prostatectomy if the rectum is to be successfully displaced backward and out of danger.

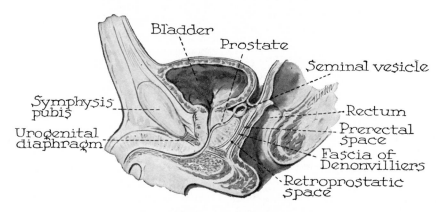

FIG. 455. Denonvilliers' fascia.

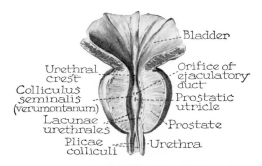

Bladder

Urethral crest

Colliculus seminalis (verumontanum)

Lacunae urethrales

Plicae colliculi

Orifice of ejaculatory duct

Prostatic utricle

Prostate

Urethra

FIG. 456. The prostatic urethra. A frontal section is made so that the posterior aspect of the urethra is seen.

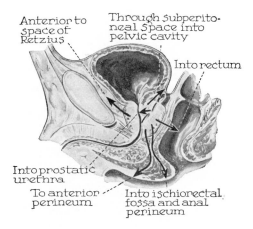

Anterior to space of Retzius

Through subperitoneal space into pelvic cavity

Into rectum

Into prostatic urethra

To anterior perineum

Into ischiorectal fossa and anal perineum

FIG. 457. The arrows indicate the possible paths of extension and rupture of a prostatic abscess.

Vessels. The blood supply of the prostate is derived from the inferior vesical and the middle rectal (hemorrhoidal) arteries. The prostatic plexus of veins is joined in front by the deep dorsal vein of the penis. As these veins pass backward they extend around the junction of the prostate and the bladder and are joined by numerous vesical veins. They continue backward, lateral to the seminal vesicles and below the ureter, and terminate in the internal iliac vein. The lymph vessels end in the internal iliac and the sacral lymph glands.

Prostatic Urethra. The prostatic part of the urethra is about 1 inch long and is the widest and the most dilatable part (Figs. 440 and 456). It passes almost perpendicularly from the neck of the bladder, slightly forward through the prostate, and emerges a little above its apex where it becomes continuous with the second or membranous part. It is fusiform in shape, but on transverse section appears crescentic, owing to the presence of a prominent verticle ridge on the posterior wall called the *urethral crest*.

On each side of this crest a gutter is formed; this is called the *prostatic sinus* and appears as a groove into which numerous small ducts of the prostate open.

The highest point or summit of the urethral crest is called the *seminal colliculus* (*verumontanum*) and lies over the middle of the prostatic urethra. This colliculus bifurcates as it fades away.

Opening onto the colliculus is a diverticulum called the *prostatic utricle;* through this a probe may be passed for about ½ inch into the substance of the prostate. This tiny structure is the homologue of the uterus and the vagina. It is of practical importance because it may catch the end of a catheter or a small bougie and impede its passage.

The *ejaculatory ducts* open into the urethra by minute slitlike orifices at the sides of the mouth of the utricle. There is much clinical interest concerning the prostatic urethra. A seminal vesiculitis (verumontantitis) may cause obliteration or constriction of the ejaculatory ducts. If such an inflammation travels through the openings of the ejaculatory ducts, an epididymitis may result. In chronic urethral infections the prostatic duct may also be involved and obstructed. If the infection travels by way of the prostatic opening, a prostatic abscess may result. The seminal vesicles are also involved in gonorrheal infections of the prostatic urethra via the ejaculatory ducts.

The internal and the external urinary sphincters of the bladder govern the outflow of urine. *The internal (vesical) urinary sphincter* is derived from the outer and the middle muscle layers of the bladder. These are the fibers which are destroyed in the operation of prostatectomy. *The external (urethral) urinary sphincter* is derived from the *sphincter urethrae membranaceae* (p. 602); this is the muscle which compensates and controls urinary flow when the internal sphincter is torn during prostatectomy.

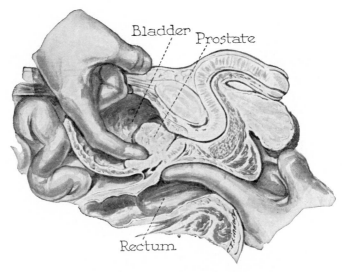

FIG. 458. Suprapubic prostatectomy. One finger is placed into the bladder and another finger is placed into the rectum so that the gland is defined completely and removed through the bladder.

SURGICAL CONSIDERATIONS

PROSTATIC ABSCESS

This condition follows a prostatitis and may appear as a single large abscess or as several small foci. The path of least resistance is toward the urethra, and many prostatic abscesses may rupture here (Fig. 457). The dense pelvic fascia which invests the prostate usually resists the progress of the

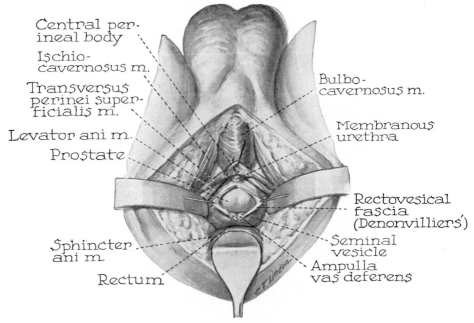

FIG. 459. Perineal prostatectomy. Denonvilliers' fascia has been incised, and the prostate gland is exposed.

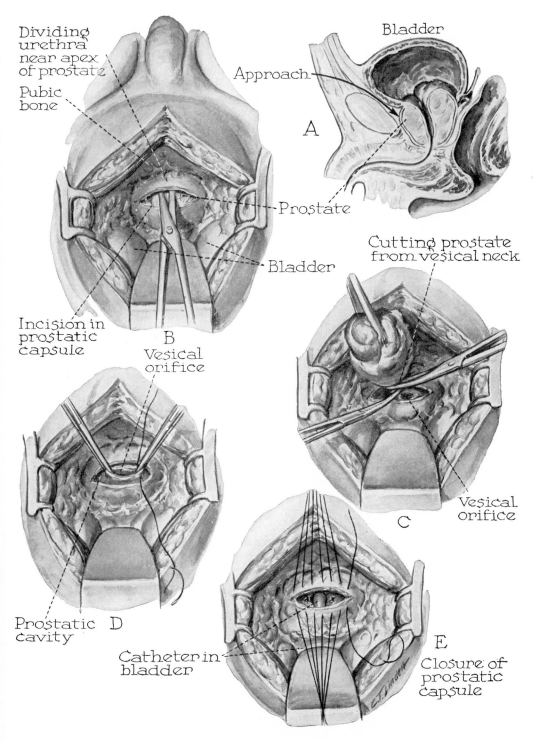

Dividing urethra near apex of prostate

Pubic bone

Bladder

Approach

A

Prostate

Bladder

Incision in prostatic capsule

B

Vesical orifice

Cutting prostate from vesical neck

C

Vesical orifice

Prostatic cavity

D

Catheter in bladder

E

Closure of prostatic capsule

FIG. 460. Retropubic prostatectomy. (A) The approach through the space of Retzius is indicated by the arrow. (B) Exposure and mobilization of the gland. (C) Enucleation and removal of the prostate. (D) Appearance after removal of the gland. (E) Closure.

abscess upward through the peritoneum and into the pelvic cavity; the strong urogenital diaphragm resists its spread downward to the perineum. However, it can reach the perineum by pointing toward the rectum where it comes into contact with a thin rectovesical fascia. The abscess may follow this fascia through the space between the urogenital diaphragm and the anus into the perineum; the pus also may erode through the rectovesical fascia and rupture into the rectum. A periprostatic infection can lie lateral to the gland, invade the levator ani muscle and reach the ischiorectal fossa. A rare path of spread is anteriorly through the pubovesical ligaments and into the space of Retzius.

PROSTATECTOMY

Four accepted methods of removal of the prostate gland have been described: suprapubic prostatectomy, transurethral resection, perineal prostatectomy and retropubic prostatectomy.

The suprapubic prostatectomy requires exposure through the bladder (Fig. 458). There are many who find fault with this approach because the gland lies entirely outside of the bladder; the bladder is entered, the enucleation is done blindly and hemorrhage may be difficult to control. In addition, it does not permit complete removal of a carcinomatous gland which has invaded the capsule.

The transurethral resection operation is well adapted to smaller glands, median bars and serves as a palliative procedure for obstruction due to carcinoma. However, in the hands of excellent resectionists, the scope of the operation is much greater, and the results are good; hence, some outstanding urologists remain most enthusiastic about it. The morbidity may be prolonged by the necrosing of tissue electrically treated; in a fairly large percentage of resections the procedure has to be repeated.

Perineal prostatectomy is a surgical operation in which the gland is removed under direct vision; hemorrhage can be controlled more readily (Fig. 459). It is applicable in the removal of a malignant prostate which has invaded the capsule. It requires a thorough knowledge of perineal anatomy and a highly skilled and trained surgical team. In

inexperienced hands, a persistent fistula may result, the rectum may be injured or complete incontinence may be an annoying sequela.

Retropubic Prostatectomy. Millin, of London, has described a new approach in the operation of retropubic prostatectomy (Fig. 460). Although the space of Retzius has been considered the potential danger area, nevertheless this operation takes place directly through this space. The skin incision extends from the symphysis to the umbilicus in the midline, and the rectus muscles are separated. The preprostatic fat which occupies the space of Retzius is identified. The bladder is retracted upward, and an incision is made into the prostatic capsule. The gland is enucleated to the vesicle neck, the prostate is peeled off of the bladder, and the prostatic arteries are ligated. A catheter is introduced from the meatus and into the bladder. This operation too has its antagonists and protagonists.

No one operative procedure will meet the requirements of every case; therefore, all the methods must be known and included in the armamentaria of the surgeons who do this type of work.

PELVIC VISCERA IN THE FEMALE

EMBRYOLOGY

Before the sex of the embryo is determined, 4 parallel tubes grow caudally in the subperitoneal tissue of the posterior abdominal wall (Fig. 461). They are the right and the left müllerian (paramesonephric) ducts and the right and the left wolffian (mesonephric) ducts. They terminate in that anterior part of the cloaca known as the urogenital sinus. The wolffian duct predominates in the male and gives rise to the spermatic duct, the epididymis, the vas deferens and the ejaculatory duct (p. 537). The müllerian duct predominates in the female and becomes the fallopian tubes, the uterus and the vagina.

The cephalic ends of Müller's (paramesonephric) ducts open into the body cavity, but the caudal ends, having crossed the wolffian ducts, fuse with each other and form a single tube which opens into the urogenital sinus.

The cranial ends of these ducts become the fallopian tubes; their intermediate parts fuse to form the uterus, and the caudal ends fuse and form the upper part of the vagina. To meet its fellow in the midline, the intermediate part of the duct must pull away from the side wall of the pelvis and in so doing pulls a peritoneal fold with it; this fold becomes the broad ligament of the uterus. Therefore, the broad ligament is the "mesentery of the müllerian duct." In the male, Müller's duct almost entirely disappears, with the exception of its caudal extremity, which forms the prostatic utricle, and the cephalic extremity, which forms the appendix testis (sessile hydatid). The wolffian duct only persists at its extremities in the female.

At its cephalic end it forms longitudinal tubules of the epoophoron and the paroophoron. The transverse tubules of these vestigial bodies occupy the broad ligament in the vicinity of the ovaries.

The caudal extremity of the wolffian duct may persist as a tubular remnant, known as the duct of Gartner, which is embedded in the lateral wall of the cervix and the vagina.

The ovary originally is a retroperitoneal abdominal organ, as is the testicle, but in

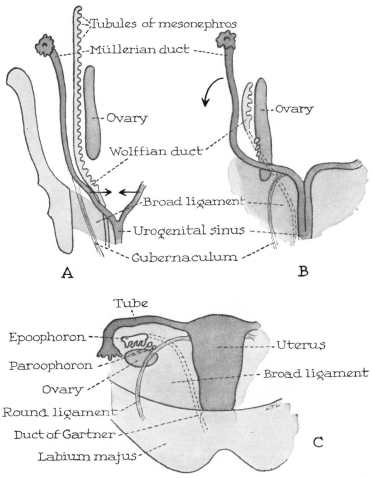

Fig. 461. Development of the female pelvic viscera. (A) Two wolffian and two müllerian ducts are present. (B) The wolffian ducts do not persist in the female. (C) The cranial ends of the müllerian ducts become the fallopian tubes, the intermediate parts fuse to form the uterus, and the caudal ends fuse and form the upper part of the vagina. In the female, the wolffian duct persists only at its extremities; at its cephalic end, the epoophoron and the paroophoron are formed; at its caudal end, the duct of Gartner may persist.

the adult it becomes a pelvic organ. The gubernaculum of the ovary is attached caudally to the skin, which later becomes the labium majus; in its course the gubernaculum becomes attached to the side of the uterus. In the male, the gubernaculum testis passes through the inguinal canal and into the scrotum, pulling with it a processus vaginalis and the testis; in the female, the gubernaculum ovarii passes through the inguinal canal into the labium majus, followed by a similar processus vaginalis which is called the canal of Nuck. As the ovary descends into the pelvis it draws its nerve and vascular supply across the external iliac vessels.

In its fully developed state the gubernaculum in the female becomes the ligament of the ovary and the round ligament of the uterus (Fig. 463 A). These 2 ligaments are practically continuous at their site of uterine attachment, which is just below the uterine tube. The round ligament of the uterus parallels the subperitoneal course taken by the vas deferens in the male; it crosses the side wall of the pelvis and the external iliac vessels, then turns around the inferior epigastric artery, passes through the inguinal canal and

ends in the labium majus, which is the homologue of the scrotum. The ovary may descend abnormally; in such instances it follows the gubernaculum into the labium majus; this is known as an ectopic ovary.

THE 6 LIGAMENTOUS SUPPORTS

The 6 ligamentous supports of the female pelvic viscera are the broad, the round, the uterosacral, Mackenrodt's, the ovarian and the infundibulopelvic ligaments (Figs. 462 and 463).

Broad Ligaments. Each broad ligament of the uterus is a thick, mesenterylike fold which passes from the lateral margin of the uterus to the lateral wall of the pelvis. It is a structure of great importance because of its relation to the uterine tube, the uterine and the ovarian vessels and the ovary. The 2 layers of the broad ligament are triangular in shape when placed on a stretch. Medially, its 2 layers separate to envelope the uterus, and inferiorly and laterally they separate to cover the floor and the side wall of the pelvis (Fig. 466). Superiorly, these 2 layers become continuous with each other and form a free upper border, which in the normal pelvis

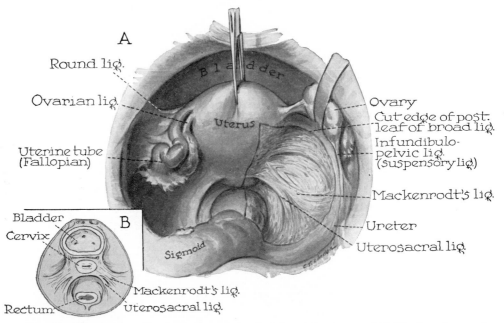

FIG. 462. The 6 ligamentous supports of the female pelvic viscera. (A) The broad, round, ovarian, infundibulopelvic, uterosacral and Mackenrodt's ligaments are shown from behind. On the right the posterior leaf of the broad ligament has been removed to show the structure of the ligaments. (B) Transverse diagrammatic section to show the formation of Mackenrodt's ligament.

is more anterior than superior. The inner four fifths of the free upper border is occupied by the fallopian tube, and the shorter lateral one fifth extends beyond the tube from the fimbriated end to the wall of the pelvis as the infundibulopelvic ligament. The 2 layers pass in opposite directions at their lines of attachment to the lateral pelvic wall and floor to become continuous with the general peritoneal lining of the pelvic cavity. Between the layers of the broad ligament the extraperitoneal connective tissue is located; this is the parametrium. In addition to the uterine tube, the round ligament of the uterus, the ovarian ligament, the epoophoron and the uterine and the ovarian vessels also are found between the two layers of the broad ligament.

Two secondary ligaments originate from it. Passing posteriorly is a fold, the *mesovarium,* which contains the ovary and the ovarian ligament. The *mesosalpinx* is that portion of the broad ligament which lies immediately below the uterine tube between it and the ovary.

The round ligaments of the uterus are not duplications of peritoneum but are true ligamentous fibromuscular cords. They pass from the superolateral angle of the uterus to the internal inguinal ring, representing the lower part of the gubernaculum; they are enclosed between the serous layers of the broad ligaments (Fig. 463). Usually they raise a ridge on the anterior aspect of the broad ligament and occasionally may be accompanied by a persistent tubular prolongation of abdominal peritoneum known as the canal of Nuck. They pass horizontally and extend outward to the wall of the lesser pelvis, pass forward under the peritoneum and cross the obliterated hypogastric artery, the external iliac vessels and the psoas major muscle. They then cross the pelvic brim to reach the internal inguinal ring through which they enter the inguinal canal. Each round ligament leaves the external inguinal ring and terminates in the labium majus where it ends by breaking up into fine fibrous strands. The function of the round ligaments is to draw the uterus forward after it has been displaced backward by a pregnant uterus or a distended bladder. Once returned to its normal forward position, the intra-abdominal pressure on the posterior surface of the uterus maintains its position. Should the round ligaments fail to function, intra-abdominal pressure presses the fundus of the uterus downward and into the vagina. This in turn puts a greater strain on the other supporting ligamentous structures and results in prolapse of the uterus.

The infundibulopelvic ligament (suspensory ligament of the ovary) extends from the tubal end of the ovary to the lateral pelvic

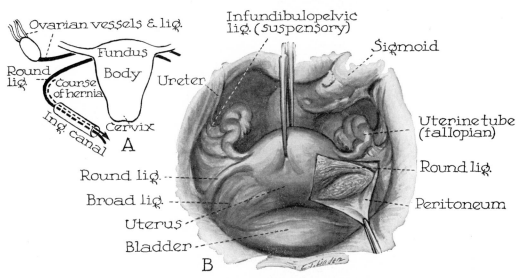

FIG. 463. Ligamentous supports of the female pelvic viscera. (A) The division of the gubernaculum into the ovarian and the round ligaments. (B) The structures seen from above and in front. The anterior leaf of the left broad ligament has been reflected forward.

The ovarian vessels & nerves travel in the infundibulopelvic ligament!!

wall; it is the lateral one fifth of the broad ligament and is not occupied by the fallopian tube. It passes upward from the ovary, crosses the external iliac vessels and becomes lost in the fascia and the peritoneum covering the psoas major muscle. The ovarian vessels and nerves travel in this ligament.

The uterosacral ligaments are 2 short, fibromuscular cords which pass backward from the posterior aspect of the upper end of the cervix on each side of the rectum and end in the sacrum. They lie directly in contact with the peritoneum and form ridges called recto-uterine folds in the lateral walls of the recto-uterine pouch. Following inflammatory conditions, these ligaments may shorten and overaccentuate the anteflexion of the uterus. The function of the uterosacral ligaments is to hold the cervix up and back. If they fail to function (congenital weakness, loss of tonus from pregnancies, etc.), the cervix is displaced downward and forward; this permits a backward displacement of the corpus so that the axis of the uterus and the vagina coincide. Intra-abdominal pressure then forces the uterus into the vagina (prolapse).

Mackenrodt's ligaments (cardinal or transverse cervical ligaments) are situated lateral to the cervix and the vagina and are continuous on each side with the corresponding uterosacral ligaments. They are the bases of the broad ligaments. Blood vessels, especially veins, make up the chief components of this ligament. They are a condensation of parametrial tissue which helps suspend the cervix and the uterus to the pelvic walls (Fig. 462 B). When the cardinal ligaments become stretched, the uterus drops to a lower level.

The ovarian ligament is a rounded fibromuscular cord which is enveloped between the 2 layers of the broad ligament and may be seen through the peritoneum as it passes along a line separating the mesosalpinx from the mesovarium. It extends from the uterine (lower) pole of the ovary to the lateral aspect of the uterus; here it is attached between the fallopian tube and the round ligament of the uterus. The ovarian and the round ligaments of the uterus together represent the gubernaculum of the ovary, the entire cord being subdivided into ovarian and uterine parts (Fig. 463 A).

UTERUS

The uterus is a pear-shaped muscular organ that is intermediate in position between the bladder, the rectum and the broad ligaments (Figs. 464 and 465). It is 3 inches long, 2 inches at its widest part and 1 inch at its thickest part; it is flattened in front where it is in contact with the bladder, but is convex behind. Its lower third is cylindrical, but the remaining upper two thirds widens gradually toward the free end. It is lined with mucous membrane and is invested partially by peritoneum. The uterine (fal-

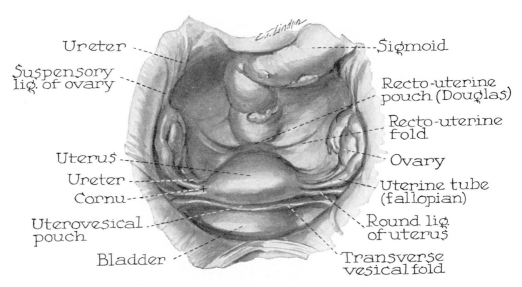

FIG. 464. The uterus as seen from above.

lopian) tubes enter at its widest part, the broad ligaments are attached to its side margins, and the ligament of the ovary and the round ligament of the uterus are attached just below the tubes.

The uterus is divided into three parts: a base or fundus; a main portion, the body or corpus; and the larger lower prolongation known as the neck or cervix, which projects into the vagina. The cervix is demarcated from the corpus by a slight constriction called the isthmus. The fundus and the body form the upper 2 inches, and the cervix forms the lower inch.

The fundus is the dome-shaped uppermost end which rises above the tubes. It is broad in its transverse diameter, and the fallopian tubes form a junction, called the cornua or horns, with it at its lateral margins.

The corpus narrows as it approaches the cervix, and when inspected from the front, it appears to be triangular in shape. The anterior surface of the corpus, which has also been referred to as the ventral or inferior surface, is covered by visceral peritoneum, which is reflected to the upper surface of the bladder at the junction of the body and the cervix of the uterus. This reflection of peritoneum forms a potential space known as the uterovesical pouch. The posterior (dorsal or superior) surface is covered by peritoneum which extends downward beyond the corpus to cover the cervix from which it is reflected to the front of the rectum. The space thus formed is known as the rectouterine excavation (cul-de-sac of Douglas or Douglas' pouch). The lateral margins of the uterus extend from the fallopian tubes above to the uterosacral ligaments below; they are devoid of peritoneum, since these margins give attachments to the diverging layers of the broad ligaments (Fig. 466). The round ligament of the uterus is attached in front of the origin of the fallopian tube, and the uterine and the ovarian vessels are situated below and behind it. The ligament of the ovary is attached to the intestinal surface of the uterus, but the round ligament is attached to the vesical surface. These structures lie between the opposed layers of the broad ligaments as the latter pass toward the lateral pelvic walls.

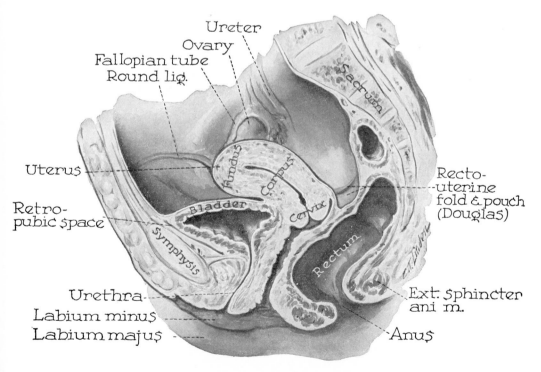

FIG. 465. The uterus as seen in sagittal section. The organ is divided into 3 parts: a fundus, a corpus and a cervix.

A fatty fibrous tissue fills the spaces between the broad ligaments. This tissue is called the *parametrium* and is most abundant near the cervix and the vagina, where it becomes continuous with the extraperitoneal tissue of the pelvic wall and floor.

The cervix is the narrower cylindrical segment of the uterus; it enters the vagina through the anterior vaginal wall and lies at right angles to it. Since it pierces the vagina, it is divided into supravaginal and intravaginal (vaginal) portions (Fig. 465). The supravaginal part lies above the ring of vaginal attachment, is covered with peritoneum posteriorly and is related to the intestines. Anteriorly, it is separated from the bladder by fatty tissue and is connected laterally with the broad ligament and the parametrium, which contains the blood vessels. The lower intravaginal (vaginal) portion is the free segment which projects through the vault of the vagina; it is covered with mucous membrane which has been reflected onto it from the upper part of the vaginal wall.

The cervix opens into the vaginal cavity through the *external os*. The os has anterior and posterior lips which are normally in contact with the posterior vaginal wall; this wall ascends to a higher cervical level than does the anterior wall and thus envelopes the inferior third of the cervix. In nulliparae, the os is a small transverse slit, the lips of which are smooth and rounded; but in multiparae it is wider, and the lips are quite irregular.

The cavity of the uterus is small when compared with the thickness of its wall. In sagittal section it is an elongated narrow cleft, but when viewed from in front is triangular in shape with all of its sides being convex inward (Fig. 469). Its normal capacity is about 3 to 8 cc. The base of the triangle is directed upward, and at its two upper corners it is continuous with the fallopian tubes; the apex of the triangle is directed downward where, at the constricted internal os (corresponding to the isthmus externally), it becomes continuous with the cervical canal. The mucous membrane of the cavity of the body of the uterus is smooth and velvety.

The canal of the cervix is spindle-shaped and about 1 inch long; it opens into the vagina at its lower end through the external os. The mucous membrane in the canal is raised into median longitudinal folds both in front and behind. Between these, in nulliparae, are secondary branching folds which pass upward and laterally. The treelike appearance has been called the arbor vitae (rugae or plicae

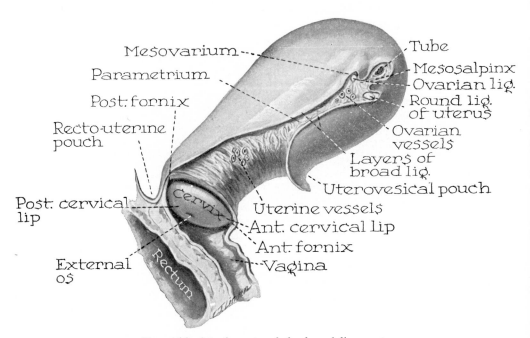

FIG. 466. Attachments of the broad ligament.

palmatae); these folds usually are absent after the first pregnancy.

The body of the uterus is the most movable part; the cervix, although mobile, is held rather firmly at either side by fascial and ligamentous bands known as *Mackenrodt's* *(cardinal) ligaments* (p. 558).

In the virgin the uterus lies with its long axis almost parallel with the superior aperture of the true pelvis and almost at right angles to the long axis of the vagina. Therefore, the fundus of the uterus is directed forward; this position is described as anteversion. Furthermore, the uterus is bent forward upon itself, producing anteflexion. It also is rotated slightly on its own axis. The position varies greatly in different individuals and is subject to change, depending on posture and the condition of the bladder and the rectum.

The structure of the uterus consists of 3 layers: an outer serous coat, a middle muscular coat and an inner lining, the mucous membrane.

The outer serous coat (perimetrium) is visceral peritoneum which consists of mesothelial cells; it is attached to the subjacent muscular coat through a thin layer of connective tissue. This attachment is firm over the fundus and the posterior part of the corpus but is much less firm over the posterior part of the cervix. *The muscular layer* is known as the *myometrium* and makes up the greater part of the organ. It consists of interlacing bundles of smooth muscle fibers which are united by connective tissue. These fibers increase in size and probably in number during the first half of pregnancy and they never regain their virginal size. *The inner lining* of mucous membrane is the *endometrium;* it is smooth and velvety and is about 2 to 5 mm. in thickness. The epithelium is columnar in type and is firmly attached to the underlying myometrium.

The endocervix also is a columnar epithelium richly provided with compound racemose glands which secrete a clear mucous; this may fill the cervical canal and act as a protective plug against uterine infection.

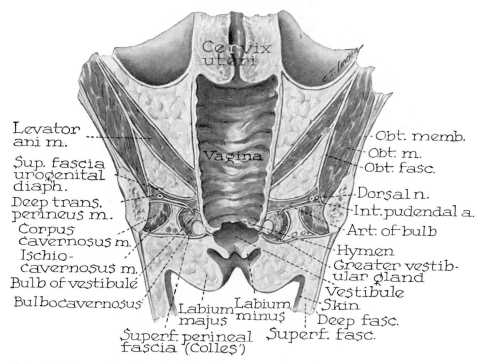

FIG. 467. The vagina, frontal section. The vagina passes through the fascia of the pelvis, between the levator ani muscles, through the urogenital diaphragm and opens onto the surface of the perineum.

Malformations. Various developmental malformations of the uterus may take place. The 2 müllerian ducts normally fuse over those parts which form the uterus and the vagina (Fig. 461). The upper or tubal portions of the ducts retain their independence as the 2 fallopian tubes. The fused uterus and the vagina are at first partitioned by a median septum which disappears later, and the double uterine and vaginal canals become converted into a single cavity. The disappearance of this median partition occurs from the vulva upward, and the degree of its absorption may vary. Therefore, a partitioned vagina with a partitioned uterus (*uterus didelphys*), a completely developed single vagina and a partitioned uterus (*uterus duplex*), or a single vagina and a single uterus (*uterus simplex*) may result. Occasionally, the ducts remain separated throughout their entire length and then 2 *entirely separate uteri and vaginae* are found. The uterus may be divided, producing the *bicornate uterus;* the cervix may be either single or double. If one müllerian duct fails to keep pace with the other, any variety of asymmetry may result.

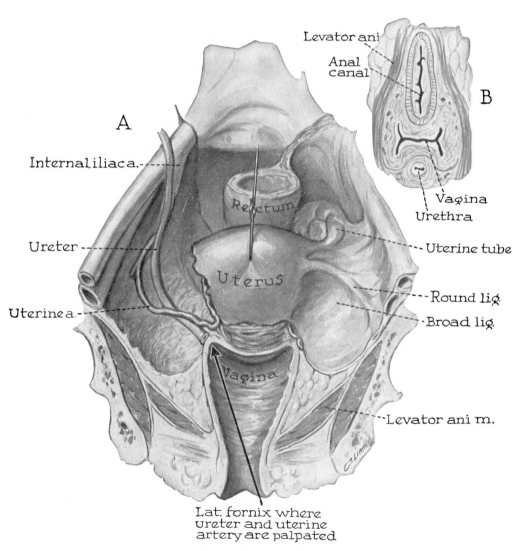

FIG. 468. The vagina. (A) Seen from in front and above. The arrow leads to the lateral fornix. (B) The "H"-shape of the upper part of the vagina seen in cross section.

VAGINA

The vagina is a flattened but distensible musculomembranous canal which usually measures about 3 inches in length. It extends from the vulva, through the urogenital diaphragm and to the region of the recto-uterine pouch of Douglas (Figs. 465, 467 and 468). If followed from above downward, it passes forward through the fascia of the pelvis, between the borders of the 2 levators and, after passing through the urogenital diaphragm, opens onto the surface of the perineum between the labia minora (Fig. 467). Therefore, it lies partly in the pelvis and partly in the perineum. Its anterior wall is 3 inches long, and its posterior wall 3½ inches long; these walls are normally in contact with each other. In transverse sections the vagina appears as a transverse slit, or in its upper part as the letter "H" (Fig. 468 B). The walls are separated where the cervix uteri projects into the vaginal cavity.

The space which exists between the intravaginal portion of the cervix and the vaginal walls is divided into anterior, lateral and posterior *fornices*. Since the posterior vaginal wall is nearly ½ inch longer than the anterior, the posterior fornix is deeper (Fig. 465). The normal nulliparous vagina is held in position as a semirigid tube by its surrounding fascia. Anteriorly, the fascia is found between the bladder and the vagina, and it stretches from the symphysis beneath the bladder to the anterior wall of the cervix. Posteriorly, fascia separates the vagina from the rectum (rectovaginal fascia). When these fascial structures are stretched or are torn during childbirth, rectoceles and cystoceles develop.

Relations. The vagina is related anteriorly, in its upper part, to the back of the bladder and the terminal parts of the ureters, and in its lower part to the urethra and the fatty areolar tissue behind and below the symphysis pubis. Posteriorly, in its upper ½ inch, it is covered with peritoneum which separates it from loops of intestines; below this it is related to the lowest part of the rectum and still lower to the perineal body which separates it from the anal canal. Laterally, the vagina is crossed by the ureters and the uterine arteries lying in the parametrium of

the lower and the inner parts of the broad ligaments; therefore, a thickened tuberculous ureter or the pulsations of the uterine artery can be felt vaginally (Fig. 468 A). At a lower level the vagina is clasped by the inner borders of the levator ani muscles which form a "sphincter" vagina; at its lowest part it is covered by the vestibular glands and the bulb of the vestibule.

Arteries. The chief artery on each side is the *vaginal artery*; this replaces the inferior vesical artery of the male (Fig. 475). It arises from the anterior division of the internal iliac artery and passes forward and medially on the levator ani to the vagina. Further arterial blood is contributed by the uterine and the middle rectal arteries and by the artery of the bulb of the vestibule.

Veins. The veins form networks in the submucous coat and on the surface. These networks are drained by veins accompanying the arteries.

Lymphatics. The lymph vessels from the upper part accompany the uterine lymph vessels to the external and the internal iliac glands; those from the middle part pass along the vaginal blood vessels to the internal iliac glands, while some of those from the lower part drain into the sacral and the common iliac glands. Other glands are associated with lymph vessels from the anal canal and the vulva; they end in the superficial inguinal glands.

Coats. The vagina has 4 coats: (1) external fascial coat of areolar tissue containing a plexus of veins; (2) a coat of nonstriated muscle; (3) a submucous coat of elastic areolar tissue which contains a dense plexus of veins, so thin-walled that it resembles erectile tissue, and (4) a mucous coat which is covered with stratified epithelium and is mucous only in name, for the vagina per se does not contain mucous glands. It is kept moist by mucous from the uterus.

UTERINE TUBES (FALLOPIAN TUBES)

The uterine tubes are the paired oviducts which convey the ovum to the uterus. Each is about 4 inches long, ¼ inch wide and is quite tortuous (Figs. 464, 466, 469). They are found in the upper border of the broad ligaments, which, therefore, form a "mesen-

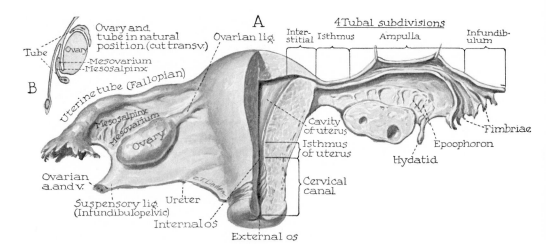

FIG. 469. Uterus, ovaries and fallopian tubes. (A) A section of the uterus has been removed so that the interior of the uterine cavity and the cervical canal can be seen. (B) Transverse section through the ovary.

tery" for the tube. Each tube emerges from the uterine wall at the junction of the corpus and the fundus uteri. Its course is at first horizontally outward and then backward; it curls around the tubal end of the ovary and overlaps its medial surface (Fig. 462). It connects with the uterine cavity through the uterine ostium and with the abdominal cavity through the abdominal ostium. The caliber of the latter is subject to great variation in different individuals.

These 4 chief *subdivisions* are recognized (Fig. 469). (1) The interstitial part is a short portion which begins at the upper angle of the uterine cavity with which it connects by a minute ostium. It is that part which passes through the uterine wall (about ½ inch thick) and appears externally at the cornu just above the uterine attachment of the round and the ovarian ligaments. (2) The isthmus is that medial inch of tube which is short and cordlike; it appears just outside of the uterus and runs a rather narrow but straight course. The lumen of the isthmus gradually increases and joins the ampulla. (3) The ampulla is that portion which is the widest and the longest subdivision of the tube; it appears to be convoluted. It is thin-walled and dilatable and constitutes the most important part of the tube. It leads into the trumpet-shaped expansion which is the in-

fundibulum. (4) The infundibulum is funnel-shaped, but the surface of the funnel is broken into numerous fingerlike processes called fimbriae, which give the free margin a fringed or ragged appearance.

From its uterine attachment to the fimbriated end, the tube is enveloped by a superior fold of broad ligament, the *mesosalpinx*. The isthmus of the tube, which has a relatively short mesosalpinx, moves with the uterus, but the ampulla and the infundibulum, with a comparatively long mesosalpinx, are nearly as mobile as the ovary.

In addition to an outer serous coat derived from the broad ligament, the tube is surrounded by a subserous layer and a muscle layer which is continuous with that of the uterus. The mucosa lining the tube is peculiar in that it is arranged in folds which are directed longitudinally. This mucous membrane is covered with a ciliated epithelium; the action of the cilia is supposed to create a stream of lymph from the peritoneal cavity into the mouth of the tube and along it to the uterus.

The *arterial blood supply* is derived from the tubal branches of the uterine and the ovarian arteries (Fig. 478). The *lymph vessels* drain to the aortic glands with the vessels to the ovary and the fundus of the uterus. The *nerve supply* is derived from the uterine and the ovarian plexuses and ultimately from 11 and 12 T and 1 L.

OVARIES

The genital gland of the female resembles a large almond, in both size and shape. It projects from the posterior layer of the broad ligament, which it draws outward to form the mesovarium (Fig. 469). It is covered with cuboidal epithelium, not peritoneum. The mesovarium is usually short and attaches only to the anterior border of the ovary. The gland is smooth and pink in young nulliparae but becomes gray and puckered in elderly women and in multiparae. This is due to the repeated discharge of ova through its surface and the resultant formation of puckering scars; in old women it becomes shrunken, wrinkled and atrophic.

The ovary lies in the peritoneal depression on the side wall of the pelvis; the depression is bounded behind by the ureter and in front by the broad ligament. In the floor of this fossa the obturator vessels and nerves are found. At the first pregnancy, the broad ligament enlarges with the uterus and carries the ovary up into the abdomen proper. After childbirth, the organ returns to the pelvis but seldom regains its former position; it may be found in any location in the dorsal part of the pelvis. It also may be prolapsed deep into the cul-de-sac, where it can be palpated vaginally, lateral to or behind the cervix.

Extremities and Surfaces. The ovary has 2 extremities and 2 surfaces. The tubal extremity, which is referred to as the upper pole, is rounded, faces superiorly and is embraced by the fallopian tube. The infundibulopelvic ligament (suspensory ligament of the ovary) attaches this pole to the peritoneum of the pelvic wall; it is derived from the upper and the lateral aspects of the broad ligament and contains the ovarian vessels. The fimbriae of the fallopian tube also are found at the upper pole of the organ. The lower (uterine) pole connects the ovary with the superolateral angle of the uterus by means of the ovarian ligament; it is about ¼ inch above the pelvic floor. The medial surface is directed inward, and since it is overlapped to a great extent by the fallopian tube, only a small part of it is exposed to the eye. The lateral surface faces outward and is in direct contact with the parietal peritoneum of the pelvic wall where this layer is depressed to form the ovarian fossa. Although pregnancy may alter the position of the ovary in multiparae, it nevertheless remains anchored at 3 places: the ovarian ligament, the mesovarium and the infundibulopelvic ligament.

Arteries. The blood supply is derived from the ovarian artery, a direct branch of the aorta, which arises just below the origin of the renal artery (Fig. 478). Unlike the corresponding artery in the male, it does not pass through the internal inguinal ring but turns medially over the pelvic inlet to enter the infundibulopelvic ligament of the ovary. Its branches reach the hilum by way of the mesovarium, but the terminal branches continue medially in the broad ligament to supply the uterine tube and the upper part of the uterus. It anastomoses with branches of the uterine artery.

Veins. Several veins arise from the hilum of the ovary but they unite to form a single or double ovarian vein. The right ovarian vein empties into the inferior vena cava, and the left joins the left renal vein.

Lymphatics. The lymph vessels follow the ovarian veins and end in the aortic lymph glands.

Nerves. The nerve supply is derived from the aortic and the renal plexuses (10 T.).

The structure of the ovary reveals 2 zones: a central medullary and an outer cortical layer or zone. The medullary zone is characterized by its numerous blood vessels within the connective tissue. The cortical layer, besides containing connective tissue, contains the essential glandular tissue in the form of graafian follicles in various stages of development.

Ureters

The ureters are expansile muscular tubes, whitish in appearance, which are approximately 10 inches long and about ¼ inch in diameter. The iliopectineal line serves as a dividing point between the abdominal and the pelvic portions of the ureters.

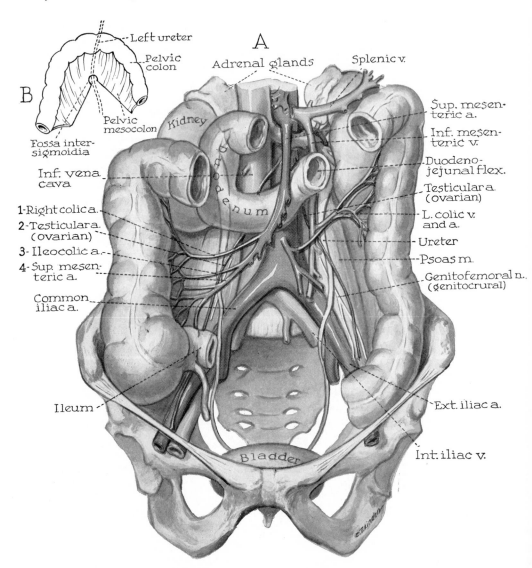

FIG. 470. The ureter. (A) The ureters are shown in their entire courses and their anatomic relationships. Four vessels cross the right ureter: the right colic, the testicular (ovarian), the ileocolic and the superior mesenteric. (B) The relation of the left ureter to the intersigmoid fossa.

RELATIONS

From above downward the ureter rests on the genitofemoral (genitocrural) nerve, the common iliac vessels on the left side, and the external iliac vessels on the right side; after passing downward on the internal iliac artery, it is related to the ligaments in the pelvis (Fig. 470). As the ureter bends into the true pelvis the ovarian (testicular) vessels gradually diverge from it. The end of the abdominal portion of the ureter is separated from the iliopectineal line by the psoas muscle and the iliac vessels. On the right side it crosses the vessels at the point of bifurcation of the common iliac artery, but on the left side it crosses the common iliac about 1 to 1.5 cm. above its bifurcation. On the left side it bears

a constant relationship to the sigmoid. It appears above the iliopectineal line at the apex of the intersigmoid fossa (Fig. 470 B). On the right side the relation of the ureter to the intestine is less constant because of the variable position of the cecum and lower loops of the ileum. The ureters are placed behind the peritoneum to which they are loosely attached.

RIGHT URETER

The *right ureter* is a little lateral to the inferior vena cava; its pelvis is covered by the second part of the duodenum. Four sets of blood vessels cross in front of it, between it and the peritoneum (Fig. 470 A). These are: the right colic artery, the testicular

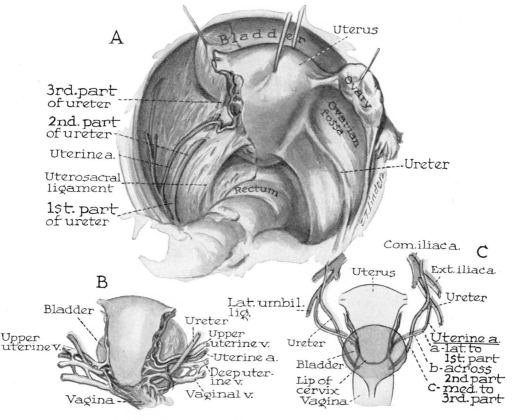

Fig. 471. The 3 parts of the pelvic ureter. (A) It is convenient to divide the pelvic portion of the ureter into 3 parts: (1) a posterior part in the uterosacral ligament, (2) an intermediate part, Mackenrodt's ligament, and (3) an anterior part in the vesico-uterine ligament. (B) The intermediate part of the ureter is surrounded on all sides by vessels, mostly veins. (C) The uterine artery is lateral to the first part, passes across the second part and is medial to the third part of the ureter.

(ovarian) artery, the ileocolic artery and the superior mesenteric artery in the root of the mesentery.

LEFT URETER

The *left ureter* is a little lateral to the inferior mesenteric vein. Its pelvis is more exposed than the right and, after appearing from behind the renal vessels, is covered only by the peritoneum. It is separated, as on the right side, at intervals from the peritoneum by the upper left colic, the testicular (ovarian) and two or more left colic vessels. Because of the vessels which cross the abdominal part of the ureter, the extraperitoneal lumbo-inguinal approach is preferable to the transperitoneal one.

THE PELVIC PART OF THE URETER

This part is divided into 3 portions (Figs. 471 and 472): (1) a pars posterior (in the uterosacral ligament), (2) a pars intermedia (in Mackenrodt's ligament) and (3) a pars anterior (in the vesico-uterine ligament).

The pars posterior of the pelvic portion of the ureter begins at the level of the sacroiliac joint. At this point the ureters are separated by a distance of 6 to 7 cm., a distance which corresponds roughly to the width of the middle of the sacrum (Fig. 420).

In this part of their course they form an arch, the convexity of which is directed laterad. After traveling about an inch, they lie from 12 to 13 cm. from each other; they reach the upper edge of Mackenrodt's ligament via the uterosacral ligaments (p. 558).

They next bend mediad and, due to the position of the uterosacral ligament on the posterior surface of Mackenrodt's ligament, they pass in an antero-inferior and medial direction into this ligament. This portion of the ureter remains attached to the lateral pelvic wall and the anteromedial aspect of the internal iliac artery. It crosses all the anterior branches of this artery, namely, the obturator and the superior vesical arteries (Fig. 472).

Medially, this portion of the ureter approaches the posterior margin of the ovary, which lies immediately anterior to the internal iliac artery; therefore, the posterior boundary of the ovarian fossa is formed by the pars posterior of the pelvic portion of the

ureter (Fig. 471 A). This part of the ureter is accompanied by the uterine artery, which lines along its anterolateral surface (Fig. 468).

The pars intermedia of the pelvic portion of the ureter is that part which runs in Mackenrodt's ligament. It extends from its entrance into the ligament as far as the vesicouterine ligament. In this ligament the ureter comes into close relationship with the cervix for a short distance, being about 1.5 cm. from it (Fig. 471 C).

In the upper portion of its course the ureter is covered by the uterine artery and vein, but in its deepest portion these vessels cross it. In its intermediate portion it is difficult to isolate because it is surrounded on all sides by vessels, mostly veins (Fig. 471 B). Caudally, the deep uterine veins and the vaginal veins are found; medially there is the uterovaginal plexus, which passes downward along the edge of the uterus and the vagina; laterally, the anastomoses between the superficial and deep uterine veins appears. Although these vessels surround the ureter, they do not directly touch it, since the ureter travels in a preformed canal to which its adventitia is attached by loose connective tissue. Therefore, in order to free this part of the ureter the dissection must be carried along the correct cleavage plane, which is between the canal of the ureter and its adventitia. If this plane is found, it is possible to dissect it without injury and unnecessary hemorrhage.

The distance from the ureter to the cervix is not constant, the average being ½ to 1 inch. It depends on the framework of vessels around the ureteral canal. If the anastomoses between the deep and the superficial veins are close to the edge of the uterus, the ureter lies near to the cervix; if the anastomoses are situated nearer to the pelvic wall, the ureter is farther away. Lateral displacement of the uterus also alters the ureteral position. If the uterus is displaced to the right, then the right ureter lies nearer to the edge of the cervix and vice versa.

The pars anterior of the pelvic portion of the ureter extends from its entrance into the vesico-uterine ligament as far as the ureteral orifice of the bladder. The veins draining the vesical plexus lie lateral to and above the ureters. The vaginal plexus is caudad and forward toward the symphysis, and the anterior vaginal wall is adjacent to it. Medially, it is bounded by the vesico-vaginal space. As it passes forward in the vesico-uterine ligament it gradually turns upward and medially; it empties into the bladder about 1.5 cm.

below the level of the anterior lip of the cervix (Fig. 471 C). This is a relationship which should be appreciated, for at times a calculus in this portion of the ureter may be felt vaginally (Fig. 468 A). As the ureter (pars intermedia) travels through a sort of canal in Mackenrodt's ligament, so does the pars anterior course through a similar canal in the

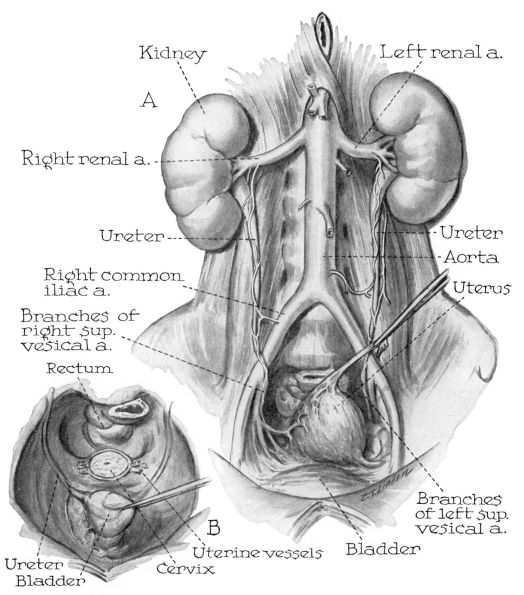

FIG. 472. The ureter. (A) The blood supply of the ureter is derived from the renal, the testicular, the colic, the vesical and the middle rectal arteries (Fig. 443 A). (B) The pelvic portion of the ureter, showing its entrance into the bladder.

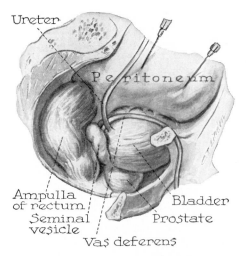

FIG. 473. The ureter in the male, seen from the right. The vas deferens crosses above the ureter as it is overlapped by the upper end of the seminal vesicle.

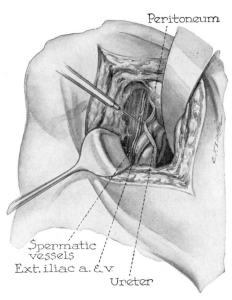

FIG. 474. Exposure of the right ureter. The illustration reveals a retroperitoneal approach. The peritoneum is retracted medially, and the relations to the surrounding vessels are demonstrated.

vesico-uterine ligament. The wall of the canal is attached to the ureter by a similar type of loose connective tissue.

The uterine artery is lateral to part one, runs across part two and is medial to part three of the ureter.

THE PELVIC PART OF THE URETER IN THE MALE

This part of the ureter crosses the beginning of the external iliac artery, passes backward and downward along the lower border of the internal iliac (hypogastric) artery and reaches the level of the ischial spine (Fig. 473). At this point it curves forward and mediad in the fat above the levator ani muscle and reaches the posterosuperior angle of the bladder. It passes through the posterior wall of the bladder at an extreme oblique angle, running medially and downward. It opens into the bladder at the upper angle of an area called the trigone. As the ureter approaches the bladder, it is under cover of the closely adherent peritoneum and at times may be seen shining through it. In the beginning of its course the internal iliac artery is above and behind it. Lateral to it are the psoas and the obturator internus muscles, the external iliac vein, the obturator nerve, the umbilical artery, and the obturator and the

inferior vesical vessels. As the ureter turns downward it lies in the fat above the levator ani muscle and beneath the peritoneum; the vas deferens crosses above it, between it and the peritoneum near the bladder. Near the bladder it is surrounded by a plexus of veins and is overlapped by the upper end of the seminal vesicle. It receives its blood supply from branches arising from the renal, the testicular, the colic, the vesical and the middle rectal arteries. Because of its great vascularity, the ureter may withstand a considerable amount of surgical trauma, and large segments of it may be mobilized without sloughing. It is for this reason that injury to it heals quickly. Its nerve supply is derived from the renal, the testicular and the hypogastric plexuses. The lymphatics end in glands nearest it in the abdomen and the pelvis.

The ureter is constricted in certain localities. The uppermost of these constrictions is about 5.5 cm. from the kidney pelvis, the next at the brim of the pelvis where the ureter crosses the common iliac artery, and the third or lowermost just outside of the ureteral orifice. A ureteral calculus usually stops at one of these constrictions as it passes down the ureter.

SURGICAL CONSIDERATIONS

Exposure of the Ureter

It may be necessary to expose the ureter for excision, the removal of stones or for repair (Fig. 474).

A number of incisions have been described (Fig. 490); however, it is agreed that this structure is approached most readily by a retroperitoneal route. The incision should be ample and allow for examination of not only the entire ureter but the kidney as well. The patient is placed in the lateral decubitus and is well arched over a kidney-rest or a sandbag. An adequate lumbo-iliac incision is made. The incision begins about the mid-dle of the 12th rib and extends downward and forward to a midpoint between the center of the iliac crest and the anterior superior iliac spine; it then passes around the anterior iliac spine and continues forward and parallel with the inguinal ligament. The external and the internal oblique muscles and the transversus abdominis muscle are incised in the direction of the skin incision; the transversalis fascia is incised; and the extraperitoneal fat is exposed.

The peritoneum is mobilized medially, and the ureter and the pelvic vessels are identified. The ureter normally remains adherent to the peritoneum when that structure is reflected toward the midline. Nevertheless, the ureter can be detached easily from the peritoneum to permit any surgical procedure or exploration which might be deemed necessary.

Neurovascular Structures

Most of the vessels supplying the structures within the pelvis lie in the extraperitoneal fatty tissue which intervenes between the peritoneum and the fascia. The nerves, at first, lie outside of the fascia and are not only retroperitoneal but, like the muscles, are also retrofascial.

ARTERIES

The arteries of the pelvis are the internal iliac (hypogastric), the superior hemorrhoidal (rectal), which is the continuation of the inferior mesenteric, and the median sacral. The ovarian artery is an exception in that it does not arise within the true pelvis but originates from the aorta at the level of the kidneys (Fig. 478).

The internal iliac artery (hypogastric) is the largest artery in the true pelvis and gives rise to all the arteries of the pelvis except the superior hemorrhoidal, the median sacral and the ovarian (Figs. 475 and 476). It is a wide vessel, smaller than the external iliac, and is about 1½ inches long. It arises as a terminal branch of the common iliac on the medial border of the psoas muscle, passes backward and downward across the medial surface of the psoas muscle and enters the pelvis. In its course it passes the sacro-iliac joint and ends near the upper border of the greater sciatic notch by breaking up into anterior and posterior divisions which supply the exterior and the interior of the pelvis. Although it is narrower in the adult than the external iliac, it is twice as wide in the fetus because of its umbilical branch which passes to the umbilicus and the placenta. After birth, the umbilical branch is patent to a point where the superior vesical arteries arise, and beyond this it becomes a fibrous cord called the lateral umbilical ligament. The ureter is in front of it; behind it lies its vein, and as it

descends subperitoneally it crosses medial to the external iliac vein and the obturator nerve (Fig. 475). At the upper border of the greater foramen, the artery divides into anterior and posterior divisions; the terminal branches from these divisions follow a pattern which is open to considerable variation.

The *posterior division* gives rise to the following 3 branches, all of which are parietal: the iliolumbar, the lateral sacral and the superior gluteal (Fig. 475).

The iliolumbar artery, located at the 5th lumbar segment, corresponds to a lumbar artery. It passes upward and laterally, first between the obturator nerve and the lumbosacral cord and, secondly, between the psoas muscle and the spinal column. Opposite the pelvic brim the artery divides into an iliac and a lumbar branch, the former ramifying the iliac fossa and the latter ascending behind the psoas to send a spinal branch into the vertebral canal via the lumbosacral intervertebral foramen. The iliolumbar vein does not descend into the pelvis with its artery but ends in back of the common iliac vein.

The lateral sacral artery passes mediad and downward in front of the sacral nerves, and each of them divides into 2. Therefore, 4 arteries pass through the anterior sacral foramina to nourish the structures in the sacral canal; they emerge through the posterior sacral foramina to supply the muscles on the back of the sacrum and the overlying skin.

The superior gluteal artery is the largest branch of the posterior division of the internal iliac artery, and its course in the pelvis is short. It passes downward and backward between the lumbosacral trunk and the 1st sacral nerve, pierces the parietal pelvic fascia and enters the gluteal region via the upper part of the greater sciatic foramen above the piriformis muscle. It travels with its vein and the superior gluteal nerve.

The *anterior division* of the internal iliac artery gives rise to 9 branches. All of the posterior branches previously described are parietal, but the anterior branches are both visceral and parietal. The 3 parietal branches are the obturator, the internal pudendal and the inferior gluteal; the 6 visceral branches are the umbilical, the superior vesical, the inferior vesical, the middle hemorrhoidal, the uterine and the vaginal.

The obturator artery passes forward and downward along the lateral wall of the pelvis and emerges through the obturator fora-

men above the obturator internus muscle. It is accompanied by its nerve and vein; the order, from above downward, is nerve, artery and vein. Converging on the nerve and after passing through the upper part of the obturator foramen, it divides into lateral and medial branches which surround the obturator foramen lying between it and the obturator externus muscle. These branches encircle the outer surface of the obturator membrane, supply the obturator externus muscle and give an acetabular branch to the hip joint. An *abnormal obturator artery*, when present, is important in the surgery of femoral hernias (p. 766). The obturator and

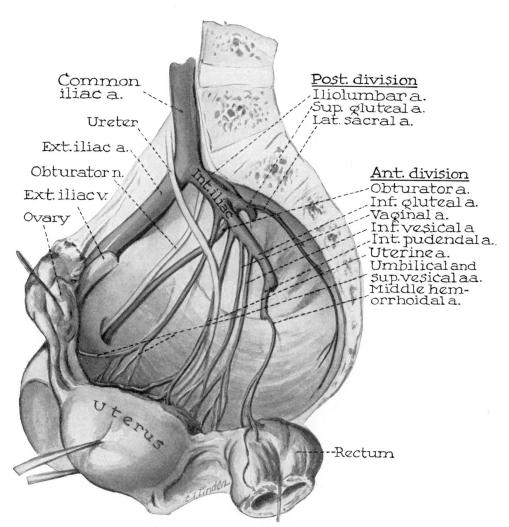

F<small>IG</small>. 475. The right internal iliac artery and its branches. The uterus and the rectum have been pulled to the left and forward.

the inferior epigastric arteries each supply pubic branches, which are small and anastomose at the back of the pubis. In 30 to 35 per cent of cases, however, the pubic branch of the inferior epigastric artery is large and replaces the obturator branch; it is called the abnormal obturator artery (Fig. 477). This apparently is attributable to an obliteration of the usual origin of the obturator artery. From its origin the abnormal artery descends into the true pelvis on the medial side of the external iliac vein and usually lies lateral to the femoral ring. If the artery is on the medial side of the ring and along the edge of the lacunar ligament, it is in a precarious location, since cutting this ligament in a strangulated femoral hernia

might sever the artery and result in profuse hemorrhage.

The internal pudendal artery travels a rather complicated course. It descends over the piriformis muscle and the sacral plexus in the interval between the piriformis and the coccygeus muscles. At this point the artery leaves the pelvis through the greater sciatic foramen and enters the buttock, where it rests on the spine of the ischium with the pudendal nerve on its medial side and the nerve to the obturator internus on its lateral side; these are covered by the gluteus maximus muscle. The artery then disappears through the lesser sciatic foramen and reaches Alcock's pudendal canal where it passes downward to gain access to the peri-

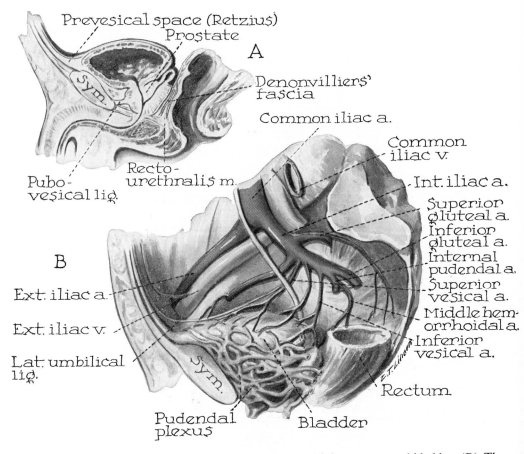

FIG. 476. The right internal iliac artery. (A) Relations of the prostate and bladder. (B) The middle hemorrhoidal vessels form the posterior boundary of the prevesical space.

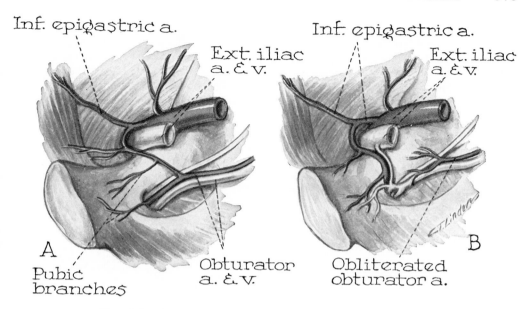

Inf. epigastric a.   Inf. epigastric a.

Ext. iliac a. & v.   Ext. iliac a. & v.

A   B

Pubic branches   Obturator a. & v.   Obliterated obturator a.

FIG. 477. The obturator arteries: (A) normal; (B) abnormal.

neum (Fig. 358). It terminates by piercing the perineal membrane and divides into the deep and the dorsal arteries of the penis or the clitoris. It supplies inferior rectal, scrotal (labial), transverse perineal, bulbar, penile and clitoral branches.

The inferior gluteal artery is the terminal and largest branch of the anterior division. It passes downward and backward, pierces the fascia in front of the piriformis muscle and continues between the 1st and the 2nd, or the 2nd and the 3rd sacral nerves. It leaves the pelvis through the lower part of the greater sciatic foramen and appears in the buttock between the piriformis and the gemellus superior. Its branches in the pelvis are only twigs to the surrounding structures.

The umbilical artery passes downward and forward along the side wall of the pelvis in front of the obturator nerve; it is in contact with the bladder when it is full but is some distance from it when it is empty. It proceeds upward from the bladder to the umbilicus, being covered by peritoneum. In the pelvis it is crossed by the ureter and the vas deferens (ligamentum teres in the female). It gives off the superior vesical artery; beyond that point its lumen becomes obliterated, and then it is

known as the lateral umbilical ligament (Fig. 476 B). Under that name it ascends out of the pelvis in the extraperitoneal tissue of the anterior abdominal wall to reach the umbilicus. The umbilical artery has no accompanying vein; the umbilical vein which accompanies the fetal arteries in the umbilical cord leaves them at the umbilicus, continues to the liver and becomes the round ligament of the liver.

The superior vesical arteries may arise as 2 or 3 branches from the umbilical artery. They supply the superior aspect of the bladder and may give off the artery to the vas deferens.

The inferior vesical artery is small; in the male it arises a little below the obturator artery. It passes forward to reach the bladder and supplies the seminal vesicles, the prostate and the posterior and the inferior parts of the bladder. It gives off a long slender branch called the *artery of the vas deferens* which supplies and accompanies the vas as far as the testis.

The vaginal artery replaces the inferior vesical artery of the male. It is larger than the latter and arises a little below the obturator artery, descends and divides into branches which pass to the vagina; other branches pass onward to the posterior and the lower parts of the bladder.

The middle hemorrhoidal (rectal) artery travels in a leash of veins that forms the posterior limit of the retropubic space. It usually arises from the internal pudendal artery but may arise with the inferior vesical. It passes medially to the rectum, ramifies its walls and sends twigs forward to the vagina or to the seminal vesicles and the prostate gland. With the veins and a condensation of extraperitoneal areolar tissue, it constitutes the rectal stalk or the lateral rectal ligament.

The uterine artery is a large vessel which arises near the lower end of the anterior division of the internal iliac. It may be divided conveniently into the following parts: (1) descending, (2) horizontal and (3) ascending (Fig. 478).

The descending part represents its course on the lateral pelvic wall which corresponds to the posterior edge of the ovarian fossa. Since this part is associated with the parietal

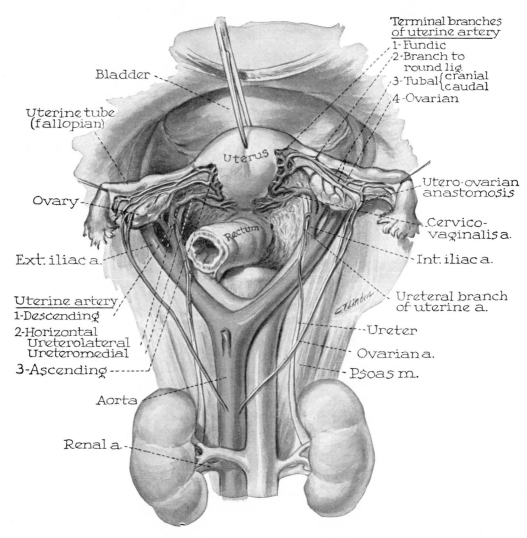

FIG. 478. The uterine artery. This vessel may be divided into 3 parts: (1) descending, (2) horizontal and (3) ascending. The tubes and the ovaries have been retracted outward to show the entire course of the uterine and the ovarian arteries.

wall, it is known as the parietal portion, and it is here that the artery may best be isolated from its surrounding tissues.

The horizontal part is the parametrial portion; it crosses the ureter and is related to Mackenrodt's ligament. This part may be subdivided into ureterolateral and uretero-mesial portions, depending on its relation to the ureter.

The ascending part is the para-uterine portion; it extends upward along the edge of the uterus and with the accompanying veins it forms a definite vascular cord in the parametrium.

The first branch of the uterine artery is the ureteral branch which is given off where the artery crosses the ureter; it passes upward along the ureter. At or just after crossing the ureter, a second uterine branch, the cervicovaginal artery, is given off. This branch supplies the posterior and the anterior walls of the cervix and the vagina; it lies within the cervical and the vaginal septa of the surrounding connective tissue. The uterine branches proper are given off from part three (ascending part).

At the tubo-uterine junction the uterine artery divides into its 4 terminal branches: (1) The fundic branches, which pass medially, penetrate the musculature of the uterus and supply the fundus. (2) The branch to the round ligament is the smallest branch; it passes forward beneath the tube at the cornu and accompanies the round ligament along its course in the inguinal canal. This vessel anastomoses with a branch from the inferior epigastric. (3) The tubal branch extends from the ligament of the ovary into the mesosalpinx and divides into cranial and caudal branches. The cranial branch extends along the underside of the tube within the mesosalpinx and supplies branches to both the tube and the ampulla. The caudal branch lies in the lower portion of the mesosalpinx near the hilus of the ovary and bends around the upper extremity of the ovary to reach the infundibulopelvic ligament where it anastomoses with the ovarian artery. The cranial and the caudal branches anastomose via small vessels which cross between the layers of the broad ligament. (4) The ovarian branch arises beneath the ligament of the ovary, extends along the ventral side of the ligament, passes to the hilus of the ovary, gives off numerous branches and then joins the ovarian artery.

The location of the uterine artery is important because of the great number of surgical procedures performed in this region. It is especially important where it crosses the

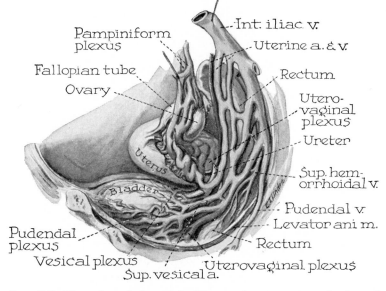

FIG. 479. The veins of the pelvis. These veins anastomose freely and form many venous plexuses on and in the walls of the pelvic viscera.

ureter. This crossing is near the level of the internal os about 1 or 2 cm. from the lateral border of the cervix. At this point the ureter may be injured when the artery is ligated.

The ovarian artery is homologous to the internal spermatic artery in the male. It arises from the aorta below the origin of the renal artery and passes downward and laterally on the posterior abdominal wall (Fig. 478). Unlike the corresponding artery in the male, it does not pass to the deep inguinal ring but turns medially over the pelvic inlet, coursing over the psoas muscle and crossing the external iliac vessels. It enters the infundibulo-pelvic ligament and reaches the ovarian hilus by way of the mesovarium. Its terminal branches continue medially in the broad ligament and supply the tube and the upper part of the uterus. It anastomoses freely with branches of the uterine artery. This vessel also crosses the ureter but in a different direction than the uterine artery. It crosses at an acute angle at the entrance of the true pelvis where it lies in front of the ureter; distal to this point the ovarian artery and the ureter separate. The vessel proceeds along the lateral border of the ureter until the latter dips into the true pelvis at the terminal line.

VEINS

The chief veins of the pelvis are the 2 internal iliac veins and their tributaries. Besides these there are the superior hemorrhoidal (rectal) and the median sacral veins, and in the female there is a pair of ovarian pampiniform plexuses (Fig. 479). The veins of the pelvis are thin-walled, accompany the arteries and anastomose freely, thus forming many venous plexuses on and in the walls of the viscera from which the visceral veins arise. These plexuses are the rectal, the vesical, the prostatic, the uterine and the vaginal. They are not closed systems, but since they anastomose freely, the plexus of one organ communicates with the plexus of a neighboring viscus. It has been stated that the pelvic viscera lie within a basket woven of large, thin-walled, venous plexuses among which the arteries thread their way.

Internal Iliac Veins. This is the widest vein of the pelvis. It is short and is formed by the confluence of the venae comitantes of the superior gluteal artery and most of the veins that accompany the other branches of the internal iliac artery. It commences immediately above the greater sciatic foramen, passes forward and slightly upward out of the pelvis and ends on the medial surface of the psoas muscle. It joins the external iliac vein to form the common iliac vein. The internal iliac artery is below and in front of it, and the sacro-iliac joint and the lumbosacral trunks are above and behind it; medially, it is separated from the intestines by peritoneum, and laterally it is related first to the pelvic wall and the obturator nerve and then to the psoas muscle (Fig. 360).

Uterine Plexus. The veins of the uterus constitute one of the most important of the plexuses. The uterine plexus completely encircles the ascending portion of the artery and continues downward along the sides of the vagina as far as the external genitalia. The uterovaginal plexus lies enclosed in the compact connective tissue of the cervical and the vaginal septa as it continues upward to the edge of the uterus. These veins, like the vaginal, are chiefly on the sides of the organ where they surround the nutrient arteries. They arise in the cavernous venous spaces in the uterine wall and leave the lateral aspect of the organ at about the level of the cervix; here, they form a plexus which surrounds the ureter. The uterine veins anastomose with those of the vagina to form the uterovaginal plexus. The trunks from this plexus converge into the internal iliac vein or into one of its main tributaries. The vaginal venous plexus is massed at the sides of the vagina and communicates with the vesical, the rectal and the uterine plexuses. A vaginal vein arises on each side and accompanies the vaginal artery to the internal iliac vein.

Vesical Venous Plexus. In the female the vesical venous plexus lies on the surface of the bladder; it is densest around the neck and the upper part of the urethra, where it receives the dorsal vein of the clitoris. It drains into the vaginal plexus. In the male the plexus lies on the surface of the bladder, chiefly below, behind and around the seminal vesicles. It empties into the internal iliac vein by large vesical veins that accompany the inferior vesical artery.

Prostatic Venous Plexus. This dense network lies on the front and the sides of the prostate between its capsule and its fascial sheath (Fig. 454). Anteriorly, it receives the deep dorsal vein of the penis; superiorly, it is continuous with the vesical plexus, into which its blood is drained. The rectal venous plexuses have been discussed elsewhere (p. 462).

Ovarian Vein. This vein arises at the pelvic brim from the pampiniform plexus, which surrounds the ovarian artery in the pelvis. It accompanies this artery in the abdomen and ends, on the left side, in the left renal vein; on the right side it passes directly into the inferior vena cava.

Testicular Vein. In the male this vein arises from the pampiniform plexus at or near the deep inguinal ring and accompanies the artery into the abdomen. The left testicular vein ends in the left renal vein, and the right ends in the inferior vena cava a little below the level of the renal vein. Many believe that this arrangement of the left testicular vein predisposes this side to the formation of varicoceles.

Medial Sacral Vein. This vein is formed from the junction of the venae comitantes which travel with the median sacral artery. It usually passes along the right side of the artery and ends in the left common iliac vein.

Inferior Vena Cava. This vessel is formed by the junction of the 2 common iliac veins on the right side of the 5th lumbar vertebra (Fig. 480). It ascends along the right side of the abdominal aorta and continues upward in a groove on the posterior surface of the liver. It perforates the diaphragm between the right and the median portions of its central tendon. After inclining forward and mediad for about 1 inch, it pierces the fibrous pericardium, passes behind the serous pericardium and opens into the lower and the back part of the right atrium.

The relations of the abdominal portion of the inferior vena cava are as follows: *In front,* from below upward, it is related to the right common iliac artery, the mesentery, the right internal spermatic artery, the inferior part of the duodenum, the pancreas, the common bile duct, the portal vein and the posterior surface of the liver, which partly overlaps and occasionally surrounds it completely. *Behind,* it is in relation with the vertebral column, the right psoas major muscle, the right diaphragmatic crus, the right inferior phrenic, suprarenal, renal and lumbar arteries, the right sympathetic trunk and the right celiac ganglion, and the medial part of the right suprarenal gland. Relations on the *right side* are with the right kidney and ureter; on the *left side,* with the aorta, the right diaphragmatic crus and the caudate liver lobe.

Anomalies of the inferior vena cava are not infrequent because of the complicated mode of development of this structure. It should be recalled that embryologically 3 parallel channels—the posterior cardinal, the supracardinal and the subcardinal veins—develop bilaterally. It is from this complicated arrangement that the various anomalies result. A persistence of the subcardinal vein rather than the supracardinal below the level of the kidneys leads to retrocaval ureter. Gladstone states that a large ascending vein on the left side of the abdomen represents a left inferior vena cava; he further states that a double inferior vena cava is about twice as frequent as is a single left one. In double vena cava either vein may be the larger one, and both may communicate below with the com-

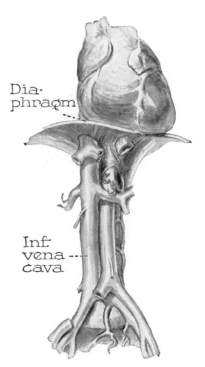

FIG. 480. The inferior vena cava.

mon iliac veins on their respective sides. Numerous other connections of these venous channels have been recorded. So-called "absence" of the vena cava has been reported. Of course, this refers to the hepatic portion of the inferior vena cava. The infrarenal or the suprahepatic portions apparently are never absent. Cases of so-called absence of the hepatic portion of the vena cava have been reported by Kaestner, Dwight and Neuberger. Other authors such as Huseby and Boyden and Effler, Greer and Sifers have reported quite extensively on the subject and can be referred to.

LYMPHATICS

The lymph glands and the lymph vessels of the female pelvis occupy rather constant positions (Fig. 481). The afferent lymph vessels from the skin and the subcutaneous tissue of the perineum, with the superficial afferent vessels from the inferior extremity, drain into a small group of lymph glands which are situated on either side of the upper part of the great saphenous vein. This group is known as the *superficial subinguinal glands*.

An adjacent group of glands, the *super-ficial inguinal glands,* about 10 to 20 in number, are situated just below the inguinal ligament and also receive perineal vessels, including those from the anus and the vulva. Into this latter group, the afferent lymphatics of the abdominal wall below the level of the umbilicus also pass.

The efferent vessels from both groups (superficial inguinal and superficial subinguinal) converge toward the saphenous opening in the deep fascia of the thigh; through this they drain into the *deep subinguinal glands*. This group usually numbers about 3 or 4 glands and is situated on the medial side of the femoral vein; they receive afferent vessels from the clitoris and associated structures.

The highest gland in this group has been called the gland of Rosenmüller or the node of Cloquet. It is located in the femoral ring; should it become inflamed, it might be mistaken for a strangulated femoral hernia.

This group as a whole is continuous with an extensive chain of parietal pelvic glands which are related to the common iliac artery and its branches. These iliac glands have been subdivided into 3 groups: the external

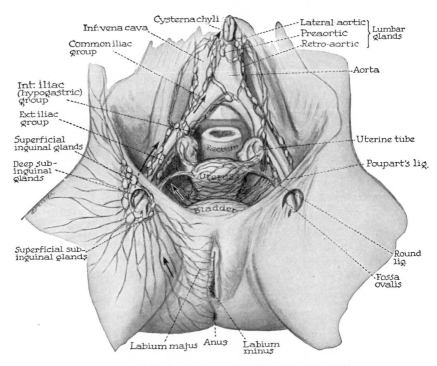

FIG. 481. The lymphatic system of the female pelvis.

iliac, the internal iliac (hypogastric) and the common iliac. All of these connect by numerous anastomoses. Their efferent vessels pass upward to a group of lumbar glands which, because of their position in relation to the abdominal aorta, are called the preaortic, the retro-aortic and the lateral aortic glands. The efferent vessels of these glands end in the cysterna chyli of the thoracic duct opposite the 2nd lumbar vertebra.

Lymph Vessels. The lymph vessels of the pelvic organs end mainly in the hypogastric and the iliac glands, but a small number may travel to the aortic, and a few may reach the inguinal glands. Those from the *bladder* pass to the external iliac, the hypogastric and the common iliac glands, and those from the urethra and the intrapelvic part of the ureter drain directly into the hypogastric group. The efferent lymph vessels from the *cervix* and the major portion of the *vagina* drain with those of the urinary bladder into the 3 groups of pelvic glands. However, those from the lowermost part of the vagina descend to join

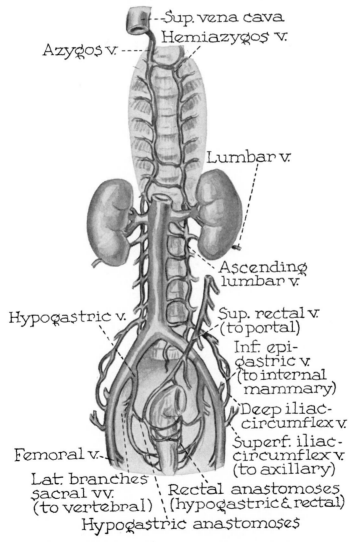

FIG. 482. Numerous collateral venous channels are available when the inferior vena cava becomes obstructed; this illustration depicts some of these possibilities.

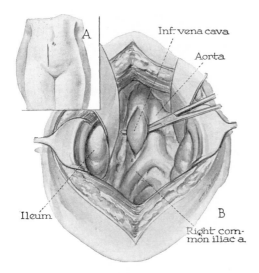

Inf. vena cava

Aorta

A

Ileum

B

Right common iliac a.

FIG. 483. Ligation of the inferior vena cava.

those of the vulva and pass to the superficial inguinal group. The majority of the lymph vessels from the fundus and the cervix of the *uterus* pass laterad in the broad ligament and become continuous with the ovarian lymph vessels which ascend, with the ovarian blood vessels, to the aortic glands. However, some of these may pass to the hypogastric and the other iliac groups. The efferent vessels of the *fallopian tubes* join those of the uterus and the ovaries. The vessels from the *rectum* pass upward to glands of the sigmoid mesocolon and then to the aortic group. Those from the *anal canal* end in the hypogastric glands, and those from the anus pass forward with those of the perineum to the inguinal group.

Malignant neoplasms of the female genital tract drain into the iliac and the aortic glands and therefore are not palpable superficially; cancerous processes which affect the vulva, the perineum, the anus and the lowermost portions of the vagina may cause easily felt enlargements of the superficial inguinal glands. However, there is a rare exception to this rule, since lymph drainage from the fundus of the uterus may travel along the lymphatics of the round ligament through the inguinal ring and to the superficial inguinal glands. Since the surgery of cancer is the surgery of the lymph drainage, it is important to visualize this system when at-

tempting to do a radical removal of cancer and its extensions.

SURGICAL CONSIDERATIONS

LIGATION OF THE INFERIOR VENA CAVA

Ligation or obstruction of the inferior vena cava can be understood only if one has a picture of the numerous collateral venous channels that are available when this structure becomes obstructed (Fig. 482). Although the collateral channels are numerous, these may not be sufficiently developed to allow survival following sudden and total obstruction of the vessel at or above the level of the renal veins. In contrast with this, sudden and total ligation of this vessel below the level of the renal veins is compatible with life. The degree of morbidity and disability following this differs according to various authors. The operation has been performed to prevent pulmonary emboli. The chief superficial channel for collateral circulation is from the femoral vein through the superficial epigastric and then via the thoracoepigastric vein to the lateral thoracic or some other tributary of the axillary vein.

Other available channels from the femoral to the subclavian vein are by way of the inferior and the superior epigastrics, between the circumflex iliac and the lumbar veins, between the hypogastric and the inferior mesenteric veins, as well as numerous lumbar and vertebral venous plexuses. The ascending lumbar veins communicate below with the common iliac vein, with the lateral sacral veins, with the middle sacral vein when it is present, and with the hypogastric and the iliolumbar veins; in the abdomen they connect with lumbar and vertebral plexuses, especially at the level of the renal veins or with the left renal vein itself, and above with the azygos and the hemiazygos systems. Naturally, the availability of these pathways varies according to their variational anatomy. Numerous other channels have been described. For further study one may refer to the works of Northway and Buxton and of Keen.

The inferior vena cava may be approached and ligated either transperitoneally or extraperitoneally (Fig. 483).

The transperitoneal operation is accomplished through a long lower right rectus incision which extends from the symphysis to well above the umbilicus (Fig. 483 A). The peritoneal reflection is incised along the paracolic gutter of the cecum and the ascending colon, which are reflected medially to the midline. The right ureter and the right ovarian vessels are identified. It is best to ligate the right ovarian veins and artery. The vena cava is identified easily and is doubly ligated about the level of the 4th lumbar vertebra. The cecum and the ascending colon are replaced into their normal positions, and peritonization is accomplished.

The extraperitoneal approach may be accomplished through a lateral incision similar to that used in lumbar sympathectomy. The inferior vena cava is identified easily; great caution should be used when ligating this vessel because of possible injury to lumbar veins. These latter veins are 4 in number, on either side of the vena cava, and may be injured while passing the ligatures under the major venous trunk. Injury to these veins obscures the field and makes structure identification most difficult. This type of hemorrhage is hard to control and may result in annoying hematomas.

LIGATION OF THE ILIAC VESSELS

Ligation of the Common Iliac Artery. The indications for this operation are injury, aneurysms of the external iliac artery, or preliminary to amputations about the hip joint.

The collateral circulation takes place in the following ways:

1. The inferior mesenteric artery above anastomoses with the visceral branches of the internal iliac artery below.

2. The ovarian artery above anastomoses with the uterine and the vesical arteries below.

3. The middle sacral artery above anastomoses with the lateral sacral branch of the internal iliac artery below.

4. The internal mammary, the lower intercostal and the lumbar arteries above anastomose with the inferior epigastric below.

The operation may be done either intraperitoneally or extraperitoneally.

The intraperitoneal method is done with the patient in the high Trendelenburg position. A low rectus incision is used. The bowel is packed off and retracted so that the posterior parietal peritoneum is exposed and opened over the artery. The veins lie behind the artery on the right side, but behind and medial on the left. The vessel is doubly ligated, and at times severed; the peritoneum is sutured.

The extraperitoneal method usually is done through an incision about 1 inch above and parallel with the inguinal ligament; it extends upward to the tip of the 11th rib (Fig. 484). The abdominal muscles are divided; the peritoneum is exposed and is pushed forward and mediad until the vessel is located. The inner

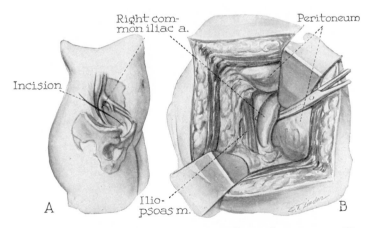

FIG. 484. The extraperitoneal approach to the common iliac artery. (A) The incision extends from the 11th rib to 1 inch above and parallel with the inguinal ligament. (B) The peritoneum is pushed forward and medially, and the vessel is isolated.

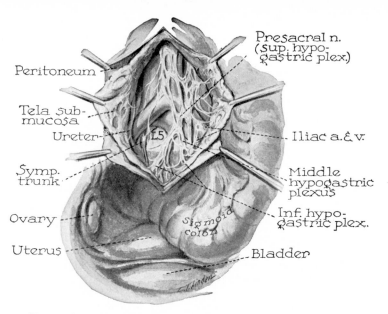

Peritoneum

Tela sub-
mucosa

Ureter

Symp.
trunk

Ovary

Uterus

Presacral n.
(sup. hypo-
gastric plex.)

L5

Iliac a. & v.

Middle
hypogastric
plexus

Inf. hypo-
gastric plex.

Sigmoid
colon

Bladder

FIG. 485. The superior hypogastric plexus (presacral nerve).

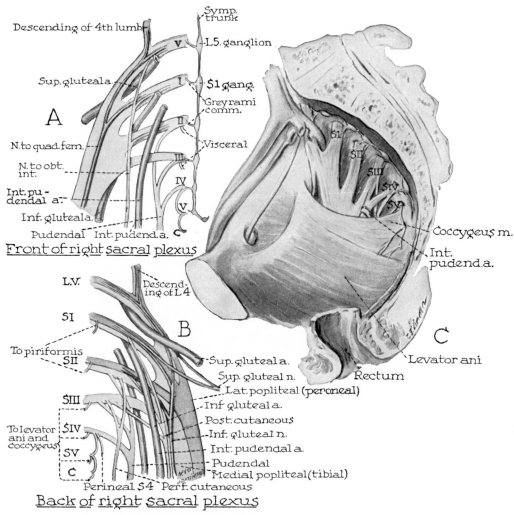

Descending of 4th lumb.

Sup. gluteal a.

A

N. to quad. fem.

N. to obt.
int.

Int. pu-
dendal a.

Inf. gluteal a.

Pudendal   Int. pudend. a.

Front of right sacral plexus

Symp.
trunk

L5. ganglion

S1 gang.

Grey rami
comm.

Visceral

Coccygeus m.

Int.
pudend. a.

Levator ani

Rectum

L.V.

SI

To piriformis
SII

SIII

To levator   SIV
ani and
coccygeus   SV

C

Perineal S4

B

Descend-
ing of L 4

Sup. gluteal a.
Sup. gluteal n.
Lat. popliteal (peroneal)
Inf. gluteal a.
Post. cutaneous
Inf. gluteal n.
Int. pudendal a.
Pudendal
Medial popliteal (tibial)
Perf. cutaneous

Back of right sacral plexus

FIG. 486. The sacral plexus: (A) seen from in front; (B) seen from
behind; (C) relations to musculature.

border of the psoas major muscle is used as the chief muscular guide.

Ligation of the Internal Iliac (Hypogastric) Artery. This is done for malignant growths in the pelvis which produce hemorrhage, for gluteal aneurysm and at times for excision of the rectum.

The collateral circulation is carried out in the following way:

1. Communication between the 2 internal iliac arteries.

2. Communications between the internal iliac artery and the inferior mesenteric.

The ureter lies anterior, the vein behind, and the lumbosacral trunk still more posterior.

The operation is similar to the one described for ligation of the common iliac artery.

Ligation of the External Iliac Artery. The indications for this operation are usually femoral aneurysm, and hemorrhage from the femoral artery or its branches.

The collateral circulation takes place in the following way:

1. Branches of the internal iliac artery above anastomose with branches of the external iliac artery below.

2. Arteries of the anterior abdominal wall above anastomose with branches of the inferior epigastric artery below; the femoral, the superficial epigastric, the circumflex iliac and the external pudendal vessels also anastomose with the anterior abdominal wall vessels above.

This operation may be done either through a transperitoneal or an extraperitoneal route.

The transperitoneal operation is conducted through a vertical low rectus incision with the patient in high Trendelenburg position. The intestines are packed off, and the peritoneum overlying the vessel is incised; the ligature is passed preferably from within outward so that the ureter which crosses the artery near its origin can be avoided. The vein is located to the medial side of the artery. On the left side, the mesocolon overlies the artery.

The extraperitoneal operation is done through a similar incision described above for exposure of the common or the internal iliac artery. When the peritoneum is reached, it is wiped medially until the artery is exposed. The femoral nerve lies lateral, the

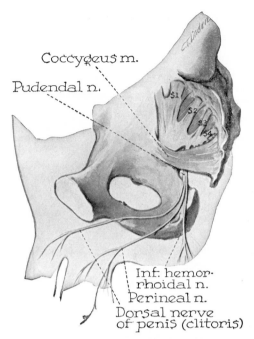

FIG. 487. The pudendal nerve.

external spermatic branch of the genitofemoral nerve anterior, and the vein posterior to the artery above but medial to it below.

NERVES

Superior Hypogastric Plexus. The autonomic nerves below the bifurcation of the aorta, where the intermesenteric nerves join to form the superior hypogastric plexus, is known to the surgeon as the *presacral nerve* (Fig. 485). This plexus or nerve supplies the bladder, the rectum and the internal genitalia, except the ovary and part of the fallopian tube.

As these fibers pass caudally they diverge and form the bilateral inferior hypogastric plexus (hypogastric nerve). Between the superior and the inferior plexuses, a rather inconstant, middle hypogastric plexus may be present in front of the promontory of the sacrum. The inferior hypogastric plexus fibers pass downward and laterad, then forward over the lateral surface of the ampulla of the rectum to join the pelvic plexus (Frankenhäuser). The nervi erigentes also add other fibers to the pelvic plexus. The plexus is quite large and supplies the rectum, the anal canal, the uterus, the vagina, the urethra and the urinary bladder. In the lower lumbar and upper sacral areas, the 3 hypogastric plexuses are situated deep in the retroperitoneal connective tissue. The autonomic nerve trunk of the superior and the middle hypogastric plexuses is located a little to the left of the midline. This is an important relationship in the operation of presacral neurectomy. The autonomic fibers which supply the ovary are not derived from the sacral ganglion nerves but arise from the renal and the aortic plexuses. They accompany the ovarian vessels as they pass in the suspensory ligament of the ovary.

The muscles which form the walls and the floor of the pelvis minor receive their innervation from the ventral divisions of the last lumbar nerve and the sacral nerves.

The sacral plexus is formed by L 4 and 5 and S 1, 2, 3 and 4 (Fig. 486). The portion of L 4 which does not join the lumbar plexus runs downward medial to the psoas muscle to join L 5, thus forming the lumbosacral cord or trunk. This nerve is joined by S 1, and the resulting broad nerve cord is further joined by S 2 and part of S 3. It lies in front of the piriformis muscle and behind the parietal pelvic fascia. The piriformis muscle separates the sacral plexus from the lateral part of the sacrum. Anteriorly, it is covered by the parietal pelvic fascia, which separates it from the internal iliac (hypogastric) vessels above and from their lateral sacral, the inferior gluteal and the internal pudendal branches below. Still more anteriorly, the rectum is related to the lower part of the plexus. The branches of the plexus are the following:

1. The superior gluteal nerve (L 4, 5 and S 1) passes backward above the piriformis into the gluteal region; it supplies the gluteus medius and minimus and the tensor fasciae latae muscles.

2. The inferior gluteal nerve (L 5 and S 1, 2) passes backward below the piriformis and supplies the gluteus maximus muscle.

3. The nerve to the quadratus femoris (L 4, 5 and S 1) enters the gluteal region below the piriformis.

4. The nerve to the obturator internus (L 5 and S 1, 2) travels in company with the internal pudendal vessels and enters the gluteal region below the piriformis muscle.

5. The posterior cutaneous nerve of the thigh (S 1, 2, 3) passes below the piriformis muscle and enters the gluteal region behind the sciatic nerve.

6. The sciatic nerve (L 4, 5 and S 1, 2, 3) constitutes the continuation of the nerve cord which has been formed within the pelvis. It leaves the pelvis through the lower part of the greater sciatic foramen.

7. The pudendal nerve (S 2, 3, 4) is accompanied by the internal pudendal vessels and the nerve to the obturator internus (Fig. 487). It passes through the greater sciatic foramen between the piriformis and the coccygeus muscles to gain entrance to the ischiorectal fossa. It divides into 3 branches: (1) the inferior hemorrhoidal nerve, (2) the perineal nerve and (3) the dorsal nerve of the penis (clitoris).

8. The nerve to the piriformis (S 2, 3) is a branch of the plexus.

9. The pelvic splanchnics (S 2, 3, 4) form a group which runs forward on the levator ani muscle and joins the branches of the pelvic plexus on the walls of the pelvic viscera. Small ganglia are situated at the points of this junction; they are distributed to the pelvic viscera and constitute the sacral part of the parasympathetic system.

10. The perforating cutaneous nerve (S 2, 3) runs between the adjoining borders of the coccygeus and the levator ani muscles and supplies the skin of the lower and the medial parts of the buttock.

The coccygeal plexus is formed by part of S 4 and the whole of S 5 plus the coccygeal nerve. It lies on the pelvic surface of the coccygeus muscle and supplies muscular branches to the levator ani, the coccygeus and the external sphincter ani. After being joined by S 5, the coccygeal nerve pierces the coccygeus muscle and supplies the skin in the neighborhood of the coccyx.

LUMBAR SYMPATHETIC CHAIN

After a rather thorough study of the anatomy of the lumbar sympathetics, Yaeger and Cowley have come to the conclusion that this chain is the most variable portion of the entire sympathetic system and one of the most variable structures in the human body (Fig. 488). With this in mind, one should not look upon the lumbar sympathetic chain as it is usually presented in diagrams, namely, as a ganglion resting on the body of each of the first 4 lumbar vertebrae on the right and the left sides. In 1937, Livingston stated that the variations in this structure are so common that it is ridiculous to state that given ganglia were removed. Atlas stated that the fusion of the lumbar sympathetic tissue is so erratic that it is impossible to designate lumbar ganglia on a numerical basis. Yaeger and Cowley made a series of 19 anatomic studies. They could not find a sympathetic ganglion on the first lumbar vertebra on the right side in 9 instances nor on the left side in 6 instances; in 4 other instances a ganglion could

not be found on either side of the 1st lumbar vertebra. They further reported that the number of lumbar ganglia ranged from 2 to 5, the average on each side being 3. The rami to a ganglion varied from 2 to 7; no two chains were similar in their entire series, and no pattern of variation could be established. The direction of the rami varied from cephalad to transverse to caudad. Therefore, it is to be concluded that the identification of a specific ganglion is unreliable according to the direction of its rami. The most constant and largest of the lumbar ganglia and hence the most easily identified even by palpation

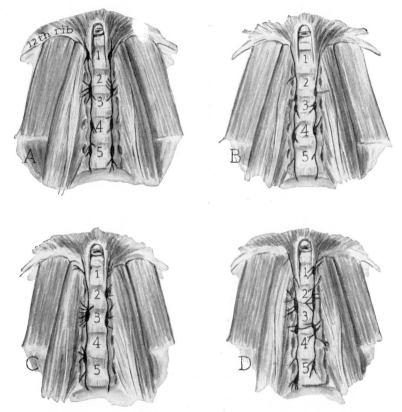

FIG. 488. The lumbar sympathetic nervous system (after Yaeger and Cowley). This has been shown to be one of the most variable portions of the sympathetic nervous system in the human body. (A) Four ganglia rather symmetrically placed on both sides in corresponding positions to the lumbar vertebrae. This is usually described as the typical arrangement but has been found to be the most atypical. (B) No ganglia are noted on either side of L 1 and almost all of L 2. Three ganglia appear on either side. (C) No ganglia appear overlying L 1 on either side or below the level of L 3 on the left. (D) The rami radiate in all directions, and there are intercommunications between the right and the left trunks.

was found to be associated with the 2nd lumbar vertebra, usually at its lower end. If a ganglion is present at the 1st lumbar vertebra, it usually is not seen because it is covered by the medial lumbocostal arch. The sympathetic tissue overlying the 4th lumbar vertebra usually is obscured by the common iliac vessels.

SURGICAL CONSIDERATIONS

LUMBAR SYMPATHETIC BLOCK

This procedure has become quite popular in the treatment of thrombo-embolic phenomena of the inferior extremities. Oschner and DeBakey have done much to popularize and standardize it. The procedure may be performed either in the lateral decubitus or with the patient in the prone position. Intracutaneous wheals are made approximately 2 fingersbreadth lateral to the spinous processes of the 1st, the 2nd, the 3rd and the 4th lumbar vertebrae (Fig. 489). A needle is inserted vertically through each wheal until it reaches the transverse process of the corresponding vertebra. Then the direction of the needle is changed, either superiorly or inferiorly and toward the midline. The needle can be advanced another 2 fingersbreadth so that its point comes to lie against the lateral surface of the body of the vertebra in the retroperitoneal space. Usually 1 per cent procaine solution is injected.

LUMBAR SYMPATHECTOMY

This operation has been recommended for vasospastic conditions of the lower extremities, for megacolon, hyperhidrosis and chronic ulcers; it may be done either extraperitoneally or transperitoneally.

The retroperitoneal approach can be accomplished through one of many skin incisions. A commonly used incision begins at the lower border of the 12th rib at the outer edge of the sacrospinalis group of muscles and extends downward parallel with the muscles to the crest of the ilium. It then curves forward along the brim of the pelvis for about 5 or 6 inches (Fig. 490 A). The lumbodorsal fascia is divided, and the oblique and the transverse abdominal muscles are separated from the sacrospinalis and the quadratus lumborum muscles. Between the peritoneum and the transversalis fascia, the iliohypogastric and the ilio-inguinal nerves usually are identified and protected. The abdominal muscles are cut along the iliac crest. The peritoneum is separated from the quadratus lumborum and the iliopsoas muscles by blunt dissection; the ureter is identified, and the peritoneum and the overlying viscera are retracted toward the midline (Fig. 490 B). The

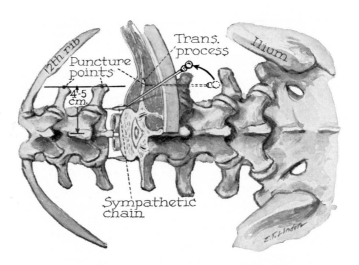

FIG. 489. Lumbar sympathetic block. Diagrammatic presentation of the injection of the lumbar sympathetic chain. The arrow indicates the change in direction of the needle after it comes into contact with the left transverse process.

removal of the 2nd, the 3rd and the 4th lumbar ganglia with their connecting trunks is similar to that described in the next paragraph.

The transperitoneal approach utilizes a lower rectus incision; the patient is placed in the Trendelenburg position, and the intestines are packed into the upper abdomen (Fig. 491 A). The lateral peritoneal attachment is incised on the left, and the sigmoid, with its mesentery, is reflected toward the midline (Fig. 491 C). This exposes the left sympathetic chain; the ureter, the aorta and the left common iliac artery are identified and protected. The genitofemoral nerve usually is seen extending obliquely downward over the psoas muscle. The ganglia lie just beneath the edge of the aorta in the gutter between the psoas muscle and the vertebrae. The approach to the right lumbar ganglionated chain is similar to that on the left, but the incision is made lateral to the inferior vena cava and continues downward over the right common iliac vein and into

the pelvis (Fig. 491 B). The small intestines, the cecum, the ascending colon and the ureter are retracted to the right. The nerve trunk on this side bears the same relation to the vena cava and the common iliac vein that it bears to the aorta and the common iliac artery on the left. The vena cava is retracted to the left. Lumbar veins overlying or beneath the sympathetic trunk may be injured during exposure and obscure the field. To dissect the chain it is best first to locate the 4th lumbar ganglion. It lies beneath the margin of the left common iliac artery and near the aortic bifurcation. It is grasped with a hemostat and freed from the surrounding areolar tissue and sympathetic rami. The trunk is dissected and severed above the 2nd lumbar ganglion. The connecting sympathetic trunk is removed with the ganglia.

PRESACRAL (SUPERIOR HYPOGASTRIC) NEURECTOMY

This operation has been done for intractable pain in the uterus, the bladder or the

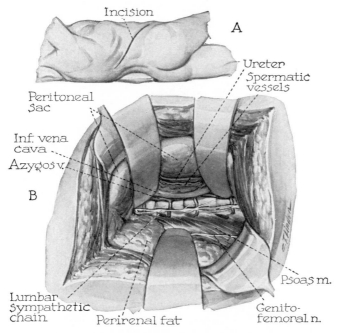

FIG. 490. Lumbar sympathectomy (retroperitoneal approach). (A) The incision extends from the 12th rib to the brim of the pelvis. (B) The peritoneum has been retracted forward, and the lumbar sympathetic chain is found in a gutter formed by the psoas muscle and the lumbar vertebrae.

rectum, and for the relief of spasms of the bladder resulting from spinal cord disease or injury. Removal of the presacral nerves usually causes the loss of power of ejaculation, but the powers of erection and orgasm is not impaired.

The operation is done through a low rectus incision (Fig. 492 A). The intestines are packed upward, and the bifurcation of the aorta is sought. The posterior peritoneum is incised above the aortic bifurcation, and the peritoneal margins are carefully dissected laterally and retracted (Fig. 492 B). The superior hemorrhoidal vessels (inferior mesenteric), if visible, usually are retracted to the left, and the presacral nerves are exposed

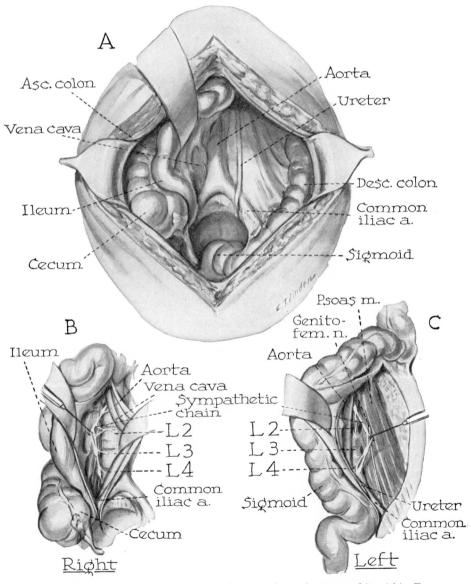

Fig. 491. Lumbar sympathectomy (transperitoneal approach). (A) Exposure through a low rectus incision. (B) Incision into the posterior parietal peritoneum lateral to the inferior vena cava for exposure of the right lumbar sympathetic chain. (C) Incision into the posterior parietal peritoneum placed lateral to the sigmoid for exposure of the left lumbar sympathetic chain.

where they lie in the loose connective tissue in this area. The hollow of the sacrum, between the common iliac arteries, lodges the continuation of these nerves. At times it may be necessary to ligate the middle sacral artery. The left common iliac vein lies medial to the artery and should be protected during this entire procedure; as a rule, the right ureter is exposed. The nerves are picked up as they cross the aortic bifurcation and are freed downward. The communicating rami are severed, and the entire plexus is removed. All primary fibers should be severed. The peritoneal incision is closed, and the operation is concluded.

SURGICAL CONSIDERATIONS OF THE UTERUS AND THE ADNEXAE

HYSTERECTOMY

Subtotal (Supravaginal) Hysterectomy. This operation commonly is performed for benign lesions or extensive inflammatory disease.

A low midline incision is made, and the round ligaments are severed on both sides about 1 inch away from the cornual end of the uterus (Fig. 493); these severed ends are ligated. This step opens the broad ligaments so that an anterior vesical flap of peritoneum can be formed. If the adnexae are to remain, an avascular area is found in the broad ligament close to the uterus; this is entered with either a curved hemostat or the finger. Clamps are applied to the tube and the ovarian ligament adjacent to the uterus. These structures are cut between clamps, and the clamps are replaced by transfixion sutures. If one desires to remove the tube or the ovary, the end of the tube is grasped and reflected medially. Clamps are applied to the infundibulopelvic ligament, and an incision is made between these; they also are replaced by transfixion sutures. The uterine vessels are clamped and severed at approximately the corpocervical junction; the cervix is coned. The cervical stump is closed transversely with interrupted sutures.

Peritonization is accomplished in the following way (Fig. 493 F): a stitch is placed in the (1) posterior cervical wall, then grasps

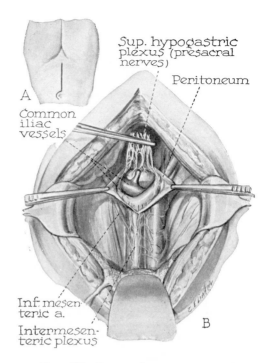

FIG. 492. Presacral neurectomy. (A) Incision. (B) An incision has been placed into the posterior parietal peritoneum at the bifurcation of the aorta. The nerves are severed and dissected downward.

(2) the tube or the infundibulopelvic ligament, as the case may be, then (3) the round ligament and finally (4) the anterior vesical flap which has been mobilized. When this flap is tied, one side of the cervical stump is peritonized and supported. A similar 4-bite stitch is placed on the opposite side. Peritonization is completed by a few interrupted sutures which grasp the posterior cervical wall and the anterior vesical flap.

Panhysterectomy. The steps of this procedure may be similar to those for subtotal hysterectomy until the uterine vessels are ligated (Fig. 494). After this step, the operator examines the region of the cervix to determine the length of the cervix and the position of the bladder. The latter is pushed downward, usually by gauze dissection. This is continued downward and forward until the thumb and the index finger can compress the vaginal wall below the cervix. The peri-

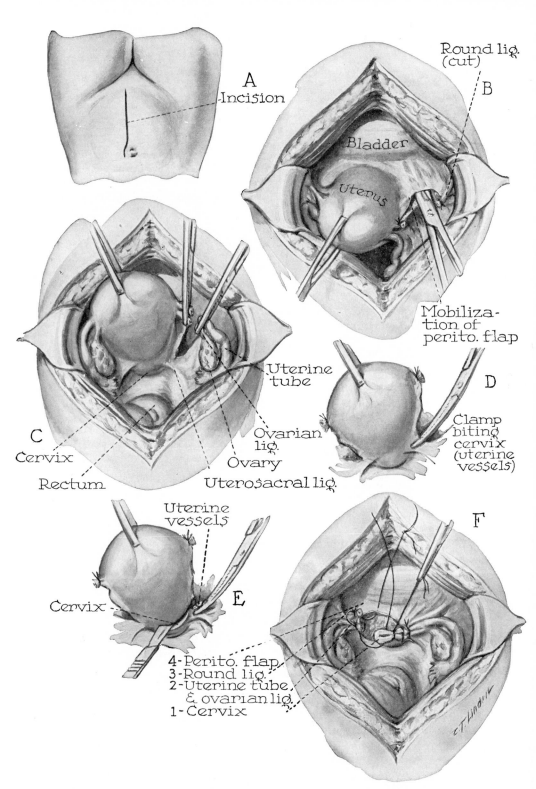

FIG. 493. Subtotal (supravaginal) hysterectomy. (A) The lower midline incision extends to the left of the umbilicus if necessary. (B) The round ligaments are severed and tied, and a peritoneal (vesical) flap is formed. (C) The tubes and the ovarian ligaments are severed and tied. (D) Clamps bite into and slide off of the cervix; in this way the uterine vessels are secured. (E) The uterine vessels are severed, and the cervix is coned and cut across. (F) Peritonization.

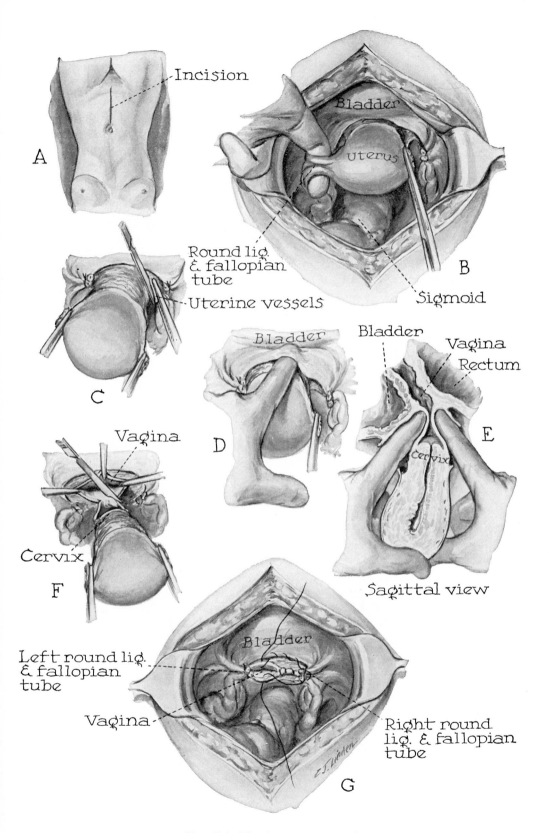

A — Incision

B — Bladder, Uterus

Round lig. & fallopian tube

Uterine vessels

Sigmoid

C

D — Bladder

E — Bladder, Vagina, Rectum, Cervix

Sagittal view

F — Vagina, Cervix

G — Bladder

Left round lig. & fallopian tube

Vagina

Right round lig. & fallopian tube

FIG. 494. (*Caption on next page.*)

toneum on the posterior cervical wall is incised and dissected downward until the cervix can be palpated through the vaginal vault. The vagina is entered, and the vaginal vault is divided as close to the cervix as possible. After freeing the cervix from the vagina, the anterior and the posterior vaginal walls are approximated. During the closure, the round ligaments, the tubes and the utero-ovarian ligaments are anchored to the angles of the vaginal vault. All raw surfaces are carefully peritonized.

SALPINGECTOMY AND SALPINGO-OOPHORECTOMY

Removal of the fallopian tubes and the ovaries usually is done for inflammatory involvement, cysts, neoplasms, ectopic pregnancies, etc.

Salpingectomy. After exposing the tube, clamps are applied to the outer margin of the mesosalpinx (Fig. 495). It is important that these clamps be placed as close to the tube as possible so that the vascular supply of the ovary is not interfered with. The mesosalpinx is cut, and the uterine cornu is excised. The latter is closed, and the hemostats on the mesosalpinx are ligated. Peritonization is accomplished by suturing the posterior leaf of the broad ligament to the posterior surface of the uterus.

Salpingo-oophorectomy. When both the tubes and the ovary are to be removed, the clamps are applied to the infundibulopelvic ligament, which contains the ovarian vessels (Fig. 496). The remainder of the procedure is the same as that described for salpingectomy.

SURGERY FOR RETRODISPLACEMENT OF THE UTERUS

Many operations have been devised to correct the retrodisplaced uterus. The usual procedures performed are the Gilliam, the Baldy-Webster, the Olshausen and the Coffey.

Gilliam Operation. After opening the abdomen, a clamp is used to grasp the round ligaments about 1 inch from the cornua of the uterus; the clamp is withdrawn through the aponeurosis, the muscle and the peritoneum. The same is done on the other side. Then these knuckles of ligaments are pulled well up through the defects, bringing the uterus into an anterior position; they are anchored to the aponeurosis with a few interrupted sutures. Although this is one of the most popular operations for retrodisplacement, some authorities are of the opinion that the procedure is faulty, since it does not retain the cervix in its normal position; also, it is dangerous because of the possibility of strangulation of a loop of intestines in the pocket formed between the round ligament and the anterior abdominal wall.

Baldy-Webster Operation. In this procedure, an avascular area in the mesosalpinx is sought by stretching the tube and the ovary (Fig. 497). The clamp is placed through this area immediately beneath the utero-ovarian ligament, and the round ligament is grasped about 1½ inches from the cornua of the uterus. Then the knuckle of round ligament is brought posteriorly through this perforation; the same is done on the opposite side. The loops of the 2 ligaments are approximated on the posterior surface of the uterus and sutured; each suture includes the uterine wall.

FIG. 494. Panhysterectomy. (A) A long midline incision extends to the left and above the umbilicus. (B) The vesico-uterine peritoneum is incised transversely. The round ligaments may or may not be grasped with the fallopian tubes and the utero-ovarian ligaments. The finger has perforated an avascular area in the left broad ligament. (C) The uterine vessels are clamped and cut; this permits downward displacement of the ureter. (D) The bladder is separated from the cervix by blunt dissection. (E) The anterior and the posterior dissections are completed below the cervix. (F) Amputation across the vaginal vault is done as close to the cervix as possible. (G) Closure of the vaginal vault with apposition to it of the round and the utero-ovarian ligaments.

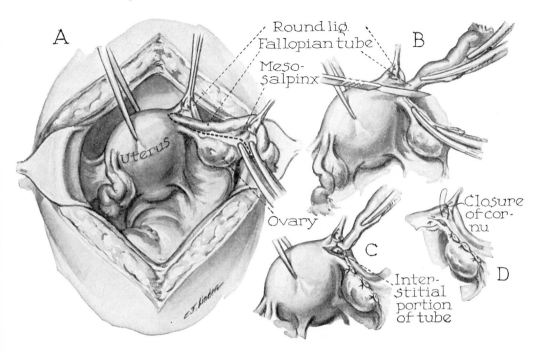

FIG. 495. Salpingectomy.

Olshausen Operation. The round ligament is picked up by a suture which is carried beneath it about 1½ inches from the cornua of the uterus; the same is done on the opposite side. The uterus is brought forward to a point corresponding to its normal anterior position, and the sutures previously introduced are carried through the peritoneum,

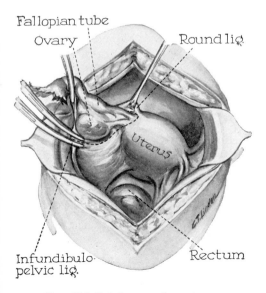

FIG. 496. Salpingo-oophorectomy.

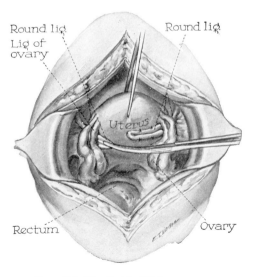

FIG. 497. The Baldy-Webster operation for retrodisplaced uterus.

the recti muscles and the aponeurosis about ½ inch to each side of the median incision. The sutures are tied. This operation also has a disadvantage in that it leaves 2 apertures between the ligaments and the anterior abdominal wall; through these openings loops of intestines or omentum may become strangulated.

Coffey Operation. In this procedure, the folded excess loop of round ligament is sutured to the anterior surface of the uterus. This suture begins about 1 inch below the uterine end of the round ligament and extends upward toward the cornu of the uterus. At times, the anterior leaf or broad ligament is used to peritonize the sutured area.

Male Perineum

EMBRYOLOGY

In the embryo, the endodermal alimentary tract ends as a blind receptacle called the cloaca; this has an anterior diverticulum called the allantois (urachus). The mesonephric duct (adult vas deferens) grows caudally and opens into the anterior part of the cloaca (Fig. 498). The ureter develops as an outpouching of the mesonephric duct, the two for a period ending in one terminal duct. This common duct subsequently is absorbed into the wall of the bladder and the prostatic urethra, with the result that the ureter and the vas deferens eventually have separate openings. A mesodermal septum (urorectal septum) divides the cloaca into an anterior, urogenital part and a posterior, intestinal part. The cloaca has a sphincter, also divided into an anterior portion, which becomes the superficial transversus perineus, the bulbospongiosus, the ischiocavernosus and the urogenital diaphragm; the posterior part of the sphincter becomes the external sphincter ani. One nerve, the pudendal, supplies the cloacal sphincter as well as the skin of the region around it; its accompanying artery, the pudendal, nourishes this region. The bladder and the rectum receive their nerve supply through the pelvic splanchnic nerve and the hypogastric plexus.

The perineum is a lozenge-shaped space which is bounded by the pubic symphysis, the rami of the pubes and the ischia, the ischial tuberosities, the great sacrotuberous ligament, the edges of the great gluteal muscles and the coccyx (Fig. 499). If a transverse line is drawn across the space between the anterior extremities of the ischial tuberosities, directly in front of the anus, it divides the perineum into two parts. The anterior part forms a nearly equilateral triangle which measures approximately 3¼ inches on all sides and is known as the anterior or the urogenital triangle. The posterior part is also somewhat triangular; it contains the rectum and the ischiorectal fossae and is called the anal triangle. The bony framework of the perineum may be felt more or less distinctly, and in thin subjects the sacrotuberous ligament may even be made out beneath the

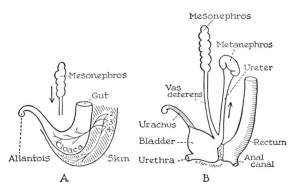

FIG. 498. Embryology of the male urogenital system. (A) An early stage; a cloaca is present. (B) A later stage; the cloaca has been divided by the urorectal septum.

597

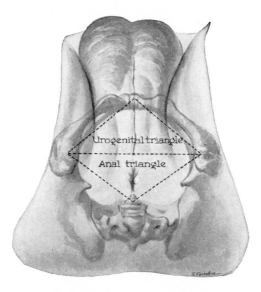

FIG. 499. The male perineum.

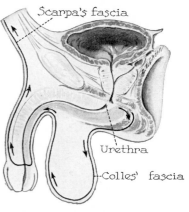

FIG. 500. Colles' fascia. This fascia is the deep layer of superficial fascia; on the anterior abdominal wall it is called Scarpa's fascia. This fascia determines the direction of spread of extravasated urine.

gluteus maximus muscle. The superficial areas of the perineum depend on the posture of the body. When the thighs are brought together, it is very limited and then is represented only by a narrow groove which contains the anus and the roots of the scrotum and the penis. The region is wider in the female because of the greater size of the pelvic outlet. In the midline of the perineum a cutaneous ridge, the median raphe, can be followed from the front of the anus forward over the scrotum and along the lower surface of the penis. This raphe marks that line along which the floor of the urethra was completed and where the two halves of the scrotum fused during their development.

UROGENITAL TRIANGLE

This is the anterior triangle of the perineum or the genitourinary part. It is bounded in front by the pubic symphysis, on the sides by the rami of the pubis and the ischium, and posteriorly by a line drawn between the anterior parts of the ischial tuberosities.

The superficial fascia consists of 2 layers: an outer fatty layer and an inner membranous layer. The *superficial fatty layer* of the superficial fascia is continuous with the superficial fat of the rest of the body and contains small cutaneous vessels and nerves. The farther downward this layer is traced the scarcer becomes the fat, so that over the scrotum the

fat entirely disappears and gives place to a thin layer of involuntary muscle fibers. These constitute the dartos muscle and are responsible for the rugosity of the scrotal skin which is caused by their contraction. The *deep layer of superficial fascia* is not fatty but membranous and is continuous with a similar layer of fascia in the lower part of the anterior abdominal wall. In the anterior abdominal wall it is called Scarpa's fascia but changes its name in the perineum to the fascia of Colles; it is found only over the urogenital triangle (Fig. 500). Its attachments are to the fascia lata, the pubic arch and the base of the perineal membrane. It is prolonged over the penis and the scrotum and so forms a covering for the testis and the spermatic cord.

The arrangements and the attachments of this fascia are important because they determine the direction in which extravasated urine will spread after rupture of the cavernous portion of the urethra. The fascia has a median septum which attaches to the perineal muscles, but this septum is not complete, and fluid may pass through it from side to side. Urine under Colles' fascia following rupture of the urethra may extend downward as far as the lower border of the urogenital diaphragm because at this point it fuses with the base of the diaphragm. Laterally, it may extend through the median septum as far as the attachment of the fascia to the conjoined ischiopubic rami; upward, it may extend over the scrotum and the penis and onto the anterior abdominal wall. Once the fluid has reached the anterior abdominal wall it can extend downward and over the inguinal ligament until it is held up by the attachment of Scarpa's fascia to the fascia lata approximately 1 inch below and parallel with the inguinal ligament.

THE SUPERFICIAL PERINEAL POUCH

The superficial perineal pouch is a compartment in the urogenital part of the perineum which is bounded inferiorly (a floor) by Colles' fascia and superiorly (a roof) by the urogenital diaphragm (perineal membrane) (Fig. 501). The pouch is closed behind by the fusion of its roof and floor, and on each side by the attachments of the walls to the margins of the pubic arch. Above, however, it remains open and communicates with the cellular interval which is situated between Scarpa's fascia and the anterior rectus sheath. Should the urethra rupture into this space, it would fill the posterior part of the pouch and then spread into the scrotum and the penis and, if allowed to continue, would ascend in front of the symphysis pubis and so reach the anterior abdominal wall.

The contents of the superficial perineal compartment consist of the roots or fixed portions of the corpora cavernosa of the penis and the urethra, their overlying ischiocavernosus and bulbocavernosus muscles, the superficial transverse perineal muscles and those branches of the internal pudendal vessels and nerves which pierce the inferior fascia of the urogenital diaphragm to reach this space.

The 2 roots of the corpora cavernosa of the penis arise from the midportion of the ischiopubic rami, run obliquely upward and forward and adhere to the periosteum of the descending rami of the pubes and to the inferior surface of the urogenital diaphragm (p. 602). Each cavernous body is covered by the ischiocavernosus muscle.

Superficial Perineal Muscles. On each side, the following 3 superficial perineal muscles lie in the superficial perineal pouch (Fig. 502).

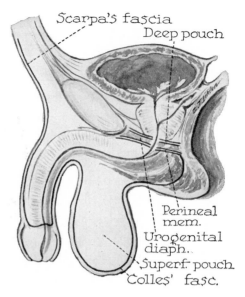

FIG. 501. The superficial and the deep perineal pouches.

1. *The superficial transverse perineal muscle* lies at the base of the pouch and extends from the ischial tuberosity to the central point of the perineum. The 2 transverse muscles act together to steady the perineal body during defecation and to fix it during contractions of the external sphincter and the bulbospongiosus.

2. *The ischiocavernosus muscle* is applied to the crus and arises close to the superficial transverse perineal muscle; it covers the free surface of the crus into which it is inserted anteriorly. The 2 ischiocavernosus muscles compress the crura against the pubic arch and so obstruct the venous return of the corpora cavernosa.

3. *The bulbocavernosus (bulbospongiosus) muscle* arises from the perineal body and from a median raphe which separates the 2 halves of the muscles on the inferior surface of the bulb. Therefore, it is a bilateral structure. The most posterior fibers of this muscle pass to the perineal membrane, the intermediate fibers of the 2 sides meet on the dorsum of the corpus spongiosum, and the most anterior fibers meet on the dorsum of the penis where they blend with the fascia of the penis. This muscle acts as a sphincter which empties the bulb and part of the spongy urethra and also compresses the bulb

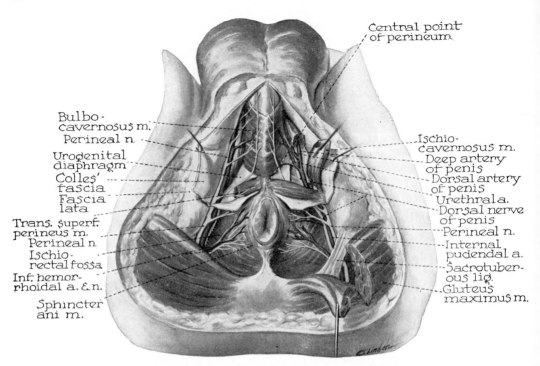

FIG. 502. The superficial perineal pouch and its contents. Colles' fascia has been incised and reflected to reveal the contents of this pouch.

against the perineal membrane, thereby constricting the corpus spongiosum.

All the superficial perineal muscles are supplied by the perineal branch of the pudendal nerve. The perineum on each side of the corpus cavernosum urethra is traversed by nerves and vessels which are small branches of the pudendal trunks. They supply the sur-

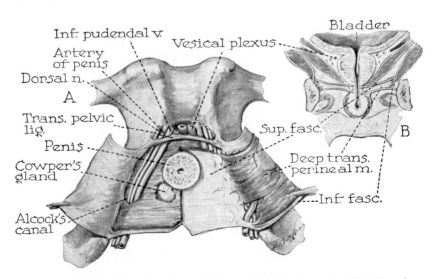

FIG. 503. The deep perineal pouch (urogenital diaphragm): (A) Seen from below. The inferior layer of fascia has been retracted, and the muscle has been left intact; on the opposite side the deep transverse perineal muscle has also been reflected, exposing the superior layer of fascia. (B) Frontal section.

rounding structures in the superficial perineal compartment.

DEEP PERINEAL POUCH
(UROGENITAL DIAPHRAGM)

The urogenital diaphragm is a musculo-membranous diaphragm which is stretched tightly across the pubic arch and is attached

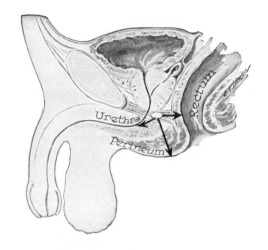

FIG. 504. The bulbo-urethral gland (Cowper). The gland is situated between the layers of the urogenital diaphragm. If the gland suppurates, it may evacuate into the urethra, the perineum or the rectum.

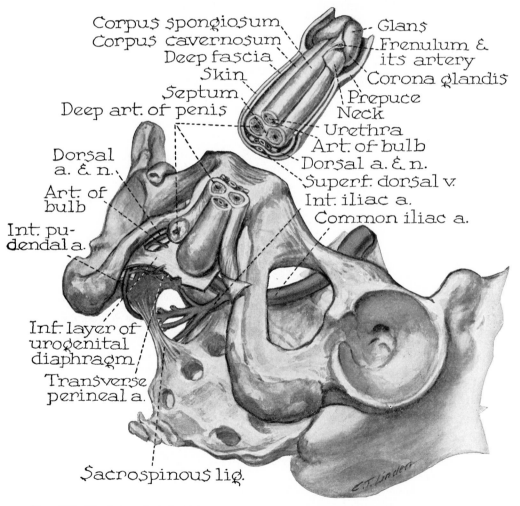

FIG. 505. The internal pudendal artery. This artery gives rise to the dorsal artery of the penis, the deep artery of the penis and the artery to the bulb. The dorsal nerve of the penis accompanies the internal pudendal artery.

to the ischiopubic rami (Figs. 501, 502 and 503). It separates the perineum from the pelvis and consists of 2 layers of fascia with 2 muscles between them. The 2 fascial layers are the superior (upper) and the inferior (lower) layers; the 2 muscles are the sphincter urethrae membranaceae and the deep transverse perineal. The space which is created by these 2 layers of fascia and is filled by the 2 muscles is known as the deep perineal pouch or compartment.

The inferior fascial layer of the urogenital diaphragm also has been referred to as the superficial layer of the triangular ligament and the perineal membrane. It covers the lower surface of the sphincter urethrae and the deep transverse perineal muscle. Its lower surface is largely covered by the root of the penis, and each side is attached to the side of the pubic arch. Its posterior border is fused with the posterior border of the superior fascia of the urogenital diaphragm and the membranous layer of superficial fascia.

In the midline, the fused borders are continuous with a fatty fibromuscular nodule called the *perineal body*. Anteriorly, this fascia presents a thickened free margin known as the transverse perineal ligament; between this ligament and the inferior ligament of the pubis there is an oval interval through which the deep dorsal vein of the penis passes into the pelvis to enter the venous network around the prostate (Fig. 452).

The membrane is pierced by several structures which enter the superficial perineal pouch: (1) the urethra pierces it in the midline about 1 inch below the symphysis pubis; it is accompanied on either side by the small ducts of the bulbo-urethral glands opening into the spongy portion; (2) the artery to the bulb of the penis pierces the membrane a little to either side of the urethra; (3) the internal pudendal artery; (4) the dorsal nerve to the penis pierces the membrane close to its lateral attachment and under cover of the anterior part of the crus.

The superior or upper layer of perineal fascia is derived from the parietal pelvic fascia. It is a loose layer of fibrous tissue which covers the pelvic surface of the sphincter urethrae and the deep transverse perineal muscles. On each side it is attached to the obturator fascia. The apex of the prostate rests on it, and it is continuous with the fascial sheath of that viscus. The urethra, emerging from the prostate, pierces it in the midline.

The deep perineal muscles are one sheet of muscle which is divided into 2 parts, namely, a deep transverse perineal and a sphincter urethrae (Fig. 511). The *sphincter urethrae (membranaceae) muscle* arises from the pubic arch on a level with the urethra. As the fibers approach the median plane some of them pass behind the membranous part of the urethra, and some in front of it; they blend with the corresponding fibers of the opposite side. The *deep transverse perineal muscle* is the posterior part of the muscle just described. It is small and passes below and behind the membranous part of the urethra.

Both muscles are supplied by 2 delicate twigs from the perineal nerve. When the sphincter vesicae (internal sphincter) is destroyed after prostatectomy, the sphincter urethrae is the only muscle left but is perfectly competent to control urination.

The deep perineal pouch is that space which is enclosed by the superior and the inferior fasciae of the urogenital diaphragm. It is separated from the superficial perineal pouch by the perineal membrane and from the anterior part of the pelvis by the fibrous tissue which forms the sheath of the prostate and contributes to the formation of the perineal body. This pouch contains the (1) two muscles just described (sphincter urethrae and the deep transverse perineal), (2) the membranous part of the urethra, (3) the bulbo-urethral gland, (4) the internal pudendal artery and the artery to the bulb of the penis and (5) the dorsal nerve of the penis.

The membranous portion is the shortest part of the urethra, being about ½ inch long, and lies about 1 inch below the pubic symphysis (Fig. 510). It is continuous above with the prostatic and below with the spongy urethra. The prostatic and the membranous portions of the urethra are directed downward and forward, but the spongy part curves upward and forward in the bulb of the penis before it turns down in the corpus spongiosum. The membranous urethra is the least dilatable and the narrowest part with the exception of the external orifice. If this part of the urethra ruptures proximal to a stricture in the cavernous portion, extravasation of urine results into the deep perineal compartment from which an exit can be found only through one or the other of the fascial sheaths of the urogenital diaphragm. If urine breaks through the inferior fascia, it passes into the superficial perineal pouch and forward onto the abdomen in front of the pubis. However, if the extension is through the superior fascia, or if there is an extraperitoneal rupture of the bladder, the extravasated urine enters the interval above the median puboprostatic ligaments and extends forward into the retropubic space of Retzius. From there it ascends in the anterior abdominal wall between the transversalis fascia and the parietal peritoneum.

The bulbo-urethral glands (Cowper) are 2 small pea-sized bodies which lie posterolateral to the membranous urethra and under cover of its sphincter muscle (Figs. 504 and 509). They are located between the layers of the urogenital diaphragm. Their ducts, which are about 1 inch long, pass through the urethral openings in the perineal membrane and open into the floor of the spongy portion of the urethra. Each gland receives a branch of the bulbo-urethral artery. They are involved in gonorrheal inflammation of the cavernous urethra and may give rise to abscesses which can be felt through the rectum. Such suppurations may evacuate into the urethra, the perineum or the rectum.

The internal pudendal artery is a branch of the internal iliac artery and passes forward from the pudendal canal deep to the inferior layer of the urogenital diaphragm (Fig. 505). It lies under cover of the pubic arch and has the dorsal nerve of the penis to its lateral side. In its course it passes through the pelvis, the gluteal region and the perineum and is accompanied throughout by its 2 veins. Under cover of the anterior part of the crus penis it pierces the inferior layer of the urogenital diaphragm, enters the superficial pouch and divides into the dorsal artery of the penis and the deep artery of the penis. The deep artery of the penis pierces the medial side of the crus penis and runs forward in the substance of the corpus cavernosum which it supplies. The dorsal artery of the penis runs upward between the bone and the commencement of the crus to gain the dorsum of the penis. The internal pudendal artery gives rise to the *artery to the bulb*; this vessel runs medially on the surface of the deep transverse perineal muscle, pierces the perineal membrane and ends in the bulb. It supplies a small twig to the bulbo-urethral gland. It pierces the perineal membrane, enters the bulb of the penis and runs onward through the whole length of the corpus spongiosum, supplying its substance.

The dorsal nerve of the penis arises from the pudendal nerve in the pudendal canal (Fig. 505). It accompanies the internal pudendal and the dorsal arteries, which lie to its medial side, and supplies the corpus cavernosum penis, the glans and the skin of the penis.

The anterior prolongation of the ischiorectal fossa is the deepest space in the anterior perineum. It runs forward toward the pubes, between the superior fascia of the urogenital diaphragm, the anterior portion of the levator ani, and the mesial surface of the obturator internus muscle (p. 531).

The central point of the perineum is marked by a fibromuscular node lying between the anorectal junction and the apex of the sphincters, and the bulbocavernosus muscle (Fig. 502). It is also a point of insertion for the recto-urethral and the superficial transverse perineal muscles and for the levator fibers which are associated with the support of the prostate (Fig. 502). This point is an excellent guide, since it unites the urogenital diaphragm and the anus with their substratum of levators. It affords the proper perineal approach to the deeper pelvic structures.

External Genitalia

PENIS

The penis has a posterior fixed part or root and an anterior mobile portion called the body. It is composed of 3 fibroelastic cylinders which are filled with spongy or erectile tissue. These cylinderlike masses are the right and the left corpora cavernosa and the corpus spongiosum (urethrae) (Fig. 505).

Corpora Cavernosa. The 2 roots of the corpora cavernosa of the penis arise from the midportion of the ischiopubic rami, pass obliquely upward and forward, hugging the periosteum of the descending rami of the pubes and the inferior surface of the urogenital diaphragm. Each is covered by the ischiocavernosus muscle. The corpora are united, side by side, in the body of the penis, but at its root they are separate and assume the name of crura, each of which tapers to a point posteriorly. **The corpus spongiosum,** which is much more slender, lies along the lower surface of the united corpora cavernosa and is traversed lengthwise by the longest of the 3 divisions of the urethra. Anteriorly, at the end of the penis, it enlarges to form the *glans* of the penis, in which the anterior ends of the corpora cavernosa are embedded.

Body. The body of the penis is formed by the union of all the cavernous masses; it begins at the apex of the urogenital diaphragm and is attached to it by connective tissue bands. The corpora cavernosa lie side by side on the dorsum, and the corpus spongiosum lies ventrally. The corpus spongiosum terminates posteriorly in a large, free bulbous sac known as the *bulb of the urethra* (Fig. 511). This latter structure overlaps the junction of the membranous and the cavernous divisions of the urethra posteriorly.

SUPERFICIAL STRUCTURES

Prepuce. The skin of the penis is continued forward as the prepuce (foreskin) (Fig. 506). The skin is devoid of hair, and the fascia is devoid of fat. The prepuce is a fairly dense portion of skin which forms a cuff or

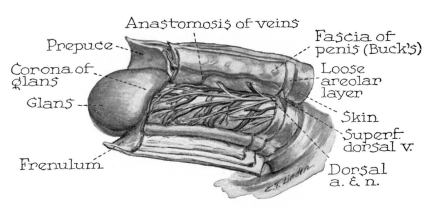

FIG. 506. The superficial structures of the penis. The penis has 3 superficial encircling coats: the skin, the loose areolar subcutaneous tissue and the fascia of the penis (Buck's). These have been reflected in the drawing.

hood covering the glans. Within the cavity of the prepuce the modified skin contains sebaceous glands which secrete smegma.

Frenulum. On the under aspect of the glans a well-defined fold of skin called the frenulum passes forward and is attached to the prepuce. The subcutaneous tissue of the penis, a continuation of Colles' fascia, is very loose in texture and is traversed by the superficial dorsal vein. The looseness of these tissues gives mobility to the penis and explains the ease with which blood or urine may extravasate, producing tremendous swellings of the organ. The superficial lymphatics accompany the superficial dorsal vein and enter the subinguinal lymph nodes. These become involved in infections about the prepuce and the glans.

Buck's Fascia. Beneath the subcutaneous layer, the penis is invested by a thin fibrous membrane known as the fascia of the penis (Buck's fascia). This fascia envelops the body of the penis and the corona of the glans to the root of the penis. It is adherent on each side in the groove between the corpora cavernosa and the corpus spongiosum.

The suspensory ligament of the penis is a thickened, triangular, fibroelastic band. It is fixed above to the lower part of the linea alba and the upper part of the symphysis pubis; below, it splits to form a sling for the penis at the junction of its fixed and mobile parts where it blends with the fascia of the penis.

The deep dorsal nerve, arteries, veins and lymph vessels run beneath Buck's fascia and along the dorsum of the penis. Encircling branches of the veins drain the corpora cavernosa and the corpus spongiosum, and encircling arteries send twigs to the same structures.

The deep dorsal vein passes between the intrapubic ligament and the urogenital diaphragm to the prostatic venous plexus. On the dorsum of the penis a pair of dorsal nerves pass lengthwise beneath the deep fascia; between these there is a pair of dorsal arteries, and between these the deep dorsal vein lies in the median plane (Figs. 505 and 506).

The superficial dorsal vein, also median, lies in the superficial fascia and is the one

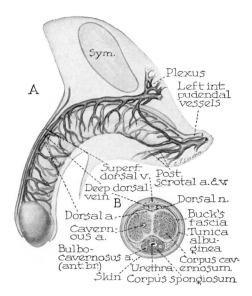

Fig. 507. The venous drainage of the penis. (A) Lateral view of the relations between the superficial and the deep dorsal veins. (B) Cross section showing relations of vessels to the fasciae.

which is seen through the skin. It should be noted that the veins are not left and right, as are the arteries and the nerves, but are median, either superficial or deep.

The superficial dorsal vein receives tributaries from the skin and the prepuce and terminates posteriorly by dividing into right and left branches which drain into the external pudendal veins in the thigh (Fig. 507). The deep dorsal vein begins by the union of several twigs from the glans and the prepuce. It runs backward in the median line, passes between the 2 layers of the suspensory ligament and enters the pelvis after passing below the inferior pubic ligament. It ends by joining the venous plexus which surrounds the prostate.

The dorsal arteries of the penis are the terminal branches of the internal pudendal. They pass forward in the interval between the corpora cavernosa and reach the dorsum of the penis. Here the 2 arteries lie one on each side of the deep dorsal vein (Fig. 505). The dorsal nerve lies lateral to the artery; both vessels and nerves are enclosed between the 2 layers of the suspensory ligament of the penis. These vessels supply the body of the

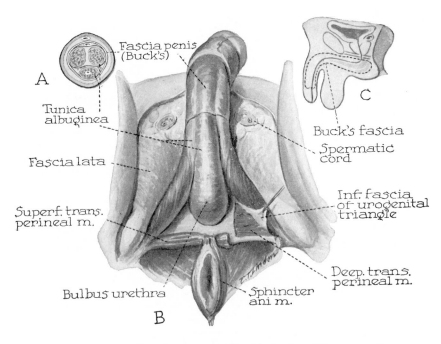

FIG. 508. The tunica albuginea and Buck's fascia: (A) cross section, (B) relations to the urogenital diaphragm, (C) sagittal view.

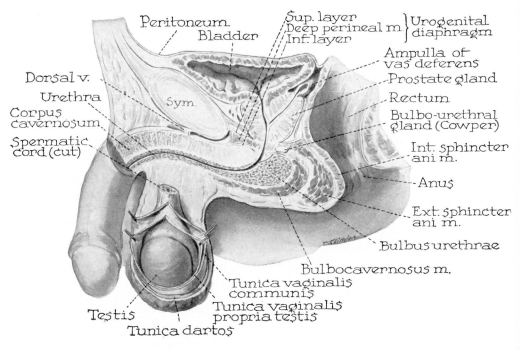

FIG. 509. The male urethra. The urethra is divided into prostatic, membranous and penile parts. The relations of each part are shown in sagittal section.

penis and terminate in the glans. The *deep artery* of the penis pierces the medial aspect of the anterior part of the crus and runs forward in the corpus cavernosum penis.

Each **dorsal nerve** of the penis is a terminal branch of the pudendal nerve. It supplies branches to the corpus cavernosum, the glans and the skin of the penis.

Tunica Albuginea. Each erectile body is surrounded by a distensible elastic fibrous tissue called the tunica albuginea, the trabeculae of which surround blood spaces (Fig. 508). Where the corpora are applied against each other, the albuginea forms a median partition called the septum of the penis. It is difficult at times to differentiate or separate Buck's fascia from the tunica albuginea.

URETHRA

The urethra is a fibro-elastic structure which measures about 8 inches in length and is divided by the superior and the inferior fasciae of the urogenital diaphragm into 3 parts: prostatic, membranous and spongy (Fig. 509). The part above the superior fascia travels through the prostate, the part between the 2 urogenital diaphragm fasciae constitutes part 2, and the part beyond the inferior fascia (perineal membrane) traverses the corpus spongiosum.

The prostatic urethra is the widest and most dilatable portion of the urethra and travels almost perpendicularly; it is about an inch in length. On transverse section it appears crescentic because of the presence of a prominent vertical ridge on its posterior wall, the *urethral crest* (Fig. 510). The gutter to each side of this crest is known as the *prostatic sinus*. The urethral crest rises to a summit, the *colliculus,* and bifurcates below as it disappears. Opening onto the colliculus is a diverticulum called the *prostatic utricle,* through which a probe can be passed for about ½ inch into the substance of the prostate. On its lips open the much finer orifices of the *ejaculatory ducts.* Onto the floor of each prostatic sinus the prostatic ducts appear as several dozen small openings.

The membranous urethra passes through the urogenital diaphragm and its 2 fasciae. It is approximately ½ inch long and has no surrounding tissue proper. Behind it on each

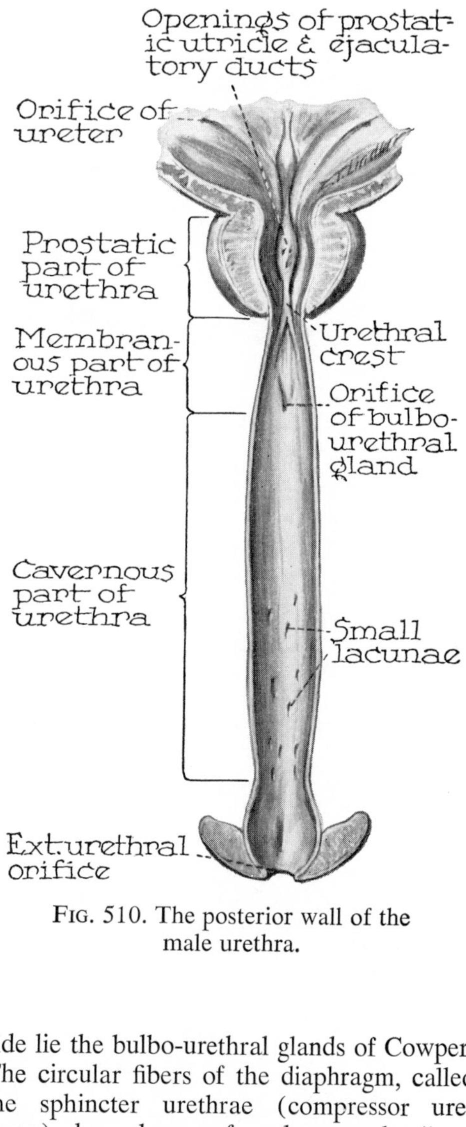

FIG. 510. The posterior wall of the male urethra.

side lie the bulbo-urethral glands of Cowper. The circular fibers of the diaphragm, called the sphincter urethrae (compressor urethrae), have been referred to as the "cut-off" or "shut-off" muscle; it has a sphincter-like action and is a voluntary muscle supplied by the perineal branch of the internal pudendal nerve. Like the sphincter ani, also supplied by the pudendal nerve, it is in constant contraction.

The spongy, penile or cavernous urethra traverses the bulb, the body and the glans of the corpus spongiosum penis. It is the longest portion of the urethra and extends from the inferior layer of fascia of the urogenital diaphragm to the external meatus. After piercing the urogenital diaphragm it enters the

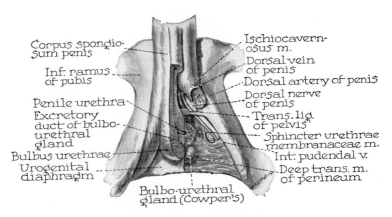

Corpus spongio-sum penis
Inf. ramus of pubis
Penile urethra
Excretory duct of bulbo-urethral gland
Bulbus urethrae
Urogenital diaphragm

Ischiocavern-osus m.
Dorsal vein of penis
Dorsal artery of penis
Dorsal nerve of penis
Trans. lig. of pelvis
Sphincter urethrae membranaceae m.
Int. pudendal v.
Deep trans. m. of perineum

Bulbo-urethral gland (Cowper's)

FIG. 511. The penile portion of the urethra after it pierces the urogenital diaphragm.

bulb about 1 cm. in front of its rounded posterior extremity (Fig. 511). In its passage it lies nearer the dorsal aspect. Its lumen is dilated both in the bulb and in the glans, the latter dilatation being known as the terminal (navicular) fossa. The bulbous portion of the urethra forms the most dependent part of the perineal curve. The bulbo-urethral glands of Cowper open into this portion of the urethra at its lower or posterior wall. The external orifice is the narrowest part and at times requires incision to permit the passage of instruments which may pass easily through the remainder of the urethra. The passage of a sound is a simple procedure in a normal urethra, if the beak is kept in contact with the urethral roof after the navicular fossa has been passed. Once the level of the membranous portion has been reached, little difficulty is encountered in entering the bladder except

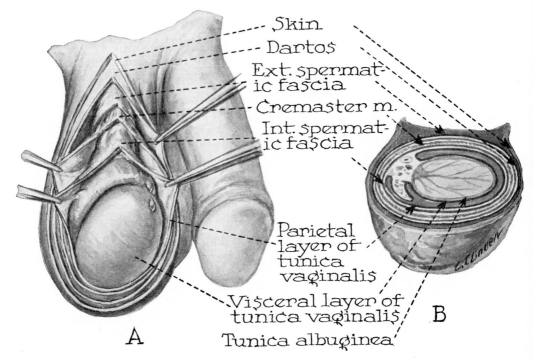

Skin
Dartos
Ext. spermat-ic fascia
Cremaster m.
Int. spermat-ic fascia

Parietal layer of tunica vaginalis
Visceral layer of tunica vaginalis
Tunica albuginea

A   B

FIG. 512. The scrotum and its 6 associated layers: (A) side view; (B) schematic cross section.

in pathologic conditions which involve either the urethra or the prostate gland.

SCROTUM

The scrotum is a pendulous purselike bag of skin and fascia in which the testes are found (Fig. 512). It has a bilateral origin, being derived from right and left labioscrotal folds. In the female, these folds remain separated as the labia majora, but in the male they fuse behind the penis to form the scrotum. A vestige of the fusion of the 2 sides of the scrotum remains as the median raphe, which is continued into the perineal skin behind the scrotum and along the lower aspect of the penis anteriorly.

The skin of the scrotum forms a single pouch. It is delicate in texture, darker in color than the surrounding region and quite distensible. Its rugosity, which varies with temperature, is produced by the *dartos muscle* which lies immediately subjacent.

Fascia. *The superficial fascia* in the scrotum is entirely devoid of fat and is largely replaced by the thin sheet of muscle just mentioned, the dartos. This muscle sends a median partition across the scrotum which separates the testes from each other; however, the septum is incomplete superiorly. It is a laminated thin sheet of involuntary muscle which is platysmalike, since it is intimately adherent to the skin, causing it to wrinkle. It contracts with cold and relaxes with heat, its tonicity decreasing with age. Sympathetic nerve fibers supply it.

In the wall of each scrotal chamber there are, besides skin and dartos, 3 complete layers which are derived from the anterior abdominal wall. They are, named from without inward: the external spermatic fascia, the cremaster muscle and the internal spermatic fascia. These provide additional coverings or coats for each testis.

The external spermatic fascia, which is derived from the external oblique aponeurosis, appears as a small layer of areolar tissue situated directly under the dartos. Though the skin and the superficial fascia are common to both halves of the scrotum, the 3 additional layers are confined to each corresponding side because of the septum produced by the dartos muscle.

The cremaster muscle is derived from the internal oblique. Its muscle loops reach the testicle as thin strands. By their contraction the testis is drawn toward the subcutaneous

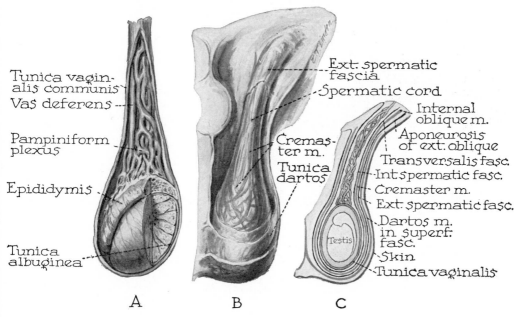

FIG. 513. The testis. (A) A section of the gland has been removed to show its relations to the epididymis and the tunica albuginea. (B) and (C) Coverings of the spermatic cord and the testis.

inguinal ring and produces the cremasteric reflex.

The internal spermatic fascia is derived from the transversalis fascia. It is composed of loose connective tissue and closely invests the elements of the cord and the testicle.

The tunica vaginalis testis is developmentally a portion of the peritoneum. It is a serous membrane and, like all other serous membranes, has parietal and visceral layers; these are separated by a capillary interval which contains a film of fluid which keeps the surfaces moist. The parietal layer lines the wall of the scrotum and is closely adherent to the internal spermatic fascia. At the back of the scrotum it is reflected forward and becomes continuous with the visceral layer. The latter covers the epididymis and then the testis itself. In inguinal herniae of long standing, the coats of the testis and the spermatic cord become thickened and may be separated and displayed, but in normal individuals, although the dartos and the tunica vaginalis are identified easily, the external spermatic fascia, the cremaster and the internal spermatic fascia have a tendency to become fused and are defined less easily.

TESTIS

This gland appears as an oval body with flattened sides; it lies in the scrotum with its long axis oblique, its upper pole tilted forward. It varies in size, but its average dimensions are 1½ inches in length, 1 inch in anteroposterior diameter, and a little less than that from side to side. The vas deferens and the epididymis are applied to its posterior border (Fig. 513). On each side and anteriorly, it is enveloped by the tunica vaginalis which, under normal conditions, forms a completely closed sac. The visceral layer of this tunic is closely adherent to the testis and becomes continuous with the parietal layer at the upper and the lower poles and along the posterior part of both sides of the gland. On the lateral aspect it is reflected onto the medial side of the epididymis, thus forming the underlying sinus of the epididymis, which partially separates the body of the epididymis from the testis (Fig. 514).

The tunica albuginea is a pearly white coat which forms a complete fibrous covering deep to the tunica vaginalis. At the posterior border of the gland it becomes thicker, forming the *mediastinum testis*. From this

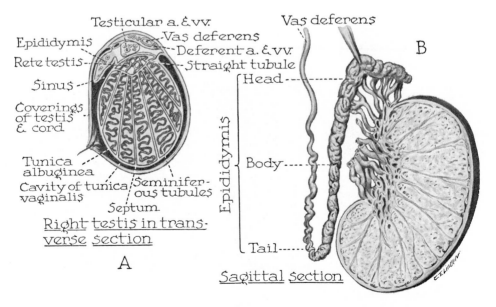

FIG. 514. The internal structure of the testis. (A) Transverse section of the right testis. (B) Teased sagittal section.

mediastinum, incomplete fibrous septa pass inward to subdivide the gland into lobes. Convoluted seminiferous tubules lie in the lobes and pass backward into the mediastinum testis, where they unite and form a network called the *rete testis*. From this network about 20 efferent ductules (vasa efferentia) arise; they emerge from the upper pole of the testis and enter the head of the epididymis.

The epididymis is applied to the upper pole and the posterior border of the testis. It tapers from above downward and is subdivided into a head, a body and a tail. The head of the epididymis is enlarged and fits like a cap on the upper pole of the testis, to which it is attached by the efferent ductules. The body is separated from the testis by the sinus of the epididymis, and the tail or lower end is attached only by areolar tissue near its lower end. Within the head, the efferent ductules unite to form the canal of the epididymis, which is coiled up within the body and the tail. When unraveled, it measures almost 20 feet in length. This duct emerges from the tail as the vas (ductus) deferens which ascends, medial to the epididymis, and enters the spermatic cord. The body and the tail of the epididymis can be separated easily from the testicle, but the head must be severed at its efferent ductules.

SPERMATIC CORD

This appears as a long, rounded bundle which extends from the deep inguinal ring to the posterosuperior border of the testicle (Figs. 513, 514 and 515). Within the abdomen its constitutent parts are widely sepa-

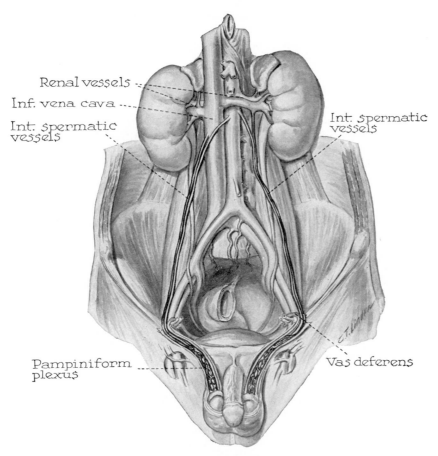

FIG. 515. The blood supply of the testis and the constituents of the spermatic cord.

rated, but from the deep inguinal ring to the testis they are wrapped together by the coverings of the cord. It is encased in 3 fibrous coats derived from the abdominal wall during the descent of the testis, namely, a continuation of the external abdominal oblique (the external spermatic fascia), a continuation of the internal abdominal oblique (the cremaster muscle), and a continuation of the transversalis fascia (the internal spermatic fascia). Plus this, the 2 inner layers of the abdominal wall, namely peritoneum and preperitoneal fat, are also present. In the fatty layer run the duct, the vessels and the nerves of the testis, and the vessels and the nerves of the epididymis. These constituents of the cord assemble at the internal inguinal ring lateral to the inferior epigastric artery, pass through the inguinal canal and descend in the scrotum to the testis. The cord lies behind the internal oblique laterally and in front of it medially. As it emerges from the superficial inguinal ring it passes over the pubic tubercle and covers it; hence, when one attempts to feel the tubercle, it is first necessary to displace the cord.

The constituents of the spermatic cord are:

1. Continuations of the 2 inner layers of the abdominal wall (processus vaginalis peritonei and the preperitoneal fatty areolar tissue).

2. Structures associated with the testicle (vas deferens and artery, veins, lymphatics and nerves).

3. Vessels and nerves associated with the vas deferens and the epididymis.

The processus vaginalis peritonei (funicular process of peritoneum, tunica vaginalis testis) is a tubelike process of peritoneum, the upper part of which lies in front of the vas; it is obliterated before birth or within a month thereafter to become a fibrouslike thread (Fig. 282). Its lower part remains patent and is invaginated from behind by the testis, changing its name to the tunica vaginalis testis.

The preperitoneal fatty areolar tissue is an extension of the extraperitoneal abdominal fat which surrounds the processus vaginalis and forms a covering for the structures which pass to and from the testis. This layer is the surgeon's landmark to the underlying "sac" in inguinal hernia operations. The adipose tissue in this layer diminishes as one proceeds down the cord; thus, no fat is found in the scrotum.

The vas deferens (ductus deferens) is the structure which conveys spermatozoa from the testis to the urethra; it is as long as an adult femur. It starts in the tail of the epididymis, of which it is the prolongation; the pathologic changes of one affects the other. It is the only hard structure in the spermatic cord; hence, it can be identified easily; the firmness is due to a thick muscular coat. It has a tiny lumen and is dilated at its two extremities, which are the only thin-walled portions of the vas. It first ascends behind the testis along the medial border of the epididymis, continues through the scrotum and the inguinal canal as the posterior constituent of the spermatic cord, then winds around the lateral side of the inferior epigastric artery and descends to the posterolateral angle of the bladder, and thence to the urethra (Fig. 515). The vas is subperitoneal throughout its entire course. Normally, it is bluish white in color, resembling cartilage. Because of its posterior relationship, the sac of an indirect inguinal hernia usually lies anterior to it.

ARTERIES

There are *two* arteries in the spermatic cord, namely, the testicular and the deferential arteries (Fig. 515).

The testicular (internal spermatic) artery is the larger and supplies the testis. It arises from the abdominal aorta in the lumbo-iliac region and joins the cord at the abdominal inguinal ring. In the cord it is surrounded and hidden by the spermatic group of veins. It lies in front of the vas.

The artery of the vas deferens is a slender branch of the inferior vesical artery which passes along the vas to supply it and the epididymis.

VEINS

The pampiniform plexus represents the veins of the testis and the epididymis; they number about a dozen. This anastomosing plexus receives its name from its resemblance to a vine. The veins ascend in 3 longitudinal groups. The anterior group surrounds the testicular artery, and the middle surrounds the vas; the posterior group runs alone. As the veins ascend they decrease in number but increase in size and finally end at or near the deep inguinal ring as the *testicular vein,* which continues upward over the posterior wall of the abdomen. The right vein ends in the inferior vena cava, the left joins the left renal vein. In the lower part of the abdomen they are frequently double. On the right, the vein empties into the inferior vena cava near the renal pedicle; on the left, it enters the renal vein almost at a right angle. This fact explains the increased incidence of varicoceles on the left side as compared with the right.

LYMPHATICS

The lymphatics of the cord and the testicle follow the spermatic vessels throughout their course and end in the external iliac glands or the lumbar nodes about the aorta and the inferior vena cava.

In addition to the structures just discussed, a *cremasteric artery* exists; it arises from the inferior epigastric artery close to the deep inguinal ring and supplies the coverings of the cord.

NERVES

The genital branch of the *genitofemoral nerve* (L 1 and 2) supplies the cremaster muscle and a sensory branch to the tunica vaginalis. *Sympathetic fibers* from the renal and the aortic plexuses carried by the testicular artery, and from the pelvic plexus carried by the artery to the vas, supply branches to the testis (T 10) and to the epididymis (T 11, 12 and L 1).

SURGICAL CONSIDERATIONS

VARICOCELECTOMY

A varicocele is a dilatation and varicose condition of the spermatic veins (pampiniform plexus). It is more common on the left than on the right side (p. 611). The veins usually involved are the anterior group which surround the testicular artery. To perform

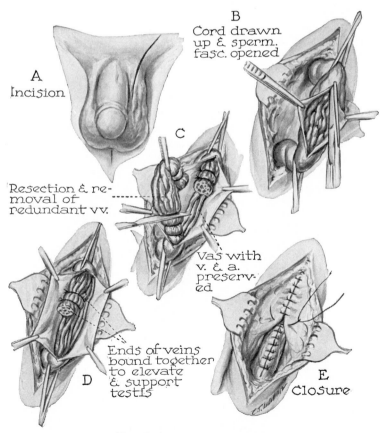

A
Incision

B
Cord drawn up & sperm. fasc. opened

C

Resection & removal of redundant vv.

Vas with v. & a. preserved

D
Ends of veins bound together to elevate & support testis

E
Closure

FIG. 516. Varicocelectomy.

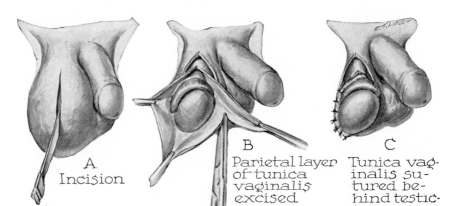

A
Incision

B
Parietal layer
of tunica
vaginalis
excised

C
Tunica vag-
inalis su-
tured be-
hind testic-
le

Fig. 517. Hydrocelectomy.

the operation an incision is made low in the inguinal region (Fig 516). The spermatic cord is located at the external inguinal ring and drawn into the wound. The coverings of the cord are incised, and the veins are exposed; two thirds of the veins involved are doubly ligated, and the intervening segment is removed. The ends of the severed veins are brought together, thus supporting the testicle. It is important to make certain that at least one large vein or group of veins remains so that some return venous flow is preserved.

HYDROCELECTOMY

This operation is done for a collection of fluid which is found between the layers of the tunica vaginalis (vaginal hydrocele). Other types of hydrocele have been described (p. 370). The usual operation performed is the so-called "bottle" operation (Fig. 517). The incision is made through the skin, the dartos and the superficial fascia; it is placed directly in the scrotum and over the hydrocele. The testicle with its tunica vaginalis is exposed, the fluid is aspirated, and the tunica is opened. The parietal layer of the tunica vaginalis is excised partially, but enough is permitted to remain so that it may be everted and sutured behind the testicle and the spermatic cord. In this way, the secreting surface faces outward.

CIRCUMCISION

Before the operation is attempted, the prepuce should be freed from the glans, since adhesions might be present and result in an unsatisfactory operation or injury to the glans. The redundant prepuce is placed on tension and amputated parallel with the corona. The redundant inner layer is mucous membrane and should be excised. The remaining tissue is folded back and sutured to the skin of the shaft of the penis. An alternate method of dorsal slit may be utilized (Fig. 518).

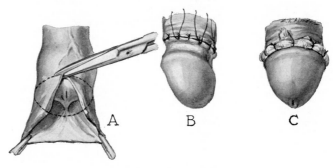

A   B   C

Fig. 518. Circumcision.

CHAPTER 36

Female Perineum

The perineum is a region at the inferior end of the trunk which is situated between the thighs and the lower part of the buttocks. It is a diamond-shaped space at the angles of which are found the inferior pubic (arcuate) ligament above, the tip of the coccyx below, and the ischial tuberosities at each side. The pubic arch and the sacrotuberous ligaments form its sides, but the latter are hidden by the gluteus maximus muscles. If a line is drawn from the anterior part of one ischial tuberosity in front of the anus to the anterior part of the other tuberosity, this diamond-shaped area becomes conveniently divided into an anterior urogenital triangle and a posterior anal triangle (Fig. 519). The anal triangles are about the same in both sexes, but the urogenital triangles differ. On the surface the urogenital triangle is bounded by the mons veneris in front, by the gluteal region (buttocks) behind and by the femoral region (thigh) at each side.

THE UROGENITAL REGION

EXTERNAL GENITALIA

The mons veneris is a cushionlike eminence on the front of the pubes; it is produced by a collection of fatty tissue under the skin (Figs. 519 and 520). It is covered with hair which ceases abruptly as the mons merges with the anterior abdominal wall.

Pudendum (Vulva). This collective term includes the labia majora, the labia minora, the body and the glans of the clitoris and the vaginal orifice. It extends from the pubes above to a point in front of the anus below.

The labia majora are homologous to the halves of the scrotum in the male; the line of the intervening vestibular or pudendal cleft between the 2 labia corresponds to the scrotal raphe. In mulliparae these labia are in contact with each other, and are therefore the only visible part of the external genitalia. Each labium is a broad rounded cutaneous

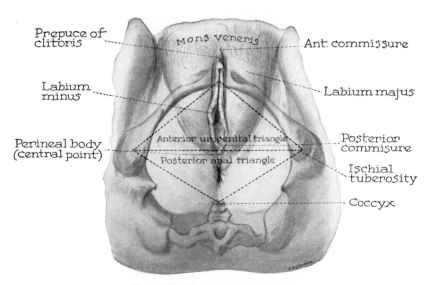

FIG. 519. The female perineum.

615

fold which lies lateral to the labium minus and covers a long fingerlike process of fat. The two large labia are united below the mons veneris (mons pubis) and form the *anterior commissure*; they are connected posteriorly and form a narrower and less distinct *posterior commissure*. The outer convex surface is covered by ordinary skin and hair and is provided with numerous sebaceous glands, but the inner surface, which lies against the opposite labium, possesses a more delicate skin with large sebaceous follicles. The elevation of the labium is produced by the presence of a diverticulum of fat which is a continuation of the superficial fat of the inguinal region. This fatty fingershaped process is demarcated from the surrounding fat in which it is embedded; it rests against the deep layer of superficial fascia.

The labia minora (nymphae) are cutaneous folds which lie medial to the labia majora (Fig. 520). The minor lips enclose the vestibule, and in the young they are commonly concealed by the approximated majora. In older women and multiparae they are not infrequently pendulous and externally visible; they are shorter and thinner than the labia majora and become highest near their anterior end. The anterior extremities each split into two layers, the upper of which meet

above the clitoris to form the *prepuce;* the lower layers become attached to the inferior aspect of the glans of the clitoris and form its *frenulum.* The labia minora diminish in size as they pass posteriorly and blend with the labia majora. In front of the posterior commissure they are connected by a transverse fold of skin, the frenulum of the labia (fourchet). Immediately anterior to and above this fold, between it and the posterior limit of the vaginal orifice, a shallow depression is formed which is known as the *fossa navicularis.* These labia are hair-free and resemble mucous membrane.

The clitoris is the female penis and lies at the apex of the vestibule. Only a small part of the body and the glans are visible when the labia minora are retracted, since the labia and the mons hide the greater part of this structure.

The vestibule of the vagina is the cleft which exists between the labia minora. It is a fissure which is placed anteroposteriorly and into which the urethral orifice opens above and the vaginal orifice below. On each side, the entrance of the two minute ducts of the corresponding Bartholin glands are found.

The urethral orifice also has been referred to as the external urinary meatus; it appears as a vertical slitlike or ovoid opening about

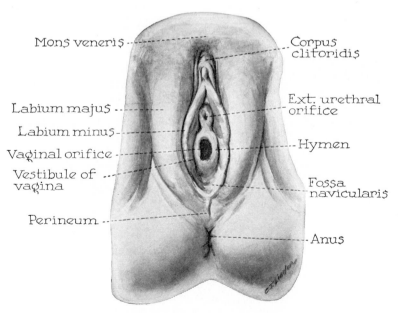

FIG. 520. The female external genitalia.

4 or 5 mm. in diameter. It is about 1 inch below the clitoris, and the mucous membrane around its margin is somewhat prominent and puckered. A group of minute glands appear at each side of the lower part of the urethra and represent the homologue of the prostate gland in the male. On each side they group themselves to employ a common para-ure-thral duct (Skene's) which passes downward in the submucous coat and opens at the sides of the orifice. They are of clinical importance because they may harbor infections.

The vaginal orifice is nearer the posterior end of the vestibule, and in the virgin is par-tially closed by the *hymen*. The latter is a duplication of mucous membrane which, after rupture, is represented by irregular projec-tions into the vaginal orifice known as the hymenal caruncles (carunculae myrti-formes). The hymen is usually a thin vascu-lar fold of mucous membrane which varies in shape and thickness and presents a central opening which can be stretched sufficiently to admit one examining finger without tearing. Whether the hymen is intact or torn, it never-theless persists anteriorly as a membranous band as it approaches and joins the tissues forming the urethral floor at the meatus. These bands become stretched and pull on the floor of the meatus when the vaginal in-troitus is dilated by digital examination or

coitus. This is a feature of diagnostic im-portance especially in dyspareunia.

The superficial perineal fascia divides into 2 definite layers in the urogenital diaphragm: a superficial fatty layer and a deeper mem-branous one (Fig. 521). This arrangement is a continuation of the 2 layers of superficial fascia of the anterior abdominal wall, namely, the superficial fatty layer of Camper and the deeper membranous layer of Scarpa.

The superficial layer of the superficial fas-cia is part of the general adipose panniculus which covers the entire body. Posteriorly it is continuous with the adipose tissue which fills the ischiorectal fossa, and anteriorly it is carried upward in front of the pubis as Camper's fascia. Where it covers the labia, the fat is replaced by a very thin layer of involuntary muscle fibers which is the homo-logue of the dartos muscle in the male scro-tum; laterally, it leaves the perineum and becomes continuous with the fatty tissue of the thighs.

The deep layer of superficial perineal fas-cia is membranous and is a continuation of Scarpa's fascia of the abdomen but changes its name in this region to Colles' fascia. It is found only in the anterior half of the peri-neum and ends behind at a transverse line which joins the ischial tuberosities. At the side of the anterior urogenital triangle it ends

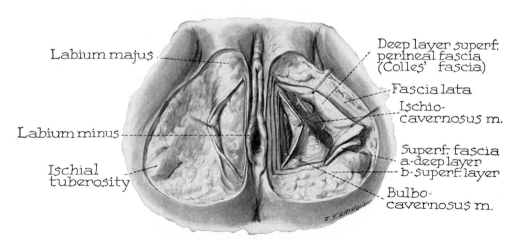

FIG. 521. The superficial anatomy of the urogenital region. On the right side (reader's left) the superficial layer of superficial fascia has been incised longitudinally to expose the continuation of the superficial inguinal fascia which appears as a fatty diverticular process; this process accounts for the labial elevation. On the left side (reader's right) the 2 layers of superficial fascia and the superficial musculature are demonstrated.

by becoming firmly attached to the ischio-pubic rami and the ischial tuberosities. On the same plane, but laterally placed, is the fascia lata of the thigh; the deep layer of superficial fascia joins the fascia of the uro-genital diaphragm behind.

The superficial perineal pouch is a space or compartment which exists between the perineal membrane (p. 599) and the deep layer of the superficial perineal fascia. This space is bounded inferiorly by the membran-ous layer of fascia which forms its floor; it is bounded superiorly by the perineal mem-brane which forms its roof, and laterally by the side of the pubic arch between the at-tachments of these 2 membranes. It is closed posteriorly by their fusion. Anteriorly, how-ever, the pouch remains open and is con-tinuous with that interval which exists be-tween the superficial fascia of the anterior abdominal wall and the aponeurosis of the external oblique muscle, the interval being filled with areolar tissue. Each half of the pouch contains a crus of the clitoris, the bulb of the vestibule, the greater vestibular gland and the superficial perineal muscles, nerves and vessels (Fig. 522). Through the com-partment and in vertical directions, in the median plane, pass the terminal portions of the urinary and the genital tracts.

The only portion of the clitoris which is visible when the labia are retracted is the small end known as the glans and a small part of its body. The other constituents of this erectile tissue, with the investing muscu-lature, are in the superficial perineal com-partment and are brought into view only when the deep layer of the superficial peri-neal fascia and the inferior perineal fascia are incised. The crus of the clitoris corre-sponds to the crus penis, although much diminished in size. Like the male structure, it is covered by the ischiocavernosus muscle. The crura are continuous with the corpora cavernosa at the lower part of the pubic symphysis; the crura are large in comparison with the corpora. On the symphysis each crus passes backward and laterally to taper at a point near the lower end of the ischium. It lies on the lower surface of the perineal mem-brane along the side of the pubic arch whose perineal surface is grooved to accommodate it. It is adherent to both the bone and the membrane and is hidden by the overlying ischiocavernosus muscle. The laterally placed corpora cavernosa fuse anteriorly to form the small unpaired body of the clitoris. This is bent upon itself and tapers distally where it is covered by the glans. The clitoris is supplied with a suspensory ligament which passes upward to the symphysis and onto the anterior abdominal wall. The glans, like

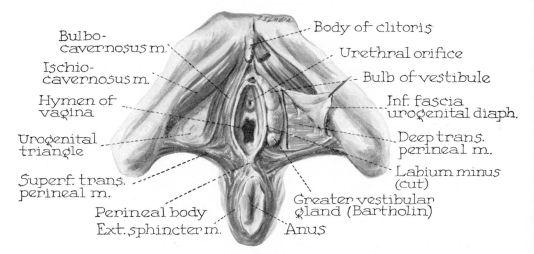

Bulbo-cavernosus m.
Ischio-cavernosus m.
Hymen of vagina
Urogenital triangle
Superf. trans. perineal m.
Perineal body
Ext. sphincter m.

Body of clitoris
Urethral orifice
Bulb of vestibule
Inf. fascia urogenital diaph.
Deep trans. perineal m.
Labium minus (cut)
Greater vestibular gland (Bartholin)
Anus

FIG. 522. Deeper dissection of the urogenital region. The contents of the superficial peri-neal pouch are shown. On the reader's right the inferior fascia of the urogenital diaphragm has been incised to show the relation of the deep transverse perineus muscle.

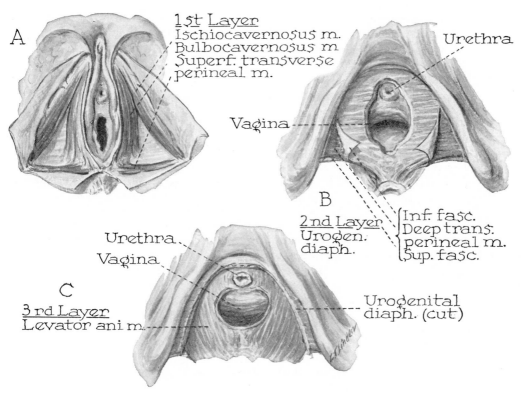

A

1st Layer
Ischiocavernosus m.
Bulbocavernosus m
Superf. transverse
perineal. m.

Urethra

Vagina

B

2nd Layer
Urogen.
diaph.

Inf. fasc.
Deep trans.
perineal m.
Sup. fasc.

Urethra

Vagina

C

3rd Layer
Levator ani m.

Urogenital
diaph. (cut)

FIG. 523. The 3 layers of the perineal musculature. (A) The first layer with its 3 superficial muscles. (B) The urogenital diaphragm. This diaphragm consists of an inferior layer of fascia, a deep transverse perineus muscle and a superior layer of fascia. The inferior fascial layer has been incised to show the relations. The deep transverse perineus muscle continues upward as the sphincter urethrae muscle. (C) The third layer consists of the puborectal portion of the levator ani muscle; it is necessary to cut through the urogenital diaphragm to visualize this structure.

the homologous male organ, has a frenum and a prepuce.

The bulb of the vestibule corresponds to the bulb of the penis, but because of the presence of the vagina, it has become a bilateral structure (Fig. 522). These appear as 2 oblong masses of erectile tissue which lie on the inferior aspect of the perineal membrane and in contact with the lateral walls of the vagina. They are covered by the bulbocavernosus muscles, and where they are in close contact with the Bartholin glands they are rounded. In front where they pass to the sides of the urethra and unite near the body of the clitoris they are pointed. The 2 halves are united in front of the urethra by a venous plexus called the pars intermedia.

The muscles which cover the bulb are the superficial and deep transverse perineal muscles plus the external sphincter of the anus converge to a central point. This is a musculotendinous point which is located in the midline of the perineum, anterior to the anus at the posterior limit of the superficial perineal compartment. The fibers of this musculotendinous portion, plus the tissue between the anal and the vaginal canals, constitute the *perineal body*.

The greater vestibular glands (Bartholin) correspond to the bulbo-urethral (Cowper's) glands of the male but differ in position and in the termination of their ducts. They are about 1 cm. in length and lie on the side of the lowest part of the vagina under cover of the posterior part of the bulb. The long axis of the gland is transverse. The duct follows an oblique course, passing anteromedially and opening into the vestibule, one on each side of the fossa navicularis. Their orifices are macroscopically visible just external to the hymen near the middle of the vaginal orifice (Figs. 520 and 522).

The normal Bartholin glands are not palpable, since they are covered by the bulb of the vestibule. However, when diseased, they are enlarged and become palpable at the junction of the posterior and the middle thirds of the vagina.

MUSCULATURE OF THE PERINEUM AND THE PELVIS

It is helpful to consider the perineal muscles as being arranged in 3 separate strata or layers (Fig. 523). There is a superficial layer which consists of 3 muscles: the superficial transverse perineal, the bulbocavernosus and the ischiocavernosus. The middle layer (urogenital diaphragm) consists of the sphincter of the urethra and the deep transverse perineal plus its fascia; the deep layer is the levator ani and the coccygeus, which have been discussed elsewhere (p. 532).

The superficial transverse perineal mus-cle lies along the base of the urogenital diaphragm, is at times difficult to define and even may be absent. It is a slender fasciculus which originates from the ramus of the ischium close to the tuberosity, passes medially and inserts into the perineal body, at which point it fuses with its fellow of the opposite (Fig. 523). Posteriorly, it lies against the external sphincter of the anus; anteriorly, it almost reaches the posterior wall of the vagina. If visible, it is a good surgical landmark, since the pudendal nerve and artery wind around its posterior border to turn upward and reach the urogenital region. At this point the nerve may be blocked for surgical and obstetric procedures, as well as for the relief of pruritus vulvae.

The ischiocavernosus muscle arises from the medial aspect of the ischium close to its tuberosity, extends forward over the crus and becomes aponeurotic. As these fibers pass upward they ensheath and insert into the medial and the inferior surfaces of the crus and extend as far forward as the body of the clitoris. These 2 muscles compress the crura, thereby retarding the outflow of blood and assisting in the production of an erec-

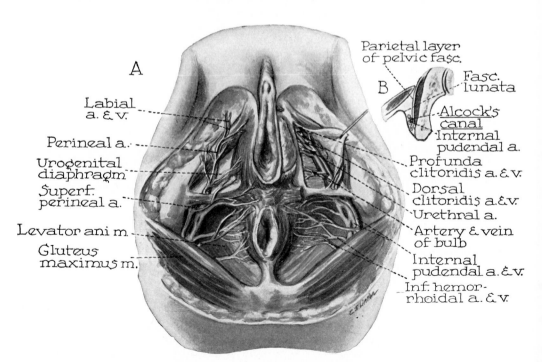

FIG. 524. The internal pudendal artery and its branches.

tion of the clitoris. They are smaller than the corresponding muscles of the male.

The bulbocavernosus muscle has also been referred to as the bulbospongiosus and the sphincter vaginae. In the male, the bulbo-cavernosus is a single structure, but in the female it is halved symmetrically by the vesti-bule, and each side becomes closely related to the lateral surface of the vestibular bulbs. The fibers originate from the central tendi-nous point, separate, pass forward on the walls of the vestibule and converge toward the midline in front, where they are attached to the body of the clitoris; they cover the bulbs of the vestibule and act as constrictor muscles of the erectile tissue, as does the ischiocavernosus.

The 3 superficial perineal muscles are supplied by the perineal branch of the pu-dendal nerve.

UROGENITAL DIAPHRAGM

The urogenital diaphragm (triangular lig-ament) consists of 2 layers of fascia with 2 intervening muscles. The lower layer of fas-cia is the inferior layer, and the upper layer constitutes the superior fascia. The interposed muscles are the deep transverse perineal and the sphincter urethrae membranaceae. The space between the 2 layers of fascia not only contains the deep transverse perineal muscles but also encloses the space which is called the second or the deep compartment of the perineum (Figs. 522 to 525).

The inferior layer (perineal membrane) of the urogenital diaphragm is the more superficial of the 2 fascial layers and forms the roof of the superficial and the floor of the deep perineal compartments; laterally, it at-taches to the ischiopubic rami. Medially, it is attached to the sides of the vagina; pos-teriorly, the 2 halves of the membrane join behind the vagina; their posterior borders fuse with the posterior borders of the fascia above the deep transversus and the mem-branous layer of the superficial fascia. This fusion closes the deep perineal pouch pos-teriorly. Anteriorly, the halves meet in front of the vagina and the urethra, and their borders fuse with the anterior borders of the fascia above the sphincter urethrae. The fused anterior borders are thickened to form a band called the transverse ligament of the perineum; this is separated from the inferior ligament of the pubis by an oval interval which transmits the dorsal vein of the clitoris. The inferior layer of fascia is pierced in the midline by the urethra, the vagina, to either

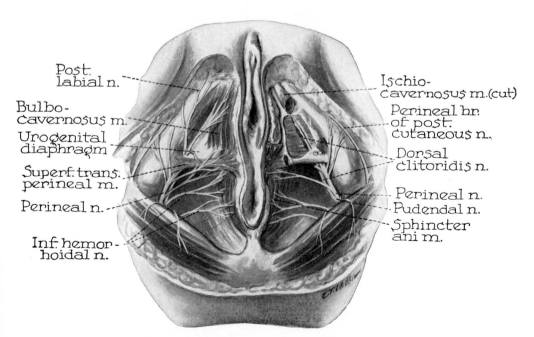

FIG. 525. The pudendal nerve and its branches.

side by the internal pudendal vessels and the pudendal nerves, and by branches of these to the erectile tissue of the bulb, the crus and the glans.

The superior layer of the urogenital diaphragm (upper lamina) also has been referred to as the deep layer of the triangular ligament (Fig. 509). It forms the roof of the deep perineal compartment and the floor of the anterior extension of the ischiorectal on either side of the midline. It is derived from the parietal layer of the pelvic fascia. Anteriorly conjoined with the inferior layer, it forms the transverse ligament of the pelvis; behind, it again becomes continuous with the inferior layer around the deep transverse perineal muscles and by means of this fusion attaches to the deep layer (Colles') of superficial fascia. At the sides it meets the obturator fascia. Medially and above, it joins the fascial coverings on the under surface of the levator ani muscle.

The deep perineal compartment is the pouch which exists between the 2 layers of deep fascia of the urogenital diaphragm of the perineum. It contains the deep transverse perineal muscle, the sphincter muscle surrounding the membranous portion of the urethra, and the pudendal vessels and nerves (Fig. 524).

The sphincter muscle of the membranous urethra (sphincter urethrae membranaceae) is not named entirely correctly, since it would indicate that it is related only to the urethra, but in reality it sends fibers to the vaginal and the anal canals as well. The muscles arise on each side from the ischiopubic rami, and as they approach the midline, an anterior group passes to the urethra, almost reaching the inferior margin of the symphysis pubis. More posteriorly, a group becomes implanted into the urethra; similarly, a group of fibers is related to the vagina; the postvaginal group crosses transversely behind the vaginal canal between it and the anus.

The deep transverse perineal muscle is the backward continuation of the sphincter urethrae (Figs. 522 and 523). It appears as a triangular prolongation which passes backward deep to the coccygeal extension of the external anal sphincter and surrounds the anal canal. The fibers of the two sides, which

originate at the junction of the ischial and the pubic rami, are inserted into the tip of the coccyx. While both of these muscles may have some sphincteric function, the main function of the urogenital musculature is to support the pelvic organs. They are supplied by the perineal nerve.

Between the 2 layers of fascia the following structures are found: the membranous urethra, the sphincter urethrae, the vagina, the internal pudendal arteries, arteries to the bulb and the dorsal nerve to the clitoris. In the female the greater vestibular glands (Bartholin) do not lie between the 2 layers of fascia but beneath the inferior layer so that the ducts (bulbo-urethral glands) do not have to pierce this fascia as they do in the male.

Ischiorectal Fossa. In the urogenital half of the perineum and above the superior layer of urogenital fascia a fat-filled ischiorectal fossa (anterior recess) extends forward for 2 inches on either side. This space resembles a triangular prism. The lateral boundary is formed by the parietal fascia which covers the obturator internus muscle; the superior boundary is the inferior fascia of the pelvic diaphragm which covers the undersurface of the levator ani muscle, and the inferior boundary is the superior fascia of the urogenital diaphragm.

PELVIC DIAPHRAGM

This diaphragm consists of the levator ani and the coccygeus muscles plus the fascia which invests their perineal and pelvic surfaces. From the pelvic wall on either side these muscles pass downward toward the midline, where they fuse or surround the terminal portions of the anus, the vagina and the urethra (Fig. 430). The inferior layer of fascia which covers this muscular diaphragm also is referred to as the anal or the ischiorectal fascia; the superior layer is called the visceral layer of diaphragmatic fascia (p. 531).

The internal pudendal artery leaves the lesser pelvis to enter the gluteal region by passing through the lower part of the greater sciatic foramen between the piriformis and the coccygeus muscles (Fig. 524). After turning around the spine of the ischium it reaches the anal part of the perineum by passing through the lesser sciatic foramen. Then it passes along the lateral wall of the ischiorectal fossa, where it is accompanied by its venae comites and the pudendal nerve. In this location the artery lies in an aponeurotic canal known as Alcock's canal (Fig. 524 B). In the fossa the artery at each side gives off the inferior hemorrhoidal artery, which passes medially through the fatty tissue of the fossa to supply the anus and the anal canal. It also supplies the superficial fascia, the skin of the perineum and the skin and the musculature of the gluteal region.

The main stem of the vessel continues upward, leaves the anal triangle and enters the urogenital triangle. It supplies the following branches (Fig. 524): small posterior labial branches which are distributed to the skin and the fatty tissue of the labia; the perineal artery arises within the ischiorectal fossa, passes forward and mesialward to enter the superficial perineal pouch by passing either over or under the perineal muscle (within this compartment it supplies the 3 muscles of the superficial pouch, namely, the ischiocavernosus, the bulbocavernosus and the superficial transverse perineal); the clitoridal branch of the perineal artery enters the deep perineal compartment by piercing the base of the urogenital diaphragm, continues forward in the substance of the urethral sphincter muscle which it supplies and ends in terminal branches known as the deep and the dorsal arteries of the clitoris. These branches also supply the erectile tissue of the superficial perineal compartment.

The dorsal vein of the clitoris occupies a groove in the medial line, with the dorsal artery and nerve lying on each side of it; it corresponds to the deep dorsal vein of the penis. It takes origin in the glans, passes backward and, at the root of the clitoris, passes between the transverse ligament of the perineum and the inferior pubic ligament; it continues upward into the pelvis to join the plexus of veins on the wall of the vagina in the region of the neck of the bladder. Communication is also made with the internal pudendal vein.

The pudendal nerve is the chief source of innervation to the muscles and the skin of the perineum (Fig. 525). The nerve on each side represents a smaller part of the pudendal plexus (the larger part constituting the sciatic nerve). It is derived from the anterior rami of S 2, 3 and 4 and accompanies the internal pudendal artery and vein, leaving the pelvis through the greater sciatic foramen and entering the ischiorectal fossa through the lesser sciatic foramen. As the nerve enters the ischiorectal fossa it gives off the *inferior hemorrhoidal nerves,* which accompany the vessels of the same name medialward to supply the external sphincter ani muscle and the skin around the anus. Near the posterior margin of the urogenital diaphragm, the pudendal nerve divides into its two terminal branches, namely, the perineal nerve and the dorsal nerve of the clitoris.

The perineal nerve sends superficial branches forward; they enter the superficial perineal compartment as the *posterior labial nerves.* These are accompanied by the arteries of the same name to the skin of the labia and the anterior part of the perineum. The deep division of the nerve is muscular and supplies the muscles in the anal and the urogenital portions of the perineum. In the anal triangle, fibers are sent to the levator ani and the external anal sphincter; the nerve then pierces the base of the urogenital diaphragm, enters the deep perineal compartment and supplies the deep transverse perineal muscles and the urethral sphincter. Other fibers supply the superficial transverse perineal, the ischiocavernosus and the bulbocavernosus.

The dorsal nerve of the clitoris enters the deep compartment at the anterior end of Alcock's canal. It is accompanied by the dorsal artery; it traverses this space and pierces the inferior fascia of the urogenital diaphragm to travel forward on the dorsum of the clitoris to the glans. It supplies the erectile tissue. The integument of the perineum has an additional nerve supply which will be discussed with the individual nerves appearing in this region.

ANAL TRIANGLE

This triangle is bounded behind by the coccyx, on each side by the ischial tuberosities and the sacrotuberous ligament, which are overlapped by the lower borders of the gluteus maximus muscles (Fig. 519). In the midline, it contains the lower part of the anal canal and the external sphincter ani muscle; on each side it includes the ischiorectal fossae.

Ischiorectal Fossa. Each ischiorectal fossa is prismatic in shape and lies below the lateral part of the pelvic diaphragm (Fig. 432). Its roof is formed by the levator ani; the origin of that muscle from the fascia covering the parietal pelvic muscles separates the fossa from the pelvic cavity. Its lateral wall is formed by the lower part of the obturator internus muscle and its fascia. In the posterior part of this wall the fascia interrupts communications with the gluteal region through the lesser sciatic foramen. Posteriorly, the fossa is limited by the sacrotuberous ligament; anteriorly, the base of the perineal ligament intervenes between the fossa and the urogenital triangle. The medial wall is formed by the anal canal and the levator ani muscle. Anteriorly, the fossa does not end at the base of the urogenital diaphragm but continues forward, laterally, between the urogenital and the pelvic diaphragms into the urogenital part of the perineum. The cavity is about 2 inches long, 2 inches deep and 1 inch wide. Under the skin is a large fat pad which fills the fossa. This fat fulfills an important supporting function, since it assists in holding the rectum in place. Should it disappear, as occurs in wasting diseases, the rectum may prolapse and protrude through the anus.

The deep fascia is not directly under the skin in this region because of the intervening fat. This fascia was studied in detail by Elliot Smith who gave it the name of "fascia lunata" (Fig. 524 B). Medially, it covers the levator fascia (anal fascia) and ends at the lower end of the levator; laterally, it covers the obturator fascia and is attached to the ischium. The internal pudendal vessels and nerves are between these two layers. Therefore, it has been argued that Alcock's canal is not formed by a division of the obturator fascia but is really that space that exists between the obturator fascia and the fascia lunata. Anteriorly, the fascia fuses with the urogenital diaphragm; superiorly, it arches

upward, at which point it is called the tegmentum (Fig. 430). The space which exists between this tegmen and the apex of the fossa is called the suprategmental space; it is devoid of fat.

Hiatus of Schwalbe. The levator ani arises from the pubic bone anteriorly, the ischial spine posteriorly and the obturator fascia between these 2 points. At times, however, it arises from the tendinous ring which is attached only to the bone in front and behind and not to the fascia between. This results in a space between its 2 points of origin. This gaping space is known as the hiatus of Schwalbe (Fig. 432). The practical importance of the hiatus is that a process of pelvic peritoneum may be pushed through it into the suprategmental space, resulting in a hernia into the ischiorectal fossa. The coverings of the hernia would be the tegmentum of the fascia lunata, the ischiorectal fat pad and the skin.

The external sphincter ani muscle surrounds the margin of the anal canal and consists of 3 parts: subcutaneous, superficial and deep. The subcutaneous portion of the external sphincter is the only muscle which surrounds the anal orifice proper. The superficial and deep portions of the muscle surround the anal canal. The adjacent fibers of the deep external sphincter intermingle with those of the puborectal portion of the levator ani. Partial division of the muscle usually leaves a competent sphincter, but a complete perineal tear results in a sphincteric incontinence. The muscle has been described in detail elsewhere (p. 458).

The anococcygeal body consists of the posterior fibers of the external sphincter ani, a backward extension of the deep perineal muscles and the median strip of the pubococcygeal part of the levator ani (Fig. 502). It is an important unit in the perineum, and injury to it may result in the loss of the essential elements of visceral suspension and support.

SURGICAL CONSIDERATIONS

VAGINAL HYSTERECTOMY

This operation is usually done for procedentia and for prolapse of moderate degree associated with cystocele and rectocele (Fig. 526). Prolapse of the uterus results from a failure of the supporting structures to hold the uterus in place. These supporting structures are: the round ligaments, the utero-sacral ligaments, the bases of the broad ligaments, (Mackenrodt), the pelvic floor and the fascia surrounding the vagina.

Vaginal hysterectomy is performed in the following way: the lips of the cervix are sewed together or grasped with a tenaculum for the purpose of traction (Fig. 527). A circular incision is made around the cervix in such a way that the bladder is not injured. The anterior vaginal wall is freed, and the bladder is dissected off of the anterior surface of the cervix until the vesico-uterine peritoneum is identified.

With the bladder retracted upward, the vesico-uterine peritoneum is opened, and the index and the middle fingers of the left hand are introduced into the peritoneal cavity (Fig. 527 C). The fingers depress the fundus, and the peritoneal opening is extended laterally on each side as far as the broad ligament. The fundus is delivered as the fingers in the peritoneal cavity push the peritoneum forward over the pouch of Douglas. An incision is made over this finger, and the peritoneal cavity is entered posterior to the cervix.

The peritoneum is incised as far as the uterosacral ligaments on each side. These ligaments are clamped, divided and ligated. Then hemostats are placed at the top of the broad ligament in the region of the cornu of the uterus, and they grasp the round ligament and the adnexal attachments. Similar clamps are placed at the base of the broad ligament; these secure the uterine vessels. The tissue between these clamps is divided. It is best to carry this out on the left side first and replace the clamps by transfixion sutures (Fig. 527 F). Then the uterus can be rotated outward so that it remains attached only on the right side, and a similar procedure is carried out here.

The peritoneum of the pouch of Douglas and the bladder are approximated by interrupted sutures; the stump of the adnexae remains extraperitoneal. The vaginal flaps are closed by interrupted sutures, and a slight

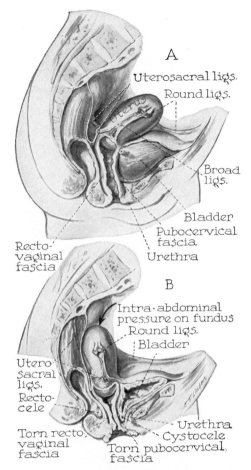

FIG. 526. Descent of the uterus, cystocele and rectocele. (A) Normal uterine supports. (B) Failure of the normal uterine supports.

opening is permitted to remain for drainage, if desired.

REPAIR OF CYSTOCELE
(ANTERIOR COLPORRHAPHY)

The limits of the bladder should be identified by a sound or a catheter placed in the urethra and carried down toward the cervix. Also, the presence or the absence of a urethrocele should be noted. Through a short transverse incision a cleavage plane is found between the vaginal wall and the bladder (Fig. 528). The vaginal wall is dissected laterad on each side and separated from the underlying musculofascial tissue; this tissue

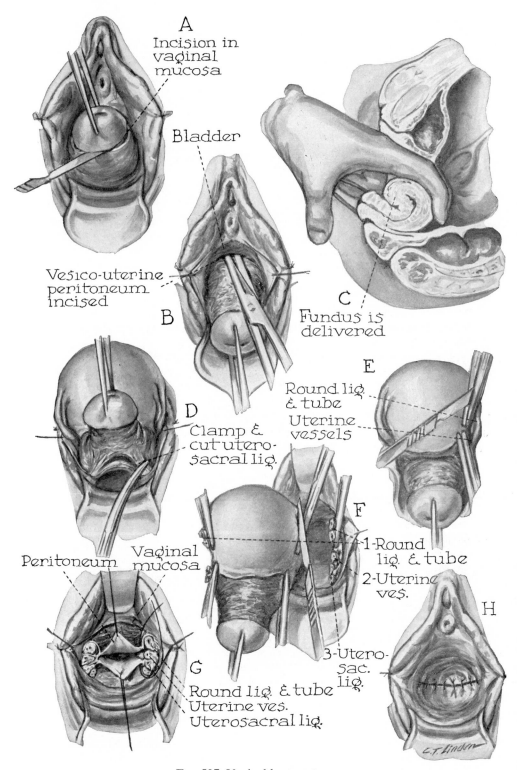

A
Incision in
vaginal
mucosa

Bladder

Vesico-uterine
peritoneum
incised

B

C
Fundus is
delivered

D
Clamp &
cut utero-
sacral lig.

E
Round lig.
& tube
Uterine
vessels

F
1-Round
lig. & tube
2-Uterine
ves.
3-Utero-
sac.
lig.

Peritoneum   Vaginal
mucosa

G
Round lig. & tube
Uterine ves.
Uterosacral lig.

H

FIG. 527. Vaginal hysterectomy.

is chiefly the urogenital diaphragm (Fig. 528 C). The bladder is separated from the cervix, and the pillars on each side are cut; this permits upward displacement of the bladder (Fig. 528 D).

Mattress-type sutures are placed from side to side in the tissue of the urogenital diaphragm but are placed lateral to the urethra. With the bladder held in an upward direction, sutures are placed through the lateral musculofascial tissue and through the uterus. In this way, the herniation of the bladder is corrected. The redundant vaginal flaps are trimmed and approximated with interrupted sutures.

REPAIR OF RECTOCELE
(PERINEORRHAPHY)

Clamps are applied slightly within the mucocutaneous junction on each side at the carunculae myrtiformes (Fig. 529). Outward

traction is made on the clamps, and the skin and the mucous membrane are divided along this line. The posterior vaginal wall is separated from the rectal wall. This dissection is carried in an upward direction and extends above the upper margin of the rectocele. The puborectal portions of the levator ani muscles are identified and sutured; thus, a musculofascial bridge which keeps the herniated rectum in place is formed. The uppermost suture grasps the undersurface of the vaginal wall. If the torn fascia of the urogenital diaphragm is visible, this too is sutured as a separate layer over the levator. Skin sutures are placed.

POSTERIOR COLPOTOMY

This is usually used in the treatment of pelvic abscess or as a diagnostic method in ruptured ectopic pregnancy. Tenacula are applied to the cervix to pull it upward and

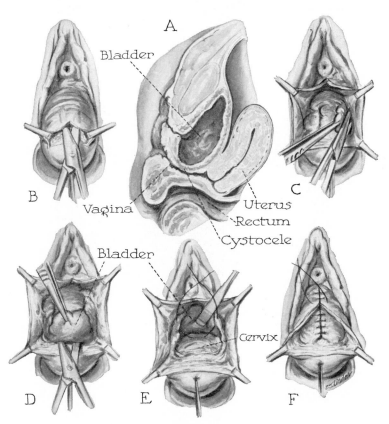

FIG. 528. Repair of a cystocele. (A) Sagittal view of the cystocele. (B through F) The repair.

forward, and an incision about 1½ inches in length is made in the mucous membrane at the junction of the posterior vaginal wall and the cervix (Fig. 530). The underlying tissue is divided with scissors, the points of which are directed toward the cervix. When the abscess cavity has been entered, a finger is inserted to explore, and the opening is enlarged sufficiently so that drainage may be instituted.

Vesicovaginal Fistulae

Birth injuries, surgery, radium burns and carcinoma are the chief causes of such fistulae. Reich and Wilkey have described a combined gynecologic and urologic technic to treat this condition. The cystoscopist passes a ureteral catheter into the bladder via the urethra and then through the fistula into the vagina (Fig. 531). An incision is made in the vaginal wall, and the bladder is freed. A purse-string suture is placed and tightened

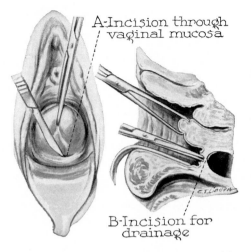

A-Incision through vaginal mucosa

B-Incision for drainage

Fig. 530. Posterior colpotomy. (A) The cervix is drawn upward, and an incision is placed in the vaginal mucosa. (B) A sagittal section showing the location of pus or blood in the recto-uterine cul-de-sac (Douglas).

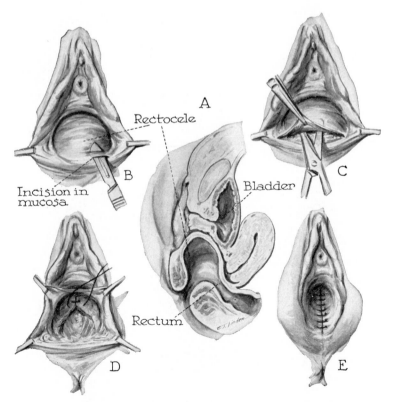

A

Rectocele

Incision in mucosa.

B

Bladder

C

Rectum

D

E

Fig. 529. Repair of a rectocele. (A) Sagittal view of the rectocele. (B through E) The repair.

simultaneously with upward withdrawal of the catheter. Reinforcing sutures and repair complete the procedure.

RECTOVAGINAL FISTULAE

These fistulae may result from carcinoma of the cervix or the rectum, the repair of a complete perineal laceration, and operations for abscesses and fistulae-in-ano. Smaller fistulae above the level of the sphincter ani may be closed according to the technic of V. C. David. A circular incision is made around the fistula, and the fistulous tract is inverted into the rectum (Fig. 532).

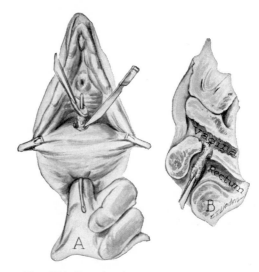

FIG. 532. Repair of a rectovaginal fistula.

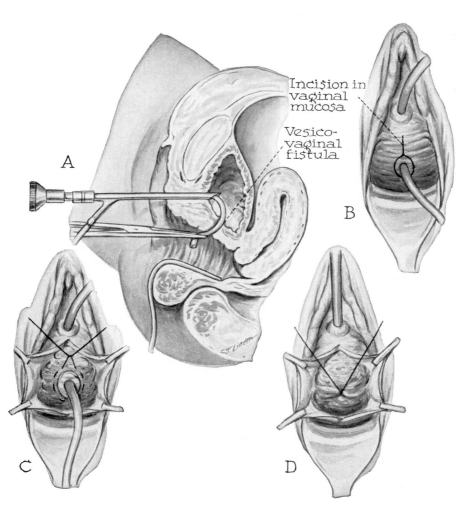

FIG. 531. Repair of a vesicovaginal fistula.

Shoulder

The shoulder is divided topographically into the axillary, the pectoral, the deltoid and the scapular regions.

The cutaneous nerve supply of this region is derived from the supraclavicular, the axillary, the medial antibrachial cutaneous, the medial brachial cutaneous and the intercostobrachial nerves (Fig. 533).

AXILLARY AND PECTORAL REGIONS

AXILLA

The axilla is an anatomic pyramid situated between the medial side of the upper arm and the upper lateral side of the chest wall. Since it is pyramidal in shape, it consists of 4 walls, an apex and a base.

Walls. The four walls are the anterior, the posterior, the medial and the lateral (Fig. 534). The *anterior* (*pectoral*) *wall* is composed of a superficial layer (pectoralis major muscle with its enveloping fascia) and an inner or deeper layer (pectoralis minor and subclavius muscles with their enveloping clavipectoral fascia). The *posterior* (*scapular*) *wall* is formed by the scapula, which is covered by the subscapularis, the latissimus

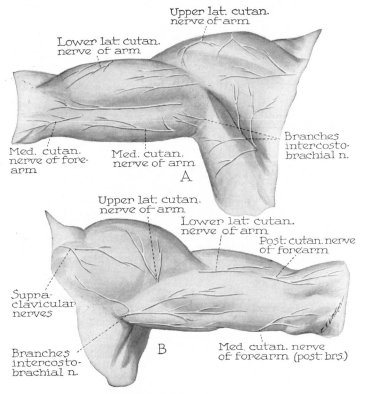

FIG. 533. The cutaneous nerve supply of the shoulder:
(A) anterior view; (B) posterior view.

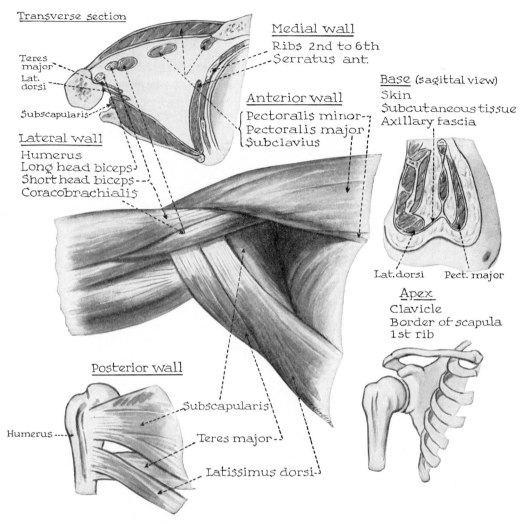

FIG. 534. The 4 walls of the axilla. The axilla is pyramidal in its shape; hence, it has an anterior (pectoral) wall, a posterior (scapular) wall, a medial (costal) wall and a lateral (humeral) wall. The various walls and views are depicted.

dorsi and the teres major muscles. The *medial (costal) wall* consists of the upper ribs (2nd to 6th) and the serratus anterior muscle; the *lateral (humeral) wall* is formed by the humerus (bicipital groove). This groove lodges the long head of the biceps tendon, and its lips give attachment to the muscles of the anterior and the posterior axillary walls. The long head of the biceps tendon is covered by the short head of the biceps and the coracobrachialis.

Apex. The axillary apex is blunted and triangular and is bounded by 3 bones: anteriorly by the *clavicle,* posteriorly by the upper border of the *scapula* and medially by the *first rib.*

Base. The base of the axilla is made up of skin, subcutaneous tissue and *axillary fascia,* the latter extending from the lower border of the pectoralis major muscle to the latissimus dorsi (Fig. 535). Occasionally, a small strip of muscle extends from the latissimus dorsi to the structures deep to the pectoralis major; this forms the anomalous axillary arch.

PECTORAL REGION

Fasciae. There are 2 fasciae in the pectoral

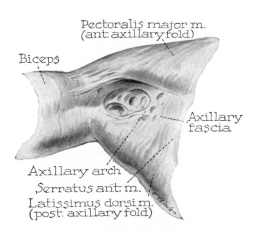

FIG. 535. The axillary fascia.

region, namely, the pectoral fascia proper and the clavipectoral fascia (Fig. 536).

The pectoral fascia proper (Fig. 536 B) is attached above to the anterior superior aspect of the clavicle; it passes down to ensheath the pectoralis major muscle and then blends with the axillary fascia in the floor of the axilla. Medially, it is attached to the sternum and is continuous below and medially with the serratus anterior and the external oblique muscles. Laterally, it blends with the fascia of the arm.

The clavipectoral fascia lies deep to the pectoral fascia proper (Fig. 536). Vertically,

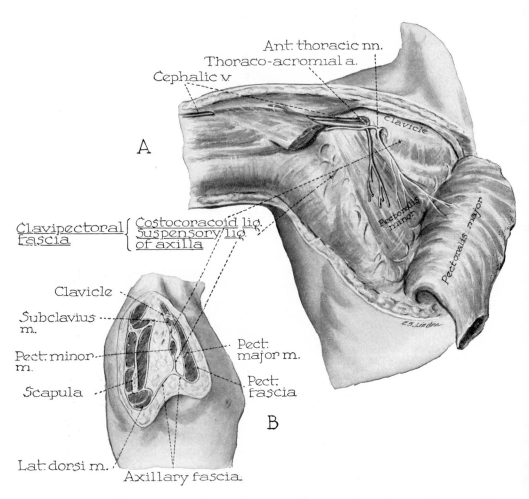

FIG. 536. The clavipectoral fascia. (A) Seen from in front after reflecting the pectoralis major muscle. (B) Sagittal section; the pectoral fascia is also shown.

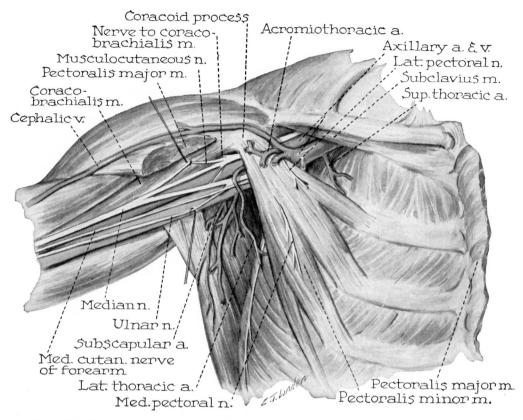

Coracoid process
Nerve to coraco-brachialis m.
Musculocutaneous n.
Pectoralis major m.
Coraco-brachialis m.
Cephalic v.
Acromiothoracic a.
Axillary a. & v.
Lat. pectoral n.
Subclavius m.
Sup. thoracic a.
Median n.
Ulnar n.
Subscapular a.
Med. cutan. nerve of forearm
Lat. thoracic a.
Med. pectoral n.
Pectoralis major m.
Pectoralis minor m.

FIG. 537. The pectoralis minor muscle and its relations. The pectoralis major muscle has been reflected, and the clavipectoral fascia has been removed. The axillary vein lies medial to the axillary artery, and the brachial plexus appears to be wrapped around the artery.

it extends from the clavicle above to the dome of the axillary fascia below, thereby acting as a *suspensory ligament* for the axillary fascia. It is interrupted in its vertical path by the subclavius and the pectoralis minor muscles, both of which it separates and encloses. That portion of the clavipectoral fascia which lies between the subclavius and the pectoralis minor muscles is called the *costocoracoid ligament (membrane)*; it is attached laterally to the coracoid process and medially to the 1st and the 2nd costal cartilages. The suspensory ligament is that part of the clavipectoral fascia which lies between the pectoralis minor and the axillary fascia. The costocoracoid ligament is pierced by the cephalic vein, which drains into the axillary vein; the thoraco-acromial artery, a branch of the axillary artery; the anterior

thoracic nerves to the pectoral muscles; and lymph vessels from the upper outer quadrant of the breast.

Muscles. *The pectoralis minor muscle* is the key structure to the axillary and the pectoral regions; its position and relations to the brachial plexus and the axillary vessels are important surgically (Fig. 537). The pectoralis minor is a triangular muscle which has its origin from the 3rd, the 4th and the 5th ribs near their costochondral junctions, and its insertion on the medial border of the coracoid process of the scapula. The coracoid lies 1 inch below the clavicle, barely covered by the anterior border of the deltoid muscle. The pectoralis minor is covered by the pectoralis major, which lies on the same plane as the deltoid muscle.

The deltopectoral groove is situated be-

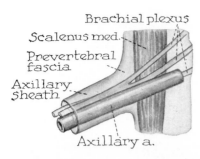

FIG. 538. The axillary sheath. The prevertebral layer of deep cervical fascia gives off a fascial process which is continuous down the arm as the axillary sheath.

tween the deltoid and the pectoralis major muscles.

The cephalic vein runs in this groove, crosses the anterior surface of the pectoralis minor muscle and pierces the costocoracoid membrane before emptying into the axillary vein. The cephalic vein is an important surgical guide to the axillary vein and the axillary artery, and it acts as a compensatory vein when the axillary can no longer function.

Axillary Sheath. If the pectoralis minor muscle is severed and reflected downward with its clavipectoral fascia, the axillary vessels and the brachial plexus do not immediately come into view because they are covered by a connective tissue layer known as the axillary sheath; this is a lateral prolongation of the prevertebral layer of fascia traveling down the arm as far as the elbow (Fig. 538). The fascia passes over the scalenus muscles, the brachial plexus and the subclavian artery. On leaving the neck, on their way to the axilla, these vessels and nerves pierce this fascia and carry a tubular sheath of it along with them.

VEINS

The axillary vein is the first structure to appear following incision into the axillary sheath (Fig. 537). It is formed by the junction of 3 veins of the superior extremity: the 2 vena comites of the brachial artery (the brachial veins) and the basilic vein, which pierces the deep fascia in the middle of the arm. The axillary vein begins at the lower border of the teres major muscle and con-

tinues to the outer border of the 1st rib, where it becomes the subclavian vein. The latter joins the internal jugular to form the innominate vein. Sometimes the union of the basilic and the brachial veins does not take place until the clavicle is reached; in such instances a single-trunk axillary vein may not exist or may be very short.

When the arm is abducted, the vein covers the axillary artery and conceals it. This intimate relationship between the artery and the vein explains the not-too-infrequent appearance of arteriovenous aneurysms in this region. The tributaries of the axillary vein correspond to the branches of the axillary artery.

ARTERIES

The axillary artery is a continuation of the subclavian and is about 6 inches in length (Fig. 537). It starts at the outer border of the 1st rib and ends at the lower border of the teres major muscle, where it becomes the brachial artery. The pectoralis minor muscle divides the axillary artery into 3 parts (Fig. 539). The first part lies proximal to the pectoralis minor muscle under the costocoracoid membrane and has one branch, the highest or superior thoracic artery. The second part lies behind the pectoralis minor muscle, is the shortest part and has 2 branches, the thoraco-acromial and lateral thoracic arteries. The third part lies distal to the pectoralis minor muscle, is the longest part and has 3 branches: the subscapular, the anterior humeral circumflex and the posterior humeral circumflex arteries. It is well to remember that part *one* has *one* branch; part *two* has *two* branches and part *three* has *three* branches.

The superior thoracic artery is the first branch of the axillary artery and the only branch of part one. It is usually small, runs medially and supplies the muscles of the first two intercostal spaces.

The thoraco-acromial artery arises from the second part as a very short trunk but is of considerable size. Winding around the upper border of the pectoralis minor muscle, it pierces the costocoracoid membrane and divides into 4 branches: the pectoral, the acromial, the deltoid and the clavicular. The deltoid branch accompanies the cephalic vein in the deltopectoral groove.

The lateral thoracic artery also arises from the second part of the axillary artery, but it follows the lower border of the pectoralis minor muscle to the chest wall. It does not accompany the long thoracic nerve, as is commonly thought. The latter is found with the terminal part of the subscapular artery.

The subscapular artery is the largest branch of the axillary artery. It arises near the lower border of the subscapularis muscle, along which it descends accompanied by its venae comites (Fig. 537). The subscapular artery supplies the posterior axillary wall (subscapularis, teres major and latissimus dorsi muscles). Although it is the vessel of the posterior wall, it terminates on the medial wall (serratus anterior muscle). Branches of this artery accompany the nerve supply to the subscapularis, the teres major and the latissimus dorsi muscles. The nerve to the latissimus dorsi muscle is the thoracodorsal; hence, that part of the subscapular artery which runs with it is called the *thoracodorsal artery*. The terminal branches of the subscapular artery send twigs to the serratus anterior muscle, and here the artery is accompanied by the nerve supply to that muscle (the long thoracic nerve). The subscapular artery also gives rise to the circumflex scapular artery, which passes through the triangular space on its way to the dorsum of the scapula.

Anterior and posterior circumflex humeral arteries form an arterial ring around the surgical neck of the humerus. The anterior lies behind the biceps and the coracobrachialis muscles, and the posterior accompanies the axillary nerve through the quadrilateral space to reach the deep aspect of the deltoid muscle (Fig. 565). The 3 branches of the third part of the axillary artery may arise from a common trunk.

Brachial Plexus

To visualize the brachial plexus as a whole, it must be followed from its origin in the neck, through the axilla and into the superior extremity (Figs. 540 and 541).

The following facts should be kept in mind to understand the brachial plexus: (1) It is made up of the anterior rami of the 5th to the 8th cervical nerves and the 1st thoracic nerve, with communications from the 4th cervical and the 2nd thoracic. (2) The plexus is arranged so that 5 rami (roots) = 3 trunks = 6 divisions = 3 cords = nerve supply (branches) to the upper extremity. (3) The roots and the trunks lie in the neck; the divisions are behind the clavicle, and the cords and the branches are in the axilla. (4) The roots and the trunks are in relation to the subclavian artery; the cords are in relation to the first and the second parts of the axillary artery. (5) The cords become branches at the lower border of the pectoralis minor muscle (third part of the axillary artery).

The 5th and the 6th cervical roots join to form the upper trunk; the 7th cervical forms the middle trunk; and the 8th cervical and the 1st thoracic form the lower trunk. Each trunk divides into an anterior and a posterior division. The 3 posterior divisions join to form the posterior cord; the anterior divisions of the upper and the middle trunk unite to form the lateral cord; and the anterior division of the lower trunk continues alone as the medial cord. Branches arise from the roots, the trunks and the cords; no branches have their origin from the divisions.

Branches. The branches (Fig. 541) arising from the *roots* are: dorsal scapular (to the rhomboids), C 5; long thoracic (to the serratus anterior), C 5, 6 and 7; muscular branches (to the 3 scalenii and longus coli muscles). The branches arising from the *trunks* are: suprascapular (to the supraspinatus and the infraspinatus), C 5 and 6; subclavius (to the subclavius), C 5 and 6. The branches arising from *cords* are as follows: from the *lateral* cord, the lateral anterior thoracic (to the pectoral muscles), C 5, 6 and 7; the musculocutaneous (to the biceps, the coracobrachialis and the greater part of the brachialis), C 5, 6 and 7; the lateral head of the median, C 5, 6 and 7. From the *medial* cord arise the medial anterior thoracic (to the pectoral muscles), C 8 and T 1; the medial head of the median, C 8 and T 1; the ulnar, C 8 and T 1; medial cutaneous nerve of the forearm, C 8 and T 1; medial cutaneous nerve of the arm, T 1.

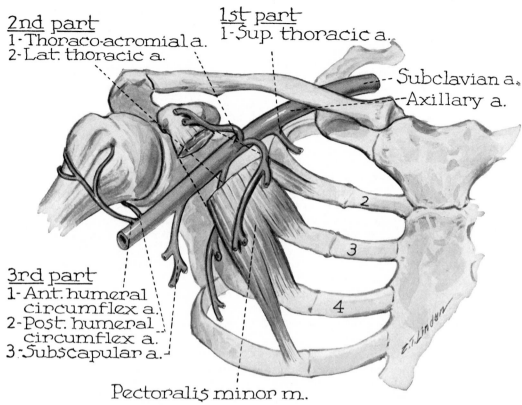

2nd part
1- Thoraco-acromial a.
2- Lat. thoracic a.

1st part
1- Sup. thoracic a.

-- Subclavian a.
-- Axillary a.

2

3

4

3rd part
1- Ant. humeral
    circumflex a.
2- Post. humeral
    circumflex a.
3- Subscapular a.

Pectoralis minor m.

FIG. 539. The pectoralis minor muscle divides the axillary artery into 3 parts.

FIG. 540. The brachial plexus. The "formula" for the plexus may be presented as follows: 5 rami (roots) = 3 trunks = 6 divisions = 3 cords = the nerve supply (branches) to the superior extremity.

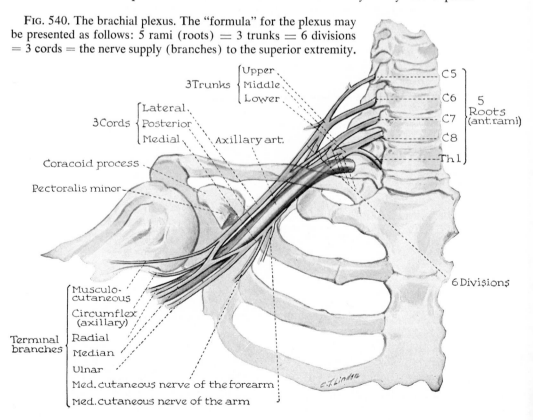

3 Trunks { Upper / Middle / Lower

3 Cords { Lateral / Posterior / Medial

Axillary art.

Coracoid process

Pectoralis minor

C5
C6
C7
C8
Th1

5 Roots (ant. rami)

6 Divisions

Terminal branches { Musculo-cutaneous / Circumflex (axillary) / Radial / Median / Ulnar / Med. cutaneous nerve of the forearm / Med. cutaneous nerve of the arm

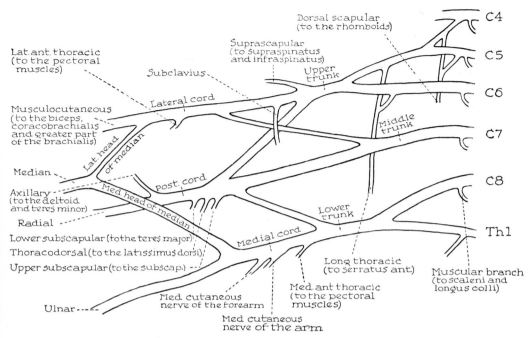

Lat. ant. thoracic
(to the pectoral
muscles)

Subclavius

Dorsal scapular
(to the rhomboids)

Suprascapular
(to supraspinatus
and infraspinatus)

Upper
trunk

C4

C5

C6

Lateral cord

Musculocutaneous
(to the biceps,
coracobrachialis
and greater part
of the brachialis)

Middle
trunk

Lat. head
of median

C7

Median

post. cord

C8

Med. head of median

Axillary
(to the deltoid
and teres minor)

Lower
trunk

Radial

Th1

Lower subscapular (to the teres major)

Medial cord

Thoracodorsal (to the latissimus dorsi)

Upper subscapular (to the subscap.)

Long thoracic
(to serratus ant.)

Muscular branch
(to scaleni and
longus colli)

Ulnar

Med. cutaneous
nerve of the forearm

Med. ant. thoracic
(to the pectoral
muscles)

Med. cutaneous
nerve of the arm

FIG. 541. Diagram showing the construction of the brachial plexus.

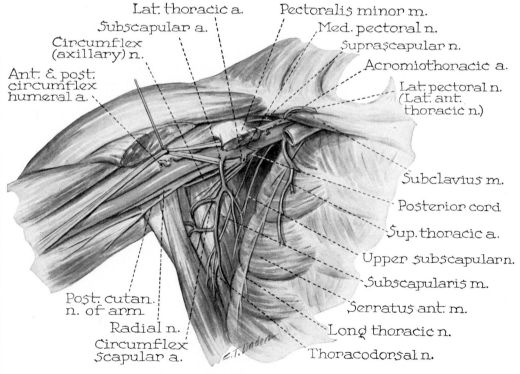

Lat. thoracic a.

Subscapular a.

Circumflex
(axillary) n.

Ant. & post.
circumflex
humeral a.

Pectoralis minor m.

Med. pectoral n.

Suprascapular n.

Acromiothoracic a.

Lat. pectoral n.
(Lat. ant.
thoracic n.)

Subclavius m.

Posterior cord

Sup. thoracic a.

Upper subscapular n.

Subscapularis m.

Serratus ant. m.

Long thoracic n.

Thoracodorsal n.

Post. cutan.
n. of arm

Radial n.

Circumflex
scapular a.

FIG. 542. Relations of the brachial plexus. The pectoralis minor muscle and the axillary vein have been removed; the lateral and the medial cords of the brachial plexus are retracted upward.

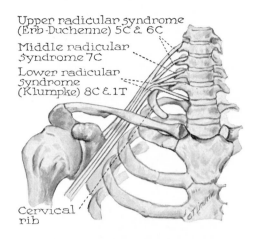

Upper radicular syndrome
(Erb-Duchenne) 5C & 6C

Middle radicular
syndrome 7C

Lower radicular
syndrome
(Klumpke) 8C & 1T

Cervical
rib

FIG. 543. Three types of brachial
plexus palsy.

From the *posterior* cord arise the radial, C 5, 6, 7 and 8 and T 1; axillary (to the deltoid and the teres minor), C 5 and 6; thoraco-dorsal (to the latissimus dorsi), C 6, 7 and 8; upper subscapular (to the subscapular), C 5 and 6; and lower subscapular (to the teres major), C 5 and 6.

Relation of Brachial Plexus to Axillary Artery. The brachial plexus arises in the neck and takes a downward course; the axillary artery travels upward from the chest (Figs. 537 and 542). Therefore, the plexus lies lateral to the subclavian artery. The 3 cords of the plexus are placed around the second part of the axillary artery and in this way receive their names. Thus, the lateral cord lies lateral to the artery, the medial lies medial to the artery, and the posterior behind it. Since all the nerves lie lateral to the artery in the neck, it must follow that the medial cord crosses the artery to assume its medial position. This it does by running behind part one of the axillary artery. Most of the branches of the plexus are grouped around the third part of the artery. The musculo-cutaneous nerve lies lateral to the median nerve, and both of these lie lateral to the artery. In the groove between the axillary artery and vein 2 nerves are found: the medial cutaneous nerve of the forearm and the deeper lying ulnar nerve. Because of this arrangement these nerves usually are

confused with each other. The medial cutaneous nerve of the arm passes along the medial border of the vein. The axillary and the radial nerves separate the axillary artery from the subscapular muscle, and the radial nerve alone separates the artery from the latissimus dorsi and the teres major muscles.

SURGICAL CONSIDERATIONS

BRACHIAL PLEXUS PALSY

Brachial plexus lesions are divided into those lesions which involve the entire plexus or only the upper, the middle or the lower portions (Fig. 543). When the *entire plexus* is involved, either from injury or pressure, the following features are noted: complete anesthesia of the lower part of the arm, the forearm and the hand, and flaccid paralysis of the superior extremities, with eventual wasting of the muscles.

Erb-Duchenne (upper arm) paralysis is the most common type of nerve injury occurring at birth; it involves the 5th and the 6th cervical nerves. It may occur during the course of a complicated delivery, with marked downward traction on the head, resulting in a widening of the angle between the head and the shoulder. The injury usually is located where the 5th and the 6th cervical nerves join to form the upper trunk of the plexus; this is known as Erb's point and is the spot where 6 nerves meet, namely, the 5th cervical root, the 6th cervical root, the anterior division of the upper trunk, the posterior division of the upper trunk, the suprascapular nerve and the nerve to the subclavius muscle. The hand hangs at the side in internal rotation with the forearm pronated and the fingers and the wrist flexed. This is referred to by some as the "head-waiter's tip hand." External rotation and abduction are lost at the shoulder, as are flexion and supination of the forearm. The clinical appearance is produced by a paralysis of the abductors and the lateral rotators of the shoulder (deltoid, supraspinatus and infraspinatus) plus a paralysis of the flexors of the elbow (biceps, brachialis and brachio-radialis); a weakness of the adductors and the medial rotators of the shoulders (pectoralis major, teres major, latissimus dorsi, subscapularis) also results. The pronator teres, the supinator, the flexors of the wrist and the thenar muscles may be slightly involved.

The middle arm type lesion (middle radicular syndrome) involves the 7th cervical nerve and produces a paralysis of the entire radial nerve except its branch to the brachioradialis; there is also a paralysis of the coracobrachialis.

Klumpke (lower arm) paralysis is usually the result of upward traction on the shoulder. It also may result from injuries or during breech presentations when the arms are placed over the head. The lesion involves the 8th cervical and the 1st thoracic nerves. It results in a paralysis of the intrinsic muscles of the hand and a paralysis of the flexors of the digits. A "claw" hand results. There is also diminished sensation over the medial side of the arm, the forearm and the hand.

LIGATION OF THE AXILLARY ARTERY

If the axillary artery is ligated above the origin of the thoraco-acromial, the collateral circulation is the same as that of the third part of the subclavian artery. When ligated at its lower limit, the following arteries are involved in the collateral supply: the subscapular, the transverse scapular, the transverse cervical, the internal mammary, the intercostal, the thoraco-acromial, the lateral thoracic and the anterior and the posterior humeral circumflex.

The axillary artery may be ligated in its first part (above the pectoralis minor muscle) or in its third part (below the pectoralis minor muscle).

Ligation of the *first part* can be accomplished by an incision extending just below the clavicle from the coracoid process to the sternoclavicular joint (Fig. 544). The clavicular portion of the pectoralis major muscle is incised through its whole thickness, and the pectoralis minor is retracted downward. The costocoracoid membrane is divided along the upper border of the pectoralis minor, care being taken not to injure the axillary vein. The axillary artery is now exposed with the vein on its inner side and the

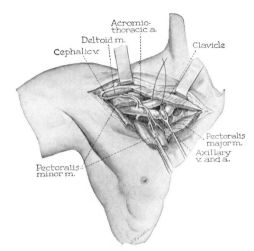

FIG. 544. Ligation of the first part of the axillary artery.

cords of the brachial plexus outside and behind it. To accomplish the ligation it may be necessary to lower the arm, since the vein overlies and conceals the artery when the arm is abducted.

The third part of the axillary artery is superficial and is easier to approach. The incision is an upward prolongation of an incision placed over the brachial artery. The coracobrachialis muscle is exposed and drawn outward with the musculocutaneous nerve. The basilic vein, which joins the brachial venae comites to form the axillary vein, is found on the inner side of the artery. The cords of the brachial plexus are disposed around all sides of the artery and must be identified and retracted out of the way.

DELTOID AND SCAPULAR REGIONS

It is well to study the scapula in the discussion of the deltoid and the scapular regions, since this bone presents many bony surgical landmarks and gives attachment to the muscles in this region.

SCAPULA (SHOULDER BLADE)

The scapula (shoulder blade) is a flat, triangular bone which lies on the posterolateral aspect of the thorax opposite the 2nd to the 7th ribs. It has 3 borders, 3 angles, 2 surfaces and 2 processes (Figs. 545 and 546).

Borders. The 3 borders are the superior, the medial and the lateral.

The superior border is the shortest; it inclines laterally and downward from the superior angle, where the levator scapulae is inserted. The suprascapular notch is located at its lateral part and is converted by the suprascapular ligament into a foramen which transmits the nerve of the same name. Since this border gives attachment only to the small omohyoid muscle, it remains thin and sharp.

The medial (vertebral) border is the longest and is quite thick; it gives insertion to the second layer of back muscles (rhomboid minor, rhomboid major and levator scapulae).

The lateral (axillary) border is the thickest of the 3. It extends from the inferior

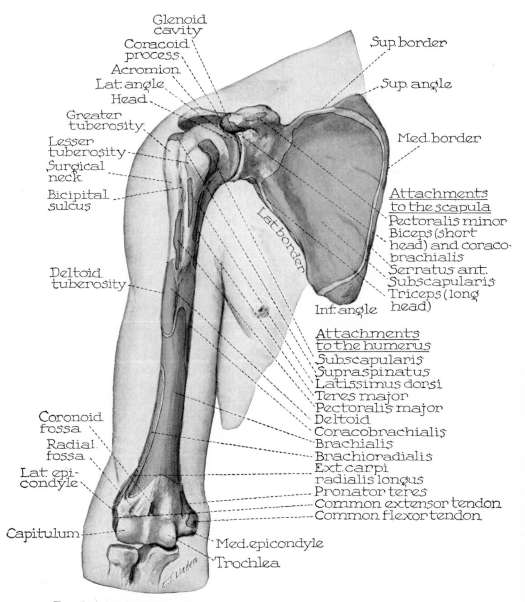

Glenoid cavity
Coracoid process
Acromion
Lat. angle
Head
Greater tuberosity
Lesser tuberosity
Surgical neck
Bicipital sulcus
Deltoid tuberosity
Coronoid fossa
Radial fossa
Lat. epicondyle
Capitulum

Sup. border
Sup. angle
Med. border

Lat border

Inf. angle

Attachments to the scapula
Pectoralis minor
Biceps (short head) and coraco-brachialis
Serratus ant.
Subscapularis
Triceps (long head)

Attachments to the humerus
Subscapularis
Supraspinatus
Latissimus dorsi
Teres major
Pectoralis major
Deltoid
Coracobrachialis
Brachialis
Brachioradialis
Ext. carpi radialis longus
Pronator teres
Common extensor tendon
Common flexor tendon

Med. epicondyle
Trochlea

FIG. 545. Muscle attachments to the scapula and the humerus (anterior view). Origins are represented in red, and insertions in blue.

angle upward, laterally and forward to the glenoid cavity; at its upper end is the triangular impression known as the infraglenoid tubercle for the attachment of the long head of the triceps.

Angles. The 3 angles are the superior, the inferior and the lateral. The obtuse *superior angle* is situated between the superior and the medial borders. It is covered by the trapezius and, therefore, is difficult to feel. The acute *inferior angle* is located between the medial and the lateral borders and is an important anatomic and surgical landmark; fortunately, it is felt easily at the level of the 7th intercostal space when the extremity hangs at the side. The *lateral angle,* located between the superior and the lateral borders, forms the shallow glenoid cavity, which articulates with the head of the humerus and displays above its apex a slightly roughened area (the supraglenoid tubercle) for the origin of the long head of the biceps.

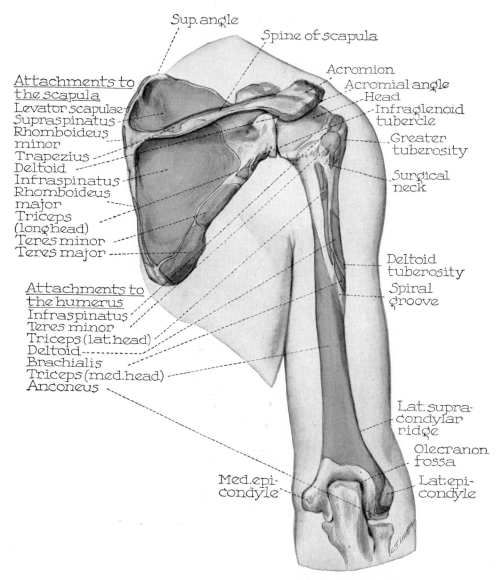

Fig. 546. Muscle attachments to the scapula and the humerus (posterior view). Origins are represented in red, and insertions in blue.

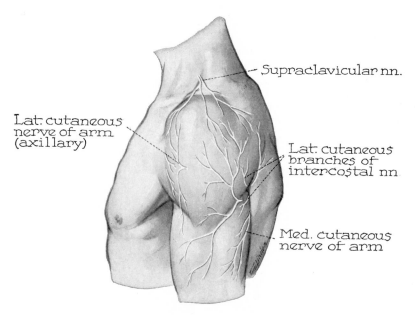

FIG. 547. Cutaneous nerve supply of the deltoid region.

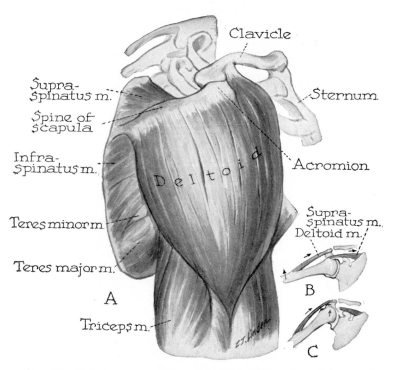

FIG. 548. The deltoid muscle. (A) Origin and insertion of the muscle. (B) The supraspinatus muscle initiates abduction of the arm, and this is continued by the deltoid muscle. (C) With a torn supraspinatus muscle, abduction cannot be started by the deltoid unless at first the arm is pushed away from the body.

Surfaces. The 2 surfaces are the dorsal and the costal (ventral). The *dorsal surface* is unequally subdivided by the spine of the scapula into the smaller supraspinous and the larger infraspinous fossae. Transverse grooves for the circumflex scapular artery are noted over this surface. The *costal surface* is hollow and forms the floor of the subscapular fossa, which is deepest opposite the spine. This area is covered by the serratus anterior and the subscapularis muscles.

Processes. The 2 processes are the coracoid and the acromion.

The coracoid process projects from the lateral part of the superior border of the bone and sharply bends forward and laterally at a right angle. The lateral border of this process gives attachment to the coraco-acromial ligament, which helps the acromion form an arch above the head of the humerus. The tip of the coracoid gives origin to the coracobrachialis and the short head of the biceps muscles. Although this tip is covered by the anterior fibers of the deltoid, it can be felt on deep pressure through the lateral boundary of the infraclavicular fossa about 1 inch below the clavicle.

Acromion Process. The spine of the scapular terminates laterally as the acromion process, which projects laterally at first and then bends sharply forward to form the acromial angle. The entire upper surface and borders of the acromion are palpable subcutaneously. Immediately in front of the shoulder joint it gives attachment to the lateral end of the coraco-acromial ligament.

MUSCULAR ATTACHMENTS, VESSELS, NERVES AND BURSAE

Deltoid Region. *The skin* over the deltoid region is thick. Fibrous septa extend from the skin into the fibrous investments of the deltoid muscle. This area is supplied above by the supraclavicular nerves and below by the cutaneous branches of the axillary nerve and the intercostal nerves (Fig. 547).

The deep fascia covering the deltoid invests the muscle and sends many septa be-

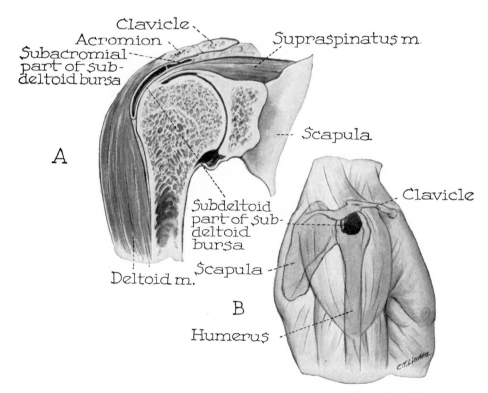

FIG. 549. The subdeltoid bursa. (A) The bursa has 2 parts: a subacromial and a subdeltoid. (B) Surface projection of the subdeltoid part of the bursa.

tween its fasciculi. In front it is continuous with the fascia covering the pectoralis major muscle, and it becomes thick posteriorly, where it is continuous with the fascia covering the infraspinatus muscle. It is continuous below with the deep fascia of the arm and is attached above to the clavicle, the acromion process and the spine of the scapula.

The deltoid muscle is large, thick and triangular and covers the shoulder joint in front, behind and laterally (Fig. 548). It has a wide V-shaped origin from the lateral third of the clavicle (anterior border), the acromion (tip and lateral border) and the crest of the spine of the scapula (lower border). The fibers converge and are inserted into a roughened area called the deltoid tuberosity, which is located about halfway down the lateral aspect of the humerus. It is the great abductor of the arm. Most au-

thorities agree that the first 15° of abduction of the arm are effected by the supraspinatus muscle, but the deltoid continues and maintains it (Fig. 548 B and C). The clavicular fibers aid in flexion and internal rotation, and the posterior fibers aid in extension and external rotation. The muscle is supplied by the axillary (circumflex) nerve from C 5 and 6.

The subdeltoid (subacromial) bursa is one large bursa with subacromial and subdeltoid subdivisions (Fig. 549). The subacromial division lies between the deep surface of the acromion above and the tendon of the supraspinatus muscle below. The subdeltoid division lies between the deltoid muscle and the upper and lateral aspect of the humerus. These two subdivisions usually communicate but occasionally are separated by a thin partition. The bursa does not nor-

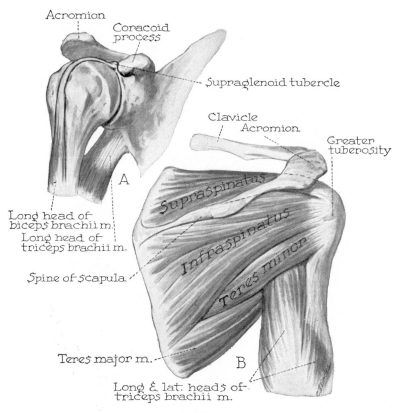

FIG. 550. The muscles of the scapular region. (A) The relations of the long head of the biceps and the long head of the triceps brachii muscles. (B) The supraspinatus, the infraspinatus and the teres minor muscle insert on the greater tuberosity.

mally communicate with the shoulder joint but may do so when the bursal floor (supraspinatus tendon) is torn.

The long head of the biceps muscle arises by a round tendon from the supraglenoid tubercle on the scapula and passes through the shoulder joint (Fig. 550). Although it is intrascapular, it remains extrasynovial, since it receives a tubular sheath from the synovial membrane. The tendon and its acquired synovial sheath pass through the intertubercular sulcus (bicipital groove) and are held in this groove by a thickened part of the capsule, which is called the transverse humeral ligament and is attached to both tubercles. Should this ligament be torn, the tendon of the biceps becomes displaced to the medial side of the lesser tubercle. The tendon strengthens the upper part of the joint and keeps the head of the humerus against the glenoid cavity.

The short head of the biceps and the coracobrachialis muscles arise together from the coracoid process of the scapula. The coracobrachialis is slender, descends along the medial margin of the biceps and is inserted into the medial part of the humerus. The short head of the biceps muscle is the medial and is discussed elsewhere (p. 655).

Scapular Region. Three muscles, the supraspinatus, the infraspinatus and the teres minor, are attached to the greater tuberosity (Fig. 550). The shoulder joint is bounded above by the supraspinatus muscle, below by the long head of the triceps brachii, behind by the tendons of the infraspinatus and the teres minor, and in front by the tendon of the subscapularis.

The supraspinatus muscle arises from the medial two thirds of the floor of the supraspinous fossa. The fibers pass laterally under the acromion and end in a short, stout tendon inserted into the top of the greater tuberosity of the humerus. The supraspinatus is covered by the trapezius, the coraco-acromial arch and the deltoid. Its tendon is closely adherent to the capsule of the shoulder joint. This muscle initiates the action of abduction, which is then continued by the deltoid (Fig. 548). In cases of injury to the suprascapular nerve, the supraspinatus and the infraspinatus muscles are paralyzed; in such cases the patient cannot initiate abduction but can

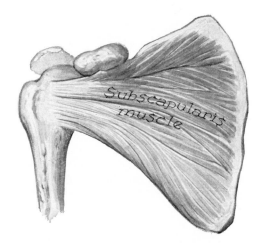

FIG. 551. The subscapularis muscle.

carry out this action if he starts it with the hand of the other arm or swings the arm away from the side of the body by a quick movement.

The infraspinatus muscle arises from the whole of the floor of the infraspinous fossa and is inserted into the greater tuberosity a little behind the supraspinatus. Its tendon is closely adherent to the capsule of the shoulder joint, and its lateral part is covered by the deltoid. At times a small bursa is found between its tendon and the capsule of the shoulder joint; if present, it may communicate with the joint. This muscle is a lateral rotator of the arm.

The teres minor muscle is small and lies along the lower border of the infraspinatus. It arises from an elongated flat impression on the dorsum of the scapula and is inserted into the back of the greater tuberosity of the humerus slightly behind the infraspinatus. As it approaches its insertion it is separated from the teres major by the long head of the triceps brachii (Fig. 550 B). It is adherent to the capsule of the shoulder joint and acts as an abductor and a lateral rotator of the arm.

The greater tuberosity of the humerus is reserved for the insertion of the three "SIT" muscles: the *Supraspinatus* on the anterior impression, the *Infraspinatus* on the middle impression and the *Teres minor* on the posterior impression. These muscles aid in lateral rotation of the arm.

The subscapularis muscle is thick and wide

and arises from the ventral surface of the scapula (Fig. 551). It does not reach the vertebral border of the scapula because this is reserved for insertion of the serratus magnus muscle. Its fleshy fibers converge on a stout tendon which is closely adherent to the capsule of the shoulder joint and is inserted into the lesser tuberosity of the humerus; this tendon is seen when the joint is opened posteriorly. As the muscle proceeds to its insertion, it passes under an arch formed by the coracoid process and the conjoined origin of the short head of the biceps and the coracobrachialis muscles. The subscapularis is an adductor and internal rotator of the arm. If it is cut vertically, it will be noted that the muscle does not arise from the part of the subscapular fossa which is near the joint; the muscle only passes over this part and is separated from it by a loose tissue which contains the subscapularis bursa. At this site the bursal wall and the joint capsule are in contact. The bursa facilitates the movement of

the subscapularis on the front of the head and the neck of the humerus. An opening between the bursa and the joint tends to weaken the capsule, and at this point the head of the humerus may burst through in dislocations.

The tendons of the supraspinatus, the infraspinatus, the teres minor and the subscapularis converge and fuse with the capsule of the shoulder joint to form a common tendon, capsule "cuff" (Figs. 552 and 553). The *subdeltoid (subacromial) bursa* lies on this "cuff" and the greater tuberosity; it is covered by the deltoid muscle, the acromion process and the coraco-acromial ligament.

THE SHOULDER JOINT

The shoulder joint is a ball-and-socket joint (enarthrodial) (Figs. 552 and 553). The ball is the head of the humerus, and the socket is the glenoid cavity of the scapula. In no other joint are the movements so free and varied. The ligaments do not maintain

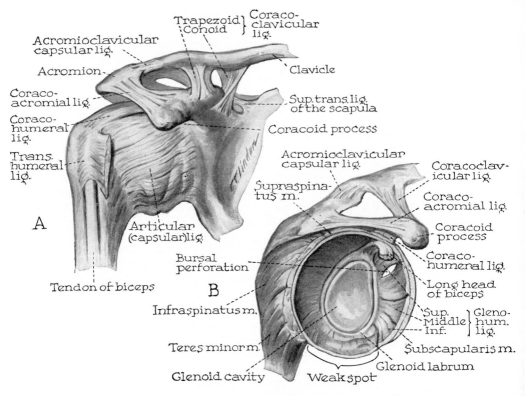

FIG. 552. Five ligaments surround the shoulder joint proper: (A) seen from in front; (B) lateral view with the humerus removed.

the joint surfaces in apposition; when only the ligaments remain, the humerus can be separated from the glenoid cavity for almost 1 inch. The joint is protected above by an arch formed by the coracoid process, the acromion and the coraco-acromial ligament; this prevents upward displacement of the joint.

The ligaments of the shoulder joint proper are five in number: (1) the articular (capsular), (2) the coracohumeral, (3) the gleno-humeral (superior, middle and inferior), (4) the transverse humeral and (5) the glenoidal labrum (Fig. 552).

The articular capsule (capsular ligament) completely encircles the shoulder joint and is attached above to the circumference of the glenoid cavity beyond the glenoid labrum; below, it is attached to the anatomic neck of the humerus. This capsule, or ligament, is so remarkably loose and lax that it has no action in keeping the bones in contact. It is strengthened above by the supraspinatus tendon, below by the long head of the triceps brachii, behind by the tendons of the infraspinatus and the teres minor, and in front by the tendon of the subscapularis. The weakest part of the capsule is its lower portion, this being partially due to the lax folds which are visible when the arm is adducted. Because of this weakness, dislocations of the head of the humerus take place through this inferior part of the capsule, downward and into the axilla. When such a dislocation occurs, the circumflex vessels and the nerves may be injured.

There are usually 3 openings in the capsule: the *first* is anterior and below the coracoid process and establishes a communication between the joint and the bursa beneath the tendon of the subscapularis (Fig. 553). When this aperture (subscapular bursa) is large, a dislocation may take place through it rather than the inferior aspect of the shoulder joint. The *second* aperture is not constant; if present, it is situated at the posterolateral part of the capsule and permits protrusion of the synovial membrane to form a bursa under cover of the infraspinatus muscle. The *third* aperture is in the groove between the tubercles of the humerus; this permits passage of the long tendon of the biceps brachii. The tendon is enclosed in a

tubular prolongation of synovial membrane which surrounds it and lines the bicipital groove (Fig. 553 B). The articular capsule cannot extend onto the lesser and the greater tuberosities because the subscapularis, the supraspinatus, the infraspinatus and the teres minor muscles insert here; however, it does extend inferiorly down to the surgical neck.

The coracohumeral ligament is a broad band which strengthens the upper part of the articular capsule. It passes from the lateral border of the coracoid process to the front of the greater tubercle of the humerus, where it blends with the tendon of the supraspinatus. The ligament is connected intimately to the capsule by its hind and lower borders; its anterior and upper borders present a free edge which overlaps the capsule.

The glenohumeral ligament consists of 3 parts (Fig. 552 B). They constitute 3 bands which are thickenings of the anterior part of the capsular ligament and have been referred to as the superior, the middle, and the inferior glenohumeral ligaments. They may be thick enough to bulge into the joint and raise ridges on the synovial membrane.

The transverse humeral ligament is a broad band which passes from the lesser to the greater tubercle of the humerus. It is limited to that portion of the bone which lies above the epiphyseal line and converts the intertubercular groove into an intertubercular canal in which the long head of the biceps brachii is located.

The glenoid labrum is a dense fibrocartilaginous lip attached to the rim of the glenoid cavity; it aids in deepening the socket. It is somewhat triangular in shape and becomes continuous above with the tendon of the long head of the biceps brachii.

The synovial membrane lines the capsular ligament and is prolonged onto the glenoid labrum and over the neck of the humerus to the articular margin. It supplies the long tendon of the biceps with a sheath which is prolonged into the bicipital groove. It becomes reflected upward and is continuous with the joint lining beneath the ligament to form bursae which have been described previously (p. 644).

Relations Around the Shoulder Joint (Fig. 553). *Anteriorly,* the subscapularis muscle and its bursa separate the axillary vessels and nerves from the joint. *Above,* the supraspinatus and the coraco-acromial ligament form an overhanging arch; the subacromial bursa is beneath this arch and the deltoid muscle. *Posteriorly,* there are the infraspinatus and the teres minor muscles. *Inferiorly,* there are the long head of the triceps, the posterior circumflex vessels and the circumflex nerve, which lie in the quadrilateral space, and that part of the subscapularis which arises alongside of the lateral margin of the scapula.

The circumflex (axillary) nerve and the posterior circumflex vessels separate the teres major and the latissimus dorsi from the inferior portion of the subscapularis muscle. Passing through the joint and over the head of the humerus is the long tendon of the biceps, which is excluded from the joint cavity proper by its synovial sheath. The deltoid overlaps the joint anteriorly, poste-

riorly, laterally and above but does not come into contact with the capsule because it is separated by the coracoid process, the coraco-acromial ligament, the subacromial bursa and the muscles which attach to the tuberosities.

Scapular Anastomoses. Around large joints throughout the body there occur free arterial anastomoses; these are situated close to the bones which take part in the articulation. The shoulder joint is no exception to this rule (Fig. 554). The anterior and the posterior *circumflex humeral arteries* form an anastomosing circle around the upper end of the humerus and a free anastomosis on both the costal and the dorsal surfaces of the scapula.

The scapular anastomosis takes place in the following way: the *suprascapular artery* (transverse scapular) is distributed to both supraspinous and infraspinous fossae, and

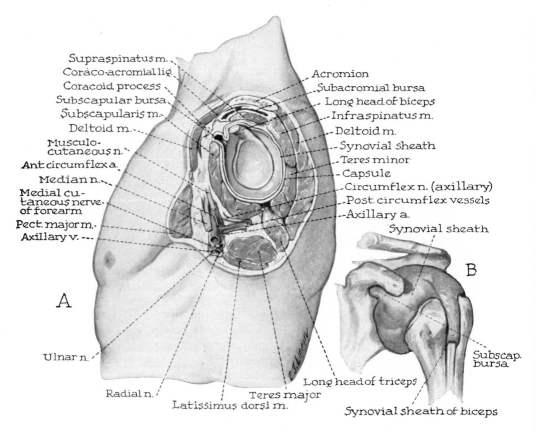

FIG. 553. Relations around the shoulder joint: (A) seen from the left side with the humerus removed; (B) the synovial sheath.

the deep branch of the *transverse cervical artery* passes downward along the medial border of the scapula. These two arteries are branches of the subclavian via the *thyrocervical trunk*.

Both the *subscapular artery,* which passes downward along the lateral border of the scapula, and the *circumflex scapular artery,* which arises from the subscapular, are distributed to the infraspinous fossa; both are derived from the third part of the axillary. Since the suprascapular and the transverse cervical arteries are derived from the first part of the subclavian, and since the subscapular and the circumflex scapular are derived from the third part of the axillary, the scapular anastomosis connects these 2 widely separated vessels. On the thoracic wall the intercostal arteries anastomose with the transverse cervical, the highest thoracic, the lateral thoracic and the scapular arteries.

Nerves and Movements. The *nerve supply* to the shoulder joint is derived from the suprascapular, the upper subscapular and the circumflex (axillary) nerves.

Since the shoulder is a ball-and-socket joint, movements in every direction are permitted. *Flexion* (forward movement) is produced by the pectoralis major, the coracobrachialis, the anterior part of the deltoid and the biceps. *Extension* (backward movement) is produced by the latissimus dorsi, the teres major and minor, the posterior part of the deltoid, the infraspinatus and the long head of the triceps. *Abduction* is brought about by the deltoid and the supraspinatus; *adduction* by the subscapularis, the pectoralis major, the teres major and minor, the latissimus dorsi, the coracobrachialis and the long head of the triceps. The force of gravity aids this latter movement. *Circumduction* (a combination of movements) is accomplished by combining the 4 preceding movements. *Medial rotation,* which is much stronger than lateral rotation because of the number of muscles brought into play, is produced by the pectoralis major, the anterior part

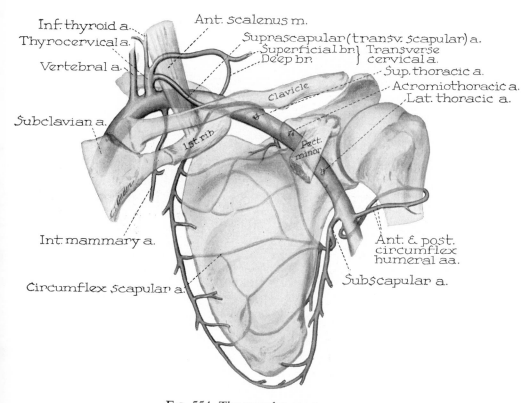

FIG. 554. The scapular anastomoses.

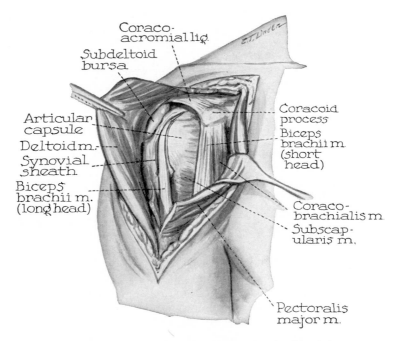

FIG. 555. The anterior approach to the shoulder joint.

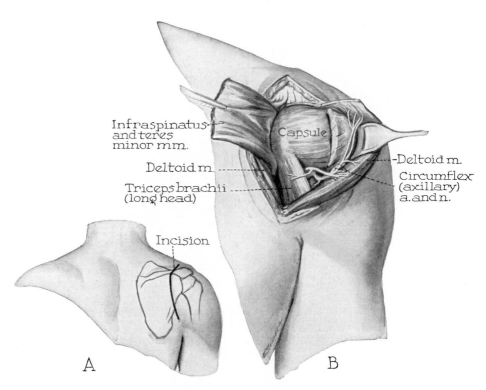

FIG. 556. The posterior approach to the shoulder joint. (A) Incision. (B) Exposure.

of the deltoid, the subscapularis, the latissimus dorsi and the teres major. The *lateral rotators* are the infraspinatus, the teres minor and the posterior part of the deltoid.

SURGICAL CONSIDERATIONS

SURGICAL APPROACH TO THE SHOULDER JOINT

Many approaches to the shoulder joint have been described, but the 3 used most frequently will be discussed here.

The anterior approach is the method described by Ollier and is the most popular of the 3 (Fig. 555). It gives access to the subdeltoid bursa and the upper part of the humerus as well as the joint. The incision is made in the deltopectoral groove, beginning at the coracoid process and extending about 5 inches down the arm. The cephalic vein is exposed and retracted in a downward direction, and the deltoid muscle is retracted laterally. The joint capsule is hidden by the muscles which attach to the tuberosities: the subscapularis to the lesser tuberosity, and the "SIT" muscles (*Supraspinatus, Infraspinatus* and *Teres minor*) to the greater tuberosity. The capsule can be exposed by detaching the muscles from their respective tuberosities or by detaching the tuberosities themselves. Through this approach the vessels and the nerves are avoided.

The posterior approach has been described by Kocher (Fig. 556). Although it is more difficult than the anterior, some authorities state that it gives better exposure of the joint. The incision is curved and commences over the acromioclavicular joint; it extends backward along the inner border of the acromion, then over the junction of the acromion with the spine of the scapula and ends about 2 inches above the posterior axillary fold.

A finger is inserted beneath the deltoid muscle, separating it from the deeper muscles. The deltoid is cut away from the spine of the scapula to the acromioclavicular joint, leaving about ¼ inch of muscle attached to the scapular spine. The cut deltoid is retracted laterally, and by gentle traction the circumflex vessels and the nerve can be exposed without injury. The infraspinatus, the teres minor, the teres major and the long and the lateral heads of the triceps are now visible, as is the upper posterior aspect of the humeral shaft. If further exposure of the posterior aspect of the shoulder capsule is desired, the supraspinatus, the infraspinatus and the teres minor are divided near their insertions and retracted medially.

The superior approach is used rarely, being reserved for cases where bony union of the humerus with the scapula is desired. Through this method the action of the deltoid muscle usually is sacrificed.

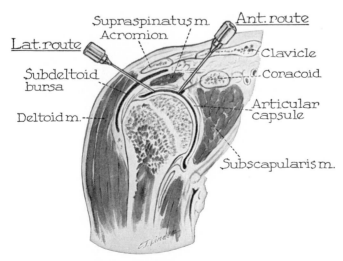

FIG. 557. Aspiration of the shoulder joint. A frontal section showing 2 routes of approach (anterior and lateral).

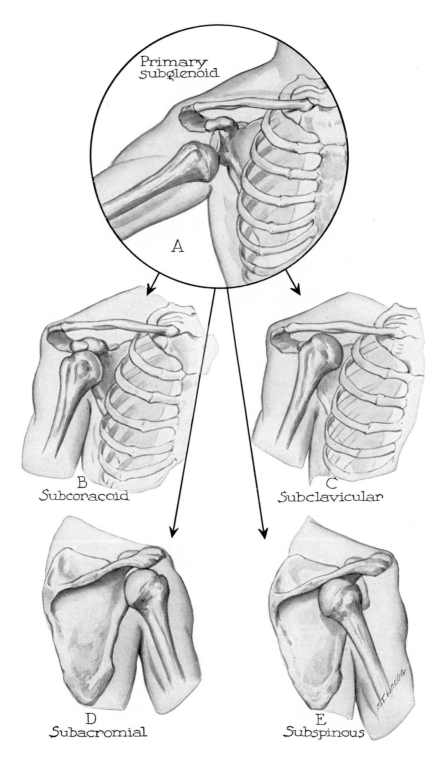

FIG. 558. Dislocations of the shoulder. Primarily, a shoulder dislocation
assumes a subglenoid position, but then it may pass anteriorly (subcoracoid
or subclavicular) or posteriorly (subacromial or subspinous).

RUPTURE OF THE SUPRASPINATUS TENDON

This usually takes place close to the greater tuberosity, and most authorities are of the opinion that it is the most common cause of traumatic subdeltoid bursitis. Codman has devised a saber-cut incision which affords the necessary exposure. It passes posteriorly from the acromioclavicular joint, over the top of the shoulder and continues through the superficial soft structures. The acromion and its attached deltoid are then retracted laterally, and the superior aspect of the shoulder joint comes to view. The tendons overlying the humeral head and the capsule can be inspected, and the extent of supraspinatus tendon injury determined. The arm is placed in abduction, and a groove is cut in the anatomic neck of the humerus in which the edge of the tendon will be placed. Drill holes are made through the lateral edge of this groove, and fascia lata or a similar type of suture laces the tendon in place.

ASPIRATION OF THE SHOULDER JOINT

It may become necessary to withdraw fluid from this joint for diagnostic or therapeutic purposes. There are 2 methods for aspirating this joint: anterior and lateral (Fig. 557).

The anterior method is accomplished by placing the needle just lateral to the tip of the coracoid process and passing it in a backward and outward direction.

The lateral method is accomplished by placing the needle just lateral to the angle formed by the junction of the spine of the scapula with the acromion. The needle is then passed inward until the joint cavity is reached. Fluid in the shoulder joint can follow the long head of the biceps and present a swelling on the anterior surface of the arm, or it can communicate with the subacromial bursa; it may escape through the weak areas of the capsule. At times, effusions in this joint pass under the deltoid muscle and appear at either the anterior or the posterior border of the muscle.

DISLOCATIONS OF THE SHOULDER

This is the most frequent of all dislocations because of the shallowness of the glenoid fossa and the disproportion between the head of the humerus and the glenoid cavity.

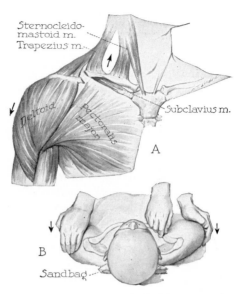

FIG. 559. Fracture of the clavicle. (A) The usual displacement. (B) Reduction in the recumbent position.

The capsule is protected by muscles in front and in back, and above by the coracoacromial arch; below, the capsule remains unprotected. The latter is the weakest part, and here the head of the humerus leaves the joint (Fig. 558). A primary subglenoid position results as the head tears through this weak point; the humeral head enters the axilla in front of the triceps. From this position it may pass either anterior or posterior and assume one of the following positions:

Anterior. If anterior, a *subcoracoid* dislocation results, and the humeral head lies below the coracoid process and the pectoralis minor muscle; three fourths of all shoulder dislocations are of this type. In *subclavicular* (anterior) dislocations, the head lies under the clavicle and the pectoralis major muscle, a rare occurrence.

Posterior. The posterior positions are: *subacromial,* where the head rests on the posterior angle of the acromion, the supraspinatus is stretched or torn, and the infraspinatus is relaxed; *subspinous,* in which the head travels from the subglenoid position in a posterior direction and comes to rest on the posterior aspect of the neck of the scapula, the subscapularis muscle usually being torn.

Luxatio erecta is a rare form of dislocation in which the head of the humerus remains below the glenoid cavity, with the arm pointing in an upward direction along the side of the head. As the head continues to pass downward, it comes to lie on the serratus anterior muscle.

Many methods and modifications for the treatment of dislocations of the shoulder have been described. One of the oldest and most widely used is Kocher's method. It is accomplished by 3 movements: the wrist is moved outward until the arm assumes a position of external rotation; external rotation and flexion at the elbow are maintained by moving the elbow forward and inward until the arm is nearly horizontal; the arm is rotated inward, and the hand is brought to the opposite shoulder. By external rotation, the first movement, tension is relieved on the posterior scapular muscles, and the rent in the capsule is widened; in the second movement, relaxation of the tense but untorn portion of the capsule is obtained, and the head of the humerus is permitted to enter the socket; in the third movement, the head of the humerus is brought into contact with the glenoid fossa.

Recurrent (Habitual) Dislocation of the Shoulder Joint. Following a traumatic dislocation, a weak point is left; this might result in recurrent dislocation from trivial trauma. Other authorities are of the opinion that structural weaknesses besides those in the inferior aspect of the capsule are the cause, and that all shoulder dislocations, therefore, do not start originally as a subglenoid variety.

NICOLA OPERATION

An incision is made from the clavicle, above the coracoid, through the anterior border of the deltoid. The long head of the biceps is freed by dividing the transverse humeral ligament, below which the biceps is divided; the upper end is brought through a hole in the head of the humerus. This is united with the lower end. The capsule and other structures are repaired as the last stage of the operation.

FRACTURED CLAVICLE

The clavicle is fractured more frequently than any other bone in the body. The usual location of such a fracture is at the junction of the middle and outer thirds of the bone (Fig. 559). The medial fragment is tilted upward by the contractions of the sternocleidomastoid and the trapezius muscles, and the lateral fragment is displaced downward by the contractions of the pectoralis, the teres major and the weight of the arm.

Treatment of a fractured clavicle may be bothersome because direct splinting of the bone is difficult. All methods of closed reduction aim at pushing the shoulder backward until the 2 fragments are placed in apposition (Fig. 559 B). The recumbent position aids such reduction because the muscles are relaxed, and the displacement due to the weight of the arm is relieved.

Arm (Brachial Region)

SURFACE ANATOMY

The arm in the adult appears to be flattened from side to side because of grouping of the anterior and the posterior arm muscles (Fig. 560). The fullness anteriorly is produced by the fleshy belly of the biceps brachii; this is lost under the deltoid muscle. Over the posterior aspect of the arm the fullness is produced by the triceps brachii muscle; this fades into a flattened distal appearance, produced by the triceps tendon.

The medial bicipital sulcus (groove) commences in front of the posterior axillary fold and descends along the inner aspect of the arm to its lower third, where it bends obliquely forward to the center of the elbow. It separates the biceps and the coracobrachialis muscles in front from the triceps behind. The groove indicates the course of the brachial vessels, the median nerve and the basilic vein.

The lateral bicipital sulcus (groove) does not stand out as well as the medial. It commences at the middle of the arm near the insertion of the deltoid muscle and ends at the bend of the elbow. In its lower part it separates the biceps muscle from the brachioradialis and the radial extensor muscles; the cephalic vein ascends in this sulcus.

The cutaneous nerve supply is depicted in Figure 561.

FASCIA

The arm, or brachium, is completely invested by a deep fascia called the *brachial aponeurosis*. This is a sleeve of tough fascia which is continuous with that of the forearm (Fig. 562). It is fixed at each side of the arm by the intermuscular septa, which are attached along the outer and the inner margins of the humerus. The lateral intermuscular septum extends from the lateral epicondyle to the deltoid tubercle; the medial extends from the medial epicondyle to the insertion of the coracobrachialis muscle (in the middle of the shaft of the humerus). This fascial arrangement divides the arm into anterior and posterior compartments, which also serve to limit inflammatory exudates and hemorrhagic effusions. However, it is possible for such fluids to pass from one compartment into another by following those structures which pierce the intermuscular septa.

MUSCLES

ANTERIOR COMPARTMENT

In the anterior (flexor) compartment 3 muscles are found: the biceps, the coracobrachialis and the brachialis (Fig. 563).

The biceps muscle (biceps brachii) arises by 2 tendinous heads: the long and the short.

The long head is lateral and arises from the supraglenoid tubercle on the scapula. Its tendon passes through the cavity of the shoulder joint ensheathed by synovial membrane; it emerges from under the transverse ligament and occupies the bicipital groove.

In the middle of the arm, the long head joins the belly of the *short head,* which arises from the tip of the coracoid process. This head shares its origin on the coracoid process with the coracobrachialis muscle. The tendon of the biceps is inserted into the posterior part of the radial tuberosity. The bicipital aponeurosis (lacertus fibrosis) has been discussed elsewhere (p. 676).

Since this 2-headed muscle crosses 2 joints, the shoulder and the elbow, it acts on both; at the shoulder joint its action holds the head of the humerus firmly in contact with the glenoid cavity, and at the elbow it is the strongest supinator of the forearm when the elbow is flexed. Since it is a flexor and a supi-

nator, it may be stated that the biceps is the muscle that "puts a corkscrew in and pulls the cork out."

The coracobrachialis muscle runs parallel

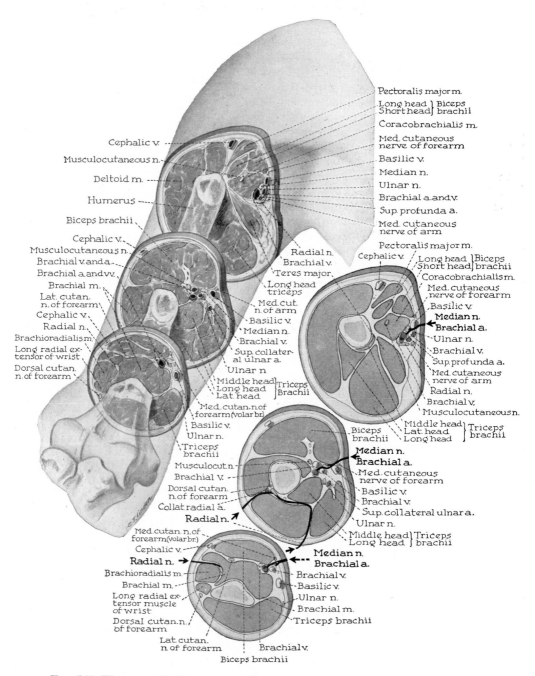

FIG. 560. The arm. Multiple cross sections are shown, and to the side of these the surgical approaches to the neurovascular structures are indicated by arrows.

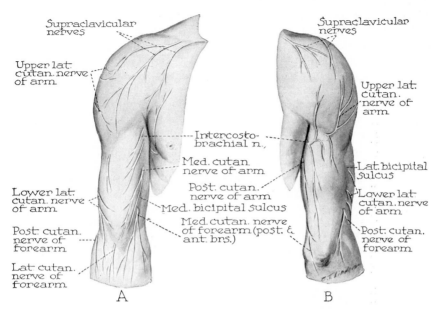

FIG. 561. Surface anatomy and cutaneous nerve supply of the arm:
(A) the anterior aspect; (B) the posterior aspect.

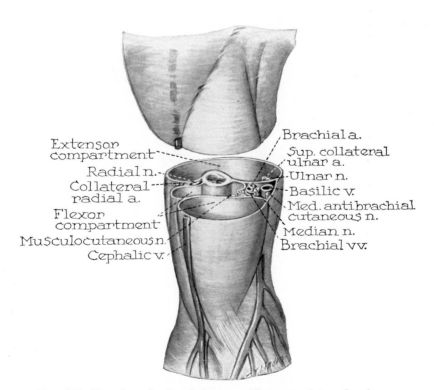

FIG. 562. The deep fascia of the arm. The musculature has been removed. This fascia is known as the brachial aponeurosis; it divides the
arm into the anterior (flexor) and the posterior (extensor) compartments.

with and medial to the short head of the biceps. As its name suggests, it originates from the coracoid process and inserts at about the middle of the medial side of the humerus. It aids in flexion and adduction of the arm.

The brachialis muscle has its origin by means of 2 limbs which pass to either side of the deltoid tuberosity. The posterior limb passes up into the spiral groove; the anterior extends upward between the insertions of the deltoid and the coracobrachialis. The muscle crosses in front of the elbow joint and inserts into the anterior aspect of the coronoid process of the ulna. It is the most powerful flexor of the elbow joint.

POSTERIOR COMPARTMENT

The triceps muscle fills the posterior (extensor) compartment of the arm. As its name implies, it has 3 heads: lateral, medial and long (Fig. 564).

The lateral head arises from the posterior surface of the humerus, proximal to the radial groove, and from the lateral intermuscular septum. This head is covered at its upper and by the posterior fibers of the deltoid muscle, but the remainder is superficial. This head converts the spiral groove into a tunnel.

The medial head arises from the posterior surface of the shaft of the humerus, distal to the radial groove, and from the median intermuscular septum. It is covered by the other 2 heads, except for its lower fibers which become superficial.

The long head is tendinous and arises from a tubercle situated below the glenoid cavity (infraglenoid tubercle). This head is

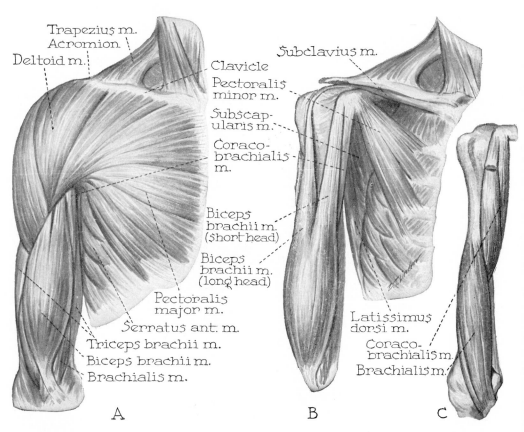

FIG. 563. The muscles of the flexor compartment of the arm: (A) seen from in front with the intact deltoid; (B) the deltoid has been removed; (C) the deep musculature.

superficial throughout and passes between the teres major and the teres minor muscles to form the triangular and the quadrangular spaces. The fibers of the triceps muscle are inserted by a common tendon into the proximal surface of the olecranon. It is separated from the posterior ligament of the elbow joint by a small bursa. This muscle is the powerful extensor of the forearm.

Quadrangular Space. This space does not actually exist, but its boundaries must be artificially separated before it can be visualized. As seen from behind, it is bounded by the teres minor muscle above, the teres major below, the long head of the triceps medially and the surgical neck of the humerus laterally (Fig. 565). The boundaries of the space as seen from in front are the same with the

exception of the teres minor, which is replaced by the subscapularis as the upper boundary. The circumflex (axillary) nerve and the posterior circumflex humeral vessels pass backward through the space immediately below the capsule.

Triangular Space. This space is formed by the teres minor above and the teres major below; the long head of the triceps forms its base (Fig. 565). Although of little importance, the space acts as a landmark for the circumflex scapular vessels which pass through it.

NERVES

The circumflex (axillary) nerve supplies an articular twig to the capsule of the shoulder joint, muscular branches to the deltoid

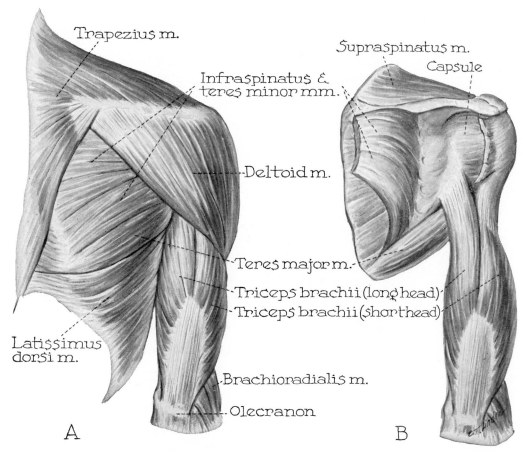

FIG. 564. The triceps muscle: (A) superficial view; (B) deep view.

and the teres minor, and cutaneous branches to the skin over the lower half of the deltoid (Fig. 565). It arises from the posterior cord of the brachial plexus and descends between the axillary artery and the subscapularis muscle (Fig. 540). It winds around the lower border of the subscapularis muscle, passes backward with the posterior humeral circumflex vessels through the quadrangular space and divides into anterior and posterior branches. The articular twig originates from the trunk of the nerve in the quadrangular space and enters the joint from below. The posterior branch supplies the nerve to the teres minor, curves around the posterior border of the deltoid and supplies this muscle; it continues as the *lateral cutaneous nerve* of the arm. The anterior branch of the nerve continues around the humerus with the posterior circumflex artery and ends near

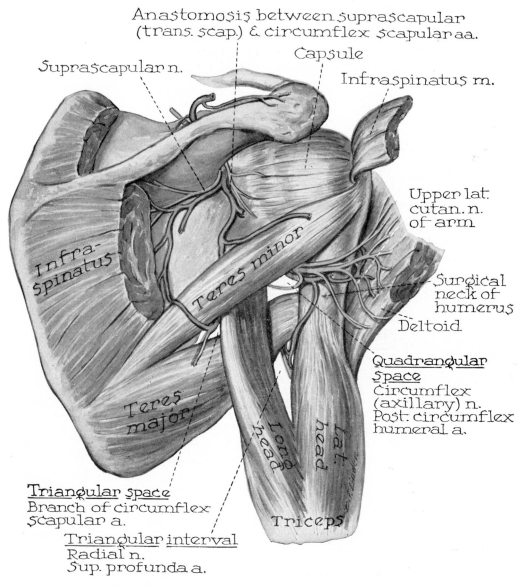

FIG. 565. The quadrangular and the triangular spaces.

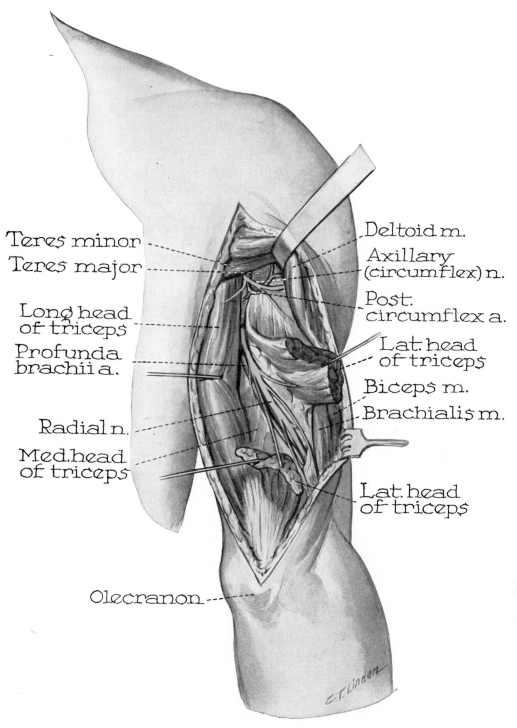

Teres minor

Teres major

Long head
of triceps

Profunda
brachii a.

Radial n.

Med. head
of triceps

Olecranon

Deltoid m.

Axillary
(circumflex) n.

Post.
circumflex a.

Lat. head
of triceps

Biceps m.

Brachialis m.

Lat. head
of triceps

FIG. 566. The radial nerve.

the anterior border of the deltoid, supplying this muscle (Fig. 565). It also distributes a few fine twigs to the skin.

The radial (musculospiral) nerve travels through the posterior compartment of the arm, the "tunnel," and the anterior compartment (Figs. 560 and 566). The course of the nerve is more vertical than spiral, being spiral in only a small portion of its middle third; in its upper and lower thirds it is almost perpendicular. In the *posterior compartment* of the arm the nerve appears as a continuation of the posterior cord of the brachial plexus. It lies on the long head of the triceps and appears below the lower border of the teres major muscle with the profunda brachii artery which accompanies it. It then enters the fascial plane between the long and the lateral heads of the triceps. The so-called "tunnel" is the musculospiral groove; its roof is the lateral head of the triceps, and its floor is the humerus proper. The radial nerve in this part of its course is in contact with the humerus. In its almost vertical descent through the "tunnel," it separates the lateral from the medial head of the triceps and supplies both. The nerve gains access to the *anterior compartment* by piercing the lateral intermuscular septum at the junction of the lower and the middle thirds of the humerus. It then passes vertically between the supinator longus (brachioradialis) and the brachialis, where it descends vertically (Fig. 566). In the region of the lateral epicondyle it divides into its 2 terminal branches: the posterior interosseous and the radial nerves.

SURGICAL CONSIDERATIONS OF THE RADIAL NERVE

For exposure of the nerve in the *posterior compartment,* an incision is made 3 cm. below the acromion and is continued for 5 cm. past the middle of the humerus; this is in a line with the olecranon. The incision is carried through the deep fascia. At its upper end 3 muscular structures may be identified: the posterior border of the deltoid muscle, and the long and the lateral heads of the triceps. The deltoid muscle is retracted laterally, and the 2 heads of the triceps are separated in their fascial planes. It may be necessary to

incise a small part of the deltoid for more adequate exposure. After separating the 2 heads of the triceps, a glistening aponeurosis (the teres major muscle) is exposed. Distal to this an incision is made in a loose areolar sheath which reveals the nerve and its accompanying vessels.

For exposure of the nerve in its course through the "tunnel," an incision is made extending from a point 3 cm. above the level of the insertion of the deltoid directly downward for 12 cm. This incision is carried through the triceps, separating the fibers longitudinally until the aponeurosis on its deep surface is seen. This aponeurosis is incised, and the nerve is exposed beneath it.

The exposure of the radial nerve in the *anterior (flexor) compartment* is shown in Figure 562 (p. 657).

ARTERIES AND VEINS

The posterior circumflex humeral artery arises from the axillary artery a short distance below the subscapular, passing backward through the quadrangular space with the circumflex nerve (Fig. 565). Winding around the surgical neck of the humerus, it is distributed to the deep surface of the deltoid muscle. Some of its terminal branches are distributed to the surrounding muscles, the shoulder joint and the skin.

The anterior circumflex humeral artery is smaller than the posterior circumflex humeral artery. It passes anteriorly around the surgical neck of the humerus and makes an arterial circle by joining the posterior humeral circumflex.

The brachial artery is subject to striking variations as are other vessels in the body, particularly the arteries affecting the extremities. I must repeat that the description given herein is the most common and the most accepted pattern of the vessel under discussion. The brachial artery is considered to be a direct continuation of the axillary artery. It commences at the lower border of the teres major muscle and terminates about 1 inch below the transverse skin crease of the elbow, where it divides into 2 branches: a larger ulnar and a smaller radial.

The pulsations of the artery can be felt along the medial bicipital groove throughout the length of the arm until the vessel disappears behind the lacertus fibrosus.

The brachial artery lies successively on *3 muscles, gives 3 main branches,* is in contact with *3 important nerves* and is associated with *3 veins* (Fig. 567).

The 3 muscles which constitute the floor upon which the brachial artery runs are (from above downward): the long head of the triceps, the coracobrachialis and the brachialis. To cross the muscles in the above order, the vessel must pass downward and laterally; this it does, its course corresponding to the inner border of the biceps muscle.

The 3 main branches of the brachial artery are the profunda brachii, the superior ulnar collateral and the inferior ulnar collateral.

The profunda brachii is a large vessel arising from the upper part of the brachial artery, sometimes as high as the teres major muscle. It passes downward, backward and outward between the long and the medial heads of the triceps muscle; it is the companion vessel of the radial nerve (Fig. 566). An important ascending branch arises from the upper part of the vessel and anastomoses with the posterior humeral circumflex artery, thus connecting the axillary and the brachial vessels. Having traversed the musculospiral groove, the profunda brachii reaches the lateral intermuscular septum and divides into anterior and posterior branches. The anterior branch follows the radial nerve through the intermuscular septum, passes in front of the lateral epicondyles and anastomoses with the radial recurrent artery. The posterior branch continues downward behind the intermuscular septum, in back of the lateral epicondyle and anastomoses with the posterior interosseous recurrent artery. In this way a complete arterial circle is formed around the lateral epicondyle (Fig. 578).

The superior ulnar collateral artery has also been called the inferior profunda artery. It arises near the middle of the arm and is the companion vessel of the ulnar nerve (Fig. 567). It pierces the medial intermuscular septum, enters the posterior compartment and passes behind the medial epicondyle. It anastomoses with the posterior ulnar recurrent artery.

The inferior ulnar collateral artery has been called the anastomotica magna. It arises about 2 inches above the termination of the brachial artery and passes inward behind the median nerve. It passes in front of the medial epicondyle, anastomoses with the anterior ulnar recurrent artery and forms an arterial circle around the medial epicondyle. These 2 arterial circles of the epicondyles in turn are connected by a branch of the inferior ulnar collateral artery which passes transversely across the back of the humerus; hence its name "anastomotica magna." In this way the rich anastomoses are formed around the elbow joint (Fig. 578).

The 3 important nerves which are associated with the brachial artery are the radial, the ulnar and the median (Fig. 567). The medial cutaneous nerve of the forearm lies to the medial side of the artery and, although not as important as the other 3, it still may cause annoying cutaneous manifestations if involved or injured.

The radial nerve is associated with the artery only in its upper part immediately below the lower border of the teres major muscle. Here it lies behind the artery, separating it from the long head of the triceps muscle.

The median nerve is related closely to the brachial artery throughout its entire course. In the upper arm it lies lateral to the vessel but, as it descends, it crosses in front of the artery in the region of the midarm. At times the nerve crosses behind the vessel. As it continues downward, it comes to lie on the medial side of the artery in the lower arm and elbow region.

The ulnar nerve passes downward on the medial side of the brachial artery, lying between it and the basilic vein. In the middle of the arm the nerve pierces the medial intermuscular septum and leaves the vessel. It should be noted that the median and the ulnar nerves make a "nonstop trip" through the arm, giving off no branches.

The 3 veins which are associated with the brachial artery are its *2 vena comites* (brachial veins) and the *basilic.* The basilic vein ascends in the groove on the medial side of the biceps muscle superficial to the deep fascia and medial to the artery. Halfway up the arm the basilic vein pierces the

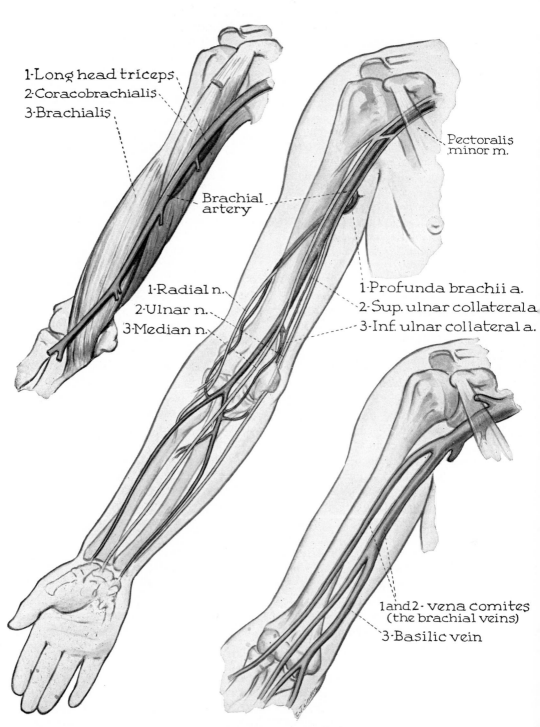

1·Long head triceps
2·Coracobrachialis
3·Brachialis

Pectoralis minor m.

Brachial artery

1·Radial n.
2·Ulnar n.
3·Median n.

1·Profunda brachii a.
2·Sup. ulnar collateral a.
3·Inf. ulnar collateral a.

1and2· vena comites
(the brachial veins)
3·Basilic vein

FIG. 567. The brachial artery lies successively on 3 muscles, gives 3 main branches, is in contact with 3 important nerves and is associated with 3 veins.

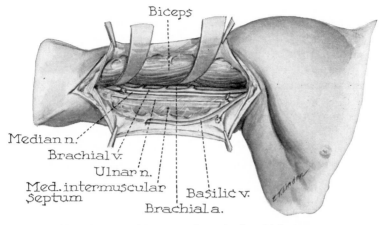

Fig. 568. Medial approach to the brachial artery.

deep fascia and becomes more intimately related to the brachial artery. At a variable point, it joins the 2 brachial veins to form the axillary. The brachial veins pass one on each side of the brachial artery and make many venous contacts around the artery as they ascend.

Relationships Around the Brachial Artery. These relationships are best described in thirds (Fig. 560).

In the *proximal third,* the brachial artery lies medial to the humerus and can be compressed laterally against this bone. It is overlapped laterally by the coracobrachialis muscle, from which it is separated by the median nerve. Both the medial cutaneous nerve of the forearm and the ulnar nerve lie to its medial side and separate it from the basilic vein. Posterior to the artery is the radial nerve, which separates the vessel from the long head of the triceps muscle.

The *middle third* of the artery may be compressed backward and laterally against the bone. The vessel is overlapped by the medial border of the biceps muscle and is crossed from lateral to medial by the median nerve. The ulnar nerve is medial, but about the middle of the arm it passes posteriorly to reach the posterior compartment of the arm. Posteriorly, the artery lies on the brachialis and the insertion of the coracobrachialis muscles. The basilic vein and the medial cutaneous nerve of the forearm are separated from the vessel by the deep fascia.

In the *distal third,* the brachial artery lies

in front of the humerus and can be compressed backward against it. The biceps tendon overlaps it. The median nerve is medial to it; the ulnar nerve has passed into the posterior compartment.

SURGICAL CONSIDERATIONS OF THE BRACHIAL ARTERY

The bifurcation of the brachial artery is not constant and may take place at a high level in the arm. Such a bifurcation may be troublesome as well as embarrassing when attempting to ligate the vessel for hemorrhage distal to the bifurcation.

Ligation. The usual indications for ligation of the brachial artery are wounds, secondary hemorrhage, and hemorrhage from the deep palmar arch. Ligation may be done either at the middle of the arm or at the bend of the elbow.

Ligation at the middle of the arm is accomplished in the following way (Fig. 568). The arm is placed in abduction, and the hand in supination. If the arm is allowed to lie on a flat surface, the triceps muscle may be pushed upward and be mistaken for the biceps. Dissection through this distorted area exposes the superior ulnar collateral artery and the ulnar nerve instead of the brachial artery and the median nerve. The incision is made in the line of the artery along the medial edge of the biceps muscle. The basilic vein and the medial cutaneous nerve of the forearm may be identified superficial to the deep fascia at this level. If seen, they are drawn to one side. The deep fascia is incised, and the inner fibers of the biceps muscle are identified and retracted upward. The artery is found lying on the triceps muscle, with the median nerve in front of it. The nerve is isolated and protected. The brachial artery with its 2 venae comites are exposed; the artery is isolated from its companion veins and ligated.

The *collateral circulation* differs when the brachial artery is ligated above or below the profunda brachii (Fig. 566). If ligated *above*

the profunda brachii, the circumflex humeral vessels above anastomose with the profunda brachii below. If ligated *below* the profunda brachii, the profunda brachii above anastomoses with the vessels around the elbow joint below.

HUMERUS

The humerus is a long cylindrical bone which articulates with the scapula above and with the radius and the ulna below (Fig. 569).

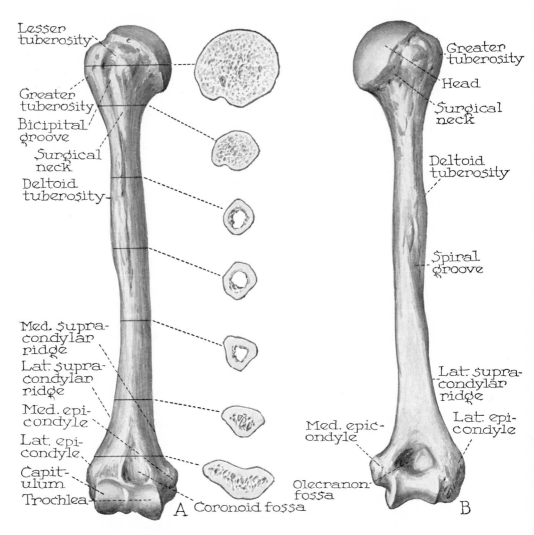

FIG. 569. The right humerus. (A) Seen from in front. The different shapes of the humerus are depicted in cross section taken at the various identified levels. (B) The posterior view.

The head of the humerus forms a third of a sphere. It is covered with cartilage which is thickest in its central part and thins toward the circumference. The head is directed medially, upward and a little backward.

The anatomic neck is a constriction which surrounds the articular cartilage and gives attachment to the capsular ligament.

Tuberosities. Projecting forward and laterally from the humeral head is a mass of bone which is divided into two unequal parts called the lesser and the greater tuberosities. The groove dividing this bony mass is the bicipital (intertubercular) sulcus; it lodges the long tendon of the biceps. To these two tuberosities attach the tendons of the muscles which hold the head of the humerus in its socket.

The greater tuberosity is the more lateral of the two and has been called the "point of the shoulder." Although it is covered by the deltoid, it can be felt on deep pressure. It has depressions for insertion of the three "SIT" muscles (*Supraspinatus, Infraspinatus* and *Teres minor*) (p. 645). The tuberosity gradually fades and becomes continuous with the shaft of the humerus.

The lesser tuberosity is located on the front of the shaft and immediately below the anatomic neck. It is also covered by the deltoid and can be felt on deep pressure, especially during rotation of the bone. It provides attachment for the subscapularis muscle.

The surgical neck of the humerus is a fingerbreadth below the tuberosities. A region of surgical importance, it is a narrow zone encircled by the circumflex vessels and partially encircled by the circumflex (axillary) nerve. This neurovascular bundle hugs the bone and does not pierce the 4 muscles inserted into the greater and the lesser tuberosities or the 3 muscles (pectoralis major, teres major and latissimus dorsi) which insert into the medial and the lateral lips of the bicipital groove. These lips descend from the tuberosities and deepen the bicipital sulcus.

Epiphyseal Line. The surgical and the anatomic necks meet medially in the region of the quadrangular space (p. 660). Slightly above the level of the surgical neck is the epiphyseal line, which coincides with the lower margin of the humeral head on the medial side, but passes through the lowest part of the greater tuberosity on the lateral side.

The deltoid tuberosity is a roughened inverted "delta" with its apex downward. It is located about halfway down the shaft of the bone over its lateral aspect. The shallow spiral (radial) groove lies immediately behind this tuberosity and contains the radial nerve and the profunda artery.

The body or shaft of the humerus is almost cylindrical in its upper half and prismatic and flattened in its lower half. The humeral body has 3 borders: anterior, lateral and medial.

The anterior border extends from the front of the greater tuberosity to the coronoid fossa, its proximal part forming the lateral lip of the bicipital groove and its middle part the anterior margin of the deltoid tuberosity.

The lateral border extends from the back of the greater tuberosity to the lateral epicondyle. It is indistinct proximally where the lateral head of the triceps arises and it is interrupted in its midportion by the oblique groove for the radial nerve. Its distal part is the prominent lateral supracondylar ridge.

The medial border extends from the lesser tuberosity to the medial epicondyle and forms the medial lip of the bicipital groove. It is roughened in the middle for the insertion of the coracobrachialis, and its distal part becomes the medial supracondylar ridge.

The body of the humerus has three surfaces: anteromedial, anterolateral and posterior.

The anteromedial surface is situated between the anterior and the medial margins; the bicipital groove forms its proximal part.

The anterolateral surface is located between the anterior and the lateral margins, with the deltoid tuberosity slightly above its midportion.

The posterior surface, situated between the medial and the lateral margins, is occupied by the origin of the medial head of the triceps. The spiral groove begins on the posterior surface, running obliquely downward between the origins of the medial and the lateral heads of the triceps and ending below the deltoid tuberosity. The radial nerve and

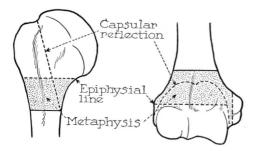

FIG. 570. Capsular reflections, epiphyses and metaphyses of the upper and the lower ends of the humerus.

its accompanying profunda vessels lie in this groove. A nutrient foramen is situated near the middle of the medial border and another is found frequently in the spiral groove.

The lower end of the humerus is divided into 2 areas: the *capitellum*, which receives the head of the radius, and the *trochlea* for the trochlear (semilunar) notch of the ulna. The capitellum is sphere-shaped, and the trochlea is spool-shaped.

The radial fossa is located immediately above the capitellum and receives the head of the radius during full flexion.

The coronoid fossa, situated immediately above the trochlea, receives the coronoid process of the ulna during flexion.

The olecranon fossa, the largest of the three fossae, is also situated above the trochlea; posteriorly, it receives the olecranon during extension.

The lateral epicondyle is placed immediately above and lateral to the capitellum; its posterior aspect is broad, smooth and easily felt subcutaneously.

The medial condyle is large and is felt easily medial to and above the trochlea; its posterior aspect presents a groove in which the ulnar nerve can be felt and rolled about.

The metaphysis represents the line of junction between the epiphysis and the diaphysis of a long bone; frequently it is the site of bone disease in the young. If part of the metaphysis is inside of the joint capsule, the disease is likely to involve the joint; conversely, joint disease may involve the shaft of the bone if the metaphysis is partly within the affected joint. Therefore, the relationship between epiphyseal lines and capsular reflections becomes clinically important. At the upper end

of the humerus, the epiphyseal line passes around the bone at the level of the lowest part of the articular surface of the head (Fig. 570). The capsule is attached to the anatomic neck above, but below it is attached to the shaft about 1 inch lower than the lowest part of the articular surface of the head. This arrangement places the metaphysis partly intracapsular. At the lower end of the bone, the epiphyseal line is represented by a horizontal line at the level of the lateral epicondyle, the medial epicondyle having a separate epiphysis. The capsule follows the coronoid and the radial fossae anteriorly, and the distal half of the olecranon fossa posteriorly. Medially and laterally, it attaches about ¼ inch from the articular margins. Therefore, the metaphysis is partly intracapsular.

Attachments to the Humerus. The following are the attachments to the humerus (Figs. 545 and 546):

To the greater tuberosity—the "SIT" muscles (*Supraspinatus, Infraspinatus* and *Teres minor*).

To the lesser tuberosity—the teres major and the subscapularis, both extending to the surgical neck.

To the anatomic neck—above and about ½ inch from it below and medially, the capsular ligament of the shoulder; the coracohumeral ligament extends onto the anterior part of the greater tuberosity.

To the bicipital groove—the transverse ligament, attached to both tuberosities, bridges across its proximal part; the pectoralis major to its lateral lip; the teres major to its medial lip; and the latissimus dorsi to the floor.

To the lateral epicondyle—the common extensor tendon, the lateral ligament of the elbow, the supinator and the anconeus.

To the medial epicondyle—the medial ligament, the common flexor tendon and the pronator teres.

To the medial margin of the shaft—the coracobrachialis.

To the lateral margin of the shaft—the lateral head of the triceps.

To the medial supracondylar ridge—the medial intermuscular septum and the pronator teres.

To the lateral supracondylar ridge—the lateral intermuscular septum, the brachio-

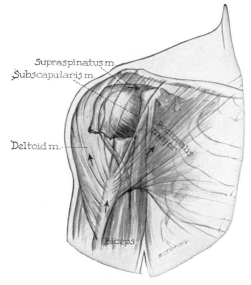

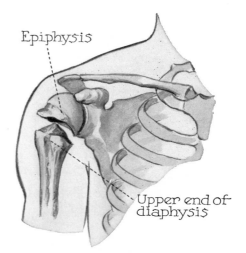

Fig. 572. Separation of the upper humeral epiphysis.

Fig. 571. Fracture of the surgical neck of the humerus. The arrows indicate the pull of the muscles which produces the deformity.

radialis and the extensor carpi radialis longus.

To the deltoid tuberosity—the deltoid muscle.

From the anteromedial and the anterolateral surfaces—the brachialis.

From the posterior surface—the medial head of the triceps.

To the radial and the coronoid fossae—the anterior ligament of the elbow; the posterior ligament attaches to the margins of the olecranon fossa on either side and to the back of the epicondyles.

SURGICAL CONSIDERATIONS

FRACTURES

Fractures of the humerus may occur at the upper end, at the shaft and at the lower end.

Fracture of the anatomic neck is intracapsular, rare and occurs mainly in older people. At times the shaft may be driven into the head of the bone, producing marked impaction. It may become necessary to treat the condition surgically, so that function is improved; or it may be necessary to remove a loose fragment.

Fractures of the surgical neck are extracapsular and usually result from direct violence; they occur mainly in young or middle-aged adults (Fig. 571). The deformity, although it may vary depending upon the relationship of the site of fracture to the insertion of muscles, remains fairly constant. The upper end of the lower fragment is carried upward toward the axilla by the pull of the deltoid, the biceps, the coracobrachialis and the triceps muscles. It is drawn medially by the pectoralis major, the teres major and the latissimus dorsi. The upper fragment is abducted by the supraspinatus. In reducing the fracture, abduction of the arm should not be performed too forcefully or too rapidly because the pectoralis major acts as a fulcrum, and the upper end of the sharp lower fragment may injure the brachial plexus. Therefore, bringing the arm forward and making traction outward and forward will release the tension of the pectoralis major and allow the lower fragment to be brought into apposition. After complete reduction, the position should be maintained in abduction, usually by means of axial traction.

Fracture of the greater tubercle can result from either direct violence or muscle pull from the attached supraspinatus, the infraspinatus and the teres minor. This type of fracture may accompany a fractured neck of the humerus or an anterior dislocation. The supraspinatus usually pulls the tuberosity upward and backward. The arm should be fixed in abduction and external rotation; if this fails, surgical correction becomes necessary.

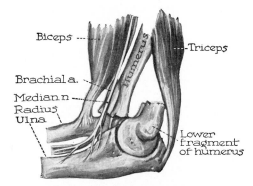

FIG. 574. Supracondylar fracture of the humerus. The close relations of the median nerve and the brachial artery to the sharp fractured fragments are shown.

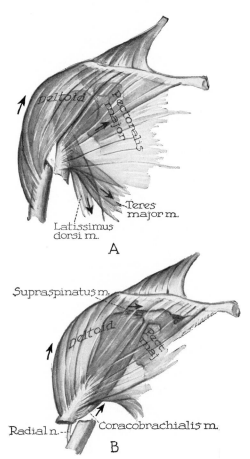

FIG. 573. Fractures of the shaft of the humerus: (A) above the insertion of the deltoid muscle; (B) below the insertion of the deltoid muscle.

Separation of the upper humeral epiphysis occurs up to the 20th year and usually is the result of the same type of injury as causes fractures of the surgical neck. Due to action of the supraspinatus, the infraspinatus and the teres minor, the upper fragment usually is abducted. Since the upper end of the diaphysis is conical, the epiphysis fits into this by a corresponding concavity (Fig. 572). This results in a cup and cone arrangement which makes reduction difficult but immobilization easy. As the child grows older, the concavity of the epiphysis gradually becomes flattened so that this is altered. Reduction and immobilization in abduction are required.

Fractures of the lesser tubercle are rare. The deformity is produced by the subscapularis, which pulls the fragments medially.

Shaft fractures may occur in the upper third of the humerus above the deltoid attachment or, more commonly, in the middle of the shaft below the deltoid attachment; hence, the displacement and the deformity vary with the site of the fracture (Fig. 573). If the fracture is situated above the insertion of the deltoid, the upper fragment is drawn medially by the muscles attached to the bicipital groove (pectoralis major, teres major and latissimus dorsi), and the lower fragment is drawn upward and laterally by the deltoid (Fig. 573 A). If the fracture is below the insertion of the deltoid, the upper fragment is pulled laterally by the deltoid and the supraspinatus, and the lower fragment is displaced medially and upward (Fig. 573 B). The relationship of the radial nerve to this fracture is important. At about the middle of the humerus and below the attachment of the deltoid muscle this nerve lies in direct contact with the bone, and a sharp bony fragment may injure it. The sensory branches of the radial nerve leave at a higher level than this site of injury; therefore, the nerve symptoms are entirely motor and will be manifested by a wrist drop. For proper reduction, normal relations between the external epicondyle and the greater tubercle should be maintained.

Supracondylar (lower end) fractures occur frequently in children and at that point where the bone is thin (the anteroposterior diameter immediately above the condyle). The lower fragment is displaced upward and

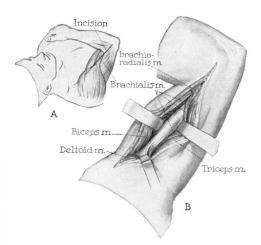

FIG. 575. Exposure of the shaft of the humerus: (A) incision and position of the arm; (B) the relations of the exposed bone to the surrounding musculature.

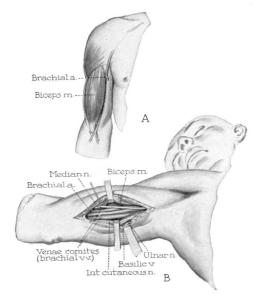

FIG. 576. Exposure of the neurovascular structures of the arm.

backward and may simulate a dislocation (Fig. 574). However, the internal condyle, the olecranon and the external condyle remain in normal relations, which would not be true in posterior dislocation of the elbow. The median nerve and vessels in the cubital fossa may be injured, and the possibility of Volkmann's ischemic contracture must be kept in mind. The importance of incising the brachial fascia, following reduction and immobilization, has been stressed (Fig. 562).

Intercondylar fractures are supracondylar and extend into the joint between the condyles, forming a T- or Y-shaped fracture. They are difficult to reduce and maintain in position.

Fractures of the epicondyle may be caused by powerful abduction and extension of the elbow or by muscular action. Involvement of the ulnar nerve must be kept in mind when the medial epicondyle is fractured. The lateral epicondyle usually is fractured by a fall on the hand; this may involve the capitulum and the trochlear surface.

Lower epiphyseal separation is usually seen in children between the ages of 5 to 10 years. The displacement is lateral and backward.

OPERATIONS ON THE SHAFT OF THE HUMERUS

Exposure of the humeral shaft is difficult because this bone is not subcutaneous anywhere, and important vessels and nerves are closely related to it. The best approach is a lateral one (Fig. 575). The lower two thirds of the shaft of the humerus is exposed through a skin incision which extends downward from the medial border of the deltoid, along the lateral border of the biceps almost to the lateral condyle of the humerus. The cephalic vein may be encountered. The deltoid is retracted laterally and the biceps medially, thus exposing the brachialis muscle. Flexion of the elbow will relax the brachialis tendon. The brachialis muscle is incised longitudinally to the bone, and the cut surfaces of the muscle are retracted laterally and medially. The radial nerve can be protected if it is retracted with the posterior part of the brachialis muscle. Thus the lower two thirds of the shaft of the humerus is exposed safely.

The neurovascular structures in the arm are approached through a medial incision which is placed in the medial bicipital groove (p. 655). The basilic vein is encountered and is retracted posteriorly (Fig. 576). The medial border of the biceps muscle is elevated and retracted anterolaterally; thus the median and the ulnar nerves and the brachial artery, with its venae comites, are exposed.

Elbow

ELBOW JOINT

The elbow joint is the articulation of the humerus with the radius and the ulna; since it permits only flexion and extension, it belongs to the hinge or ginglymus variety. The trochlea and the capitellum of the humerus articulate respectively with the trochlear notch of the ulna and the head of the radius. The trochlea of the humerus is grasped by the trochlear (semilunar) notch of the ulna, and the capitellum of the humerus rests on the upper surface of the head of the radius. Some anatomists prefer to consider the elbow joint as the result of three separate joints having one synovial cavity: namely, the humero-ulnar, the humeroradial and the superior radio-ulnar joints. Here the elbow joint will be considered as having humero-ulnar and humeroradial parts, and the superior radio-ulnar joint will be discussed as a separate joint communicating with the other two.

Ligaments. The joint is surrounded by a *capsular ligament*, thickened and reinforced at the sides to form medial and lateral ligaments; the intervening portions are known as the anterior and the posterior ligaments of the elbow (Fig. 577).

The broad, thin *anterior ligament* is attached superiorly to the radial and the coronoid fossae and the epicondyles; inferiorly, it is attached to the anterior margin of the coronoid process and the annular ligament of the radius.

The posterior ligament is placed medially and is thin and weak. Superiorly, it is attached to the floor and the medial and the lateral margins of the olecranon fossa and

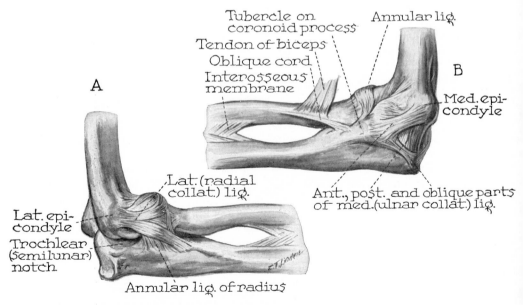

Tubercle on coronoid process

Tendon of biceps

Oblique cord

Interosseous membrane

Annular lig.

B

Med. epi-condyle

A

Lat. (radial collat.) lig.

Lat. epi-condyle

Trochlear (semilunar) notch

Ant., post. and oblique parts of med. (ulnar collat.) lig.

Annular lig. of radius

Fig. 577. Ligaments of the elbow joint: (A) the lateral aspect; (B) the medial aspect.

the epicondyles; inferiorly, it is attached to the anterior and the lateral margins of the olecranon.

The medial ligament (ulnar collateral) consists of 3 bands which pass between the internal epicondyle, the coronoid process and the olecranon. The anterior band is strong and taut in extension. The posterior part is a weak (fan-shaped) portion which becomes taut in flexion; its oblique fibers, which also have been referred to as the ligament of Cooper, deepen the socket for the trochlea of the humerus. The ulnar nerve lies on the posterior and the middle parts of this ligament as it descends from the back of the medial epicondyle into the forearm.

The lateral ligament (radial collateral) is fan-shaped and extends from the lateral epicondyle to the side of the annular ligament. It is a strong, short band, the superficial fibers of which may be continued onto the radius as the supinator. It is attached below to the annular ligament and not to the bone.

The epiphyseal line of the humerus and the radius is almost entirely intracapsular; that of the ulna is extracapsular.

The synovial membrane lines the deep surface of the capsular ligament but does not reach as high in the radial, the coronoid and the olecranon fossae as does the fibrous capsule. On the lateral side it is continuous with the synovial membrane of the superior radioulnar joint. The pads of fat which fill the coronoid, the radial and the olecranon fossae are intracapsular but extrasynovial. The anterior fat pad projects into the coronoid fossa during extension of the joint, and the posterior projects into the olecranon fossa during flexion. The synovial capsule bulges about ¼ inch below the lower margin of the annular ligament and surrounds the neck of the radius (Fig. 579).

The blood supply around the elbow joint is derived from anastomoses which constitute free communications between the brachial artery and the upper end of the radial and the ulnar arteries (Fig. 578). This, like all other periarticular anastomoses, lies close to the bone. Branches of 9 arteries take part in its formation; they are: (1) the anterior branch of the profunda brachii; this anastomoses with (2) the radial recurrent on the front

of the lateral epicondyle; (3) the posterior branch of the profunda brachii anastomoses with (4) the interosseous recurrent on the back of the lateral epicondyle. (5) The anterior branch of the supratrochlear anastomoses with (6) the anterior ulnar recurrent on the front of the medial epicondyle; (7) its posterior branch and (8) the ulnar collateral anastomose with (9) the posterior ulnar recurrent on the back of the medial epicondyle.

The nerve supply of the joint is derived from the median, the ulnar, the radial, the musculocutaneous and the posterior interosseous nerves.

Relations. Anteriorly, the brachialis muscle nearly covers the entire anterior ligament (Fig. 579). It separates the joint proper from the brachial artery, its companion veins, the biceps tendon and the median nerve. Medial to the brachialis the anterior recurrent ulnar artery is found related to the anterior ligament. Under cover of the muscles is the radial nerve, with its posterior interosseous branch accompanied by the radial recurrent artery.

Laterally, the common tendon of the extensors overlies the lateral ligament of the elbow, and the extensor carpi radialis brevis and the supinator arise from it.

Medially, the common tendon of the flexors overlies the anterior band of the medial ligament of the elbow; the flexor sublimis arises from it. The flexor carpi ulnaris overlies the posterior band, and the ulnar nerve and the posterior ulnar recurrent artery lie directly on it.

Posteriorly, the triceps and its bursa lie above the olecranon. The anconeus and the interosseous recurrent artery are at the lateral side of the olecranon. That part of the flexor carpi ulnaris which originates from the olecranon is found to its medial side. A fracture across the olecranon brings the bursa into direct communication with the joint.

Movements at the elbow joint should not be confused with those that take place at the superior radio-ulnar joint. At the elbow joint there are two movements, namely, flexion and extension. The muscles which are chiefly concerned in flexing the forearm are the biceps, the brachialis, the brachioradialis and

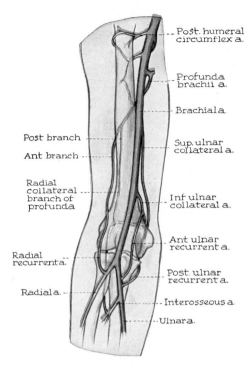

FIG. 578. Anastomoses around the elbow joint.

the pronator teres. Those which extend the forearm are the triceps and the anconeus; these are aided somewhat by the muscles arising from the lateral epicondyle. In extension, the forearm bones make an angle with the humerus. This is known as the "carrying angle" and is produced by the inner condyle of the humerus, which is set obliquely so that the axis of the elbow joint is transverse between the radius and the humerus but oblique between the ulna and the humerus. This angle disappears on full flexion, but in extension it is about 10 to 15°. The angle may be disturbed by fractures of the lower end of the humerus or by rupture of the collateral ligaments. If it is increased, the condition of cubitus valgus results; if it is obliterated, the condition of cubitus varus ensues.

ELBOW REGION

The cubital (antecubital) fossa is a triangular depression lying anterior to the elbow joint. The base of this triangle is formed by an imaginary line drawn between the hu-

meral condyle; its converging borders are the pronator teres medially and the brachioradialis laterally. At the apex the brachioradialis overlaps the pronator teres; the floor is formed by the brachialis muscle, and the deep fascia forms its room (Fig. 580).

FASCIA, VESSELS AND NERVES

The superficial veins of the cubital fossa lie in the superficial fascia. Although variable in their course and arrangement, a general plan usually can be adhered to. In this area 5 superficial veins are found: the cephalic, the basilic, the median cephalic, the median basilic and the median (Fig. 580).

The median basilic vein lies, as its name implies, medial to the basilic; the *median cephalic* lies medial to the cephalic, and the cephalic lies lateral to the basilic. The *cephalic vein* arises on the radial side of the hand, from the dorsal venous arch, passes upward and receives the median cephalic vein at the lateral epicondyle. It ascends over the lateral aspect of the biceps brachii and continues in the deltopectoral groove. It then pierces the costocoracoid membrane and terminates either in the axillary or the subclavian vein (Fig. 536).

The basilic vein arises on the ulnar side of the hand, from the dorsal venous arch, passes upward and receives the median basilic vein in front of the medial epicondyle. It ascends in the medial bicipital groove and pierces the deep fascia in the region of the middle of the arm. It continues as the axillary vein in conjunction with the two brachial veins.

The median vein commences in the palmar venous plexus, ascends on the front of the forearm and divides at the apex of the cubital fossa into the median cephalic and the median basilic veins. This division takes place soon after the entrance of its chief tributary, the profunda vein, which drains the deeper structures of the forearm.

The profunda vein drains into the median. It enters the median vein at the distal edge of the lacertus fibrosus and, in this location, may be compressed as a result of trauma or tight bandaging. Thus the vessel can become obliterated and the return venous flow from the deeper structures of the forearm

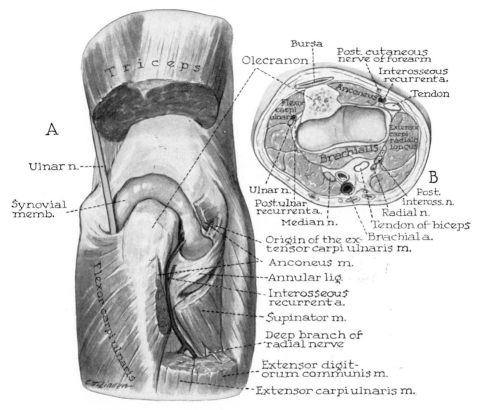

FIG. 579. The relations around the elbow joint; (A) seen from behind; (B) cross-section.

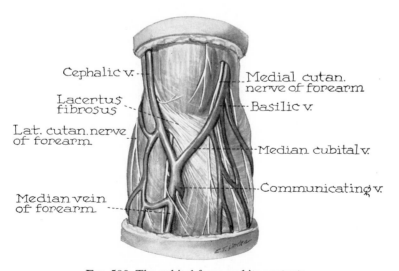

FIG. 580. The cubital fossa and its contents.

impaired. This, it is thought, is one of the contributing causes of Volkmann's contracture. For this reason, one of the treatments suggested for the condition is incision of the deep fascia to release pressure.

Lacertus Fibrosus. The bicipital fascia, or, as it is more commonly called, the lacertus fibrosus, lies deep to the superficial veins of the elbow region. It is an excellent surgical landmark (Fig. 580).

The biceps brachii is inserted into the tuberosity of the radius by means of a flat tendon. However, some of the fibers of this muscle do not pass into the formation of this tendon but continue on as a flat tendinous expansion which passes medially and distally to fuse with and become lost in the fascia of the forearm. This flat tendinous expansion is called the lacertus fibrosus; it also has been referred to as the bicipital aponeurosis. It occupies the middle of the front of the elbow region and is about ¾ inch wide.

The lacertus is the key structure of this region. The pulsations of the brachial artery can be felt immediately beneath its free medial margin. Full extension of the forearm facilitates the palpation of the artery by relaxing the bicipital fascia; the median nerve lies just medial to the brachial artery.

The lateral antibrachial cutaneous nerve is the continuation of the musculocutaneous nerve; it pierces the lacertus fibrosus, runs under the median cephalic vein, becomes superficial and divides into anterior and posterior branches which supply the skin over the anterolateral and the posterolateral aspects of the forearm (Fig. 587).

The medial antibrachial cutaneous nerve, a branch of the medial cord of the brachial plexus, divides at the middle of the arm into a volar and an ulnar branch. The volar branch passes under the median basilic vein and supplies the skin of the ulnar half of the forearm as far as the wrist.

Four structures are found on the lacertus fibrosus: the median cephalic vein, the median basilic vein, the lateral antibrachial cutaneous nerve and the medial antibrachial cutaneous nerve (or the branches of these nerves).

When the lacertus fibrosus is cut and reflected, the underlying brachial artery and median nerve are exposed (Fig. 581). The brachial artery and its venae comites are just medial to the biceps tendon, and the median nerve in turn is medial to the artery. The radial nerve can be found lateral to the biceps tendon in a compartment between the brachioradialis and the brachialis muscles. The groove between these muscles may be difficult to determine, owing to the absence of a well-marked septum. The usual

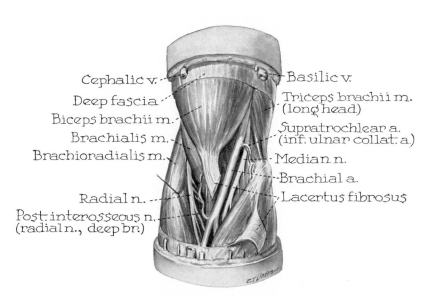

FIG. 581. The cubital fossa and its contents after cutting the lacertus fibrosus.

error is to open the interval immediately between the brachialis and the biceps muscles, thereby exposing the musculocutaneous nerve instead of the radial. Therefore, it is advisable to hug the lateral border of the biceps tendon and seek the interval between the brachioradialis muscle and the biceps tendon. Lateral retraction of the brachioradialis will expose the radial nerve where it divides into superficial and deep branches.

The brachial artery can be felt along the medial bicipital groove throughout the length of the arm until it disappears behind the lacertus fibrosus. It passes through the cubital fossa under the lacertus fibrosus and divides into a larger ulnar and a smaller radial artery. This division takes place at the level of the coronoid process of the ulna and the neck of the radius. These structures are located about 1 inch below the distal elbow crease.

The ulnar and the median nerves give off no branches in the arm; they make a "non-stop" trip through it. The ulnar nerve lies medial to the brachial artery until it reaches the middle of the arm, where it pierces the medial intermuscular septum to reach the posterior compartment. The superior ulnar collateral artery accompanies it at this point. The nerve passes to the back of the medial epicondyle and then on into the forearm. The median nerve lies lateral to the brachial artery at its beginning but crosses it obliquely and then lies medial to it in the cubital fossa. This crossing usually takes place in front of the artery.

POSTERIOR OR OLECRANON REGION

The olecranon region includes the posterior soft parts of the elbow; the joint coverings are thin, and the articular extremities of the bones are felt easily (Fig. 582).

A knowledge of the surface landmarks in this region is essential. Both of the humeral epicondyles are subcutaneous and readily

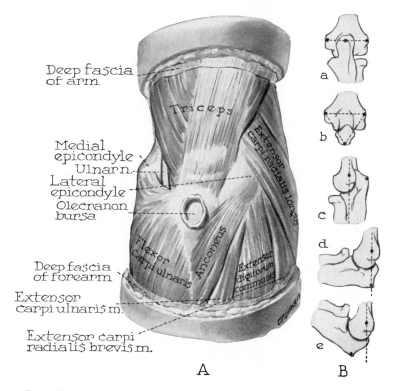

FIG. 582. The posterior or olecranon region: (A) bony and muscular landmarks; (B) the varying bony relationships in flexion and extension.

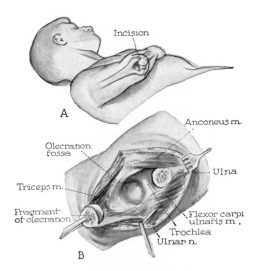

A

Incision

Anconeus m.

Olecranon
fossa

Ulna

Triceps m.

Fragment
of olecranon

Flexor carpi
ulnaris m.

Trochlea

Ulnar n.

B

FIG. 583. The posterior "U" approach to the elbow joint: (A) incision; (B) the resulting wide exposure of the joint following division of the olecranon.

palpable, but the medial epicondyle is the more prominent. A rather deep but narrow medial para-olecranon groove separates the medial epicondyle from the olecranon. The ulnar nerve can be felt passing through the posterior aspect of this groove. The lateral epicondyle is palpated most easily with the arm semiflexed, but when the arm is in full extension, this condyle is hidden in a small depression bounded by the anconeus muscle medially and the extensor carpi radialis muscle laterally. In the region of the para-olecranon groove the joint capsule and the synovia are nearest to the surface.

When the forearm is extended, the intercondylar line is horizontal and passes through the proximal border of the olecranon (Fig. 582 B). However, when the forearm is flexed, the olecranon becomes prominent and appears below the horizontal level of the intercondylar line. When the forearm is flexed to a right angle, the olecranon lies on the same plane as the posterior surface of the shaft of the humerus. In this last-mentioned position it forms the apex of an inverted triangle, the base of which is located at a line drawn between the epicondyles of the humerus. In full flexion of the forearm, the olecranon is carried

downward and lies anterior to the articular end of the humerus.

Distal to the lateral epicondyle and in a depression which marks the site of the humeroradial joint, the projecting head of the radius can be felt, especially on rotary movements produced through supination and pronation. With the forearm flexed, the head of the radius lies about 1 inch anterior to the lateral epicondyle, the interval separating them being occupied by the capitellum of the humerus. With the forearm in complete extension, a distinct depression appears immediately proximal to the head of the radius; this corresponds to the lateral and the posterior parts of the radiohumeral joint. An effusion in this joint obliterates this depression.

The skin over the back of the elbow is thicker than that over the front; it moves with great freedom over the underlying parts.

The olecranon bursa is situated between the dorsal surface of the olecranon process, the tendinous expansion of the triceps muscle and the skin (Fig. 582). Enlargements or involvements of this bursa result in the condition known as "miner's elbow," which is associated with constant bruising as is produced when working in small and confined spaces.

The tendon of the triceps brachii is situated proximal to the joint line where it inserts into the olecranon.

The anconeus muscle is the only muscle which legitimately belongs to this posterior elbow region; throughout its extent it is palpable in the lateral olecranon groove.

The flexor carpi ulnaris muscle arises from the medial epicondyle and the medial surface of the olecranon.

The ulnar nerve reaches the elbow behind the medial intermuscular septum and can be palpated in the medial olecranon groove. It lies in contact with the periosteum under an expansion of the triceps tendon. The nerve leaves the para-olecranon region between the heads of origin of the flexor carpi ulnaris muscle. It may be drawn from its bed and brought around the medial epicondyle to a more protected position during surgery.

The arteries of the back of the elbow are part of a network made up of the collateral branches of the brachial, the radial and the ulnar trunks which serve as a collateral anastomosis when the main brachial trunk is involved (p. 673).

SURGICAL CONSIDERATIONS

SURGICAL APPROACH TO THE ELBOW JOINT

There are many approaches to the elbow joint; each has its advantages and disadvantages. Some authorities believe that the lateral approach is the safest. The medial approach is hazardous. A posterolateral approach has also been used. Herein described is a posterior approach, using a U-shaped (MacAusland) incision. It begins at the external epicondyle of the humerus, extends downward and medially, crosses the ulna 2 inches distal to the dip of the olecranon and continues up to the medial epicondyle (Fig. 583). The resulting flap is dissected upward, and the olecranon, with the attached triceps tendon, is exposed. The ulnar nerve is isolated and retracted medially, and the lateral expansions of the triceps tendon are divided transversely. The olecranon is divided with an osteotome and is retracted upward with its muscle attachment. The lateral and the medial muscles in this region are stripped subperiosteally and retracted. A wide exposure results.

DISLOCATION OF THE ELBOW

Dislocation of the elbow involves one or both bones of the forearm and may be backward, forward, lateral or medial. With these injuries, the ulnar and the radial collateral ligaments and the articular capsule usually are torn, and either condyle may be fractured.

Posterior dislocation of both bones is the most common type; it usually results from a fall on the outstretched hand (Fig. 584). The fibers of the brachialis muscle attaching to the coronoid process usually are torn. If the dislocation is complete, the head of the radius lies behind the lateral epicondyle, and the distal end of the humerus falls into the cubital fossa. As a result of this, the arm and the forearm are semiflexed and at an angle of about 120°. The olecranon projects

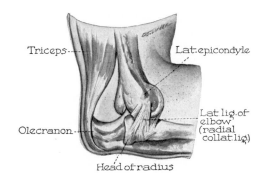

FIG. 584. Posterior dislocation of both bones of the forearm.

posteriorly as a hump; the normal relations between the humeral condyle and the olecranon are changed, and the olecranon is found above and behind its normal line.

Anterior dislocation of both bones is rare. It results from trauma to the olecranon when the elbow is flexed. The olecranon then lies anterior to the trochlea.

Lateral and *medial* dislocations are also quite rare and occur from falls on the pronated and outstretched hand.

ARTHROPLASTY OF THE ELBOW

This operation forms an artificial joint and is indicated when an ankylosis is present in a poor position (complete extension). Two longitudinal posterior incisions are made, passing on each side of the olecranon. A single posterior incision also has been used. The 2 incisions are deepened down to the bony structure; the musculospiral nerve is located through the radial incision. The ulnar nerve is found behind the internal condyle of the humerus and is protected. The soft parts are retracted, and the ankylosed joint is exposed. The lower end of the humerus is removed in such a way that a convex rounded end results. The ulnar end is removed, but its end remains concave. It may or may not be necessary to include the radial head in the arthroplasty. Fascia and fat flaps are formed from the radial and the ulnar aspects of the arm and the forearm and are placed over the ends of the bones; these flaps are sutured to the capsule and the periosteum. If no capsule remains, or if it is destroyed, the flaps are sutured to the surrounding soft tissues. The wounds are closed,

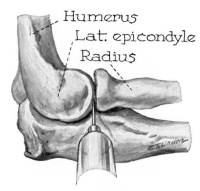

Humerus
Lat. epicondyle
Radius

FIG. 585. Aspiration of the elbow joint.

and the elbow is immobilized at a right angle. Fascia lata transplants also have been used and sutured to the capsule.

ASPIRATION OF THE ELBOW JOINT

The part of the joint which is closest to the surface lies posteriorly between the head of the radius and the lateral condyle of the humerus (Fig. 585). The joint should be flexed to a right angle and the forearm placed in a position of semipronation. The head of the radius is palpated, and the needle is inserted just proximal to it in a forward and anterior direction. If the joint is distended with fluid or pus, the capsule bulges to either side of the triceps and can be drained easily.

FRACTURE OF THE OLECRANON PROCESS

This injury results from direct or muscular violence and is characterized by a transverse type of fracture. The deformity is brought about by the triceps muscle, which pulls the olecranon upward. Flexion of the elbow further separates the fragments. The treatment of a fractured olecranon process may be nonoperative, with the arm in complete extension, or surgical, with the fragments held together by wire placed posterior to the long axis of the ulna.

Forearm

The forearm (Fig. 586) is that part of the upper extremity which is between the elbow and the wrist. The anterior (volar) region contains those structures which are anterior to the plane of the radius and the ulna; these include the internal and the external muscle groups which arise from the medial and the lateral epicondyles, respectively. The posterior (dorsal) region contains the extensor muscle group, which composes the bulk of this region. When the forearm is in full supination, it appears as a cone which is flattened anteroposteriorly. Muscle masses which arise from the humeral epicondyles increase its transverse diameter near the elbow. Distally, the forearm loses its bulk because of the transition of the fleshy muscles into their respective tendons. The shafts of the radius and the ulna can be felt superficially in the distal part of the forearm.

The cutaneous nerve supply to the forearm is derived from the lateral and the medial cutaneous nerves ventrally, and the lateral, the medial and the posterior nerves dorsally (Fig. 587).

The deep fascia of the forearm is a continuation of the deep fascia of the arm. It is strengthened around the olecranon by expansions from the triceps brachii and reinforced anteriorly by the lacertus fibrosus. At the wrist the deep fascia is continuous with the transverse and the dorsal carpal (annular) ligaments. From its deep surface arise intermuscular septa which extend to the radius and the ulna, and also form compartments for the various muscle groups which are to be described (Fig. 588).

ANTERIOR (VOLAR) REGION

Muscles. The muscles of the volar aspect of the forearm occupy 3 planes or floors which, from above downward, are as follows (Fig. 589):

FIRST FLOOR (SUPERFICIAL). This consists of 4 muscles which have a common origin from the medial epicondyle of the humerus. They pass obliquely down the forearm, with the exception of the flexor carpi ulnaris, and are supplied by the median nerve.

The pronator teres, although a powerful pronator of the forearm, is also a flexor. It is the most lateral and most obliquely placed muscle of the group. In addition to its origin from the medial epicondyle, it has a small deep head of origin from the coronoid process of the ulna. This deep head separates the median nerve from the ulnar artery; the nerve lies between the superficial and the deep heads, and the artery lies behind both heads (Fig. 590). It inserts on the lateral surface of the middle of the radius.

The flexor carpi radialis muscle becomes tendinous about the middle of the forearm; it is inserted into the bases of the 2nd and the 3rd metacarpals and produces flexion and radial deviation of the hand.

The palmaris longus muscle becomes tendinous at about the middle of the forearm, but its tendon is longer and narrower than the tendon of the flexor carpi radialis. It passes anterior to the transverse carpal (anterior annular) ligament and inserts into the palmar fascia. Its contraction tenses the palmar fascia and flexes the hand.

The flexor carpi ulnaris is placed most medially; the digitorum sublimis may be

681

mistaken for it. It inserts onto the pisiform bone. Contraction of this muscle produces flexion and adduction (ulnar) of the hand.

SECOND FLOOR. The second-floor muscle, the *flexor digitorum sublimis,* lies deep to the preceding muscle tendons and to their ulnar side. It has an extensive origin which is part humeral, part ulnar and part radial. The ulnar and the radial origins are bridged by a fibrous band through which the median

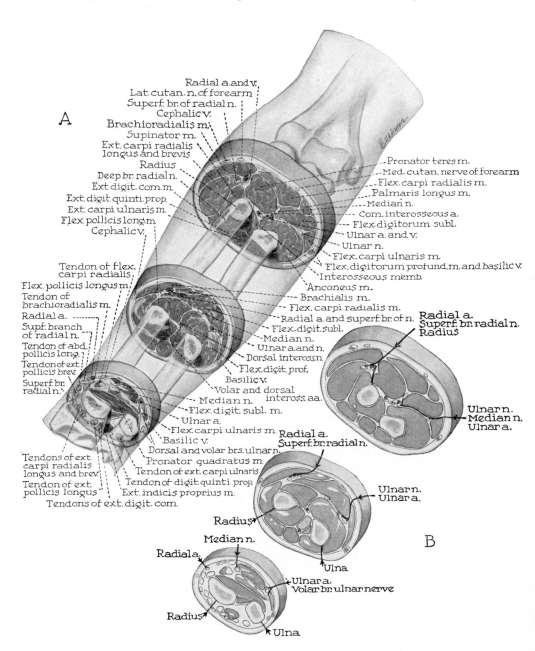

FIG. 586. The right forearm. (A) Cross section study of the relations of the forearm. (B) The arrows indicate the proper surgical cleavage planes utilized in approaching the neurovascular structures.

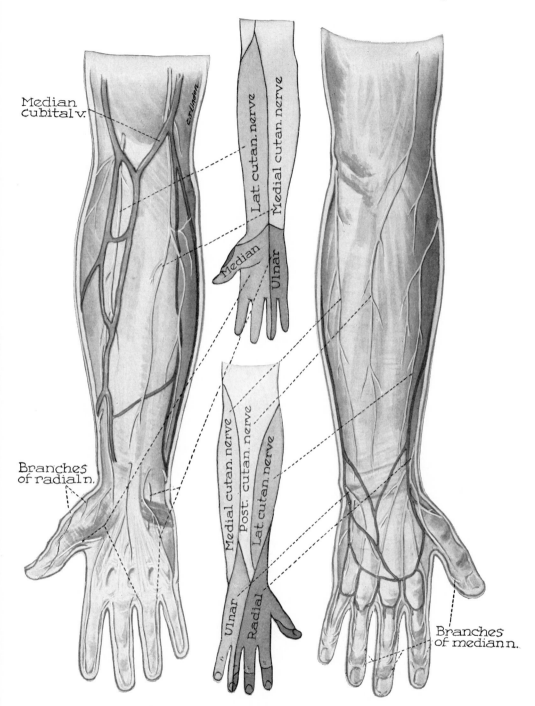

FIG. 587. The cutaneous nerve supply of the dorsal and the volar aspects of the forearm.

nerve and the ulnar artery pass to enter the space between the second-floor and the third-floor musculature. The individual tendons of this muscle start in the lower third of the forearm; they do not lie side by side but pass 2 above and 2 below. The 2 above travel to the 3rd and the 4th fingers, and the 2 below pass to the 2nd and the 5th fingers. The entire muscle is supplied by the median nerve. The splitting of these tendons and their insertions into the borders of the middle phalanges is discussed elsewhere (p. 721).

THIRD FLOOR. The third floor (deep) consists of 3 muscles: the flexor pollicis longus, the flexor digitorum profundus and the pronator quadratus. They form a covering for the radius and the ulna, and it is upon this that the nerves and the arteries of the front of the flexor region of the forearm travel.

The flexor pollicis longus muscle arises from the anterior surface of the radius between the oblique line above and the pronator below. It inserts at the base of the terminal phalanx of the thumb.

The flexor digitorum profundus muscle arises from the volar and the medial surfaces of the ulna between the pronator quadratus and the brachialis muscles. Unlike the sublimis, the tendons of the profundus lie alongside of the tendon of the flexor pollicis longus as they pass beneath the transverse carpal ligament to insert into the bases of the distal phalanges.

The pronator quadratus lies at the distal

end of the forearm but is behind the flexor tendons and sheaths, the median nerve and the radial vessels. It originates from the distal fourth of the anterior surface of the ulna, and inserts into the distal fourth of the anterior surface of the radius and a triangular area on the medial side of the radius in front of the interosseous membrane. It pronates the forearm.

All of the muscles previously discussed are supplied by the median nerve with the exception of the flexor carpi ulnaris and the ulnar half of the flexor digitorum profundus (4th and 5th fingers); as the word "ulnaris" suggests, these muscles are supplied by the ulnar nerve.

Nerves. The ulnar nerve enters the forearm by passing between the 2 heads of the flexor carpi ulnaris and continues downward on the flexor digitorum profundus (Figs. 590 and 591). In the wrist it is overlapped by the tendon of the flexor carpi ulnaris. It supplies the ulnar half of the flexor digitorum profundus and the flexor carpi ulnaris. It descends vertically near the medial border of the flexor digitorum sublimis and can be exposed by splitting the septum between the sublimis and the flexor carpi ulnaris.

The median nerve enters the forearm between the superficial and the deep heads of the pronator teres, passes through the sublimis arch and continues downward on the flexor digitorum profundus. It clings to the deep surface of the flexor digitorum sublimis and in the wrist is overlapped by the tendon of the palmaris longus. It supplies all the

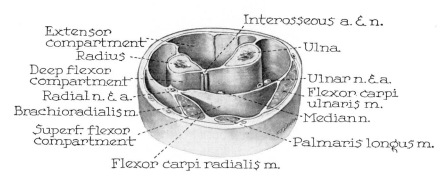

Extensor compartment
Radius
Deep flexor compartment
Radial n. & a.
Brachioradialis m.
Superf. flexor compartment

Interosseous a. & n.
Ulna
Ulnar n. & a.
Flexor carpi ulnaris m.
Median n.
Palmaris longus m.

Flexor carpi radialis m.

FIG. 588. The deep fascia of the right forearm. The section is taken at the middle of the forearm and shows the fascial spaces and compartments formed for the muscles, the vessels and the nerves.

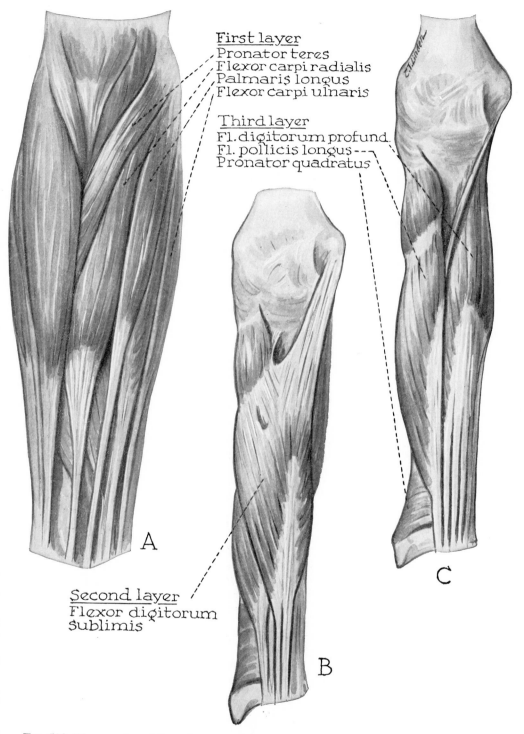

First layer
Pronator teres
Flexor carpi radialis
Palmaris longus
Flexor carpi ulnaris

Third layer
Fl. digitorum profund.
Fl. pollicis longus
Pronator quadratus

Second layer
Flexor digitorum
sublimis

A

B

C

FIG. 589. The muscles of the volar aspect of the forearm. These muscles occupy 3 layers
or floors, which can be divided into superficial, middle and deep groups.

forearm flexors except those already mentioned. That branch of the median nerve which supplies the deep flexors is called the anterior interosseous nerve. As the nerve descends, it clings to the undersurface of the flexor digitorum sublimis and appears at its lateral border.

The radial nerve divides in the region of the lateral epicondyle into superficial and deep branches. The superficial (sensory) branch descends beneath the brachioradialis muscle; it approaches the radial artery in the middle of the forearm and then leaves it to pierce the deep fascia and supply the skin of the dorsum of the hand and the wrist. The deep (dorsal interosseous) branch

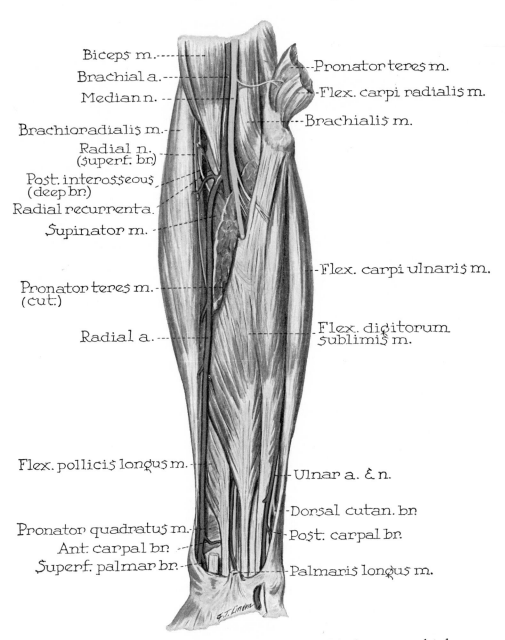

Biceps m.

Brachial a.

Median n.

Brachioradialis m.

Radial n. (superf. br.)

Post. interosseous (deep br.)

Radial recurrent a.

Supinator m.

Pronator teres m. (cut.)

Radial a.

Flex. pollicis longus m.

Pronator quadratus m.

Ant. carpal br.

Superf. palmar br.

Pronator teres m.

Flex. carpi radialis m.

Brachialis m.

Flex. carpi ulnaris m.

Flex. digitorum sublimis m.

Ulnar a. & n.

Dorsal cutan. br.

Post. carpal br.

Palmaris longus m.

FIG. 590. The blood vessels and the nerves of the right forearm as related to the flexor digitorum sublimis.

is mainly motor and reaches the back of the forearm by winding around the neck of the radius through the supinator muscle, which makes a tunnel for it (Fig. 593). At the lateral side of the shaft of the radius, the nerve passes between the superficial and the deep muscles of the back of the forearm and innervates them.

Arteries. In the upper forearm, the *ulnar artery* is separated from the median nerve by the deep (ulnar) head of the pronator teres; in the mid-forearm, it descends obliquely behind the flexor digitorum sublimis and on the flexor digitorum profundus (Figs. 590 and 591). At the wrist it is closely related to the ulnar nerve, which lies medial to it. Both the artery and the nerve are overlapped by the flexor carpi ulnaris. Its

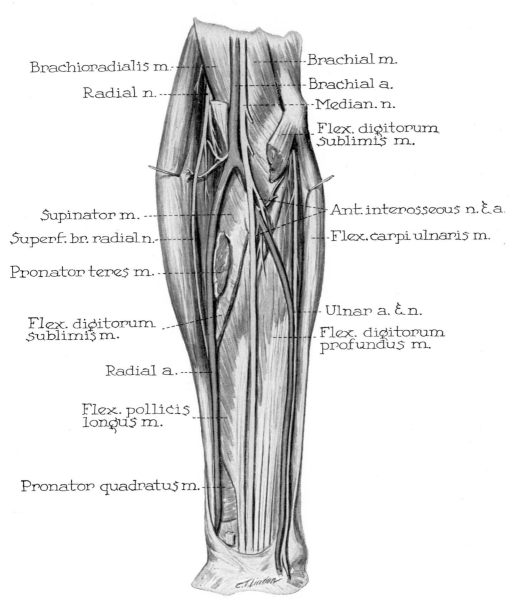

Brachioradialis m.

Radial n.

Supinator m.

Superf. br. radial n.

Pronator teres m.

Flex. digitorum Sublimis m.

Radial a.

Flex. pollicis longus m.

Pronator quadratus m.

Brachial m.

Brachial a.

Median. n.

Flex. digitorum Sublimis m.

Ant. interosseous n. & a.

Flex. carpi ulnaris m.

Ulnar a. & n.

Flex. digitorum profundus m.

FIG. 591. The blood vessels and the nerves as related to the deep flexors of the right forearm.

branches are the anterior and the posterior ulnar recurrent arteries and, more distally, the common interosseous, which immediately divides into volar (anterior) and dorsal (posterior) branches.

The radial artery is unique in that no muscle crosses it; therefore, it lies quite superficial and can be ligated almost anywhere in the forearm. However, it is true that in the upper forearm it is overlapped by the brachioradialis but, as it continues distally, it lies on the supinator, the pronator teres, the flexor digitorum sublimis, the flexor pollicis longus and the pronator quadratus in the order named. No motor nerve crosses it.

SURGICAL CONSIDERATIONS

EXPOSURE OF THE RADIAL NERVE

This nerve is injured easily because of its close relation to the humerus. A posterior approach usually is utilized. The incision begins about the middle of the posterior border of the deltoid muscle and extends almost to the olecranon. The deep fascia is incised, and the space between the long and the lateral heads of the triceps is identified. These are separated, and through this space the nerve with its accompanying profunda artery emerges from the axilla; it passes in the musculospiral (radial) groove. The lateral head of the triceps can be severed, and the nerve can be followed in its groove to the lateral region of the arm.

LIGATION OF THE ULNAR ARTERY

Ligation of the ulnar artery per se is rarely done. It may be ligated at any site along its course, but usually this is done in its lower two thirds. The course of the artery in its lower two thirds can be visualized along a line which corresponds to the lower two thirds of a line drawn from the medial epicondyle to the pisiform bone. The skin incision is placed along this imaginary line. The superficial veins are ligated, and the deep fascia is incised. The artery will be found under the flexor carpi ulnaris tendon, which can be drawn medially. The vessel is surrounded by its venae comites; the ulnar nerve is medial. This neurovascular bundle is covered by a layer of fascia which not only binds it down to the surface of the flexor digitorum profundus but also binds the structures to each other. Therefore, it is dangerous to place a hemostat without first identifying and dissecting the nerve. In the upper half of the forearm, the vessel lies more deeply, being placed beneath the muscle mass which consists of the flexor carpi ulnaris and the flexor digitorum sublimis. The intermuscular cleavage plane existing between these muscles should be opened. The vessel will be found here and can be followed proximally.

LIGATION OF THE RADIAL ARTERY

Ligation of the radial artery may be done anywhere along its course, which corresponds to a line drawn from the middle of the elbow fold (cubital fossa) to the inner side of the front of the styloid process of the radius. The lower two thirds of the radial artery may be exposed through a skin incision which is placed in the line of the artery and is of sufficient length for adequate exposure. The superficial veins are ligated, and the deep fascia is divided along the edge of the brachioradialis muscle. In the upper part of the forearm, the muscle is retracted laterally so that the artery is exposed with its venae comites as they pass over the pronator teres. The radial nerve approaches the vessels and lies close to them for a short distance in the middle of the forearm, but proximal to this there is a slight interval which separates them. The nerve should be guarded. In the lower part of the forearm the vessels are exposed immediately under the deep fascia.

POSTERIOR REGION

The subcutaneous border of the ulna, which can be palpated from the olecranon to the wrist, separates the extensor muscles of the forearm from the flexors. Such a palpable bony ridge may be utilized as an excellent surgical landmark and guide.

MUSCLES, NERVES AND VESSELS

The muscles of the back of the forearm are divided into superficial and deep groups (Fig. 592). The superficial group has 6 muscles, and the deep group has 5.

The 2 muscles which belong to the superficial group which do *not* originate from the lateral epicondyle are the brachioradialis and the extensor carpi radialis longus; those which *do* originate from the lateral epicondyle are the extensor carpi radialis brevis, the extensor digitorum communis, the extensor digiti quinti proprius and the extensor carpi ulnaris. These latter 4 superficial muscles have a common origin by means of a tendon which is attached to the lateral epicondyle.

The deep group of muscles consists of the supinator, the abductor pollicis longus, the extensor pollicis brevis, the extensor pollicis longus and the extensor indicis.

The brachioradialis muscle (radial nerve) lies more toward the front of the forearm than on the back. It originates from the upper two thirds of the lateral supracondy-

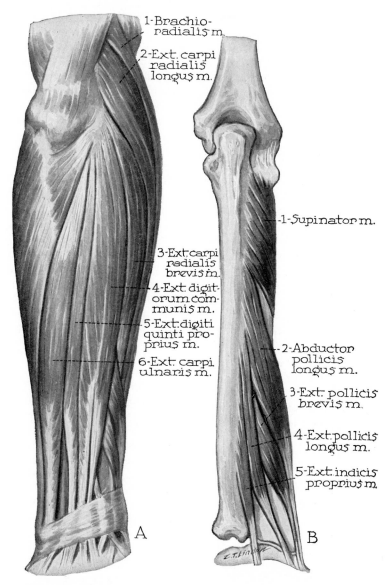

1-Brachio-
radialis m.

2-Ext. carpi
radialis
longus m.

-1-Supinator m.

3-Ext. carpi
radialis
brevis m.

4-Ext. digit-
orum com-
munis m.

5-Ext. digiti
quinti pro-
prius m.

6-Ext. carpi
ulnaris m.

2-Abductor
pollicis
longus m.

3-Ext. pollicis
brevis m.

4-Ext. pollicis
longus m.

5-Ext. indicis
proprius m.

A

B

FIG. 592. The muscles of the back of the right forearm. (A) The superficial group consists of 6 muscles. (B) The deep group consists of 5 muscles.

lar ridge, and about halfway down the forearm is converted into a flat tendon which inserts into the lateral surface of the distal end of the radius. Its fleshy part overlaps the brachialis and descends in front of the lateral epicondyle. It forms the lateral boundary of the cubital fossa. The principal action of the brachioradialis is to flex the forearm; it helps to initiate supination when the forearm is prone and helps to initiate pronation when the forearm is supine.

The extensor carpi radialis longus muscle (radial nerve) is closely associated with the brachioradialis. It arises from the distal third of the lateral supracondylar ridge and, as it descends, it passes over the lateral epicondyle deep to the brachioradialis. At first it is lateral to the radius but it gains the dorsal surface about halfway down the forearm. It has a long tendon which is continued downward toward the wrist, where it passes under cover of the extensor retinaculum and inserts into the base of the 2nd metacarpal bone (Fig. 627). It aids in extension and abduction of the hand at the wrist and is a slight flexor of the forearm.

The extensor carpi radialis brevis muscle (posterior interosseous nerve) arises from the common extensor origin on the lateral epicondyle and passes downward; at first it is overlapped by the extensor carpi radialis longus but more distally is medial to it. Its tendon begins at the middle of the forearm and passes under cover of the extensor retinaculum through a compartment which it shares with the longus (Fig. 632). It is inserted into the base of the 3rd metacarpal bone. Both radial extensors act as their names indicate: extension and abduction of the wrist.

The extensor digitorum communis muscle (posterior interosseous nerve) arises from the common extensor origin at the lateral epicondyle; it passes downward medial to the extensor carpi radialis brevis. In the distal part of the forearm, its fleshy belly ends in a tendon which passes under cover of the extensor retinaculum and then divides into 4 tendons for the fingers. Over the dorsum of the hand the individual tendons diverge and proceed onward to the fingers, where they are inserted into the middle and the distal phalanges. These tendons are connected to each other by oblique bands. As a result of this, complete extension of an individual finger at the metacarpophalangeal joint is impossible so long as the other fingers are kept flexed. The manner of insertion of these tendons is discussed elsewhere.

The extensor digiti minimi (quinti proprius) muscle (posterior interosseous nerve) is a slender muscle which arises in common with the extensor digitorum and at first seems to be part of it. It lies along the medial side of the extensor digitorum, but its tendon passes through a special compartment in the extensor retinaculum. The tendon splits into two parts, the lateral being joined by the tendon of the little finger from the extensor digitorum. It forms the dorsal extensor expansion for the little finger and is an extensor of all the joints of the little finger.

The extensor carpi ulnaris muscle (posterior interosseous nerve) arises by means of the common extensor origin from the lateral epicondyle and remains fleshy until it reaches the wrist joint, where it becomes tendinous. It occupies the groove on the back of the distal end of the ulna, passes through the most medial compartment of the extensor retinaculum and inserts into the base of the 5th metacarpal. It is an extensor of the wrist and aids the flexor carpi ulnaris in adducting the hand.

The anconeus muscle (radial nerve) does not really belong to the superficial group of extensor muscles, but it is convenient to consider it with this group. It originates from the posterior aspect of the lateral epicondyle and is narrow and tendinous; its fibers soon diverge and become inserted into the lateral aspect of the olecranon and the adjoining part of the posterior surface of the ulna. It covers the posterior aspect of the annular ligament of the radius, thus helping to separate the head of the bone from the surface. Its action assists the triceps in extension of the forearm.

If the extensor digitorum communis and the extensor digiti minimi are divided transversely about their middle, the following structures are exposed: the posterior interosseous vessels, the posterior interosseous nerve and the deep muscles of the back of the forearm (Fig. 593 A).

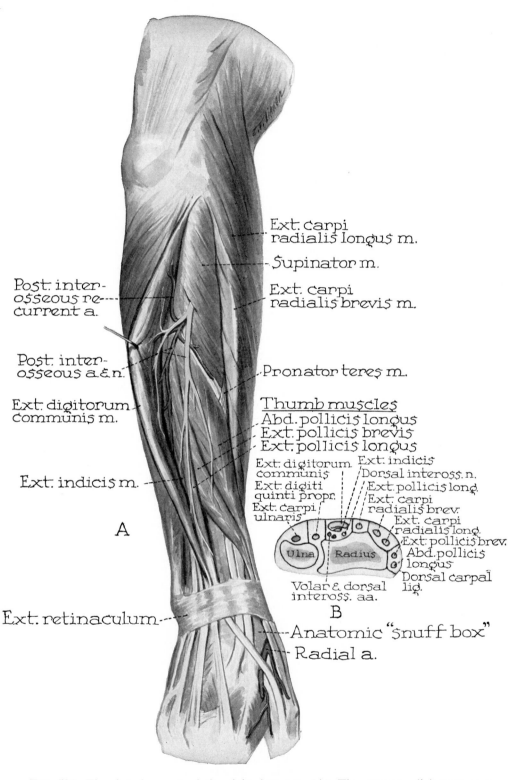

Ext. carpi
radialis longus m.

Supinator m.

Ext. carpi
radialis brevis m.

Post. inter-
osseous re-
current a.

Post. inter-
osseous a.&n.

Pronator teres m.

Ext. digitorum
communis m.

Thumb muscles
Abd. pollicis longus
Ext. pollicis brevis
Ext. pollicis longus

Ext. digitorum   Ext. indicis
communis   Dorsal inteross. n.
Ext. digiti   Ext. pollicis long.
quinti propr.   Ext. carpi
Ext. carpi   radialis brev.
ulnaris   Ext. carpi
                      radialis long.
                      Ext. pollicis brev.
Ulna   Radius   Abd. pollicis
                      longus
                      Dorsal carpal
Volar & dorsal   lig.
inteross. aa.

Ext. indicis m.

A

B

Ext. retinaculum

Anatomic "snuff box"

Radial a.

FIG. 593. The dorsal aspect of the right forearm. (A) The extensor digitorum communis muscle has been retracted to expose the posterior interosseous nerve and artery. The
anatomic "snuff box" is shown. (B) A cross section of the extensor retinaculum and the 6
compartments which it forms.

At a variable point in the region of the lateral epicondyle, the radial nerve divides into two branches: sensory (superficial) and motor nerves.

Posterior Interosseous Nerve. The motor nerve is the posterior interosseous (deep radial) nerve. The level at which branches of nerves originate may be variable, but the side from which nerves originate is quite constant. A motor nerve leaves from that side of the nerve which is nearest the muscle to which it is distributed; hence, we may speak of "sides of safety" and "sides of danger." Since the radial nerve supplies the extensor muscles, its branches arise laterally, and, therefore, it is safe to dissect on the medial side of this nerve. The reverse is true of the median nerve.

The posterior interosseous nerve winds around the radius in the substance of the supinator muscle, which creates a muscular tunnel for the nerve. The nerve emerges from the posterior surface of the supinator a little above its lower border and in this way gains access to the fascial plane between the superficial and the deep groups of extensor muscles of the forearm.

In its course the nerve is accompanied by the posterior interosseous vessels; they pass across the dorsal surface of the abductor pollicis longus muscle and under cover of the extensor digitorum. At about the middle of the forearm the nerve reaches the extensor pollicis longus and at this point leaves the posterior interosseous vessels and descends over the back of the interosseous membrane. It is accompanied by the anterior interosseous vessels and passes under the extensor pollicis longus and the extensor indicis. The posterior interosseous nerve supplies all the muscles in this region with the exception of the brachioradialis, the extensor carpi radialis longus and the anconeus. The latter are innervated by the radial nerve itself. The nerve terminates on the back of the wrist joint in a slight elevation which sends branches to this joint and to the intercarpal joints.

The posterior interosseous artery arises from the common interosseous artery near the upper border of the interosseous membrane. It passes backward between the radius and the ulna above the upper border of the membrane and appears on the back of the forearm between the supinator and the abductor pollicis longus (Fig. 593 A). It travels in the fascial plane between the superficial and the deep group of extensor muscles with the posterior interosseous nerve and reaches the back of the wrist; its lower part is so slender that it seldom can be traced below the middle of the forearm. It ends by taking part in the anastomosis about the wrist joint. A recurrent branch (the interosseous recurrent artery) passes upward to take part in an anastomosis about the elbow joint.

The supinator muscle (posterior interosseous nerve) should not be confused with the supinator longus muscle (Figs. 592 and 593 A). The term "supinator muscle" means the supinator brevis; the term "supinator longus" has been used for the brachioradialis. The supinator (brevis) arises from the lateral epicondyle of the humerus and the supinator fossa of the ulna. Its fibers pass backward and laterally around the posterior and the lateral aspects of the upper part of the radius and are inserted into the anterior, the lateral and the posterior aspects of that bone. This muscle inserts as far down as the insertion of the pronator teres. The more the radius is pronated, the tighter and more twisted becomes the supinator. Its action is to untwist itself, and this it does by supination.

The abductor pollicis longus muscle (posterior interosseous nerve) arises from the posterior surfaces of both bones of the forearm and from the interosseous membrane. This origin approximately covers the second quarter of the ulna and the middle third of the radius. At the junction of the middle and the lower thirds of the forearm, its tendon emerges between the extensor digitorum and the extensor carpi radialis brevis. Having come to the surface, it crosses the 2 radial extensors (extensor carpi radialis brevis and radialis longus) and is accompanied closely by the extensor pollicis brevis. It passes under the extensor retinaculum and is inserted into the radial side of the base of the metacarpal bone of the thumb. As its name suggests, it is an abductor of the thumb and also slightly assists in abduction of the hand.

The extensor pollicis brevis muscle (posterior interosseous nerve) is placed along the distal border of the preceding muscle. It arises from a small area on the posterior surface of the radius and from the interosseous membrane. Its tendon is associated closely with that of the abductor pollicis longus and accompanies it under the extensor retinaculum. It is inserted by a delicate tendon to the dorsum of the base of the proximal phalanx of the thumb. It extends the proximal phalanx of the thumb; in a small number of cases it is absent.

The extensor pollicis longus muscle (posterior interosseous nerve) arises from the ulna and the interosseous membrane, below the origin of the abductor pollicis longus, and takes an oblique course across the carpus. It is inserted into the base of the distal phalanx of the thumb. It is an extensor of all the joints of the thumb and plays a part in initiating supination of the forearm.

The extensor indicis (proprius) muscle (posterior interosseous nerve) is a special extensor for the index finger, arising from the ulna and the interosseous membrane immediately below the preceding muscles. It passes downward and laterally to the extensor retinaculum, under which it travels in company with the tendons of the extensor digitorum. It terminates by joining the dorsal expansion of the index tendon of that muscle and it lies on the medial side of the most lateral tendon of the common extensor. Its action is to extend all the joints of the index finger.

EXTENSOR RETINACULUM LIGAMENT

The extensor retinaculum (dorsal carpal or posterior annular) ligament is a specialized part of the deep fascia of the forearm which passes obliquely across the back of the limb (Fig. 593). It is about 1 inch wide, has 4 borders and 2 surfaces and is longer than the flexor retinaculum but not as strong. The extensors are not able to spring away from the wrist as are the flexors. The ligament acts as a strap which binds the extensor tendons down and holds them in place and, being obliquely placed, does not interfere with pronation or supination at the wrist.

Its *inferior border* is continuous with the deep fascia of the hand; the *superior* is continuous with the deep fascia of the forearm; the *medial* border is attached to the triquetrum (cuneiform) and pisiform; and the *lateral* is attached to the lower inch of the anterior border of the radius. In this way it forms an annular ligament for the head of the ulna. The retinaculum is not attached to the lower end of the ulna by its medial border; hence, there is no interference with the movements of the radius around the ulna.

The dorsal or *superficial surface* of the extensor retinaculum is crossed by veins draining the dorsal carpal arch; this arch usually lies across the lower part of the back of the hand but is inconstant in position and shape. The arch gives origin to the basilic and the cephalic veins and receives tributaries from 3 dorsal metacarpal veins. Four cutaneous nerves cross superficial to the extensor retinaculum: the dorsal branch of the ulnar nerve, the superficial branch of the radial, and terminations of the posterior branches of the medial and the lateral cutaneous nerves of the forearm.

Five septa, springing from the deep surface of the extensor retinaculum, are attached to the head of the ulna and to the ridges on the back of the lower end of the radius, thus forming 6 compartments for the extensor tendons (Fig. 593 B). In this respect it is unlike the flexor retinaculum, which forms only one large compartment for the flexor tendons. Each compartment transmits 1 or 2 tendons and is lined with a synovial sheath which envelopes the tendon or tendons. Attached to the deep surface of the extensor retinaculum are the *6 compartments* with their enclosed structures. The first compartment is located on the lateral side of the distal end of the radius; it contains the tendons of the abductor pollicis longus and the extensor pollicis brevis. The second compartment contains the extensors carpi radialis longus and brevis; compartment three contains the extensor pollicis longus. The fourth compartment lies over a rather wide but shallow groove at the medial part of the back of the distal end of the radius and contains the tendons of the extensor digitorum as well as the extensor indicis. Deep to these enclosed tendons this compartment also contains the terminal parts of the posterior interosseous nerve and the anterior interosseous artery. The fifth compartment is situated in the interval that exists between the distal ends of the radius and the ulna and it contains the tendon of the extensor digiti minimi. The sixth is the most medial compartment and is marked by a groove over the dorsum of the distal end of the ulna; it encloses the tendon of the extensor carpi ulnaris.

Eight synovial sheaths surround 9 tendons, since each tendon has a synovial sheath of its own, with the exception of the extensor digitorum and the extensor indicis which have a common sheath. The proximal ends of the sheaths are deep to the extensor retinaculum or slightly proximal to it. The sheaths of the abductor pollicis longus and the 3 extensors of the carpus extend to the insertions of these muscles. The sheaths of the extensors of the digits usually end about midlength down the hand. At times the abductor pollicis and the extensor pollicis brevis may have a common sheath. Three oblique bands unite the 4 tendons proximal to the knuckles; hence, the independent action of the fingers is restricted. No one finger can be held in flexion while the others pass into extension.

EXTENSOR (DORSAL) REGION OF THE FOREARM AND THE HAND (DORSUM)

This entire area (muscular) is innervated by the *radial nerve. No motor nerves are found on the dorsum of the hand.* No muscles originate from the dorsum of the hand, and no tendons insert into the dorsum of the carpal bones (Fig. 593).

Skin. Over the lateral posterior aspect of the forearm, the skin is supplied by the lateral cutaneous nerve of the forearm; this is the terminal branch of the musculocutaneous nerve, which becomes cutaneous at the lateral border of the biceps about 1 inch above the elbow (Fig. 580). It divides into anterior and posterior branches, which pass in front of the elbow; they then descend on the front and the back of the radial side of the forearm, the anterior reaching the thenar eminence and the posterior ending at the wrist joint. The medial cutaneous nerve of the forearm is a direct branch of the medial cord of the brachial plexus (Fig. 587). Like the lateral, it too divides into anterior and posterior branches, which descend in front of the elbow and then on the front and the back

of the ulnar side of the forearm to the wrist. The large strip of skin which passes down the middle of the back of the forearm is supplied by the posterior cutaneous nerve of the forearm, a branch of the radial; it becomes cutaneous about 2 inches above the lateral epicondyle, supplies the back of the forearm as far as the wrist and, in most instances, reaches the dorsum of the hand.

The skin of the dorsum of the hand is supplied by the radial nerve and the dorsal branch of the ulnar nerve. The radial nerve winds around the radius, deep to the brachioradialis tendon, about 3 inches above the wrist, and continues downward superficial to the extensor retinaculum; it supplies the skin over the lateral two thirds of the dorsum and sends digital branches to the thumb, the index finger and the radial side of the middle finger. The dorsal branch of the ulnar nerve winds around the ulna about 3 inches above the wrist, descends superficial to the extensor retinaculum and supplies the rest of the skin, namely, that over the dorsum of the hand, the little and the ring fingers, and the ulnar side of the middle finger.

The cutaneous patterns of distribution are variable. The dorsal digital nerves usually do not extend beyond the proximal interphalangeal joints; hence, the rest of the dorsum of each finger receives its nerve supply from the palmar digital nerves.

Fascia. *The superficial fascia* contains an irregular dorsal venous arch which receives digital veins. From its ulnar and radial extremities, respectively, the basilic and the cephalic veins arise and continue upward in the superficial fascia.

The deep fascia is part of a strong layer which forms a tubular investment around the muscles of the forearm. At the olecranon, at the posterior margin of the ulna and at the lateral distal end of the radius it is connected to the periosteum. It separates the extensor from the flexor muscles by a septum which passes along the posterior margin of the ulna. However, on the radial side the separation between extensors and flexors is not developed as definitely. Furthermore, it sends partitions between the individual muscles.

At the dorsal aspect of the wrist the fascia is strengthened greatly by transverse fibers; this forms the *dorsal carpal ligament (pos-*

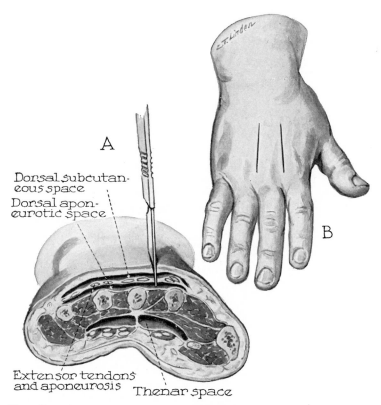

A

Dorsal subcutan-
eous space

Dorsal apon-
eurotic space

B

Extensor tendons
and aponeurosis   Thenar space

FIG. 594. The subcutaneous and the subaponeurotic spaces of the
dorsum of the hand. The drainage of these spaces is indicated.

terior annular or *extensor retinaculum*),
which can be likened to a postage stamp,
having 4 borders and 2 surfaces (Fig. 632).

The fascia over the dorsum of the hand
reveals the *superficial lamina,* a thin layer
under the superficial fascia and above the
tendons of the extensor muscles; on both
sides of the hand it blends with the fascia of
the volar aspect.

The intertendinous lamina is a connecting
membrane which lies between the tendons
of the extensor digitorum. It is very thin in
the white race but thick in the Negro; it is
a rudimentary tendon plate.

The dorsal interosseous lamina lies above
the dorsal interosseus muscles and dips down
to fuse with the periosteum of each metacarpal bone.

**Anatomic Snuffbox (La Tabatière Ana-
tomique of Cloquet).** On the dorsum of the
hand, the hollow at the base of the thumb
is called the "anatomic snuffbox" (Fig. 593).
It is bounded anteriorly by the abductor pol-

licis longus and the extensor pollicis brevis;
posteriorly, by the extensor pollicis longus.
Its floor is formed by the navicular (scaphoid), the trapezium and the articulation between the latter and the first metacarpal
bones. The radial artery lies in this "box"
on its way to the first interosseous space. A
vein lies superficial to the artery and is called
the cephalic vein of Treves; fine branches of
the radial nerve are also found here. The
vein is closer to the skin; the artery lies
deeper and on the lateral ligament of the
bones which form the floor. When ligating
the radial artery it is best to avoid opening
the sheath of the tendons to the thumb or the
scaphoid trapezial joint.

SURGICAL CONSIDERATIONS

Infections of the dorsum of the hand may
involve either the subcutaneous or the subaponeurotic spaces (Fig. 594). The dorsal
subcutaneous space may become involved in
boils or carbuncles; these infections are su-

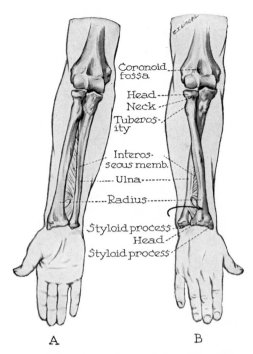

Coronoid
fossa

Head
Neck
Tuberos-
ity

Interos-
seous memb.

Ulna

Radius

Styloid process
Head
Styloid process

A   B

FIG. 595. The radius and the ulna: (A) in supination; (B) in pronation.

perficial to the extensor tendons and the aponeurosis. The dorsal subaponeurotic space infection is uncommon. It may result from perforating dorsal wounds which have pierced the dorsal aponeurosis or may follow an osteomyelitis of the metacarpal or carpal bones. Infections can reach this space from other spaces via the lumbrical sheath. The dorsum almost always becomes edematous in palmar infections because of the loose connective tissue on the back of the hand which is rich in lymphatics; actual suppuration and primary involvement of this space is rare. When pus collects here, it is limited proximally by fibrous partitions at the base of the metacarpals and distally by similar partitions at the metacarpophalangeal joints. Treatment consists of establishing drainage of the abscess through one or more incisions running parallel with the extensor tendons, on the dorsum. The hemostat which opens the space should be placed between the tendons.

RADIUS AND ULNA

The radius and the ulna form the bony framework of the forearm, the radius lying to the lateral and the ulna to the medial side of the superior extremity. These 2 bones articulate above with the humerus and below with the carpal bones of the wrist (Fig. 595). They also articulate with each other at their upper and lower extremities and are firmly united by the ligaments of the radio-ulnar joints and the interosseous membrane. They are so arranged that the radius supports the entire hand and can revolve on a longitudinal axis around the ulna. This action takes place at the radio-ulnar joints and provides the movements of pronation and supination. The ulna, which does not enter into the wrist joint, is the more important bone at the elbow joint; the radius has only a secondary role in the latter location.

RADIUS

The proximal end of the radius has a head, a neck and a radial tuberosity.

The head of the bone is a cup-shaped disk, the upper surface of which is concave and articulates with the capitellum humeri. It is covered by hyaline cartilage, and its circumference articulates with the radial notch of the ulna. Although it is embraced by the annular ligament, the ligament is not attached to it. This disklike head can be felt easily from the posterior aspect of the limb. If the limb is passively extended, a depression becomes visible over the posterior aspect of the elbow on its lateral side. The radial head can be felt in the lower part of it and can be made to rotate within the annular ligament when the hand is alternately pronated and supinated. In the upper part of this depression, the back of the lateral epicondyle of the humerus is palpable, and between these two bony projections the line of the radio-humeral joint is located.

The neck is that constricted portion of the radius which supports the head; it marks the point at which the brachial artery divides into radial and ulnar arteries.

The tuberosity is placed on the medial side below the neck; anteriorly, it is smooth, and a bursa is located here. It is rough posteriorly for the insertion of the biceps tendon.

The shaft of the radius reveals a roughened area over its lateral aspect for the insertion of the pronator teres. The interosseous membrane is attached to the interosseous border of the shaft but does not extend as high as the radial tuberosity.

The **metaphysis** of the upper end of the radius has the following relationships: since the epiphysis is formed by the head of the bone and the capsule is attached to the neck, the metaphysis or the joint may extend to one or the other very readily.

The distal end of the radius, the widest and bulkiest part of the bone, presents 5 notches, a styloid process, a dorsal tubercle and an ulnar notch.

The styloid process is present over the lateral aspect as a downward prolongation which is partially obscured in life by the tendons of the abductor pollicis longus and the extensor pollicis brevis. These tendons should be kept relaxed when the bone is being examined. The styloid processes are of great importance in the diagnosis of fractures of the radius; the radial styloid normally projects about ¼ inch distal to the ulnar styloid.

The dorsal radial tubercle of Lister is the most prominent of the ridges over this area and usually can be felt, since it is grooved obliquely by the tendon of the extensor pollicis longus.

The medial surface is concave and smooth and articulates with the head of the ulna.

The lateral surface is about ½ inch wide and extends onto the ulna and to the styloid process.

The posterior surface is convex and reaches farther down than the anterior; the dorsal tubercle is located about its center. Shallow grooves lateral to the tubercle lodge the tendons of the extensor carpi radialis longus and brevis, and a narrow oblique groove at the medial side of the tubercle marks the tendon of the extensor pollicis longus. A wide, shallow groove medial to this lodges the tendons of the extensor digitorum and the extensor indicis.

The anterior surface is smooth and slightly concave, being limited distally by a thick ridge which can be felt above the wrist and laterally by a sharp edge which separates it from the lateral surface.

The distal or carpal surface is concave, smooth and divided into a lateral and a medial area. The lateral area is triangular and articulates with the scaphoid bone, and the medial area is square and articulates with the lunate bone.

The lower epiphyseal line passes around the bone on the level with the upper margin of the ulnar notch; it does not join the shaft until the 20th year.

The metaphysis in this region has the following relationships: the epiphysis is represented by a horizontal line at the level of the upper part of the ulnar notch, and the capsule is attached very close to the articular margin all the way around. Therefore, the metaphysis is entirely extracapsular. Both bone and joint diseases are more limited than they would be if the upper metaphysis were involved.

Ulna

The ulna is the medial and longer bone of the forearm. Its proximal end presents an olecranon, a coronoid process and radial and trochlear notches.

The olecranon is easily palpable posteriorly, and in extension the upper edge of this process is on the same level as the epicondyle of the humerus. It gives insertion to the tendon of the triceps.

The coronoid process projects forward and ossifies with the shaft; its anterior aspect is covered by and gives insertion to the brachialis muscle.

The radial notch is located over the lateral surface, is concave and articulates with the head of the radius. Its inferior and posterior borders give attachment to the annular ligament.

The trochlear notch (incisura semilunaris) is a wide concavity bounded by the olecranon and the coronoid; it articulates with the trochlea.

The shaft of the ulna tapers as it passes distally; the posterior border of the shaft is subcutaneous in its whole length from the posterior aspect of the olecranon to its styloid process.

The distal end of the ulna presents a head and a styloid process.

The head is small and rounded, and its distal surface articulates with the triangular articular disk. The head of the ulna can be grasped between the fingers and the thumb when the flexors and the extensors are re-

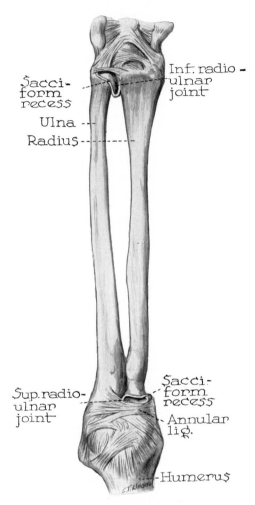

Inf. radio-ulnar joint

Sacci-form recess

Ulna

Radius

Sup. radio-ulnar joint

Sacci-form recess

Annular lig.

Humerus

FIG. 596. The superior and the inferior radio-ulnar joints.

of the articular surface for the radius; the capsule is attached to the margins of the articular surface, except laterally, where it is a little proximal to the radial articular surface. Therefore, the metaphysis in this location is partly intracapsular, and diseases of the bone or the joint may spread in either direction.

RADIO-ULNAR JOINTS

The radius and the ulnar are united at proximal and distal radio-ulnar joints. There is an intermediate "joint" where the bodies of the 2 bones are united by the oblique cord, the interosseous membrane, and the posterior layer of the fascia which covers the pronator quadratus (Fig. 596).

The interosseous membrane of the forearm is a fibrous sheath which stretches across the interval between the 2 bones of the forearm and is attached to the interosseous border of each. It begins about 1 inch below the radial tuberosity and extends to and blends with the capsule of the inferior radio-ulnar joint. Its fibers pass downward and mediad from the radius to the ulna, so that shocks transmitted to the radius from the hand are passed on to the ulna and then to the humerus. Over the anterior surface of this membrane and from its upper three quarters the flexor pollicis longus and the digitorum profundus arise; the anterior interosseous vessels lie between them and perforate the membrane near its lower end. The pronator quadratus lies on the lower one fourth. The posterior surface gives origin to the abductor pollicis longus, the extensors pollicis brevis and longus, and the extensor indicis. The supinator lies on its anterior part, the anterior interosseous vessels and the posterior interosseous nerve on its lower part. The oblique cord is a slender band arising from the tuberosity of the ulna and extending downward and laterally; it attaches to the radius immediately below its tuberosity. This cord crosses the open space between the bones of the forearm above the upper border of the interosseous membrane. The posterior interosseous vessels pass backward through the gap which exists between this cord and the interosseous membrane.

Superior (Proximal) Radio-ulnar Joint. This joint is considered with the elbow joint

laxed, and in some individuals it presents a conspicuous prominence in full pronation.

The styloid process projects downward from the posteromedial aspect of the head and is felt best when the hand is in full supination.

The upper and the lower metaphyses have the following relations: at the upper end, the epiphysis may be variable but it usually is represented as a flake of bone on the upper surface over its whole extent. Therefore, this epiphysis is entirely extracapsular, so that the metaphysis and part of the diaphysis are related to the capsular line. At the lower end, the epiphysis is represented by a horizontal line at the level of the upper extremity

because they have a common synovial cavity, and the lateral ligament of the elbow joint is connected to the annular ligament of the superior radio-ulnar joint (Fig. 596). At this joint the medial part of the head of the radius fits into the radial notch of the ulna.

The annular ligament forms a collar for the head of the radius; this collar retains the

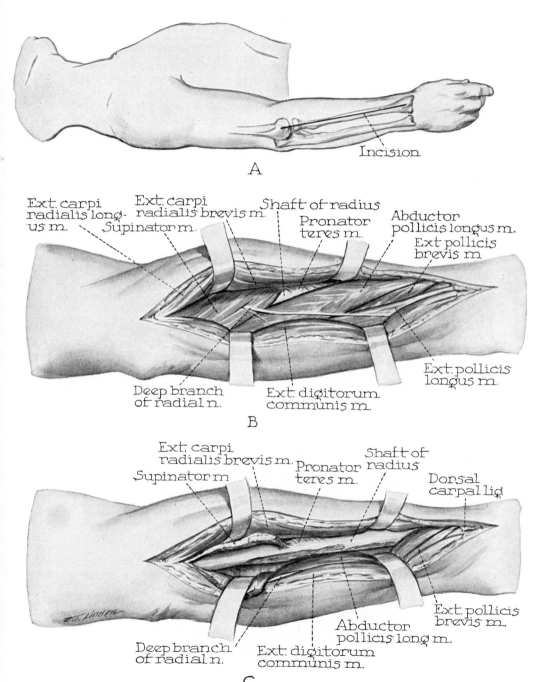

FIG. 597. Exposure of the shaft of the radius: (A) incision; (B) relations of the deep branch of the radial nerve (dorsal interosseous); (C) the exposed shaft of the radius.

radial head in the radial notch of the ulna. This ligament forms four fifths of a circle which is attached to the anterior and the posterior margins of the notch. It is narrower below than above; hence, the head of the radius cannot be pulled downward and out. The lower border of the ligament is free; this allows the head of the radius to rotate during pronation and supination.

The synovial membrane of the joint lines the deep surface of the annular ligament and is continuous with that of the elbow joint, so that the joint cavities communicate freely. It lines the deep surface of the annular ligament and bulges slightly below it, producing a sacciform recess which encircles the neck of the radius.

Inferior (Distal) Radio-ulnar Joint. This is a synovial joint formed by the head of the ulna where it articulates with the ulnar notch of the radius laterally and the articular disk inferiorly (Fig. 596). Union is maintained by the articular disk and is aided by a weak capsular ligament passing between the margins of the articular surfaces.

The articular disk is a thick triangular fibrocartilaginous plate. Its apex is related to the depression at the base of the ulnar styloid process, and its base to the lower border of the ulnar notch of the radius. Its anterior and posterior margins blend with the corresponding ligament of the radiocarpal joint. Although it usually is a complete plate, it may be perforated. When this occurs, the joint cavities and the synovial membranes of the inferior radio-ulnar and the radiocarpal (wrist) joints become continuous.

The capsular ligament is weak, possessing feeble anterior and posterior ligaments which invest the anterior, the posterior and the superior aspects of the joint. It is continuous with the capsular ligament of the wrist joint.

The synovial membrane lines the capsular ligament and the upper surface of the articular disk. It projects upward to form a small cul-de-sac (recessus sacciformis) in front of the lower end of the interosseous membrane. The joint is supplied by the anterior and the posterior interosseous nerves and vessels.

Movements of the Radio-ulnar Joints. The *rotary* movements of these joints take place around a vertical axis which passes through the center of the head of the radius above and the ulnar attachment of the triangular articular disk below.

Supination, the position in which the bones of the forearm are parallel and the thumb points laterally, is produced mainly by the supinator, the biceps and the brachioradialis.

In *pronation* the radius crosses in front of

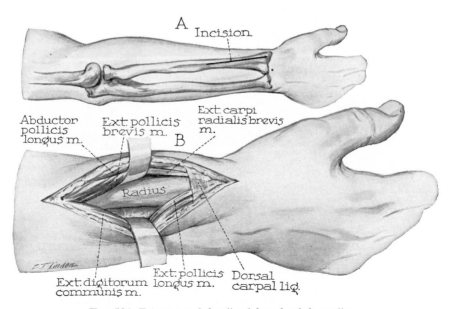

Fig. 598. Exposure of the distal fourth of the radius.

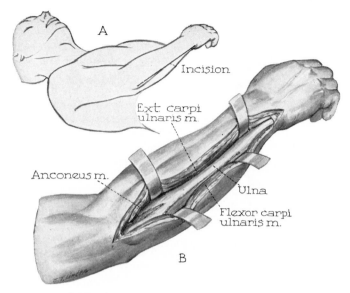

FIG. 599. Exposure of the shaft of the ulna.

the ulna, the upper end remaining lateral and the thumb pointing medially. Supination is the strongest movement, due to the strength of the biceps. Starting from the supine position, the upper limb can be rotated so that the palm, originally directed forward, can be directed successively medially, backward and laterally, moving through an arc of 270°. However, the greater part of that movement is not pronation but medial rotation at the shoulder joint. Pronation alone can move through an arc of about 130°.

SURGICAL CONSIDERATIONS

EXPOSURE OF THE SHAFT OF THE RADIUS

This is accomplished through an incision over the dorsal aspect of the forearm (Fig. 597). The deep fascia is divided, and the extensor digitorum communis is retracted. This exposes the supinator muscle and the deep branch of the radial nerve (dorsal interosseous) piercing it. The supinator is divided longitudinally to the bone and retracted with the muscles of the thumb. The extensor carpi radialis brevis is retracted in the opposite direction, and the shaft of the radius is exposed.

EXPOSURE OF THE DISTAL FOURTH OF THE RADIUS

Exposure of the distal fourth of the radius is accomplished through an incision, about 3 or 4 inches long, extending upward and medially along the dorsal aspect of the bone (Fig. 598). The deep fascia and the dorsal carpal ligament are incised, exposing the extensor digitorum communis muscle, the extensor pollicis longus tendon, the extensor pollicis brevis muscle, the abductor pollicis longus muscle and the tendon of the extensor carpi radialis brevis; a small part of the radius also is visible. The abductor pollicis longus, the extensor pollicis brevis and the tendon of the extensor carpi radialis brevis are retracted laterally, and the extensor digitorum communis and the tendon of the extensor pollicis longus are retracted medially. This will expose the distal fourth of the radial shaft.

EXPOSURE OF THE SHAFT OF THE ULNA

In the exposure of the shaft of the ulna, the location of the incision depends on the part of the bone requiring exposure (Fig. 599). The incision is located somewhere on a line drawn between the olecranon and the ulnar styloid. The flexor carpi ulnaris is retracted medially, and the extensor carpi ulnaris and the anconeus are retracted laterally. These muscles must be stripped off of the bone with an osteotome. Thus the shaft of the ulna can be exposed in its entire length.

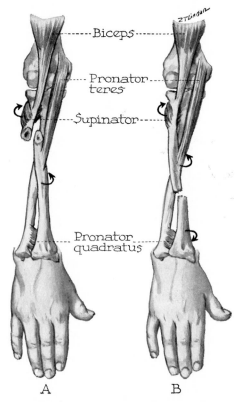

FIG. 600. Fractures of the radius in relation to the pronator teres muscle: (A) fracture above the insertion of the pronator teres; (B) fracture below the insertion of the pronator teres.

FRACTURES OF THE FOREARM

Fractures of the forearm present many problems in mechanics because of the complicated system of muscles which control movements of the hand and the fingers. For practical purposes some anatomists consider the ulna a downward extension of the arm which is associated with motion and strength of the elbow, and the radius an upward extension of the hand concerned with motions of the hand and the wrist. Therefore, the principal articulation of the ulna is with the humerus, and that of the radius is at the wrist. It is well known that the head of the radius may be removed from its articulation with the humerus without causing any disability to the elbow. The 2 forearm bones are joined by the interosseous membrane, the fibers of which run from the ulna to the radius in an upward direction.

If *both bones* of the forearm are fractured, the membrane has a tendency to pull the ulna toward the radius. In the important motions of pronation and supination, the ulna remains fixed and the radius rotates around it so that when the hand is in full pronation the radius comes to lie immediately over the ulna, crossing it a little above its middle. The distance between the bones is greatest in semipronation.

The pronator teres muscle is the important landmark in fractures of the forearm. It is located a little above the middle of the radius, and it must be determined whether the fracture is above or below its insertion (Fig. 600). In a fracture of the radius *above* the insertion of the pronator teres, the upper fragment of the radius is pulled into supination by the supinator brevis and the biceps; the lower fragment is fully pronated. In such a fracture the biceps also will accomplish some flexion of the proximal fragment. In fractures *below* the attachment of the pronator teres, the supinator brevis and the pronator teres will equalize each other between pronation and supination in the upper fragment, and the lower fragment will be in full pronation.

The correct position for a radius fractured above the insertion of the pronator teres is with the elbow flexed and the hand supinated. In fractures below the pronator teres, the thumb up (midprone) position is used with flexion at the elbow. In this position the palm of the hand faces the chest. The important rule in all fractures of the radius above the position of a Colles' fracture is to keep the elbow flexed, otherwise it will be impossible to maintain the forearm in any given position of rotation.

Where both the radius and the ulna are fractured, the broken ends of bone are usually drawn together by the supinators and the pronators, and the interosseous space is narrowed. The lower fragments may be displaced laterally or anteroposteriorly with overriding. Shortening of the forearm results.

The upper part of the *shaft of the ulna* may be fractured; this usually is associated with anterior dislocation of the head of the radius due to the fact that the annular (orbicular) ligament also may be torn. This is so common an occurrence that in all fractures

of the upper part of the ulna, radial dislocation should be ruled out. Fractures along
other parts of the ulnar shaft are usually
transverse and occur in the distal third of
the bone, where muscle masses are replaced
by tendons. Marked displacement usually is
absent because of the splinting effect of the
intact radius. However, there is a tendency
toward a narrowing of the interosseous space;
this is brought about by a pull from the pronator quadratus muscle upon the lower
fragment.

FRACTURE OF THE HEAD AND THE NECK OF THE RADIUS

This usually occurs in adults from indirect
violence, such as a fall on the palm. Such
a fracture produces interference with flexion
and rotation of the forearm; these movements may produce crepitus. Reduction is
brought about by pressure and flexion, and
fixation is maintained in supination and flexion. Excision may be necessary. Fracture of
the neck of the radius usually results from
indirect violence, the fracture occurring between the head and the bicipital tuberosity.
The treatment may be open or closed reduction.

COLLES' FRACTURE

Colles' fracture involves the lower end of
the radius; it is nearly transverse and within
1 inch of the articular surface of the bone. It
produces a deformity due to dorsal displacement of the distal fragment and volar displacement of the proximal. Usually it is due
to a fall on the extended hand, and the typical sign is the "silver fork" deformity, in
which there is a prominence on the back
of the wrist and a lateral displacement of
the hand toward the radial side. This is not
present if the fracture is impacted or incomplete. If proper reduction has been accomplished, the surface markings can be
made out even in the presence of swelling.
Normal relations should exist between the
styloid processes, and a uniform line should
be present along the forearm through the
wrist and to the hand.

A reverse Colles' fracture is called Smith's
fracture. This usually is produced by a fall
on the back of the hand with the wrist flexed.

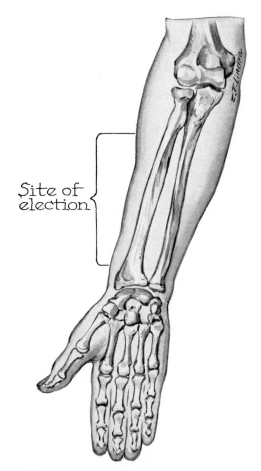

FIG. 601. Site of election in forearm
amputations.

Epiphyseal separation may be confused
with a Colles' fracture. It is common in children and may occur at any time up to the
18th or the 20th year. Since the radius takes
the brunt of the injury in falls on the outstretched hand, separation of the distal ulnar
epiphysis is rare.

AMPUTATIONS

The site of election in forearm amputations
is at the junction of the lower and the middle
thirds. However, any site above this junction to within 3 or 4 inches of the elbow will
produce a good stump (Fig. 601). A short
forearm stump is difficult to fit because the
biceps muscle pushes the limb socket when
the elbow is flexed.

In amputations of the forearm, anterior
and posterior U-shaped incisions are made

through the skin and the superficial fascia, thus outlining the flaps. The vertical incisions are carried through the muscles to the bone. The muscles on the anterior and the posterior aspects of the forearm are divided to the bone, and the periosteum is freed and retracted upward. The interosseous membrane is cut transversely at approximately the saw line, the soft parts are retracted, and the bones are sawed. Attempt is made to ligate separately the radial, the ulnar, and the anterior and the posterior interosseous arteries. The median, the ulnar and the radial nerves are cut short. The muscles and the deep fascia are closed over the bone ends, and the skin is closed with interrupted sutures.

Wrist

The wrist is the link between the forearm and the hand. It contains the soft parts, the bones and the joints in that area which includes the carpus, the distal extremities of the radius and the ulna, and the bases of the metacarpals. The radiocarpal, the midcarpal and the carpometacarpal joints are located in the wrist, and it is in this region that the tendons of the forearm cross on their way to insert onto the carpus. The tendons are held close to the wrist bones by thickenings of the deep fascia which form ligaments.

CARPAL BONES

There are 8 small carpal bones which are arranged in 2 rows: proximal and distal.

Each row consists of 4 bones which have received their names according to their general appearance. The proximal row, named from lateral to medial, consists of the navicular (scaphoid), the lunate (semilunar), the triquetrum (cuneiform) and the pisiform. The distal row, named from lateral to medial, presents the greater multangular (trapezium), the lesser multangular (trapezoid), the capitate (os magnum) and the hamate (unciform) (Fig. 602).

These 8 bones are more or less cubical in shape and, therefore, have 6 surfaces: proximal, lateral, distal, medial, palmar and dorsal. Of these, only 2 surfaces, the anterior and the posterior, are roughened by the attach-

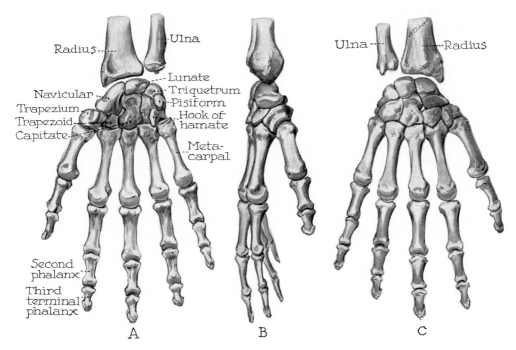

FIG. 602. The carpal bones: (A) seen from in front; (B) seen from the radial side; (C) seen from behind.

705

ments of the ligaments. The remaining 4 surfaces, which articulate with adjacent bones, remain smooth and are entirely or partly covered with cartilage. The lateral surfaces of the lateral bones and the medial surfaces of the medial bones also receive ligamentous bands and are also roughened.

The navicular (boat-shaped) bone does not withstand an indirect blow well. Such a blow may be received by falling on the palm of the hand in radial deviation. The bone is not adapted to receive such trauma because of its curved shape and obliquely curved axis. However, if the fall occurs, with the hand in ulnar deviation, only the proximal part of the bone is exposed to trauma. The navicular is the most commonly fractured of all the carpals.

The tubercle of the scaphoid can be felt through the skin at the base of the thenar eminence and in line with the radial side of the middle finger. At times it forms a visible protrusion, but it usually is concealed by the tendon of the flexor carpi radialis, which inserts on it and can be felt when that muscle is relaxed. The distal transverse crease at the front of the wrist crosses this tubercle and the pisiform bone.

The lunate (moon-shaped) is the middle bone of the proximal row; its distal articular surface, with a part of the distal scaphoid articular surface, lodges the head of the capitate bone. It is the carpal bone which is dislocated most frequently.

The triquetrum (triangular-shaped) articulates with the articular disk, and by means of a specialized surface it also articulates with the ulnar collateral ligament. This arrangement permits the triquetrum, with the pisiform on its volar aspect, to glide toward the ulna in ulnar flexion. The remainder of the proximal surface of the bone is nonarticular. The scaphoid, the lunate and the triquetral bones form the carpal articular surface in the radiocarpal joint.

The pisiform (pea-shaped) bone is located at the base of the hypothenar eminence on the medial side of the front of the wrist. Many anatomists consider it a sesamoid bone in the tendon of the flexor carpi ulnaris. When this tendon is relaxed, the bone can be moved about on the palmar surface of the triquetrum, thus revealing an isolated facet for the pisiform. The latter bone does not enter into the radiocarpal joint.

The trapezium (greater multangular) is the most radially placed bone of the distal row. This and the scaphoid can be palpated in the "anatomic snuffbox," the hollow at the lateral side of the wrist which is situated between the styloid process of the radius proximally and the base of the metacarpal of the thumb distally. In this location the radial artery crosses these bones, and its pulsations can be felt here.

The trapezoid and the trapezium are placed distally to the capitate. With the exception of the pisiform, the trapezoid is the smallest of the carpal bones, and it has been likened to a Chinese boot.

The capitate (headlike) is the largest of the carpal bones; it is centrally placed and appears most prominent. It has a head, a neck and a body. The head occupies the deep concavity on the medial side of the first row of bones, and the body below supports the 2nd, the 3rd and the 4th metacarpal bones. It is the head of the capitate which transmits the force of a fall upon the hand to the radius through the navicular and the lunate bones.

The hamate (hooklike) bone presents a projecting process, the hook of the hamate, which can be identified through the skin. It can be felt in the ball of the little finger about 1 inch below and lateral to the pisiform and in a line with the ulnar border of the ring finger. The interval between the hook and the pisiform allows the passage of the ulnar artery and nerve.

The carpus is cartilaginous at birth. Complete ossification takes place between the 20th and the 25th years. The capitate, which is the largest of the carpal bones, begins to ossify during the 1st year; with the exception of the pisiform, which undergoes ossification about the 12th year, all the carpal bones are in the process of ossification by the 8th year. As a whole, the bones of the carpus are fitted closely together but permit a certain amount of movement, thereby giving a degree of flexibility to the wrist. The proximal surface of the carpus reveals that the pisiform has been placed in front of the triquetrum, leaving only 3 bones of the proximal row in the articulation with the wrist joint above and the distal row of carpal bones below. The

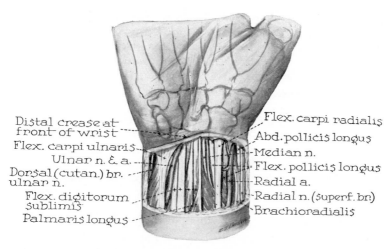

Distal crease at front of wrist
Flex. carpi ulnaris
Ulnar n. & a.
Dorsal (cutan.) br. ulnar n.
Flex. digitorum sublimis
Palmaris longus

Flex. carpi radialis
Abd. pollicis longus
Median n.
Flex. pollicis longus
Radial a.
Radial n. (superf. br.)
Brachioradialis

FIG. 603. The distal skin crease of the wrist.

widened distal end of the scaphoid supports 2 bones: the trapezium and the trapezoid. The distal surface of the carpus, on the other hand, is quite irregular, since 5 metacarpal bones must articulate with 4 distal carpal bones. The 4th and the 5th metacarpals articulate with the hamate. The carpus as a whole forms a surface which is concave from side to side on its palmar aspect and convex over its dorsum; the extremities of this concavity give attachment to the flexor retinaculum (transverse carpal ligament)

(p. 708). This ligament, plus its bony attachment, forms the osteofascial tunnel for the flexor tendons of the fingers.

DISTAL SKIN CREASE

The distal skin crease of the wrist is always visible and is an excellent landmark (Fig. 603). It crosses the tip of the styloid process of the radius and the lower part of the lunate bone. It has the following features: it marks the *proximal border* of the transverse carpal ligament and the *proximal row* of the

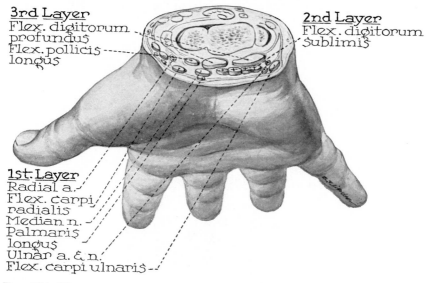

3rd Layer
Flex. digitorum profundus
Flex. pollicis longus

2nd Layer
Flex. digitorum Sublimis

1st. Layer
Radial a.
Flex. carpi radialis
Median n.
Palmaris longus
Ulnar a. & n.
Flex. carpi ulnaris

FIG. 604. The structures which are located proximal to the distal skin crease of the wrist. These structures are considered as lying in 3 layers.

carpal bones. It is bisected by the tendon of the palmaris longus (the clenched fist renders this tendon prominent). The median nerve lies immediately beneath the tendon of the palmaris longus; therefore, we may say that the median nerve bisects the crease. The flexor carpi radialis tendon crosses its lateral third, and the flexor carpi ulnaris is at the extreme medial end of the crease.

It is interesting to flex the index finger and observe the wrist. Although the index is placed radially, the tendon produces movements on the ulnar side of the wrist. This illustrates the point that all the tendons of the flexor digitorum sublimis and the profundus lie on the ulnar side of the wrist; therefore, these tendons lie between the ulnar and the median nerves.

Structures That Are Proximal to the Distal Skin Crease. These structures will be remembered more easily if they are discussed and visualized in layers or planes (Fig. 604).

The first layer of structures consists of, from lateral to medial: the radial artery, the flexor carpi radialis tendon, the palmaris longus tendon, the median nerve, the flexor carpi ulnaris and the ulnar artery and nerve.

The radial artery, after crossing the pronator quadratus, comes in contact with the lower end of the radius. It then lies on the skeletal plane, and in this region it is covered only by skin, superficial and deep fascia. Therefore, this is the correct site to feel the pulse. The artery is no longer in relation to the major portion of the radial nerve, since the latter leaves it by winding around the radial border of the forearm deep to the brachioradialis tendon. The artery disappears deep to the abductor pollicis longus tendon.

The flexor carpi radialis tendon lies between the radial artery and the median nerve. As it passes distally, it pierces the deep fascia (flexor retinaculum), making a private tunnel for itself. In its course it travels over the tubercle of the scaphoid bone and may be used as a guide to this latter structure.

The palmaris longus tendon is not always present, but if it is, it crosses at a point which is in the middle of the wrist and, therefore, bisects the distal skin crease. It crosses in front of the flexor retinaculum and continues into the palm as the palmar aponeurosis; it lies immediately above the median nerve. If this tendon is absent, the nerve is more exposed to injury; hence, this tendon might be considered as the "roof" or "protector" of the median nerve.

The median nerve is behind the flexor digitorum sublimis in the forearm, but in the region of the wrist it appears at the lateral border of and somewhat above this muscle. It is differentiated from the surrounding tendons by the fact that numerous small vessels (vaso nervorum) are noted distinctly on its surface. At the wrist it lies directly behind the palmaris longus tendon, the deep

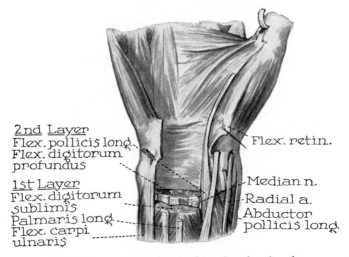

2nd Layer
Flex. pollicis long.
Flex. digitorum
profundus

1st Layer
Flex. digitorum
sublimis
Palmaris long.
Flex. carpi
ulnaris

Flex. retin.

Median n.
Radial a.
Abductor
pollicis long.

FIG. 605. Deep dissection in the wrist, showing the arrangement of the tendons.

fascia intervening between the palmaris longus and the nerve; the latter usually clings to this deep fascia. At times a small "median artery" accompanies it.

The flexor carpi ulnaris tendon lies at the medial extremity of the distal skin crease. It forms a "roof" and protection for the ulnar nerve and artery and acts as a guide to the pisiform bone. The muscle does not become entirely tendinous, but as far as the wrist, distinct muscular fibers of the flexor carpi ulnaris accompany the tendon, so that it is really half tendon and half muscle.

The ulnar artery and nerve are both protected by the overlying flexor carpi ulnaris tendon. They are bound together closely by connective tissue, and it is extremely difficult to ligate the artery in this region without incorporating the nerve.

The second layer consists of the *flexor digitorum sublimis.* This group of 4 tendons lies between the median and the ulnar nerves, and, as they pass forward into the palm, the tendons of the middle and the ring fingers are placed somewhat in front of those for the index and the little fingers (Fig. 605).

The third layer consists of the flexor digitorum profundus and the flexor pollicis longus. The 4 tendons of the *flexor digitorum profundus* enter the hand by passing behind the sublimis. The tendon for the index finger separates from the remainder of the muscle about halfway down the forearm and represents a large structure. These 4 tendons do not lie 2 upon 2, as do the tendons of the flexor digitorum sublimis, but they all lie in the same plane (Fig. 605). The *flexor pollicis longus* tendon lies in the same plane as the flexor digitorum profundus but is easily separated from it, since it travels in its own synovial sheath. It is found immediately beneath and lateral to the median nerve. At the extreme lateral (radial) margin of the wrist, the tendons of the abductor pollicis longus and the extensor pollicis brevis are found. They form the anterior margin of the "anatomic snuffbox" (p. 695).

Structures That Are Distal to the Distal Skin Crease. The *transverse carpal ligament* has been referred to as the anterior annular ligament and the flexor retinaculum. It is a specialized portion of the deep fascia of the forearm which assumes the form of a tough

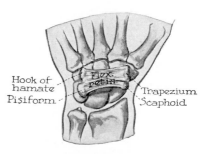

FIG. 606. The flexor retinaculum (transverse carpal ligament). Its attachments to the 4 end bones of the carpus are shown.

fibrous band stretching across the arch formed by the carpal bones. It attaches to the 4 end bones of the carpus, namely, the navicular (scaphoid) and the greater multangular (trapezium) laterally, and the pisiform and the hamate medially (Fig. 606).

The arched carpal bones and the transverse carpal ligament form an osseofibrous tunnel called the *carpal tunnel.* Proximally, the ligament is continuous with the deep fascia of the forearm; distally, it merges with the palmar fascia.

The structures *superficial* to the transverse carpal ligament are the palmaris longus tendon, the ulnar nerve and artery, the superficial branch of the radial artery and the cutaneous nerves and veins.

The structures passing *deep* to the transverse carpal ligament are the median nerve, the flexor digitorum sublimis, the flexor digitorum profundus and the flexor pollicis longus.

Unnecessary confusion seems to exist between the volar carpal ligament and the transverse carpal ligament. The *volar carpal ligament* is a fascial process which passes from the pisiform bone and the flexor carpi ulnaris medially to the palmar surface of the transverse carpal ligament laterally. In this way it forms the roof of a tunnel for the ulnar artery and nerve, the floor of the tunnel being formed by the medial border of the transverse carpal ligament. The median nerve, the flexor digitorum sublimis, the flexor digitorum profundus and the flexor pollicis longus cross under the ligament. The flexor carpi radialis goes through the ligament, creating in this way a fibrous tunnel for itself.

JOINTS

RADIOCARPAL (WRIST) JOINT

This is the joint which exists between the forearm and the hand, the other joints in this region being known as the intercarpal joints (Fig. 607). The proximal surface of the radiocarpal joint is formed by the concave lower articular surface of the radius and the articular disk. The distal surface is formed by the convex scaphoid, the lunate and the triquetral bones. Union is maintained by a capsular ligament which is strengthened by the anterior and the posterior radiocarpal, and the lateral and the medial ligaments of the wrist.

The capsular ligament is of moderate strength and is attached close to the margins of the articular surfaces.

The anterior and the posterior ligaments only moderately strengthen their respective aspects of the capsule. The fibers of these ligaments pass obliquely downward and medially from the front and the back of the proximal row of carpal bones and to the capitate. Therefore, during pronation and supination of the forearm, the radius drags the carpal bones after it.

The lateral (radial collateral) ligament passes from the radial styloid process to the tuberosity of the navicular and the greater multangular. The radial artery crosses it.

The medial (ulnar collateral) ligament extends from the styloid process of the ulna to the pisiform and the triquetrum.

The synovial membrane lines the interior of the capsular ligament, the inferior surface of the articular disk and the 2 interosseous ligaments which complete the carpal surface. It does not communicate with the intercarpal joints. The blood supply is derived from the carpal branches of the radial, the ulnar and the interosseous arteries and the recurrent branches of the deep palmar arch. The nerve supply of the radiocarpal joint is derived from the anterior and the posterior interosseous nerves and the dorsal and the deep branches of the ulnar nerve.

The active movements at the wrist joint are flexion, extension, abduction (radial deviation), adduction (ulnar deviation) and circumduction, the last being produced by a combination of the preceding movements. Rotation of the carpus and the hand around a vertical axis cannot be performed actively. Movements are checked in some cases by ligaments and tendons. When the fingers are flexed, the stretched extensor tendons do not allow full flexion of the wrist. Abduction is less free than adduction because the styloid of the radius meets the carpus.

INTERCARPAL JOINTS

In the carpus there are 2 joint cavities: the pisiform and the transverse carpal (Fig. 608).

The pisiform joint is a small synovial joint which possesses a capsular ligament and a synovial membrane. Its cavity is shut off from the other joint cavities of the carpus.

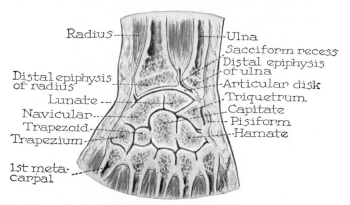

FIG. 607. The radiocarpal (wrist) joint, seen in frontal section.

The transverse carpal joint is a synovial joint which is common to the other intercarpal joints; it also has been referred to as the intercarpal or midcarpal joint. It is located between the bones of the proximal and distal rows of the wrist. These bones are connected to one another by palmar and dorsal ligaments, and at the radial and the ulnar extremities of the joint, by the lateral and the medial ligaments. The synovial membrane which lines this joint cavity is thin, not only between the two rows of bones, but also between the scaphoid and the lunate, between the lunate and the triquetral and downward between the bones of the distal row. Generally the cavity communicates with the joint cavities of the 4 medial carpometacarpal and the intermetacarpal joints. The opposed surfaces of the carpal bones, which are nonarticular, are connected to each other by interosseous ligaments.

The intercarpal joints derive their nerve supply from the anterior and the posterior interosseous nerves and the dorsal and the deep branches of the ulnar nerve. The movements at these joints supplement those at the radiocarpal joints and increase the range of movements of the hand. Between the individual bones of each row the movements are of a gliding nature and are quite limited.

Carpometacarpal and Intermetacarpal Joints

The metacarpal bone of the thumb articulates with the os trapezium by a joint which is entirely separated from the other carpometacarpal joints (Fig. 608). It is a synovial joint of the saddle variety and, because of its shape, permits a wide range of movements. The articular capsule which surrounds it is sufficiently lax to permit these movements.

The medial 4 metacarpal bones are connected to the carpus by the palmar and the dorsal ligaments and by one interosseous ligament. A medial ligament is present also; this closes the medial side of the joint of the 5th metacarpal bone. The interosseous ligament arises from the contiguous distal margins of the capitate and the hamate bones and runs to the medial side of the base of the 3rd metacarpal bone. The metacarpal bones of the fingers are united by strong ligaments and articulate with each other at their bases.

The ligaments which bind the medial 4 metacarpals together are: (1) a series of palmar and dorsal metacarpal ligaments which pass transversely between the palmar and the dorsal surfaces of the bases; (2) three interosseous ligaments which pass between the nonarticular parts of the sides of contiguous bases; (3) the deep transverse ligament of the palm, which indirectly connects the heads of the bones. Though the intercarpal, the carpometacarpal and the intermetacarpal joints are spoken of individually as having separate ligaments, these constitute one single ligament which surrounds a continuous joint cavity. (The pisiform joint and the carpometacarpal joint of the thumb possess separate capsules.) The synovial membrane lines all the ligaments and is

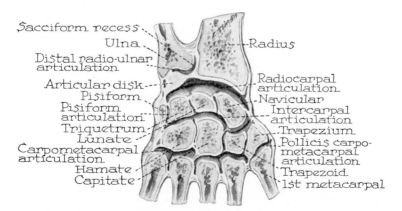

Fig. 608. The radiocarpal, the intercarpal and the carpometacarpal joints. Frontal section through the joints of the carpus.

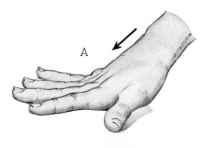

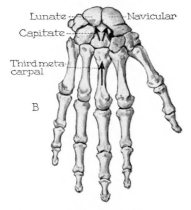

FIG. 609. The mechanism of injury to the navicular or lunate bone. The arrows indicate the direction of force following a fall on the outstretched hand.

prolonged over all the intra-articular parts of the bone that do not contain articular cartilage.

METACARPOPHALANGEAL AND INTERPHALANGEAL JOINTS

The metacarpophalangeal joints are synovial joints which form where the head of the metacarpal articulates distally with the base of the proximal phalanx and anteriorly with the palmar ligament. Union is maintained by a capsular ligament which is greatly strengthened in front by the palmar ligament and at the sides by collateral ligaments.

The capsular ligament is attached near the margin of the articular surfaces, but posteriorly it is defective, and its place is taken by the expanded extensor tendon.

The collateral ligaments are strong oblique bands which pass downward and forward from the sides of the head of the proximal bone of the joint to the sides of the base of the distal bone.

The palmar ligament is a dense fibrous plate which is the thickened palmar part of the capsular ligament. At the sides it fuses with the collateral ligaments and is connected with the deep transverse ligaments of the palm. Distally, it is attached to the base of the phalanx; proximally, it is loosely connected with the palmar surface of the metacarpal immediately above the head. It forms part of the socket and articulates with the front of the head. Its palmar surface is smooth and is covered by the flexor tendons and their synovial sheaths. In a metacarpophalangeal joint of a finger, the margins of the palmar ligament give attachment to the deep transverse ligament of the palm and partial attachment to the processes of the palmar aponeurosis.

The interphalangeal joints are similar in structure to the metacarpophalangeal joints. They are of the synovial variety and have capsular, collateral and palmar ligaments. The interphalangeal joints have ligaments corresponding to those of the metacarpophalangeal joints but, since they do not have rounded heads, they do not permit adduction or abduction.

SURGICAL CONSIDERATIONS

Injuries to the carpal bones result from falls on the outstretched palm, the force being directed from the 3rd metacarpal to the capitate and then to the navicular and the lunate (Fig. 609). Any type of injury may result; the most common is fracture of the navicular, and the next most frequent is dislocation of the lunate.

FRACTURE OF THE NAVICULAR (SCAPHOID) BONE

This fracture is more frequent than had been suspected previously. As a result of a fall on the outstretched hand, the navicular is brought directly under the radius and is pinched between it and the capitate bone. Treatment is by reduction and immobilization. Excision of the navicular, either total or partial, should be avoided, if possible, since this leaves a permanent disability.

DISLOCATION OF THE LUNATE (SEMILUNAR) BONE

Dislocation of this bone is caused by a fall on the outstretched hand which results in a momentary backward dislocation of the wrist. Since the lunate is attached more firmly to the radius and the ulna than are the other carpal bones, it does not take place in the backward dislocation; its ligamentous connection with the other carpals is torn. The backward wrist dislocation spontaneously reduces itself and, on returning, knocks the lunate forward. The proximity of the median nerve must be kept in mind, since an anteriorly dislocated lunate may produce signs of median nerve involvement. The dorsal ligament, which contains the important nutrient vessel to the bone, may be injured, and this may result in a progressive degeneration called Kienböch's disease.

DISLOCATIONS OF THE WRIST
Dislocations of the wrist are rare; they may be forward or backward, and their importance is mainly in their recognition, since they may resemble a Colles' or Smith's fracture. In dislocations the relationship between the styloid processes is preserved, but the relation of the carpal bones to these processes is altered. Dislocation usually involves the radiocarpal articulation; frequently, it is compound, and the articular edge of the radius may be fractured. True dislocation may occur from great violence, and the inferior end of the radius and the ulna then protrude, either to the dorsal or the volar surface of the wrist. In dorsal dislocation of the carpus, the deformity may resemble a Colles' fracture but it is closer to the hand. Dislocation of the inferior radio-ulnar joint is an extremely rare wrist dislocation, but it may complicate a fracture. Reduction should be accomplished by pressure on the displaced bone with supination.

ARTHRODESIS OF THE WRIST JOINT
A surgical bony ankylosis of the wrist joint

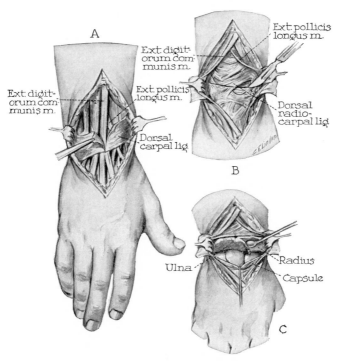

FIG 610. Arthrodesis of the wrist joint: (A) skin incision and division of the dorsal carpal ligament; (B) retraction of the extensor tendons and incision into the capsule; (C) the joint cavity is exposed, and the radius is curetted.

usually is created for flail wrist, ankylosis in a faulty position, wrist drop or arthritis (Fig. 610). The position of choice (optimum position) for ankylosis should be sought; this is a 30° extension with some degree of ulnar deviation. In this position the flexors and the extensors are in proper balance. With the hand in pronation, a dorsal incision is begun opposite the center of the 2nd metacarpal; it is continued obliquely upward, bisecting a line drawn between the styloid processes and ending about 2 inches above the radial styloid. The dorsal carpal ligament is exposed and divided, and the extensor tendons are retracted. The capsule is opened so that the proximal row of carpal bones is exposed. A small wedge may be removed from the radius, the navicular and the lunate bones, or the bony surfaces may be curetted.

AMPUTATIONS AND DISARTICULATIONS

Amputations and disarticulations at the wrist joint prevent the proper fitting of artificial hands; if possible, they should be avoided. However, there are times when carpometacarpal disarticulation is indicated; if possible, the thumb and a finger or other parts of the hand should be saved. A U-shaped incision is begun on the palmar side about ½ inch below the styloid process of the radius, passing down to the middle of the 2nd metacarpal, where it arches across the middle of the remaining metacarpals and ends about 1 inch below the styloid of the ulna. The dorsal incision is placed transversely across the carpal bones and connects with the palmar incision. The palmar flap is deepened to the flexor tendons and is reflected to the joint. The extensor tendons and ligaments are divided, the joint is traversed, and the flexor tendons and the remaining tissues are severed in similar fashion. Tendons and nerves are cut short. Some authorities advocate suturing the tendons together, but others permit them to retract. After careful hemostasis has been achieved, the wound is closed in layers.

Hand

The hand is an organ that is directed by the will and is capable of a great variety of complicated movements. These movements are possible because of the highly co-ordinated actions of its intrinsic and extrinsic muscles and its numerous joints. The thumb is all-important to the hand, since the property of apposition depends on it; without this, the functional capacity of the hand is reduced greatly.

The hand can be divided conveniently into the palmar region, the dorsal region and the phalanges.

PALMAR REGION

This region is quadrilateral in shape and contains the soft parts in front of the metacarpal bones. The "hollow" of the hand is the triangular central part which is bounded on the radial side by the thenar eminence and on the ulnar side by the hypothenar eminence. These eminences approximate

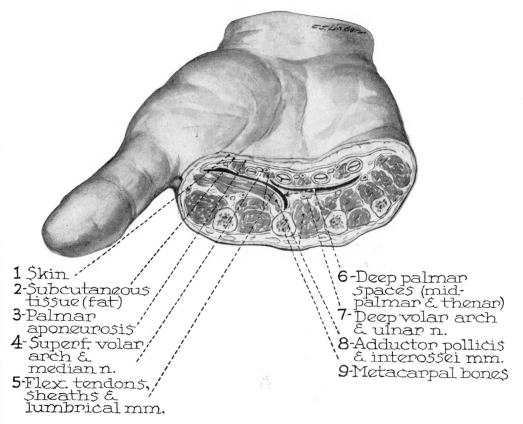

1-Skin
2-Subcutaneous tissue (fat)
3-Palmar aponeurosis
4-Superf. volar arch & median n.
5-Flex. tendons, sheaths & lumbrical mm.

6-Deep palmar spaces (mid-palmar & thenar)
7-Deep volar arch & ulnar n.
8-Adductor pollicis & interossei mm.
9-Metacarpal bones

FIG. 611. Cross section through the right hand, showing the 9 layers in the center of the palmar region of the hand.

each other as they approach the wrist. It is helpful to consider the central part of the palmar region and then to discuss the thenar and the hypothenar eminences. The central part of the palm consists of the following 9 layers, from superficial to deep (Fig. 611):

1. The skin
2. The subcutaneous tissue
3. The palmar aponeurosis
4. The superficial volar arch and the median nerve
5. The flexor tendons, their sheaths and the lumbrical muscles
6. The deep palmar spaces
7. The deep volar arch and the ulnar nerve
8. The adductor pollicis and the interosseus muscles
9. The metacarpal bones

Skin. The skin of the palm is thicker, coarser and more vascular than that of the dorsum of the hand. It is thin over the thenar eminence and especially thick over the heads of the metacarpals. It is free from hairs and sebaceous glands but is well supplied with sweat glands. Two transverse skin creases (proximal and distal) are present in the palm (Fig. 612). The proximal crease accommodates movements of the index finger and approximately marks the convexity of the superficial volar arterial arch. The distal crease accommodates movements of the medial 3 digits and marks the heads of the 3rd, the 4th and the 5th metacarpals. A vertical palmar crease which limits the thenar eminence also is present.

A series of longitudinal grooves extend from the roots of the fingers toward the palm; between these grooves are raised intervals of fatty tissue. The grooves correspond to the digital slips of palmar fascia, and the raised intervals mark the lumbrical spaces, which contain the digital vessels, the nerves and the lumbrical muscles.

The palmar region of the hand receives its cutaneous nerve supply from the following nerve branches (Figs. 612 and 614): the *palmar cutaneous branch of the median nerve* arises about 1 inch above the wrist, passes obliquely downward behind the flexor carpi radialis tendon and pierces the deep fascia between that tendon and the tendon

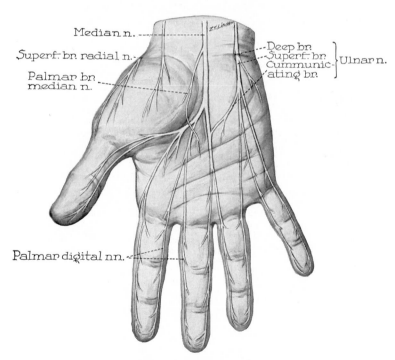

Fig. 612. The skin creases and the cutaneous nerve supply of the palmar region.

of the palmaris longus. It then descends, branching as it goes, to supply the skin of the hollow of the palm.

The palmar cutaneous branch of the ulnar nerve is very slender and at times is difficult to find. It arises at a variable point below the middle of the forearm and passes downward over the ulnar artery; it pierces the deep fascia near the wrist and supplies the skin over the medial third of the palm.

The terminal part of the radial nerve pierces the deep fascia about 2 inches above the styloid process of the radius at the lateral border of the front of the forearm. It descends, crossing the tendons that overlie the lateral surface of the distal end of the radius, and supplies the skin over the thenar eminence.

The palmar digital nerves are 7 in number; 2 arise from the ulnar nerve and are distributed to the little finger and the medial half of the ring finger. The others arise from the median nerve and are distributed to the outer 3½ digits. These nerves are accompanied by the palmar digital vessels, which are in front of them in the palm but behind them at the sides of the fingers. They supply the joints of the digits and the soft parts on the sides and the front of the fingers. Each nerve terminates at the end of the digit by dividing into 2 branches, one of which enters the pulp of the digit and the other the bed of the nail.

Subcutaneous Tissue. The skin is bound to the palmar aponeurosis by fibrous septa, between which quantities of granular fat are present. This fat constitutes the subcutaneous tissue. Over the ball of the thumb (thenar eminence) and the ball of the 5th finger (hypothenar eminence) this fat is not so plentiful or granular. Where skin creases are found, subcutaneous fat is present in small amounts or is absent entirely; hence, perforating injuries are serious in these locations.

The palmaris brevis muscle (Fig. 613) is a superficial sheet of muscle which arises from the flexor retinaculum and the ulnar margin of the palmar aponeurosis. It passes medially, superficial to the ulnar vessels and nerve, and inserts into the skin of the ulnar border of the hand. The superficial branch of the ulnar nerve supplies it. This muscle

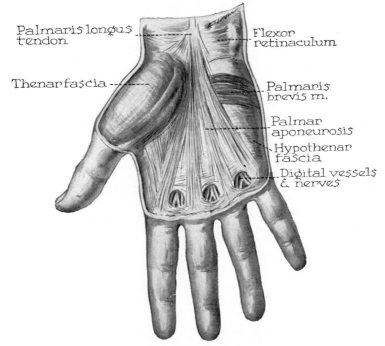

Palmaris longus tendon

Thenar fascia

Flexor retinaculum

Palmaris brevis m.

Palmar aponeurosis

Hypothenar fascia

Digital vessels & nerves

FIG. 613. The palmar aponeurosis. The triangular intermediate part is thick and strong, but the medial and the lateral parts are thin and weak.

raises the skin and the fascia over the hypothenar eminence when the fingers bend; this enables the hand to grasp more firmly.

The webs of the fingers are present over the palm of the hand but are absent on the dorsum. In these webs transverse fibers (superficial transverse ligaments) are found. These should not be confused with the superficial transverse metacarpal ligaments, which are incomplete and pass across the webs just anterior to the digital vessels and nerves.

The palmaris brevis muscle (ulnar nerve) is thin and subcutaneous and lies across the uppermost inch of the hypothenar eminence, hiding the termination of the ulnar artery and nerve. It arises from the flexor retinaculum and the palmar aponeurosis and is inserted into the skin of the ulnar border of the hand. If the palm of the hand is placed in the position of scooping up water, the skin over the hypothenar eminence is thrown into wrinkles caused by the action of the palmaris brevis. This muscle must be severed and reflected before the hypothenar fascia and muscles become visible.

The Palmar Aponeurosis. This deep palmar fascia is divided into medial, lateral and intermediate parts (Fig. 613). The medial and the lateral portions are thin and weak, and they extend over the hypothenar and the thenar eminences, respectively. The intermediate part is thick and strong and is the palmar aponeurosis proper. It is triangular in shape, with its apex placed proximally, where it becomes continuous with the palmaris longus tendon and the flexor retinaculum. Opposite the distal transverse palmar crease it divides into 4 slips, one going to each finger. Between these slips the digital vessels and nerves and the lumbrical muscles

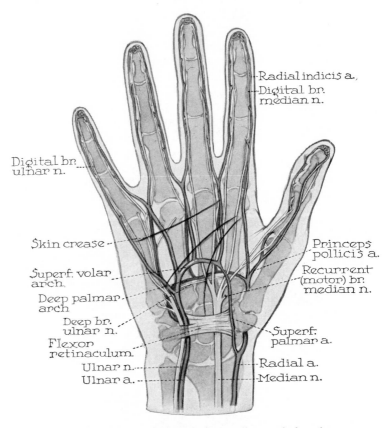

FIG. 614. The volar arches and the median and the ulnar nerves. The superficial volar arch is formed mainly by the ulnar artery and a small branch of the radial artery; the deep volar arch is formed mainly by the radial artery and a small branch of the ulnar artery.

are located. Each slip divides into 2 processes between which the flexor tendons pass. These processes diverge and attach along the inner and outer aspects of the proximal phalanges and to the proximal part of the second phalanges. They are continuous with the fibrous flexor sheath and assist in flexion; they also bind the flexor tendons to the front of the fingers. A spontaneous contracture of the palmar fascia results in a flexion of the fingers which is known as Dupuytren's contracture.

At the base of the palmar fascia the diverging slips are connected to one another by transverse fibers called the superficial transverse metacarpal ligaments. In order to avoid confusion concerning these ligaments, it is wise to recapitulate: (1) The *superficial transverse (palmar) ligament* appears in the webs of the fingers as a thin band of transverse fibers. It stretches across the roots of the 4 fingers; however, at times it is incomplete. (2) The *superficial transverse metacarpal ligament* is a part of the palmar aponeurosis which connect the diverging slips of fascia. (3) The *deep transverse metacarpal ligament* holds the heads of the metacarpal bones together on their palmar surfaces. (4) The *dorsal transverse metacarpal ligament* holds the heads of the metacarpal bones together on their dorsal aspect.

Between the 4 digital processes of the central portion of the palmar fascia are 3 intervals. These are occupied by fat in which is imbedded the digital arteries, the nerves and the lumbrical muscles. Corresponding to these intervals, in the distal part of the palm, are 3 slight elevations. If the palm is inspected, it is noticed that these elevations are bounded by 4 vertical depressions which mark the fusion of the digital processes of the palmar fascia with the fibrous sheath containing the flexor tendons. These elevations mark 3 intervals of surgical importance which have been referred to by such names as commissural spaces, lumbrical canals or web spaces. They are important because infections extending from the subcutaneous tissue of the finger to the subaponeurotic spaces of the palm must pass by way of these spaces.

The space is bounded anteriorly by the superficial transverse palmar ligament, posteriorly by the deep transverse metacarpal ligament and laterally by the digital processes of the palmar fascia which fuse with the theca (fibrous tendon sheath). Their contents are fatty tissue, lumbrical muscle and the digital vessels and nerves.

The superficial volar (palmar) arch lies immediately beneath the palmar aponeurosis and upon the branches of the median nerve (Fig. 614). It is formed by a continuation of the ulnar artery and one of the 3 branches of the radial artery (superficial palmar, princeps pollicis or radial indicis). The anastomosis between the ulnar artery and the radial branch is so complete that both ends require ligation when the arch is cut. The arch lies superficial to the flexor tendons, the lumbrical muscles and the digital branches of the median nerve in the hand. These digital vessels and nerves cross each other in their trip through the palm: hence, in the fingers the nerve lies superficial to the vessels. The medial 3½ fingers are supplied by the arch through 4 digital vessels. The branch to the 5th finger does not bifurcate but travels along the ulnar border of this finger. The other 3 digital branches bifurcate in the 2nd, the 3rd and the 4th finger webs, each being distributed to its respective finger borders. The proximal transverse palmar skin crease marks the convexity of the arch.

The median nerve enters the palm behind the transverse carpal ligament, and at the distal border of the ligament it breaks up into lateral and medial divisions (Figs. 614 and 615). The lateral division supplies the thenar muscles (recurrent branch), both sides of the thumb and the radial side of the index finger. The digital branch to the index finger supplies a branch which innervates the first lumbrical muscle. There are 2 medial divisions; both bifurcate to supply the adjacent sides of the index, the middle and the ring fingers. From the first of these divisions the nerve supply to the second lumbrical is derived. Therefore, the motor part of the median nerve supplies 5 muscles: the 3 thenar muscles (abductor pollicis brevis, opponens pollicis and flexor pollicis brevis) and the 2 lateral lumbricals (lumbricals 1 and 2). The sensory fibers of the median nerve supply the lateral 3½ fingers and the corresponding part of the palm.

Flexor Tendons, Their Sheaths and the Lumbrical Muscles. As the *flexor tendons* (*sublimis, profundus* and *pollicis*) pass under the transverse carpal ligament and into the palm they are provided with 2 sheaths: a fibrous and a synovial.

The fibrous sheaths of the thumb and the little finger are similar in construction to those of the middle 3 fingers. With the underlying bone, they form strong osteofascial tunnels which retain the tendons in place. A pair of tendons (sublimis and profundus) pass under each fibrous flexor sheath. The sheaths attach to the lateral and the medial borders of the phalanges. In front of the joints they are pliable and thin, but in front of the bodies of the proximal and the middle phalanges the fibers are curved transversely and are strong. These structures (flexor retinaculum, palmar aponeurosis and fibrous flexor sheaths) constitute a single continuous fibrous plate, the main function of which is to hold the tendons in position and to increase their efficiency. The arrangement of the fibrous flexor sheaths converts part of the tendon sheaths into cul-de-sacs. Directly beneath these resisting bands, the space is restricted greatly, so there is little or no room for pus. On the other hand, toward the finger end in front of the second joint and also in front of the metatarsophalangeal joint, dilatations in which pus may collect exist. In contradistinction to the arrangement in the foot, the palmar aponeurosis gives no fibrous extension to the thumb. The wide range of motion of the thumb is due to this fact and is characteristic of the human hand.

The synovial or mucous sheath is a lubricating device in tubular form which ensheaths a tendon. These are necessary for the flexor tendons, since they rub on the back of the flexor retinaculum during flexion of the wrist, and during extension they rub against the carpal bones and the anterior margin of the lower end of the radius. Therefore, these tendon sheaths act as bursae. The sheath forms a sac which is closed at both ends and is made up of glistening, endothelial-lined membranes (Fig. 616).

Each within its sheath has or did have a mesotendon (which is a double layer of synovial membrane attaching the tendon to the wall of the sheath and carrying vessels to it. It is attached to the side of the tendon which has least friction. The flexor tendons (sublimis, profundus and pollicis) must have these sheaths, first, where they pass through the osseofibrous carpal tunnel and, then, where they pass through the osseofibrous digital tunnel. Therefore, there are carpal synovial and digital sheaths. However, in the thumb the sheath is always in continuity, but that of the 5th finger may fail to unite in about 10 per cent of the cases and thus be

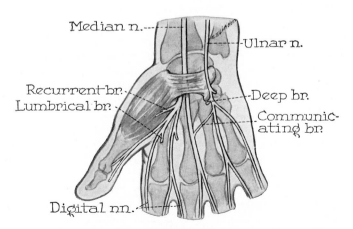

FIG. 615. Distribution of the median nerve. The median nerve has both sensory and motor fibers. Its motor fibers supply 5 muscles of the hand, namely, the 3 thenar thumb muscles and the first 2 lumbricals.

identical with that of the other fingers. The sheaths of the index, the middle and the ring fingers remain separate (Figs. 617 and 618). The carpal sheaths of the 4 sublimis and the profundus tendons become one and are then known as the common *flexor (carpal) sheath;* this has a laterally placed meso-tendon.

The digital synovial sheaths of fingers 2, 3 and 4 extend from the neck of the meta-carpal bone to the base of the third phalanx, where the profundus tendon ends. Over the middle third of these metacarpal bones the corresponding tendons have no sheaths. The common flexor synovial sheath extends for about ½ to 1 inch above and below the flexor retinaculum. The sheaths investing the tendons to the 5th finger as a rule continue proximally without interruption to join the common flexor sheath at the wrist. This common flexor sheath, with its extension along the little finger, is called the *ulnar bursa.* The tendon of the thumb has a sheath which extends from the base of the last phalanx to 1 inch beyond the proximal border of the wrist joint; this is called the *radial bursa.* These two bursae have been discussed elsewhere (p. 736); they may be separate or they may communicate with each other. Should they communicate, an infection can spread easily from one sheath to the other. Thus, in a tenosynovitis of the thumb, the infection may extend along the sheath and infect the sheath of the little finger via such a communication. The radial and the ulnar bursae lie on the front of the carpus and are separated from the wrist and the intercarpal joints only by ligaments. Therefore, these joints may become infected from such suppurative processes.

Certain portions of the original meso-tendons of the flexors may remain as tri-angular folds, *vincula,* which pass between the tendons and the phalanx. The blood ves-sels run in the vincula to the tendons as they would in any mesentery.

Scheldrup has described certain variations in tendon sheath patterns in the hand and has worked out their frequency statistically; these are represented in Figure 619. It is his opinion that the generally accepted anatomic pattern is present in 71.4 per cent of cases. He has described 8 separate and different types of anastomoses. These are important to keep in mind, since they may alter the spread of infection in tenosynovitis.

Opposite the base of the proximal phalanx the sublimis tendon divides so that the profundus tendon can pass to its insertion into the volar aspect of the base of the distal phalanx. The slips of the sublimis tendon insert into the volar surface of the base and the sides of the middle phalanx (Fig. 620).

The lumbrical muscles are 4 fleshy muscles that arise from the tendons of the flexor digitorum profundus and insert into the radial side of the tendinous expansions of the extensor digitorum communis of the medial 4 fingers (Fig. 621). They are peculiar in that they arise from flexor tendons and insert into extensors.

Each lumbrical muscle passes to the radial side of the corresponding finger and is accompanied by the digital vessels and nerves. They lie behind the vessels and the nerves and on the deep transverse metacarpal ligament; the interossei lie behind this ligament. The lateral 2 lumbricals arise by single heads

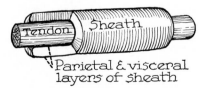

FIG. 616. Arrangement of a tendon sheath.

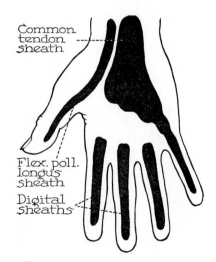

FIG. 617. The synovial sheaths.

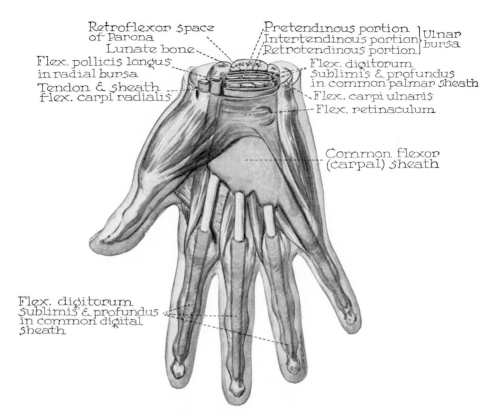

Retroflexor space of Parona

Lunate bone

Flex. pollicis longus in radial bursa

Tendon & sheath flex. carpi radialis

Pretendinous portion
Intertendinous portion
Retrotendinous portion
} Ulnar bursa

Flex. digitorum sublimis & profundus in common palmar sheath

Flex. carpi ulnaris

Flex. retinaculum

Common flexor (carpal) sheath

Flex. digitorum sublimis & profundus in common digital sheath

FIG. 618. Arrangement of the flexor tendon sheaths in the fingers, the hand and the wrist. The ulnar bursa has been divided into its 3 component parts.

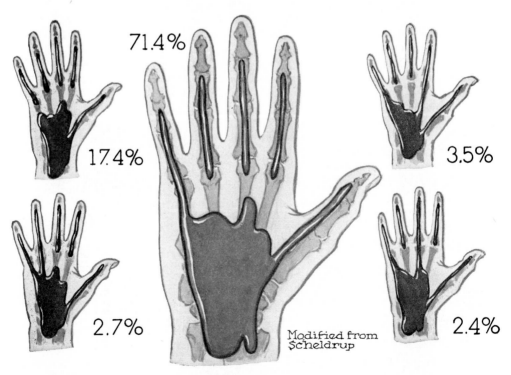

71.4%

17.4%

2.7%

3.5%

2.4%

Modified from Scheldrup

FIG. 619. Some of the variations in tendon sheath patterns and their statistical frequencies according to Scheldrup.

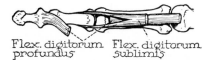

Flex. digitorum   Flex. digitorum
profundus   sublimis

FIG. 620. Insertion of the flexor tendons. The sublimis separates, and the profundus perforates.

from the radial sides and the volar surfaces of the deep tendons of the index and the middle fingers. The medial two each arise by 2 heads from adjacent sides of the tendons of the middle, the ring and the little fingers.

These slender muscles end in delicate tendons which pass backward across the lateral surface of the metacarpophalangeal joint and connect with the expansion of the extensor tendon. It is inserted with the tendon of an interosseous muscle into the base of a terminal phalanx. They flex the finger at the metacarpophalangeal joints but extend them at the 2 interphalangeal joints through the medium of the extensor expansions.

The action of the muscle is interesting, since in suppurative tenosynovitis of the flexor tendons and their sheaths, complete loss of function may result; yet often the patient can flex the metacarpophalangeal joint by means of the lumbrical muscles. The lateral 2 lumbricals are supplied on their superficial surface by the median nerve. The medial two are supplied on their deep surface by the deep branch of the ulnar nerve. The lateral two arise by single heads, and the medial lumbricals arise by double heads. This fact is important because it explains the formation of a fibrous septum which divides

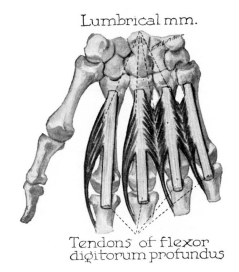

Lumbrical mm.

Tendons of flexor
digitorum profundus

FIG. 621. The 4 lumbrical muscles.

the palm into midpalmar and thenar spaces.

Any fibrous septum (partition) which extends from the palmar aponeurosis deep into the palm is interrupted by the double-headed lumbricals which are associated with the 4th and the 5th fingers. However, such a lamina can be carried back on the lateral side of the belly of the 2nd lumbrical throughout its entire extent and insert onto the 3rd metacarpal bone. In this way a fibrous partition is formed which passes from the undersurface of the palmar aponeurosis to the 3rd metacarpal bone. This fibrous septum is the fascial investment of the 2nd lumbrical muscle (Fig. 622). Such a partition also could be associated with the 1st lumbrical muscle,

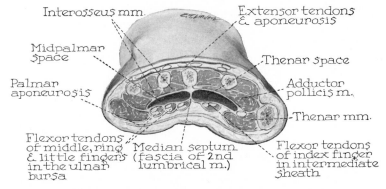

Interosseus mm.   Extensor tendons
                                                   & aponeurosis

Midpalmar
space

Palmar
aponeurosis   Thenar space

                                                   Adductor
                                                   pollicis m.

                                                   Thenar mm.

Flexor tendons
of middle, ring   Median septum   Flexor tendons
& little fingers   (fascia of 2nd   of index finger
in the ulnar   lumbrical m.)   in intermediate
bursa   sheath

FIG. 622. Fascia of the lumbrical muscles. The fascia of the second lumbrical forms the fibrous septum which separates the thenar from the midpalmar space.

but because of the greater mobility of the 2nd digit, the fibrous tissue associated with its lumbrical is lax and thin and forms no barrier across the palm. In this way 2 spaces are formed: a middle palmar and a thenar.

Deep Palmar Spaces. These spaces exist between the deep flexor tendons and the lumbrical muscles on the palmar side, and also between the interosseous fascia covering the metacarpal bones and the interosseous muscles dorsally (Fig. 623 A). Localization of pus in this space and the spread of dyes when injected under pressure indicates that it is divided into two compartments. The work of Kanavel and Spaulding has shown that the lumbrical fascia of the second lumbrical passes to the lateral side of the muscle, thereby producing one complete anteroposterior septum which passes from the palmar aponeurosis to the 3rd metacarpal bone

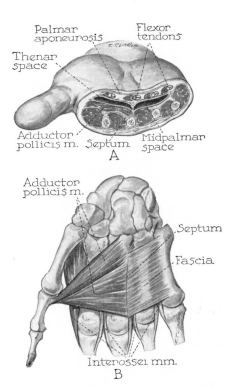

FIG. 623. The 2 palmar spaces. (A) The thenar space is laterally placed, and the midpalmar space is medial. (B) The posterior boundaries of the 2 spaces.

(Fig. 622). This septum divides the deep palmar space into two: a thenar space laterally and a midpalmar space medially.

The thenar space lies under the outer half of the hollow of the palm; it has a roof, a floor and lateral and medial walls. The roof is made up of the flexor tendons, the lumbricals of the 2nd digit, and the thenar muscles. The floor is formed by the 2 heads of the adductor pollicis, particularly its transverse head (Fig. 623 B). The medial wall is made up of the fibrous septum (fascia of the 2nd lumbrical muscle), and the lateral wall is formed by the flexor pollicis longus tendon and its synovial sheath. This space may be mapped out on the hand proximally from the distal border of the anterior annular ligament to the transverse palmar crease distally. The 1st lumbrical sheath extends as a distal diverticulum of the space (Fig. 638).

The midpalmar space lies in the inner half of the hollow of the hand; it has a roof, a floor and lateral and medial walls. The roof is made up of the flexor tendons and the lumbricals of the medial 3 digits. The floor consists of the dense fascia covering the medial 2½ metacarpal bones and their corresponding interosseous muscles. The lateral wall is made up of the fibrous septum described above and separates it from the thenar space. The medial wall is made up of the hypothenar muscles, which are separated from the midpalmar space by the attachment of the palmar aponeurosis, which passes to the 5th metacarpal bone. Distally, the space extends almost to the level of the distal palmar crease; proximally, it reaches the level of the distal margin of the transverse carpal ligament (Fig. 639).

The midpalmar space is connected potentially with the so-called Parona's retroflexor space (Figs. 618 and 624). It has been referred to as the forearm space and has the following boundaries: anteriorly, the flexor digitorum profundus (ulnar bursa) and the flexor pollicis longus in its synovial sheath (radial bursa); posteriorly, the pronator quadratus and the interosseous membrane; proximally, it is continuous with the intermuscular spaces of the forearm; distally, it reaches the level of the wrist; and laterally, the space extends to the outer and the inner borders of the forearm. It is along these lateral borders that the space is drained by incisions.

The Deep Volar Arch. Two arteries take part in the formation of the deep volar arch: the radial and the deep branch of the ulnar (Fig. 614).

The radial artery plays the chief part in its formation. On leaving the forearm, the radial artery winds around the radial side of the wrist and crosses the dorsal surface of the navicular and the trapezium (greater multangular). It then passes through the anatomic snuffbox (abductor pollicis longus, extensor pollicis brevis and extensor pollicis longus) to gain entrance to the proximal end of the first interosseous space. It continues medially and, in the palm, appears between the oblique and the transverse heads of the adductor pollicis. It turns medially and joins the deep branch of the *ulnar artery* at the base of the 5th metacarpal bone.

The arch thus formed passes across the metacarpal bones immediately distal to their bases. The deep arch is about a fingerbreadth nearer the wrist than is the superficial; its convexity is directed toward the fingers. The deep branch of the ulnar nerve lies in its concavity. This arch lies deep to the flexor tendons and upon the volar interosseous muscles.

Three arteries usually arise from the radial: the superficial palmar, which supplies the thenar eminence; the princeps pollicis to the thumb; and the radial indicis, which passes along the lateral aspect of the index

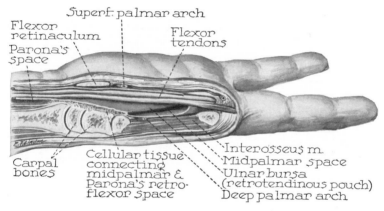

FIG. 624. The retroflexor space of Parona.

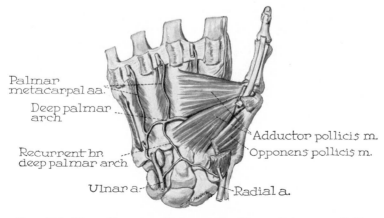

FIG. 625. The adductor pollicis muscle. The radial artery divides its origin into 2 heads: a transverse and an oblique.

finger. The deep arch usually supplies the 3 palmar metacarpal arteries, which pass between the fingers and unite with the digital branches of the superficial arch.

The ulnar nerve enters the palm between the volar carpal and the transverse carpal ligaments (Fig. 614). It divides into superficial and deep branches in the region of the hamate bone. The *superficial branch* supplies sensory fibers to the little finger and the ulnar side of the ring finger. The *deep branch* is motor; it supplies all the muscles of the palm of the hand, with the exception of the 5 supplied by the median nerve (p. 719). Therefore, the deep branch of the ulnar nerve supplies the 3 hypothenar muscles, the 7 interosseous muscles, the medial 2 lumbricals (3 and 4) and the adductor pollicis. This branch passes to the medial side of the hook of the hamate bone and dips into the palm through the cleft between the abductor and the flexor of the little finger. It runs transversely across the palm and is accompanied by the deep volar arch. As it crosses, it lies behind the flexor tendons and on the interossei and it terminates in the adductor pollicis. Since it supplies most of the muscles of the hand which are responsible for the fine movements of the hand, it has been called the "musician's nerve."

Adductor Pollicis Muscle. The triangular adductor pollicis muscle lies in the depth of the palm and arises from the palmar border of the 3rd metacarpal and its corresponding carpal bone, the capitate (Fig. 625). The radial artery divides the origin of the muscle into 2 heads: a transverse (distal) and an oblique (proximal) head. It inserts into the base of the 1st phalanx of the thumb. Although the muscle lies deep in the palm, its distal edge is subcutaneous and can be exposed by removing the skin and the fascia of the 1st interdigital web. It forms the floor of the thenar space. Its contraction draws the thumb across the palm and thus keeps the thumb and the palm approximated to each other. This action should not be confused with the action of the opponens, which approximates the tip of the thumb to the tip of the 5th finger.

The interosseous muscles are 7 in number: 4 dorsal and 3 palmar. They are supplied by the deep branch of the ulnar nerve (Fig. 626). The 4 *dorsal* interossei arise by double heads from the adjacent sides of the 5 metacarpals. On the palmar surface, the adductor pollicis arises from the 3rd metacarpal and inserts into the thumb. This leaves only the 2nd, the 4th and the 5th metacarpals free, and so it is that these give rise to the single heads of the 3 palmar interossei.

The interossei insert into the bases of the proximal phlangeal and the extensor expan-

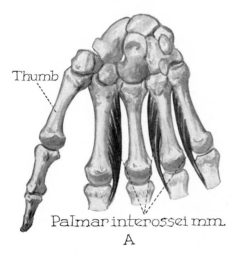

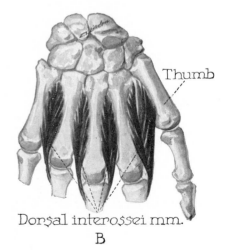

Thumb — Palmar interossei mm.
A

Thumb — Dorsal interossei mm.
B

FIG. 626. The interossei: (A) the 3 palmar interossei; (B) the 4 dorsal interossei.

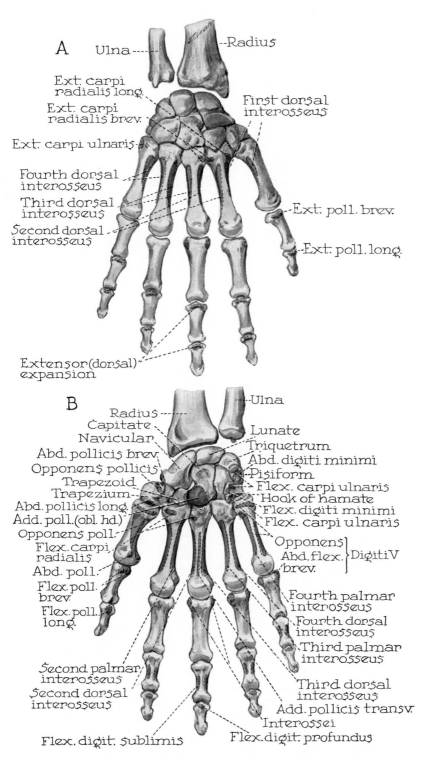

A

Ulna ---- --Radius

Ext. carpi
radialis long.
Ext. carpi
radialis brev.

First dorsal
interosseus

Ext. carpi ulnaris -

Fourth dorsal
interosseus
Third dorsal
interosseus
Second dorsal
interosseus

- Ext. poll. brev.

- Ext. poll. long.

Extensor (dorsal)
expansion

B

Radius --- --Ulna
Capitate
Navicular
Abd. pollicis brev.
Opponens pollicis
Trapezoid
Trapezium -
Abd. pollicis long.
Add. poll. (obl. hd.)
Opponens poll.
Flex. carpi
radialis
Abd. poll.
Flex. poll.
brev.
Flex. poll.
long.

Lunate
Triquetrum
Abd. digiti minimi
Pisiform
Flex. carpi ulnaris
Hook of hamate
Flex. digiti minimi
Flex. carpi ulnaris

Opponens
Abd. flex. } Digiti V
brev.

Fourth palmar
interosseus
Fourth dorsal
interosseus
Third palmar
interosseus

Second palmar
interosseus
Second dorsal
interosseus

Third dorsal
interosseus
Add. pollicis transv.
Interossei

Flex. digit. sublimis
Flex. digit. profundus

FIG. 627. The metacarpal bones. The origins of the muscles are
shown in red; the insertions, in blue.

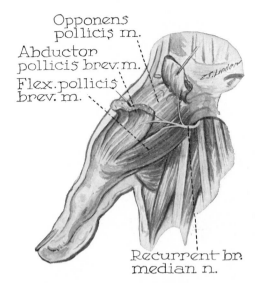

Opponens
pollicis m.

Abductor
pollicis brev.m.

Flex.pollicis
brev. m.

Recurrent br.
median n.

Fig. 628. The 3 thenar (thumb) muscles. These are the abductor pollicis brevis, the flexor pollicis brevis and the opponens pollicis. The last lies in a deeper plane than the other 2. The recurrent branch of the median nerve supplies this entire group.

sions. Since their tendons pass backward and across the metacarpal joints to reach their insertions, they aid in flexing these joints. They are inserted by means of the extensor expansions into the bases of the terminal phalanges and aid in extending the interphalangeal joints. However, their main action is abduction and adduction. The dorsal interossei are abductors, and the palmar interossei are adductors.

An injury to their nerve supply, the deep branch of the ulnar nerve, produces a characteristic deformity of the hand. When the interossei are paralyzed, they no longer can act as flexors of the metacarpophalangeal joints. Then the extensors are unopposed and bend the fingers backward at these joints; neither can the interossei act as extensors of the interphalangeal joints. Therefore, the flexors bend the fingers forward at these interphalangeal joints. The result is a typical *main en griffe* or "claw hand."

The interossei pass dorsal to the deep transverse metacarpal ligament; this ligament separates them from the lumbricals. The dorsal metacarpal ligament joins the heads of the metacarpal bones of the fingers together posteriorly. With the deep transverse ligament it forms 3 osseofibrous tunnels between the 4 fingers in which the palmar and the dorsal interosseus muscles lie.

Metacarpal Bones. The 5 metacarpal bones form the skeleton of the palm, articulate with the distal row of the carpus and diverge slightly as they extend distally to articulate with the phalanges; each has a base, a shaft and a head.

The proximal ends (*bases*) are somewhat expanded and present articular surfaces; proximally, these articulate with the carpal bone, and at the sides there are one or more articular surfaces for articulation with each other (Fig. 627). There are distinguishing features on the bases: the second is notched for the trapezoid, the medial margin of the notch articulates with the capitate, and the lateral boundary articulates with the trapezium. The base of the 3rd metacarpal articulates with the capitate; it has a short styloid process extending upward from its dorsolateral part. The fourth base is cuboidal and articlulates with the hamate and slightly with the capitate bones. The fifth has a tubercle on its medial side and a metacarpal facet on its lateral side.

The shafts of the bones are 3-sided, each presenting a flat surface toward the dorsum and a smooth ridge toward the palm of the hand. Each shaft is curved longitudinally, with a palmar concavity and is prismatic on transverse section, revealing dorsal, lateral and medial surfaces. The anterior border of the 3rd metacarpal body is almost monopolized by the transverse head of the adductor pollicis. The 2nd, the 4th and the 5th bodies present the attachments of the 3 palmar interossei. The anteromedial and the anterolateral surfaces of the 5 digits give origin to the 2 heads of the 4 dorsal interossei.

The heads of the medial 4 metacarpal bones are convex and smooth distally, and they articulate with the phalanges and the palmar ligaments which are attached to the shafts immediately above the heads. At these metacarpophalangeal joints the prominences of the knuckles are formed by the distal aspects of the heads of the metacarpal bones.

The first metacarpal bone (thumb) is usually discussed alone because it is the shortest and most movable of all. Its dorsal surface is the same breadth throughout and shows no sign of the flattened triangular areas which differentiate the dorsal aspect of the shaft of the other metacarpal bones. The base of this bone is saddle-shaped and articulates with the trapezium.

Thenar and Hypothenar Eminences. *The 3 thenar (thumb) muscles* are the abductor pollicis brevis and the flexor pollicis brevis, which are superficial, and the opponens pollicis, which lies deeper. They all are supplied by the recurrent branch of the median nerve (Fig. 628). These muscles lie to the radial side of the flexor pollicis longus tendon and make up the thenar eminence. They are supplied by the recurrent branch of the median nerve, which turns back after appearing from under the distal margin of the transverse carpal ligament. Since the deep fascia is very thin over this area, this important nerve is almost subcutaneous and is unprotected. A guide to it is the superficial palmar branch of the radial artery, which lies medial to it. The 3 thumb muscles arise together from the transverse carpal ligament and the lateral carpal bones (navicular and greater multangular).

The abductor pollicis brevis muscle forms the upper or lateral part of the ball of the thumb. It is inserted into the lateral side of the base of the proximal phalanx of the thumb. Its action pulls the thumb directly forward so that it comes to lie at right angles to the plane of the palm.

The flexor pollicis brevis muscle is medial to the abductor and inserts with it. Its action produces flexion at the metacarpophalangeal joint of the thumb.

The opponens pollicis muscle is visible only after the other two have been divided. Its fibers spread out and insert into the lateral half of the palmar surface of the first metacarpal bone. At times it is separable into superficial and deep laminae. Its action brings the metacarpal bone of the thumb across the palm of the hand, and also rotates it medially so that the pad of the tip of the thumb faces and comes into contact with the pads of the tips of the other fingers. This action should not be confused with adduction (p. 726).

The nerve to these muscles is seen after the superficial muscles are reflected. It is a

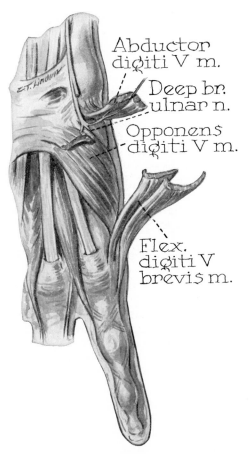

FIG. 629. The 3 hypothenar muscles. Theses are the abductor, the flexor and the opponens digiti quinti. They are supplied by the deep branch of the ulnar nerves.

short branch which, having given off superficial twigs to the flexor brevis and the abductor, passes between these two to enter the opponens.

The three muscles are segregated from the central space of the palm by a fascial sheet which passes dorsally (under the muscles) from the radial edge of the palmar aponeurosis and attaches to the first metacarpal bone. Therefore, pus formed among these muscles shows no tendency to spread to the palm. Incisions into this space should be placed laterally to avoid the median nerve.

The 3 muscles of the hypothenar eminence correspond to those of the thenar group and are the abductor digiti quinti, the flexor digiti quinti and the opponens digiti quinti (Fig.

629). They are supplied by the deep branch of the ulnar nerve. These 3 muscles originate from the transverse carpal ligament and from the medial 2 carpal bones (pisiform and hamate).

The abductor digiti quinti muscle inserts into the medial side of the base of the proximal phalanx of the little finger. By its action it abducts the little finger from the axial line of the middle finger.

The flexor digiti quinti muscle is inserted with the abductor. It is partly fused with the abductor and sometimes it is partly incorporated in the opponens. By its action it flexes the metacarpophalangeal joint of the little finger.

The opponens digiti quinti muscle lies on a deeper plane and is inserted into the whole length of the medial part of the front of the 5th metacarpal bone. The deep branch of the ulnar nerve enters from the lateral side of the hypothenar eminence; hence, incisions into this space are made along the medial side. The space is separated from the central space of the palm by a septum similar to that described under the thenar eminence. This septum attaches to the 5th metacarpal bone.

DORSAL REGION OF THE HAND

The surface anatomy of this region reveals the extensor tendons as being both visible and palpable over the dorsum of the hand. The metacarpal bones can be felt easily.

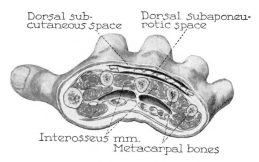

FIG. 631. The dorsal subcutaneous and the subaponeurotic spaces

In contrast with the palmar surface of the hand, the dorsal surface is covered with skin of finer texture which has numerous sebaceous glands and short hairs. The cutaneous nerve supply is derived from the dorsal rami of the ulnar, the radial and the dorsal antibrachial cutaneous nerves (Fig. 630).

The dorsal subcutaneous space is a rather extensive area of loose areolar tissue within definite boundaries (Fig. 631). If infected, pus can spread quite readily over the entire dorsum of the hand.

The dorsal subaponeurotic space (Fig. 631) should not be confused with the dorsal subcutaneous space. Over the dorsum of the hand the extensor tendons are united by oblique bands, thus forming an aponeurotic sheet; this is attached on each side to the 2nd and the 5th metacarpal bones. The dor-

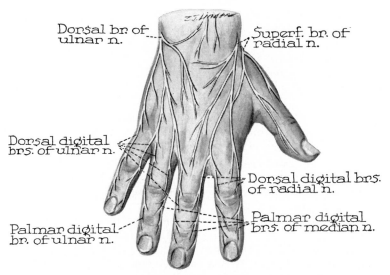

FIG. 630. The cutaneous nerve supply of the dorsum of the hand.

sal subaponeurotic space lies between this sheet and the interosseous muscles; it is filled with loose connective tissue. Pus in this space is limited distally at the metacarpophalangeal joints and proximally at the bases of the metacarpal bones.

The extensor digitorum communis is enclosed with the extensor indicis in a synovial sheath which is in a compartment of the extensor retinaculum. It divides into tendons which diverge to the fingers (Fig. 632). On the dorsal surface of the proximal phalanx each tendon expands to form the dorsal extensor expansion, which is inserted into the bases of the middle and the distal phalanges (Fig. 633). It is supplied by the posterior interosseous nerve and, as its name suggests, it extends the phalanges and the hand.

The extensor carpi radialis longus tendon is crossed by the extensors of the thumb; it is enclosed in a synovial sheath, with the ex-

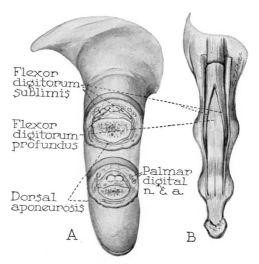

FIG. 633. Diagrammatic presentation of the anatomy of a finger: (A) cross sectional study; (B) the superficial and the deep flexor tendons.

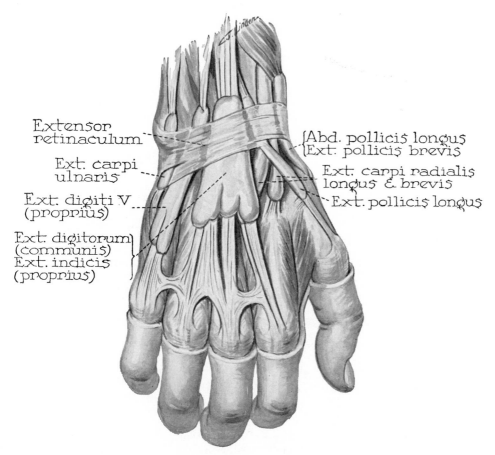

FIG. 632. The tendons of the dorsum of the wrist and the hand.

tensor carpi radialis brevis, under the extensor retinaculum.

The extensor digiti minimi tendon is ensheathed in the compartment of the extensor retinaculum that lies between the radius and the ulna. It is inserted with the tendon from the extensor digitorum to the little finger.

The extensor carpi ulnaris tendon also is enclosed in a synovial sheath and is inserted into the base of the 5th metacarpal bone.

PHALANGES (FINGERS)

The hand has a thumb and 4 fingers. Some authorities prefer to refer to the thumb as the first of 5 digits, but this is a matter of convenience rather than one of argument. The construction of all 5 fingers is essentially the same, except that the thumb has 2 phalanges and the other fingers have 3. The thumb also has a short thick metacarpal associated with it which adds to its strength and mobility.

Skin. The skin of the flexor surface of the digits is thick, contains some subcutaneous fat, is only slightly mobile and is devoid of hair follicles. That over the dorsum is thinner, more mobile and has very little subcutaneous fat. The *transverse flexor creases* do not indicate the exact positions of the underlying joints. The proximal digital crease is distal to the metacarpophalangeal joint. The middle crease is a good guide to the joint, since it lies directly opposite it; the distal crease is somewhat proximal to the distal interphalangeal joint. Therefore, the only digital transverse crease that can be used as an exact landmark of the joint is the middle one. These creases are bound closely to the underlying flexor tendon sheaths by fibrous tissue strands. The amount of fat is minimal or even entirely absent beneath them; hence, a penetrating wound at the crease is likely to penetrate the underlying synovial sheath.

The subcutaneous tissue over the flexor surface is made up of fibrous tissue enclosing small amounts of fat. These septa connect the skin to the fibrous layers of the tendon

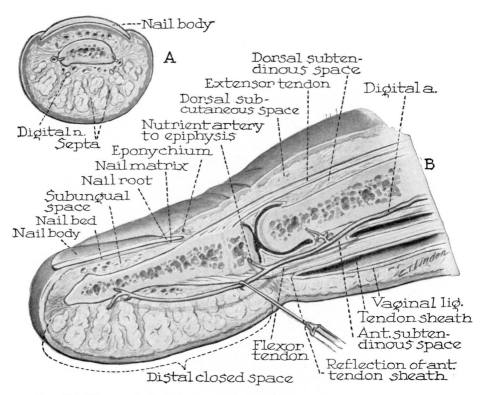

FIG. 634. The terminal phalanx and the distal closed space: (A) cross section; (B) longitudinal section.

sheath below and to the periosteum in the terminal phalanges. The last-named relationship is important in the treatment of a felon (p. 739). The digital vessels and nerves run in this subcutaneous tissue layer.

Distal Closed Space. The important distal closed space can be understood if the arrangement of the subcutaneous tissue is visualized properly (Fig. 634). In the distal phalanx the subcutaneous tissue is arranged in such a way that it consists of a number of strong fibrous septa which radiate from the periosteum to the skin. In the compartments thus formed between these septa, fatty tissue is found. Therefore, the distal four fifths of the phalanx is converted into a closed space and, together with the diaphysis, receives its blood supply from the 2 palmar digital arteries which are found anterolateral to the bone. If a transverse section of the distal closed space is studied, it will be seen that dense connective tissue separates the subungual space or nail bed from the anterior

closed space. The epiphysis receives its blood supply from the digital arteries before those vessels enter the closed space (Fig. 635 B). If inflammatory exudates and edema occur within this space, the tension rises, shuts off the blood supply, and a necrosis of the diaphysis occurs. Even after the age of 20 and after union of the epiphysis and the diaphysis, necrosis usually is limited to the diaphyseal region alone, and new bone may grow from the epiphyseal end.

The phalanges are the bones of the fingers. There are 14 in all, 3 (proximal, middle and distal) for each finger and 2 for the thumb. They are built on the same general plan as the metacarpals but are shorter, the distal phalanx being the shortest of all and having a rough distal end which underlies the tips of the fingers. The distal ends of the terminal phalanges are neither weight-bearing nor force-transmitting. The surface under the fingernail is smooth; the surface under the finger pad is rough, owing to the attachment

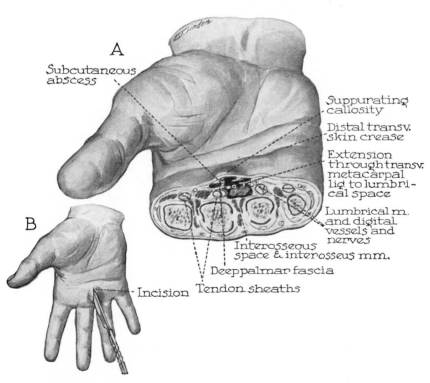

Fig. 635. Suppurating callosity and web space infections: (A) path of extension of a suppurating callosity to a web (lumbrical) space; (B) incision into the abscess.

of the fibrous bands which bind the skin to it. The dorsal aspect of the proximal and the middle phalanges is smooth, rounded and covered by the extensor expansions. The palmar surfaces take part in the floor of the osseofibrous tunnel in which the flexor tendons run. The borders of the middle phalanx are more prominent because they receive the attachment of the slips for the insertion of the flexor digitorum sublimis tendon. The bases of the proximal phalanges articulate with the rounded knuckles and, therefore, are concave.

The common volar digital arteries arise from the convexity of the superficial volar arch and give off digital branches which sup-

ply contiguous sides of the thumb and the fingers as well as the distal part of their dorsal surfaces (Fig. 614). The proximal part of the dorsum of the fingers receives its arterial supply via the *dorsal digital arteries,* which arise from the dorsal metacarpal arteries from the dorsal carpal arch. On the fingers, the digital arteries and nerves run side by side in contact with the fibrous flexor sheath, not with the phalanges. Each of these vessels gives off a branch to the epiphysis of the terminal phalanx before entering the anterior closed space. The branches ramify across the anterior aspect of the phalanx, sending nutrient vessels to the bone.

The digital nerve lies anterior or antero-

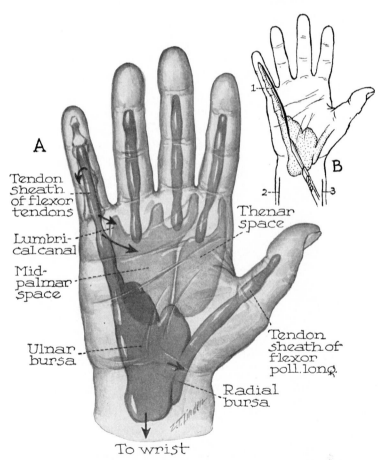

FIG. 636. Infection of the ulnar bursa. (A) This bursa is usually infected as a result of extension from an infected tendon sheath of the 5th finger. The arrows indicate the possible paths of extension from the infected ulnar bursa to surrounding structures. (B) Combined digital and palmar incision. Accessory incisions are shown to drain Parona's retroflexor space.

medial to its fellow artery. The distribution of these nerves has been discussed elsewhere.

SURGICAL CONSIDERATIONS

WEB SPACE INFECTIONS AND SUPPURATING CALLOSITY

Web space infections may start as a *suppurating callosity* which spreads down toward the commissural or web space (Fig. 635). The pus tends to spread backward or laterally. It can spread from one web to another and thus may involve 3 web spaces without going deeply. Since there are deficiencies in the palmar aponeurosis between its digital prolongations, the infection can burrow backward so that a "collar button" abscess is formed. Adequate drainage can be instituted by making an incision through the web between the fingers and continuing into the palmar aspect of the hand.

TENOSYNOVITIS

Tenosynovitis, or infection, in the tendon sheath of the little finger and the thumb is discussed under ulnar and radial bursae infections. Tenosynovitis of the middle, the ring and the index fingers has a tendency to remain localized, since the sheath ends in the region of the heads of the metacarpal bones. The incision which drains a digital tenosynovitis should be made at the side of

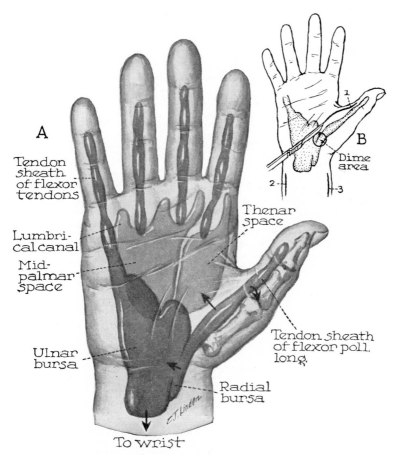

FIG. 637. Infection of the radial bursa. (A) This bursa is usually infected as a result of extension from an infected tendon sheath of the thumb. The arrows indicate the possible paths of spread from the infected radial bursa to surrounding structures. (B) The incisions used in the treatment of an infected radial bursa and flexor pollicis longus tendon.

the sheath and at the site of the known infection. The incision is carried along the shaft of the proximal and the middle phalanges but usually leaves that part which is over the joint untouched to prevent herniation of the tendon.

INFECTION OF THE ULNAR BURSA

Infection of the ulnar bursa usually results from an extension of an infection in the flexor tendon sheath of the little finger (Fig. 636). Perforating wounds, an infected midpalmar space and infections of the tendon sheath of the middle or the ring fingers may also spread to this bursa. In the last case, the pus breaks through the proximal end of the synovial sheath, passes along the lumbrical muscle into the midpalmar space and from there secondarily involves the ulnar bursa. An infection of the ulnar bursa may

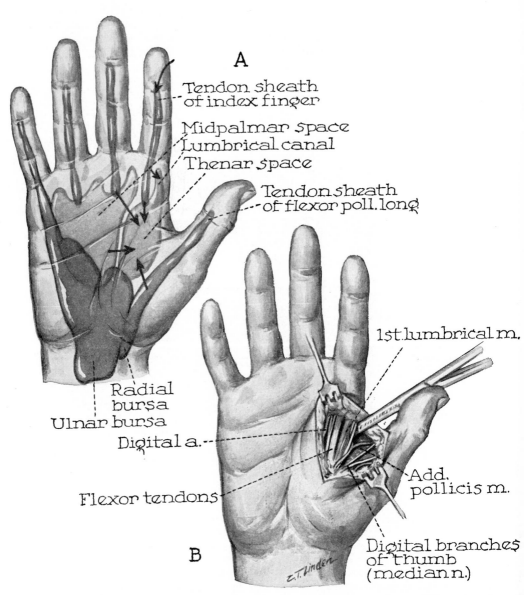

A

Tendon sheath
of index finger

Midpalmar space
Lumbrical canal
Thenar space

Tendon sheath
of flexor poll. long

1st. lumbrical m.

Radial
bursa
Ulnar bursa
Digital a.

Add.
pollicis m.

Flexor tendons

B

Digital branches
of thumb
(median n.)

FIG. 638. The infected thenar space. (A) The arrows indicate the possible paths of extension into the thenar space. (B) Drainage of the infected thenar space.

spread to the underlying bone or joint, to the lumbrical canal, to the middle palmar space, to the radial bursa or into the wrist.

Since this condition usually results from extension of a tenosynovitis of the little finger, the treatment of the latter should be carried out first as described on p. 735. The incision is placed either on the lateral or the medial side of the finger and is carried down into the palm and into the hypothenar emi-

nence (Fig. 636 B). The tendon sheath may be absent between the little finger tendon sheath and the ulnar bursa. This should be kept in mind in order to avoid contaminating a healthy bursa. The combined palmar and digital incision makes it possible to drain both the tendon sheath of the 5th finger and the ulnar bursa at the same time. It extends to the flexor retinaculum. If the infection has extended into the forearm, an incision is

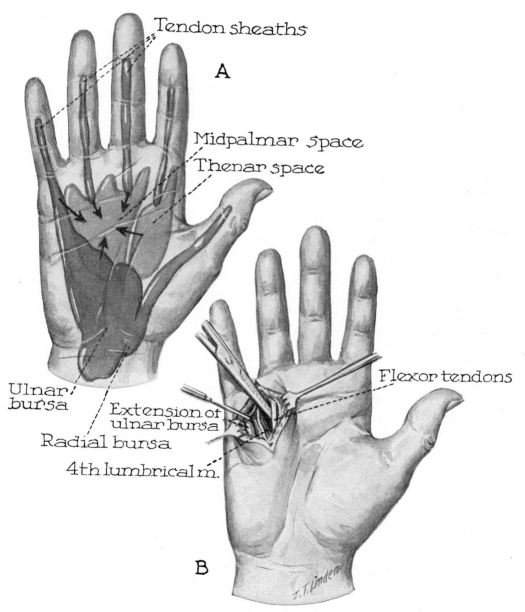

FIG. 639. The infected midpalmar space. (A) The arrows indicate the possible paths of extension into the midpalmar space. (B) Drainage of the infected midpalmar space.

placed along the ulna. Accessory incisions on the radial side may be necessary sometimes for through-and-through drainage of Parona's retroflexor space.

INFECTIONS OF THE RADIAL BURSA

Infections of the radial bursa usually arise from an infected tendon sheath of the flexor pollicis longus, an infected ulnar bursa or an infected thenar space (Fig. 637). The infection may spread from the flexor pollicis longus to the interphalangeal joint, the bone, the ulnar bursa, the thenar space or under the anterior annular ligament and into the wrist. The incision for an infected radial bursa and flexor pollicis longus tendon starts as an anteromedial incision at the distal volar skin crease and extends through the thenar eminence down to within 1½ inches of the anterior annular ligament, *but no farther*

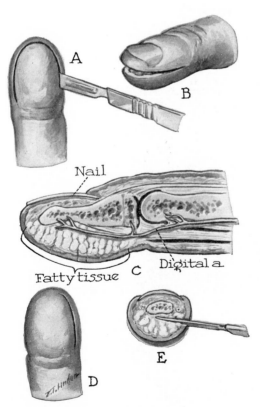

FIG. 640. Felon. (A) and (B) "Fishmouth" type of incision. (C) Closed space arrangement of the distal phalanx. (D) and (E) "Hockey-stick" type of incision.

(Fig. 637 B). This precaution is taken because the motor branch of the median nerve to the thenar muscles is in this region (the dime area) (p. 728). The bursa itself should be drained in the forearm via the approach described under ulnar bursitis; this permits drainage of both bursae and, unlike the approach from the radial side, involves no risk to the radial artery.

INFECTIONS OF THE THENAR SPACE

Infections of the thenar space occur as a result of a perforating wound directly into the space or following a tenosynovitis of the index or the middle finger, abrasions of the thumb, radial bursitis and midpalmar space abscesses (Fig. 638). Abscesses of this space occasionally have been reported following osteomyelitis of the 1st, the 2nd or even the 3rd metacarpal bones. When it follows a tenosynovitis of the index finger, as it usually does, the cellulitis of the tendon sheath extends downward and bursts through the proximal end of the sheath; it then comes to lie in the loose areolar tissue around the lumbrical muscle which guides it into the thenar space. The pus lies anterior to the adductor muscle of the thumb, and ballooning of the web between the thumb and the index finger becomes visible. The treatment is immediate incision and drainage, the incision being placed along the anterior border of the lateral side of the 2nd metacarpal bone or along the web between the thumb and the index finger (Fig. 638 B). A hemostat is placed into the space between the flexor tendons and the adductor pollicis. Pus may accumulate behind the adductor muscle, and an incision placed as described above can drain both anterior and posterior adductor partitions of the thenar space. The hemostat which is placed into the thenar space should not be thrust past the middle metacarpal bone because the fascial septum may be perforated and the midpalmar space contaminated.

INFECTIONS IN THE MIDPALMAR SPACE

Infections in the midpalmar space occur from a tenosynovitis involving one or any of the 3 medial digits, from an infected ulnar bursa or from osteomyelitis of the underlying metacarpals. The condition also may be caused by extension from an infected thenar space, direct penetrating wounds or from infections of one of the medial 3 web spaces traveling along a lumbrical muscle (Fig. 639). When the midpalmar space is involved, the concavity of the palm is lost. Since direct attack on the space would endanger too many structures, effective drainage can be obtained via a lumbrical space by opening a web between the ring and the middle finger or the ring and the little finger (Fig. 639 B). In this way a hemostat can be placed beneath the flexor tendons and into the midpalmar space. It should not be thrust past the middle metacarpal bone, since this in turn may involve the thenar space.

Felon (Whitlow)

Felon (whitlow) is an infection of the anterior closed space of the finger; it is extremely painful, common and dangerous. The connective tissue arrangement (Fig. 640 C) accounts for the fact that if pus develops here, it has no means of escape and produces marked pressure. This shuts off the blood supply and causes early necrosis. Since the epiphysis (base of the bone) receives its blood supply from vessels which do not pass through this space, it does not become necrotic, as does the rest of the bone, and new bone can grow from it, especially in the young. A "hockey stick" incision or "fish mouth" type of incision may be used to establish adequate drainage and open these spaces (Fig. 640). Incisions of this type place the scar away from the very sensitive tactile surface of the finger. A midline incision is an error, since the drainage produced would be inadequate, the tactile sense interfered with and the flexor tendon sheath possibly could be involved.

Paronychia

Paronychia is an acute infection involving the subepithelial tissue at the side of the nail. If incised and drained early, no ill effects result, but, if neglected, the infection may spread along the side and the base of the nail, forming a so-called "run around." The pus may lodge beneath the overlying epithelium (eponychium) and then travel under the nail itself, forming a subungual abscess. In the treatment of paronychia, a lateral incision should be made over the

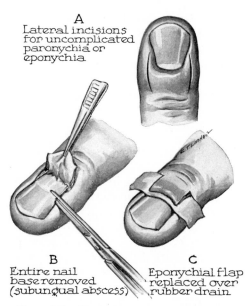

A Lateral incisions for uncomplicated paronychia or eponychia.

B Entire nail base removed (subungual abscess)

C Eponychial flap replaced over rubber drain.

Fig. 641. Treatment of uncomplicated and complicated paronychia.

point of maximum tenderness; bilateral incisions should be used if the infection has run around the nail (Fig. 641). If a subungual abscess results, an eponychial flap is raised, and the nail bed is removed, for the nail acts as a foreign body in the subungual abscess cavity. The distal portion of the nail is not removed, as it protects the underlying sensitive tissue.

Fractures of the Metacarpal Bones

The metacarpal bones frequently are fractured when the fist is clenched and a blow is struck. McNealy and Lichtenstein have emphasized the important points regarding the mechanism and the treatment of hand fractures.

In *metacarpal bone fractures exclusive of the thumb,* a typical deformity results, which is characterized by shortening of the bone due to bowing of the fragments. This results in a dorsal projection at the fracture site and volar displacement of the metacarpal head because of the action of the interosseus muscle which flexes the proximal phalanx. The distal fragment of the metacarpal bone is attached to the proximal phalanx through the metacarpophalangeal joint and is drawn into a flexed position. An inverted-V deformity is typical for fractures of the metacarpal bones and requires immobilization on a straight dorsal splint. This removes the deformity and restores the normal horizontal contour to the dorsum of the hand. The 3rd and the 4th metacarpal bones are splinted laterally by their adjacent metacarpals, but the 2nd and the 5th, lacking such support, require lateral splinting in addition to the dorsal.

The usual deformity in *fractures of the first metacarpal* (*thumb*) is adduction of the distal fragment and abduction of the proximal. The treatment for such fractures is abduction, which overcomes the contraction of the abductor muscles and maintains the web of the thumb.

In a *Bennett's fracture* (fracture of the base of the first metacarpal), abduction may fail to restore the alignment of the bones and, in addition to abduction, traction may be necessary.

DISLOCATION OF THE METACARPOPHALANGEAL JOINTS

Dislocation of the metacarpophalangeal joints occurs frequently because of their ball-and-socket arrangement.

Dislocation of the thumb occurs usually after a fall which produces forceful dorsiflexion on the hyperextended hand. This results in a tear in the glenoid (volar accessory) ligament and permits the phalanx to pass backward. The resultant deformity is typical, as the proximal phalanx comes to rest on the dorsal aspect of the thumb metacarpal. The head of the metacarpal is caught between the tendons of the flexor pollicis brevis and the flexor pollicis longus. Because of this, reduction cannot be accomplished with traction alone, but the joint must be hyperextended almost to a right angle, followed by pressure at the proximal end of the phalanx to force it over the head of the metacarpal. Should this fail, it becomes necessary to make an incision and enlarge the opening in the capsule so that reduction may be accomplished.

Dislocations of the middle and the distal phalanges occur quite frequently and usually are produced by a blow struck at the tip of the finger. They may be accompanied by a fracture and, since the extensor tendon usually is ruptured at its insertion into the base of the terminal phalanx, a "dropped finger" or "loose ball finger" results. The extensor tendon does not retract because of its attachment along its lateral expansion.

FRACTURES OF THE PHALANGES

Distal Phalanx. In fractures of the distal phalanx, the distal part of the bone is not subject to pull of either intrinsic or extrinsic muscles; therefore, displacement is minimal,

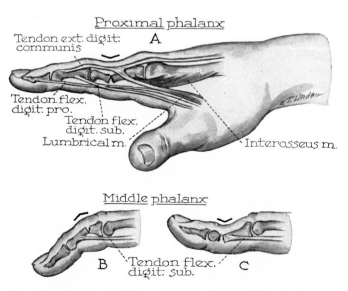

FIG. 642. Fractures of the proximal and the middle phalanges.

even if crushing is marked. The fingernail may be used as a suitable splint, and the fragments can be molded into place. Fractures involving the *proximal* portion of the *terminal* phalanx are affected by the pull of the flexor digitorum profundus and the extensor digitorum communis. This is the same injury described under "dropped finger." Hyperextension usually aligns the fragments and can be maintained by some such splint as described by Lewin.

Middle Phalanx. The deformity and the treatment of fractures of the middle phalanx depend on whether the fracture is proximal or distal to the insertion of the flexor digitorum sublimis. If it is distal, then flexion of the proximal fragment and dorsal displacement of the distal fragment result (Fig. 642 C). When the fracture is proximal to the tendon insertion, flexion of the distal frag-

ment, with the proximal fragment in an extended position, results (Fig. 642 B). Therefore, a fracture distal to the tendon insertion produces a V-shaped deformity, but a fracture proximal to the tendon insertion produces an inverted V-shaped deformity. A straight splint will correct the deformity in a fracture proximal to the tendon insertion, and a curved volar splint will correct the deformity found in a fracture distal to the tendon insertion.

Proximal Phalanx. In fractures of the proximal phalanx, flexion of the proximal fragment is produced by the pull of the interosseous and the lumbrical muscles, and dorsal displacement is brought about by the action of the lumbrical muscles (Fig. 642 A). This results in a V-shaped deformity which can be corrected by a curved splint, which approximates the broken ends of the bone.

Hip

The pelvifemoral region is that area in which the lower extremity is firmly bound to the pelvis by powerful muscles and ligaments. For study it can be divided conveniently in the gluteal (hip) region and the hip joint.

GLUTEAL REGION

BOUNDARIES AND SUPERFICIAL STRUCTURES

The gluteal region is roughly quadrilateral in shape and is bounded above by the iliac crest, below by the gluteus maximus, medially by the lateral margin of the sacrum and the coccyx and laterally by the tensor fasciae latae muscle (Fig. 643).

Iliac Crest and Spine. *The iliac crest is* palpable because of its subcutaneous posi-

tion. If the anterosuperior iliac spine is located and the fingers then run backward over the iliac crest they reach a definitely palpable *posterosuperior iliac spine* at which point the iliac crest ends. Below this, the posterior border of the innominate bone is continued vertically for about 1 inch to the postero-inferior iliac spine at which point it turns abruptly forward to form the great sciatic notch (Fig. 422). This notch continues to the ischial spine, where a shallow indentation is formed known as the *small (lesser) sciatic notch*. Therefore, the ischial spine separates the greater and the lesser sciatic notches. Below the latter the bone ends in a stout projection known as the *ischial tuberosity*. The sacrospinous and the sacrotuberous ligaments

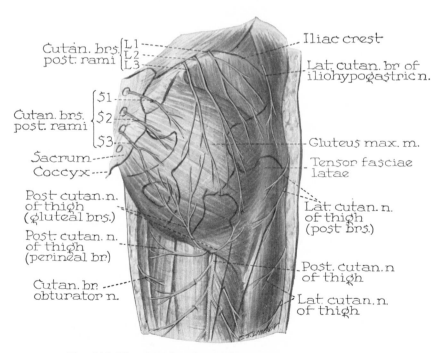

FIG. 643. The gluteal region and its cutaneous nerve supply.

convert the greater and the lesser sciatic notches into foramina.

The buttock (natis) forms a smooth rounded elevation which is separated from its fellow by a deep fissure called the natal cleft. It is limited inferiorly by another groove called the fold of the buttock. The bulging of the buttock is caused by a thick layer of fat and the lower part of the large gluteus maximus muscle.

The superficial fascia has the same general characters as it has in other parts of the body but is peculiar in this region in that it is loaded with fat, and the numerous small cutaneous nerves may be difficult to locate. This fat is particularly present in the female. The fascia thickens over the upper and the lower margins of the gluteus maximus and is tough and stringy over the ischial tuberosity

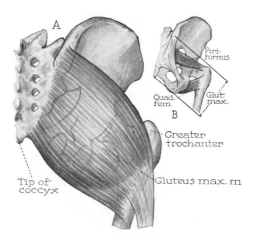

FIG. 644. The gluteus maximus muscle: (A) the origin and the insertion of the muscle; (B) the muscle outlined on the pelvifemoral bony framework.

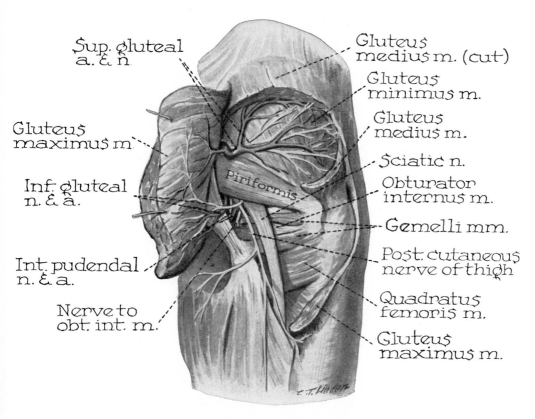

FIG. 645. The structures lying deep to the gluteus maximus muscle. The muscle has been severed and reflected medially to expose its deep surface; its nerve and blood supplies are also shown. The structures associated with the suprapiriformic and the infraperiformic spaces are shown.

where it forms a most efficient cushion upon which the body weight presses while in a sitting posture.

The cutaneous nerves are numerous and difficult to find, but the small arteries which accompany them may act as guides (Fig. 643). These nerves are derived partly from the posterior primary rami and partly from the anterior primary rami of the spinal nerves. Three twigs arise from the first 3 lumbar nerves, and 3 from the first 3 sacral nerves. From the anterior primary rami of the spinal nerves are derived the lateral cutaneous branch of the iliohypogastric, the lateral cutaneous branch of the last thoracic, twigs from the posterior branch of the lateral cutaneous nerve of the thigh which terminates over the greater trochanter, branches from the posterior cutaneous nerve of the thigh and, finally, twigs from the perforating cutaneous branch of the fourth sacral.

The superficial lymph vessels of the gluteal region join the lateral lymph glands of the superficial inguinal group.

DEEP FASCIA

The deep fascia is strongly attached to the iliac crest. Where it overlies the gluteus medius muscle it appears as a dense, opaque pearly white sheet. However, when it reaches the upper border of the gluteus maximus, it splits into 2 layers which enclose the muscle. Its appearance over the maximus is not thick and opaque, as over the medius, but in marked contrast appears thin and transparent. It sends septa into the muscle and thus divides it into coarse bundles.

MUSCLES

Gluteus Maximus. This muscle is rhomboidal in shape and is the most massive in the body; it is also the coarsest, heaviest and strongest muscle (Fig. 644). Being associated with the upright posture of the biped, it is especially well developed in man. It arises from the posterior part of the gluteal surface of the ilium, the dorsal aspect of the sacrum and the coccyx, and the posterior surface of the sacrotuberous ligament. From this extensive origin the bundles proceed obliquely downward and forward toward the upper part of the shaft of the femur, but only a part of the muscle is inserted into the bone. Three quarters of it is inserted into the iliotibial tract; the lower deep fibers attach to the gluteal tuberosity. It should be noted that the lower border of the muscle does not run parallel with the fold of the buttock but crosses it obliquely, being above its medial part and below its lateral part. The lower border extends from the tip of the coccyx and across the ischial tuberosity to the shaft of the femur (Fig. 644 B). The tuberosity is covered by the muscle when one stands erect, but it is uncovered when one sits down. It was not the plan of the body to have fleshy muscle support weight; therefore, there is a thick mass of stringy fibrous tissue between the tuberosity and the skin when one is sitting. The upper border of the muscle may be indicated by a line which runs parallel with the lower border and extends outward from the posterosuperior iliac spine to a point 2 inches above the greater trochanter. This muscle is the great extensor of the thigh, bringing the bent thigh into line with the body. Therefore, it is important in walking, going up an incline or rising from the sitting posture, which it does by pulling the pelvis backward. The blood supply is derived from the inferior gluteal artery. Many important structures lie beneath the deep surface of the gluteus maximus muscle, and to understand them the piriformis muscle may be used as a guide (Fig. 645). The lower border of this muscle can be indicated on the skin by a line joining the midpoint between the posterosuperior iliac spine and the tip of the coccyx to the top of the greater trochanter. If an incision is made through the gluteus maximus along this "piriformis line," and if the incision is carried to the greater trochanter until its bony resistance is felt, the proper cleavage plane will be found. It is wise to relax the gluteus by extending and rotating the thigh laterally, so that a finger may be inserted through the incision and moved about.

Three subgluteal synovial bursae are usually found beneath the muscle in the following locations: (1) between the muscle and the ischial tuberosity, (2) between the muscle and the greater trochanter and (3) between the gluteus and the upper part of the vastus lateralis. The bursa between the maximus and the ischial tuberosity may enlarge in those who follow sedentary occupations; such a bursa has been referred to as "weaver's bottom." This bursa is usually small and may be absent. However, the bursa which exists between the muscle and the greater trochanter is normally quite large.

For orientation in the region which lies subgluteally (gluteus maximus) it is important to utilize two units as key structures, namely, the piriformis muscle and the greater sciatic foramen, which has been called the "door to the gluteal region." The piriformis muscle itself enters the region via this door; some vessels and nerves enter the region *above* the piriformis (suprapiriformic), while others pass *below* the muscle (infrapiriformic), but all enter through the greater sciatic foramen. Some structures which enter this great door may disappear at once through the lesser sciatic foramen. The obturator internus is the only structure which enters the gluteal region by way of the lesser sciatic foramen.

The piriformis muscle arises within the pelvis by 3 digitations from the anterior surface of the 2nd, the 3rd and the 4th segments of the sacrum, these fibers arising between the anterior sacral foramina. *Outside* of the pelvis this muscle arises from the upper part of the greater sciatic notch and from the sacrotuberous ligament. The fibers pass through the greater sciatic foramen, continue laterally forward and insert into the highest point of the greater trochanter. The muscle is chiefly an extensor and lateral rotator of the femur. It receives its nerve supply from the sacral plexus (S 1).

Nerves and Vessels of the Infrapiriformic and the Suprapiriformic Spaces

Infrapiriformic Space. The structures which enter at the lower border of the piriformis are from lateral to medial, the sciatic nerve (which hides the nerve to the quadratus femoris), the nerve to the gluteus maximus (inferior gluteal nerve), the posterior cutaneous nerve of the thigh, the inferior gluteal artery, the nerve to the obturator in-

ternus, the internal pudendal vessels and the internal pudendal nerve (Fig. 645).

Sciatic Nerve. This (L 4, 5; S 1, 2, 3) is the largest nerve in the body; it is broad and flat (Fig. 679). As it appears from under cover of the piriformis it runs downward to the thigh. At first it lies on the ischium and then crosses successively the gemelli and the obturator internus, the quadratus femoris and the adductor magnus. The posterior cutaneous nerve of the thigh passes on the superficial aspect of the sciatic. The sciatic continues downward deep to the long head of the biceps; in its course it passes midway between the ischial tuberosity and the greater trochanter. It is the most lateral structure in the infrapiriformic region, having a "side of danger" and "a side of safety." Its lateral side is the "side of safety" along which dissection may take place without harm. However, its medial side is its "side of danger" from which branches spring to the hamstring muscles.

The inferior gluteal nerve (L 5; S 1, 2) is the nerve supply to the gluteus maximus muscle. Arising from the sacral plexus, it enters the gluteal region through the lower part of the greater sciatic foramen and enters the deep surface of the muscle.

The posterior cutaneous nerve to the thigh (S 1, 2, 3) passes deep to the gluteus maximus and medial to the sciatic nerve (Fig. 645). It is purely sensory and has been referred to as the "small sciatic" nerve. Its gluteal branch turns around the lower border of the gluteus maximus, and its perineal branch passes lateral to the ischial tuberosity to supply the scrotum or the labium majus. The main nerve continues downward to the middle of the thigh, subfascially, and ends on the calf.

The inferior gluteal artery divides into numerous terminal branches as soon as it appears beneath the lower border of the piriformis (Fig. 645). These branches are distributed to the neighboring musculature, and a small branch accompanies the sciatic nerve; it anastomoses with branches which join the trochanteric and the crucial anastomoses. The *crucial anastomosis* establishes a connection between the internal iliac and the femoral arteries. The cross is formed by

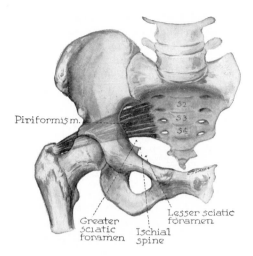

Piriformis m.

Greater
sciatic
foramen

Ischial
spine

Lesser sciatic
foramen

FIG. 646. The piriformis muscle.

horizontal arms from the transverse branches of the circumflex femoral artery, the upper limb from the descending branches of the inferior gluteal artery, and the lower limb from the ascending branch of the first perforating artery.

The nerve to the obturator internus, the internal pudendal artery and the pudendal nerve run only a small part of their course in the gluteal region; the artery lies between the 2 nerves. They emerge from the pelvis through the greater sciatic foramen, cross the spine of the ischium and the sacrospinous ligament and enter the lesser sciatic foramen to disappear from view. The nerve to the obturator internus is placed most laterally and supplies a twig to the gemellus superior. The internal pudendal artery with a companion vein on each side crosses the tip of the spine.

Suprapiriformic Space. The structures which enter along the upper border of the piriformis muscle are the superior gluteal vessels and the superior gluteal nerves (Fig. 645). The *superior gluteal nerve* (L 4, 5; S 1) passes in the interval between the gluteus medius and the minimus. It supplies both of these muscles and ends in the tensor fasciae latae. Therefore, it supplies the 3 abductors and the medial rotators of the hip joint, namely, the gluteus medius, the gluteus minimus and the tensor fasciae latae. The *superior*

gluteal artery is a branch of the posterior division of the internal iliac (hypogastric) artery. As soon as it passes above the upper border of the piriformis muscle it supplies a superficial branch which is distributed to the gluteus maximus. The remaining deep branch breaks up into upper and lower branches which follow the middle and the inferior gluteal lines in the interval between the gluteus medius and the minimus.

The Glutei Medius and Minimus Muscles. These are really two parts of a single muscle, since they are common in shape, direction of fiber action, nerve and blood supply (Fig. 645). Therefore, it is unusual to find a fascial plane between them, although at times such an ill-defined plane may be present.

The gluteus medius arises from the area between the middle gluteal line and the iliac crest. Its fibers converge to form a flattened band, partly fleshy and partly tendinous, which inserts into the greater trochanter of the femur. A small bursa separates this tendon from the anterior part of the trochanter.

The gluteus minimus is covered by the preceding muscle. It arises from the gluteal surface of the ilium between the middle and the inferior gluteal lines, its fibers converge and become inserted into the anterior surface of the greater trochanter. It is intimately connected near its insertion with the capsule of the hip joint and is separated from the trochanter major by a small bursa. These muscles are supplied by the superior gluteal nerve and arteries.

The tensor fasciae latae muscle (N. superior gluteal, L 4, 5; S 1) arises from the forepart of the lateral lip of the iliac crest and the subjacent bony surface and is invested by fascia lata. It lies over the anterior borders of the gluteus medius and minimus. Its fibers pass downward and backward to become inserted into the fascia lata a little below the greater trochanter. This part of the fascia lata is known as the iliotibial band (tract) (Fig. 694). It is an extensor of the knee, acting through the iliotibial band and a medial rotator of the thigh.

Two Gemelli and Obturator Internus Muscles. These muscles constitute a 3-headed muscle plate which occupies the interval between the quadratus femoris and the piriformis (Figs. 645 and 646).

The obturator internus arises from almost the entire pelvic surface of the hip bone below the level of the obturator nerve (Fig. 651). It makes a right-angle turn as it passes through the lesser sciatic foramen and is separated from the margin of the foramen by a bursa. Its tendon passes across the posterior surface of the ischium and the capsule of the hip joint to reach the anterior facet on the upper border of the greater trochanter.

The superior gemellus arises from the ischial spine, and the *inferior gemellus* from the ischial tuberosity. They are associated with the upper and the lower borders of the obturator internus tendon, and the three together have been referred to as the *tricipital tendon.*

The quadratus femoris is an oblong muscle which is continuous at its origin and insertion with the adductor magnus. By some it is considered as an upper extension of this latter muscle, the division between the two not always being clearly evident. It arises from the lateral border of the ischial tuberosity, passes laterally and becomes inserted into a rounded prominence on the trochanteric crest of the femur. Its upper border lies edge to edge with the inferior gemellus.

The 2 gemelli, the obturator internus and the guadratus femoris, are closely related to the capsular ligament of the hip joint and act as lateral rotators of the thigh. However, when the thigh is flexed the position of the greater trochanter is altered so that the piriformis and the obturator internus and the gemelli become abductors. The nerve supply of the obturator internus and the superior gemellus comes from the nerve to the abturator internus, but the inferior gemellus and the quadratus femoris are supplied by the nerves to the quadratus.

The obturator externus muscle is visible in this region, but it is better to study its origin when the medial side of the thigh is discussed (Fig. 429). It winds backward below the hip joint, its tendon passing obliquely upward and laterally on the back of the neck of the femur to become inserted into the trochanteric fossa.

HIP JOINT

The hip joint is an excellent example of the ball-and-socket variety of joints (Figs. 647 and 648). Although it does not allow as free a range of movement as that which

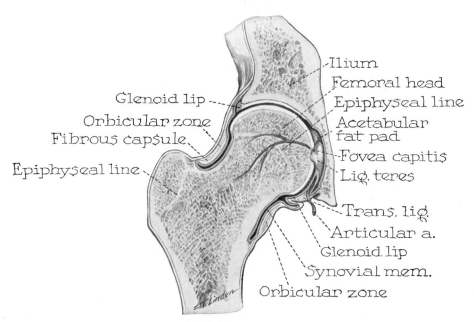

Fig. 647. The hip joint seen in frontal section.

takes place in the shoulder joint, the loss in this respect is counterbalanced by a gain in stability and strength. The head of the femur forms the ball; the acetabulum, which is deepened by the transverse acetabular ligament and the acetabular labrum, forms the socket.

ACETABULUM AND HEAD OF THE FEMUR

The ball (femoral head) forms two thirds of a sphere. However, this sphere is not perfect, since it is flattened above where the acetabulum rests most heavily upon it. It is covered by cartilage over its globoid surface as far as its junction with the femoral neck.

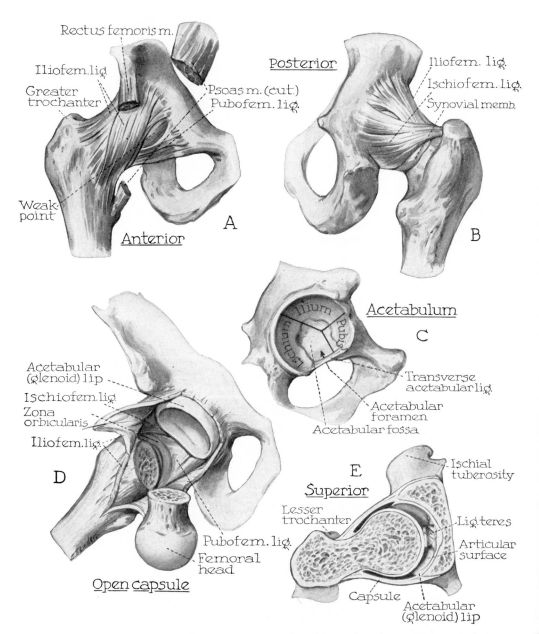

FIG. 648. The hip joint. Five different views showing the relations between the acetabulum, the ligaments, the head of the femur and the synovial membranes.

A small depression called the *fovea capitis* is located a little behind the summit of the head; it lodges the femoral attachments of the ligamentum teres through which the head receives a small arterial supply. At birth the proximal end of the femur is entirely cartilaginous. The neck is ossified by an extension from the diaphysis; as it forms, it divides the cartilage into two parts. The more proximal of these parts forms the head. A center of ossification appears in the head early in the 1st year and unites with the neck during the 20th year. The more distal part forms the greater trochanter, which begins to ossify in the 3rd year and joins the shaft about the 19th year.

In order to increase the power and the mobility of the inferior extremity, the neck of the femur is inclined to the shaft at an angle which is about 125° in the adult and 160° in the child. This has been known as the angle of inclination.

The acetabulum (acetum; L. = vinegar cup) lies at the point of union of the ilium, the ischium and the pubis. This cup-shaped cavity is deficient below where it forms a gap called the *acetabular notch,* which is bridged over by the *transverse acetabular ligament* and the glenoid lip, thus being converted into a *foramen* for the entrance of vessels and nerves. The remainder of the peripheral part of this cup is horseshoe shaped; since it articulates with the femur, it is covered with cartilage. The floor of the acetabulum, which is called the acetabular fossa, is covered by a small fat pad (haversian) which in turn is covered by synovial membrane.

The acetabular lip (labrum acetabulare, glenoid labrum) is a firm fibrocartilaginous ring which is fixed to the rim of the acetabulum; it deepens the cavity of the acetabulum and narrows its mouth. It fits closely on the head of the femur and has a suckerlike action which exerts an important influence in retaining it in place. Therefore, although the hip joint has been opened, it is not easy to pull the head of the femur out of the acetabulum. Both surfaces of the lip are covered with synovial membrane; its free margin is thin, but at its attachment at the acetabular ring it becomes much thicker. Inferiorly, where it bridges the acetabular notch, it is called the transverse acetabular ligament.

The epiphysis of the head of the femur encircles the articular margin and lies entirely within the synovial capsule. The ilium, the ischium and the pubis contribute to the articular part of the acetabulum. This synostosis is completed about the 16th year.

LIGAMENTS

The capsular ligament is exceedingly strong and surrounds the joint on all sides. It is attached proximally around the acetabulum and grasps the neck of the femur distally. The anterior part of the distal attachment occupies the whole length of the trochanteric line and the roof of the greater trochanter; it is very firm and strong. Posteriorly, it falls short of the trochanteric crest by about ½ inch; therefore, its attachment to the neck of the femur is weak. The fibers of this ligament run in two different directions, the majority passing obliquely from the hip bone to the femur. However, other fibers lie at right angles to the oblique ones, and these constitute the *zona orbicularis* (Figs. 648 and 649). They are circular fibers and are more distinct in the posterior part of the capsule; they encircle the neck of the femur posteriorly and below but are lost toward the upper and the anterior part of the capsule.

Since the ilium, the pubis and the ischium take part in the formation of the acetabulum, capsular fibers proceed from each of these bones to the femur; they are known as the iliofemoral, the pubofemoral and the ischiofemoral ligaments (Fig. 648). These are thickened portions of the capsule which have been given special names.

The iliofemoral, or inverted Y-shaped ligament of Bigelow, is placed over the front of the joint and is the thickest and most powerful part of the capsule. It is attached above to the antero-inferior iliac spine immediately below the origin of the straight head of the rectus femoris. As it passes downward it divides into two bands which are separated by a narrow interval. The upper band extends to the upper part of the intertrochanteric line, and the lower to the lower part of the same line. It is thicker at its sides than in the mid-

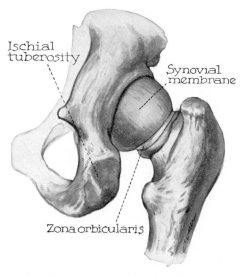

Ischial
tuberosity

Synovial
membrane

Zona orbicularis

FIG. 649. The synovial membrane and
the zona orbicularis of the hip joint seen
from behind.

dle, which accounts for its "Y" appearance. The thinner central portion is perforated by an articular twig from the ascending branch of the lateral femoral artery. This ligament is approximately ¼ inch thick and is one of the strongest ligaments in the body, its only rival being the interosseous sacro-iliac ligament. Bigelow has stated that a strain varying from 250 to 750 pounds is required for its rupture. It is rarely torn in hip dislocations.

The pubofemoral ligament arises from the pubic bone and the obturator membrane and is inserted with the lower limb of the iliofemoral ligament. Above, between these 2 ligaments, there is usually a gap through which the subpsoas bursa communicates with the joint.

The ischiofemoral ligament is a weak band which arises from the ischium below the acetabulum and passes upward and lat-

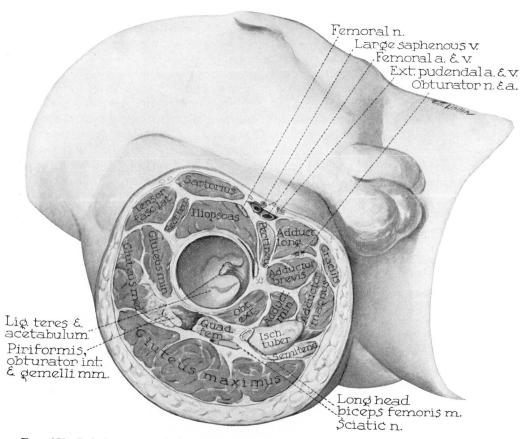

Femoral n.
Large saphenous v.
Femoral a. & v.
Ext. pudendal a. & v.
Obturator n. & a.

Sartorius
Tensor fasc. lat.
Gracilis
Iliopsoas
Pectineus
Adduct. long.
Gluteus min.
Gracilis
Gluteus med.
Adductor brevis
Adduct. min.
Adductor magnus
Lig. teres &
acetabulum
obt. ext.
Piriformis,
obturator int.
& gemelli mm.
Quad. fem.
Isch. tuber.
Gluteus maximus
Semitend.
Long head
biceps femoris m.
Sciatic n.

FIG. 650. Relations around the right hip joint. The femur has been removed, and the acetabulum is viewed from the right side.

erally to blend with the posterior part of the capsule.

When one stands erect with the toes turned out, the articular cartilage on the head of the femur is directed forward. Its lateral part is protected by the iliofemoral ligament, and its medial part by the pubofemoral ligament; however, the intermediate part has no covering ligament; hence, it is the "weak point" which is commonly perforated (Fig. 648 A). However, passing over this weak point is the tendon of the psoas muscle which provides some protection. Muscle fibers do not withstand pressure by underlying bone; therefore, in such locations they give place to tendons. This is true of the psoas tendon. Furthermore, tendons which pass over bony prominences require bursae to diminish friction and to facilitate a free movement. The psoas bursa which commonly communicates with the joint between the iliofemoral and the pubofemoral ligaments is no exception to this rule. In front of this tendon lies the femoral artery. The femoral nerve, which is lateral, lies in front of the iliacus muscle; the femoral vein, which is medial, lies in front of the pectineus muscle (Fig. 651).

The synovial membrane lines all parts of the interior of the hip joint except where articular cartilage or fibrocartilage is found

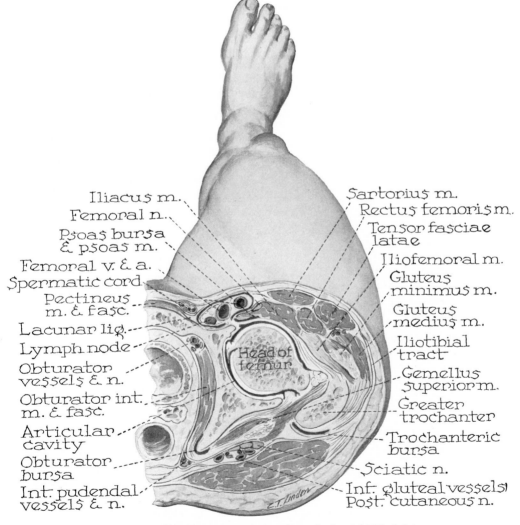

FIG. 651. Transverse section through the right hip joint.

(Figs. 647, 648 B and 649). This last statement is true of all synovial joints. The membrane lines the neck of the femur completely in front and as far as the obturator externus tendon behind; it stretches across the acetabular fossa. In front of the femoral neck and below it, the membrane is thrown into several loose folds which are called retinacula and in which arteries run onto the neck of the femur. As the membrane protrudes posteriorly between the free lower border of the fibrous capsule and the neck, it forms a bursa for the tendon of the obturator externus. Therefore, an incision made above this tendon usually will enter the joint, but one made below usually will miss it.

The ligamentum teres or ligament of the head of the femur consists mainly of synovial membrane; it has the form of a flattened triangular band. It is attached above to the fovea on the head of the femur, and below it blends with the transverse ligament. Most anatomists believe that it does not play a major part in holding the femur in the acetabulum. The Weber brothers showed the importance of the part played by atmospheric pressure rather than the ligamentum teres. They suspended a cadaver and divided all the muscles and ligaments around the joint, and the head of the femur did not pull free. If an opening was made into the acetabulum to allow the entry of air, the lower limb immediately fell off. On closing the opening with the finger the limb could again be kept in position. The ligament is tense when the semiflexed limb is adducted or rotated outward. It acts as a "mesentery," since it carries an artery to the femoral head.

VESSELS

The arteries that supply the hip joint are derived from the gluteal, the circumflex and the obturator arteries. Wolcott is of the opinion that the anastomosis between the ligamentum teres vessel, the capsular artery and the nutrient artery of the shaft does not take place until the ossification of the head of the femur is practically, if not entirely, completed.

At this time the vessels of the three systems unite by penetrating the thinned-out cartilage area at the fovea, thus establishing the anastomosis. The ligamentum teres circulation, he believes, is a closed one in so far as the femoral head is concerned, until such an anastomosis takes place.

NERVES

The nerves are derived from the nerves to the quadratus femoris, the femoral via the nerve to the rectus femoris, the anterior division of the obturator nerve, and occasionally the accessory obturator nerve.

MOVEMENTS

The depth with which the femoral head enters its socket would have made only flexion and extension possible, but, owing to the length of the femoral neck, greater freedom of movement is permitted.

Flexion is much greater in the flexed than in the extended position because in this position the capsule is looser. In full extension the head of the femur tends to leave the acetabulum, and the articular surfaces may be separated by 1 or 2 centimeters. Flexion

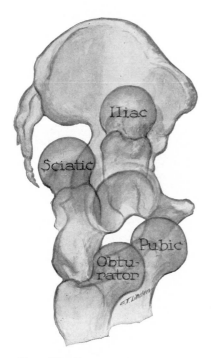

FIG. 652. Traumatic dislocation of the hip joint.

is limited by the sides coming in contact with the anterior abdominal wall. The muscles which produce flexion are the psoas, the rectus femoris, the sartorius, the pectineus, the anterior part of the gluteus medius and the minimus.

In extension the articular surfaces are held in close contact; rotation and abduction are not as free as in flexion. Extension is limited by the iliofemoral (Bigelow) ligament. The muscles which produce extension are the gluteus maximus, the hamstrings and the posterior part of the adductor magnus.

Abduction is very slight in extension, being checked by the "Y" and the pubocapsular ligaments. It is produced by the gluteus medius, the minimus, the upper part of the maximus, the tensor fasciae latae and the sartorius.

Adduction is produced by the adductors, the gracilis and the pectineus; it is checked by the other limb, but, if in flexion, by the "Y" ligament.

Rotation. The extent of rotation is about 90°. *Internal rotation* is produced by the anterior part of the gluteus medius and minimus, the tensor fasciae latae and the iliopsoas and is limited by the ischiocapsular ligament. *External rotation* is produced by the obturator externus, the obturator internus, the gemelli, the piriformis, the quadratus femoris, the posterior parts of the glutei, the adductors and the sartorius, and in the flexed condition by the iliopsoas.

RELATIONS

The relations are the following (Figs. 650 and 651):

1. *Anteriorly,* the psoas and the femoral artery, the iliacus, the femoral nerve, the pectineus and the femoral vein.

2. *Laterally,* the rectus femoris in front of the iliofemoral ligament and the gluteus minimus.

3. *Inferiorly,* the obturator externus crosses below the head and runs behind the neck of the femur.

4. *Posteriorly,* the piriformis, the obturator internus, the gemelli, the upper border of the quadratus femoris and the sciatic nerve.

SURGICAL CONSIDERATIONS

TRAUMATIC DISLOCATIONS OF THE HIP

Since the hip is firmly stabilized by the powerful muscles and the strong capsule which are associated with it, traumatic dislocations are rather infrequent. The weak point of the joint is at its lower part where a portion of the acetabular rim is deficient. However, when dislocations do occur, they may be posterior, anterior or central (Fig. 652).

In a posterior dislocation the head of the femur is forcefully pushed against the posterior part of the capsule which it tears; it then passes upward and backward and may occupy an iliac or sciatic position. Hence, two types of posterior dislocations have been described, namely, the iliac variety and the sciatic variety. In the latter the head of the femur lies below the tendon of the obturator internus muscle; in the iliac variety the femoral head lies on the dorsum of the ilium and can be felt in the buttock. The iliofemoral ("Y") ligament usually is not torn, since it is the strongest part of the capsule, but the posterior portion of the capsule usually is torn. The sciatic nerve may be damaged, and the short rotator muscles of the femur, particularly the obturator internus, also may be injured.

In the anterior dislocation the head of the femur is forced through the inferomedial aspect of the joint and passes medially and forward; it may come to rest on the obturator foramen (obturator variety) or may continue still more anteriorly to reach a position beneath the pubis (pubic variety). In the obturator variety the femoral head rests on the obturator externus muscle. In the pubic variety the femoral head is found in front of the horizontal ramus of the pubis opposite the iliopectineal eminence. The iliopsoas and the pectineal muscles, as well as the obturator and the femoral nerves, may be injured.

A central dislocation of the head of the femur penetrates through the acetabulum and has been referred to as the intrapelvic variety. Usually, a radiating type of fracture of the acetabulum results with a depression of the socket.

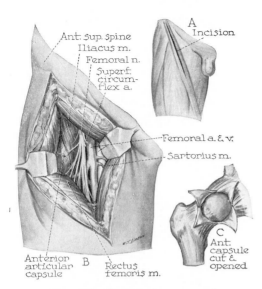

FIG. 653. The anterior approach
to the hip joint.

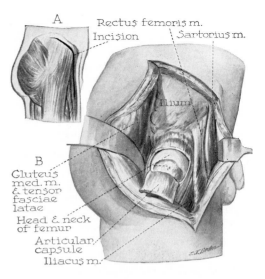

FIG. 654. The anterior iliofemoral approach to the hip joint (Smith-Peterson).

SURGICAL APPROACHES TO THE HIP JOINT

Numerous approaches have been described for exposure of the hip joint. However, only 4 of these will be discussed in this section: the anterior, the anterior iliofemoral, the lateral and the posterior.

The anterior approach to the hip joint commences with a 5-inch or 6-inch skin incision which extends from the anterior superior iliac spine downward along the sartorius muscle (Fig. 653). The superficial and the deep fasciae are incised, and the upper third of the sartorius and the rectus femoris muscles are exposed. In this region the superficial circumflex iliac vessels are seen and may require ligating. The sartorius and the iliopsoas muscles are retracted medially, and the femoris muscles laterally. This exposes the anterior capsule of the hip joint. The femoral nerve lies on the medial aspect of this capsule and should be retracted medially. The capsule is opened in a longitudinal direction; if greater exposure of the joint is needed, a transverse incision into the capsule is added at the end of the longitudinal one.

The anterior iliofemoral approach to the hip joint has been described by Smith-Peterson (Fig. 654). This exposes the anterior and the lateral aspects of the hip joint. The incision commences at about the middle of the iliac crest, curves forward to the anterior superior iliac spine and then continues distally and somewhat laterally for about 5 inches. The superficial and the deep fasciae are incised, and the gluteus medius and the tensor fasciae latae muscles are severed about ¼ inch from the iliac crest. These muscles are stripped subperiosteally downward and backward. At times the lateral cutaneous nerve is seen and retracted medially. The capsule is now exposed and is incised transversely, care being taken to avoid injuring the iliofemoral ligament which is on the anterior aspect of the capsule. If greater exposure of the hip joint is needed, the ligamentum teres can be cut, and the femur rotated externally so that the head of the femur is dislocated. Rapid closure may be accomplished by replacing the periosteum against the ilium and suturing the severed muscles to the crest of the ilium.

The lateral approach to the hip joint can be accomplished through a "U"-shaped incision as described by Ollier (Fig. 655). (Watson-Jones described a lateral approach through a curved incision.) The "U"-shaped incision commences at the anterosuperior iliac spine, continues distally below the greater trochanter, across the femur, then posteriorly and upward and ends midway between the greater trochanter and the pos-

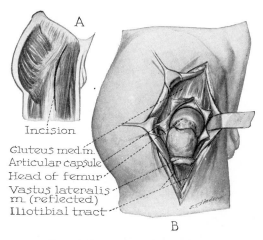

Incision
Gluteus med.m.
Articular capsule
Head of femur
Vastus lateralis
m. (reflected)
Iliotibial tract

FIG. 655. The lateral approach
to the hip joint.

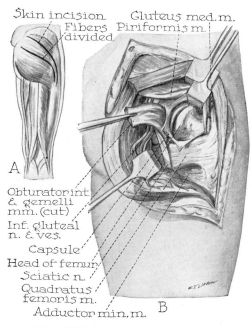

Skin incision   Gluteus med.m.
Fibers   Piriformis m.
divided

Obturator int.
& gemelli
mm. (cut)
Inf. gluteal
n. & ves.
Capsule
Head of femur
Sciatic n.
Quadratus
femoris m.
Adductor min. m.

FIG. 656. The posterior approach
to the hip joint.

terosuperior iliac spine. The gluteus medius
muscle is separated posteriorly, and the tensor fasciae latae muscle anteriorly down to
the greater trochanter. The greater trochanter is removed with an osteotome and, with
its attached muscles, is displaced proximally.
The incision is extended posteriorly by separating fibers of the gluteus maximus muscle
so that adequate exposure is attained. The
exposed capsule is incised longitudinally
along the superior surface of the femoral
neck.

The posterior approach to the hip joint
may be accomplished by means of a posterior
curved incision described by Kocher. This
incision begins at the posterosuperior iliac
spine, extends outward and downward 1 inch
distal to the greater trochanter (Fig. 656).
The superficial and the deep fasciae are incised, and the gluteus maximus muscle is
divided about 1 inch distal to the posterior

iliac spine. The aponeurotic insertion of the
gluteus maximus is separated from the trochanter. Then the muscle is retracted proximally and distally, thus exposing the sciatic
nerve and the external rotator muscles of the
hip joint. The hip is rotated outward; the
tendons of the superior gemellus, the obturator internus and the inferior gemellus muscles are divided about ½ inch from their
insertions. After retracting these latter muscles medially, and the piriformis muscle proximally, the posterior articular capsule will
be exposed. The capsule is incised longitudinally and transversely, thereby exposing
the posterior aspect of the head and the neck
of the femur.

Thigh

The thigh extends from the hip to the knee (Fig. 657). The spine of the pubis and the anterosuperior iliac spine, with the inguinal ligament stretched between these 2 points, is the dividing line between the thigh and the abdomen. The upper boundary of the thigh posteriorly is the transverse gluteal fold; the lower thigh boundary has been set at a level 3 fingerbreadths above the base of the patella.

The contour is conical and oblique in a downward and inward direction; this obliquity is more marked in the female. The muscles stand out boldly in the well-developed male, but in the female the thigh is rounded more uniformly, due to the greater amount of subcutaneous fat.

FRONT OF THE THIGH

NERVES, FASCIA, VESSELS AND LYMPH GLANDS

The skin of the thigh is thicker over the lateral aspect.

The cutaneous nerves of the front of the thigh are (Fig. 658):

1. *The ilio-inguinal nerve* (L 1), which is located close to the pubic spine and to the outer side of the spermatic cord. It supplies the skin of the scrotum and the root of the penis in the male, as well as that part of the thigh in contact with the genitals. It supplies the labium majus in the female.

2. *The lumbo-inguinal nerve* (femoral branch of the genitofemoral, L 1, 2) is small and supplies a limited area below the middle of the inguinal ligament. It is a slender nerve and not easily found. It pierces the deep fascia a little lateral to the saphenous opening.

3. *The lateral cutaneous nerve* of the thigh (L 2, 3) appears behind the lateral end of the inguinal ligament. It divides into anterior and posterior branches which supply the skin of the lateral aspect of the thighs as far down as the knee; it helps in the formation of the patellar plexus. The posterior branch supplies the anterior part of the buttocks.

4. *The intermediate cutaneous nerve* of the thigh (L 2, 3) supplies the skin over the anterior aspect of the thigh by means of lateral and medial branches, which end in the patellar plexus.

5. *The medial cutaneous nerve* of the thigh (L 2, 3) supplies the medial aspect of the thigh and ends in the patellar plexus.

The superficial fascia of the lower limb is the same as that of the body generally. Therefore, it has 2 layers, a fatty superficial layer of superficial fascia, which is a continuation of Camper's fascia of the abdomen, and a deep membranous layer of superficial fascia, which is a continuation of Scarpa's fascia of the abdomen. The latter is attached to the deep fascia of the thigh about a finger's breadth below the inguinal (Poupart's) ligament; more medially, it attaches along a line which runs parallel with and lateral to the spermatic cord. This line runs from the pubic tubercle to the pubic arch.

If urine or other fluids pass into the anterior part of the perineum, they cannot encroach upon the medial side of the thigh because of the attachment of the membranous layer of superficial fascia from the pubic tubercle to the pubic arch. However, they can ascend between the membranous layer and the deep fascia of the abdominal wall. Upon reaching the abdominal wall they cannot descend the front of the thigh because of the connection of the mebranous layer and the fascia lata (deep fascia).

Internal Saphenous Vein. In the superficial fascia the subcutaneous vessels, the nerves and the lymph glands are found. Of

practical importance is the internal saphenous vein (saphena magna, great or long
saphenous vein) (Fig. 659). In the thigh it
usually is concealed by the surrounding fat,
but it is seen easily in the leg; hence, its
name (saphes = easily seen). This vein origi-

nates at the inner side of the *dorsal venous
arch* of the foot and passes upward in front
of the internal malleolus. It continues to
ascend behind the inner border of the tibia
as far as the posterior surface of the internal
condyle of the femur. From here it takes a

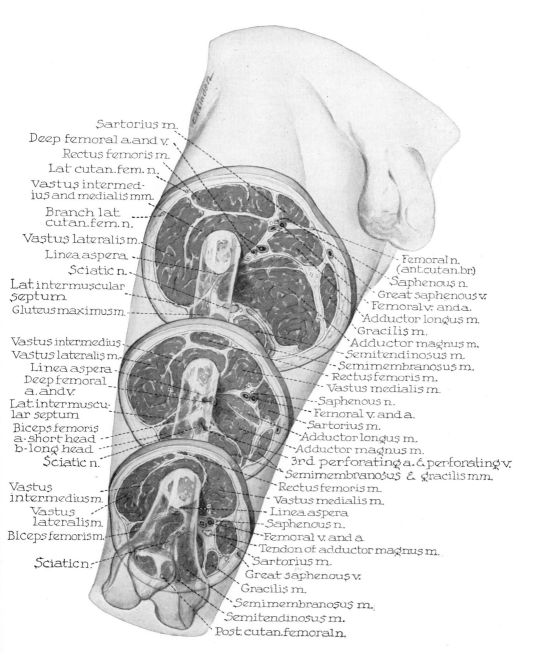

Sartorius m.
Deep femoral a. and v.
Rectus femoris m.
Lat. cutan. fem. n.
Vastus intermed-
ius and medialis mm.
Branch lat.
cutan. fem. n.
Vastus lateralis m.
Linea aspera
Sciatic n.
Lat. intermuscular
septum
Gluteus maximus m.

Vastus intermedius
Vastus lateralis m.
Linea aspera
Deep femoral
a. and v.
Lat. intermuscu-
lar septum
Biceps femoris
a - short head
b - long head
Sciatic n.

Vastus
intermedius m.
Vastus
lateralis m.
Biceps femoris m.

Sciatic n.

Femoral n.
(ant. cutan. br)
Saphenous n.
Great saphenous v.
Femoral v. and a.
Adductor longus m.
Gracilis m.
Adductor magnus m.
Semitendinosus m.
Semimembranosus m.
Rectus femoris m.
Vastus medialis m.
Saphenous n.
Femoral v. and a.
Sartorius m.
Adductor longus m.
Adductor magnus m.
3rd. perforating a. & perforating v.
Semimembranosus & gracilis mm.
Rectus femoris m.
Vastus medialis m.
Linea aspera
Saphenous n.
Femoral v. and a.
Tendon of adductor magnus m.
Sartorius m.
Great saphenous v.
Gracilis m.
Semimembranosus m.
Semitendinosus m.
Post. cutan. femoral n.

FIG. 657. The thigh.

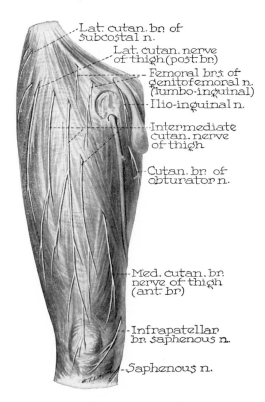

Lat. cutan. br. of
subcostal n.

Lat. cutan. nerve
of thigh (post. br.)

Femoral brs. of
genitofemoral n.
(lumbo-inguinal)

Ilio-inguinal n.

Intermediate
cutan. nerve
of thigh

Cutan. br. of
obturator n.

Med. cutan. br.
nerve of thigh
(ant. br)

Infrapatellar
br. saphenous n.

Saphenous n.

FIG. 658. The cutaneous nerve supply
of the anterior region of the thigh.

straight upward course along the medial aspect of the thigh to the fossa ovalis where
it empties into the femoral vein (sapheno-
femoral junction.

Entering the long saphenous vein are 2
veins which run almost parallel with it. One
enters from the antero-external aspect of the
thigh and is called the *anterior (lateral superficial) saphenous;* the other from the
postero-internal aspect of the thigh is called
the *posterior (medial superficial) saphenous.*

Three additional veins enter the long saphenous; they are the *superficial external
pudic,* the *superficial epigastric* and the
superficial circumflex iliac. Each of these is
accompanied by its corresponding artery; the
arteries are branches of the femoral artery.
Some of the superficial tributaries may empty
directly into the femoral instead of the internal saphenous vein; therefore, they do not

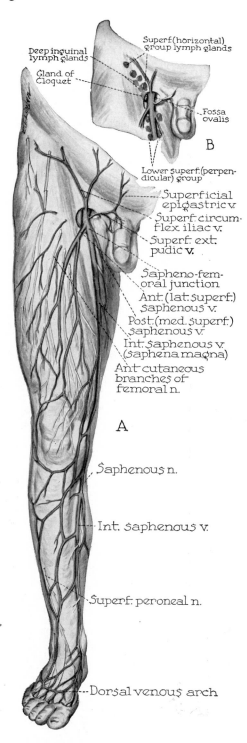

Superf. (horizontal)
group lymph glands

Deep inguinal
lymph glands

Gland of
Cloquet

Fossa
ovalis

B

Lower superf. (perpen-
dicular) group

Superficial
epigastric v.

Superf. circum-
flex iliac v.

Superf. ext.
pudic v.

Sapheno-fem-
oral junction

Ant. (lat. superf.)
saphenous v.

Post. (med. superf.)
saphenous v.

Int. saphenous v.
(saphena magna)

Ant. cutaneous
branches of
femoral n.

A

Saphenous n.

Int. saphenous v.

Superf. peroneal n.

Dorsal venous arch

FIG. 659. (A) The internal saphenous
vein. (B) The inguinal lymph glands.

serve as absolute guides; hence, the femoral vein may be ligated by mistake.

At times the term "accessory saphenous" is seen in many of the standard texts. The term usually seems to mean a lesser saphenous vein that ends high in the greater saphenous. Whether this designates a medial or a lateral vein is still not clear. Daseler and his co-workers have worked extensively in this field and can be referred to. The *valves* in the great saphenous vein vary tremendously in number and are also variably placed. However, according to Kampmeier and Birch, one is typically located at the mouth of the great saphenous vein. Variations are present not only in the valves but also in the veins themselves. Some are of the opinion that the variations in the greater saphenous vein are in direct relation to the veins entering it at its upper end. The most typical pattern is described here. As they pass upward, the greater and the lesser saphenous veins communicate with each other and with the deep veins of the limb. Especially those of the leg communicate by means of so-called communicating or perforator veins, which are so arranged that blood normally passes from the superficial to the deep-set (Fig. 660). Incompetence of some of their valves is regularly associated with varicose veins and, under these conditions, permits the blood flow to reverse.

The superficial external pudic (pudendal) vessels pass medially over the spermatic cord in the male and the round ligament of the uterus in the female. The deep external pudic vessels run under the spermatic cord or the round ligament; the internal pudic vessels reach the external genitals within the pelvis.

The superficial epigastric vessels arise about 1 cm. below the inguinal ligament. The vein usually enters the saphenous opening, but the artery pierces the deep fascia lateral to the opening.

Lymph Glands. In this region a number of lymph glands will be encountered (Fig. 659 B). They are subdivided as follows:

Superficial Group:

1. An upper (horizontal) group lies parallel with the inguinal ligament below the

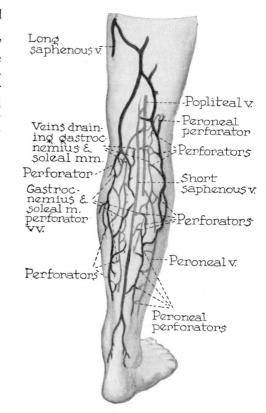

Fig. 660. A composite representation of the communicating and the perforating veins on the back of the leg.

attachment of Scarpa's fascia to the fascia lata. They drain the regions supplied by the 3 superficial inguinal blood vessels (anterior abdominal wall below the navel, the penis, the scrotum, the vulva, the vagina, the anus, the perineum and the buttock).

2. A lower (perpendicular) group is placed on both sides of the upper end of the long saphenous vein. This group receives the superficial lymph vessels of the lower limb, except those from the lateral side of the foot and the posterolateral area of the leg which enter the popliteal glands. Lymphangitis from septic conditions of the toes produces enlargement of this set of glands.

Deep Group: The deep inguinal lymph glands receive the deep lymph vessels of the lower limb. They are 4 or 5 in number and

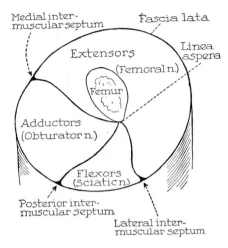

FIG. 661. The septa of the thigh. The 3 main intermuscular septa of the thigh (lateral, medial and posterior) form fascial compartments for the 3 main groups of muscles (extensors, flexors and adductors).

lie beneath the deep fascia close to the upper part of the femoral vein. The most proximal gland of this group (gland of Cloquet) lies in the femoral canal (p. 766). The efferents from the popliteal glands end in these glands, and they in turn drain into the external iliac lymph glands.

DEEP FASCIA (FASCIA LATA)

The structures discussed to this point lie in the superficial fascia. Beneath this is the deep fascia (fascia lata). This fascia attaches above and below to all the bony and the ligamentous structures available.

Above, it is attached completely around the limb, to the anterior superior iliac spine, the inguinal ligament, the pubic bone (body), the pubic arch, the ischial tuberosity and the sacrotuberous ligament. Posteriorly, the fascia lata becomes the gluteal fascia and is attached to the sacral spines and the iliac crest and ends as the fascia lata at the anterior superior iliac spine.

Below, the fascia lata attaches to the periosteum of the patella, the medial and the lateral condyles of the tibia and the head of the fibula. Thus it completely surrounds

the thigh as a tight-fitting sleeve. Posteriorly, it continues as the popliteal fascia. The fascia lata is much stronger laterally than medially because of the iliotibial tract which fuses and runs with it. This tract is a conjoined tendon for the insertion of the gluteus maximus and the tensor fasciae latae into the deep fascia of the thigh. The fascia lata provides septa which separate the various groups of muscles of the thigh. Each septum inserts at the linea aspera (Figs. 657 and 661). Thus each group is enclosed in a separate fascial compartment. Since there are 3 main groups of muscles (extensors, flexors and adductors) there are 3 main septa:

1. *The lateral intermuscular septum* separates the extensors from the flexors and extends from the deep surface of the fascia lata to the femur along the linea aspera as far as the lateral epicondyle.

2. *The medial intermuscular septum* separates the extensors from the adductors. This septum is much thinner than the lateral; it forms the floor of Hunter's canal (p. 772).

3. *The posterior intermuscular septum* separates the adductors from the flexors. This septum which originates from the deep surface of the fascia lata is associated with the connective tissue surrounding the sciatic nerve. There are also separate fascial compartments for the individual muscles as well as the larger compartments for the muscle groups.

Fossa Ovalis. The fascia lata has numerous small openings for the passage of the vessels and the nerves and one large opening, the fossa ovalis for the internal saphenous vein (Fig. 662). This opening is not quite as well marked as the average textbook picture would lead us to believe. Although present and demonstrable, it may be quite indistinct. It is a little more than 1 inch long, a little less than 1 inch wide and appears about 1 inch below the medial end of the inguinal ligament. When well developed its upper, lateral and lower boundaries are well defined and together form a sharply curved edge, the falciform margin. Its medial border is poorly defined and blends with the pectineus fascia. The falciform margin has an upward and medial prolongation, the superior cornu, and a downward and medial prolongation, the inferior cornu. The superior cornu passes in front of the femoral vessels and attaches to the pubic spine. The inferior cornu passes behind the saphenous vein and blends with the pectineus fascia. The fossa ovalis is covered by a loose areolar and fatty tissue, the fascia cribrosa, which fills the fossa.

INGUINOFEMORAL (SUBINGUINAL) REGION

This region extends from the inguinal ligament above to the level of the apex of the femoral (Scarpa's) triangle below. It also includes the area from the tensor fasciae latae muscle laterally to the pectineus muscle medially.

Femoral Triangle. The femoral triangle of Scarpa (femoral trigone) lies directly below the inguinal ligament which forms its base (Fig. 663). Laterally, it is bounded by the

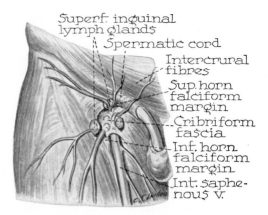

FIG. 662. The fossa ovalis.

medial border of the sartorius muscle, and medially by the medial border of the adductor longus muscle. The floor of the triangle is formed, lateral to medial, by the

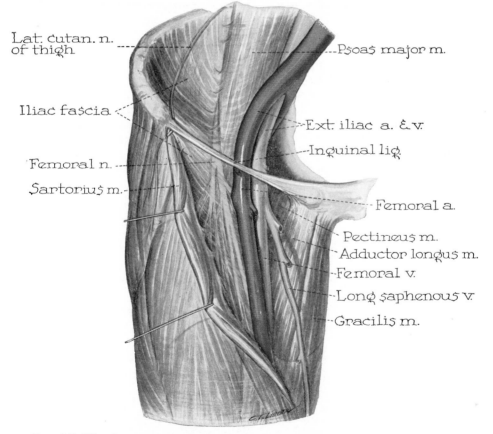

FIG. 663. The femoral triangle of Scarpa and its contents. The roof (fascia lata) of the triangle has been removed, and the relations of the femoral nerve and vessels to the iliac fascia are shown.

iliacus, the pectineus and the adductor longus muscles. The adductor longus forms part of the floor as well as the medial boundary. The roof is formed by the fascia lata. When the roof of the triangle is removed, the contents, namely, the femoral nerve, the artery and the vein, become visible.

The femoral sheath can be understood by studying the fascial relations in the false pelvis and following them into the thigh (Figs. 664 and 665). The fascia which covers the iliopsoas muscle is the iliopsoas fascia. It extends from the iliac crest laterally to the pelvic brim medially. The femoral nerve lies behind it, but the femoral vein and artery lie upon it. The iliopsoas muscle and its fascia pass behind the inguinal ligament on their way to the thigh. The iliac part of the fascia comes in direct contact with the inguinal ligament since no structures intervene; however, that part of the fascia which covers the psoas muscle cannot touch the inguinal ligament because the femoral artery and vein lie on the fascia, separating it from the ligament. The femoral vessels thus leave the pelvis and enter the thigh, and the psoas fascia continues behind the vessels to become continuous with the pectineus fascia. It has been stated that the fascia lata "takes its origin" from the inguinal ligament; hence, the iliac part of the iliopsoas fascia fuses with the fascia lata, but it is impossible for the psoas part of the fascia to touch

the fascia lata because of the interposed femoral artery and vein. Therefore, the fascia lata lies in front of the vessels, and the continuation of the iliopsoas fascia (pectineus fascia) lies behind them. The femoral vessels (not the nerve) are thus wrapped in a downward prolongation of the extraperitoneal fatty areolar tissue which becomes the femoral sheath. The anterior wall of this sheath is formed by a continuation of transversalis fascia; this lines the deep surface of the anterior abdominal wall. The posterior wall of the sheath is formed by that part of the iliopsoas fascia which lies behind the femoral vessels. The sheath ends about 1½ inches below the inguinal ligament by blending with the adventitial coats of the femoral vessels. Two anteroposterior septa divide the sheath into 3 compartments. Separate longitudinal incisions may be made over each compartment to identify the contents. The femoral artery occupies the lateral compartment, the femoral vein occupies the middle compartment, and in the medial compartment, also called the *femoral canal* (p. 766), are found the main lymph vessels of the lower limb.

The femoral artery, a continuation of the external iliac artery, bisects the inguinal ligament (midinguinal point) and is therefore the ventral structure running through the femoral triangle (Fig. 666). To locate the *nerve to the pectineus muscle (femoral*

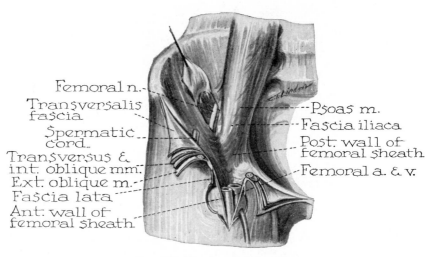

FIG. 664. The femoral sheath.

nerve) one must retract the femoral artery medially and the femoral nerve laterally. It is of fair size and descends downward and inward to disappear deep to the femoral artery or between it and the deep femoral artery. This is the only motor nerve that crosses the femoral artery in Scarpa's triangle, and since it does so posteriorly it is in a protected position.

Branches of the Femoral Artery. Several superficial branches arise from the femoral artery. The superficial circumflex iliac and the superficial epigastric arteries have been described (Fig. 666). The superficial external pudendal passes medially in front of the femoral vein and then crosses to the spermatic cord. The deep external pudendal artery arises a little over 1 inch below the inguinal ligament, runs medially but behind the femoral vein and in front of the pectineus and the adductor longus muscles. It pierces the fascia lata and is distributed to the scrotum or the labium majorum.

As the femoral artery travels through Scarpa's triangle it crosses its trimuscular floor. However, it is separated from each of these muscles in the following way: (1) from the psoas by its sheath and by the nerve to the pectineus, (2) from the pectineus by a fat pad which contains the profunda vessels, and (3) from the adductor longus by the femoral vein.

The profunda femoris artery is a large vessel which usually arises from the posterolateral aspect of the femoral artery. It may arise as high as the level of the inguinal ligament, in which case 2 main arteries appear to enter the limb. The profunda femoris artery is almost as large as the femoral artery proper. The profunda leaves the triangle by passing behind the adductor longus, which separates it from the femoral vessels proper. It then lies on the adductor magnus, where it ends as the fourth perforating artery. The lateral and the medial circumflex arteries spring from the profunda near its origin.

The lateral circumflex artery passes laterally among the branches of the femoral nerve, sometimes separating this nerve into superficial and deep sets of branches. It leaves the triangle by passing under cover of the sartorius muscle. It divides into 3

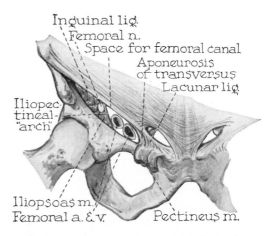

FIG. 665. The femoral sheath and its associated structures as seen from below.

branches: (1) an ascending branch, which ends with the nerve to the tensor fasciae latae; (2) a transverse branch, which anastomoses with the medial circumflex artery; and (3) a descending branch, which is associated with the nerve to the vastus externus (vastus lateralis).

The medial circumflex artery passes through the floor of the triangle between the pectineus and the iliopsoas muscles and terminates in the buttocks at the lower border of the quadratus femoris. The femoral artery leaves the apex of Scarpa's triangle to enter the subsartorial (adductor) canal of Hunter (p. 772).

The femoral vein is a large vessel and is a direct continuation of the popliteal vein. It begins at an opening in the adductor magnus, ascends through the subsartorial canal of Hunter and the femoral triangle and ends behind the inguinal ligament, where it becomes the external iliac vein. Below, it lies posterolateral to the artery, but in the greater part of its course it lies posteriorly, except in the upper part of the thigh, where it lies to the medial side of the femoral artery. It receives the long saphenous vein as its main tributary and other smaller tributaries, some of which correspond to the artery. At the apex of Scarpa's triangle a definite order of structures exists (Fig. 667), from before backward: the femoral artery, the femoral vein, the adductor longus muscle, the profunda vein and the profunda artery. Hence, a stab or a bullet wound at the apex of Scarpa's triangle could penetrate all 4 of these vessels in succession.

The femoral nerve is the nerve of the anterior compartment of the thigh. It arises within the abdomen from the lumbar plexus and forms a thick nerve (Fig. 668). In the false pelvis it lies deep in the groove between the psoas and the iliacus and enters the femoral triangle by passing behind the inguinal ligament. In the thigh it is lateral to the femoral artery, from which it is separated by a small part of the psoas muscle and the femoral sheath. About 1 inch below the inguinal ligament it breaks up into a "cauda

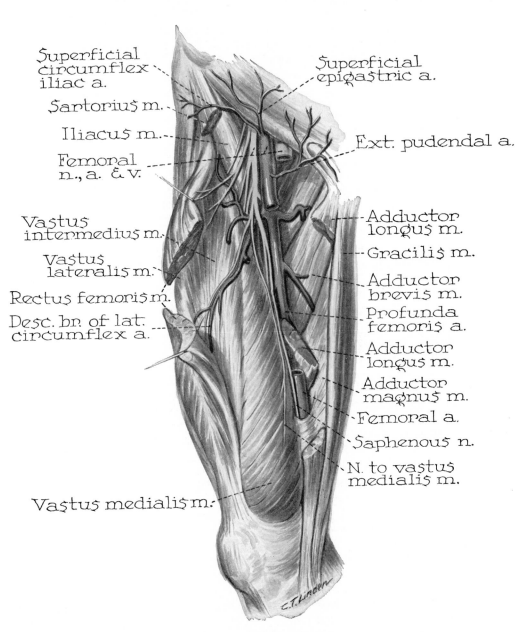

Fig. 666. The femoral artery.

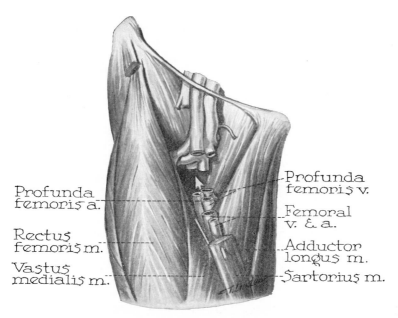

Profunda
femoris a.

Rectus
femoris m.

Vastus
medialis m.

Profunda
femoris v.

Femoral
v. & a.

Adductor
longus m.

Sartorius m.

FIG. 667. The relations of the femoral artery
and vein in the femoral triangle.

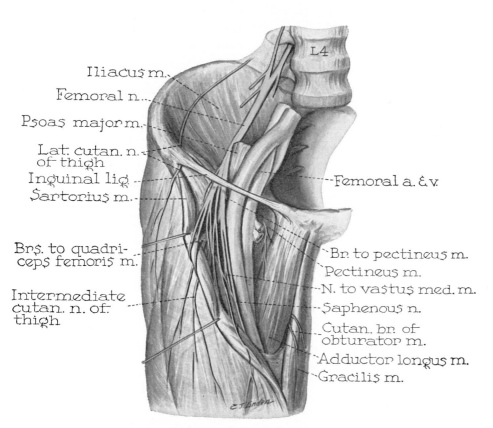

L4

Iliacus m.

Femoral n.

Psoas major m.

Lat. cutan. n.
of thigh

Inguinal lig.

Sartorius m.

Brs. to quadri-
ceps femoris m.

Intermediate
cutan. n. of
thigh

Femoral a. & v.

Br. to pectineus m.

Pectineus m.

N. to vastus med. m.

Saphenous n.

Cutan. br. of
obturator m.

Adductor longus m.

Gracilis m.

FIG. 668. The femoral nerve.

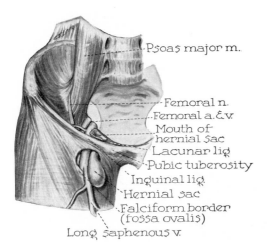

FIG. 669. Femoral hernia.

equina"—like a leash of muscular and cutaneous nerves. The muscular branches pass to the pectineus, the sartorius and the quadriceps femoris. The cutaneous branches constitute the medial cutaneous and the intermediate cutaneous nerves of the thigh and the saphenous nerve. Two of these branches closely follow the artery on its lateral side and into the subsartorial canal: the saphenous nerve, which is sensory, and the nerve to the vastus medialis, which is motor. The nerve supply to the quadriceps femoris is through 4 separate nerves, one to each head: the rectus femoris and the 3 vasti. Articular nerves arise from these 4 muscular branches. The nerve to the rectus femoris sends a slender branch to the hip joint, and the nerves to the vasti send filaments through the muscles to the knee joint.

SURGICAL CONSIDERATIONS

Surgical Anatomy and Repair of a Femoral Hernia

In a femoral hernia the abdominal contents enter the femoral ring, pass through the femoral canal and leave through the fossa ovalis (Fig. 669). In so doing, the abdominal contents push the parietal peritoneum, the extraperitoneal fat and the femoral septum on ahead. The femoral canal is only about ½ inch in length; therefore, it is more of an anatomic landmark than a true canal or surgical structure.

The femoral ring has the following boundaries:

Anterior: the inguinal ligament
Posterior: the pectineus fascia and muscle
Lateral: the femoral vein
Medial: the lateral sharp edge of the lacunar (Gimbernat's) ligament

With these boundaries kept in mind one readily comprehends the danger of cutting lateral to a femoral hernia (femoral vein).

Surgical Repair. The surgical repair of a femoral hernia may be accomplished through a subinguinal approach or an inguinal approach.

The subinguinal approach usually is performed through a vertical incision placed directly over the protruding mass (Fig. 670). The incision is deepened until a fatty mass is seen below the fatty areolar layer. If the falciform margin is well developed it can be severed; otherwise, one proceeds directly to the femoral ring where the neck of the sac is freed. The extraperitoneal fat is incised, and the sac (peritoneum) is located and opened. If the femoral ring is so small and tight that strangulation is produced and the contents cannot be reduced, more room can be gained by cutting the lacunar ligament. If viable, the contents are reduced, and the sac is ligated and excised. The usual method of repair is one in which the inguinal ligament is sutured to the fascia of the pectineus muscle. The femoral vein must not be encroached upon.

The inguinal approach opens the inguinal canal, as in the repair of an inguinal hernia. The transversalis fascia is incised, and the neck of the femoral hernia sac is located in the extraperitoneal fatty layer just proximal to the femoral ring. The sac is drawn into the inguinal canal; it is handled in the routine manner. Both the femoral ring and the inguinal canal are closed by placing sutures which approximate the conjoined tendon and the inguinal ligament to Cooper's ligament.

Ligation of the Femoral Artery in the Femoral Triangle

The femoral artery is situated in a superficial position in the femoral triangle of Scarpa (Fig. 671). The femoral vein lies in close proximity to the artery. The artery is easily ligated in this location because of its superficial position and because of the ease with which it can be separated from the femoral vein, since each vessel is situated in its own compartment within the femoral sheath. Collateral circulation is maintained through anastomoses between the superior and the inferior gluteal vessels and the first perforating branch of the deep (profunda) femoral artery.

Ligation of the artery at the apex of the femoral trigone can be accomplished through an incision placed directly over the vessel. The sartorius muscle is identified and re-

tracted laterally; the vessel is isolated just before it enters the subsartorial (adductor) canal of Hunter. Collateral circulation is maintained by anastomoses around the knee joint, where the branches of the profunda femoris artery anastomose with the branches of the popliteal artery.

MUSCULATURE OF THE THIGH

Since the thigh is capable of performing 4 principal types of movements it is well to consider the musculature in 4 parts (Fig. 650):

1. Adductors (obturator nerve)

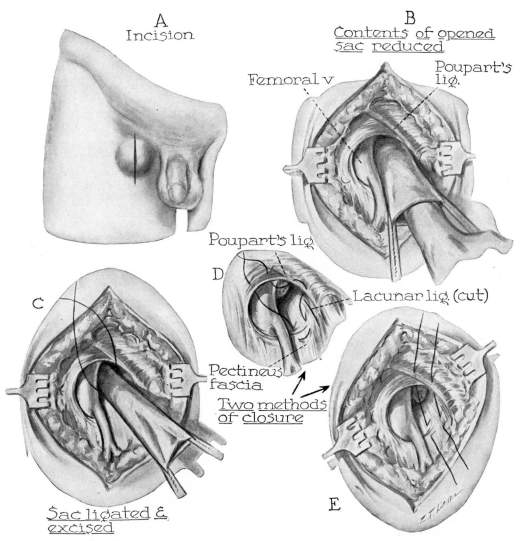

FIG. 670. The anatomy involved in the repair of a femoral hernia.

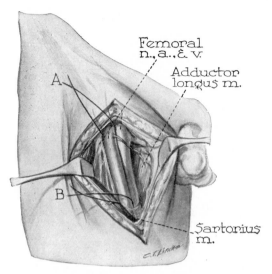

FIG. 671. Exposure and ligation of the femoral artery in the femoral triangle.

2. Abductors (superior gluteal nerves) (see p. 746)

3. Extensors, anterior femoral muscles, (femoral nerve)

4. Flexors, posterior femoral muscles, (sciatic nerve)

ADDUCTOR (OBTURATOR) GROUP

The adductor region has been referred to as the obturator region, since it is supplied by the obturator nerve. In this region, which is situated on the medial aspect of the thigh, are found 6 muscles: 3 adductors (longus, brevis and magnus) plus 3 other muscles: the pectineus, the gracilis and the obturator externus (Fig. 672).

These muscles constitute a group which is interposed between the extensor group in front and the flexor group behind. The adductor muscles *arise* from the bones around the obturator foramen and the obturator membrane; they *insert* from the trochanteric fossa of the femur above to the medial surface of the tibia below (Fig. 683).

The pectineus muscle can be exposed after having identified the femoral triangle; it makes up part of the floor of this triangle. It arises from the superior ramus of the pubis, runs downward and backward to become inserted into the posterior aspect of the proximal part of the femoral shaft just below

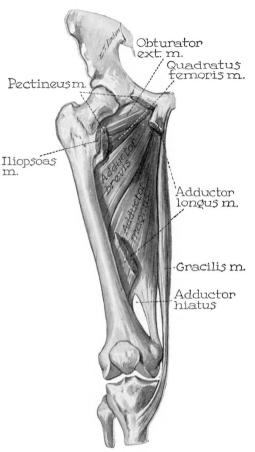

FIG. 672. The adductor group of muscles. Six muscles constitute this group: the 3 adductors (longus, brevis and magnus), the pectineus, the gracilis and the obturator externus.

the lesser trochanter. This muscle is peculiar in that it has a double nerve supply (Fig. 673). The medial part is supplied by the obturator nerve; the lateral half, by the femoral nerve. Because of this, some anatomists believe that the muscle has a double origin and should be divided into medial and lateral parts. Although the greater part of the muscle is supplied by the nerve to the pectineus (Fig. 673) (femoral nerve), it is still considered one of the adductors in the obturator group.

The adductor longus muscle lies on the same plane as the pectineus; therefore, it also makes up part of the floor of Scarpa's triangle. It arises by a flattened tendon from the body of the pubis in the angle between the crest of the pubis and the symphysis pubis. If the thigh is abducted, its tendon becomes prominent and palpable and acts as a guide to the pubic tubercle. Extending downward and laterally, its fibers spread out into a rather broad thin aponeurosis which inserts into the medial lip of the linea aspera. It lies between the pectineus and the gracilis. (The adductor brevis may be seen behind and between the pectineus and the adductor longus muscles.) It is the most anterior of the 3 adductor muscles. If it is divided near its origin and turned down, its nerve and blood supply are seen entering its deep surface. The muscle which is exposed by reflecting the adductor longus is the adductor brevis.

The adductor brevis, a large muscle, is covered with fat on its anterior surface. In this fat lies the anterior division of the obturator nerve. (The posterior division of the nerve lies behind the adductor brevis.) The anterior division of the nerve supplies the adductor longus and the brevis, the gracilis and the hip joint. Also running in this fat is the deep branch of the femoral artery (profunda femoris) with its accompanying veins. The adductor brevis arises from the front of the pubis below the adductor longus and runs downward, backward and laterally. It inserts into the linea aspera above and behind the adductor longus, reaching almost as high as the lesser trochanter. Its upper border lies against the obturator externus. If the adductor brevis is cut near its origin and turned downward the adductor magnus is seen.

The adductor magnus muscle, largest and most posterior of the 3 adductors, rises from the inferior ramus of the ischium and the outer part of the inferior surface of the ischial tuberosity. It inserts on the linea aspera extending upward along the linea aspera's lateral continuation, the gluteal tuberosity, and downward on its medial continuation, the medial epicondylar line. The fibers which arise from the ischial tuberosity pass almost vertically downward to insert by means of a short tendon into the adductor tubercle which is located on the medial condyle of the femur.

At the insertion of the muscle a series of

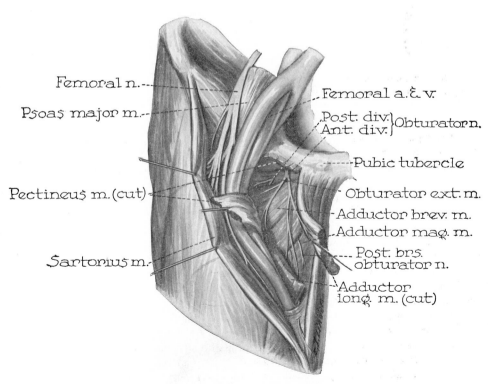

FIG. 673. The obturator nerve.

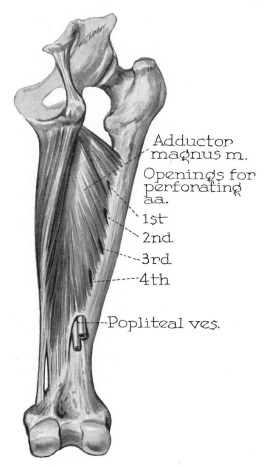

Adductor magnus m.

Openings for perforating aa.

1st

2nd

3rd

4th

Popliteal ves.

FIG. 674. The adductor magnus muscle and its 4 osseo-aponeurotic openings.

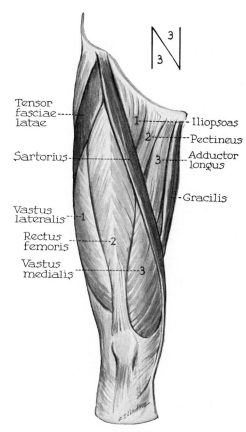

Tensor fasciae latae

Sartorius

Vastus lateralis

Rectus femoris

Vastus medialis

Iliopsoas

Pectineus

Adductor longus

Gracilis

FIG. 675. The extensor group of muscles. To identify immediately the entire musculature of the front of the thigh, the letter "N" can be constructed, using the tensor fasciae latae, the sartorius and the gracilis. Three muscles lie above the sartorius (iliopsoas, pectineus and adductor longus), and 3 muscles lie below the sartorius (vastus lateralis, rectus femoris and vastus medialis).

osseo-aponeurotic openings are formed by tendinous arches which attach to the bone (Fig. 674). The upper openings, usually 4 in number, are small and give passage to the perforating branches of the profunda femoris artery. The lowest opening is the largest and is called the *adductor hiatus*. Through it the femoral vessels enter the popliteal fossa. The upper border of the adductor magnus lies close to the lower border of the obturator externus; the posterior border of the adductor magnus is in relation to the hamstring muscles and the sciatic nerve (Fig. 679).

The obturator externus muscle arises from the medial margin of the obturator foramen and from the lateral surface of the obturator membrane (Figs. 429 and 672). The fibers converge and pass behind the neck of the femur. The obturator vessels lie between the

muscle and the obturator membrane. The anterior branch of the obturator nerve reaches the thigh by passing in front of the muscle, the posterior branch by piercing it. It is the powerful lateral rotator of the thigh and is seen best after division of the pectineus muscle.

The gracilis muscle is the most superficial muscle on the medial side of the thigh. It is thin and straplike and arises from the margin of the upper part of the pubic arch and the adjoining part of the body of the pubis. It passes behind the medial epicondyle of the femur and inserts into the upper part of the

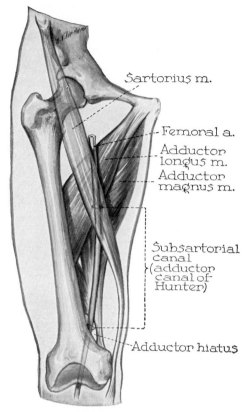

Sartorius m.

Femoral a.

Adductor longus m.

Adductor magnus m.

Subsartorial canal (adductor canal of Hunter)

Adductor hiatus

FIG. 676. The subsartorial (adductor) canal of Hunter.

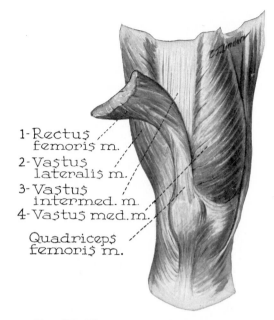

1-Rectus femoris m.

2-Vastus lateralis m.

3-Vastus intermed. m.

4-Vastus med. m.

Quadriceps femoris m.

FIG. 677. The quadriceps femoris muscle.

to the tendons of the gracilis and the semitendinosus and inserts in front of them (Fig. 695 B). It flexes, abducts and laterally rotates the hip while flexing and medially

medial surface of the tibia. When the hamstring muscles are paralyzed, flexion of the leg is accomplished by the gracilis and the sartorius muscles.

EXTENSOR (ANTERIOR) GROUP

The extensor group of muscles is the *femoral nerve group*. This group has been referred to as the flexors of the hip, but usually they are called the extensors of the knee. The group consists of the sartorius, the quadriceps femoris, the iliopsoas and the pectineus (Fig. 675).

The sartorius muscle is the longest muscle in the body, its fleshy part usually measuring over 18 inches in length. It arises mainly from the anterosuperior iliac spine, then crosses the upper third of the thigh obliquely and descends almost vertically to the posterior part of the medial side of the knee. It passes forward and ends in a thin tendon which is inserted into the upper part of the medial surface of the tibia. It is superficial

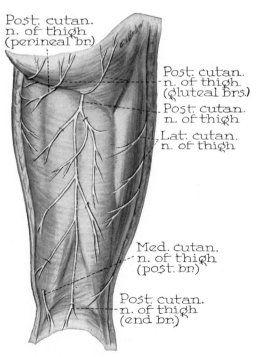

Post. cutan. n. of thigh (perineal br.)

Post. cutan. n. of thigh (gluteal brs.)

Post. cutan. n. of thigh

Lat. cutan. n. of thigh

Med. cutan. n. of thigh (post. br.)

Post. cutan. n. of thigh (end br.)

FIG. 678. The cutaneous nerve supply of the posterior aspect of the thigh.

rotating the knee joint. In this way it brings about the position which the tailor assumes at work. It forms the lateral boundary of the femoral triangle and the roof of the subsartorial (adductor) canal of Hunter.

The subsartorial (adductor) canal of Hunter is an intermuscular canal that is situated on the medial aspect of the middle third of the thigh. It extends from the apex of Scarpa's triangle to the opening in the

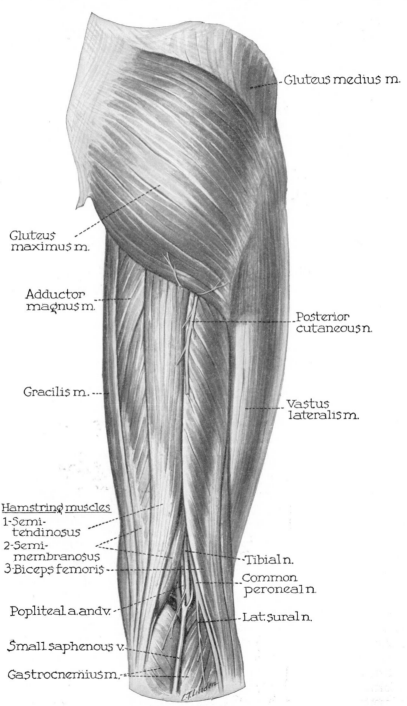

FIG. 679. The hamstring muscles.

adductor magnus muscle, which has been referred to as the adductor hiatus (hiatus tendineus) (Fig. 676). It is called Hunter's canal because it was here that John Hunter ligated the femoral artery for popl'teal aneurysm. The canal is bounded laterally by the vastus medialis; posteriorly, a floor is formed by the adductor longus proximally and the

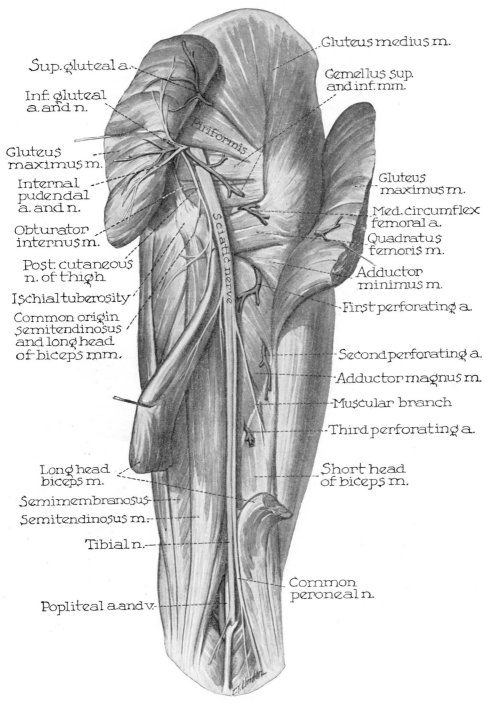

Sup. gluteal a.

Inf. gluteal a. and n.

Gluteus maximus m.

Internal pudendal a. and n.

Obturator internus m.

Post. cutaneous n. of thigh

Ischial tuberosity

Common origin semitendinosus and long head of biceps mm.

Long head biceps m.

Semimembranosus

Semitendinosus m.

Tibial n.

Popliteal a. and v.

Piriformis

Sciatic nerve

Gluteus medius m.

Gemellus sup. and inf. mm.

Gluteus maximus m.

Med. circumflex femoral a.

Quadratus femoris m.

Adductor minimus m.

First perforating a.

Second perforating a.

Adductor magnus m.

Muscular branch

Third perforating a.

Short head of biceps m.

Common peroneal n.

E. H. Linden

FIG. 680. The deeper structures of the posterior aspect of the thigh.

adductor magnus distally. The roof of the canal is formed by the sartorius muscle with a strong layer of deep fascia, which lies under the sartorius.

This fascia has been called the *subsartorial fascia* (fascia vasto-adductoria). It stretches from the fascial coverings of the adductors to the fascial coverings of the vastus medialis. Since the anterior surface of the adductor longus and the magnus are covered by the medial intermuscular septum, this septum forms the floor of the canal. The femoral vessels and the saphenous nerve traverse the canal.

Before incising the subsartorial fascia in order to expose the femoral artery, one should endeavor to expose a fine subsartorial nerve plexus. This lies immediately beneath the sartorius and is formed by branches of the obturator, the long saphenous and the internal cutaneous nerves. Once the subsartorial fascia is incised, the most superficial structures in the canal will be found, namely, the long saphenous nerve, which crosses the artery from without inward and gives off a small twig to the subsartorial plexus.

To the outer side of the long saphenous nerve another nerve is found, the nerve to the vastus medialis muscle. The femoral artery is situated directly beneath the long saphenous nerve. The artery is separated from the floor of Hunter's canal by the femoral vein. The vein is posterior to the artery in the upper part of the canal but posterolateral to it in the lower part.

The adductor longus muscle separates the femoral vessels from the profunda vessels (Fig. 667). The femur and the vastus medialis are anterolateral to the femoral artery, and the sartorius is anteromedial. Near the lower end of the canal the femoral artery gives off the descending genicular artery (superior geniculate anastomotica magna). This vessel supplies a superficial branch which accompanies the saphenous nerve, an articular branch which takes part in the anastomosis around the knee joint, and muscular branches.

The quadriceps femoris muscle is composed of 4 parts: the rectus femoris and the 3 vasti (medialis, lateralis and intermedius) (Figs. 675 and 677). The rectus femoris arises from the ilium, and the 3 vasti arise from the shaft of the femur. The rectus femoris is placed over the anterior aspect of the thigh and is quite distinct from the others, except at its insertion. The vasti clothe the front and the sides of the shaft of the femur and are more or less blended with each other; therefore, they are difficult to separate.

The rectus femoris is the most superficial of the 4 and lies between the 2 vasti; it covers the vastus intermedius. Since it is the only portion of the quadriceps which arises from the innominate bone, it acts as a flexor of the hip joint as well as an extensor of the knee. The rectus arises by 2 heads: a straight head from the anterior inferior iliac spine and a reflected head which arises from the impression on the ilium immediately above the acetabulum. The latter is under cover of the gluteus minimus. The 2 heads unite in front of the hip joint, and the muscular belly which results passes down in front of the thigh and inserts into the common extensor tendon. If the gluteus medius and minimus are displaced backward and the rectus femoris forward, the hip joint is exposed. By this approach no motor nerves are encountered. After being crossed by the sartorius, the rectus femoris becomes superficial and forms a well-rounded elevation in front of the thigh which is seen best when the knee is extended. It is safe to dissect along the lateral side of the rectus femoris, since its nerve, from the femoral, enters its medial side.

The vastus lateralis arises from the lateral part of the linea aspera and from its upward lateral continuation (the gluteal tuberosity), as well as its downward lateral continuation (the lateral epicondylar line). This muscle is best seen after the rectus femoris has been severed about its middle and dissected upward and downward. It forms the greater part of the fleshy muscle mass on the lateral side of the thigh and is recognized, since its superficial stratum is a glistening aponeurosis. It overlaps the vastus intermedius and is partly blended with that muscle. It gains attachment to the patella by means of the common tendon of insertion. The descending branch of the lateral femoral circumflex artery is accompanied by the nerve to the vastus lateralis. This then is the best guide to the anterior border of the muscle.

The vastus medialis is intimately connected with the vastus intermedius, and difficulty may be found in separating the two. It originates from the medial lip of the linea aspera and from its medial upward continuation (the spiral line) and its medial downward continuation (the medial epicondylar line); its lowermost fibers arise from the tendon of the abductor magnus muscle. The muscle covers the medial surface of the femur. Its lowest fibers, which run almost horizontally, form the fleshy mass which can be seen medial to the upper part of the patella in the living. It is inserted into the common tendon and into the medial border of the patella and, like the vastus lateralis, gives off a fibrous expansion to the capsule of the knee joint.

The vastus intermedius arises from and covers the anterior and the lateral surfaces of the shaft of the femur. Although the vastus medialis covers the medial aspect of the femur, no muscle originates from this surface; hence, the bone is almost bare. It is a large fleshy muscle covered laterally and medially by the vastus lateralis and the medialis and is covered above by the rectus femoris. It is inserted into the deep aspect of the common tendon.

The quadriceps as a whole acts as a powerful extensor of the knee joint, but in addition to this the rectus femoris part of the quadriceps acts as a flexor of the hip joint.

The articularis genu consists of a few of the deepest bundles of the vastus intermedius. It arises from the front of the femur and is inserted into the synovial membrane of the knee.

Where the common tendon plays across the front of the lower end of the femur a sesamoid bone (the *patella*) develops. The portion of the tendon distal to the patella is called the *patellar ligament*. The patella does not lie in front of the knee joint but rather in front of the end of the femur (p. 789).

It is well to keep the following picture in mind, so that the anterior thigh musculature may be quickly visualized:

1. The "N" arrangement in which the sartorius makes up the oblique line with 3 muscles placed above it (iliopsoas, pectineus and adductor longus) and 3 muscles below it (vastus lateralis, rectus femoris and vastus medialis) (Fig. 675).

2. The adductor brevis is located in the interval between the pectineus and the adductor longus; the adductor magnus is located in the interval between the longus and the gracilis; the gracilis lies immediately behind and inserts deep to the sartorius (Fig. 666).

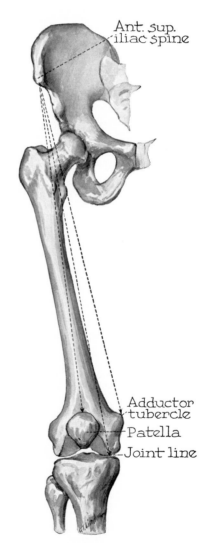

Fig. 681. Methods of measuring the length of the femur.

FLEXOR (POSTERIOR) GROUP

The posterior aspect of the thigh derives its cutaneous nerve supply in the following way: medially, it is supplied by the anterior cutaneous rami of the femoral nerve; poste-riorly, by the posterior femoral cutaneous nerve; and, laterally, by the lateral femoral cutaneous nerve (Fig. 678).

The posterior thigh compartment contains the 3 hamstring muscles, namely the semi-

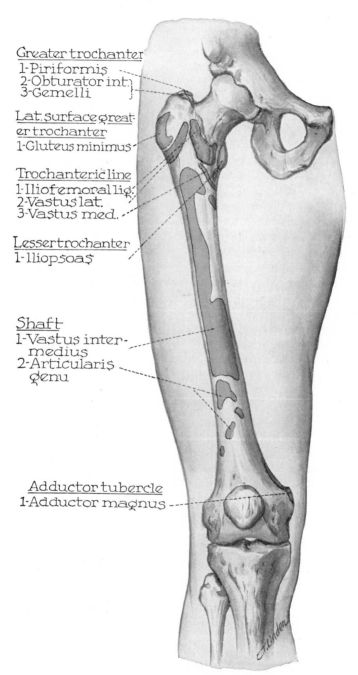

Greater trochanter
1-Piriformis
2-Obturator int.
3-Gemelli

Lat. surface greater trochanter
1-Gluteus minimus

Trochanteric line
1-Iliofemoral lig.
2-Vastus lat.
3-Vastus med.

Lesser trochanter
1-Iliopsoas

Shaft
1-Vastus inter-medius
2-Articularis genu

Adductor tubercle
1-Adductor magnus

FIG. 682. The femur seen from in front. Muscle origins are shown in red; insertions, in blue.

membranosus, the semitendinosus and the biceps femoris (Figs. 679 and 680). The compartment also contains the sciatic nerve and its 2 terminal branches—the tibial and the common peroneal. A hamstring muscle is one that arises from the ischial tuberosity and inserts into one of 2 bones of the leg; it is supplied by the tibial division of the sciatic nerve. Although it covers the femur, it has no attachments to it. The long head of the

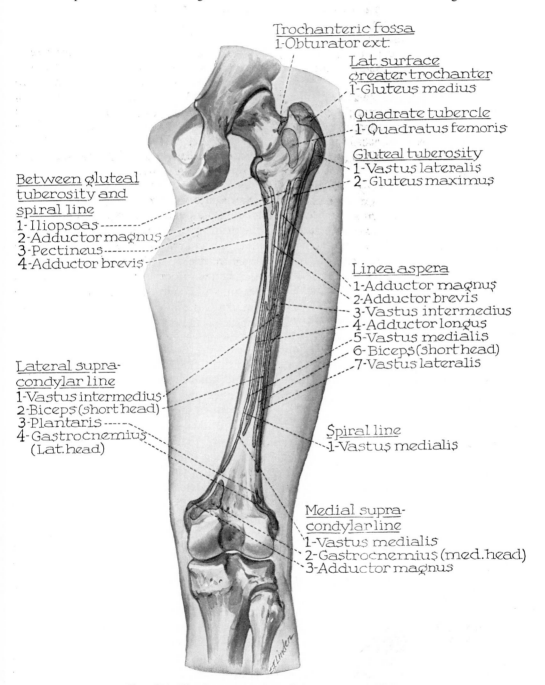

Trochanteric fossa
1-Obturator ext.

Lat. surface
greater trochanter
1-Gluteus medius

Quadrate tubercle
1- Quadratus femoris

Gluteal tuberosity
1-Vastus lateralis
2- Gluteus maximus

Between gluteal
tuberosity and
spiral line
1- Iliopsoas
2-Adductor magnus
3-Pectineus
4-Adductor brevis

Linea aspera
1-Adductor magnus
2-Adductor brevis
3-Vastus intermedius
4-Adductor longus
5-Vastus medialis
6-Biceps(short head)
7-Vastus lateralis

Lateral supra-
condylar line
1-Vastus intermedius
2-Biceps (short head)
3-Plantaris
4-Gastrocnemius
(Lat.head)

Spiral line
1-Vastus medialis

Medial supra-
condylar line
1-Vastus medialis
2-Gastrocnemius (med.head)
3-Adductor magnus

FIG. 683. The femur seen from behind. Muscle origins
are shown in red; insertions, in blue.

biceps femoris meets these prerequisites, but the short head does not; hence, this is an exception to the rule. It is interesting also to note that the adductor magnus muscle arises from the ischial tuberosity, inserts onto the tibia and is supplied by the tibial division of the sciatic nerve; therefore, it meets the 3 prerequisites of a hamstring and should be considered as such. For convenience sake, however, it should be discussed with the adductor group.

Since the **short head of the biceps femoris** does not meet these 3 prerequisites, it is not really a hamstring but belongs to the muscle plate of the gluteus maximus. It is supplied by the peroneal division of the sciatic nerve (Fig. 680).

The long head of the biceps femoris arises from the lower and the inner impression of the back part of the tuberosity of the ischium by means of a tendon common to it and the semitendinosus; it also arises from the lower part of the sacrotuberous ligament. Its 2 heads unite just above the knee joint to form a common tendon. As the muscle bundles pass downward and medially, they lie on the surface of the semimembranosus. The common tendon inserts into the lateral side of the head of the fibula and forms the upper and the lateral boundaries of the popliteal fossa. The common peroneal nerve descends along its medial border. In addition to its action as a flexor of the knee joint and extensor of the hip, it is a lateral rotator.

The semitendinosus, so named for the great length of its tendon of insertion, arises from the lower and the medial impression of the ischial tuberosity by a tendon common to it and the long head of the biceps femoris. It inserts into the upper part of the medial surface of the tibia just below the gracilis muscle. It is a medial rotator of the tibia on the femur.

The semimembranosus, so named for its membranous tendon of origin, arises by this thick tendon from the upper and the outer impression on the ischial tuberosity above and lateral to that of the biceps femoris and the semitendinosus. It passes downward and medially, at first deep to the conjoined tendon of the biceps and the semitendinosus, and then is overlapped subsequently by the laterally placed muscles. It inserts on the medial condyle of the tibia.

Nerves and Vessels. The sciatic nerve leaves the pelvis through the greater sciatic foramen, passes through the gluteal region and the upper part of the thigh. It ends at about the middle of the thigh by dividing into lateral and medial popliteal nerves. In the thigh the adductor magnus muscle is anterior to the nerve, and the long head of the biceps muscle crosses behind it from medial to lateral. It sends branches to the semitendinosus, the semimembranosus, the long head of the biceps and the adductor magnus via the medial popliteal nerve. The short head of the biceps muscle is supplied by the lateral popliteal nerve (Fig. 680).

Perforating branches of the profunda femoris artery enter the posterior aspect of the thigh through openings found in the adductor magnus muscle. These vessels continue posteriorly to supply the vastus lateralis muscle and the hamstrings. The first perforating artery enters into the "crucial anastomosis," and the 3rd and the 4th perforating vessels anastomose with muscular rami from the popliteal artery.

FEMUR

The femur or the thigh bone is the longest, the largest and the heaviest bone in the body, being about a quarter of the entire height of the individual. The femur is more liable to inequality than is the tibia or the fibula; hence, the relative length of the lower limb is equal in only 10 per cent of individuals. The measurements of the length of the femur are taken from the anterosuperior iliac spine to either the adductor tubercle or the lower limits of the medial condyle (joint line) (Fig. 681). The upper border of the patella also has been used as a distal point in measuring this length; but, since it is movable, it is not as accurate as the other two. The bone consists of proximal and distal ends and a shaft (Figs. 682 and 683). The distal end is larger and close to its fellow femur, but the proximal ends are separated by the width of the pelvis. The shaft is thinnest in the middle and enlarges toward the ends, especially distally.

PROXIMAL END

The proximal end consists of a head, a neck, the greater and the lesser trochanters, the trochanteric fossa, the trochanteric line, the trochanteric crest and the quadrate tubercle.

Head. The rounded head forms two thirds of a sphere, which is directed medially, upward and forward and is gripped firmly by the labrum acetabulare beyond its maximum diameter. Therefore, it is much more secure in its socket than is the head of the humerus, which forms only one third of a sphere. In the erect posture the upper aspect of the head is pressed against the iliac part of the acetabular articular surface. The head is covered with hyaline cartilage and presents a depression or pit which gives attachment of the ligament of the head (ligamentum teres); this depression is located a little below and behind the central point.

Neck. The neck of the femur, about 1½ inches long, is triangular in shape; its apex supports the head of the femur, and its base becomes continuous with the shaft. It is placed obliquely and unites the head to the shaft and the trochanters. It thickens toward each end, especially the shaft end, which it joins at an angle of about 125° in the adult, but is more obtuse in the child. This angle is known as the "vertical neck-shaft angle." Since the neck of the femur is directed upward, inward and forward, another angulation results which is forward and is known as the "declination angle"; it is normally of about 12°. Any alteration of these angles results in deformity and disability. In reality, the neck of the femur is the medially curved upper extremity of the shaft, but the presence of the greater trochanter hides this. It is separated from the shaft by the trochanteric line in front and the trochanteric crest behind.

The trochanteric line presents a roughened edge produced by the attachment of the powerful iliofemoral ligament. Its upper end is at the front of the greater trochanter, and its lower end is continuous with a faint ridge called the *spiral line,* which winds around the lesser trochanter to the back of the shaft.

The trochanteric crest crosses the posterior aspect of the bone and continues into the lesser trochanter below. A small rounded tubercle (quadrate) about its middle gives insertion to the quadratus femoris muscle.

The trochanteric fossa is small and is located at the junction of the posterior part of the neck and the medial side of the great trochanter; the obturator externus muscle inserts here.

The greater trochanter is a fixed process which lies in line with the lateral aspect of the shaft and can be felt through the skin about one hand's breadth below the iliac crest. The muscles attached to it produce the rotatory movements of the thigh. It should be looked upon as the traction epiphysis of the gluteus medius and minimus as well as the piriformis, the obturator internus and externus, and the gemelli. When the gluteus medius contracts it draws this trochanter upward, medially and backward. Its upper and posterior borders are free, and its highest point is located at its posterosuperior angle. The anterior and the lateral aspects of this trochanter would be continuous with the corresponding aspects of the shaft except for the presence of a rough line which marks the site of fusion of the trochanter and the shaft. If a chisel is driven along the upper border of the femoral neck it would remove the greater trochanter approximately at this rough fusion line.

The lesser trochanter is a blunt-shaped pyramidal process which is directed backward and medially from the junction of the lower and the posterior part of the neck of the femur with the shaft; it is not palpable. It gives attachment to the tendon of the iliopsoas and has been considered the traction epiphysis for that structure.

The quadrate tubercle is an ill-defined protrusion which is situated about the center of the trochanteric crest; it gives insertion to the quadratus femoris muscle.

The epiphyseal line of the femoral head corresponds to its articular margin (Fig. 684). Anteriorly, the capsule is attached to the spiral line; therefore, the whole neck is intracapsular. Posteriorly, the capsule is attached about a finger's breadth medial to the intertrochanteric crest, the neck being partly intracapsular and partly extracapsular. The metaphysis is entirely intracapsular. Since the site of election for the occurrence of bone disease, especially in the young, is in the metaphysis, if the metaphysis is inside the joint capsule the disease is likely to invade the joint. On the other hand, if the disease is primarily in the joint it may affect the shaft of a bone, if the metaphysis is partly within the affected joint.

DISTAL END

The distal end of the femur reveals lateral and medial condyles and epicondyles, a patellar surface, the intercondylar notch and line, the adductor tubercle and the pit and the groove for the popliteus muscle.

The condyles make up nearly the entire distal end and give it an irregular cuboidal shape. They coalesce in front but are separated behind by the deep intercondylar notch. The top of the tibia and the semilunar cartilages of the knee joint articulate with the posterior surfaces of the condyles when the knee is bent, but with their inferior surfaces when the knee is straight.

The lateral condyle is broader than the medial. The lateral epicondyle is the eminence which is situated on the posterior part of the

lateral surface of the lateral condyle. A *pit* for the origin of the popliteus muscle is below this epicondyle. The *groove* for the tendon of the popliteus muscle passes upward and backward from this pit close to the articular margin.

The medial condyle is farther from the side of the shaft than is the lateral. It is narrower and more curved. When the shaft is held vertically it projects to a lower level than the lateral, but in the natural oblique position of the bone the lower surfaces of both condyles are in the same plane. Immediately behind and above its center its rough medial surface presents the *medial epicondyle* to which the medial ligament of the knee is attached. Immediately above this is the *adductor tubercle* for the insertion of the strong tendon of the adductor magnus.

The intercondylar notch is bounded by the opposed surfaces of the condyles and separates them behind and below. This notch is occupied by the cruciate ligament. Its floor slopes upward and backward to a horizontal ridge called the *intercondylar line,* which separates it from the popliteal surface of the shaft.

The patellar (trochlear) surface is convex from above downward and concave from side

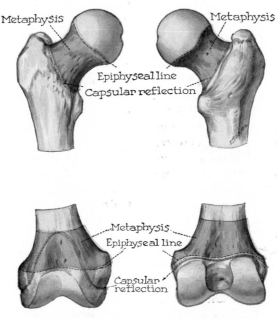

FIG. 684. The femoral epiphyseal lines.

to side; it is situated on the anterior aspect of the lower extremity and extends farther upward on the lateral condyle than on the medial. It is separated from the articular surfaces of the tibia by grooves on either side in which the semilunar cartilages of the knee rest when the joint is fully extended. The patella articulates with it when the knee is straight but is drawn off when the knee is bent; in the latter position its margin can be felt through the tendon of the quadriceps.

The sides of the condyles and the adductor tubercles are felt quite easily in the living person.

The epiphysis at the lower end of the femur is represented by an irregular horizontal line at the level of the upper limit of the articular surface in front and behind, which crosses the middle of the adductor tubercle (Fig. 684). The capsule may be outlined posteriorly to the articular margin, and laterally and medially about 2 inches proximal to the articular margin. Therefore, the metaphysis is intracapsular only in front.

SHAFT

The shaft or body of the femur is bowed slightly forward; its middle two thirds are circular on cross section, but its upper and lower extremities are oblong, the lower border being the larger. In the erect posture the shaft is oblique, since the distal ends of the femora are in contact with each other; but the proximal ends are separated by the pelvis and by the necks of the femora. Each shaft in its middle third reveals anterior, medial and lateral surfaces which are separated by rather ill-defined lateral and medial borders; a well-marked posterior border known as the linea aspera is easily discernible.

The linea aspera is a broad rough line that stands out boldly from the back of the middle two thirds of the femoral shaft. It bifurcates both above and below into divergent lines. The upper lines are the spiral line and the gluteal tuberosity; the lower ones are the medial and the lateral epicondylar lines.

The spiral line passes upward and medially and becomes continuous with the trochanteric line.

The gluteal tuberosity ascends to the side of the greater trochanter where it becomes continuous with the epiphyseal line. The lesser trochanter projects from a triangle bounded by these two lines.

The medial and the lateral epicondylar lines descend from the linea aspera to the epicondyle and give rise to the boundary of a flat triangular area which is limited below by the intercondylar line. This area is known as the *popliteal surface*. The medial epicondylar line turns abruptly so that the adductor tubercle, which is placed about ½ inch above the medial epicondyle, is easily palpable. The medial aspect of the shaft is devoid of muscular attachments.

Attachments to the Femur (Figs. 682 and (683):

To the head: the ligamentum teres

To the neck: the capsule of the hip joint

To the trochanteric line: the iliofemoral ligament, the vastus lateralis and the medialis

To the trochanteric fossa: the obturator externus

To the greater trochanter: to the medial surface the obturator internus, the gemelli and the piriformis; to the upper border the piriformis; to the anterior surface the gluteus medius

To the quadrate tubercle: the quadratus femoris

To the lesser trochanter: the iliopsoas

To the gluteal tuberosity: the gluteus maximus and the vastus lateralis

To the spiral line: the vastus medialis

To the area between the gluteal tuberosity and the spiral line from lateral to medial: the adductor magnus, the adductor brevis, the pectineus and the iliopsoas

To the linea aspera, lateral to medial: the vastus lateralis and the intermedius from the lateral lip, the lateral intermuscular septum and the short head of the biceps. From the medial lip, the adductor magnus, the brevis and the longus: the medial intermuscular septum and the vastus medialis

From the lateral supracondylar line: the vastus intermedius, the lateral septum, the short head of the biceps, the plantaris and the lateral head of the gastrocnemius

From the medial supracondylar line: the adductor magnus, the medial septum, the vastus medialis, and the medial head of the gastrocnemius

From the shaft (anterior and lateral surfaces): the vastus intermedius and the articularis genu

From the lateral condyle: the anterior cruciate ligament of the knee, the popliteus, and the lateral ligaments of the knee

From the medial condyle: the posterior cruciate ligament, and the medial ligament of the knee

The fascia lata attaches to both condyles

SURGICAL CONSIDERATIONS

FEMORAL VEIN LIGATION AND THROMBECTOMY (Fig. 685)

Recently, Allen, Linton and others have advocated interruption of the superficial femoral vein and removal of thrombi. This is done as a prevention for pulmonary embolism. A skin incision is made along the course of the pulsating femoral artery on the involved side (Fig. 685 A). The artery overlies the vein in this region, and when the former is retracted laterally the superficial

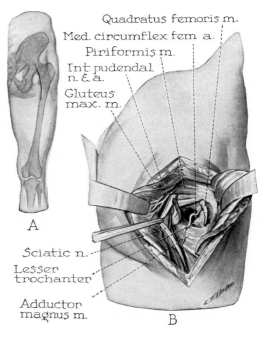

FIG. 686. Approach to the lesser trochanter of the femur.

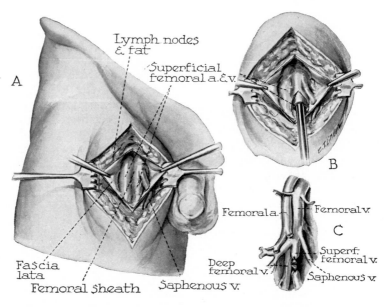

FIG. 685. Ligation of the superficial femoral vein: (A) incision and exposure; (B) removal of thrombus by suction; (C) ligation and division.

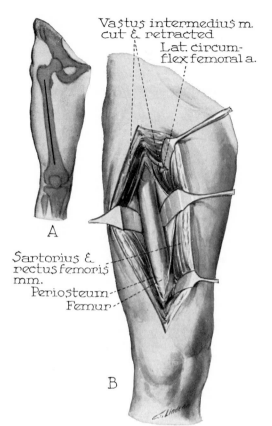

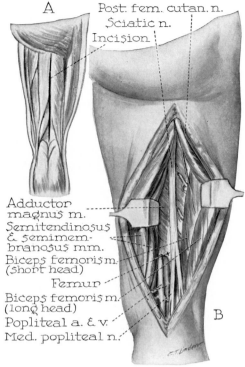

FIG. 687. The anterior approach to the shaft of the femur.

FIG. 688. The posterior approach to the shaft of the femur.

femoral vein is exposed. After identifying the deep femoral vein, the superficial femoral vein is incised, and the thrombus is removed; then it is ligated and divided (Figs. 685 B and 685 C).

APPROACH TO THE LESSER TROCHANTER OF THE FEMUR (Fig. 686)

Exposure of the lesser trochanter of the femur is accomplished through an incision which extends from the upper end of the trochanter midway between it and the midsacral line downward for about 2 or 3 inches (Fig. 686). This incision is deepened through the thickened fatty layer until the deep fascia is exposed. The gluteus maximus is incised in its thickened portion. The sciatic nerve is retracted medially, and the quadratus femoris

muscle is either divided or retracted upward. The iliopsoas tendon can be stripped off of the lesser trochanter, and this will result in an excellent view of the latter.

APPROACHES TO THE SHAFT OF THE FEMUR

The shaft of the femur may be surgically approached anteriorly, posteriorly, laterally or medially.

The anterior approach is accomplished through an incision which is made over the greater extent of the femoral shaft in a line situated between the anterosuperior iliac spine and the middle of the patella (Fig. 687). The rectus femoris and the vastus lateralis are separated along the intermuscular septum. The vastus intermedius is incised in the line of its fibers until the femur is reached. Subperiosteal dissection exposes the anterior and the lateral aspects of the femur.

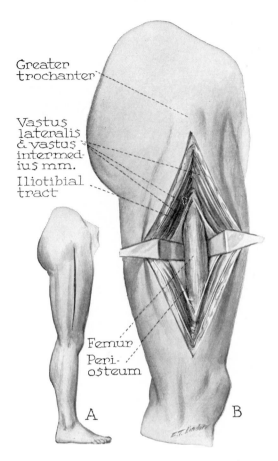

Greater trochanter

Vastus lateralis & vastus intermedius mm.

Iliotibial tract

Femur
Periosteum

A

B

FIG. 689. The lateral approach to the shaft of the femur.

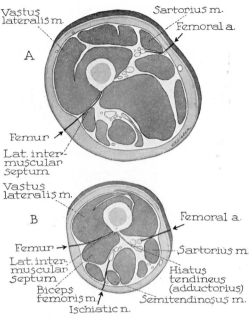

Vastus lateralis m.

Sartorius m.

Femoral a.

A

Femur
Lat. intermuscular septum

Vastus lateralis m.

B

Femoral a.

Femur
Lat. intermuscular septum
Biceps femoris m.
Ischiatic n.

Sartorius m.

Hiatus tendineus (adductorius)
Semitendinosus m.

FIG. 690. Cross sections of the lateral and the medial approaches to the shaft of the femur: (A) in the upper third; (B) in the lower third.

The posterior approach is accomplished through a long incision which is placed over the posterior aspect of the thigh in the line of the shaft of the femur (Fig. 688). The posterior femoral cutaneous nerve should be avoided. The long head of the biceps femoris muscle with the posterior femoral cutaneous nerve is retracted laterally; the semimembranosus and the semitendinosus muscles are retracted medially. The sciatic nerve and the popliteal artery and vein are now identified. The sciatic nerve is retracted laterally and the popliteal vessels medially so that the adductor magnus muscle and the short head of the biceps femoris muscle can be stripped subperiosteally from the femur; it is necessary to ligate the perforating arteries to accom-

plish this. The posterior two thirds of the lower aspect of the femoral shaft is thereby exposed.

The lateral approach commences with a longitudinal skin incision which is placed along a line extending from the greater trochanter to the external femoral condyle (Figs. 689 and 690). The iliotibial tract, the vastus lateralis and the vastus intermedius muscles are divided in the direction of their fibers. The exposed periosteum is incised longitudinally, freed anteriorly and posteriorly, thereby exposing the lateral aspect of the shaft of the femur.

The medial approach for exposure of the lower half of the femoral shaft begins with a skin incision which is placed along the adductor tendon and extends well above and below the adductor tubercle (Fig. 691). The deep fascia is freed, and one attempts to avoid entering the synovial membrane of the knee joint. The sartorius muscle is retracted posteriorly, and the tendon of the adductor magnus muscle is identified. The saphenous nerve is protected as it courses along the undersurface of the sartorius muscle. The large neurovascular bundle is retracted posteriorly.

The adductor magnus tendon and the vastus medialis muscle are retracted anteriorly. At this point the posterior surface of the femur, as it lies in the popliteal space, is exposed.

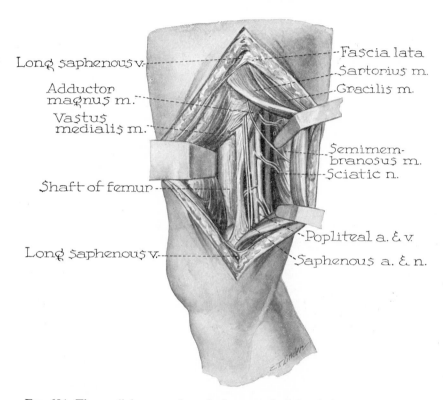

Fig. 691. The medial approach to the lower end of the shaft of the femur.

Knee

The region that constitutes the knee is bounded above by an imaginary line drawn around the thigh at a level of approximately 3 inches above the base of the patella. The inferior extent of the knee is at the tibial tuberosity.

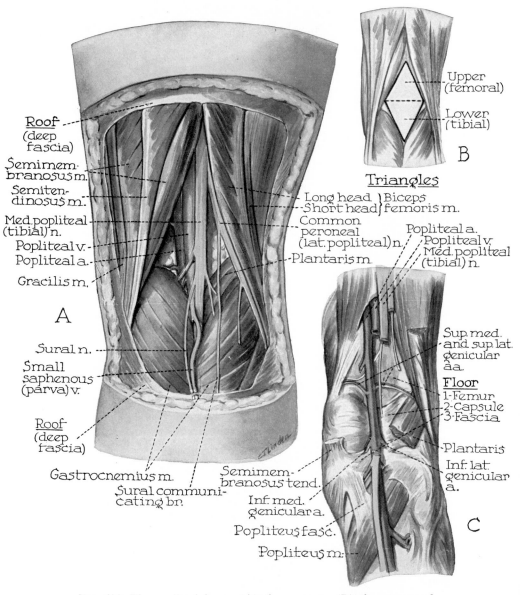

FIG. 692. The popliteal fossa: (A) the contents; (B) the upper and the lower triangles; (C) the deeper structures.

786

POPLITEAL (POSTERIOR) REGION

This region corresponds to the posterior aspect of the knee (Fig. 692). The popliteal fossa or space is lozenge-shaped and has a floor, a roof and lateral boundaries. It consists of an upper (femoral) and a lower (tibial) triangle.

The roof of the space is formed by the deep fascia, which is composed of circularly arranged fibers acting as a restraining or retinacular ligament for the hamstrings. It is pierced near its center by the small saphenous vein which passes between the 2 heads of the gastrocnemius muscle; deep to it is the cutaneous branch of the medial popliteal nerve (tibial). A transverse incision made through this deep fascia will require little or no suturing, since it approximates itself; however, a longitudinal incision will gape.

The floor of the fossa is formed by the lower end of the femur, the posterior part of the capsule of the knee joint and the popliteus muscle with its strong fascia.

The popliteus fascia is an expansion from the tendon of the semimembranosus muscle, which passes downward and outward and covers the *popliteus muscle* (Figs. 692 C and 695 B, 695 C). It attaches to the popliteal line of the tibia. The popliteal vessels lie on it and end at its lower border. The popliteus muscle arises within the capsule of the knee joint from the lateral aspect of the lateral condyle of the femur and is inserted into the posterior aspect of the tibia above the popliteal (soleal) line. Its tendon of origin passes downward and backward, separating the lateral semilunar cartilage from the lateral ligament of the joint. It emerges through the inferolateral aspect of the posterior part of the capsular ligament. It is a flexor of the leg and also acts as a medial rotator of the tibia when the knee is flexed. The medial (tibial) popliteal nerve supplies it.

The femoral (upper) triangle has the semimembranosus, overlaid by the semitendinosus on its medial side and the biceps femoris muscle on its lateral side (Fig. 692 B).

The tibial (lower) triangle is smaller, and its sides are formed by the 2 heads of the gastrocnemius muscle, together with the very variable plantaris muscle which lies laterally.

NERVES AND VESSELS

The contents of the popliteal fossa are arranged mainly as nerve, vein and artery:
1. The lateral and the medial popliteal nerves and their branches
2. The popliteal vein and its tributaries
3. The popliteal artery and its branches
4. The posterior cutaneous nerve
5. Fat and lymph glands

Popliteal Nerves. The tibial and the com-

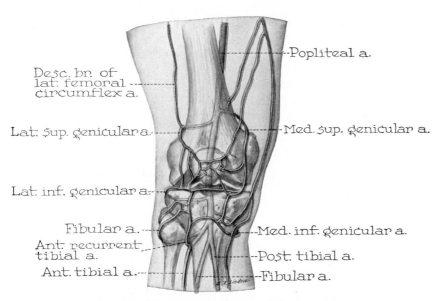

FIG. 693. The anastomosis around the knee joint.

mon peroneal nerves are the terminal branches of the sciatic nerve.

The tibial (internal or medial popliteal) nerve enters the fossa at the upper angle lateral to the popliteal vessels, runs a straight course to the lower angle of the space and is superficial to the vessels. It lies immediately beneath the deep fascia. In its course through the space it crosses superficial to the vessels from lateral to medial. It supplies the muscles of the space, namely, the lateral and the medial heads of the gastrocnemius, the soleus, the plantaris and the popliteus. Only one of these, the medial head of the gastrocnemius, lies medial to the nerve. Because of this anatomic fact it is safer to dissect on the medial side where the nerve has only one branch.

The sural nerve is a cutaneous branch which arises from the tibial nerve and descends on the surface of the gastrocnemius muscle. It supplies small branches to the integument of the calf and the back of the leg, and in the lower third is joined by the sural communicating branch from the lateral (common peroneal) popliteal nerve (Fig. 692 B). The sural nerve travels in company with the short saphenous vein. Three small articular branches usually are present; they supply the knee joint. The close relationship between the tibial nerve and the popliteal vessels explains nerve involvement and pain in popliteal aneurysm.

The common peroneal (lateral or external popliteal) nerve generally separates from the sciatic at about the middle of the thigh, enters the popliteal fossa from the lateral side and passes downward and laterally, closely associated with and appearing from behind the biceps femoris. It follows the biceps tendon to its insertion and leaves the popliteal fossa between that tendon and the lateral head of the gastrocnemius. This relationship is important and must be kept in mind when a biceps tenotomy is contemplated. The nerve continues downward behind the head of the fibula and winds around the lateral aspect of the fibular neck to pierce the origin of the peroneus longus muscle. It ends by dividing into the superficial (musculocutaneous) and the deep (anterior tibial) peroneal nerves. The common peroneal nerve gives off no muscular branches but does give a lateral cutaneous nerve of the calf (lateral

sural), a sural communicating nerve (anastomotic peroneal) and usually 3 genicular branches which accompany the genicular vessels and supply the ligaments and the synovial membranes of the knee joint.

Popliteal Vessels. *The popliteal vein* is formed by the junction of the anterior and the posterior tibial veins at the lower border of the popliteus muscle (Fig. 695 A). It ascends through the popliteal space to the aperture in the adductor magnus muscle, where it becomes the femoral vein. In its trip through this space it lies superficial to the artery but crosses it from medial to lateral. The popliteal vein and artery are bound together by a fascial tube similar to the arrangement in the region of the femoral artery and vein; hence, neither can be displaced without interfering with the other.

The small saphenous vein (parva) passes over the calf of the leg superficial to the enveloping fascia but pierces the deep fascia in the lower part of the popliteal space. It divides into 2 branches: one enters the popliteal vein, and the other communicates with the great saphenous vein.

The popliteal artery is the continuation of the femoral artery; it commences at the opening in the adductor magnus. It passes downward between the condyles of the femur and leaves the fossa at its distal angle to end at the distal border of the popliteus muscle where it divides into the anterior and the posterior tibial arteries (Fig. 693). It appears to run laterally as well as downward because of the inclination of the long axis of the femur. In addition to its terminal branches, the artery gives 3 paired branches which arise at different levels. They are:

1. *The superior genicular arteries* (lateral and medial), which originate at the level of the femoral condyle and wind around the femur proximal to these condyles. They are in close contact with the bone and anastomose anteriorly (Fig. 693).

2. *The middle genicular arteries* enter the knee joint through the posterior ligament and are chiefly muscular and articular, being distributed to the gastrocnemii and the intracapsular structures.

3. *The inferior genicular arteries* (lateral and medial) wind around the front of the knee and pass under cover of the tibial and

the fibular collateral ligaments. They anasto- mose with each other deep to the patellar ligament; they take place also in the anas- tomosis around the knee joint. Since no branches are given off in the upper part of the popliteal artery, this portion is most ac- cessible for ligation.

The anterior (*deep*) *relations* of the artery are, the popliteal surface of the femur, the oblique posterior ligament of the knee joint, and the popliteus muscle covered by its fascia. A rather thick fat pad separates the artery from the femur, but the vessel lies in direct contact with the oblique posterior lig- ament of the knee joint. *Posteriorly,* the ar- tery is separated from the fascial roof of the popliteal space by its accompanying veins and the medial popliteal nerve.

The lymph glands of the popliteal space lie under the deep fascia. They receive the lymph from the skin of the outer side of the leg and the foot, and from the deep structures of the foot via the lymph vessels which ac- company the anterior and the posterior tibial vessels. They also receive lymph from the knee joint. All the efferent vessels from the glands pass with the popliteal vein and then with the femoral vein to the deep inguinal lymph glands. It should be noted that the cor- responding glands in the upper limb, namely, the supratrochlear, lie superficial to the deep fascia.

A rich vascular anastomosis exists around and above the patella and on the ends of the femur and the tibia in the region of the knee joint (Fig 693). The arteries that take part in this anastomosis are the 2 lateral and the medial genicular branches of the popliteal, the descending branch of the lateral femoral circumflex artery and the anterior recurrent tibial artery. Superficially, these vessels are distributed between the fascia and the skin; the deeper vessels lie on the lower end of the femur and the upper end of the tibia, supply- ing the soft tissues around these structures and sending branches into the interior of the knee joint.

KNEE JOINTS

The knee joints constitute a synovial joint of the hinged variety. It is the largest and the most complicated joint in the body (Figs. 694, 695 and 696). Three bones take part in it: the femur, the tibia and the patella. In the human the fibula is entirely excluded from it. Originally, in primitive life there were 3 joint cavities in this location, which now have merged into one. One is situated between the medial condyle of the femur and the tibia, one between the lateral condyle of the femur and the tibia, and one between the patella and the femur. These may be referred to as the medial and the lateral condylar articula- tions and the patellar articulation. The condy- lar articulations are subdivided further into upper and lower parts by the medial and the lateral menisci (semilunar fibrocartilages).

In all positions of this joint the patella is in contact with the femur, and the femur with the tibia. These bones do not interlock, and their areas of contact are large; the ligaments and the surrounding muscles are strong. Therefore, dislocation of this joint is un- common.

PATELLA

The patella is a small sesamoid bone in the tendon of the quadriceps femoris. It is roughly triangular in shape, the inferior angle represents the apex, and the upper border represents the base. The lateral and the me- dial borders are rounded. Its anterior surface is easily felt through the skin, from which it is partly separated by the subcutaneous pre- patellar bursa. The femoral articular surface is divided by a vertical ridge into a larger lateral and a smaller medial area. Below the articular surface the bone is roughened and is nonarticular, and the lower half of this area covers the posterior aspect of the apex. This bone usually begins to ossify between the 3rd and the 5th years, and the process is usually completed by puberty.

If one stands erect with the feet together and the toes pointed forward (the anatomic position), it will be noted that the ball of the big toes, the medial malleoli and the knees of the two sides touch each other; the tibiae are parallel but the femora are not. The latter are set obliquely; although in contact at the knee joint, they are separated above by the width of the pelvis. The rectus femoris and the vastus intermedius are attached to the upper border (base) of the patella; when they contract they pull obliquely upward. The vastus medialis and the vastus lateralis are continuous with each other at their patellar attachments and occupy the space between the rectus femoris and the vastus intermedius. The vastus medialis is attached to the upper two thirds of the medial border of the patella and only slightly to its upper border; the vastus lateralis is attached to the whole length of the upper border and only slightly to the lateral border. The vastus medialis draws the patella medially, and the vastus lateralis pulls it upward but not laterally. A transverse incision above the patella will incise successively the skin, the fat, the fascia lata, the rectus tendon, the tendons of the vasti lateralis and the medialis, the tendon of the vastus intermedius, and the synovial joint capsule. If the quadriceps is relaxed, as when the heel is placed on a chair, the patella may be moved medially and laterally, and the posterior articular surface may be palpated. As the position is changed from extension to one of flexion, one can feel the patella glide lat-

erally onto the under aspect of the lateral condyle of the femur, thus leaving the trochlea and the entire under aspect of the medial femoral condyle exposed, except for a tiny strip which bounds the medial border of the intercondylar notch. This tiny strip articulates with a vertical facet on the medial part of the posterior surface of the patella.

LIGAMENTS AND CARTILAGES

Like other movable joints, the knee has a fibrous as well as a synovial capsule.

The capsular ligament is thin, wide and membranous at the back but thicker and shorter at the sides. It is absent in front, where it is replaced by the patella, the ligamentum patellae below the patella, and the tendon of the quadriceps above it.

The femoral attachments of the capsular ligament are to the sides of the condyles about ¼ inch from the articular margin, to the back of the femur along the inter condy-

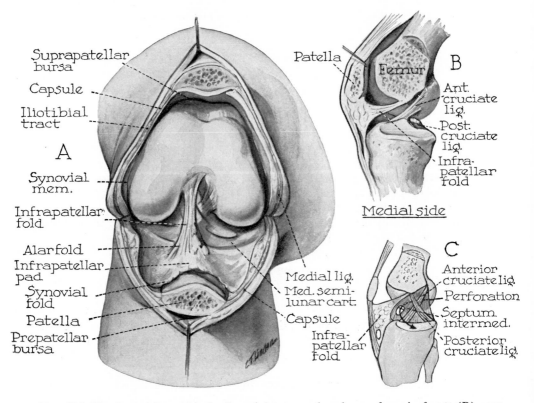

FIG. 694. The knee joint: (A) the knee joint opened and seen from in front. (B) seen from the medial side; (C) the arrow shows the relations between the septum and the perforation.

lar line and immediately above the articular margin of the condyles.

Its tibial attachments are to the posterior surfaces and the sides of the condyles about ¼ inch below the articular margin; also to the anterior surfaces of the condyles along the oblique lines that begin near the articular margins of the sides and pass to the sides of the tubercle of the tibia.

The capsule is strengthened by expansions from surrounding muscles, which for the most part are closely attached to it. However, on the anterolateral aspect there is a definite interval which is occupied by fat, vessels and nerves. The heads of the gastrocnemius and the plantaris overlie the posterior part of the capsule opposite the femoral condyles. The medial head is separated from it by a bursa; the lateral head and the plantaris are partly attached to it; the popliteus, after it emerges through the capsule, derives some fleshy fibers of origin from it. At the back of the medial femoral condyle there is usually a hole in the ligament through which the synovial

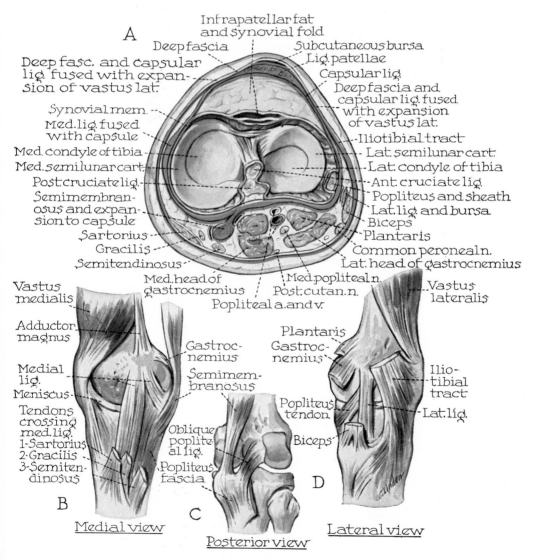

FIG. 695. The right knee joint showing the ligaments, the capsule, the synovial membrane and the relations. The capsule is colored green; the synovial membrane, blue.

membrane becomes continuous with the bursa under the medial head of the gastrocnemius (Fig. 694 C). The tendon of the popliteus perforates the capsular ligament opposite the lateral condyle of the tibia. The ligament is also perforated by articular vessels and nerves. The capsule is overlaid by and incorporated with the tendinous expansions of the lateral and the medial vasti (Fig. 695).

The patellar ligament (ligamentum patellae) is a strong fixed band about 3 inches long and 1 inch wide. It is attached above to the lower border of the patella and below to the tubercle of the tibia; this attachment extends about ½ inch farther down on the inner side (Fig. 697 A). The ligament constitutes the insertion of the quadriceps extensor into the tibia. It is separated from the skin by a bursa. Its superficial fibers are directly con-

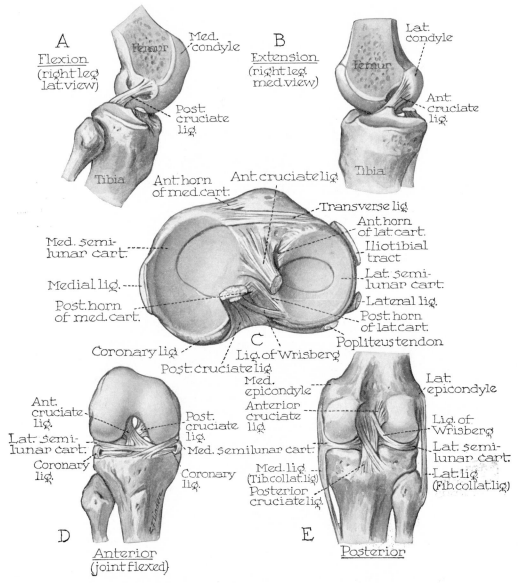

FIG. 696. The ligaments and the cartilages of the right knee joint.

tinuous over the patellar surface with the central part of the common tendon of the quadriceps femoris; the deep surface is separated from the synovial membrane by loose fatty tissue called the *infrapatellar pad of fat* (Fig. 694). A bursa also separates it from the upper part of the tibia. This bursa is crescentic and, when enlarged or inflamed, has extensions which pass upward along the sides of the ligament.

The lateral ligament of the knee (fibular collateral ligament) is a rounded cordlike band which is approximately 2 inches long. It extends from the lateral epicondyle of the femur above to the head of the fibula below (Figs. 695 and 696). Although its upper part is fused with the underlying part of the capsule, most of it is separated from the capsule by fatty tissue in which the inferior lateral geniculate vessels and nerves run. As the ligament crosses the lateral aspect of the knee joint the tendon of the popliteus muscle intervenes between it and the lateral semilunar cartilage (meniscus). The biceps tendon which is superficial to the lower part of the ligament is split in two by it.

The medial ligament of the knee (tibial collateral ligament) is broad and straplike and, unlike the lateral, is closely applied to the bone. It extends from the medial epicondyle of the femur above to the upper fourth of the shaft of the tibia below. Opposite the interval between the femur and the tibia it is closely fused with the capsular ligament (Fig. 695 A). It is attached to the medial meniscus. Three tendons cross it: those of the sartorius, the gracilis and the semitendinosus (Fig. 695 B). A bursa separates these from the ligament. The tendon of the semimembranosus extends forward and under the ligament to gain its insertion into the medial condyle of the tibia.

The 2 collateral ligaments are strong structures and prevent lateral movements at the knee joint. If they are stretched or torn, the integrity of the joint usually is lost.

The 3 ligamentous extensions of the semimembranosus are: the oblique popliteal ligament, the popliteus fascia and the deep fascia of the inner side of the leg.

The oblique popliteal ligament (oblique posterior ligament) strengthens the capsule posteriorly (Fig. 695 D). It passes upward and outward from the semimembranosus tendon and blends with the capsule. The popliteal vessels lie upon it; it is perforated by the azygos geniculate artery. The popliteus fascia is the second expansion from this tendon and passes downward and outward to cover the popliteus muscle. It gains attachment to the popliteal line of the tibia. The popliteal vessels lie upon it and end at its lower border. The third expansion continues as the deep fascia of the inner side of the leg.

The cruciate ligaments of the knee are 2 powerful cordlike structures which are so named because they cross each other like the limbs of the letter "X" (Figs. 694, 695 and 696). The crucial arrangement is seen, whether viewed from the front, the sides or the back. These ligaments have been designed to prevent forward and backward displacements of the tibia on the femur. It requires great violence to tear one of them, but, when torn, great disability is caused by the forward and backward gliding of the tibia upon the femur. These ligaments are covered in front and at the sides by synovial membrane and are related posteriorly to the capsular ligament from which they are separated by fat.

The anterior cruciate ligament extends upward, backward and laterally from the anterior part of the intercondylar area of the tibia to the posterior part of the medial surface of the lateral condyle of the femur. It is tense in extension and prevents backward sliding of the femur and forward displacement of the tibia. When the knee is flexed its 2 points of attachment are approximated, and the ligament is relaxed. It prevents hyperextension of the knee joint.

The posterior cruciate ligament is tense in flexion; it passes upward, forward and medially from the posterior part of the intercondylar area to the anterior part of the lateral surface of the medial condyle of the femur. It prevents forward gliding of the femur and backward displacement of the tibia during flexion. The anterior ligament passes backward and outward, but the posterior passes inward and forward. When the knee joint is opened from the inner side, the posterior cruciate ligament is seen first.

The semilunar cartilages (menisci) are 2

crescentic plates of fibrocartilage which lie on the circumferential portion of the articular surfaces of the tibia (Fig. 694, 695 and 696). They deepen these areas for the reception of the condyles of the femur; since they are elastic, they act as buffers which diminish shocks passing up the limbs. Their distal surfaces are flat, but the proximal are concave for reception of the femoral condyles. In the fetus, both surfaces of the menisci are covered with synovial membrane, which helps to attach their peripheral margins to the tibia; but, as the result of continued pressure, they are devoid of this synovial covering in the adult. Each cartilage has 2 fibrous extremities, which are called horns; these are attached to the intercondylar area on the proximal surface of the tibia. The cartilages are thick toward the circumference of the joint; the lateral cartilage is a little thicker than the medial. Both thin out toward the center where they end as a fine, free, concave edge. They do not cover the entire extent of the condylar surfaces of the tibia.

The lateral semilunar cartilage is nearly circular in outline, and its horns are fixed to the tibia close together. The anterior horn attaches to the front of the intercondylar eminence behind the anterior cruciate ligament with which it blends. The posterior horn attaches to the back of the intercondylar eminence and in front of the posterior end of the medial cartilage. The peripheral margin is adherent to the capsular ligament but to a lesser extent than the medial cartilage; this is due to the fact that the popliteus tendon and its bursal sheath separate part of the margin from the capsule. As a result of the presence of this popliteus tendon, the lateral semilunar cartilage is less fixed in position; therefore, it is able to adapt itself more easily to sudden twisting movements of the knee joint. The firmer fixation of the medial semilunar cartilage renders it much more liable to injury. A fibrous band leaves the posterior horn and passes upward along the posterior cruciate ligament to become attached to the medial condyle of the femur. This band has been called the *ligament of Wrisberg* (Fig. 696 C). It is well to remember that in flexion and extension the tibia and the cartilages move on the femur, but in rotatory movements the femur and the cartilages move on the tibia.

The medial semilunar cartilage is "C"-shaped and adapts the upper surface of the medial condyle of the tibia to the curvature of the medial condyle of the femur. It is wider behind than in front; while its peripheral borders are thick, its central border thins out into a fine edge. Its anterior horn attaches to the anterior part of the intercondylar area in front of the anterior cruciate ligament; its posterior horn becomes attached to the posterior part of the intercondylar area in front of the posterior cruciate ligament. Its periphery is adherent to the capsule and therefore to the medial ligament of the knee.

The transverse ligament of the knee is a fibrous band which stretches across the anterior part of one semilunar cartilage to the corresponding part of the other. By means of this connection the movements of one cartilage are partly controlled and partly accompanied by the other. Some authorities believe that the transverse ligament may be considered the continuation of the peripheral fibers of each meniscus; the more central fibers attach to the tibia. Therefore, if any force acts on the periphery of the meniscus while the central part is fixed, it will tear longitudinally along the line between these inner and outer sets of fibers. This will result in the condition known as a *"bucket handle" tear of the cartilage*. The medial cartilage is the one usually affected.

The relationship of the medial ligament of the knee (tibial collateral ligament) to the medial meniscus is clinically important. It is responsible for the fact that injuries to the medial meniscus are more frequent than to the lateral. The lateral is free to move slightly, but even this slight degree of mobility is sufficient to provide for its safety. The medial, on the other hand, is fixed at one point by the tibial collateral ligament; because of this firm fixation, it is prone to injury. The medial ligament of the knee consists of long and short fibers; the short ones are on the deep surface of the ligament at its posterior part and are attached to the margin of the medial meniscus, thereby binding the meniscus to the tibia. Passing between these 2 sets of fibers of this ligament is the tendon of the semimembranosus muscle. By this arrangement the back part of the medial meniscus is firmly fixed. Therefore, excessive rotation of the femur on the tibia tears the movable front part away from the back which is firmly anchored.

On the nonarticular area of the upper surface of the tibia, the structures from before backward are: the transverse ligament, the anterior horn of the medial semilunar cartilage, the anterior cruciate ligament, the anterior horn of the lateral semilunar cartilage, the intercondylar tubercle, the posterior limb of the lateral semilunar cartilage, the posterior horn of the medial semilunar cartilage,

and the posterior cruciate ligament (Fig. 695 A).

The coronary ligaments are the deeper portions of the capsule which unite the semilunar cartilages to the tibia and the femur respectively. Those fibers which extend to the tibia are shorter, since the cartilages follow the movements of this bone more closely than those of the femur.

INTERIOR OF THE KNEE JOINT AND THE SYNOVIAL MEMBRANE

When the knee joint is laid open the semilunar cartilages, the cruciate ligaments and

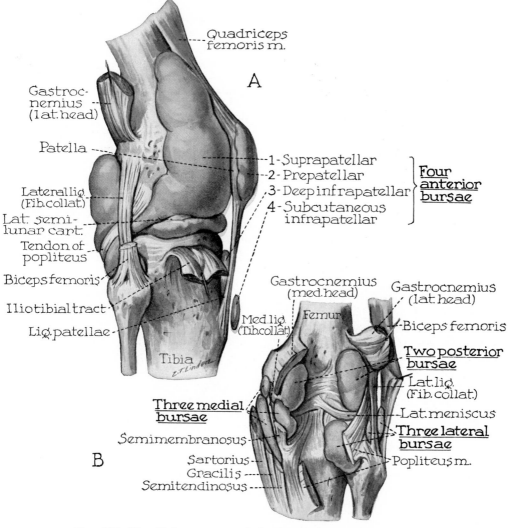

FIG. 697. The 12 bursae around the knee joint: (A) lateral view of the right knee joint; (B) posterior view.

the synovial membrane, including its infrapatellar fold, becomes visible (Figs. 694, 695 and 696).

The infrapatellar synovial fold (ligamentum mucosum) is the first structure to be seen. This is a triangular fold of synovial membrane which is pinched upward. Its apex is attached to the most anterior part of the intercondylar notch of the femur, and the base extends from below the articular surface of the patella to the anterior intercondylar area on the tibia (Fig. 694 A). Its sides are prolonged in a fringelike arrangement which forms the alar folds into which fat extends. Knee joint injuries may result in bruising of these fringes. Its base is related to the infrapatellar fat pad which covers the deep surface of the ligamentum patellae; its borders, the alar folds, remain free.

The synovial membrane lines the capsular ligament but leaves the capsule posteriorly to pass forward around the cruciate ligament (Fig. 695 A). The complexity of the synovial membrane may be simplified if we recall that developmentally the joint possessed 3 synovial cavities: a patellar and 2 condylar. The partition which separated the condylar from the patellar cavity disappeared, leaving only its vestigial alar folds. In prenatal life a partition called the intercondylar septum exists which separates the condylar cavities from each other. The lower border of this septum is attached to the intercondylar area on the upper aspect of the tibia. The posterior half of its upper border is attached to the intercondylar notch of the femur, and the anterior half of its upper border is free and extends from the intercondylar notch of the femur to the patella just below its articular surface.

During development a perforation appears in this septum which extends backward to the anterior cruciate ligament (Fig. 694 C). In this way the intercondylar septum is divided into an anterior part, the infrapatellar fold, and the posterior part which is associated with the anterior and the posterior cruciate ligaments. The infrapatellar fold has been described previously. After these developmental changes have taken place fluid may pass from one condylar cavity to the other, either by way of the patellar cavity that is over the infrapatellar folds or via the hole in

the intercondylar septum between the infrapatellar folds and the anterior cruciate ligament. It will be remembered that each condylar cavity is divided into upper and lower compartments by the semilunar cartilages. These two parts communicate around the free concave borders of the cartilages.

BURSAE

Since there were 3 primitive cavities in the knee joint, 3 bursae remain in the adult which communicate these cavities with the joint. They are the bursae which lie deep to the tendons of the quadriceps femoris, the popliteus, and the medial head of the gastrocnemius (Fig. 697).

Suprapatellar Bursa. The bursa which lies deep to the quadriceps femoris tendon is known as the suprapatellar bursa. This bursa lies between the anterior surface of the lower part of the femur and the deep surface of the quadriceps femoris muscle. It extends about 3 fingerbreadths above the upper border of the patella when the limb is in extension. It almost always communicates with the knee joint, and for this reason it is removed in excision of the joint for tuberculosis; however, it may become shut off from the rest of the joint by adhesions. It rests on a layer of fat which allows it to glide freely when the knee joint is in motion. Through apertures in the back of the capsule it often communicates with bursae under the head of the gastrocnemius and the bursa of the semimembranosus.

The popliteus bursa is situated between the popliteus tendon and the lateral condyle of the femur. It separates the popliteus tendon from the lateral semilunar cartilage, the lateral tibial condyle and the superior tibiofibular joint. This bursa is a tube of synovial membrane, which is situated around the popliteus tendon similar to the one around the long head of the biceps at the shoulder joint. It communicates with the knee joint both above and below the semilunar cartilage; in some instances it communicates with the superior tibiofibular joint.

The gastrocnemius bursa is situated deep to the medial head of the gastrocnemius muscle. Although this bursa does not always communicate with the medial condylar cavity, it communicates with a bursa deep to the semimembranosus. In this way it may bring the semimembranosus bursa and the knee joint into communication. At times a bursa may exist under the lateral head of the gastrocnemius muscle. An incision may be extended upward on the tibia to within ¼ inch of its articular margin and still not open the synovial cavity except posteriorly where the popliteal bursa lies.

The relationship between the synovial membrane and the cruciate ligaments is as if the 2 ligaments have pushed into the joint from behind, carrying the synovial membrane before them. Therefore, the posterior cruciate ligament has no covering on its posterior aspect, but the anterior cruciate ligament is covered anteriorly. A small diverticulum of synovial membrane is situated between the two and acts as a bursa during movements of the knee joint. Although the synovial membrane lines those portions of the capsular ligament which lie behind the condyles, it does not come into relation with the middle part of the deep surface of the posterior ligament, since it is held away from it by the cruciate ligaments. The posterior cruciate ligament may be exposed from behind without opening into the synovial cavity; the infrapatellar fold also may be exposed from in front without entering the cavity.

The infrapatellar fat pad fills the interval between the patella, the femur and the tibia. It adapts itself to the various forms which that recess assumes during movements of the joint. It is extra-articular and extrasynovial and is of a semifluid nature. A parapatellar incision close to the patella encounters this pad in its thickest portion; if the incision is placed more laterally, easier access is gained, since only the thin alar folds are encountered.

Three bursae, which communicate with the knee joint, have been discussed already. All told, however, 12 bursae are situated around this joint: 4 of these are anterior, 2 posterior, 3 medial and 3 lateral (Fig. 697).

The 4 anterior bursae are:

1. *The suprapatellar bursa:* this has been thoroughly discussed with the 3 bursae which communicate with the joint.

2. *The prepatellar bursa* is associated with the condition known as housemaid's knee. It is subcutaneous and lies in front of the lower half of the patella and the upper half of the patellar ligament. The term "housemaid" is used, because in scrubbing the floor the hands rest upon the floor, bringing the bursae into contact with the ground. This constant rubbing causes an inflammation known as bursitis. The bursa then becomes large and because of its weight drops below its normal position.

3. *The subcutaneous infrapatellar bursa* is situated between the skin and the lower end of the ligamentum patellae (front of the tibial tuberosity).

4. *The deep infrapatellar bursa* is situated between the deep aspect of the lower end of the ligamentum patellae and the tibia.

The 2 posterior bursae are located between each head of origin of the gastrocnemius and the capsule of the joint. They often communicate with the joint. The bursa which is present between the medial head of the gastrocnemius and the capsule sends a prolongation between the gastrocnemius and the semimembranosus muscles. If it is enlarged it forms a swelling at the inner side of the popliteal space, which is referred to as an enlarged semimembranosus bursa.

The 3 medial bursae are: One which separates the sartorius, the gracilis and the semitendinosus from the tibial collateral ligament. The two others separate the tendon of the semimembranosus from the tibial collateral ligament medially and the head of the tibia laterally. The semimembranosus tendon is placed between the ligament medially and the condyle of the tibia laterally.

The 3 lateral bursae are:

1. Between the biceps femoris tendon and the fibular collateral ligament

2. Between the popliteus tendon and the lateral condyle of the femur

3. Between the fibular collateral ligament and the popliteus tendon

The nerve supply is rich around the knee joint. It is supplied by 3 branches each from the femoral, the lateral and the medial popliteal nerves and an additional twig from the obturator nerve.

Movements. Flexion, extension and rotation constitute the active movements at the knee joint.

Flexion is accompanied by some degree of flexion of the hip joint; the movements of the tibia and the femur on one another combine sliding, rolling and rotating actions. When one is in a resting upright position the knee joints are not fully extended, and the attitude is maintained by the balanced tone of the flexor and the extensor muscles.

The movement of *extension* is completed by a movement of lateral rotation of the tibia on the femur; the latter action locks the joint and renders all ligaments tense, with the exception of the anterior fibers of the posterior cruciate ligament. This locking mechanism enables the fully extended knee to become subjected to severe strains without becoming injured.

Rotation is impossible when the knee is fully extended and any attempt to produce pure rotation in this position results in injury. Flexion is accompanied in its initial stages by medial rotation of the tibia on the femur. When the knee is flexed to a right angle a considerable range of rotation is allowed, but when it is slightly flexed only a small amount of abduction and adduction can be produced, provided that the foot is placed on the ground.

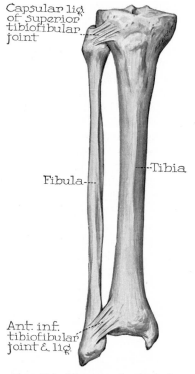

FIG. 698. The superior and the inferior tibiofibular joints.

TIBIOFIBULAR JOINTS

The fibula articulates with the tibia at both of its ends. Therefore, superior and inferior tibiofibular joints are formed (Fig. 698). The superior forms a small synovial joint, but the inferior is a syndesmosis.

The superior tibiofibular joint is formed where the head of the fibula articulates with the postero-inferior surface of the lateral condyle of the tibia. These bones are united by a capsular ligament. The tendon of the popliteus and its synovial pouch cross the upper and back part of the joint. The pouch sometimes is continuous with the synovial membrane of the joint through a hole in the capsule, and in this way the joint indirectly communicates with the knee joint. The lateral ligament of the knee and the tendon of the biceps cross the upper surface of the joint.

Some fibers of the biceps tendon extend to the tibial condyle and thus form an additional ligament for the joint. Since the uppermost fibers of the extensor digitorum longus and the peroneus longus arise from the lateral condyle of the tibia, they cross in front of the joint. It is supplied by twigs from the nerve to the popliteus and from the recurrent branch of the lateral popliteal (common peroneal) nerve. It permits gliding movements which take place during the separation and the approximation of the lower ends of the tibia and the fibula in dorso- and plantarflexion of the ankle joint.

Inferior Tibiofibular Joint. These bones are held together by ligaments which do not enclose a cavity. The joint is formed between a convex fibular surface and a corresponding concave tibial one. However, the bones are not in contact with each other because the interosseous ligament not only binds them but separates them. At times this ligament does not quite reach the lateral border of the distal end of the tibia, and in such cases there is a narrow strip above the lateral border which is covered with cartilage for articulation with the uppermost part of the facet of the lateral malleolus. This joint is constructed firmly; the strength of the ankle joint largely depends on its integrity. The antero-inferior and the postero-inferior tibiofibular ligaments (anterior and posterior liga-

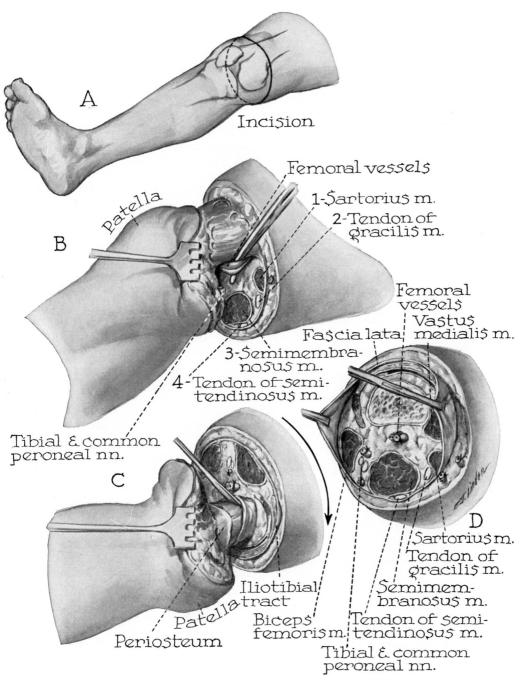

FIG. 699. Supracondylar amputation. (A) A circular incision is placed at the level of the upper border of the patella. (B) The 4 medial muscular structures have been severed, and the femoral vessels are identified. (C) The periosteum is incised and dissected 2 inches cephalad to the skin incision. (D) The fascia lata is approximated.

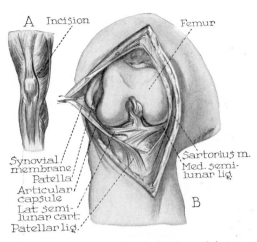

FIG. 700. Exposure of the knee joint.

ments of the lateral malleolus) hide the interosseous ligament. They are strong, flat bands that pass upward and medially from the front and the back of the uppermost part of the lateral malleolus to the distal end of the tibia. The posterior ligament is continuous inferiorly with the transverse ligament. The transverse tibiofibular ligament is attached along the whole length of the posterior border of the tarsal surface of the tibia and to the malleolar fossa of the fibula. Superiorly, it is continuous with the postero-inferior ligament, and its deep surface is in contact with a facet on the talus. The joint derives its nerve supply from the anterior tibial nerve and a long filament from the nerve to the popliteus that descends through the interosseous membrane.

SURGICAL CONSIDERATIONS

SUPRACONDYLAR AMPUTATION

The author described a supracondylar amputation in 1942. The procedure is accom-

plished through a simple circular incision placed on a level of the upper border of the patella (Fig. 699). The internal saphenous vein is isolated and severed. This acts as a guide to the sartorius muscle. Four structures are identified and divided over the medial aspect of the lower end of the thigh. They are: the sartorius muscle, the gracilis tendon, the semimembranosus muscle and the semitendinosus tendon. Laterally, the tensor fasciae latae and the biceps femoris tendon are divided. The femoral vessels and the sciatic nerve are isolated, ligated and divided at the lower aspect of the thigh. The attachment of the quadriceps femoris muscle to the linea aspera is severed. The bone is sawed from 2 to 3 inches above the level of the skin incision. The fascia and the skin are approximated.

EXPOSURE OF THE KNEE JOINT

Numerous approaches have been described for exposure of the knee joint; only one approach will be discussed here, since the others can be found in any standard text on orthopedic surgery.

The procedure herein described is the *anteromedial approach*. This is accomplished through a long incision which begins at the medial border of the quadriceps tendon about 3 inches above the patella (Fig. 700). It extends distally and medially, curving around the patella to the tibial tuberosity. The dissection is carried between the quadriceps tendon and the vastus medialis muscle. The capsule and the synovial membrane are divided about ½ inch from the inner border of the patella and the patellar ligament. The patella is turned to the outer side of the lateral condyle of the femur; this exposes the lower end of the femur, the cruciate ligaments, the semilunar cartilages and the articular surface of the patella.

Leg

The 2 bones that are found in the leg are the tibia and the fibula (Figs. 708 and 709). These bones furnish attachments for the thigh muscles and the leg muscles (Fig. 701).

The cutaneous nerve supply of the anterior aspect of the leg is derived from the cutaneous rami of the medial crural branch of the saphenous nerve and from the cutaneous branches of the lateral popliteal nerve (Fig. 702). The lower lateral aspect of the leg is supplied by the superficial peroneal nerve. The cutaneous nerve supply of the posterior aspect of the leg is supplied by the end of the posterior cutaneous nerve of the thigh, the posterior branch of the medial cutaneous nerve of the thigh, the cutaneous branch of the lateral popliteal (common peroneal) nerve, branches of the saphenous nerve and the cutaneous branch of the medial popliteal (tibial) nerve, which is derived from the sural nerve.

DEEP FASCIA

This fascia does not form a complete investment for the leg; it is absent over the subcutaneous part of the medial surface of the tibia (Fig. 703). It is attached to the anterior border of the tibia, then sweeps laterally and around the front to the back of the leg, to reach the tibia again at its postero-medial border, where it attaches. Its strength and density vary in different parts of the leg.

By sending inward 2 partitions which attach to the fibula it divides the leg into lateral, anterior and posterior compartments. The anterior intermuscular septum attaches to the anterior border of the fibula and separates the extensor muscles of the anterior compartment of the leg from the peroneal muscles. The posterior intermuscular septum is interposed between the peroneal muscles

and the muscles on the back of the leg; it is attached to the posterior border of the fibula.

A deep layer of fascia (lamina profunda) arises from the posterior intermuscular septum and attaches to the medial border of the tibia. This layer divides the posterior compartment into a superficial and a deep compartment. In this way, the 3 muscular compartments are formed. The anterior compartment contains the extensor muscles and the anterior tibial artery and nerve. The lateral compartment contains the peroneal muscles and the superficial peroneal nerve. The posterior compartment contains the flexor muscles and the posterior tibial vessels and nerve.

The deep fascia becomes thinner as it passes toward the distal part of the leg. In the region of the ankle it again becomes thickened to form fascial bands. These bands are called retinacula; their function is to retain the tendons in position when the muscles which move the joint are in action (Fig. 715).

The superior extensor retinaculum (transverse ligament) is a band of fascia about 1½ inches wide which stretches across the front of the leg from the tibia to the fibula. At its medial end the ligament splits to enclose the tendon of the tibialis anterior muscle. In this way a special compartment is made which is invested with a synovial sheath for the tendon of this muscle. To its lateral side, the tendons of the extensor hallucis longus, the extensor digitorum longus and the peroneus tertius muscles pass behind the retinaculum in a common compartment. This is not provided with a synovial sheath. The anterior tibial vessels and nerve lie posterior to the extensor hallucis longus as they pass behind the retinaculum.

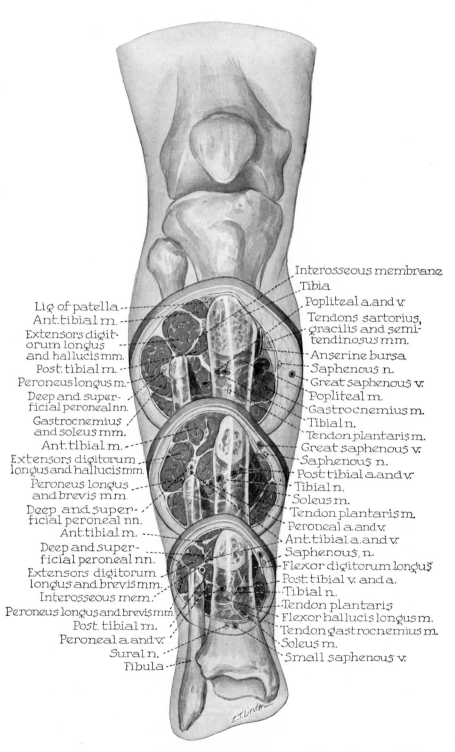

Lig. of patella
Ant. tibial m.
Extensors digit-
orum longus
and hallucis mm.
Post. tibial m.
Peroneus longus m.
Deep and super-
ficial peroneal nn.
Gastrocnemius
and soleus mm.
Ant. tibial m.
Extensors digitorum
longus and hallucis mm.
Peroneus longus
and brevis mm.
Deep and super-
ficial peroneal nn.
Ant. tibial m.
Deep and super-
ficial peroneal nn.
Extensors digitorum
longus and brevis mm.
Interosseous mem.
Peroneus longus and brevis mm.
Post. tibial m.
Peroneal a. and v.
Sural n.
Fibula

Interosseous membrane
Tibia
Popliteal a. and v.
Tendons sartorius,
gracilis and semi-
tendinosus mm.
Anserine bursa
Saphenous n.
Great saphenous v.
Popliteal m.
Gastrocnemius m.
Tibial n.
Tendon plantaris m.
Great saphenous v.
Saphenous n.
Post. tibial a. and v.
Tibial n.
Soleus m.
Tendon plantaris m.
Peroneal a. and v.
Ant. tibial a. and v.
Saphenous n.
Flexor digitorum longus
Post. tibial v. and a.
Tibial n.
Tendon plantaris
Flexor hallucis longus m.
Tendon gastrocnemius m.
Soleus m.
Small saphenous v.

FIG. 701. Cross sections of the right leg at its upper, middle and lower thirds.

The inferior extensor retinaculum (cruciate ligament) lies distal to the ankle joint. It is a Y-shaped ligament which extends from the lateral part of the calcaneum mediad and splits, thus giving it the semblance of the letter "Y" (Fig. 714 C). The upper limb of the Y passes to the medial malleolus, and the lower limb passes to the deep fascia on the medial side of the foot. The tibialis anterior has a separate synovial sheath under this retinaculum, as has the extensor hallucis. The extensor digitorum and the peroneus tertius have a common sheath under the lower retinaculum.

MUSCLES

The muscles of the leg consist of 3 groups: (1) the anterior (extensor) group, all of which are supplied by the anterior tibial (deep peroneal) nerve; (2) the posterior (flexor) group, all of which are supplied by the posterior tibial nerve; (3) the lateral peroneal (evertor) group, which is supplied by the superficial peroneal (musculocutaneous) nerve. Since the fibula is on a plane posterior to that of the tibia, the anterior compartment faces laterally as well as anteriorly (Fig. 704).

ANTERIOR (EXTENSOR) GROUP (ANTERIOR COMPARTMENT)

If one thinks of the tibia, the large toe and the 4 remaining toes, it would naturally follow that 4 muscles constitute this group. They are: the tibialis anterior, the extensor hallucis longus, the extensor digitorum longus and the extensor tertius (Fig. 704 A and B).

The tibialis anterior (tibialis anticus) arises from the upper half of the lateral surface of the tibia and from the interosseous membrane. Its tendon begins at about the middle of the leg and follows the anterior border of the tibia, crossing the bone directly in front of the medial malleolus. It passes through the medial compartments of the extensor retinacula, crosses the ankle joint, the talus and the navicular, and finally is inserted into the medial aspect of the cuneiform bone and the adjoining part of the base of the first meta-

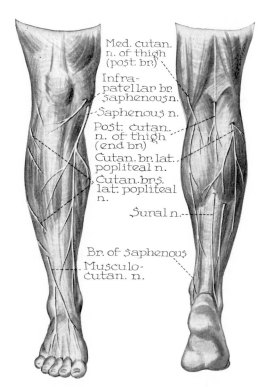

FIG. 702. The anterior and the posterior cutaneous nerve supply of the leg.

tarsal. Its action is dorsiflexion (extension) and inversion of the foot. It is separated above from the extensor digitorum longus and below from the extensor hallucis longus by a septum of deep fascia which leads to the cellular interspace; this space contains the neurovascular structures.

The extensor hallucis longus is the long extensor of the big toe. It is a thin muscle which is placed between the tibialis anterior and the extensor digitorum longus. Its upper portion is hidden by the 2 last-named muscles, but as it passes downward, it reaches the surface between them. It arises from the middle two fourths of the anterior surface of the fibula and from the interosseous membrane. It is accompanied by the extensor digitorum longus as it passes behind the upper extensor retinaculum; in the lower retinaculum it is lined with an independent synovial sheath. As it passes over the ankle joint, it crosses the anterior tibial vessels and nerves, so that its tendon comes to lie medial to the dorsalis pedis artery (Fig. 722). It is the only muscle which crosses the phalanx of the great toe on its dorsal aspect. Its action is indicated by its name—extension of the great toe; it aids also in dorsiflexion (extension) of the foot.

The extensor digitorum longus muscle arises as a long thin sheath of muscle from the upper three fourths of the anterior surface of the fibula and the interosseous membrane. Its tendon passes behind the superior retinaculum and in front of the ankle joint. It passes under the inferior retinaculum and

divides into 4 slips which diverge from each other to reach the lateral 4 toes. Each tendon inserts into the middle and distal phalanges of the lateral 4 toes. Each tendon also receives a tendon of the extensor brevis digitorum, which passes onto the dorsum of each toe and broadens into a dorsal expansion (p. 829). This is inserted in a fashion similar to the dorsal expansion of the fingers. The muscle is an extensor of the toes and a dorsiflexor of the foot.

The peroneus tertius is not a peroneal muscle but rather is a part of the extensor

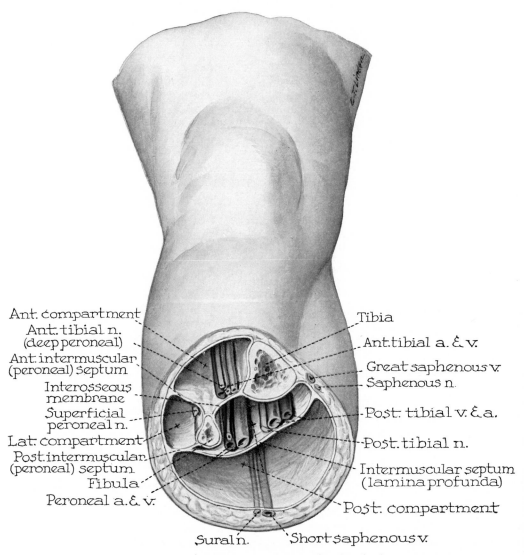

Ant. compartment
Ant. tibial n. (deep peroneal)
Ant. intermuscular (peroneal) septum
Interosseous membrane
Superficial peroneal n.
Lat. compartment
Post. intermuscular (peroneal) septum
Fibula
Peroneal a. & v.
Sural n.

Tibia
Ant. tibial a. & v.
Great saphenous v.
Saphenous n.
Post. tibial v. & a.
Post. tibial n.
Intermuscular septum (lamina profunda)
Post. compartment
Short saphenous v.

FIG. 703. The deep fascia of the leg: cross section showing the 3 compartments.

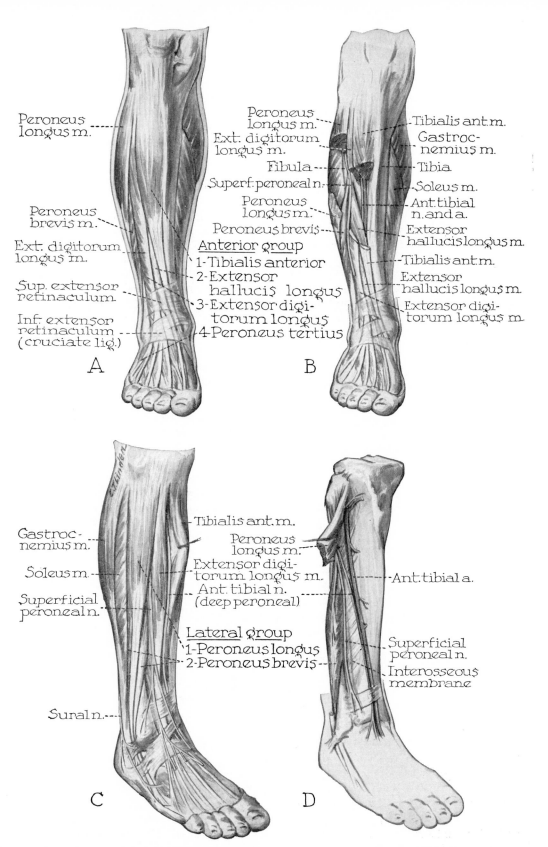

Peroneus longus m.

Peroneus brevis m.

Ext. digitorum longus m.

Sup. extensor retinaculum

Inf. extensor retinaculum (cruciate lig.)

A

Peroneus longus m.

Ext. digitorum longus m.

Fibula

Superf. peroneal n.

Peroneus longus m.

Peroneus brevis

Anterior group
1-Tibialis anterior
2-Extensor hallucis longus
3-Extensor digitorum longus
4-Peroneus tertius

Tibialis ant. m.

Gastroc-nemius m.

Tibia

Soleus m.

Ant. tibial n. and a.

Extensor hallucis longus m.

Tibialis ant. m.

Extensor hallucis longus m.

Extensor digitorum longus m.

B

Gastroc-nemius m.

Soleus m.

Superficial peroneal n.

Sural n.

C

Tibialis ant. m.

Peroneus longus m.

Extensor digitorum longus m.

Ant. tibial n. (deep peroneal)

Lateral group
1-Peroneus longus
2-Peroneus brevis

Ant. tibial a.

Superficial peroneal n.

Interosseous membrane

D

FIG. 704. The muscles of the anterior and the lateral groups of the leg: (A) the anterior group; (B) deeper dissection showing vessels and nerves; (C) the lateral group; (D) deeper dissection showing vessels and nerves.

digitorum longus. It is small and is not always present. Some anatomists consider it the lowest quarter of the extensor digitorum longus. It ends in a slender tendon which fails to reach the toe but gains attachment somewhere along the dorsum of the 5th metatarsal. The action of this muscle is to dorsiflex the foot and to aid the true peroneal muscle in eversion.

Nerves and Vessels. The *anterior tibial (deep peroneal) nerve* is one of the two terminal branches of the lateral popliteal nerve (common peroneal) (Fig. 704). It arises on the lateral side of the neck of the fibula under cover of the peroneus muscle, pierces the anterior intermuscular septum and then usually passes between the extensor digitorum longus and the fibula to enter the anterior compartment of the leg. In the upper two thirds of the anterior compartment, it lies very deep between the muscles, having the extensor longus muscle to its lateral side and the tibialis anterior to its medial side. In the distal third, where fleshy muscle bellies give place to tendons, it comes closer to the surface. At first, the nerve is in front of the interosseous membrane, with the anterior tibial vessels to its medial side. As it descends, it passes onto the front of the artery. In the distal third of the leg, the nerve lies on the tibia, with the vessels usually to its medial side again. The extensor hallucis longus, at first on the lateral side of the nerve, crosses in front of it and the vessels just above the ankle; it lies medial to them at the ankle, thus separating them from the tibialis anterior muscle. The nerve leaves the anterior compartment by passing downward deep to the anterior annular ligament, where it continues with the dorsalis pedis artery. It supplies the 4 muscles of the anterior compartment.

The anterior tibial artery begins on the posterior surface of the leg, where it arises from the popliteal artery at the lower border of the popliteus muscle (Fig. 704). It is accompanied by 2 venae comitantes which run with the artery and send interlacing veins around it. The artery enters the anterior compartment of the leg by piercing the upper part of the interosseous membrane. In the upper half of its course, the vessel is situated

deeply, with the nerve lying on the interosseous membrane between the tibialis anterior and the extensor digitorum longus. In the lower part of its course, the artery lies on the shaft of the tibia and is overlapped by the extensor hallucis longus. After passing behind the superior extensor retinaculum, it becomes superficial in the interval between the tendons of the extensor hallucis longus and the extensor digitorum longus. In front of the ankle joint, the artery continues as the dorsalis pedis artery (Fig. 722). Branches of this vessel take part in the anastomoses around the knee and the ankle joints. A straight line drawn from the medial side of the neck of the fibula to a point midway between the 2 malleoli marks the course of the anterior tibial artery.

LATERAL (PERONEAL) GROUP (LATERAL COMPARTMENT)

This group is made up of 2 muscles on the lateral aspect of the leg—the peroneus longus and the brevis; they are evertors (Fig. 704). The peronei fill the lateral crural compartment and are separated from the extensor flexor compartment by the anterior and the posterior intermuscular septa, respectively.

The peroneus longus arises from the upper two thirds of this compartment, and the **peroneus brevis** from the lower two thirds, thus overlapping each other in the middle third. Both muscles pass downward, the brevis being covered by the longus, until they reach the posterior aspect of the lateral malleolus, where the tendon of the brevis is in direct contact with the bone. Here, the tendons are held down by a thickening of the deep fascia, the superior peroneal retinaculum. They are provided with a common synovial sheath. They continue to pass below the malleolus and lie on the lateral aspect of the calcaneum, becoming separated from each other by the peroneal tubercle. At this point, they are held in place by the inferior peroneal retinaculum, and here each possesses a synovial sheath of its own. The tendon of the peroneus brevis passes above the tubercle to be inserted into the dorsal aspect of the tubercle on the base of the 5th metatarsal bone. The tendon of the peroneus longus passes below the peroneal tubercle, medial and forward across the sole of the foot to become inserted into the lateral aspect of the medial cuneiform and the adjoining part of the base of the first metatarsal bone.

Both of these muscles are supplied by the musculocutaneous (superficial peroneal) nerve.

Actions. When the foot is off the ground,

the peroneal muscles produce eversion. A most important function of the peroneus longus is to maintain the transverse arch of the foot. By their ability to draw the foot to the lateral side, the peroneal muscles balance the medial pull exerted by the tibialis posterior and the long flexors of the toes.

The musculocutaneous (superficial peroneal) nerve arises from the lateral popliteal

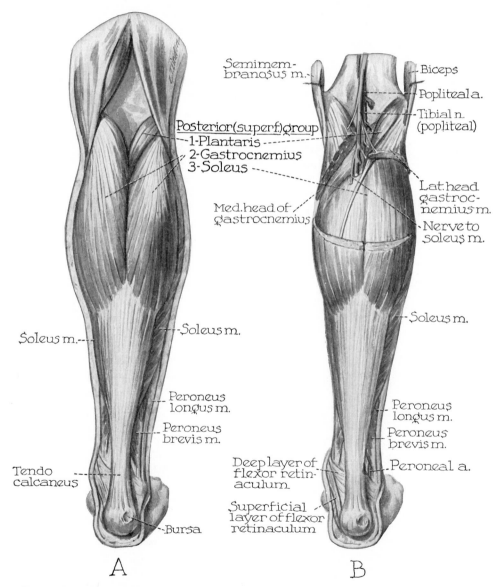

Fig. 705. The superficial posterior group of calf muscles. (A) The relations of the plantaris, the gastrocnemius and the soleus are shown. (B) The 2 heads of the gastrocnemius have been cut to show the plantaris tendon and the soleus muscle.

nerve on the lateral side of the fibular neck (Fig. 704). It proceeds downward and forward in the substance of the peroneus longus muscle and then between the peroneus brevis and the anterior intermuscular septum. At the junction of the middle and the lower thirds of the leg, it passes through the deep fascia to become cutaneous. Plus its muscular and cutaneous branches, it gives off a communicating branch on the dorsum of the foot to the sural nerve. The anterior border of the peroneus brevis acts as a guide to this nerve, since it travels with it to the surface, a variable distance above the subcutaneous area of the fibula.

POSTERIOR (FLEXOR) GROUP (POSTERIOR COMPARTMENT)

This group of muscles is supplied by the posterior tibial nerve, which also has been referred to as the tibial nerve and as the medial popliteal nerve. The muscles are divided into superficial and deep groups (Fig 705).

The superficial muscles are the gastrocnemius, the plantaris and the soleus; they

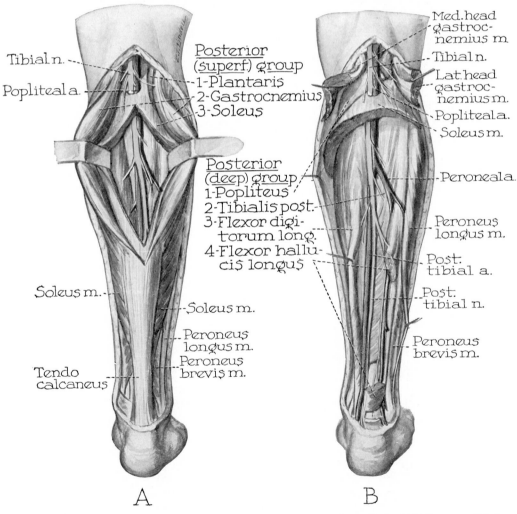

Tibial n.
Popliteal a.

Posterior (superf.) group
1-Plantaris
2-Gastrocnemius
3-Soleus

Posterior (deep) group
1-Popliteus
2-Tibialis post.
3-Flexor digitorum long.
4-Flexor hallucis longus

Soleus m.

Tendo calcaneus

Soleus m.

Peroneus longus m.
Peroneus brevis m.

Med. head gastrocnemius m.
Tibial n.
Lat. head gastrocnemius m.
Popliteal a.
Soleus m.

Peroneal a.

Peroneus longus m.

Post. tibial a.

Post. tibial n.

Peroneus brevis m.

A   B

FIG. 706. The superficial and the deep groups of the calf muscles: (A) the superficial group consists of 3 muscles; (B) the deep group consists of 4 muscles.

join to form the stout tendo calcaneus, which is inserted into the back of the calcaneus (Figs. 705 and 706).

The gastrocnemius arises from the femur by 2 heads (Fig. 705 A). The medial head arises from the back of the femur above the medial condyle; the lateral head arises from the lateral aspect of the lateral condyle. There is an asymmetry between the origins of these 2 heads. This muscle accounts for the fullness of the calf, since the 2 muscle bellies broaden as they descend. The muscle bellies do not blend with each other but are separated by a groove in which the sural nerve and the short saphenous vein are found. The lateral head often contains a small sesamoid bone called the fabella, which usually is noted on the x-ray film opposite the lateral condyle. The common tendon of the 2 heads joins the tendon of the soleus to form the tendo calcaneus; this takes place a short distance below the middle of the leg. The muscle acts as a plantar flexor of the foot and as a flexor of the knee.

The soleus has a rather extensive horseshoe-shaped origin from the upper third of the posterior aspect of the fibula and from the soleal line on the back of the tibia (Fig. 705 B). In its upper half, this muscle is covered by the bellies of the gastrocnemius, but where the common tendon of the latter begins, the belly of the soleus projects beyond its margins, becoming superficial. The tendon of this muscle develops on its superficial aspect and joins the deep surface of the tendo calcaneus. It is a plantar flexor of the foot.

The plantaris is a small muscle about 3 or 4 inches long, with a very long tendon, which at times may be over 12 inches; it may be absent. Because of this long narrow tendon, it has been referred to as "the freshman's nerve." It arises from the lateral supracondylar line of the femur and passes downward between the gastrocnemius and the underlying soleus. It reaches the inner side of the tendo achillis, with which it blends. It may have a separate insertion into the os calcis; its action is to aid the gastrocnemius.

The tendo calcaneus is the most powerful tendon in the body. It narrows as it descends,

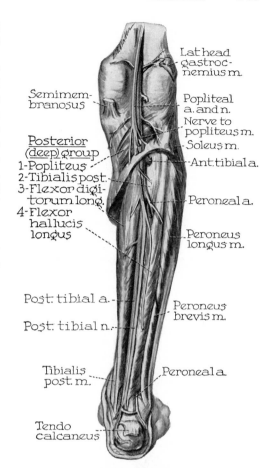

FIG. 707. The posterior tibial nerve and the posterior tibial and peroneal arteries.

but near the heel it expands again and inserts into the middle portion of the posterior surface of the calcaneum. The fleshy fibers of the soleus are continued downward on its deep surface almost to the heel. A small bursa separates the tendon from the calcaneum.

The deep group of muscles consists of the popliteus, the flexor hallucis longus, the flexor digitorum longus and the tibialis posterior.

The popliteus arises from the lateral aspect of the lateral condyle of the femur, within the capsule of the knee joint. The tendon pierces the posterior part of the capsule of the joint, and its fibers fan out to obtain insertion into the posterior aspect of the tibia

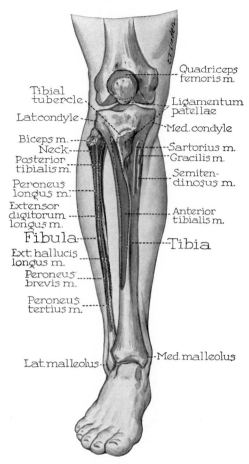

Tibial
tubercle.
Lat.condyle
Biceps m.
Neck
Posterior
tibialis m.
Peroneus
longus m.
Extensor
digitorum
longus m.
Fibula
Ext. hallucis
longus m.
Peroneus
brevis m.
Peroneus
tertius m.
Lat. malleolus

Quadriceps
femoris m.
Ligamentum
patellae
Med.condyle
Sartorius m.
Gracilis m.
Semiten-
dinosus m.
Anterior
tibialis m.
Tibia
Med. malleolus

FIG. 708. The tibia and the fibula seen
from in front. The muscular origins are
presented in red; the insertions, in blue.

above the soleal line (Figs. 706 and 707).
It is mainly a flexor of the knee joint. A
strong fascia covers the posterior surface of
the popliteus muscle; this tendon can be
traced upward and medially to the medial
side of the knee, where it becomes continuous
with the tendon of the semimembranosus.

The flexor hallucis longus is the long flexor
of the big toe. It arises chiefly from the posterior surface of the fibula, below the origin
of the soleus. The muscle belly is bulky and
overlaps and largely conceals the fleshy part
of the tibialis posterior. At the ankle joint, it
passes through a separate space in the laciniate ligament, being separated from the flexor
digitorum longus by the tibial nerve and the
posterior tibial vessels (Fig. 706 B). It inserts

into the terminal phalanx of the great toe and
is a powerful invertor as well as a flexor of
the big toe.

The flexor digitorum longus arises from
the posterior surface of the tibia, below the
popliteus muscle and medial to the vertical
ridge. After passing through the split tendon
of the flexor brevis muscle, it inserts into the
terminal phalanges of the 4 outer toes. It
flexes the toes, draws the pillars of the arches
of the foot together and also supports the
arch.

The tibialis posterior muscle originates
from the interosseous membrane and the
adjoining parts of the posterior surfaces of
the tibia and the fibula (Fig. 706). This
attachment to the interosseous membrane
does not reach as high as the attachments
to the bone. The upper end of the muscle is
bifid, the anterior tibial vessels piercing the
membrane between these 2 parts. As it passes
distally, it inclines medially under cover of
the flexor digitorum longus and becomes a
strong flattened tendon which grooves the
back of the medial malleolus under cover of
the flexor retinaculum. Its tendon enters the
sole and is inserted chiefly into the tuberosity
of the navicular bone and the cuneiform
bone. Some slips of the tendon also are inserted into other bones of the foot. The
muscle is a plantar-flexor and invertor of
the foot.

Vessels and Nerves. This region contains
2 main arteries and 1 main nerve (Fig. 707).
The arteries are the posterior tibial and its
largest branch, the peroneal; the nerve is the
posterior tibial.

The posterior tibial nerve lies between the
2 arteries, being closely applied to the lateral
side of the posterior tibial artery. All 3 travel
distally behind the fascia covering the posterior tibial muscle, and when this muscle
passes to a medial position, they continue
their course on the skeletal plane. The nerve
takes a straight course and crosses the posterior tibial artery to gain its lateral side. It
supplies the 3 deep muscles and the deep part
of the soleus muscle and then ends deep to
the flexor retinaculum (laciniate ligament)
by dividing into medial and lateral plantar
nerves.

The posterior tibial artery is the larger of

the 2 terminal branches of the popliteal artery. It begins at the upper border of the soleus and ends deep to the flexor retinaculum by dividing into the medial and the lateral plantar arteries. The flexor hallucis longus muscle lies laterally, and the flexor digitorum longus lies medially; the fascia covering the posterior tibial muscle, the shaft of the lower end of the tibia and the capsule of the ankle joint all lie anteriorly. When the fascia is relaxed by inverting the foot, the pulsations of the artery can be felt about a finger's breadth from the medial malleolus.

The peroneal artery arises from the posterior tibial artery before the latter is crossed by the tibial nerve. It descends first behind the fascia covering the tibialis posterior muscle deep to the flexor hallucis longus; then it continues downward behind the fibula and the ankle joint to end on the lateral surface of the calcaneus as the lateral calcanean artery.

TIBIA

The tibia, or shin bone, is the medial and the larger of the 2 bones of the leg (Figs. 708 and 709). It presents a proximal end, a shaft and a distal end.

The proximal end is the larger of the two, its transverse diameter is wider, and it is bent slightly backward. It consists of a tubercle, lateral and medial condyles, an intercondylar area and eminence, fibular facets and a groove for the semimembranosus. This massive prismatic upper end is broader from side to side than from before backward, and it is curved so that it overhangs the posterior surface of the shaft. Being so greatly expanded, it provides a good weight-bearing surface for the lower end of the femur.

The tubercle (tuberosity) is seen in front of and below the condyles, about 1 inch from the top. Its lower half is rough for the attachment of the ligamentum patellae; above, it is a smooth area separated by a bursa from this ligament. This prominence is felt easily subcutaneously. In the kneeling position, the body rests on the lower part of this tubercle, the front of the condyles, the ligamentum patellae and the lower part of the patella.

The 2 condyles are felt readily at the sides of the bone and make up most of the proxi-

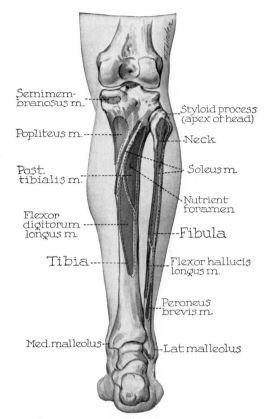

Fig. 709. The tibia and the fibula seen from behind. The origins are presented in red; the insertions, in blue.

mal end of the tibia. Anteriorly, they are united above the tubercle, but posteriorly they are separated by a wide and shallow notch. Over their superior surfaces they are covered with cartilage; they articulate centrally with the condyle of the femur and peripherally with a corresponding semilunar cartilage. Between these articular surfaces is the intercondylar area, which rises in its center to form the intercondylar eminence.

The medial condyle is larger than the lateral, and its articular surface is more concave. Over its posteromedial aspect, the groove for the insertion of the semimembranosus is found.

The lateral condyle extends farther out from the shaft and presents the facet for the head of the fibula over the postero-inferior surface. On the back and above and medial to this facet is the shallow groove for the popliteus tendon; on the front of the condyle is a raised impression for the attachment to the posterior part of the iliotibial tract. Over the lateral surface is a curved ridge which gives attachment to the strong deep fascia of the leg.

The shaft is thick and strong above but gradually tapers as it is traced downward to the junction of its middle and lower thirds, where it again becomes slightly expanded. It is distinctly prismatic in shape; because of this, it has anterior, lateral and medial borders and posterior, medial and lateral surfaces (Fig. 710).

The anterior border, which may be felt as the shin, extends from the tubercle above to the front of the medial malleolus below; it is somewhat indistinct in its lower third.

The lateral (interosseous) border is sharply defined in its middle third and extends from the fibular facet above, to the fibular notch below; the interosseous membrane is attached to it.

The medial border is rounded and less distinct from the lateral; it can be traced from the lower part of the medial condyle to the back of the medial malleolus.

The lateral surface is located between the anterior and the interosseous borders and is slightly concave in its upper two thirds to accommodate the origin of the anterior tibialis muscle. The lower third is in relation to the tendons of the extensor muscles; it is convex.

The medial surface is wide and smooth; it is subcutaneous except at its upper end, where tendons are inserted.

The posterior surface is located between the medial and the interosseous borders and encroaches on the lateral aspect near its upper end.

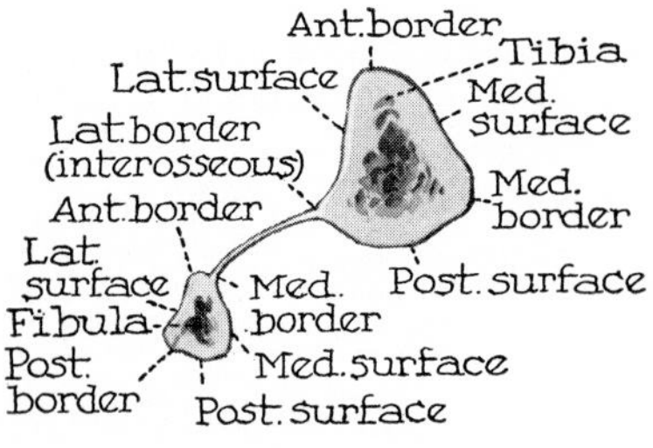

FIG. 710. Diagram of a cross section of the tibia and the fibula, showing the bony borders and surfaces.

The soleal (popliteal) line appears as a rough ridge which crosses this border obliquely from the fibular facet to the medial margin. Extending downward from this line is the *vertical line,* to the lateral side of which is found a large foramen for the nutrient artery.

The distal end of the tibia presents 5 surfaces, a medial malleolus and a fibular notch. The *medial surface* is subcutaneous and continues below as the medial malleolus. The *anterior surface* is rounded and covered with extensor tendons. The *posterior surface* also is rounded and is grooved on the malleolus for the tibialis posterior. The *inferior (tarsal) surface* is quadrilateral and wider in front than behind; it is slightly concave from behind forward and convex from side to side. It articulates with the upper surface of the talus. The *lateral surface* is occupied by a triangular depression known as the *fibular notch.* The *medial malleolus* can be palpated without difficulty. It lies a little anterior to the lateral malleolus and does not extend as far downward. Its apex gives attachment to the deltoid ligament of the ankle joint, and its posterior aspect is grooved by the tendon of the tibialis posterior. Its lateral surface articulates with the talus.

The epiphysis of the lower end is represented by a horizontal line about a ¼ inch above the broad lower end of the bone. The metaphysis is separated by the whole thickness of the epiphysis. Diseases of the tibia, either in the upper or the lower end, are unlikely to affect the joint because of epiphyseal and the capsular relationships.

Attachments to the Tibia (Figs. 708 and 709):

To the intercondylar area: the anterior horn of the medial semilunar cartilage and the anterior cruciate ligament.

To the intercondylar eminence: the anterior horn of the lateral semilunar cartilage to the front, and the posterior horn to the back.

To the intercondylar area: the posterior horn of the medial cartilage and the posterior cruciate ligament.

To the medial condyle: the semimembranosus.

To the tibial tubercle: the ligamentum patellae.

To the shaft: the tibialis anterior from the lateral condyle and two thirds of the lateral sulcus. From the upper part of the medial surface, the sartorius, the gracilis, the semi-tendinosus and the medial ligament of the knee.

To the soleal line: the popliteus and the tibialis posterior from the upper two thirds of the lateral area of the posterior surface.

From the vertical line: the fascia covering the tibialis posterior and the flexor digitorum longus from the upper two thirds of the area medial to the vertical line.

To the anterior and the medial borders: the fascia of the leg and the superior extensor retinaculum to the lower part of the anterior border.

To the interosseous border: the interosseous membrane.

To the fibular notch: the interosseous tibiofibular ligament and the inferior tibiofibular ligaments to the lower parts of its anterior and posterior margins. The anterior ligament of the ankle to the anterior border of the tarsal tibial surface, and the posterior ligament of the ankle and the transverse tibiofibular ligament to the posterior border.

To the medial malleolus: the deltoid ligament, the flexor retinaculum and the inferior extensor retinaculum.

FIBULA

The fibula is the lateral of the 2 bones of the leg; it is slender and is attached above and below to the lateral aspect of the tibia. It can be divided conveniently into proximal and distal ends and a shaft.

The proximal end consists of a head, a neck and a styloid process. The *head* appears as an irregular cuboidal area which has on its upper surface a triangular facet which articulates with the lateral condyle of the tibia. Projecting upward from its postero-lateral aspect is the blunt-shaped *styloid process (apex)*, to the top of which the short lateral ligament of the knee joint is attached. The fibular head can be felt through the skin on the posterolateral aspect of the knee, below the level of the joint. The lateral popliteal (common peroneal) nerve can be felt and rolled by the fingers on the back of this head, although it is separated from it by the uppermost fibers of the soleus muscle. The *neck* is that constricted portion just below the head where the lateral popliteal nerve divides over its lateral side.

The shaft reveals 3 borders, 3 surfaces and a crest (Fig. 710). The *interosseous border* is ill defined on the medial side of the anterior border; it extends from the neck to the apex of a rough triangle on the medial side of the distal end. It provides attachment for the interosseous membrane. The *anterior border* is sharp and distinct in its lower half, but it may be masked and joined with the interosseous border in its upper fourth. The *posterior border* is blunt but well defined and extends from the neck to the medial margin of the back of the lateral malleolus.

The *lateral (peroneal) surface* is situated between the anterior and the posterior borders; it faces laterally above but becomes twisted so that below it faces directly backward. The *anterior (extensor) surface* is that strip which is situated between the anterior and the interosseous borders. It is very narrow proximately but is wider distally. The *posterior surface* is situated between the posterior and the interosseous borders and is subdivided into 2 parts by the medial crest. The *medial crest* is at times the most prominent ridge on the bone. It begins at the neck and ends inferiorly by continuing into the interosseous border a few inches above the distal end. This crest is closely related to the peroneal artery.

The distal end of the bone may be considered the *lateral malleolus*. It is pyramidal in shape and compressed from side to side. It presents 4 surfaces, of which the medial reveals a triangular facet for articulation with the lateral surface of the talus. The *lateral surface* is smooth and convex and palpable subcutaneously. It forms the lateral prominence of the ankle and extends to a slightly lower level than the medial malleolus. The *anterior surface* is narrow and not sharply defined from the lateral. The *posterior surface* presents a longitudinal groove for the tendons of the peroneus longus and the brevis. The *medial surface* reveals a large articular area for the talus.

Attachments to the Fibula (Figs. 708 and 709):

To the head: the capsule of the superior tibiofibular joint. The arcuate ligament of

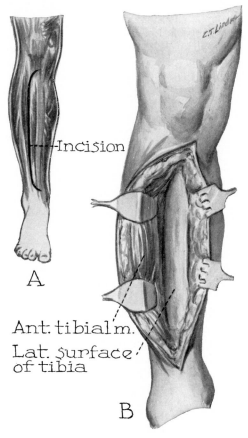

FIG. 711. Surgical approach to the tibia.

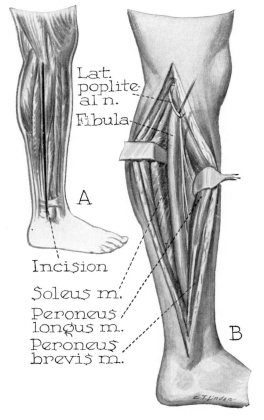

FIG. 712. Surgical approach to the fibula.

the knee to the styloid process, the lateral ligament of the knee and the biceps in front of that process, the muscles and their fasciae which arise from the upper part of the shaft and also arise from the adjoining part of the head and the fascia lata.

From the shaft: from the anterior surface, the extensor digitorum longus, the peroneus tertius and the extensor hallucis longus; from the posterior surface, the soleus and the flexor hallucis longus. From the lateral surface, the peroneus longus and the brevis. From the anterior border, the anterior intermuscular septum and the superior extensor retinaculum.

To the lateral malleolus: the anterior inferior tibiofibular ligament, the anterior talofibular ligament and the calcaneofibular ligament. The posterior inferior tibiofibular ligament, the superior peroneal retinaculum, the posterior talofibular ligament and the

transverse tibiofibular ligament to the malleolar fossa.

The epiphyses of the fibular appear as bulbous ends at both extremities. The capsules are attached to the articular margins, and the metaphyses are entirely extracapsular. The epiphyseal line at the lower end is at the level of the ankle joint. This anatomic point is important, since a disease of the ankle joint may spread to the shaft of the fibula and vice versa.

SURGICAL CONSIDERATIONS

APPROACHES TO TIBIA AND FIBULA

The tibia can be approached along its exposed medial surface (Fig. 711). The saphenous nerve and the great saphenous vein should be avoided.

The fibula is exposed in such a way that

the superficial (musculocutaneous) peroneal nerve is avoided (Fig. 712). The proximal and the middle thirds can be approached through an incision along the line of the posterior intermuscular septum. The upper third of the shaft can be approached through an incision between the adjoining borders of the soleus and the peroneus longus muscles. The common peroneal (external popliteal) nerve must be protected where it winds around the neck of the fibula. In the middle third, a lateral incision is made through the interval be-

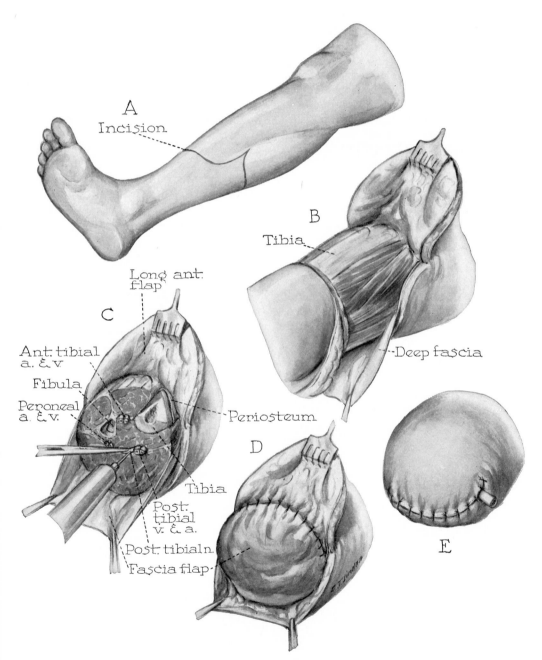

A
Incision

B
Tibia

C
Long ant. flap

Ant. tibial a. & v.

Fibula

Peroneal a. & v.

Periosteum

Deep fascia

D

Tibia

Post. tibial v. & a.

Post. tibial n.

Fascia flap

E

FIG. 713. Leg amputation. In C it should be noted that the fibula is cut at a higher level than the tibia; the tibia is beveled.

tween the peroneus longus and the flexor hallucis longus muscles. The distal third of the shaft is exposed just behind the anterior intermuscular septum, between the peroneus brevis and the tertius muscles.

LEG AMPUTATION

The technic for leg amputation in the middle third utilizes a long anterior flap and a short posterior flap (Fig. 713). The deep fascia is included in these flaps, and in those patients whose circulation seems to be adequate, an additional 2 or 3 inches of deep fascia is cut downward from the posterior incision so that a fascial flap remains attached. The anterior flap of skin and fascia is separated at a little higher level than that point at which the bones are to be sawed. All soft tissues are severed to the bone about 2 inches distal to the point of bone section. The tissues are separated from the bone and retracted high enough to promote free use of the saw. The periosteum is elevated upward. The fibula should be made about 1 inch shorter than the tibia, because if it is left as long as the tibia, it becomes prominent and tender, producing a stump that will be difficult to fit. The nerves are drawn down as far as possible, ligated and divided. The vascular stumps are secured, and the muscles are approximated with fascial sutures. The fascia of the posterior flap is sutured over the end of the stump so that the muscle surface is carefully covered. The anterior skin-fascia flap is pulled downward and sutured to the posterior fascial layer.

FRACTURES OF SHAFT OF TIBIA AND FIBULA

The shafts of both bones of the leg are fractured more commonly in young adults and children. If the injury is caused by indirect violence, the tibia usually breaks at its weakest point, which is the junction of the middle and the lower thirds; the fibula usually fractures at a higher level. If the cause is direct violence, the bones are broken at the same level, the fractures being transverse and at the site of injury. The lower fragment is pulled upward by the action of the calf muscles; the weight of the foot produces outward rotation.

In the treatment of these fractures, reduction may be difficult. The knee always should be flexed, to relax the calf muscles. To check on proper alignment, the inner margin of the great toe, the internal malleolus and the inner margin of the patella should all be in the same line.

Ankle

The ankle consists of the ankle joint (the tibia and the fibula proximally, and the talus distally) and those (structures which sur- round it (Fig. 714). The 2 malleoli can be felt distinctly, the lateral being less promi- nent, descending lower and lying farther back

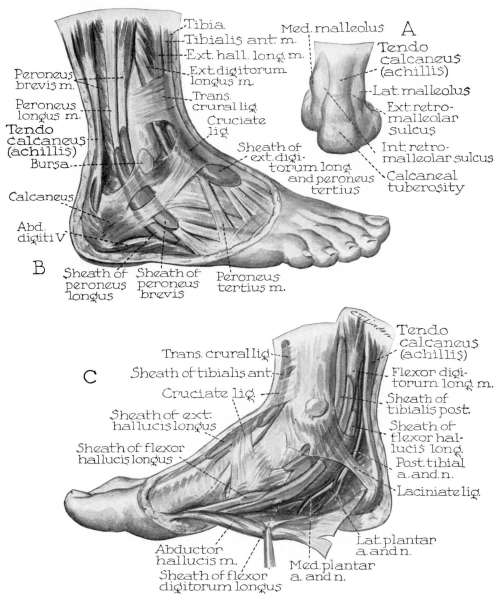

FIG. 714. The structures surrounding the right ankle: (A) seen from behind; (B) the lateral structures; (C) the medial structures.

than the medial. The tip of the lateral malleolus is about ½ inch below and behind the tip of its corresponding bony prominence. Anterior to the lateral malleolus and lateral to the tendon of the peroneus tertius is a shallow depression which indicates the level of the ankle joint. A similar depression lies between the medial malleolus and the tibialis anterior tendon. At these two points the ankle joint is very superficial, and, when fluid is present, these areas become filled and form soft projections. If the foot is forcibly plantar-flexed, the talus (astragalus) glides forward out of its socket and produces a prominence which is most apparent in front of the lateral malleolus. The medial or internal malleolus is large, flat and prominent. The ankle joint lies approximately ½ inch above the tip of the internal malleolus.

The tendo calcaneus (achillis) stands out prominently at the back of the ankle; between it and the malleoli are 2 hollowed grooves. Over the front of the ankle, the tendons of the extensor muscles stand out in bold relief, especially when the joint is flexed. From within outward, they are (Figs. 714 and 715): the tendon of the anterior tibial muscle, the extensor hallucis longus, the extensor digitorum longus and the peroneus tertius.

Above and behind the medial malleolus, the tendons of the posterior tibial and the flexor digitorum muscles are noted; the former lies closer to the bone. Behind the lateral malleolus, the long and the short peroneal tendons can be felt lying close to the edge of the fibula, the tendon of the smaller muscle being the closer to it. The interval between the medial malleolus and the calcaneus is crossed by the laciniate (internal annular) ligament, which also forms an osteo-aponeurotic canal in which are found the tendons of the flexor digitorum longus, the flexor hallucis longus and the posterior tibial muscles (Fig. 714 C).

The tendon of the tibialis posterior muscle lies immediately behind the back of the me-

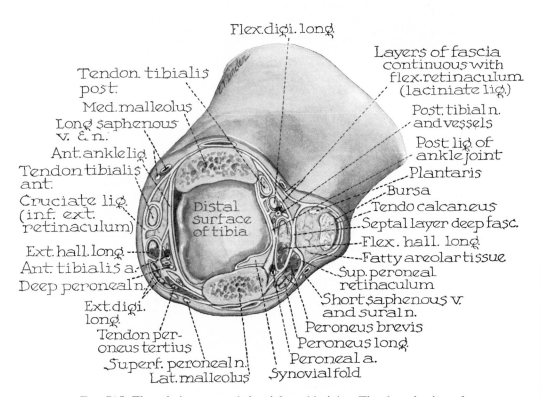

FIG. 715. The relations around the right ankle joint. The deep fascia and the ligaments are shown in blue.

dial malleolus and is succeeded by the tendons of the flexor digitorum longus and the flexor hallucis longus. The posterior tibial vessels and nerves lie between the last two named tendons. The tendons lie in close relation to the ankle joint, but the calcaneal tendon is separated from it by a considerable interval. A fairly wide space which is filled with fatty areolar tissue also exists between the flexor hallucis longus tendon and the posterior tibial vessels, so that there is little chance of damage when operating on this tendon.

The skin about the ankle is thin and loosely attached to the subjacent parts. Owing to its proximity to the underlying malleoli, it may be damaged by the pressure of a cast or a bed rest. The subcutaneous tissue varies both in quantity and character. Over the front of the ankle it is lax and free from fat; therefore, if edema is present, the skin will pit on pressure.

DEEP FASCIA

The deep fascia is strong and is directly continuous with the fascia which invests the

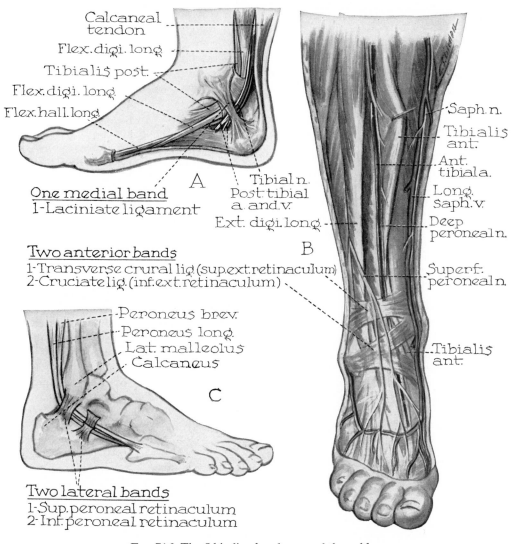

FIG. 716. The 5 binding bands around the ankle.

leg and the foot. It forms 5 definite bands (in front of and at each side of the ankle) which maintain the tendons in contact with the bones, and it assists in forming osteo-aponeurotic tunnels through which the tendons and their synovial sheaths pass.

The 5 binding bands are (Fig. 716): the 2 anterior bands, the transverse crural and the cruciate ligaments; *1* medial band, the laciniate ligament; *2* lateral bands, the peroneal retinacula.

The anterior thickening of the deep fascia has 2 divisions: an upper and a lower. The upper division, or the *transverse crural ligament,* stretches between the anterior borders of the tibia and the fibula immediately above the ankle joint. Beneath this ligament are the structures which pass from the front of the leg to the dorsum of the foot. With the exception of the tibialis anterior, which lies separately, they lie in one compartment. The

structures from medial to lateral are: the anterior tibial muscle, the extensor hallucis longus, the anterior tibial vessels, the deep peroneal nerve, the extensor digitorum longus and the peroneus tertius (Figs. 715 and 716 B). The structures which pass over the superficial surface of this ligament are: the long saphenous vein, the saphenous nerve and the superficial peroneal nerve.

The cruciate ligament is the lower division of the anterior thickening of deep fascia; it has been referred to as the inferior extensor retinaculum. It is the more important of the two. Its shape resembles the letter "Y," the stem of the letter being the lateral part of the ligament (Figs. 714, 715 and 716 B). The Y is placed on its side and lies across the dorsum of the foot close to the ankle joint. It is firmly attached to the anterior part of the upper surface of the calcaneum. The upper limb of the Y attaches to the medial malleolus; the lower part fuses with the deep fascia along the medial margin of the foot, and with the plantar fascia. The structures which pass beneath this ligament are identical with those passing under the transverse ligament. It splits to form 2 compartments. The medial of these is occupied by the tendon of the extensor hallucis longus; the lateral compartment, by the peroneus tertius and the extensor digitorum longus. Each compartment is lined with a synovial sheath. The vessels and the nerves pass deeply to the ligament. The ligament usually does not form a compartment for the tibialis anterior tendon, because the tendon runs either above or below the ligament.

The laciniate ligament (internal laterai) bridges the hollow between the medial malleolus and the calcaneus, to both of which it is attached (Fig. 716 A). It has 4 borders and 2 surfaces. Of its borders, the upper is continuous with 2 layers of fascia—the deep fascia of the leg and the strong fascia which extends between the superficial and the deep muscles of the calf. The lower border is continuous with the medial part of the plantar aponeurosis. The lateral border is attached to the tuberosity of the calcaneus; and the medial, to the medial malleolus. Of its surfaces, the superficial is related to the medial calcaneal vessels and nerves, which first pierce it and then cross it; the deep surface is re-

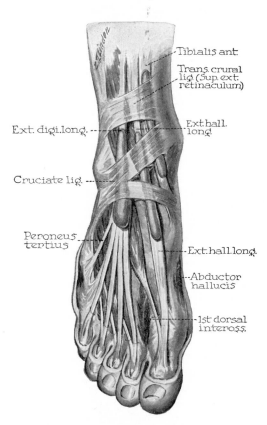

Fig. 717. The 3 tendon sheaths of the anterior aspect of the ankle.

lated to the tendons, the vessels and the nerves passing in back of the leg to the sole of the foot. These lie in a compartment, in the following order from before backward (Fig. 715): the posterior tibial tendon, the flexor digitorum longus, the posterior tibial artery with its companion veins, the posterior tibial nerve and the flexor hallucis longus. Each tendon is supplied with a synovial sheath of its own. Under the lower part of this ligament the artery and the nerve both divide into medial and lateral plantar branches.

The peroneal retinacula are 2 lateral thickened parts of the deep fascia; they also have been referred to as the external annular ligaments. They bridge the groove between the lateral malleolus and the calcaneus (Fig. 716 C). The *superior peroneal retinaculum*

extends from the calcaneus to the lateral malleolus and binds the 2 peronei, the longus and the brevis, to the back of the lateral malleolus. The brevis lies closer to the bone. The *inferior peroneal retinaculum* is attached to the outer surfaces of the calcaneus. It is divided into 2 compartments by a septum which is attached to the peroneal tubercle. The superior retinaculum forms a common compartment for the peronei, unlike the inferior retinaculum, which forms 2 compartments.

TENDON SHEATHS

The tendon sheaths around the ankle joint are mucous sheaths which are placed anteriorly, medially, laterally and posteriorly.

The anterior sheaths appear as 3 separate structures (Fig 717). They are: the sheath

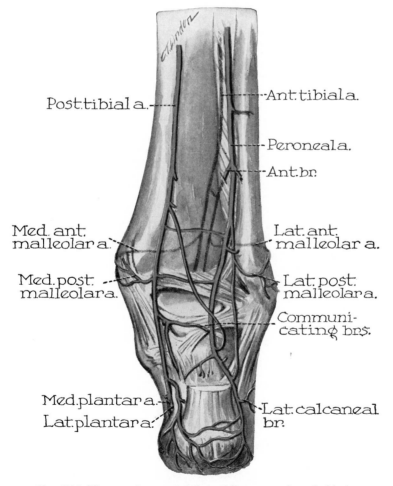

FIG. 718. The arteries around the ankle, as seen from behind.

of the tibialis anterior, which extends from the upper border of the transverse ligament to just below the ankle joint; the sheaths of the extensor hallucis longus and of the extensor digitorum longus, which extend from the malleoli to the base of the metatarsal bones.

The medial mucous sheaths are also 3 in number (Fig. 714 C): the sheath of the tibialis posterior, which extends from about 2 inches above the medial malleolus to the insertion of the tendon at the navicular tuberosity; the sheaths of the flexor hallucis longus and the flexor digitorum longus, which extend from the medial malleolus to the middle of the sole of the foot. Near the head of the metatarsal bones these tendons acquire new sheaths, resembling the arrangements seen in the fingers.

Laterally, the peroneus longus and brevis are enclosed in a sheath which extends 2 inches above the tip of the malleolus and 2 inches below it (Fig. 714 B). Above the malleolus the tendons lie together in a single sheath, but where they diverge, the sheath provides each with a separate investment.

Posteriorly, the tendo achillis has a sheath which extends about 3 inches upward from the insertion of the tendon to the calcaneus.

VESSELS

The arteries around the ankle are mainly 3 in number (Fig. 718): the anterior tibial, the posterior tibial and the peroneal.

The anterior tibial artery is continued beyond the line of the ankle joint as the dorsalis pedis (Fig. 722). Proximal to the joint line, the vessel is crossed by the tendon of the extensor hallucis longus. At a lower level it lies between the tendon of this muscle and the extensor digitorum longus. In the region of the ankle, it provides malleolar branches.

The posterior tibial artery corresponds to the center of a line which connects the internal malleolus and the most prominent part of the heel. The artery terminates opposite the lower margin of the laciniate ligament, where it divides into medial and lateral plantar arteries. The calcaneal branches supply the tissues at the medial side of the heel.

The anterior branch of the peroneal artery crosses the ankle joint in front of the interosseous ligament between the lower ends of the tiba and the fibula. The anterior and the posterior tibial arteries and the peroneal artery form an anastomotic network about the ankle and the heel regions.

ANKLE JOINT (TALOCRURAL)

The ankle joint is a synovial joint of the hinge variety which unites the foot to the leg. Its great strength and stability are ensured by surrounding powerful ligaments and tendons, as well as by a close interlocking of its articulating surfaces. Because of its hinge action, the to-and-fro movements of walking are possible. When one walks, the triceps sural (both heads of the gastrocnemius and the soleus) raises the heel from the ground and produces plantar flexion of the ankle joint. The 4 anterior crural muscles cause the foot to clear the ground, and thus produce dorsiflexion of this joint. The malleoli grasp the sides of the talus, the latter transmitting the weight of the body to the tibia. The sharp tip of the lateral (fibular) malleolus can be felt a little less than 1 inch below the level of the blunt ending medial (tibial) malleolus. Since there are no muscles at the sides of the ankle, the malleoli are subcutaneous and may be palpated readily. With the exception of the tendo calcaneus, all tendons that cross the ankle joint (4 in front and 5 behind) pass forward and become inserted into the foot anterior to the midtarsal joint.

Bones

The bones that enter into the formation of the ankle joint are the talus and the distal ends of the tibia and the fibula.

The talus articulates with the bones of the leg by 3 of its surfaces: the upper, the medial and the lateral. The bones form a deep socket which receives the upper part of the talus.

Tibia and Fibula. The roof of the joint is formed entirely by the tibia. As the 2 malleoli project downward, they grasp the talus firmly at each side, thus permitting only a slight degree of lateral or medial movement. The bones just mentioned are so intimately related with the tarsal bones and joints in the mechanics and the alignment of the ankle joint that it is impossible to isolate the ankle joint from the rest of the foot in either clinical or anatomic discussions (see Joints of the Foot, p. 838).

LIGAMENTS

Capsular Ligament. The bones that form the ankle joint are held together by a capsular ligament which is subdivided into anterior, posterior, lateral and medial ligaments (Fig. 719). (See also diagram at bottom of page 824.)

The capsule is loose in front and behind and tight at the sides. Proximally, it is attached to the margins of the articular surfaces

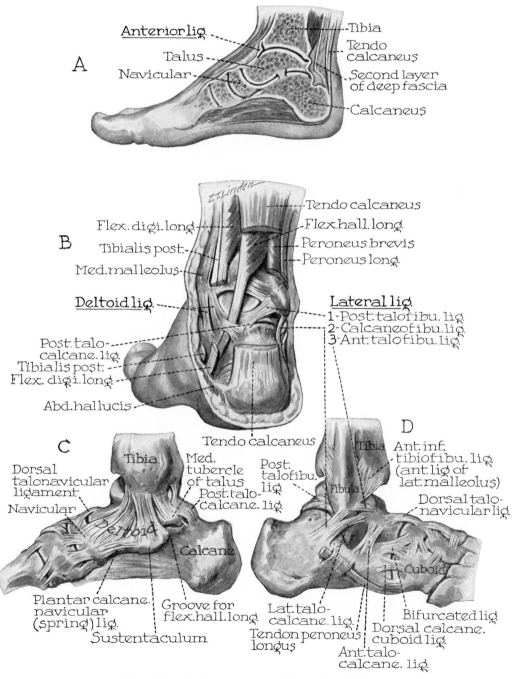

FIG. 719. The ligaments around the ankle joint.

of the tibial and the fibular epiphyses and distally to the margins of the superior articular surface of the talus except at the anterior aspect of the joint, where it extends forward to the neck of the bone. The *medial part* of this capsule is greatly thickened and is named the *deltoid ligament*. It is triangular in shape, with its apex attached above to the tip of the medial malleolus. Its base has a more extensive attachment, extending from the tubercle of the navicular, the plantar calcaneonavicular (spring) ligament, the neck of the talus and the sustentaculum tali to the body of the talus. Its medial surface is crossed by the tendons of the tibialis posterior and the flexor digitorum longus (Fig. 719 B). If the foot is everted to an extreme degree, the deltoid ligament usually tears away from the medial malleolus rather than rupturing itself. It braces the spring ligament and helps to support the head of the talus and to preserve the arch of the foot.

The lateral ligament is weaker and less complete. Most authors divide it into 3 parts (Figs. 719 B and D).

1. *The calcaneofibular ligament* extends downward and backward from in front of the apex of the lateral malleolus to the lateral surface of the calcaneus. These fibers are separated from the other fibers of the lateral ligament by some fatty and areolar tissues. The ligament is crossed by the peronei.

2. *The anterior talofibular ligament* passes horizontally forward and inward from the anterior aspect of the lateral malleolus to the lateral side of the neck of the talus.

3. *The posterior talofibular ligament* extends inward behind the joint, from the inner surface of the lateral malleolus to the posterior process of the talus. It is the strongest of the 3 bands and binds the fibula to the talus in a rigid manner.

The anterior ligament of the ankle joint is a thin wide membrane which is composed chiefly of transverse fibers. It extends from the anterior margin of the distal surface of the tibia to the dorsal surface of the neck of the talus (Fig. 719 A). A cut across the foot immediately in front of the tibia will open the ankle joint at this point.

The posterior ligament is the weakest of all the ankle ligaments. It is thin, sometimes defective and difficult to define. It extends from the posterior border of the distal end of the tibia to the posterior surface of the talus. The tendon of the flexor hallucis longus acts as a strong posterior support for the joint.

Synovial Membrane

The synovial membrane lines the capsular ligament and covers the intracapsular portion of the neck of the talus (Fig. 715). It passes up between the tibia and the fibula for about ¼ inch and extends well forward onto the neck of the talus. A puncture wound or superficial incision made in front of the joint may enter the joint cavity. The membrane is lax in front and behind where it is covered by the anterior and the posterior ligaments, at which points the capsular ligament is thin and loose. It is continuous with the synovial membrane of the distal tibiofibular joint. A joint effusion bulges the synovial membrane and the weak capsule anteriorly and posteriorly.

Vessels and Nerves

The nerves to the ankle joint are derived from the anterior and the posterior tibial nerves.

Relations (Figs. 715 and 720):

Anterior. From the medial to the lateral side lie the tibialis anterior, the extensor hallucis longus, the anterior tibial vessels, the anterior tibial nerves, the extensor digitorum

Capsular Ligament
{
Medial (Deltoid) Ligament

Lateral Ligament {
1. Calcaneofibular Ligament
2. Anterior Talofibular Ligament
3. Posterior Talofibular Ligament

Anterior Ligament

Posterior Ligament
}

longus and the peroneus tertius. The perforating branch of the peroneal vessels is found on the lateral malleolus. The inferior extensor retinaculum crosses the joint obliquely. The superficial structures which are found in this region are the branches of the musculocutaneous nerve, the superficial vessels, the long saphenous vein and the saphenous nerve on the medial malleolus.

Posterior. The tendo calcaneus is separated from the posterior ligament by an interval of fatty areolar tissue which contains small vessels. Between the joint and the tendon are found the flexor hallucis longus, the posterior tibial nerves and vessels, and the flexor digitorum longus, the latter structures being named in a lateromedial order. The vessels and the nerves are more superficial than the 2 flexors and overlap them. All of these structures are maintained in position by the flexor retinaculum.

Medial. The tibialis posterior lies on the

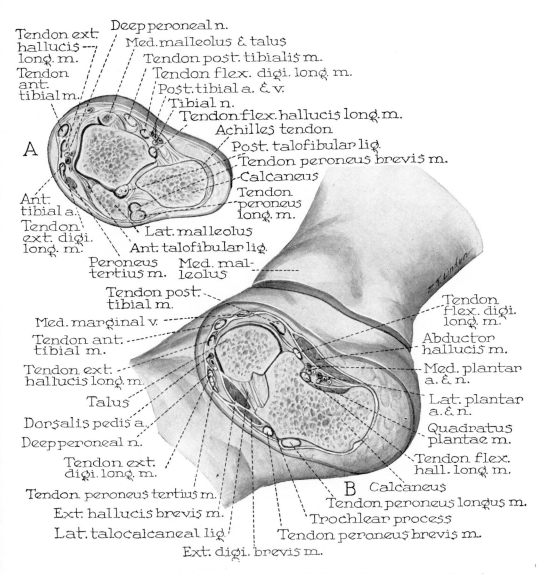

FIG. 720. Cross sections through the ankle and the foot: (A) section taken through the malleoli; (B) section taken through the calcaneus and the talus.

deltoid ligament above the sustentaculum tali, and the flexor digitorum longus lies on the attachment of that ligament to the sustentaculum. The flexor retinaculum overlies the tendon.

Lateral. The peroneus brevis lies on the posterior talofibular ligament and separates the peroneus longus from it. Its tendons are held down by a retinaculum of deep fascia; they have a common synovial sheath. The termination of the peroneal artery anastomoses with its perforating branch on this side of the joint. More superficially are the short saphenous vein and the sural nerve.

MOVEMENTS

The movements of the ankle joints involve the joints of the foot as well. Inversion and eversion of the foot are effected by plantar flexion (true flexion) and dorsiflexion (extension). Plantar flexion and dorsiflexion are effected mainly at the ankle joint between the talus, the tibia and the fibula. Dorsiflexion is limited by the lengthening of the calf muscles; if the knee is flexed, the range of movement is greater. Plantar flexion is produced by the gastrocnemius, the soleus and the flexor hallucis longus; it also is produced to a minor degree by the tibialis posterior, the peroneus longus and the plantaris muscles. When the foot is moved so that the sole faces medially, the movement is described as inversion; the contrary movement is eversion. Inversion of the foot is brought about by the action of the tibialis anterior and the tibialis posterior; eversion is accomplished by the peronei longus, the brevis and the tertius. A greater range of inversion may be produced when the ankle joint is plantar flexed; this is due apparently to an increased range of metatarsal movement. The 5 tendons which pass behind the ankle are situated too close to the axis of the joint to act on it; therefore, if the tendo calcaneus is cut, the power to plantar flex is lost.

SURGICAL CONSIDERATIONS

SYME'S AMPUTATION THROUGH THE ANKLE JOINT

This is a disarticulation with removal of both malleoli and the articular surface of the tibia. The incision passes under the heel, from the tip of the lateral malleolus to a corresponding point on the medial malleolus (Fig. 721). The distal ends of the tibia and the fibula are exposed, and these bones are sectioned about 1 cm. proximal to their articular surfaces. The terminal branches of the peroneal vessels and the posterior tibials should be preserved. The anterior tendons are united to the calcaneus tendon or to the periosteum of the tibia. This amputation provides a good end-bearing stump, but it is difficult to fit with a prosthesis without producing a wide and ugly-looking ankle.

In the *Pirogoff amputation,* the posterior portion of the calcaneus is sawed off and ap-

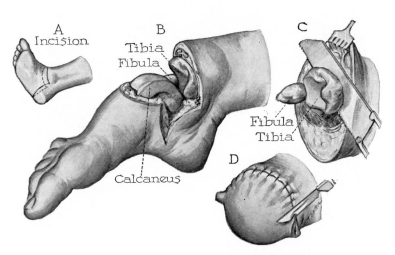

FIG. 721. Amputation through the ankle joint (Syme).

proximated to the sawed end of the tibia and the fibula. Therefore, it is a modified Syme's amputation, the only difference being that part of the calcaneus is retained and brought into contact with the divided lower ends of the tibia and the fibula.

DISLOCATIONS OF THE ANKLE JOINT

Dislocations of the ankle joint (between the talus and the tibia and the fibula) are classified according to the direction in which the foot passes: namely, backward, forward, medial, lateral or upward.

Lateral and medial displacements occur in association with Pott's fracture or fractures of the malleoli.

In forward (anterior) dislocation, the ligaments or malleoli are torn, the heel is shortened and the distance from the malleoli to the heel is diminished; the distance from the malleoli to the toes, however, is increased. The foot appears to be lengthened, the normal hollows at the sides of the tendo achillis are obliterated, and the talus may be felt in front of the tibia. The malleoli appear to lie nearer the sole.

Backward dislocation is the most frequent type; this may be associated with a Pott's fracture. It results from extreme plantar flexion of the foot which tears the ligaments. Involvement of the malleoli and the posterior articular edge of the tibia is usually present. The foot appears to be shortened, and the heel is prominent. The malleoli appear somewhat anteriorly. The distance from the malleoli to the heel is increased, while that from the malleoli to the toe is diminished.

Reduction is easy if the knee is bent to relax the tendo achillis and if proper traction and counter traction are applied.

Foot

The foot, which is triangular in outline, extends from the point of the heel to the root of the toes (Fig. 722). It is divided into the tarsus (posterior half) and the metatarsus (anterior half). The landmarks which are visible over the lateral aspect are thin in contrast with the more bulky medial markings.

LATERAL, MEDIAL AND DORSAL ASPECTS

The lateral margin of the foot rests in contact with the ground over its entire extent. Near the middle of this border, the tuberosity of the base of the 5th metatarsal bone affords a landmark for the tarsometatarsal joint (Lisfranc). If a line is constructed between the tuberosity of the base of the 5th metatarsal and the tip of the lateral malleolus, and a point just anterior to the middle of this line is marked, the cuboid midtarsal joint (Chopart) is located.

The medial aspect of the foot is arched, in contrast with the flat appearance of the lateral border. The medial border rests on the ground only at the heel and the ball of the great toe. The sustentaculum tali is located about 1 inch below the medial malleolus. A definite prominence produced by the tuberosity of the navicular bone is felt by pressing 1 inch in front of and slightly below the level of the medial malleolus. This latter tuberosity is a useful surgical guide; it is the principal point of insertion of the tibialis posterior tendon. The depression which is below and behind it is a guide to the talonavicular joint.

The dorsum of the foot reveals a very thin skin, which is much less sensitive than that on the plantar surface. The subcutaneous tissue over the dorsum is very loose, so that edema becomes quite prominent in this region. The veins are arranged in an arch, the outline of which is apparent when one is in the erect posture. The large and the small saphenous veins arise from the marginal veins of this arch. The tendons in front of the ankle can be traced over this surface to their insertions. The tendon of the extensor hallucis longus passes forward to the great toe, and the tendons of the extensor digitorum longus pass to the 4 lateral toes. A fleshy muscular mass, the extensor digitorum brevis muscle, can be felt on the posterolateral aspect of the dorsum. The tendon of the peroneus brevis muscle passes forward under the lateral malleolus to its insertion into the tuberosity of the 5th metatarsal. The dorsalis pedis artery, a continuation of the anterior tibial artery, may be indicated on the surface by a line drawn midway between the 2 malleoli to the posterior extremity of the first interosseous space. To the lateral side of this vessel is the anterior tibial nerve.

SOLE OF THE FOOT (PLANTAR SURFACE)

The skin is thicker on the sole of the foot than it is over the dorsum. It is particularly thick over those points which bear weight (heel, ball of the big toe and lateral margins of the sole). Like the palm of the hand, it is highly sensitive and contains numerous sweat glands.

The cutaneous nerves are arranged in the following way (Fig. 723): the *medial plantar nerve* supplies the 3½ digits on the big-toe side of the foot, as the median nerve supplies the 3½ digits on the thumb of the hand; the *lateral plantar nerve,* which corresponds to the ulnar nerve of the hand, supplies the remaining 1½ digits. The medial calcaneal branches of the posterior tibial nerve supply the skin under the heel.

The superficial fascia becomes thick and tough along the lateral border, on the ball of the foot and at the heel. Traversing it are small but tough fibrous bands which subdivide the fatty tissue into small lobules; these bands also connect the skin with the deep fascia.

DEEP PLANTAR APONEUROSIS (DEEP FASCIA)

The deep (plantar) fascia arrangement resembles that of the hand (Fig. 724). It lies

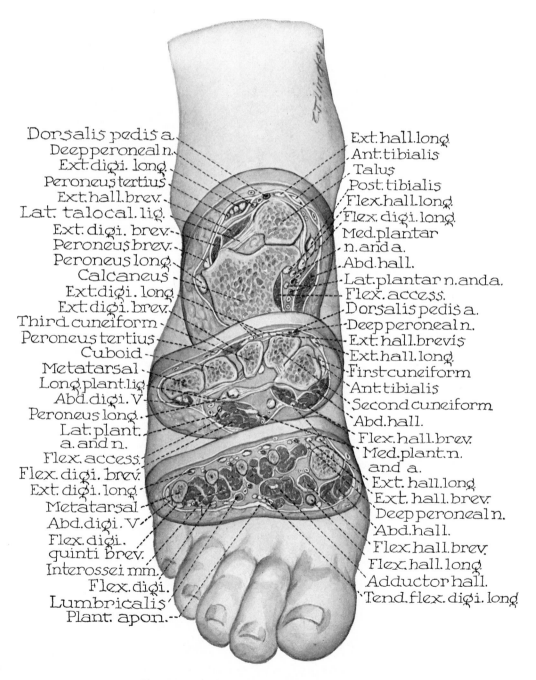

FIG. 722. The foot seen in cross-sectional views.

superficial to the vessels, the nerves, the muscles and the tendons, and consists of 3 portions: relatively thin medial and lateral parts and a very dense and strong intermediate part. This thickened strong central part is known as the plantar aponeurosis. It forms a dense fibrous sheet which is attached posteriorly to the calcaneus and widens anteriorly to divide into five slips, one for each toe. (The palmar aponeurosis of the hand divides into 4 slips, one for each finger, but none for the thumb.) Therefore, the great toe has a different relationship to this fascia than that of the thumb to the deep fascia of the palm; hence its mobility is diminished as compared with that of the thumb. The slips to the toes are connected to the fibrous flexor sheaths and to the sides of the metatarsophalangeal joints.

Fibrous Flexor Sheaths. On each toe the deep fascia is thickened to form curved plates called the fibrous flexor sheaths; these hold the flexor tendons against the phalanges. They are strong and dense opposite the phalanges but are thin and weak opposite the joints, so that movements are not hindered. These sheaths are attached to the margins of the phalanges and to the plantar ligaments and form with them a tunnel which is occupied by the long and the short flexor tendons. This tunnel is lined with the synovial sheath that envelops the tendons.

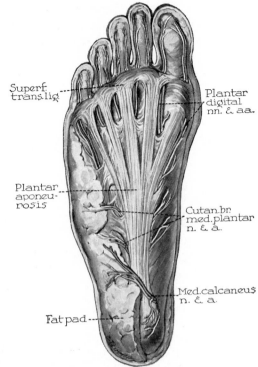

FIG. 724. The plantar fascia.

The medial division of the deep fascia covers the abductor hallucis muscle; the lateral part of the fascia extends between calcaneus and the tuberosity of the 5th metatarsal.

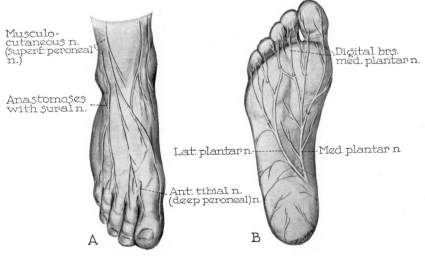

FIG. 723. The cutaneous nerve supply of the foot: (A) the dorsum of the foot; (B) the plantar surface of the foot.

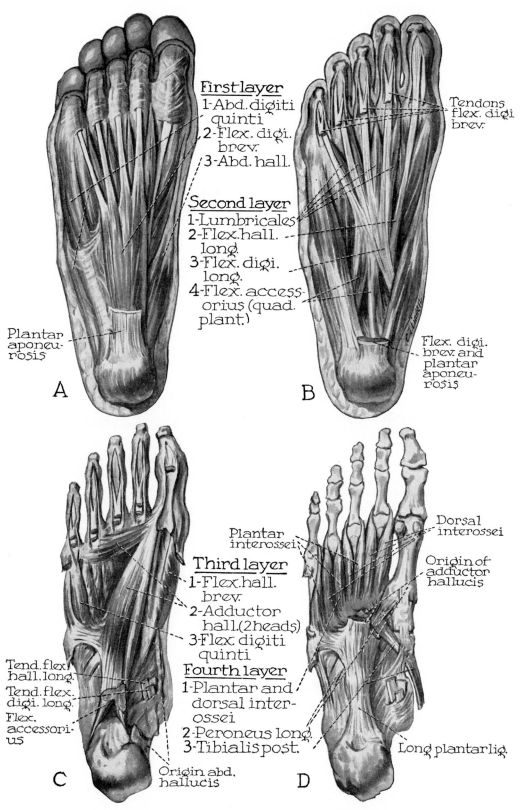

First layer
1-Abd. digiti quinti
2-Flex. digi. brev.
3-Abd. hall.

Second layer
1-Lumbricales
2-Flex. hall. long.
3-Flex. digi. long.
4-Flex. accessorius (quad. plant.)

Plantar aponeurosis

A

Tendons flex. digi brev.

Flex. digi. brev. and plantar aponeurosis

B

Plantar interossei

Dorsal interossei

Origin of adductor hallucis

Third layer
1-Flex. hall. brev.
2-Adductor hall. (2 heads)
3-Flex digiti quinti

Fourth layer
1-Plantar and dorsal interossei
2-Peroneus long.
3-Tibialis post.

Tend. flex. hall. long.
Tend. flex. digi. long.
Flex. accessorius

Origin abd. hallucis

C

Long plantar lig.

D

Fig. 725. The 4 layers of muscles and tendons of the sole of the foot.

MUSCLES AND TENDONS

The muscles and the tendons of the sole of the foot are arranged in 4 layers which are separated by fascial partitions; in these the plantar nerves and vessels run (Fig. 725). Only the muscles of the first layer cover the whole extent of the sole. The muscles of the second layer are all connected to the flexor digitorum longus tendon and form an X-shaped figure, so that on each border of the foot the first and the third layers come into contact with each other.

The First Layer of Muscles. This consists of the abductor hallucis, the flexor digitorum brevis and the abductor digiti quinti (Fig. 725 A). *The flexor digitorum brevis* divides into 4 tendons which pass to the 4 lateral toes and become inserted into the middle phalanges. *The abductor hallucis* is inserted into the medial side of the base of the proximal phalanx of the great toe, and the *abductor digiti minimi* is inserted into the lateral side of the base of the proximal phalanx of the little toe (Fig. 727). The names of these muscles indicate their actions. The lateral plantar nerve supplies the abductor digiti minimi, and the other 2 muscles are supplied by the medial plantar nerve.

The second layer of muscles consists of the flexor digitorum longus, the flexor accessorius (quadratus plantae), the lumbricales and the flexor hallucis longus (Fig. 725 B).

The tendon of the flexor digitorum longus passes forward and laterally from the medial flexor retinaculum. At first it lies on the medial side of the sustentaculum tali, and then it crosses superficial to the flexor hallucis longus tendon, which separates it from the plantar calcaneonavicular ligament. This tendon constitutes the central structure in this layer of muscles. It should be recalled that this tendon has crossed superficially to the tendon of the tibialis posterior at the back of the medial malleolus (Fig. 716 A); it now appears from under cover of the abductor hallucis and crosses superficially to the tendon of the flexor hallucis longus. Therefore, it appears superficial at 2 points —once where it crosses the tibialis posterior and again where it crosses the flexor hallucis longus. As it receives the insertion of the flexor digitorum accessorius, it divides into 4 tendons for the lateral 4 toes. These tendons resemble those of the flexor digitorum profundus in the hand, since they pass through rings made by the splitting of the fibers of the short flexor tendon and then pass on to become inserted into the distal phalanges (Fig. 725 B).

The flexor digitorum accessorius (quadratus plantae) muscle arises by 2 heads— one from each side of the calcaneus. The medial head, which is wide and fleshy, arises from the medial surface of the calcaneus. The lateral head, which is narrow and tendinous, arises from the lateral margin of the plantar surface of the bone. It inserts into the tendon of the flexor digitorum longus, in the region of the middle of the sole, and acts as a flexor of the toes (Fig. 725 B). It is supplied by the lateral plantar nerve.

The lumbricales are 4 in number and are more slender than those of the hand. They arise from the tendons of the flexor digitorum longus and proceed to the 4 lateral toes, where each is inserted into the medial side of the dorsal expansion of the corresponding extensor tendons. The lumbricalis to the 2nd toe arises from only one tendon, the tendon of the 2nd toe, but the other 3 lumbricales arise in a bipennate manner from the adjacent sides of the tendons to the 2nd and the 3rd, the 3rd and the 4th, and the 4th and the 5th toes. The 1st, or most medial, lumbricalis is supplied by the medial plantar nerve; the other 3 are supplied by the lateral plantar nerve. These muscles flex the toes at the metatarsophalangeal joints and extend them at the interphalangeal joints.

The flexor hallucis longus tendon, after supplying a slip to the tendon of the flexor digitorum longus, passes forward to the big toe, where it inserts into the base of the terminal phalanx. It crosses deeply to the tendon of the flexor digitorum longus and lies below the lateral part of the plantar calcaneonavicular ligament. Its name indicates its action; it receives its nerve supply on the back of the leg from the posterior tibial nerve.

The third layer of muscles consists of the flexor hallucis brevis, the adductor hallucis (oblique and transverse heads) and the flexor digiti quinti brevis (Fig. 725 C). The muscles of this layer are limited to the anterior part of the foot. A plan of origin of these muscles may be remembered if it is recalled that the base of each of the 5 metatarsal bones gives origin to a muscle; therefore, the 1st gives rise to the flexor hallucis brevis; the 2nd, the 3rd and the 4th to the adductor hallucis (oblique head) and the 5th to the flexor digiti quinti.

The *flexor hallucis brevis* covers the plantar aspect of the first metatarsal; its belly divides into 2 heads. The medial head is inserted, in common with the abductor hallucis, into the medial side of the base of the proximal phalanx of the hallux, and the lateral head is inserted into the lateral side of the same bone in common with the adductor (Fig. 727). A sesamoid bone usually is developed in each tendon of insertion; it flexes the first metatarsophalangeal joint. The nerve supply to this muscle derived from the medial plantar nerve.

The *adductor hallucis muscle* resembles the adductor pollicis in that it has oblique and transverse heads. It arises from the 2nd, the 3rd and the 4th metatarsal bones and is inserted in common with the lateral head of the flexor hallucis brevis. The transverse head is a small muscle bundle which is located under the heads of the metatarsal bones. It arises from the plantar ligaments of the 3rd, the 4th and the 5th metatarsophalangeal joints and is inserted in common with the preceding muscle. The nerve supply is derived from the lateral plantar nerve.

The *flexor digiti quinti brevis* is the short flexor of the little toe. It is a single fleshy muscle slip which arises from the base of the 5th metatarsal bone and the peroneus longus tendon. It inserts into the lateral side of the base of the proximal phalanx of the little toe and flexes the little toe at the metatarsophalangeal joint. It is supplied by the lateral plantar nerve.

The fourth layer of muscles consists of the interossei (plantar and dorsal), the tendon of the peroneus longus and the tendon of the tibialis posterior (Fig. 725 D).

The *interossei* are 7 interosseous muscles —3 plantar and 4 dorsal. As in the hand, the dorsal are abductors, and the plantar are adductors; but the line of action passes through the 2nd digit and not the 3rd, as in the hand. They lie between the metatarsal bones and arise from them. They abduct and adduct the lateral 4 toes to and from the middle line of the *2nd* toe and also aid in flexion of the metatarsophalangeal joints.

The 3 *plantar* interossei arise from the plantar and the medial surfaces of the lateral 3 metatarsal bones, and each is inserted onto the medial side of the corresponding toe. They are so placed that they adduct the lateral 3 toes toward the 2nd toe.

The 4 *dorsal* interossei arise by 2 heads from the dorsal parts of the sides of the metatarsal bones between which they lie. They are inserted in the following manner (Fig. 727): the 1st on the medial side of the 2nd toe, the 2nd on the lateral side of the same toe, the 3rd on the lateral side of the 3rd toe, and the 4th on the lateral side of the 4th toe. By this arrangement, they abduct the 2nd, the 3rd and the 4th toes from the midline of the 2nd toe.

The *peroneus longus tendon* runs obliquely and medially across the sole of the foot, in the groove on the plantar surface of the cuboid bone, to become inserted into the base of the 1st metatarsal bone and the adjoining part of the medial cuneiform. It is held in place by a strong fibrous sheath which is derived from the long plantar ligament. This tendon is situated below the transverse arch of the foot and, by taking the strain off the interosseous ligaments, it aids in maintaining the arch. Together with the tendon of the tibialis anterior, it forms a tendon sling for the anterior part of the tarsus. The common synovial sheath which envelops the peronei longus and brevis, behind the malleolus, commonly is continued with the synovial sheath of the longus into the sole of the foot. Therefore, any injury to either tendon in the region of the ankle may find a pathway into the sole by means of the sheath. The peroneus longus is an evertor of the foot. It is supplied by the superficial peroneal (musculocutaneous) nerve.

After the *tibialis posterior tendon* enters the sole, it divides into 2 parts. The medial is the larger part and inserts into the tuberosity of the navicular bone; the lateral part divides into slips which spread out from it to every bone of the tarsus except the talus and also to the bases of the 2nd, the 3rd and the 4th metatarsal bones (Fig. 727). The tendon lies on the plantar surface of the so-called spring ligament (calcaneonavicular) (Fig. 719 C). This muscle is an evertor and flexor of the foot. Because of its close association with the spring ligament, it is of some importance in supporting the arch. It is supplied by the posterior tibial nerve.

ARTERIES

The posterior tibial artery divides into the lateral and the medial plantar arteries at the distal border of the laciniate ligament (Fig. 726).

The lateral plantar artery is larger than the medial and is considered the continuation of the posterior tibial. It appears from under cover of the abductor hallucis muscle and, with its companion nerve, runs forward and laterally between the 1st and the 2nd layers of muscles (flexor digitorum brevis and flexor accessorius) (Fig. 726 A). It then dips deeper as it continues medially between the 3rd and the 4th layers (adductor hallucis obliquus and the interossei) (Fig. 726 B). At the back end of the first inter-

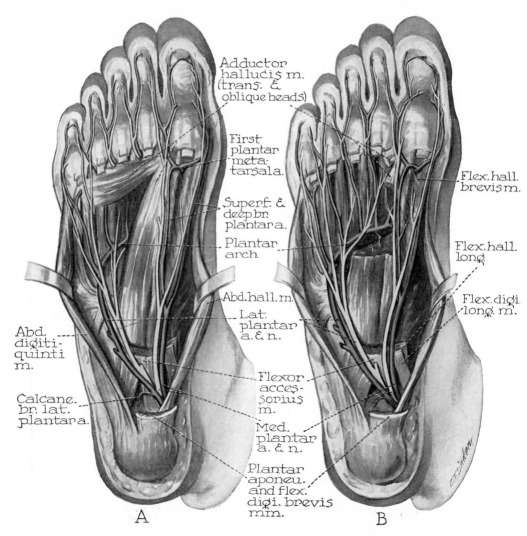

FIG. 726. The vessels and the nerves of the sole of the foot:
(A) superficial dissection; (B) deep dissection.

metatarsal space it anastomoses with the profunda branch of the dorsalis pedis artery (anterior tibial), thus forming a deep plantar arterial arch. In the first part of its course the artery gives off calcaneal branches to the skin of the heel and muscular and cutaneous branches to the skin of the sole of the foot.

The plantar arch gives off perforating branches, which pass upward through the lateral 3 intermetatarsal spaces, and plantar digital arteries to the lateral 3 clefts and the lateral side of the little toe. The arteria magna hallucis supplies the cleft between the great toe and the 2nd toe, and sends a branch to the medial side of the former; it is derived from the dorsalis pedis at its point of union with the plantar arch.

The medial plantar artery varies in size but usually is small. It is accompanied by its venae comitantes and passes along the medial side of the medial plantar nerve. It ends by joining the digital branch which the first metatarsal artery sends to the medial side of the big toe.

NERVES

The medial plantar nerve arises from the posterior tibial nerve; it corresponds to the median nerve of the hand (Fig. 726). It passes forward into the sole of the foot, under cover of the abductor hallucis muscle, accompanied by the medial plantar vessels, which are on its medial side. Reaching the lateral border of the abductor hallucis muscle, the nerve runs forward in the interval between that muscle and the flexor digitorum

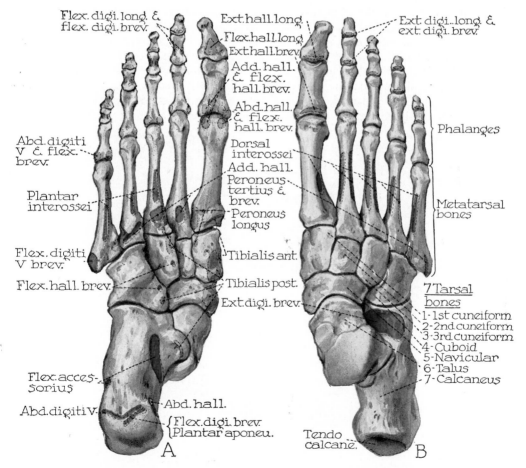

FIG. 727. The bones of the foot and the toes: (A) seen from below; (B) seen from above. The muscular origins are shown in red; the insertions, in blue.

brevis. It supplies sensory branches to the inner side of the sole of the foot, to the plantar aspect of the 3½ inner toes and to the corresponding dorsal surfaces of the last 1½ to 2 phalanges. It supplies the motor branches to 4 muscles also: the abductor hallucis, the flexor digitorum brevis, the flexor hallucis brevis and the first lumbricalis.

The lateral plantar nerve is the smaller of the 2 terminal branches of the posterior tibial nerve; it corresponds to the ulnar nerve of the hand. It reaches the outer side of the foot with its accompanying artery by passing between the flexor digitorum brevis and the quadratus plantar (between layers 1 and 2). It then divides into superficial and deep branches, which supply the outer 1½ toes and all the remaining small muscles of the foot, namely, the 3 lumbricales, all the interossei, the abductor minimi digiti, the adductor transversus and the obliques.

It should be noted that the lateral and the medial plantar vessels and nerves, plus 3 tendons, enter the sole of the foot on its medial side by passing deep to the abductor hallucis muscle; therefore, this muscle is an important landmark. It must be reflected, and the plantar vessels displaced before the flexor

hallucis longus tendon can be seen where it lies in the groove between the 2 tubercles of the talus and winds under the sustentaculum tali.

BONES

The tarsus consists of 7 tarsal bones which may be divided conveniently into a posterior row (talus and calcaneus), a middle row (navicular) and an anterior row (3 cuneiform bones and the cuboid) (Figs. 727 and 728).

The talus (astragalus, ankle bone) is discussed also in the region of the ankle joint (p. 822). It rests on the anterior two thirds of the calcaneus and has a body, a neck and a head. It lies below the tibia, sits on the upper surface of the calcaneus and is gripped by the 2 malleoli. The head of the bone is anterior and articulates with the navicular; below, it rests on the plantar calcaneonavicular (spring) ligament and the calcaneus. If the foot is inverted (so that the sole faces medially) the head of the talus is felt as a rounded prominence about 1 inch in front of the lateral malleolus. The neck is the constricted portion of the bone which is roughened by the attachment of ligaments. The

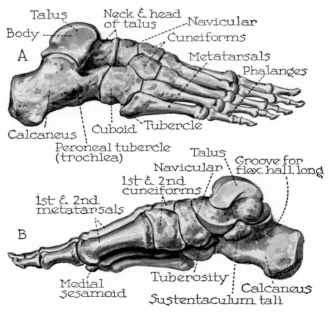

FIG. 728. Side views of the bones of the right foot:
(A) lateral view; (B) medial view.

body is hidden below by the tibia and is grasped between the malleoli at each side. The posterior surface of the body has 2 tubercles—a medial and a posterior—separated by a groove for the flexor hallucis longus tendon.

The calcaneus (os calcis) is the heel bone. It has a long, arched, anterior two thirds which supports the talus; the posterior one third forms the prominence of the heel, which rests on the ground. The anterior surface articulates with the cuboid, and the posterior third of the upper surface is saddle-shaped. The lateral surface is almost entirely subcutaneous; it is felt easily below the lateral malleolus as a wide surface that extends forward about 2 inches from the back of the heel. On the medial side, the sustentaculum tali is palpable. It is a horizontal projecting shelf which provides the bony resistance felt about a thumb's breadth below the medial malleolus.

The navicular bone (scaphoid) is on the medial side of the foot. It articulates with the head of the talus posteriorly and with the 3 cuneiforms anteriorly. On its medial side is its tuberosity, which is useful as a landmark. This tuberosity forms a prominence which is felt easily about 1 inch below and in front of the medial malleolus, midway between the back of the heel and the root of the big toe.

The 3 cuneiform bones are termed the first (medial), the second (intermediate) and the third (lateral). They articulate with the navicular posteriorly and with the first 3 metatarsals anteriorly. They are wedge-shaped, are placed side by side and articulate with each other. The lateral cuneiform articulates with the cuboid and the 4th metatarsal, while the intermediate and the medial cuneiforms grip the base of the 2nd metatarsal between them. Since the 2nd cuneiform is shorter than the other two, the base of the 2nd metatarsal articulates on its medial and lateral sides with the 1st and the 3rd cuneiforms, respectively.

The cuboid lies on the lateral side of the foot and articulates posteriorly with the calcaneus and anteriorly with the 4th and the 5th metatarsals. Its medial surface articulates with the 3rd cuneiform and the navicular,

and its plantar surface presents an oblique groove which lodges the tendon of the peroneus longus.

Webster and Roberts have stressed the importance of tarsal anomalies as the most common cause of peroneal spastic flat foot. Particularly stressed is the anomaly that consists of a calcaneonavicular bar or a talocalcaneal ridge. Therefore, these anomalies become of practical importance.

The metatarsus is composed of 5 metatarsal bones, which are numbered 1 to 5 from medial to lateral. Each bone has a head or distal end, a body or midportion and a base or proximal end. The bases of the 1st, the 2nd and the 3rd metatarsals articulate with the 3 cuneiforms, and the bases of the 4th and the 5th with the cuboid. These bases also articulate with each other; the heads articulate with the proximal phalanges. The bodies present a triangular shape on section and are concave in their long axes on the plantar surfaces. The 1st metatarsal is the shortest and the stoutest, and in the majority of people its head extends as far forward as that of the 2nd metatarsal. The metatarsal bones can be felt individually through the anterior part of the tarsus under the extensor tendons. The base of the 5th metatarsal lies proximal to the main metatarsal joint line and forms a prominent landmark on the outer margin of the foot.

The toes are numbered from medial to lateral, but the 1st toe is called the hallux, and the little toe, the digitus minimus. The bones of the toes are the *phalanges*. The big toe has 2 phalanges, but all of the others have 3: a proximal, a middle and a distal phalanx. Each proximal phalanx articulates with the head of a metatarsal bone to form the *metatarsophalangeal joint*. The middle phalanx articulates with the other two to form the *interphalangeal joints*. The proximal end of each phalanx is called its base, and its distal end is its head.

The accessory bones of the foot are of practical importance, since they may be mistaken on x-ray films for fractures. Although similar bones occur in the hand, they are so seldom seen on the x-ray film that they cannot compare in importance with those of the foot. Accessory bones have been divided into

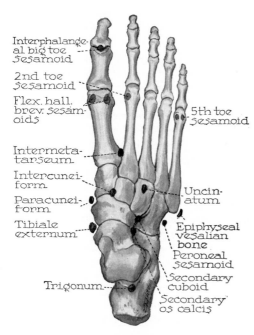

Interphalangeal big toe sesamoid

2nd toe sesamoid

Flex. hall. brev. sesamoids

Intermetatarseum

Intercuneiform

Paracuneiform

Tibiale externum

Trigonum

5th toe sesamoid

Uncinatum

Epiphyseal Vesalian bone

Peroneal sesamoid

Secondary cuboid

Secondary os calcis

FIG. 729. The accessory bones of the foot.

2 classes: (1) the sesamoids, which are regular constituents of the skeleton, and (2) the true accessory bones, which are small occasional ossicles that occur in definite sites. In the vast majority of cases they are bilateral; hence the importance of examining both feet by x-ray. They occur in about 25 per cent of human feet (Pfitzner). McGregor lists the following 20 accessory bones of the feet (Fig. 729):

1. Os tibiale externum
2. Os trigonum (accessory astragalus)
3. Os vesalianum tarsi
4. Secondary os calcis
5. Secondary cuboid
6. Astragaloscaphoid bone of Pirie
7. Intermetatarseum
8. Os intercuneiforme
9. Os paracuneiforme of Cameron and Carlier
10. Os uncinatum
11. Astragalus secundarius
12. Os subtibiale
13. Os sustentaculum proprium
14. Peroneal process of the os calcis
15. Sesanum peroneum
16. Sesamoid of the flexor hallucis brevis
17. Trochlear process of the head of the astragalus

18. Process from the middle of the upper surface of the astragalus
19. Spurs of the os calcis
20. Spurs of the phalanges

The phalangeal spurs are found on any of the distal phalanges, especially those of the great toe. They may grow from either side of the base of the phalanx and rarely, if ever, cause symptoms.

JOINTS AND LIGAMENTS

Six tarsal joints will be discussed (Fig. 730).

1. **The talocalcaneal joint** is situated between the large facet on the lower surface of the talus and the corresponding facet on the middle of the upper surface of the calcaneus. It possesses a capsular ligament which is attached to the margins of the articular areas of the 2 bones. Anteriorly, its capsule blends with the interosseous ligament, which firmly binds the 2 bones together. This ligament is attached to the inferior surface of the neck of the talus above and to the upper surface of the calcaneal joint. The capsular ligament, which is attached to the bones near its margins of the articular facet, is divided into anterior, posterior, lateral and medial talocalcaneal ligaments. They are composed of short fibers, except the anterior, which is a continuation of the interosseous talocalcaneal ligament.

2. **The talocalcaneonavicular joint** is considered the most important of the tarsal joints. It is situated between the rounded head of the talus and a socket formed for it by the posterior surface of the navicular, the upper surface of the spring ligament and the sustentaculum tali. The medial end of the ligamentum bifurcatum completes the lateral side of the socket; this ligament extends between the anterior part of the superior surface of the calcaneus and the lateral side of the navicular. This 3-boned joint conforms to a ball-and-socket variety; unlike other joints of that variety, its socket is not rigid. The joint is situated at the summit of the longitudinal arch of the foot. Its maintenance in a normal position is dependent upon the structures which protect the longitudinal arch. The plantar calcaneonavicular (spring) ligament passes between the anterior border of the sustentaculum tali and the navicular

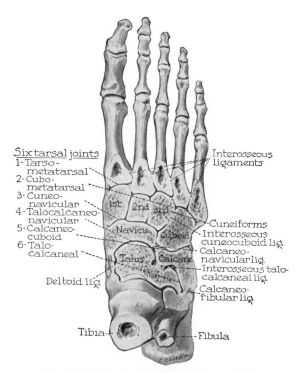

Six tarsal joints
1- Tarso-
   metatarsal
2- Cubo-
   metatarsal
3- Cuneo-
   navicular
4- Talocalcaneo-
   navicular
5- Calcaneo-
   cuboid
6- Talo-
   calcaneal

Interosseous
ligaments

1st 2nd 3rd

Navicu. Cuboid

Talus Calcane

Deltoid lig

Tibia

Fibula

Cuneiforms
Interosseous
cuneocuboid lig.
Calcaneo-
navicular lig.
Interosseous talo-
calcaneal lig.
Calcaneo-
fibular lig.

FIG. 730. The 6 tarsal joints. Some of the
associated ligaments also are shown.

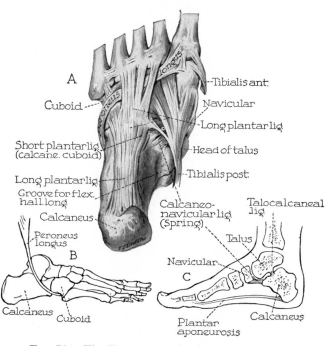

A

Cuboid

Short plantar lig.
(calcane. cuboid)

Long plantar lig.
Groove for flex.
hall. long.
Calcaneus

Peroneus
longus

B

Calcaneus

Cuboid

Tibialis ant.

Navicular

Long plantar lig.

Head of talus

Tibialis post.

Calcaneo-
navicular lig.
(Spring)

Talus

Navicular

C

Plantar
aponeurosis

Talocalcaneal
lig.

Calcaneus

FIG. 731. The ligaments and other supporting structures of the foot. (A) The right foot seen from below.
(B) The peroneus longus tendon. (C) The spring ligament and the plantar aponeurosis.

and is in contact with the inferomedial part of the head of the talus. Some authors prefer to talk about the "subastragaloid" joint, which is a large region of articulation between the talus above and the calcaneus and the navicular below and in front. The talus is not a keystone bone; since it is not wedged in between the calcaneus and the navicular, free movement is possible. In the talocalcaneal segment, the undersurface of the talus articulates with the anterior and the posterior facets of the calcaneus. The anterior talocalcaneal joint is continuous with the talonavicular joint. The 2 parts of the joint are separated by the strong interosseous talocalcaneal ligament.

3. **The calcaneocuboid joint** is a distinct joint, formed by the anterior surface of the calcaneus, which articulates with the posterior surface of the cuboid. Its cavity does not communicate with the cavities of neighboring joints. It has a capsular ligament which is strengthened inferiorly by the long and the short plantar ligaments. The long plantar ligament, which lies superficial to the short, is attached posteriorly to the plantar surface of the calcaneus as far forward as its anterior tubercle (Fig. 731). In front it attaches to the ridge of the cuboid, but some fibers are continued onward to the bases of the 3rd, the 4th and the 5th metatarsal bones and thus bridge over the groove in which the peroneus longus tendon lies. The *short plantar ligament* is attached to a groove at the undersurface of the calcaneus and to the ridge forming the posterior boundary of the groove on the cuboid.

The talocalcaneonavicular and the calcaneocuboid joints together form the *transverse tarsal joint*. This articulation plus the talocalcaneal joint are involved in the movements of inversion and eversion. The 2 joints which form the transverse tarsal joint do not communicate with each other; they lie in almost the same coronal plane. This plane is indicated by a line drawn from a point immediately behind the tuberosity of the navicular to a point ½ inch behind the base of the 5th metatarsal.

4. **The cuneonavicular joint** is formed by the navicular bone behind and the 3 cuneiforms in front. Its cavity is continuous with the joint cavity of the metatarsocuneiform and the corresponding intermetatarsal joints. When the navicular and the cuboid bones come into contact with each other, the cubocuneiform joint also is continuous with the joint cavity of the cuneonavicular. The capsular ligament of the joint is strengthened by the dorsal and the plantar ligaments.

5. **The cubometatarsal joint** articulates with the 2 lateral metatarsal bones. In this way, the joint is placed between the cuboid bone behind and the bases of the 4th and the 5th metatarsal bones in front.

6. **The tarsometatarsal joint** exists between the base of the big toe metatarsal and the first cuneiform. Like the corresponding joint of the hand, it is an independent joint with a separate synovial lining.

The tarsometatarsal joints form an oblique line which runs laterally and backward across the foot from the 1st to the 5th joints. Because of the shortness of the intermediate cuneiform, the base of the 2nd metatarsal projects farther backward between the medial and the lateral cuneiform bones, the line being interrupted at this point. The bases of the first 3 metatarsal bones articulate with the 3 cuneiform bones, and the bases of the 4th and the 5th metatarsal bones articulate with the cuboid bone. The metatarsals are attached firmly to the cuneiform and the cuboid bones by the dorsal, the plantar and the interosseous ligaments.

The metatarsophalangeal joints are formed between the heads of the metatarsal bones and the bases of the proximal row of phalanges. The capsular ligament which surrounds the joint is attached to the bone near the margins of the articular surface and is reinforced at the side to form the collateral ligaments. Its plantar part is thick, forming the so-called plantar ligament; its dorsal part is thin and is fused with the extensor tendon, so that the latter is, in effect, the dorsal ligament of the 1st metatarsophalangeal joint.

The interphalangeal joints are those which exist between the phalanges of the toes; they resemble those of the fingers. The ligaments that unite them include, in addition to the articular capsule, the collateral, the dorsal and the accessory plantar.

The ligaments which, as a rule, unite adjacent bones are the dorsal, the plantar and the interosseous (Figs. 730 and 731). The plantar ligaments situated in the concavity of the arches of the foot are stronger than the dorsal. Besides those which have been discussed already, certain ligaments require special mention:

1. *The interosseous talocalcaneal ligament* is a strong band lying in the tarsal sinus and separating the posterior talocalcaneal joint from the talocalcaneal navicular joint.

2. *The inferior calcaneonavicular,* or the so-called spring ligament, extends from the sustentaculum tali to the navicular bone (Fig. 731). It is situated under the head of the talus and is an important factor in supporting the arch of the foot.

3. *The long plantar ligament* is attached posteriorly to the undersurface of the os calcis and anteriorly to the cuboid and to the bases of the 2nd, the 3rd and the 4th metatarsals. Therefore, it converts the groove of the peroneus longus into a canal.

4. *The short plantar ligament* is about 1 inch long. It runs, under cover of the long plantar, from the front of the undersurface of the os calcis to the cuboid.

5. *The bifurcate ligament,* or the so-called "Y"-shaped ligament of Chopart, arises by its stem from the front of the upper surface of the os calcis and divides into 2 branches which pass to the upper surfaces of the cuboid and the navicular. It crosses the line of the Chopart amputation (intertarsal).

ARCHES

The feet have acquired arches for 4 main reasons: (1) to distribute the body weight properly; (2) to give elasticity and spring to the step; (3) to break the shock that results from running, walking and jumping; (4) to provide space for soft tissues which lie in the arch and thereby prevent undue pressure. The longitudinal and the transverse arches are described (Fig. 732).

The longitudinal arch is divided into 2 columns (medial column and lateral), both of which rest on a common pillar posteriorly, namely, the tuberosity of the calcaneus.

The inner, or *medial, column* of the longi-

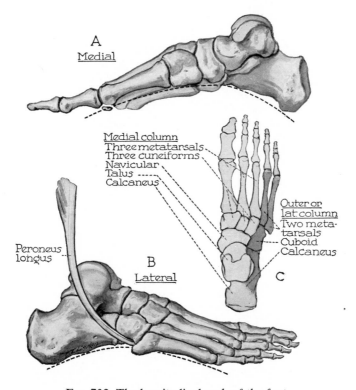

Fig. 732. The longitudinal arch of the foot.

tudinal arch is made up of the calcaneus, the talus, the navicular, the 3 cuneiforms and the 3 inner metatarsals (Fig. 732 C). This inner arch is high and is easily seen if normal; it is absent in individuals with flat feet but is increased in pes cavus. It consists of more segments than the outer arch, has more elasticity and is essentially the "arch of movement."

The outer, or *lateral, column* of the longitudinal arch is formed by the calcaneus, the cuboid and the 2 outer metatarsals. This arch is low, so that the outer border of the foot touches the ground along its entire length. The inner arch, being high, only touches the ground behind, at the tuberosity of the calcaneus, and in front, at the head of the first metatarsal bone (ball of the great toe).

The parts of the foot which normally bear the body weight and transmit it to the ground are arranged in tripod fashion, at the tuberosity of the calcaneus, the head of the 1st metatarsal and the head of the 5th metatarsal. In the young child, the arching of the foot may be masked by a plantar fat pad, so that the baby's foot looks flat.

The transverse arches are a series of arches which extend from the arch formed by the heads of the metatarsals and backward to the arch formed by the navicular and the cuboid bones. The metatarsals and the tarsal bones are arranged so that their convexity is on the dorsum and the concavity is on the plantar aspect. If the transverse arch formed by the heads of the metatarsals becomes flattened, the digital vessels and nerves which normally are protected by it are pressed upon, and pain results.

The arches must be maintained or supported by definite structures. The supporting structures are: (1) the muscles and the tendons, (2) the ligaments, (3) the fasciae and (4) the bones.

Supporting Tendons. Of the *tendons* which support the arches, 2 are important: the peroneus longus and the tibialis posterior.

The peroneus longus tendon passes down the lateral side of the leg and across the lateral side of the foot, turns at right angles on itself and continues across the sole of the foot, from lateral to medial (Figs. 731 and 732). In this part of its course it lies in a tunnel formed by the cuboid and the long plantar ligament. It is inserted into the outer side of the 1st cuneiform bone and the base of the 1st metatarsal. Therefore, it acts as a sling for the longitudinal arch, about its middle. It also forms a bolstering across the transverse arch, thus supporting it. As it abducts and everts the foot, it lowers the longitudinal arch. It is believed by some anatomists that paralysis of this muscle increases the arch.

The tendon of the tibialis posterior has its main insertion about the middle of the longitudinal arch to the undersurface of the navicular. Additional support is given to this arch, as it sends a tendinous slip into every bone of the tarsus except the talus, and also the bases of the 2nd, the 3rd and the 4th metatarsal bones. The function of the tendon of the tibialis posterior is similar to that of the peroneus longus and balances it on the inner side. It supports the spring ligament and adducts and inverts the foot.

Muscles. The muscles that support the arches do so by pulling the 2 pillars of the arches closer together or directly upward. Those muscles that adduct and invert the foot increase the longitudinal arch, while those which abduct and evert flatten it. Therefore, the long flexors of the toes and the short muscles of the foot pull the pillars together and increase the arch. The short muscles can withstand the strain better than the ligamentous structures. So powerful are these short muscles as arch maintainers that they may increase the arch and produce a pes cavus. The transverse arch is maintained mainly by the transverse head of the adductor hallucis and to a lesser degree by its oblique head.

Ligaments. The ligaments that are associated with arch support are weak over the dorsum of the foot but are powerful over the sole. All the ligaments in this region are important, but a few require special mention (Fig. 731).

The inferior calcaneonavicular (spring) ligament is an important structure in the support of the longitudinal arch. It is placed under the weakest point (the head of the talus) and thereby prevents it from sinking between the calcaneus and the navicular. When weight falls on the talus, this strong ligament gives a little but, being very elastic, pushes the head of the bone immediately back into position when the superimposed weight is removed.

The long plantar ligament is a powerful structure that is attached to the undersurface of the calcaneus and to the inferior surface of the cuboid, whence it continues forward to the bases of the 2nd, the 3rd and the 4th metatarsal bones.

The short plantar (calcaneocuboid) ligament passes obliquely forward and medially from the undersurface of the calcaneus to the posterior part of the cuboid, where the long plantar ligament conceals it. The transverse arch is maintained by the support of the plantar intertarsal and the tarsometatarsal ligaments.

The fascia also plays its part in supporting the arches. The intermediate portion of the *plantar aponeurosis* is attached to the extremities of the arch, namely, the posterior part of the calcaneus behind and the heads of all the metatarsals and the proximal phalanges in front (Fig. 731 C). In this way, it holds the extremities of the arch together.

The form of the bones also has a supporting value. They are broader in the dorsum of the foot, thus making less support necessary than if the reverse were true.

INVERSION AND EVERSION OF THE FOOT

Rotating the sole of the foot inward (inversion) around the long axis of the foot is performed by the tibialis anterior and the posterior muscles, assisted by the flexors of the toes. Rotating the sole outward (eversion) around the long axis of the foot is brought about in the following way: when the foot is plantar flexed, it is produced by the 3 peronei (longus, brevis and tertius); when the foot is dorsiflexed, the movement is performed by the extensor digitorum longus. This last statement may be verified if the foot is plantar flexed and everted strongly. In this position the strain is felt on the outer side of the leg over the perinei muscles. If the foot is everted and dorsiflexed, no strain is felt over the peronei, but the strain is taken by the extensor longus, which can be seen

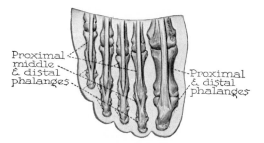

FIG. 733. The toes.

and felt. Orthopedic surgeons utilized this fact when they found that if the extensor longus digitorum were paralyzed, the foot could be everted in plantar flexion but not in dorsiflexion.

TOES

The toes or digits are numbered from the medial to the lateral side (Fig. 733). The 1st toe is called the hallux, and the 5th toe is called the digitus minimus. The bones of the toes are the phalanges. The big toe has only 2—a proximal and a distal—but the others have 3—proximal, middle and distal. Each proximal phalanx articulates with the head of a metatarsal bone and in this way forms the metatarsophalangeal joint. The middle phalanx articulates with the 2 other phalanges to form the interphalangeal joint. The proximal end of the phalanx is called its base, and its distal end is called its head. The toes are involved in various conditions which will be discussed subsequently.

SURGICAL CONSIDERATIONS

INFECTIONS OF THE FOOT

Infections of the foot are less common than those of the hand, but they can be approached and drained as effectively. Grodinsky has emphasized the clinical importance of the 4 median fascial spaces on the plantar aspect of the foot and the 2 dorsal spaces.

The 4 median plantar spaces (Fig. 734):

1. The first space is located between the plantar aponeurosis and the flexor digitorum brevis.

2. The second space is situated between the flexor digitorum brevis and the conjoined long flexor tendons and quadratus plantae.

3. The third space is found between the

flexor digitorum longus (with its associated lumbricales muscles) and the oblique head of the adductor hallucis.

4. The fourth and deepest space is situated between the oblique head of the adductor hallucis muscle and the 2nd and the 3rd metatarsal bones and their interosseous muscles. These spaces are bounded both laterally and medially by dense connective-tissue septa, along which an infection may travel from one space to another. There is nothing in the foot that corresponds to the radial and the ulnar bursae of the hand, since the sheaths of all the flexor tendons of the toes end proximal to the distal head of the metatarsal bones; the sheath of the flexor hallucis longus extends a little higher than the rest. Therefore, infections within these sheaths either may remain local or break into one of the four spaces.

Two lateral spaces have been described, but these are of little anatomic or clinical importance.

The *2 dorsal spaces,* subaponeurotic and subcutaneous, are similar to those found in the hand and are treated in the same way. Infections in any of these spaces may be the result of extension along fascial or tendon planes or may result from direct penetrating wounds into a given space.

Treatment. The 4 medial fascial spaces can be approached best from the inside of the foot, so that a scar is not left on the plantar, or weight-bearing, surface. Such an incision should be made along the inner border of the 1st metatarsal bone and should be carried between that bone and the flexor hallucis longus muscle. This incision follows the inferior surface of the bone and separates it from the flexor hallucis brevis. In this way, access is gained to the septum which forms the medial wall of all 4 spaces; the tendon of the flexor hallucis longus also is protected. At times, a counter-incision may be necessary; if so, it is made along the outer edge of the plantar surface (Fig. 734 C).

DEFORMITIES OF THE FOOT

The general term "talipes" is used to designate foot deformities. Four forms of talipes are described: equinus, calcaneus, valgus and varus (Fig. 735).

Talipes equinus is caused by a contracted tendon of Achilles, which prevents the foot from being placed squarely on the ground. The forepart of the foot is in contact with the ground; in severe forms of equinus, the foot may form almost a straight line with the leg. Usually a contracture of the plantar aponeurosis is associated with the condition; this results in a deep hollowing of the sole known as talipes cavus. The condition usu-

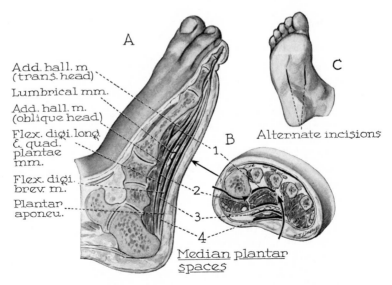

FIG. 734. The 4 plantar spaces of the foot. (A) Longitudinal section; (B) cross section; (C) alternate incisions for space drainage.

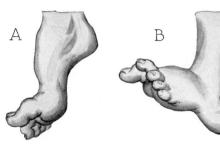
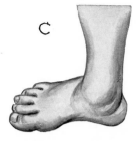
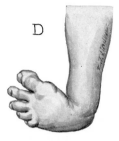

FIG. 735. Four varieties of talipes: (A) equinus; (B) calcaneus; (C) valgus; (D) varus.

ally can be corrected by stretching the calf muscles or by cutting the Achilles tendon.

Talipes calcaneus constitutes a dorsiflexion of the foot on the leg. Usually, it is caused by an involvement of the calf muscles following infantile paralysis.

In **talipes valgus,** the medial border of the foot is depressed and is in contact with the ground. If of congenital origin, the peronei are shortened, and the anterior and the posterior tibial muscles are stretched. In the acquired form, the deformity is brought about by a paralysis of the tibialis anterior and the posterior muscles.

In **talipes varus,** the foot is twisted on itself in a position of adduction and inversion. The dorsum of the foot is directed somewhat forward, and the sole is directed backward.

HALLUX VALGUS

Hallux valgus, or bunion, is a condition in which the big toe deviates laterally, and the head of the first metatarsal becomes prominent (Fig. 736). The joint surface of the head of the metatarsal pushes obliquely and laterally. An adventitious bursa, which is a bunion, usually develops over the projecting head of the bone. Numerous operations have been devised to cure this condition; however, their aim is essentially the same. The head

of the first metatarsal is reduced by removing part of its medial surface and reconstructing its articular alignment. The bursa that is present usually is dissected away, and the tendon of the extensor hallucis is displaced medially and maintained in position by suturing, so that by its contraction the great toe is kept in alignment.

HAMMER TOE

In this condition, the involved toe contracts and produces a sharp angulation. The toes that usually are involved are the 2nd or the 3rd (Fig. 737). The common extensor muscle is stretched, resulting in an elevation of the proximal phalanx but leaving the other phalanges in flexion. The proximal interphalangeal joint is flexed acutely, but the metatarsophalangeal and the distal interphalangeal joints are hyperextended. The operative correction of this condition attempts to divide the dorsal expansion of the extensor tendon which covers the dorsum of the joint. In this way the joint is opened widely, and, after division of the lateral ligament, the head of the first phalanx is dislocated into the wound and is excised.

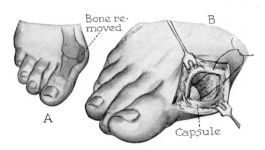

FIG. 736. Hallux valgus.

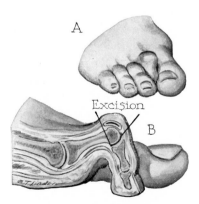

FIG. 737. Hammer toe.

Vertebral Column, Vertebral (Spinal) Canal and Spinal Cord

VERTEBRAL COLUMN

The spinal column serves many remarkable functions. It supports the weight of the head, acts as the central pillar of the body, connects the upper and the lower segments of the trunk, gives attachments to the ribs, reduces shock transmitted from various parts of the body, forms a complete tube for the reception of the spinal cord and permits a wide range of most complicated movements

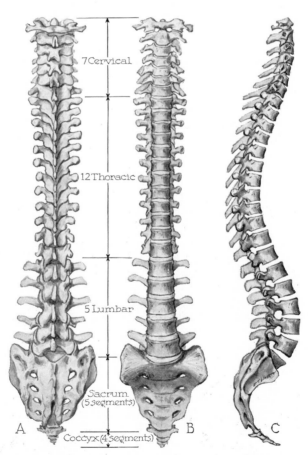

Fig. 738. The spinal column. (A) Posterior view; (B) anterior view; (C) lateral view.

846

and balancing. It consists of 33 vertebrae which are grouped according to region (Fig. 738). The movable (true) vertebrae are the 7 cervical, the 12 thoracic and the 5 lumbar. The fixed (false) vertebrae are the 5 sacral, fused in adults to form the sacrum, and usually the 4 coccygeal, fused to form the coccyx. If the bony column is examined as a whole from front or back it seems to form a straight line, but when it is seen from the side it presents definite curves.

Viewed from the side, the vertebral column reveals 4 curvatures: the cervical and the lumbar curves are convex forward; the thoracic and the sacrococcygeal curves are concave forward. At birth only the thoracic and the sacral curves exist. These early thoracic and sacral curves are called the *primary curves*. The *secondary curves* (compensatory) develop after birth; they are the cervical and the lumbar. The cervical curve results from elevation and extension of the head in infancy, and the lumbar from assumption of the erect posture when the child begins to walk. The lumbar curve is more pronounced in women than in men and in youth than after middle age.

In the midthoracic region the tips of the spines are below the level of the bodies of the corresponding vertebrae. The intervertebral foramina increase in size down to the 5th lumbar vertebra. In the sacrum they diminish from above downward. The transverse processes are in front of the articular processes in the cervical region and in line with the intervertebral foramina, but in the thoracic region they are behind both; in the lumbar region they are behind the foramina but in front of the articular processes. Viewed from in front, the bodies of the vertebrae increase in breadth from the 2nd cervical to the 1st thoracic but diminish from the 1st to the 4th thoracic. They increase from the 4th thoracic to the 1st sacral, below which they reduce rapidly in size. The transverse processes of the atlas are wide and stand out, but those of the next vertebrae are short and nearly equal in length. Those of the 7th are long, nearly as long as the 1st thoracic. They diminish gradually down to the 12th thoracic, where they are represented only by

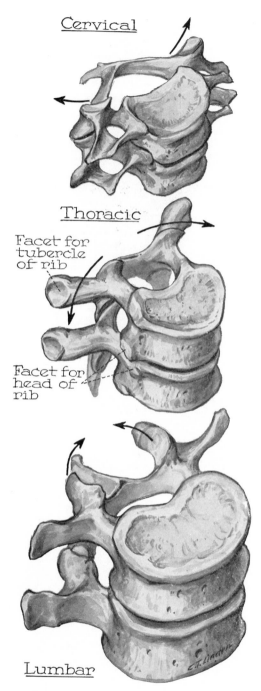

FIG. 739. The distinguishing features of the vertebrae.

tubercles. In the lumbar region they stand out again, the 3rd being the longest. The column is widest at the sacrum, and below this it diminishes, gradually at first, but

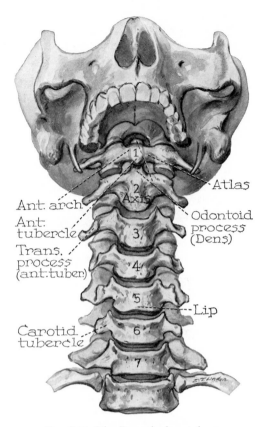

FIG. 740. The 7 cervical vertebrae.

abruptly increases at the 3rd sacral piece and becomes greatly accentuated opposite the 5th.

The vertebral column is usually about 28 inches long in men and 24 inches long in women; however, this is subject to great variations. The bodies of the vertebrae form a column for the support of the trunk and the head, the vertebral foramina provide a canal for the spinal cord and its membrane. The spines and the transverse processes provide attachments for muscles and form 3 ridges that bound a pair of grooves of which the laminae (ventral arch) form the floors. These grooves are occupied by muscles which move the vertebral column.

The thoracic vertebra consists of a short cylindrical anterior portion, called the body, the posterior aspect of which is attached to a bony arch (Fig. 739). Enclosed within these 2 portions is an opening called the *vertebral foramen.* The anterior surface of the body is convex from side to side, but the posterior surface is slightly concave. On its external surface the arch has 3 processes—one pointing backward, the *spinous process,* and the other 2 extending laterally, the *transverse processes.* The spinous processes mark the

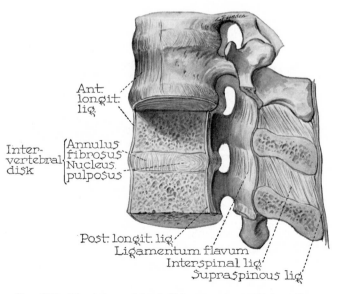

FIG. 741. The intervertebral disks seen in sagittal section.

midline of the back, and the rounded tips can be felt beneath the skin. The transverse processes give partial attachment to the ribs. Four small articular processes which interlock with similar elevations on the vertebrae above and below are found also. The *vertebral canal* formed by the series of vertebral foramina contains the spinal cord.

The lumbar vertebrae are larger than the thoracic, and their transverse processes do not give attachment to the ribs. They are distinguished by the absence of foramina in the transverse processes and also by the absence of their costal facets.

The cervical vertebrae are easily distinguished from the others by their transverse processes, which are unusually wide and contain a canal for the transmission of the vertebral artery (Fig. 740). The 7th cervical vertebra has been distinguished further by its prominent spinous process which is known as the *vertebra prominens.*

The first 2 cervical vertebrae are so markedly different from the others that they re-quire special mention. The *first* or *atlas* has no body and no spine but consists only of a pair of lateral masses united by anterior and posterior arches. It resembles a large ring. Its cavity is divided by a transverse ligament into two compartments: a larger posterior one for the spinal cord and a smaller anterior one for the odontoid process (dens) of the 2nd cervical vertebra. The upper surface of the bone reveals two smooth oval areas for articulation with the undersurface of the skull. A rocking movement of the skull, forward and backward, takes place on these areas. In turning the head from side to side the atlas moves with the skull, and the two turn on the 2nd cervical vertebra with the odontoid process as the center of rotation. The *second* cervical vertebra, also called the axis (epistropheus), differs from the others in that its body is much reduced in size, and projecting upward from it is a prominent elevation called the *odontoid process (dens).* This tooth like dens passes through a special canal in the first cervical vertebra and

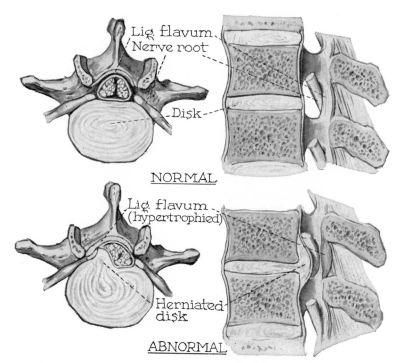

Lig. flavum.
Nerve root
Disk
NORMAL

Lig. flavum
(hypertrophied)
Herniated disk
ABNORMAL

FIG. 742. The effect of a protruded disk upon nerve roots. The normal is presented for comparison.

forms the axis of rotation for the skull and the first vertebra.

The Intervertebral Disks. Between the vertebrae there is a fibrocartilaginous disk which acts as a shock absorber. Each disk is composed of two parts: a central *nucleus pulposus,* a relic of the notochord, and an outer ring, the *annulus fibrosus* (Fig. 741). The nucleus is a very elastic semifluid tissue mass which lies more posteriorly than centrally. The annulus forms the major part of the disk and gives form and strength to it and is the main weight-bearing portion. Each disk is attached to the compact rim of the superjacent and the subjacent vertebral bodies. The nucleus has been likened to a water cushion which allows the overlying vertebrae to rock about on it, while the strong annular fibers act as stays which prevent displacement of the vertebral bodies.

When the usual stress and strain is placed on the spinal column the disks bulge in all directions but return to their normal positions when the stress has been removed. They are maintained in their positions chiefly by the anterior and the posterior longitudinal vertebral ligaments. If an unusual strain is placed upon the vertebral column, the disk proper or its nucleus may be extruded beyond its normal limits and fail to return to position (Fig. 742).

Posterior protrusion may cause root pain because of pressure of the disk on one or more of the spinal nerves; more marked protrusion may cause signs and symptoms similar to those found in transverse lesions of the cord or the cauda equina. These lesions have been mistaken for intraspinal neoplasms.

One of the most common locations for such a lesion is low in the lumbar region, and one of the most common symptoms is sciatic pain. If such an abnormal protrusion is present, it can be diagnosed by injecting Lipiodol into the subarachnoid space, since the protruded disk will impinge on the column of radiopaque oil and will indent or displace it. Complete obstructions to the passage of the oil have also been observed. After the age of 60 these disks begin to atrophy, their disappearance giving rise to the bowed back of old age.

The adjacent vertebrae articulate with each other by their bodies through the interven-

tion of the intervertebral disks and through their *articular processes*. Each vertebra has upper and lower articular processes which are arranged for the most part vertically, except in the cervical region where they are more transverse. Because of these anatomic facts, it is only possible for a vertebral dislocation without fracture to take place in the neck. Anywhere else in the spinal column a pure dislocation cannot occur, because the articular processes must break off before the body can be moved.

The adult sacrum results from the fusion of 5 sacral vertebrae which diminish in size from above downward (p. 527). It is triangular in shape, possessing a base or upper surface, an apex or lower end and dorsal, pelvic and two lateral surfaces. It is divided by paired rows of foramina on the dorsal and the pelvic surfaces into median and lateral parts. The median portion is composed of most of the parts of the 5 fused vertebrae, and the lateral part, also called the lateral masses, represents the fused costal and the transverse processes. These lateral masses contain the auricular surfaces for articulation with the ilium. The laminae of S 5 and usually S 4 fail to meet in the median plane; because of this, they form the opening to the sacral canal, called the *sacral hiatus*. The sacral canal contains the cauda equina, the filum terminale and the meninges down to the middle of the 3rd sacral vertebra (Fig. 749). At that level the meninges end, and the lower portion of the canal contains only the nerve roots of the lower sacral and coccygeal nerves, together with the coverings they acquire from the meninges. The base of the sacrum is formed by the upper surface of the 1st sacral vertebra; it is divided into a median and two lateral parts. The median part is the oval upper surface of the body of the 1st sacral vertebra, the anterior border of which forms an important forward bulging landmark called the promontory of the sacrum. Behind its posterior border is the triangular entrance to the sacral canal. The two lateral parts are called the alae, which are fan-shaped and represent the fused costal and transverse processes. Each ala is crossed by the constituent parts of the lumbosacral trunk, the iliolumbar artery, the obturator nerve and the psoas muscle. The concave anterior surface of the sacrum is crossed by 4 ridges which mark the sites where fusion took place between the bodies of the 5 sacral vertebrae before the 21st year. Lateral to these ridges, on each side, the 4 anterior sacral foramina are placed. These foramina become progressively smaller from above downward; through them the anterior rami of the upper 4 sacral nerves pass laterally.

The coccyx is that bone which results from the 3, 4 or 5 rudimentary coccygeal vertebrae that are attached to the tip of the sacrum. They are believed to represent the bony remnants of the tail of lower animals. It is triangular in shape and constitutes the terminal segment of the spine. The lateral margins of it and its tip continue to the wide origin of the sacrotuberous ligament and afford attachments to the muscles of the pelvic floor.

Ligaments. *The anterior longitudinal ligament* lies on the front of the body of the vertebrae, from the sacrum to the axis, where it is continued upward as the anterior atlantoaxial ligament (Fig. 741).

The posterior longitudinal ligament is placed on the backs of the bodies of the vertebrae inside of the spinal canal.

The ligamenta flava connect the deep surfaces of the laminae; they are made up of yellow elastic fibers.

The interspinous ligaments unite adjacent spines.

Sacralization of the 5th lumbar vertebra means the fusion of the transverse processes of the 5th lumbar vertebra with the sacrum; such a fusion may be bilateral (symmetrical) or unilateral (asymmetrical). In symmetrical sacralization the bony structure is sounder and more able to resist stress and strain, but in asymmetrical sacralization a scoliosis may result and, although not necessarily severe, may alter muscle balance, lead to arthritic changes and pain. "Lumbarization" of the first sacral vertebra is noted when this vertebra takes on lumbar characteristics. This, too, may be unilateral or bilateral.

VERTEBRAL (SPINAL) CANAL

Together the vertebral foramina make a continuous canal in the spinal column. The anterior wall is closed by the posterior sur-

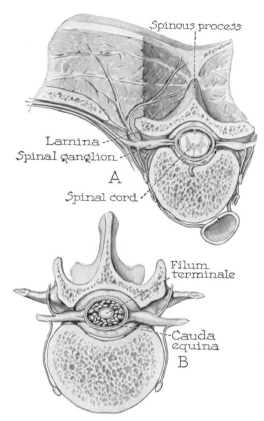

FIG. 743. The spinal meninges. Transverse section through the spinal cord and the meninges (diagrammatic). (A) Section through a thoracic vertebra. (B) Section through a lumbar vertebra.

faces of the bodies of the vertebrae and their disks; the posterior longitudinal ligament passes over these. The posterior and the lateral walls are made up of the superimposed bony arches, the interspaces which are covered behind by the ligamenta flava but remain open laterally as the intervertebral foramina. It is lined entirely by ligamentous and periosteal structures. The canal is approximately circular where it is continuous with the foramen magnum but becomes triangular through the cervical region; it becomes round again in the thoracic region and finally assumes a triangular form in the lumbar region. Within the sacrum it flattens and expands laterally, and in the flexible cervical and lumbar regions it shows distinct enlargements to accommodate the cervical and the lumbar enlargements of the spinal cord.

Spinal Meninges. These are 3 tubular fibrous membranes which are named from without inward: the dura mater, the arachnoid mater and the pia mater (Figs. 743 and 744). They are continuous with the corresponding meninges of the brain.

The space that is situated between the dura mater and the walls of the vertebral canal is called the *epidural space*; it is filled with loose areolar tissue, a semiliquid fat, a network of veins, and small arteries to the bones.

The dura is the most complicated of the 3 membranes. It is recalled that in the cranial cavity this membrane consists of two layers, namely, an outer layer constituting the lining periosteum of the skull, and an inner layer which invests the brain and by its duplications forms cranial venous sinuses. At the foramen magnum the outer layer blends with the periosteal and the ligamentous linings of the vertebral column, but the inner layer forms the dural sac which invests the more delicate meninges of the cord and the emerging nerve roots. Within the vertebral canal the dura mater forms a loose envelopelike covering outside of the arachnoid. Although firmly connected to the 2nd and the 3rd cervical vertebrae it is not intimately associated

with the periosteum elsewhere. It extends 5 vertebrae lower than the spinal cord proper; it ends at the 2nd sacral vertebra with a prolongation of it investing the filum terminale which ends at the back of the coccyx (Figs. 743 B and 745). Although firmly attached to the 2nd and the 3rd cervical vertebrae, this covering is loosely attached at the upper and the lower parts of the vertebral canal to the posterior longitudinal ligament. The anterior and the posterior nerve roots which pierce it carry tubular dural prolongations that are attached to the periosteum of the bone at the intervertebral foramina. At the level of the 2nd sacral vertebra where it ends, it forms a cul-de-sac which is pierced by the filum terminale, the latter carrying its dural prolongation and becoming attached to the coccyx.

The spinal arachnoid is a thin transparent and fragile membrane. It ends a little below the 2nd sacral vertebra; posteriorly, it is connected to the pia mater by an incomplete posterior median septum in the cervical region. The dura and the arachnoid move freely on one another in the capillary interval which exists between them.

The subarachnoid space lies between the arachnoid and the pia mater and contains

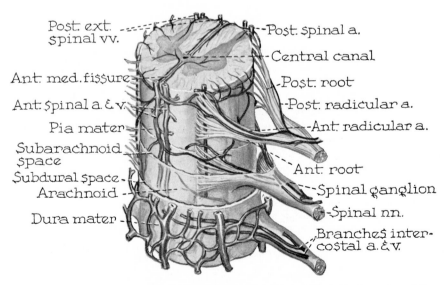

Fig. 744. A diagrammatic presentation of a section of the spinal cord and its associated vessels and spinal nerves.

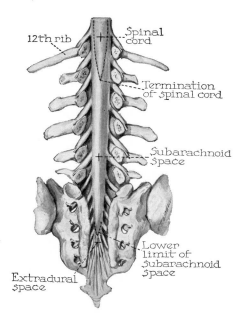

FIG. 745. Diagrammatic presentation of the levels of the termination of the spinal cord, the cauda equina, the subarachnoid space and the extradural space.

the cerebrospinal fluid. It is traversed by septa lined with flat arachnoidal cells and also by the vessels going to the brain and the spinal cord. It communicates with the corresponding intracranial space; therefore, an increase of pressure from hemorrhage or swelling in the brain may be diagnosed by lumbar puncture.

The pia mater in the vertebral canal is closely applied to the spinal cord and dips into the anterior median fissure. It is a delicate vascular membrane that is attached to the surfaces of the cord and carries blood vessels into its substance. Along the lateral side of the spinal cord the pia is attached to the dura by a thin membrane called the dentate ligament. These ligaments are 20 tooth-like processes which extend from the pia to the dura; they push the arachnoid ahead of them (Fig. 746). They leave the pia midway between the anterior and the posterior nerve roots and serve to suspend the cord in the midline. The lowest one of these ligaments is forked (Von Elsberg's forked denticulation) and is placed just above the exit of the 1st lumbar vertebra. It acts as the surgeon's guide to this nerve, giving him a nerve root

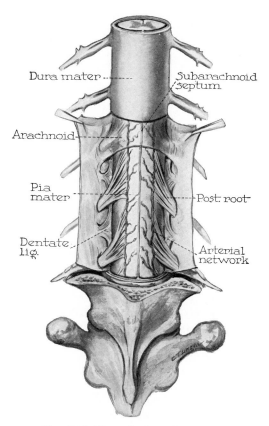

FIG. 746. The spinal cord and the meninges seen from behind.

of known number from which he may determine the position of others. The anterior and the posterior nerve roots are separated by the ligaments.

SPINAL CORD

During the first days of intra-uterine existence, a dorsal groove, the neural groove, appears on the body surface (Fig. 747). It becomes closed off from the neural canal, and from its walls the central nervous system arises. Its lumen persists as the central

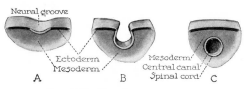

FIG. 747. Development of the spinal cord.

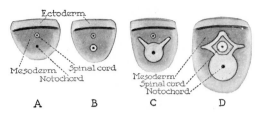

FIG. 748. Development of the neural arch of a vertebra around the spinal cord.

spinal canal. The neural canal becomes separated from the epidermal covering of the body by an ingrowth of mesoderm; anterior to the canal a solid rod of cells forms known as the notochord (Fig. 748). Around this notochord the vertebral bodies develop. Until the 4th month of intra-uterine life the spinal cord extends the whole length of the vertebral canal, but as the development proceeds, owing to the greater growth of the vertebral column, the cord extends only as far as the sacrum at the 6th month and to the lumbar vertebra at birth. However, in adults the cord extends to the upper border of the 2nd lumbar vertebra.

The spinal cord is represented as a cylindrical mass of nervous tissue which measures about 18 inches in length and about ½ inch thick (Fig. 749). In the adult it lies in the upper two thirds of the vertebral canal. Since its diameter is much less than that of the vertebral canal, the backbone can be bent and twisted without any strain being put upon the cord proper. It begins at the foramen magnum, where it is continuous with the medulla oblongata opposite a point midway between the inion and the spine of the axis. A strong glistening threadlike structure called the *filum terminale,* which is composed mainly of pia mater, attaches the end of the cord to the back of the coccyx. The filum pierces the arachnoid and the dura mater and emerges at the sacral hiatus to blend with the periosteum on the dorsum of the coccyx. In the adult the subarachnoid and the subdural, spaces extend to the body of the 2nd sacral vertebra, but the cord proper ends at the 2nd lumbar. Hence, between L 2 and S 2 there is no cord, but instead the filum terminale and the roots of the lower spinal

nerves. These roots resemble a horse's tail and therefore have been given the name of *cauda equina.* A needle that enters the subarachnoid space above L 2 may damage the spinal cord permanently, but if it enters at a lower level it would encounter only terminal nerves. The spinal cord is protected in a water cushion of subarachnoidal fluid plus its membranes and is anchored by the dentate ligaments. Opposite the 5th and the 6th cervical vertebrae and again opposite the lower 2 thoracic vertebrae, the spinal cord reveals two enlargements. These are the cervical and the lumbar enlargements that are associated with the origins of the great plexuses to the superior and the inferior extremities.

In the spinal cord the gray matter is placed centrally, and the white matter peripherally. The gray matter is "H"-shaped and contains anterior and posterior limbs known as the anterior and the posterior horns or gray columns. These divide the white matter on each side into anterior, lateral and posterior white columns. A groove in front, the anteromedian fissure, and a septum behind, the posteromedian septum, separate the right and the left sides of the white matter. The transverse limb of the "H" constitutes the gray commissure and surrounds the central canal of the spinal cord. In the thoracic region there is, in addition, a lateral horn which projects opposite the central canal.

From the large cells of the anterior horn, the fibers of the *anterior nerve roots* (motor) stream out and leave the cord at its anterolateral aspect. Opposite the tip of the posterior horn, the fibers of the *posterior nerve roots* (sensory) enter the spinal cord. This, too, further divides the white matter into 3 white funiculi (columns). The *anterior* white column lies between the anterior median fissure and the anterior nerve roots; the *lateral* white column lies between the anterior and the posterior nerve roots; the *posterior* white column lies between the posterior nerve roots and the posteromedian septum. Anterior nerve rami and their branches communicate with adjacent rami to form plexuses. Close to the vertebral column the anterior rami of nerves C 1 and 4 form the cervical plexus, those of C 5 and Th 1 the brachial

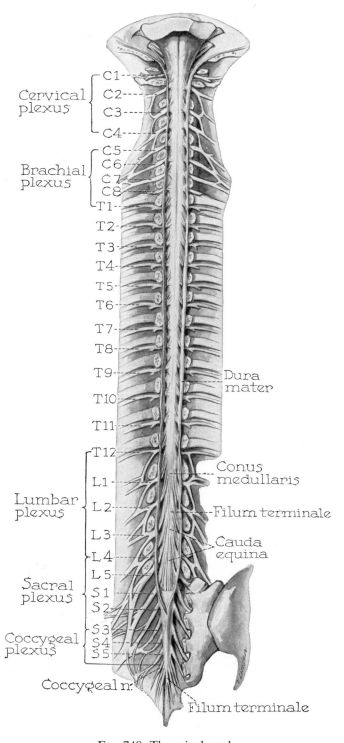

Cervical plexus
C1
C2
C3
C4

Brachial plexus
C5
C6
C7
C8
T1

T2
T3
T4
T5
T6
T7
T8
T9
T10
T11
T12

Lumbar plexus
L1
L2
L3
L4
L5

Sacral plexus
S1
S2

Coccygeal plexus
S3
S4
S5

Coccygeal n.

Dura mater

Conus medullaris

Filum terminale

Cauda equina

Filum terminale

FIG. 749. The spinal cord.

plexus, L 1 and 4 the lumbar plexus, L 4 and S 4 the sacral plexus, and S 4 and Co 1 the coccygeal plexus.

On each posterior root the *ganglion* is found, which is composed of cells giving origin to central and peripheral fibers. The ganglia of all except the sacral and the coccygeal nerves occupy the intervertebral foramina. Those of the sacral and the coccygeal nerves lie within the vertebral canal. Near the intervertebral foramen each pair of nerve roots unites to form a spinal nerve, which divides into anterior and posterior branches or primary divisions. Both of these divisions are mixed (sensory and motor) nerves. Distal to the division, the spinal nerve gives off a minute recurrent branch to the meninges and the cord, after uniting with the branch from the sympathetic trunk. Each nerve root receives a covering from the pia mater and one from the arachnoid before it meets the dura. Within the subarachnoid space the roots are bathed in cerebrospinal fluid, but outside of the space they are encased in a tubular sheath of dura which includes the ganglion on the posterior root.

The nerve fibers that constitute the white matter are divided into two main groups: (1) the ascending and (2) the descending (Fig. 750). The ascending fibers are arranged in fasciculi (tracts) which become larger as they are followed upward, because of the addition of new fibers at each ascending level. The descending fibers form fasciculi also, which become smaller as they are traced downward, since they are continually giving off fibers which are intrasegmental, establishing a pathway for local reflexes as well as connecting the gray matter at different levels. In front of and behind the central gray matter, the anterior and the posterior commissural fibers cross the median plane. They connect the two halves of the spinal cord with each other, though not necessarily at the same level, while others may join one or another of the ascending tracts after crossing the median plane.

Ascending Tracts. These ascending fibers convey afferent impulses which may or may not be associated with consciousness. They are divided into two groups: exteroceptive, which receive the initial stimulus from the outside world, and proprioceptive, which receive the initial stimuli from an internal

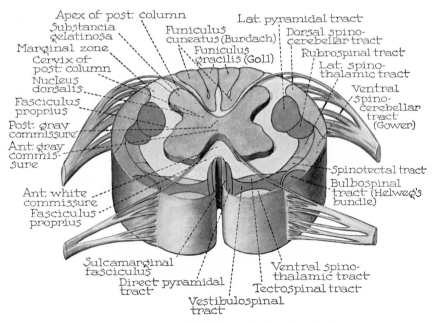

Fig. 750. Cross section of the spinal cord to indicate the various spinal tracts (diagrammatic).

source such as the muscles and the joints. It is still uncertain whether the exteroceptive paths are 2 or 3 in number. However, clinical evidence shows that painful or heat sensations ascend in the lateral spinothalamic tract, and that light touch and pressure stimuli ascend in the posterior white column, associated with some proprioceptive fibers. It has been thought that crude tactile sensibilities travel by a 4th, namely, the anterior spinothalamic tract.

The fibers which transmit painful and thermal impressions are related closely to one another; the central processes of these enter the posterior horn of the gray matter and end by arborizing round cells in that situation. They establish connections by collaterals with higher and lower segments. From these cells new fibers arise which cross the median plane and turn up in the lateral white column in the lateral spinothalamic tract. As this tract ascends it constantly receives additional fibers to the medulla oblongata where it joins the anterior spinothalamic tract and the two together from the *spinal lemniscus.*

The fibers transmitting crude tactile and pressure impressions behave similarly, but their second neurons ascend in the posterior white column for a few segments before crossing the median plane and turning upward in the anterior spinothalamic tract, which lies in the anterior white column.

The spinal lemniscus forms in the medulla oblongata by the union of the anterior and the lateral spinothalamic tracts and conveys all the thermal, painful, pressure and crude tactile sensations from the spinal nerves of the opposite side of the body. In the pons the spinal lemniscus becomes associated with the *medial lemniscus* with which it ascends through the tegmentum of the midbrain and the subthalamic region to end by arborizing around cells in the thalamus. These cells give rise to new fibers which ascend through the posterior limb of the internal capsule and reach the cerebral cortex of the postcentral gyrus.

The proprioceptive fibers convey sensations of movements, active or passive, and have their parent cells situated in the spinal ganglia. The centrally directed fibers of these ganglion cells enter the spinal cord and turn upward in the posterior white column. They constitute the *fasciculus gracilis* (Goll) and the *fasciculus cuneatus* (Burdach). Therefore, these two are identical functionally; the former is placed more medially and in the upper region and contains fibers which arise from the ganglion cells of the posterior roots of the sacral, the lumbar and the lower thoracic nerves. The fasciculus cuneatus occupies the lateral half of the posterior white column and is made up of fibers arising from the upper thoracic and the cervical nerves. In the medulla oblongata these fibers end by arborizing round cells in the gracile and cuneate nuclei. These nuclei are two masses of gray matter situated side by side in the dorsal region of the medulla oblongata. The second neuron fibers, internal arcuate fibers, pass ventrally around the central gray matter and cross the median plane where they decussate with corresponding fibers of the opposite side in the sensory decussation. They then ascend, pass through the pons and the midbrain and to the thalamus where they end. A third neuron arises in the thalamus and extends through the posterior limb of the internal capsule to the postcentral gyrus. These impressions are appreciated by consciousness.

Many fibers which originate in the spinal ganglia reach the cerebellum. They form the afferent part of the paths for spinocerebellar reflexes. On entering the spinal cord they terminate in the cells of the nucleus thoracicus, which extends throughout the thoracic segments of the spinal cord, and lie at the medial part of the base of the posterior column of the gray matter. The second neuron fibers ascend in the lateral white column of the same side. Here they are arranged in two principal groups called the posterior and the anterior spinocerebellar tracts.

Some of the posterior nerve root fibers connect with the lower visual center. These connections are brought about by the spinotectal tract. The entering fibers end in the cells of the posterior horn; the second neuron fibers cross the median plane and form a small bundle which ascends medial to the anterior spinocerebellar tract. The spinotectal tract thus formed ascends through the me-

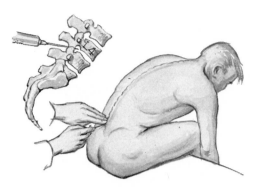

FIG. 751. Spinal (subarachnoid)
anesthesia.

dulla oblongata and the pons to the midbrain where it ends in the superior quadrigeminal body.

Descending Tracts. These are the tracts which pass downward through the spinal cord and are concerned with the production of movements, both voluntary and visceral, and also form the efferent paths for cerebellar, equilibratory, visual and other reflexes.

The cerebrospinal (pyramidal) tracts are associated with voluntary motor impulses which travel from the cortex. The cells of origin of these fibers are found in the cortex of the precentral gyrus and pass through the corona radiata where they are intercepted by fibers of the corpus callosum. They enter the posterior limb of the internal capsule and at its lower end pass as a compact bundle into the basis pedunculi of the midbrain occupying approximately the middle third. In the ventral part of the pons the tract is broken into a large number of small bundles by the nuclei pontis and the transverse fibers of the pons. In the upper part of the medulla oblongata a compact tract is re-established and forms a surface projection on the anterior aspect called the pyramid which lies lateral to the anterior median fissure. In the lower part of the medulla oblongata the majority of the fibers decussate with the fibers of the opposite side in the decussation of the pyramid and then take their final position in the middle of the lateral right column of the spinal cord.

The lateral cerebrospinal (cross pyramidal) tract becomes smaller as it passes downward, for it is constantly giving off fibers which terminate by arborizing around the large motor cells in the anterior horn. The fibers of these cells form the anterior nerve roots of the spinal nerve.

Those fibers which do not decussate in the medulla oblongata form the *anterior cerebrospinal (direct pyramidal) tract* which decends in the anterior white column close to the anterior median fissure. Before their termination these fibers also cross the median plane and end as do the fibers of the cross tract by arborizing around the large motor end cells of the anterior horn. As the fibers of the cerebrospinal tract descend they give off fibers to the motor nuclei of the cranial nerves of both sides.

The vestibulospinal tract, which is the efferent part for equilibratory reflexes, has its origin in the lateral vestibular nucleus in the pons of the medulla oblongata. It descends near the surface of the spinal cord in the anterior white column and terminates uncrossed around the motor cells of the anterior horn.

The rubrospinal tract begins in the red nucleus of the midbrain. It decussates with its fellow of the opposite side and descends through the dorsal part of the pons and the dorsolateral part of the medulla oblongata to reach the lateral white column of the spinal cord where it lies close to the lateral cerebral spinal tract. Its fibers end in association with the motor cells of the anterior horn of the same side. It is an efferent part from the cerebellum and the corpus striatum and is concerned with the maintenance of postural tone.

The tectospinal tract, together with the ascending spinotectal tract, provides a pathway for visual reflexes and begins in the superior corpus quadrigeminum of the midbrain. It decussates with its fellow of the opposite side in front of the aqueduct of the midbrain. It then passes downward in the anterior white column of the spinal cord, and its fibers end in the same manner as those of the rubrospinal tract.

ANESTHESIA

Spinal (Subarachnoid) Anesthesia. This injection produces a nerve root block. The patient may be placed in either a lateral

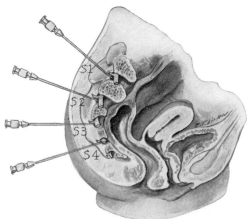

FIG. 753. Transsacral anesthesia.

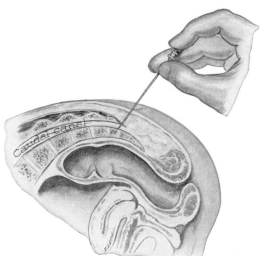

FIG. 752. Caudal anesthesia.

recumbent or a sitting position (Fig. 751). Some surgeons, particularly Babcock, prefer the space between the 1st and the 2nd lumbar vertebrae. The 4th lumbar interspace is another favorite site and is found readily by drawing an imaginary line between the crests of the ilia. Since the spinal cord per se ends at a higher level than the 4th interspace, there is little danger of striking it. The selected interspace is anesthetized, and a needle is passed through the median line. When the subarachnoid space is entered, spinal fluid escapes upon removal of the obturator.

Sacral Block Anesthesia. Lundy includes caudal and transsacral block under the term "sacral block anesthesia." This is extradural and reaches the nerves within the sacral canal.

In *caudal anesthesia* the needle is passed through the sacrococcygeal ligament and into the sacral hiatus (Fig. 752). Then the position of the needle is changed and is passed upward along the axis of the sacral canal for about 1 or 1½ inches. Then the anesthetic agent is injected. If the needle has been placed improperly, it usually fails to enter the sacral canal and passes superficial to the posterior aspect of the sacrum.

Transsacral anesthesia is produced by injecting about the sacral nerves via the posterior sacral foramina (Fig. 753). The posterosuperior iliac spine makes a good landmark for this type of anesthesia. About 1 cm. medial to and just below these spines, the second sacral foramina usually are found. The first pair of sacral foramina can be located on a line opposite the tip of the transverse process of the 5th lumbar vertebra. The distance between the foramina is approximately 1 inch.

Index

**Numerals in boldface type refer to page(s) on which
the main discussion of an item appears in the text.**